MAGILL'S

MEDICAL GUIDE

MEDICAL GUIDE

Second Revised Edition

Volume II
Fracture and dislocation — Paralysis

Medical Consultants

Karen E. Kalumuck, Ph.D.
The Exploratorium, San Francisco

Nancy A. Piotrowski, Ph.D.
University of California, Berkeley

Connie Rizzo, M.D.
Pace University

Project Editor
Tracy Irons-Georges

SALEM PRESS, INC.
Pasadena, California   Hackensack, New Jersey

Editor in Chief: Dawn P. Dawson
Project Editor: Tracy Irons-Georges
Research Supervisor: Jeffry Jensen
Photograph Editor: Philip Bader
Production Editor: Joyce I. Buchea
Page Design: James Hutson
Layout: William Zimmerman
Cover Design: Moritz Design

Illustrations: Hans & Cassady, Inc., Westerville, Ohio

Magill's Medical Guide: Health and Illness, 1995
Supplement, 1996
Magill's Medical Guide, revised edition, 1998
Second revised edition, 2002

∞ The paper used in these volumes conforms to the American National Standard for Permanence of Paper for Printed Library Materials, Z39.48-1992 (R1997).

Note to Readers

The material presented in *Magill's Medical Guide, Second Revised Edition*, is intended for broad informational and educational purposes. Readers who suspect that they suffer from any of the physical or psychological disorders, diseases, or conditions described in this set should contact a physician without delay; this work should not be used as a substitute for professional medical diagnosis or treatment. This set is not to be considered definitive on the covered topics, and readers should remember that the field of health care is characterized by a diversity of medical opinions and constant expansion in knowledge and understanding.

Library of Congress Cataloging-in-Publication Data

Magill's medical guide / medical consultants, Karen E. Kalumuck, Nancy A. Piotrowski, Connie Rizzo ; project editor, Tracy Irons-Georges.
    p. cm.
  Includes bibliographical references and index.
    1. Medicine—Encyclopedias. I. Kalumuck, Karen E. II. Piotrowski, Nancy A. III Rizzo, Connie. IV. Irons-Georges, Tracy.
RC41.M34 2001
610′.3—dc21   2001041169
ISBN 1-58765-003-7 (set)   CIP
ISBN 1-58765-005-3 (vol. 2)

First Printing

PRINTED IN THE UNITED STATES OF AMERICA

CONTENTS

CONTENTS

MAGILL'S

MEDICAL GUIDE

FRACTURE AND DISLOCATION
DISEASE/DISORDER

ANATOMY OR SYSTEM AFFECTED: Arms, bones, hands, hips, joints, knees, legs, musculoskeletal system

SPECIALTIES AND RELATED FIELDS: Emergency medicine, orthopedics

DEFINITION: A fracture is a break in a bone, which may be partial or complete; a dislocation is the forceful separation of bones in a joint.

KEY TERMS:

anesthesia: a state characterized by loss of sensation, caused by or resulting from the pharmacological depression of normal nerve function

callus: a hard, bonelike substance made by osteocytes which is found in and around the ends of a fractured bone; it temporarily maintains bony alignment and is resorbed after complete healing or union of a fracture occurs

ecchymosis: a purplish patch on the skin caused by

Types of Fracture

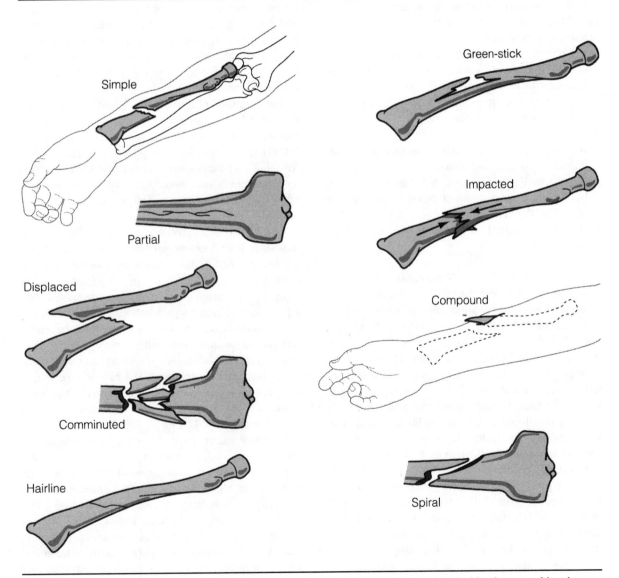

All fractures are either simple (closed) or compound (open); they are further classified by the type of break.

bleeding; the spots are easily visible to the naked eye

embolus: an obstruction or occlusion of a vessel (most commonly, an artery or vein) caused by a transported blood clot, vegetation, mass of bacteria, or other foreign material

epiphysis: the part of a long bone from which growth or elongation occurs

instability: excessive mobility of two or more bones caused by damage to ligaments, the joint capsule, or fracture of one or more bones

ischemia: a local anemia or area of diminished or insufficient blood supply due to mechanical obstruction, commonly narrowing of an artery

osteoblast: a bone-forming cell

osteocyte: a bone cell

paralysis: the loss of power of voluntary movement or other function of a muscle as a result of disease or injury to its nerve supply

petechiae: minute spots caused by hemorrhage or bleeding into the skin; the spots are the size of pinheads

prone: the position of the body when face downward, on one's stomach and abdomen

pulse: the rhythmical dilation of an artery, produced by the increased volume of blood forced into the vessel by the contraction of the heart

transection: a partial or complete severance of the spinal cord

CAUSES AND SYMPTOMS

A fracture is a linear deformation or discontinuity of a bone produced by the application of a force that exceeds the modulus of elasticity (ability to bend) of a bone. Normal bones require excessive force to fracture. Bones may be weakened by disease or other pathology such as a tumor or tumor-related disease that reduces their ability to withstand an impact. Bones respond to stresses made upon them and can thus be strengthened through physical conditioning and made more resistant to fracture. This is a normal part of training in many athletic activities.

Fractures are classified according to the type of break or, more correctly, by the plane or surface that is fractured. A break that is at a right angle to the axis of the bone is called transverse. A fracture that is similar but at an angle, rather than perpendicular to the main axis of the bone, is called oblique. If a twisting force is applied, the break may be spiral, or twisted. A comminuted fracture is a break that results

in two or more fragments of bone. If the pieces of bone remain in their original positions, the fracture is undisplaced. In a displaced fracture, the portions of bone are not properly aligned.

If bones do not penetrate the skin, the fracture is called closed, or simple. When bones protrude through the skin, the result is an open, or compound, fracture. Other types of fractures are associated with pathologic or disease processes. A stress fracture results from repeated stress or trauma to the same site of a bone. None of the individual stresses is sufficient to cause a break. If these stresses cause a callus to form, the bone will be strengthened and actual separation of fragments will not occur. A pathologic fracture occurs at the site of a tumor, infection, or other bone disease. A compression fracture results when bone is crushed; the force applied is greater than the ability of the bone to withstand it. A greenstick fracture is an incomplete separation of bone.

The diagnosis of a fracture is based on several criteria: instability, pain, swelling, deformity, and ecchymosis. The most reliable diagnostic criterion is instability. Pain is not universally present at a fracture site. Swelling may be delayed and occur at some time after a fracture is sustained. Deformity is obvious with open fractures but may not be apparent with other, undisplaced breaks.

Ecchymosis is a purplish patch caused by bleeding into skin; it will not be present if blood vessels are not broken. A definitive diagnosis is made with two plane film X rays taken at the site of a fracture and at right angles to each other. If the fracture site is visually examined and palpated shortly after the injury occurs, an accurate tentative diagnosis may be made; this should be confirmed with X rays as soon as is convenient. Occasionally, an X ray will not show undisplaced or chip fractures. If a patient experiences symptoms of pain, swelling, or ecchymosis but has a negative X ray for fracture, the site should be immobilized and X-rayed again in two to three weeks.

Fractures occur most commonly in extremities: arms or legs. Such fractures must be evaluated to determine if injuries have occurred to other tissues such as nerves or blood vessels. The presence of bruising or ecchymosis indicates blood vessel damage. The existence of peripheral pulses indicates that arteries are not injured. Venous flow is more difficult to evaluate. For a relatively short period of time, however, venous bleeding may be of lesser importance and thereby tolerated.

Dislocated Shoulder

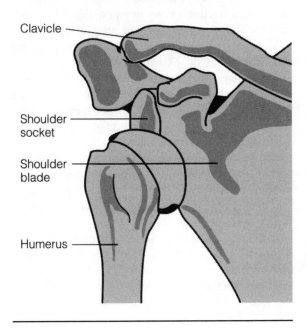

Clavicle

Shoulder socket

Shoulder blade

Humerus

Neurologic functioning may be assessed by the ability of the patient to contract muscles or sense skin touches or pinpricks. Temporary immobilization may be necessary before nerve status can be evaluated accurately.

An open fracture creates a direct pathway between the skin surface and underlying tissues. If the site becomes contaminated by bacteria, an opportunity for osteomyelitis (infection of the bone) is created. Inadequate treatment by the initial surgeon may result in skin loss, delayed union, loss of joint mobility, osteomyelitis, and even amputation.

Skin damage may or may not be related to a fracture. When skin integrity is broken over or near a fracture site, bone involvement must be assumed. The problem is infection of the fracture site; appropriate antibiotics are normally administered. If skin damage is extensive, final surgical reduction of the underlying fracture may have to be delayed until the skin is healed.

Delayed union refers to the inability of a fractured bone to heal. This is a potentially serious problem, as normal stability is not possible as long as a fracture exists. Joints may not function normally in the presence of a fracture. If a fracture heals improperly, bones may be misaligned and cause pain with movement, leading to limitations of motion. If the bones

are affected by osteomyelitis, the infection may spread to the joint capsule and reduce the normal range of motion for the bones or the joint. Amputation may become necessary if infection becomes extensive in the area of a fracture. An infection which becomes firmly established in bones or spreads widely into adjacent muscle tissue may lead to cellulitis or gangrene and may compromise a portion of an extremity. Amputation may be performed if the pathologic process cannot be treated with antibiotics.

Adequate blood supply to tissues is critical for survival. In an extremity, the maximum time limit for complete ischemia (lack of blood flow) is six to eight hours; after that time, the likelihood of later amputation increases. Pain, pallor, pulselessness, and paralysis are indicators of impaired circulation associated with a fracture. When two of these signs are present, the possibility of vascular damage must be thoroughly explored.

Dislocations occur at joints and are caused by an applied force that is greater than the strength of the ligaments and muscles that keep a joint intact. The result is a stretching deformity or injury to a joint and abnormal movement of a bone out of the joint. Accidental trauma, commonly the result of an athletic injury or automobile accident, is the most common cause of a dislocation. Joints that are frequently dislocated include the shoulder and digits (fingers and toes). Dislocations of the ankle and hip are infrequent but serious; they require immediate management. Dislocations may accompany fractures, but the two injuries need not occur together.

When dislocations are reduced, the bones of the joint are returned to normal position. Reduction is accomplished by relaxing adjacent muscles and applying traction or a pulling force to the bone until it returns to its normal position in the joint. For most dislocations of the shoulder, the victim lies in a prone position and the dislocated arm hangs down freely. Gradual traction is applied until reduction occurs. This can be accomplished by bandaging a pail to the arm and slowly filling it with water. Alternatively, a heavy book can be held by the victim and the muscles of the arm allowed to relax until the dislocation is reduced. Such treatments are usually reserved for situations in which medical assistance is unavailable. Digits are reduced in a similar manner, by gentle pulling of the end of the finger or toe. Ankle and hip dislocations are potentially more serious because these joints are more complex and have extensive blood supplies. Reduction of dislocated ankles and hips should be undertaken by qualified medical personnel in an expedited manner.

After reduction, all dislocations should be evaluated by competent medical personnel. With dislocated digits, later damage is relatively unlikely but can occur because of ligament damage sustained in the initial injury. Dislocations of the shoulder may be accompanied by a fracture of the clavicle or collar bone and may involve nerve damage in the shoulder joint. Dislocations of the ankle and hip may lead to avascular necrosis (damage to the bone as a result of inadequate blood supply) if not evaluated and reduced promptly.

TREATMENT AND THERAPY

Fractures are usually treated by reduction and immobilization. Reduction, which refers to the process of returning the fractured bones to normal position, may be either closed or open. Closed reduction is accomplished without surgery by manipulating the broken bone through overlying skin and muscles. Open reduction requires surgical intervention in which the broken pieces are exposed and returned to normal position. Orthopedic appliances may be used to hold the bones in correct position. The most common of these appliances are pins and screws, but metal plates and wires may also be employed. Orthopedic appliances are usually made of stainless steel. These may be left in the body indefinitely or may be surgically removed after healing is complete. Local anesthesia is usually used with closed reductions; open reductions are performed in an operating room, under sterile conditions using general anesthesia.

Immobilization is generally accomplished by the use of a cast. Casts are often made of plaster, but they may be constructed of inflatable plastic. It is important to hold bones in a rigid, fixed position for a sufficient length of time for the broken ends to unite and heal. The cast must be loose enough, however, to allow blood to circulate. Padding is usually put in place before plaster is applied to form a cast. Whenever possible, the newly immobilized body part is elevated to reduce the chance of swelling in the cast, which would compromise the blood supply to the fracture site and body portion beyond the cast. Casts should be checked periodically to ensure that they do not impair circulation.

The broken bone and accompanying body part must be placed in an anatomically neutral position.

This is done to minimize postfracture disability and improve the prospect for rehabilitation. The length of time that a fractured bone is immobilized is highly variable and dependent on a number of factors.

Traction may also be used to immobilize a fracture. Traction is the external application of force to overcome muscular resistance and hold bones in a desired position. Commonly, holes are drilled through bones and pins are inserted; the ends of these pins extend through the surface of the skin. Part of the body is fixed in position through the use of a strap or weights, and wires are attached to the pins in the body part to be stretched. Weights or tension is applied to the wires until the broken bone parts move into the desired position. Traction is maintained until healing has occurred.

Individual ends of a single fractured bone are sometimes held in position by external pins and screws. Holes are drilled through the bone, and pins are inserted. The pins on opposite sides of the fracture site are then attached to each other with threaded rods and locked in position by nuts. This process allows a fractured bone to be immobilized without using a cast.

Fractures of different bones require different amounts of time to heal. Further, age is a factor in fracture healing. Fractures in young children heal more quickly than do broken bones in adults. Older adults typically require even more time for healing. The availability of calcium and other nutrients also affects the speed with which a fracture heals.

Delayed union of fractures is a term applied to fractures that either do not heal or take longer than normal to heal; there is no precise time frame associated with delayed union. Nonunion refers to fractures in which healing is not observed and cannot be expected even with prolonged immobilization. X-ray analysis of a nonunion will show that the bone ends have hardened (sclerosed), that the ends of the marrow canal have become plugged, and that a gap persists between the ends of a fractured bone. Nonunion may be caused by inadequate blood supply to the fracture site, which leads to the formation of cartilage instead of new bone between the broken pieces of bone. Nonunion may also be caused by injury to the soft tissues that surround a fracture site. This damage impairs the formation of a callus and the reestablishment of an adequate blood supply to the fracture site; it is frequently seen in young children. Inadequate immobilization may also allow soft tissue to enter the fracture site, by slipping between the bone fragments, and may lead to nonunion. Respect for tissue and minimizing damage in the vicinity of a fracture, specially with open reduction, will minimize problems of nonunion. Subjecting the nonuniting fracture site to a low-level electromagnetic field will usually stimulate osteoblastic activity and lead to healing.

The epiphyseal plate is the portion of bone where growth occurs. Bony epiphyses are active in children until they attain their adult height, at which time the epiphyses become inactive and close. Once an epiphysis ceases to function, further growth does not occur. In children, a fracture involving the epiphyseal plate is potentially dangerous because bone growth may be interrupted or halted. This situation can lead to inequalities in the length of extremities or impaired range of movement in joints. Accurate reduction of injuries involving an epiphyseal plate is necessary to minimize subsequent deformity. A key factor is blood supply to the injured area: If adequate blood supply is maintained, epiphyseal plate damage is minimized.

Fractures of the spinal vertebrae are potentially very dangerous because they can cause injury to the nerves and tracts of the spinal cord. Fractures of the vertebrae are commonly sustained in automobile accidents, athletic injuries, falls from heights, and other situations involving rapid deceleration. When vertebrae are fractured, the spinal cord can be compromised. Spinal cord injury can be direct and cut all or a portion of the spinal nerves at the site of the fracture. The extent of the damage is dependent on the level of the injury. An accident that completely severs the spinal cord will lead to a complete loss of function for all structures below the level of injury. Since spinal nerves are arranged segmentally, cord damage at a lower level involves compromise of fewer structures. As the level of injury becomes higher in the spinal cord, more vital structures are involved. Transection of the spinal cord in the neck usually leads to complete paralysis of the entire body; it can cause death if high enough to cut the nerves controlling the lungs. Individuals in whom vertebral fractures and thus spinal cord injuries are suspected must have the spinal column immobilized before they are moved. Reduction of spinal cord fractures must be undertaken by a highly skilled person.

When bones having large marrow cavities such as the femur (thigh bone) are fractured, fat globules may escape from the marrow and enter the bloodstream. Such a fat globule is then called an embolus (plural is emboli). Fat emboli are potentially dangerous in that they can become lodged in the capillaries of the lungs. This causes pain and can lead to impaired oxygenation of blood, a condition called hypoxemia. About 10 to 20 percent of individuals sustaining a fractured femur also have central nervous system depression and skin petechiae (minute spots caused by hemorrhage or bleeding into the skin) in addition to hypoxemia in the two to three days after the injury. This triad of signs is called fat embolism syndrome. It is treated medically with oxygen, steroids, and anticoagulant drugs.

PERSPECTIVE AND PROSPECTS

Fractures rarely threaten a patient's life directly, and injuries to the brain, heart, circulatory system, and abdominal cavity must receive priority of treatment. It is imperative, however, not to move a patient in whom a fracture is suspected without first immobilizing the potential fracture site. This is especially true with suspected fractures of the spine. Instability may not be apparent when a patient is lying down but can become catastrophic if the person is moved without proper preparation and immobilization.

Crush injuries of the spinal cord are relatively common among victims of osteoporosis. Osteoporosis is a pathological syndrome defined by a decrease in the density of a bone below the level required for mechanical support and is frequently associated with a deficiency of calcium, problems related to calcium in the body, or a rate of bone cell breakdown that is greater than the rate of bone cell remodeling. Crush fractures occur when the bones become so weak that the weight of the upper portion of the body is greater than the ability of the vertebrae to support it. These crush injuries may occur slowly over time and cause no serious injury to the underlying spinal cord. The resulting deformity of the spine, however, impairs movement. There is no treatment for osteoporotic crush fractures of the vertebrae.

Occupational exposures may lead to fractures and dislocations. Professional athletes are clearly at increased risk for skeletal injuries. These individuals are also usually well conditioned, however, and so can withstand increased impacts and blows to the body. Many are also trained in methods that minimize the force of impact; they know how to fall properly.

The vast proportion of workers are not conditioned and are given minimal training to avoid situations that lead to fractures. Accident analysis reveals that carelessness is the most common predisposing factor. Workers operating without safety equipment such as belaying lines or belts may become overconfident. In such a situation, slips or falls can occur, and fractures result. Unsafe equipment can lead to hazardous situations and cause fractures or dislocations. Machinery that is not properly maintained can fail; parts may become detached, hit nearby workers, and cause fractures.

Recreational activities also result in fractures. Individuals who once were well conditioned may engage in sports without proper equipment and sustain fractures or dislocations. Contact sports such as football, hockey, and basketball are primary examples of such activities. Riding bicycles and motorized recreational vehicles without proper safety equipment can lead to serious skeletal injuries. Activities such as rock climbing are inherently dangerous. With proper training and use of safety equipment, accidents can be reduced or their severity minimized. The keys to avoiding fractures and dislocations when participating in recreational activities are receiving proper instruction and training, employing adequate safety equipment, and using common sense by avoiding difficult or hazardous situations that are beyond one's physical abilities or skill level.

—*L. Fleming Fallon, Jr., M.D., Ph.D., M.P.H.*

See also Bone disorders; Bone grafting; Bones and the skeleton; Fracture repair; Head and neck disorders; Hip fracture repair; Orthopedic surgery; Orthopedics; Orthopedics, pediatric; Osteoporosis; Physical rehabilitation; Spinal cord disorders; Spine, vertebrae, and disks; Wounds.

FOR FURTHER INFORMATION:

Sabiston, David C., Jr., ed. *Textbook of Surgery: The Biological Basis of Modern Surgical Practice.* 16th ed. Philadelphia: W. B. Saunders, 2001. A standard textbook of surgery which contains an extensive discussion of different types of fractures and dislocations and how they are treated. Intended for practicing professionals but can be generally understood by the layperson.

Schwartz, Seymour I., ed. *Principles of Surgery.* 7th ed. New York: McGraw-Hill, 1999. A standard textbook of surgery containing sections on fractures and dislocations. Its intended audience is practicing surgeons, and thus the language is sometimes technical. Nevertheless, the serious reader can obtain much useful detail from this work.

Way, Lawrence W., ed. *Current Surgical Diagnosis and Treatment.* 11th ed. Norwalk, Conn.: Appleton and Lange, 1998. The diagnosis and treatment of fractures and dislocations is discussed in a brief and concise format emphasizing treatment modalities. The different section authors are recognized experts in their fields. The material is accessible to the general reader, but the sections are brief.

Wilmore, Douglas W., et al., eds. *Care of the Surgical Patient.* New York: Scientific American, 1992. This book should be understandable to laypersons even though it is written for professionals. Sections in part 1 discuss fractures and dislocations. The reputation of *Scientific American* for style and clarity is evident in this book. A good source for the general reader.

FRACTURE REPAIR

PROCEDURE

ANATOMY OR SYSTEM AFFECTED: Arms, bones, hips, legs, musculoskeletal system, teeth

SPECIALTIES AND RELATED FIELDS: Dentistry, orthopedics

DEFINITION: The placement and fixation of broken portions of bones in their correct positions until they have grown together.

INDICATIONS AND PROCEDURES

A fracture is a break in a bone, either partial or complete, resulting from an applied force that is greater than the bone's internal strength. The most common causes of fractures are accidents or trauma.

Fractures are usually treated by reduction and immobilization. Reduction, which may be either closed or open, refers to the process of returning the fractured bones to normal position. Closed reduction is accomplished without surgery by manipulating the broken bone through overlying skin and muscles. Open reduction requires surgical intervention. The broken pieces are exposed and returned to their normal positions. Orthopedic appliances may be used to hold the bones in the proper position (internal fixation); the most common appliances are stainless steel pins and screws, but metal plates and wires may also be employed. These devices can be left in the body indefinitely or may be surgically removed after healing is complete. Local anesthesia is usually used with closed reductions; open reductions are performed in an operating room under sterile conditions, using general anesthesia.

After reduction, the broken bone and accompanying body part must be placed in an anatomically neutral position. Immobilization is generally accomplished by the use of a cast. Casts are usually made of plaster, but they may be constructed of inflatable plastic.

Individual ends of a single fractured bone are sometimes held in position by external pins and

Types of Fracture Repair

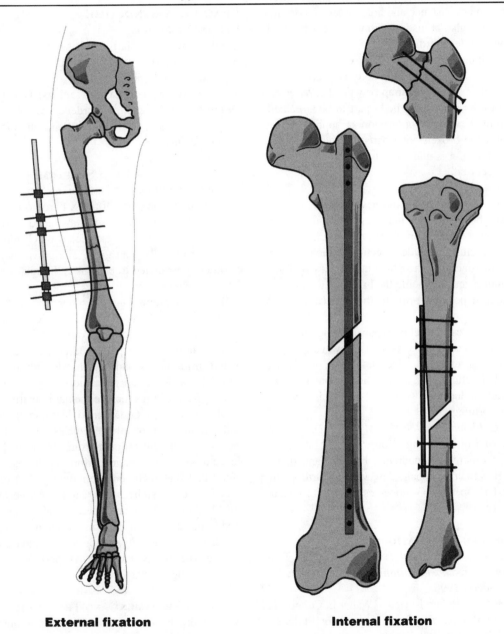

External fixation   **Internal fixation**

Severe leg fractures can be immobilized through external fixation or internal fixation. External fixation involves the use of long pins that are inserted through the bone and held in place with a steel rod on the outside of the body. Internal fixation involves the use of screws, pins, and plates that are attached directly to the bones and often left there permanently.

screws (external fixation). Holes are drilled through the bone, and pins are inserted as described above. The pins on opposite sides of the fracture site are then attached to each other with threaded rods and locked in position by nuts. This process allows a fractured bone to be immobilized without using a cast.

Traction, the external application of force to overcome muscular resistance and hold bones in a desired position, may also be used to immobilize a fracture. Commonly, holes are drilled through bones and pins are inserted; the ends of these pins extend through the surface of the skin. Part of the body is fixed in position through the use of a strap or weights. Wires are attached to the pins in the body part to be stretched. Force through weights or tension is applied to the wires until the broken bone parts are in the desired position. Traction is maintained until complete healing has occurred.

USES AND COMPLICATIONS

All broken bones must be held in position until healing takes place. The complications associated with repairing fractures include infection, which is rare, and loss of function. The potential for loss of function is minimized by placing the limb into an anatomically neutral position prior to the application of a cast.

The techniques of fracture repair have not changed radically in decades. New methods, however, are being tried. For example, electromagnetic fields are used with fractures that do not heal spontaneously. Such a field induces the growth of osteoblasts, which are bone-forming cells.

—*L. Fleming Fallon, Jr., M.D., Ph.D., M.P.H.*

See also Bone grafting; Bones and the skeleton; Dentistry; Emergency medicine; Fracture and dislocation; Hip fracture repair; Jaw wiring; Orthopedic surgery; Orthopedics; Orthopedics, pediatric; Osteoporosis; Teeth.

FOR FURTHER INFORMATION:

Browner, Bruce D. *Skeletal Trauma: Fractures, Dislocations, Ligamentous Injuries.* Philadelphia: W. B. Saunders, 1998.

Eiff, M. Patrice, Robert L. Hatch, Walter L. Calmbach. *Fracture Management for Primary Care.* Philadelphia: W. B. Saunders, 1998.

Gregg, Paul J., Jack Stevens, and Peter H. Worlock. *Fractures and Dislocations: Principles of Management.* Cambridge, Mass.: Blackwell Science, 1996.

Gustilo, Ramon B., Richard F. Kyle, and David C. Templeman, eds. *Fractures and Dislocations.* St. Louis: C. V. Mosby, 1993.

Ruiz, Ernest, and James J. Cicero, eds. *Emergency Management of Skeletal Injuries.* St. Louis: C. V. Mosby, 1995.

FRAGILE X SYNDROME
DISEASE/DISORDER

ALSO KNOWN AS: Martin-Bell syndrome

ANATOMY OR SYSTEM AFFECTED: Brain, ears, feet, genitals, hands, joints

SPECIALTIES AND RELATED FIELDS: Genetics

DEFINITION: A genetic disorder of variable expression, with mental retardation being the most common feature.

CAUSES AND SYMPTOMS

Fragile X syndrome is caused by a change in a gene located on the long arm of the X chromosome. It is a sex-linked inherited disease, transmitted from parent to child, with boys being affected much more often and more severely than girls. The prevalence of the disorder is estimated to be 1 in 1,200 males and 1 in 2,500 females.

While symptoms and their severity vary widely, common physical features of fragile X syndrome include a long, thin face, a prominent jaw and ears, a broad nose, a high palate, large testicles (macroorchidism) in males, and large hands with loose finger joints. Physical features are more subtle in females. Nonphysical features include mental impairment ranging from severe retardation to learning disabilities, with the majority of affected males demonstrating a mental impairment ranging from low-normal intelligence to severe retardation. More recent research has found that the intelligence quotients (IQs) of males with fragile X syndrome appear to decline throughout childhood. Associated behavioral symptoms include unusual speech patterns, problems with attention span, hyperactivity, motor delays, and occasional autistic-type behaviors, such as poor eye contact, hand-flapping, or hand-biting.

TREATMENT AND THERAPY

While there is no cure for fragile X syndrome, a number of possible interventions can address various symptoms. Medications can be administered to assist with attention span and hyperactivity, as well as with aggressive behavior. Schools can provide children with assistance in speech, physical therapy, and vocational planning. Early childhood special education services for children prior to school age can provide necessary early intervention that may prove most helpful if indeed the rate of learning for children with fragile X syndrome slows with age. Genetic counseling is advised for families who carry the gene.

PERSPECTIVE AND PROSPECTS

In 1969, the discovery was made of a break or fragile site on the long arm of the X chromosome. It was not until the 1980's, however, that consistent diagnoses of fragile X syndrome were made. In 1991, the responsible gene was sequenced and named the FMR-1 (fragile X mental retardation 1) gene. Cytogenetic and deoxyribonucleic acid (DNA) testing are now available to identify affected persons.

—*Robin Hasslen, Ph.D.*

See also Genetic diseases; Genetics and inheritance; Learning disabilities; Mental retardation; Motor skill development; Speech disorders.

FOR FURTHER INFORMATION:

Edlin, Gordon. *Human Genetics*. Boston: Jones and Bartlett, 1990.

Maxon, Linda, and Charles Daugherty. *Genetics: A Human Perspective*. Dubuque, Iowa: Wm. C. Brown, 1992.

Pierce, Benjamin A. *The Family Genetic Sourcebook*. New York: John Wiley & Sons, 1990.

FROSTBITE

DISEASE/DISORDER

ANATOMY OR SYSTEM AFFECTED: Hands, feet, skin and adjacent tissues

SPECIALTIES AND RELATED FIELDS: Emergency medicine, environmental health

DEFINITION: Frostbite is localized freezing of tissue, usually of extremities exposed to low temperatures and resulting in ice crystals forming within cells, thereby killing them.

KEY TERMS:

anticoagulant: a drug that reduces the clotting of the blood

basal metabolic rate: the rate at which the body burns calories and produces heat energy while the body is at rest or not active

gangrene: the death of part of the body (such as an arm or leg) caused by the death of the cells in that structure

hypothermia: the process by which the body core temperature falls below that needed for the body to function normally

hypoxia: a lack of an adequate amount of oxygen to the tissues; results in a reduction of mental and physical capabilities

maceration: the process of breaking down tissue to a soft mass, either by soaking it or through infection or gangrene

necrosis: the death of body tissue cells

sludging: an increase in red blood cell structures, known as platelets, which slows down the blood flow through vessels and promotes clotting of the blood

sympathectomy: the surgical process of removing or destroying nerves that may be afflicted by frostbite or other injury

vascoconstriction: a decrease in the diameter of vessels transporting blood throughout the body, reducing blood flow and oxygen transport

windchill: the effect of wind blowing across exposed flesh; increased heat is lost from the skin's surface, as if the air were much colder than the actual temperature indicates

CAUSES AND SYMPTOMS

The effect of cold on the human body is to reduce the circulation of blood to surface areas, such as the feet, hands, and face. This reduction restricts the amount of heat lost by the body and helps to prevent the development of hypothermia. Blood constriction may become so severe in severely chilled areas of the body, however, that circulation almost totally ceases. People with poorer circulation, such as the elderly and the exhausted, are not as resistant to low temperatures as are fit or younger people.

If the skin's temperature falls below −0.53 degree Celsius, the tissue actually freezes and frostbite occurs. Rapid freezing causes ice crystals to form within a cell. These crystals rupture the cell wall and destroy structures within the cell, effectively killing it. If freezing is slow, ice crystals form between the cells; they grow by extracting water from the cells. The tissue may be injured physically by the ice crystals or by dehydration and the resulting disruption of osmotic and chemical balance within the cells; however, tissue death following frostbite is more likely to be attributable to interruption of the blood supply to the tissue than to the direct action of freezing. Cold also damages the capillaries in the affected areas,

Frostbite

Frostbitten areas

Areas of probable gangrene

Frostbite commonly affects the hands and feet.

causing blood plasma to leak through their walls, thus adding to tissue injury and further impairing circulation by allowing the blood to sludge (to clot because of an increase in red blood cells) inside the vessels. All sensation of cold or pain is lost as circulation becomes seriously impaired. Unless the tissue is warmed quickly, the skin and superficial tissues actually begin to freeze. With continual chilling, the frozen area enlarges and extends to deeper areas. This condition is known as frostbite.

Frostbite was common among soldiers during Napoleon's campaign in Russia in the early 1800's, during World War II in Northern Europe, in the Korean War, and in fighting between Indian and Chinese troops in the Himalayas. Air crews, especially waist-

gunners in the U.S. Air Force in World War II, were particularly prone to frostbite. In 1943, frostbite injuries among these bomber crews were greater than all other casualties combined.

Polar travelers before the 1920's suffered severely from frostbite. Mountain climbers are at risk from frostbite at higher elevations. Lower oxygen availability increases the danger of frostbite because the body cannot take in sufficient oxygen in this thinner air. The resulting condition, called hypoxia, reduces mental abilities, and precautions normally taken against the cold may be either inadequate or neglected altogether. High winds, often experienced in the mountains, speed heat loss from exposed skin surfaces. This windchill can be deadly to mountaineers and often produces hypothermia. Poor appetite at high elevations reduces the energy available for the production of body heat. The insulating layer of subcutaneous fat also decreases with longer periods of time spent at higher elevations; this in turn decreases the insulation of the surface areas of the body against freezing.

Inadequate food intake while mountain climbing increases the danger of frostbite, as the body does not have enough calories to keep its temperature constant. The occurrence of hypothermia also increases the risk of frostbite as heat is drawn away from extremities to protect the body's core temperature. At higher elevations, most humans function at only about 60 percent of the physiological efficiency that they have at sea level. Women have more resistance to cold and may be less likely to experience frostbite than are men.

Frostbite at high altitudes seems to be more common for the same temperature than at lower altitudes. More red blood cells are found in the blood of persons working at higher elevations, thickening the blood and reducing circulation to the extremities. This reduced circulation lowers the temperature of these extremities. The basal metabolic rate and cardiac output of the body also decrease as one goes higher; both of these actions reduce the body's ability to keep its feet, hands, and face warm.

Blood vessels move heat from the central body core to the skin; it radiates into the air from exposed surfaces. This heat loss is greatest in the hands, feet, and head, where the vessels are close to the skin's surface. Respiration loses body heat when cold air is inhaled into the lungs and body heat warms it; this heat is lost when the air is exhaled. Evaporation, moisture leaving the skin's surface, also draws heat from the body. In low temperatures, spilling gasoline on exposed skin will create frostbite because the evaporation of the fuel draws heat away from the body quickly. Convection carries body heat away by wind currents. This windchill factor, calculated for Fahrenheit temperatures by subtracting two times the windspeed from the air temperature, determines the amount of heat energy lost from the body's surface. Conduction transfers heat from one substance to another; for example, contact between the body and snow or metal will cause the skin to lose heat. Although many people work and live in subzero temperatures, frostbite is uncommon. Nevertheless, an accident that prevents one from moving, loss of the ability to shiver in order to generate heat, or inactivity may increase the chance of developing frostbite. Frostbite can occur in any cold environment. Warning symptoms of frostbite initially include tingling and pain in the afflicted tissues. The skin may be slightly flushed before freezing. It then turns white or a blotchy blue in color and is firm and insensitive to the touch. Tissue that is painful and then becomes numb and insensitive is frozen.

TREATMENT AND THERAPY

Slight cases of frostbite, often termed frostnip or superficial frostbite, can be treated outdoors or in the field with little or no medical help. Such cases are usually reversible, with no permanent damage, as only skin and subcutaneous tissues are involved. The frozen part, although white and frozen on the surface, is soft and pliable when pressed gently before thawing. The area is often a cheek or the tip of the nose or the fingers. The frozen area, usually small, can be warmed manually. A hand is placed over the frostnipped area if it is a cheek or nose, and frozen fingers can be placed under the armpit or on a partner's bare stomach for warming. Tissue that has had only a minor amount of frostnip soon returns to normal color. A tingling sensation is felt when frostnipped tissue is thawed. After thawing, areas that have had more serious superficial frostbite become numb, mottled, or blue or purple in color and then will sting, burn, or swell for a period of time. Blisters, small ones called blebs, may occur within twenty-four to forty-eight hours. Blistering is more common where the skin is loose. Blister fluid is absorbed slowly; the skin may harden, become black (from gangrene), and be insensitive to touch. Throbbing or aching may persist for

weeks. Gangrene occurring after frostnip is essentially superficial and extends only a few millimeters deep into the tissue. In two or three months, this type of frostbite will be mostly healed. With immediate treatment, frostnipped tissue will not progress to the much more serious injury of deep frostbite.

Tissues vary in their resistance to frostbite. Skin freezes at −0.53 Celsius, while muscles, blood vessels, and nerves are also highly subject to freezing. Connective tissue, tendons, and bones are relatively resistant to freezing, which explains why the blackened extremities of a frostbitten hand or foot can be moved: The tendons under the gangrenous skin remain intact and functional.

Deep frostbite includes not only skin and subcutaneous tissue but also deeper structures, including muscle, bone, and tendons. The affected area becomes cold, mottled, and blue or gray in color and may remain swollen for months. With deep frostbite, the tissues become quite hard to the touch. One to three days after thawing, the affected area becomes quite painful. Blisters, initially small blebs and then large, coalescing ones, may take weeks to develop. The patient should not be allowed to become alarmed about his or her condition; even mild cases of frostbite have a frightening appearance during blistering. Initially, the frozen part may be painless, but shooting and throbbing pains may occur for several months after thawing. Permanent loss of tissue is almost inevitable with deep frostbite. The affected extremity has a severely shriveled look. A limb may return to almost normal over some months, however, and amputation should never be carried out until a considerable period, probably at least six to nine months, has elapsed.

In cases of frostbite, surgical intervention must be minimal. Blackened frostbitten tissue will gradually separate itself from healthy, unfrozen tissue without interference; no efforts should be taken to hasten separation. Most cases of deep frostbite seem to heal in six to twelve months, and the gangrenous tissue, if it has not become infected with bacteria, is essentially superficial. Many unnecessary amputations have been carried out because of impatience at the slow recovery rate of tissue that has suffered deep frostbite; amputation is only necessary when infection has set in and it cannot be controlled with antibiotics.

If possible, deep frostbite should be treated under hospital care, not in the field or outdoors. The deep frozen tissue should remain frozen until hospital care is available. If frozen tissues are thawed, the patient will most likely be unable to move as the pain will be severe with any movement. Walking on feet that have been thawed after being frozen will cause permanent damage; however, walking on a frozen foot for twelve to eighteen hours or even longer produces less damage than inadequate warming. As frozen tissue thaws, cells exude fluid. If this tissue is refrozen, ice crystals form and cause more extensive, irreparable damage.

Rapid rewarming is the recommended treatment for deep frostbite and is a proven method of reducing tissue loss. Rubbing the frostbitten area with the hand or snow—akin to rubbing the area with broken glass—should never be done. This treatment does not melt the intracellular ice crystals, nor does it increase circulation to the frozen area. It breaks the skin and allows infection to enter into the system. Vasodilator agents do not improve tissue survival. Local antibiotics in aerosol form can be used, but it is unwise to rely on this method alone for combating infection. Sympathectomy, the removal or destruction of affected nerves, does not improve cell survival. The use of the drug dextran early to prevent sludging has limited use and may have dangerous side effects. The use of hyperbaric oxygen or supplementary oxygen may increase the tissue tension of oxygen and save some cells partially damaged by cold injury.

Rewarming should be carried out in a water bath with water temperatures ranging from 37.7 to 42.2 degrees Celsius (100 to 108 degrees Fahrenheit). Higher temperatures will further damage already injured tissues. Rewarming in a large bathtub warms the frozen extremity more rapidly, resulting in less tissue loss in many cases, particularly where frostbite has been deep and extensive. A large container also permits more accurate control of the water temperature. If a bathtub is not available, a bucket, large wastebasket, dishpan, or other similar container can be used. During rewarming, hot water usually must be added to the bath occasionally to keep the temperature correct; in such cases the injured extremity should be removed from the bath and not returned to it until the water has been thoroughly mixed and its temperature measured. An open flame must not come into contact with the area to which heat is applied, since sensation is lost as a result of the frostbite and the tissue could be seriously burned.

For rewarming, the extremity should be stripped of all clothing, and any constricting bands, straps, or other objects that might stop circulation should be removed. The injured area should be suspended in the center of the water and not permitted to rest against the side or bottom. Warming should continue for thirty to forty minutes. The frostbitten tissues may become quite painful during this process, so it may be necessary to give painkillers to the patient in order to reduce discomfort during or after thawing of the frostbitten area. Aspirin (as well as codeine, morphine, or meperidine, if needed) may be given for pain. Aspirin or an anticoagulant increases blood circulation by reducing red blood cell platelet formation and thus reducing sludging. Phenoxybenzamine reduces vasoconstriction.

Following rewarming, the patient must be kept warm and the injured tissue elevated and protected from any kind of trauma. One should avoid rupturing blisters that have formed. Blankets or bedclothes should be supported by a framework to avoid pressure or rubbing of the injured area.

Subsequent care is directed primarily toward preventing infection. Cleanliness of the frostbitten area is extremely important. It should be soaked daily in a water bath at body temperature to which a germicidal soap has been added. If contamination of the water supply is a possibility, the bath water should be boiled and cooled before use. Dead tissue should not be cut or pulled away; the water baths remove such tissue more efficiently.

The afflicted area should be immobilized and kept sterile. Even contact with sheets can be damaging to a frostbitten limb. Sterile, dry cotton may be placed between the fingers or toes to avoid maceration. If infection appears present, as indicated by the area between the frostbitten tissue and healthy tissue becoming inflamed and feeling tender or throbbing, antibiotics such as ampicillin or cloxicillin should be given every six hours. Wet, antiseptic dressings should be applied if gangrene occurs in the damaged tissue. A tetanus toxoid booster shot, or human antitoxin if the patient has not been previously immunized against tetanus, should be given. Complete rest and a diet high in protein will help healing. Moderate movement of the afflicted area should be encouraged but should be limited to that done by a physical therapist, without assistance by the patient. Considerable reassurance and emotional support may be required by the patient, as the appearance of the frostbitten area can be alarming.

Amputation in response to infected, spreading gangrene may be needed eventually, but it should be delayed until the natural separation of dead from living tissue and bone has taken place. Radionucleotide scanning helps save frostbitten limbs. These scans accurately demonstrate blood flow in frostbitten extremities, thus predicting what tissue will survive.

PERSPECTIVE AND PROSPECTS

Frostbite is an injury that can affect anyone who works or plays under cold conditions. Increased knowledge about what causes this injury, better equipment, and techniques that minimize its effect, however, have reduced its occurrence. Advances in medical knowledge regarding how the injury occurs within the afflicted tissues have produced treatment protocols that reduce the extent of permanent injury from frostbite.

Prevention is the most effective treatment for frostbite, which can occur only when the body lacks enough heat to keep the extremities above freezing. The overall body heat deficit results from inadequate clothing or equipment, reduced food consumption, exhaustion, injury or inactivity causing a lack of body movement, or some combination of these factors. Those playing or working in a cold environment should know the conditions under which frostbite may develop. For frostnip to occur, the windchill index must exceed 1,400 and the air temperature must be below the freezing point of exposed skin (−0.53 degree Celsius). An ambient temperature of −10 to −15 degrees Celsius is usually necessary for deep frostbite to develop.

Adequate clothing—especially boots that allow circulation to occur freely, mittens (not gloves) that cover the hands, and a head covering that protects the face, ears, and neck— must be worn. Boots should be well broken in and large enough to fit comfortably with several pairs of socks. The laces at the top of the boots should not be tight. Gaiters or overboots should be worn if deep or wet snow is anticipated. Windproof or insulated pants protect the legs from cold and help keep the feet warm. Dry socks and mitten liners should be carried. Moisture greatly reduces the insulative value of clothing, so it is necessary to stay dry; if clothing becomes wet or damp, one should change into dry items. Plastic bags, worn over bare feet, provide a vapor barrier liner that is effective in helping keep one's feet dry and warm under cold conditions. Adequate ventilation avoids dampness from excessive perspiration. Dressing in layers—having several light shirts, jackets, or a windbreaker—is better than wearing only one heavy jacket.

Heat production, resulting from exercise or the protective mechanism of shivering, is just as important as clothing in maintaining body temperature. Injuries that cause the victim to go into shock or lie immobilized, even though adequate clothing may be worn, predispose the victim to frostbite.

Eating high-energy foods and taking in 6,000 or more kilocalories (Calories) a day may be necessary to keep body temperatures constant under very cold or physically demanding conditions. Adequate rest, including eight or more hours of sleep, helps to reduce fatigue, which in turn increases the body's ability to produce heat. Alcohol and tobacco should be strictly avoided. Alcohol dilates the blood vessels and, although this action temporarily warms the skin, results in increased loss of total body heat. Smoking constricts the blood vessels in the skin and so reduces heat flow to surface areas; this may be sufficient to initiate frostbite in exposed tissue. A person who has sustained frostbite in the past is usually more susceptible to more cold injury. Problems with arthritis may develop in extremities that have been frostbitten.

—*David L. Chesemore, Ph.D.*

See also Amputation; Gangrene; Hyperthermia and hypothermia; Skin; Skin disorders.

FOR FURTHER INFORMATION:

Calvert, John H., Jr. "Frostbite." *Flying Safety* 54, no. 10 (October, 1998): 24-25. Frostbite can be a painful and disfiguring injury, caused by the freezing of the moisture in one's body tissues. Steps for taking care of frostbite injuries are presented.

Phillips, David. "How Frostbite Performs Its Misery." *Canadian Geographic* 115, no. 1 (January/February, 1995): 20-21. This article explains the progression of frostbite and discusses its causes. Illustrated with photographs.

Tilton, Buck. "The Chill That Bites." *Backpacker* 28, no. 7 (September, 2000): 27. Tilton offers important information about windchill, frostbite, and appropriate attire for braving the cold.

Wilkerson, James A., ed. *Medicine for Mountaineering and Other Wilderness Activities*. 4th ed. Seattle: The Mountaineers, 1992. This book is a first-aid manual that goes beyond traditional treatment protocols. It was written for those who need information to care for serious injuries when organized medical help is not available.

FUNGAL INFECTIONS

DISEASE/DISORDER

ANATOMY OR SYSTEM AFFECTED: Immune system, nails, respiratory system, skin

SPECIALTIES AND RELATED FIELDS: Dermatology, family practice, immunology, internal medicine, microbiology, pulmonary medicine

DEFINITION: Infections caused by fungi—simple, plantlike organisms—that range from minor skin diseases to serious, disseminated diseases of the lungs and other organs; patients whose immune systems are impaired are at greater risk of serious fungal infections.

KEY TERMS:

asexual reproduction: the production of new individuals without the mating of two parents of unlike genotype, such as by budding

mycelium: a collection of threadlike fungal strands (hyphae) making up the thallus, or nonreproductive portion, of a fungus

mycosis: a disease of humans, plants, or animals caused by a fungus; the prefix *myco-* means "fungus," hence mycology (the study of fungi)

pleomorphic fungus: a fungus whose morphology changes markedly from one phase of its life cycle to another, or according to changes in environmental conditions

tinea: a medical term for fungal skin diseases, such as ringworm and athlete's foot, caused by a variety of fungi

yeast: a unicellular fungus which reproduces by budding off smaller cells from the parent cell; yeasts belong to several different groups of fungi, and some fungi are capable of growing either as a yeast or as a filamentous fungus

TYPES OF FUNGUS

The term "fungus" is a general one for plantlike organisms that do not produce their own food through photosynthesis but live as heterotrophs, absorbing complex carbon compounds from other living or dead organisms. Fungi were formerly classified in the plant kingdom (together with bacteria, all algae, mosses, and green plants); more recently, biologists have realized that there are fundamental differences in cell structure and organization separating the lower plants into a number of groups which merit recognition as kingdoms. Fungi differ from bacteria and actinomycetes in being eukaryotic, that is, in having an organized nucleus with chromosomes within the cell. One division of fungi, which is believed to be distantly related to certain aquatic algae, has spores that swim by means of flagella. These water molds include pathogens of fish and aquatic insect larvae and a few economically important plant pathogens, but none have yet been recorded as causing a defined, nonopportunistic human disease. The other division of fungi lacks flagellated spores at any stage in its life cycle. It encompasses most familiar fungi, including molds, mushrooms, yeasts, wood-rotting fungi, leaf spots, and all fungi reliably reported to cause disease in humans.

Fungi that lack flagellated stages in their life cycles are further divided into three classes and one form-class according to the manner in which the spores are produced. The first of these, the Zygomycetes (for example *Rhizopus*, the black bread mold), produce thick-walled, solitary sexual spores as a result of hyphal fusion; they are a diverse assemblage including many parasites of insects. Species in the genus *Mucor* cause a rare, fulminating, rapidly fatal systemic disease called mucormycosis, generally in acidotic diabetic patients. The Basidiomycetes, characterized by the production of sexual spores externally on a club-shaped structure called a basidium, is a large class that includes mushrooms, plant rusts (such as stem rust of wheat), and most wood-rotting fungi. There is one important basidiomycetous human pathogen (*Filobasidiella neoformans*), and a few confirmed opportunists. The Ascomycetes, including most yeasts and lichens, many plant pathogens (such as Dutch elm disease and chestnut blight), and a great diversity of saprophytes growing on wood and herbaceous material, produce sexual spores in a saclike structure called an ascus. One ascomycete, *Piedraia nigra*, regularly produces its characteristic fruiting bodies on its human host; others do so in culture. In addition, there is a form-class Deuteromycetes consisting of fungi that produce only asexual spores. Most are suspected of being stages in the life cycle of Ascomycetes, but some are Basidiomycetes or are of uncertain affinity. Human pathogens, at least as they occur on the host or in typical laboratory culture, are mostly Deuteromycetes.

Medical mycology would occupy only a single chapter in a book on the relationship of fungi to human affairs. Relatively few fungi have become adapted to living as parasites of human (or even mammalian) hosts, and of these, the most common ones cause superficial and cutaneous mycoses with annoying but scarcely life-threatening effects. Serious fungal diseases are mercifully rare among people with normally functioning immune systems.

The majority of fungi are directly dependent on green plants, as parasites, as symbionts living in a mutually beneficial association with a plant, or as saprophytes on dead plant material. One large, successful group of Ascomycetes lives in symbiotic association with algae, forming lichens. Fungi play a critical ecological role in maintaining stable plant communities. As plant pathogens, they cause serious economic loss, leading in extreme cases to famine. The ability of saprophytic fungi to transform chemically the substrate on which they are growing has been exploited by the brewing industry since antiquity and has been expanded to other industrial processes. Penicillin, other antibiotics, and some vitamins are extracted from fungi, which produce a vast array of complex organic compounds whose potential is only beginning to be explored and which constitutes a fertile field for those interested in genetic engineering.

This same chemical diversity and complexity also enable fungi to produce mycotoxins—chemicals that have an adverse effect on humans and animals. Saprophytic fungi growing on improperly stored food are a troublesome source of toxic compounds, some of which are carcinogenic. The old adage that "a little mold won't hurt you" is true in the sense that common molds do not cause acute illness when ingested, but it is poor advice in terms of long-term health.

A mycotoxicity problem of considerable medical and veterinary interest is posed by Ascomycetes of the order Clavicipitales, which are widespread on grasses. Some species of grasses routinely harbor systemic, asymptomatic infections by these fungi, which produce compounds toxic to animals that graze on them. From the point of view of the grass, the relationship is symbiotic, since it discourages grazing; from the point of view of range management, the relationship is deleterious to stock. *Claviceps purpurea*, a pathogen of rye, causes a condition known as ergotism in humans, with symptoms including miscarriage, vascular constriction leading to gangrene of the limbs, and hallucinations. Outbreaks of hallucinatory ergotism are thought by some authors to be responsible for some of the more spectacular perceptions of witchcraft in premodern times. Better control of plant disease and a decreased reliance on rye as a staple grain have virtually eliminated ergotism as a human disease in the twentieth century.

Fungi exhibit a bewildering variety of forms and life cycles; nevertheless, certain generalizations can be made. A fungus starts life as a spore, which may be a single cell or a cluster of cells and is usually microscopic. Under proper conditions, the spore germinates, producing a filament of fungal cells oriented end to end, called a hypha. Hyphae grow into the substrate, secreting enzymes that dissolve structures to provide food for the growing fungus and to provide holes through which the fungus can grow. In an asexually reproducing fungus, some of the hyphae become differentiated, producing specialized cells (spores) which differ from the parent hypha in size and pigmentation and are adapted for dispersal, but which are genetically identical to the parent. In a sexually reproducing fungus, two hyphae (or a hypha and a spore from different individuals) fuse, their nuclei fuse, and meiosis takes place before spores are formed. Spores are often produced in a specialized fruiting body, such as a mushroom.

Fungus spores are ubiquitous. Common saprophytic fungi produce airborne spores in enormous quantities; thus it is difficult to avoid contact with them in all but the most hypersterile environments. In culture, fungi (including pathogenic species) produce large numbers of dry spores that can be transmitted in

Common Fungal Infections

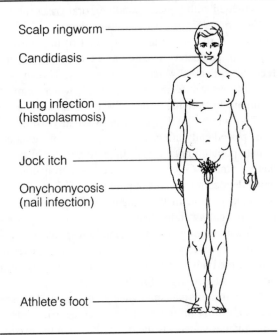

Scalp ringworm

Candidiasis

Lung infection (histoplasmosis)

Jock itch

Onychomycosis (nail infection)

Athlete's foot

the air from host to host, making working with fungi in a medical laboratory potentially hazardous.

FUNGAL DISEASES AND TREATMENTS

Human fungal diseases are generally placed in four broad categories according to the tissues they attack, and they are further subdivided according to specific pathologies and the organisms involved. The categories of disease are superficial mycoses, cutaneous mycoses, subcutaneous mycoses, and systemic mycoses.

Superficial mycoses affect hair and the outermost layer of the epidermis and do not evoke a cellular response. They include tinea versicolor and tinea nigra, deutermycete infections that cause discolored patches on skin, and black piedra, caused by an ascomycete growing on hair shafts. They can be treated with a topical fungicide, such as nystatin, or, in the case of piedra, by shaving off the affected hair.

Cutaneous mycoses involve living cells of the skin or mucous membrane and evoke a cellular response, generally localized inflammation. Dermatomycoses (dermatophytes), which affect skin and hair, include tinea capitis (ringworm of the scalp), tinea pedis (athlete's foot), and favus, a scaly infection of the scalp. Domestic animals serve as a reservoir for some cutaneous mycoses. The organisms responsible are generally fungi imperfecti in the genera *Microsporon* and *Trichophyton*. Cutaneous mycoses can be successfully treated with topical nystatin or oral griseofulvin.

Candida albicans, a ubiquitous pleomorphic fungus with both a yeast and a mycelial form, causes a variety of cutaneous mycoses as well as systemic infections collectively named candidiasis. Thrush is a *Candida* yeast infection of the mouth which is most common in infants, especially in infants born to mothers with vaginal candidiasis. Vaginal yeast infections periodically affect 18 to 20 percent of the adult female population and more than 30 percent of pregnant women. *Candida* also causes paronychia, a nailbed infection. Small populations of *Candida* are normally present in the alimentary tract and genital tract of healthy individuals; candidiasis of the mucous membranes tends to develop in response to antibiotic treatment, which disturbs the normal bacterial flora of the body, or in response to metabolic changes or decreasing immune function.

None of the organisms causing cutaneous mycoses elicits a lasting immune response, so recurring infections by these agents is the rule rather than the exception. Even in temperate climates, under modern standards of hygiene, cutaneous mycoses are extremely common.

Subcutaneous mycoses, affecting skin and muscle tissue, are predominantly tropical in distribution and not particularly common. Chromomycosis and maduromycosis are caused by soil fungi that enter the skin through wounds, causing chronic localized tumors, usually on the feet. Sporotrichosis enters through wounds and spreads through the lymphatic system, causing skin ulcers associated with lymph nodes. Amphotericin B, a highly toxic systemic antifungal agent, has been used to treat all three conditions; potassium iodide is used to treat sporotrichosis, and localized chromomycosis and maduromycosis lesions can be surgically removed.

Systemic mycoses, the most serious of fungal infections, have the ability to become generally disseminated in the body. The main nonopportunistic systemic mycoses known in North America are histoplasmosis, caused by *Histoplasma capsulatum*; coccidiomycosis, caused by *Coccidiodes immitis;* blastomycosis, caused by *Ajellomyces* (or *Blastomyces*) *dermatidis*; and cryptococcosis, caused by *Cryptococcus* (or *Filobasidiella*) *neoformans*. Similar infections, caused by related species, occur in other parts of the world.

Coccidiomycosis, also called San Joaquin Valley fever or valley fever, will serve as an example of the etiology of systemic mycoses. The causative organism lives in arid soils in the American southwest; its spores are wind-disseminated. When inhaled, the fungus grows in the lungs, producing a mild respiratory infection which is self-limiting in perhaps 95 percent of the cases. The mild form of the disease is common in rural areas. In a minority of cases, a chronic lung disease whose symptoms resemble tuberculosis develops. There is also a disseminated form of the disease producing meningitis; chronic cutaneous disease, with the production of ulcers and granulomas; and attack of the bones, internal organs, and lymphatic system. A chronic pulmonary infection may become systemic in response to factors that undermine the body's immune system. Factors involved in individual susceptibility among individuals with intact immune systems are poorly understood.

Histoplasmosis (also known as summer fever, cave fever, or Mississippi Valley fever) is even more common; 90 percent of people tested in the southern Mississippi Valley show a positive reaction to this fungus, indicating prior, self-limiting lung infection. The fungus is associated with bird and bat droppings, and severe cases sometimes occur when previously unexposed individuals are exposed to high levels of innoculum in caves where bats roost. A related organism, *Histoplasma duboisii*, occurs in central Africa. Blastomycosis causes chronic pulmonary disease, chronic cutaneous disease, and systemic disease, all of which were usually fatal until the advent of chemotherapy with amphotericin B. The natural habitat of the fungus is unclear. *Cryptococcus neoformans* occurs in pigeon droppings and is worldwide in distribution. The subclinical pulmonary form of the disease is probably common; invasive disease occurs in patients with collagen diseases, such as lupus, and in patients with weakened immune systems. It is the leading cause of invasive fungal disease in patients with acquired immunodeficiency syndrome (AIDS).

Systemic fungal diseases are notoriously difficult to treat. Chemotherapy of systemic, organismally caused diseases depends on finding a chemical compound which will selectively kill or inhibit the invading organism without damaging the host. Therefore, the more closely the parasite species is related biologically to the host species, the more difficult it is to find a compound which will act in such a selective manner. Fungi are, from a biological standpoint, more like humans than they are like bacteria, and antibacterial antibiotics are ineffective against them. If a fungus has invaded the skin or the digestive tract, it can be attacked with toxic substances that are not readily absorbed into the bloodstream, but this approach is not appropriate for a systemic infection. Amphotericin, intraconazole, and fluconazole, the drugs of choice for systemic fungal infections, are highly toxic to humans. Thus, dosage is critical, close clinical supervision is necessary, and long-term therapy may not be feasible.

PERSPECTIVE AND PROSPECTS

Medical mycology textbooks written before 1980 tended to focus on two categories of fungal infection: the common, ubiquitous, and comparatively benign superficial and cutaneous mycoses, frequently seen in clinical practice in the industrialized world, and the subcutaneous and deep mycoses, treated as a rare and/or predominantly tropical problem. Opportunistic systemic infections, if mentioned at all, were regarded as a rare curiosity.

The rising population of patients with compromised immune systems, including cancer patients undergoing chemotherapy, people being treated with steroids for various conditions, transplant patients, and people with AIDS, has dramatically changed this clinical picture. Between 1980 and 1986, more than a hundred fungi, a few previously unknown and the majority common inhabitants of crop plants, rotting vegetable debris, and soil, were identified as causing human disease. The number continues to increase steadily. Compared to organisms routinely isolated from soil and plants, these opportunistic fungi do not seem to have any special characteristics other than the ability to grow at human body temperature; however, the possibility that an opportunistic pathogen might mutate into a form capable of attacking healthy humans is worrisome.

Systemic opportunistic human infections have been attributed to *Alternaria alternata* and *Fusarium oxysporum*, common plant pathogens that cause diseases of tomatoes and strawberries, respectively. Several species of *Aspergillus*, saprophytic molds (many of them thermophilic) have long been implicated in human disease. Colonizing aspergillosis, involving localized growth in the lungs of people exposed to high levels of aspergillus spores (notably agricultural workers working with silage), is not particularly rare among people with normal immune systems, but the more severe invasive form of the disease, in which massive lung lesions form, and disseminated aspergillosis, in which other organs are attacked, almost always involve immunocompromised patients. *Ramichloridium schulzeri*, described originally from wheat roots, causes "golden tongue" in leukemia patients; fortunately this infection responds to amphotericin B. *Scelidosporium inflatum*, first isolated from a serious bone infection in an immunocompromised patient in 1984, is being isolated with increasing frequency in cases of disseminated mycosis; it resists standard drug treatment.

Oral colonization by strains of *Candida* is often the first sign of AIDS-related complex or full-blown AIDS in an individual harboring the human immunodeficiency virus (HIV). Drug therapy with fluconazole is effective against oral candidiasis, but relapse rates of up to 50 percent within a month of the cessation of drug therapy are reported. Reported rates of disseminated candidiasis in AIDS patients range from 1 to 10 percent. Invasive procedures such as intravenous catheters represent a significant risk of introducing *Candida* and other common fungi into the bloodstream of patients.

Pneumocystis carinii, the organism causing a form of pneumonia which is the single most important cause of death in patients with AIDS, was originally classified as a sporozoan—that is, as a parasitic protozoan—but detailed investigations of the life cycle, metabolism, and genetic material of *Pneumocystis* have convinced some biologists that it is actually an ascomycete, although an anomalous one that lacks a cell wall. Unfortunately, it does not respond to therapy with the antifungal drugs currently in use.

In general, antifungal drug therapy for mycoses in AIDS patients is not very successful. In the absence of significant patient immunity, it is difficult to eradicate a disseminated infection from the body entirely, making a resurgence likely once drug therapy is discontinued. Reinfection is also likely if the organism is a common component of the patient's environment.

Given the increasing number of lethal systemic fungal infections seen in clinical practice, there is substantial impetus for a search for more effective, less toxic antifungal drugs. A number of compounds, produced by bacteria and chemically dissimilar to both antibacterial antibiotics and the most widely used antifungal compounds, have been identified and are being tested. It is also possible that the plant kingdom, which has been under assault by fungi for all its long geologic history, may prove a source for medically useful antifungal compounds.

—*Martha Sherwood-Pike, Ph.D.*

See also Acquired immunodeficiency syndrome (AIDS); Athlete's foot; Candidiasis; Diaper rash; Food poisoning; Immune system; Immunodeficiency disorders; Immunology; Immunopathology; Microbiology; Mold and mildew; Nail removal; Nails; Pneumonia; Poisonous plants; Ringworm; Skin; Skin disorders.

FOR FURTHER INFORMATION:

Biddle, Wayne. *Field Guide to Germs*. New York: Henry Holt, 1995. This comprehensive book is easily accessible to the nonspecialist and includes a discussion of nearly every virus, bacterium, and fungus known to cause human and nonhuman animal disease. The history of the microbe and the treatment of diseases are included.

British Society for Antimicrobial Chemotherapy Working Party. "Antifungal Chemotherapy in Patients with Acquired Immunodeficiency Syndrome." *The Lancet* 340, no. 8820 (September 12, 1992): 648-650. Provides an overview of occurrence and therapies for the use of physicians in the British Isles. The article emphasizes candidiasis, cryptococcosis, histoplasmosis, and coccidiomycosis.

Crissey, John Thorne, Heidi Lang, and Lawrence Charles Parish. *Manual of Medical Mycology*. Cambridge, Mass.: Blackwell Scientific, 1995. This handbook discusses the diagnosis and treatment of fungal infections. Includes a bibliography and an index.

Rippon, John W. *Medical Mycology: The Pathogenic Fungi and Pathogenic Actinomycetes*. 3d ed. Philadelphia: W. B. Saunders, 1987. A standard medical mycology textbook for students of medicine and microbiology, with detailed descriptions of common mycoses and the organisms that cause them, as an aid to clinical diagnosis.

Shaw, Michael, ed. *Everything You Need to Know About Diseases*. Springhouse, Pa.: Springhouse Press, 1996. This well-illustrated consumer reference, compiled by more than one hundred doctors and medical experts, describes five hundred illnesses and conditions, their causes, symptoms, diagnosis, treatment, and prevention. Of particular interest is chapter 19, "Infection."

GALACTOSEMIA
DISEASE/DISORDER

ALSO KNOWN AS: Galactose intolerance

ANATOMY OR SYSTEM AFFECTED: Brain, eyes, kidneys, liver

SPECIALTIES AND RELATED FIELDS: Endocrinology, genetics, nutrition

DEFINITION: Galactosemia is a genetic disorder occurring in about one out of every fifty thousand births, in which the patient lacks an enzyme needed to break down galactose. Galactose is one of the components of lactose, a sugar found in milk. Galactose is also found in various fruits and vegetables. Uncontrolled galactosemia may result in cataracts, mental retardation, liver damage, and kidney damage. Severe galactosemia can be rapidly fatal if left untreated. Treatment consists of maintaining a galactose-free diet.

—*Rose Secrest*

See also Endocrine system; Endocrinology, pediatric; Genetic diseases; Lactose intolerance; Mental retardation; Nutrition.

FOR FURTHER INFORMATION:

Gracey, Michael, ed. *Diarrhea*. Boca Raton, Fla.: CRC Press, 1991.

Greenberger, Norton J. *Gastrointestinal Disorders: A Pathophysiologic Approach*. 4th ed. Chicago: Year Book Medical, 1989.

Janowitz, Henry D. *Your Gut Feelings: A Complete Guide to Living Better with Intestinal Problems*. Rev. ed. New York: Oxford University Press, 1994.

GALLBLADDER DISEASES
DISEASE/DISORDER

ANATOMY OR SYSTEM AFFECTED: Abdomen, gallbladder, gastrointestinal system

SPECIALTIES AND RELATED FIELDS: Gastroenterology, internal medicine

DEFINITION: A family of disorders affecting the gallbladder and causing abdominal pain or occasionally symptomless.

KEY TERMS:

bile: a complex solution formed by liver cells which is composed mainly of bile salts, fats, and cholesterol, which aids in fat digestion; it is secreted by the liver into a system of ducts connecting the liver, gallbladder, and intestinal tract

biliary colic: a distinct pain syndrome characterized by severe intermittent waves of right-sided, upper abdominal pain, often brought on by the ingestion of fatty foods; pain occurs when a gallstone obstructs the outflow of bile and usually resolves when the gallstone moves away from the outflow area

cholecystectomy: the surgical procedure that results in the removal of the gallbladder in its entirety; the two main techniques are the traditional open method and the laparoscopically aided method

cholecystitis: the disease that occurs when the gallbladder becomes inflamed or infected, which produces severe right-sided, upper abdominal pain, fever, and other signs of infection; a frequent indication for removal of the gallbladder

cholelithiasis: the presence of gallstones in the gallbladder

gallbladder: a muscular, walled sac located on the under surface of the liver which stores and concentrates bile; under stimulus from the intestine in response to a meal, the gallbladder contracts and expels bile into the digestive tract to aid in fat digestion

gallstones: particles that form in the gallbladder when the solubility of the components of bile is somehow altered, also resulting in the precipitation of cholesterol; the gallstones, which can grow very large, are made up mostly of cholesterol but can be pigmented or contain other substances

laparoscopic cholecystectomy: a procedure in which the gallbladder is removed with the help of a telescopic eyepiece which is attached to a tube inserted into the patient's body; the surgery is done using four small incisions and allows the patient to recover much faster than the traditional method of open surgery

CAUSES AND SYMPTOMS

Gallbladder diseases affect a large number of patients and are among the most common causes of abdominal pain. Most gallbladder problems stem from the presence of gallstones, which may be present in as many as one of every ten adults. In the past, anyone with gallstones was advised to have the gallbladder taken out, but this is no longer the case. It is now known that many people with gallstones never experience difficulty because of them.

A very common gallbladder disease is biliary colic. This is usually manifested by severe right-sided, upper abdominal pain which is fairly repetitive in nature. The pain may literally take the patient's

Location of the Gallbladder

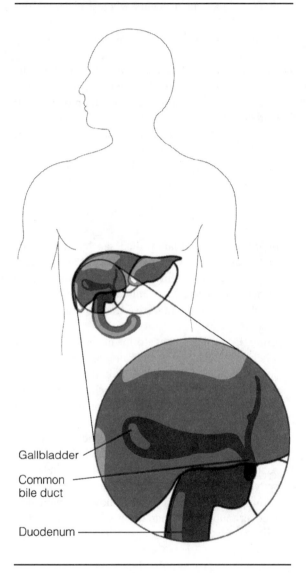

Gallbladder

Common
bile duct

Duodenum

breath away, but an episode usually lasts less than thirty minutes. The patient may also complain of right-sided shoulder or back pain, often caused by irritation of the diaphragmatic nerves, which are located just above the liver on the right side. Many people may confuse the pain of biliary colic with indigestion, because in some patients it may be experienced in the middle of the upper abdomen. This pain is almost always brought on by eating, since the gallbladder contracts in response to food in the intestinal tract. The meal triggering such an episode often is described as rich and fatty, and many patients soon learn what types of food to avoid. Biliary colic does not occur unless gallstones are present, because they tend to obstruct the outflow of bile from the gallbladder. The treatment for biliary colic usually consists of dietary manipulation, that is, the avoidance of fatty foods or other foods known to trigger the pain. Surgery is performed if the patient so desires, and removing the gallbladder should cure the problem.

When a diagnosis of gallstones is suspected, the physician will take down the patient's medical history and perform a physical examination. In most cases, however, such actions will yield no physical findings that are indicative of gallstone disease. Thus the diagnosis is usually confirmed by an imaging study of the gallbladder, in which the gallstones are either directly or indirectly visualized. The most commonly used imaging modality is the ultrasound test, which can be easily and rapidly performed with very reliable results. While the gallstones cannot actually be seen, they have a density which reflects, rather than transmits, sound waves. As a result, they create specific echoes and shadows that can be interpreted by the radiologists as gallstones. No patient should be treated for gallstone disease without such imaging to confirm the presence of gallstones.

A potentially serious type of gallbladder disease caused by gallstones is acute cholecystitis. In this condition, the outflow of bile is obstructed, usually by a gallstone that is stuck in the outflow tract, and severe inflammation and infection may develop. A patient with acute cholecystitis often complains of pain that does not go away promptly, may have chills or fever, and is usually found to have a very tender abdomen on the upper right side. The treatment of this condition is not controversial, and most physicians would probably recommend removing the gallbladder surgically. The only question remaining is whether the gallbladder should be removed immediately or electively, at a later date, if the patient recovers from acute cholecystitis with conservative management, including the use of antibiotics and the avoidance of eating until the inflammation subsides.

Inflammation and infection can also occur, although rarely, in gallbladders that do not produce gallstones. This happens in very select circumstances and is called acute acalculous cholecystitis. It usually afflicts very ill patients who have been in an intensive care unit for a long time, patients who have needed a heart-lung machine as a result of open heart surgery, or patients who are unable to eat for an extended period of time because of other problems. These patients are often fed only intravenously, which can lead to severe gallbladder problems. The exact mechanisms are not entirely known, but alterations in blood flow and an impaired ability to fight infection may play a role. Whatever the cause, the treatment often remains the same: removal of the gallbladder that does not respond to conservative therapy.

Gallstones can also move out of the gallbladder and cause serious problems. The main outflow tract of bile from the gallbladder and liver is the common bile duct, and this is a place gallstones frequently lodge. The end of this duct is surrounded by a small muscle called the sphincter of Oddi, which may not allow the passage of gallstones. If they become stuck there, they can completely obstruct the biliary system, and the patient will appear jaundiced. Removal of the gallstones will cure the problem. The presence of gallstones in the common bile duct is also associated with the development of pancreatitis, an inflammation of the pancreas which can be severe and life-threatening. Removal of the gallbladder at an appropriate time will prevent future bouts of pancreatitis.

The gallbladder can also be a source of cancer. Although cancer of the gallbladder is not common, it is estimated that one out of every one hundred gallbladders removed will contain cancer. Therefore, all specimens removed must be examined by a qualified pathologist and all reports must be reviewed in their entirety by the surgeon. If the disease is limited to a minor thickness of the gallbladder, no further therapy is needed, but if the tumor is larger, further surgery—including removal of part of the liver—may be necessary. Gallbladder cancer grows silently in many patients, and it is often not detected until late in its course.

TREATMENT AND THERAPY

Because there is no simple way to prevent gallbladder problems, surgery plays a large role in their management. Removing the gallbladder, a relatively routine operation, results in a complete cure, with acceptably low complication rates and few long-term problems. While several exciting new ways of treating gallbladder and gallstone problems have been developed, the classic and standard method of therapy for gallbladder disease has been open cholecystectomy. This procedure entails making an incision across the upper right side of the abdomen a few inches below and parallel to the bottom of the rib cage. The muscles of the abdominal wall are cut, and the abdominal cavity is opened. The gallbladder, which is usually located right under this incision, is then removed and the incision closed in layers. This method of gallbladder removal has acceptable complication rates and is relatively safe and extremely effective. It allows the surgeon to inspect the entire abdomen and rule out other problems. One must consider, however, that this procedure constitutes major surgery. Most patients need to be in the hospital for a minimum of three to five days, and there is a considerable amount of pain with this incision. These problems have prompted surgeons to find a less invasive way of removing the gallbladder, thereby achieving better pain control and reducing the length of the hospital stay and the time lost from work and other activities.

A laparoscope is an optical instrument, composed of a tube connected to a telescopic eyepiece, that allows the surgeon to perform a procedure inside the patient's body. Although it has been employed in surgeries for many years, mainly in gynecological procedures, it was adapted only recently for removal of the gallbladder, as well as in other types of surgeries. Since then, laparoscopic cholecystectomy has become a procedure that all surgeons must know in order to stay current with the profession. The laparoscope and other surgical instruments are inserted directly into

Gallstones

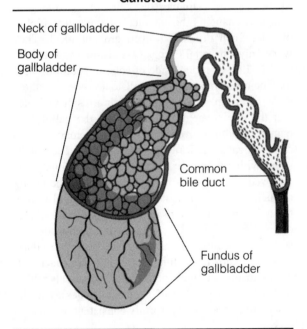

Neck of gallbladder

Body of gallbladder

Common bile duct

Fundus of gallbladder

the abdomen through several small incisions, and the gallbladder is removed without a large incision having been made. The patients are often discharged the same day of the surgery, and they return to work much faster than with the open technique.

Despite its advantages, there are some pitfalls with laparoscopic cholecystectomy, and it cannot be used for all patients. There is an increased incidence of certain injuries to other organs and bile ducts at the time of the operation because less of the area can be seen than with an open operation. In addition, patients who have had previous upper abdominal surgery are not candidates for this procedure, and for those with acute cholecystitis, severe inflammation may make this technique unsafe. For most patients, however, laparoscopic cholecystectomy can be performed easily and safely with minimal complications and excellent results. It is becoming the standard of care and will continue to change the way gallbladder surgery is performed. The laparoscope is also being used to perform appendectomies, ulcer surgeries, cancer surveillance, and all types of intra-abdominal surgery.

Radiologists and internists may play an important role in the management of gallbladder disease. In certain circumstances, the techniques performed by these specialists may be indicated for extremely ill patients who might not be able to tolerate an operation, or for whom the anesthesia might be too hazardous. Invasive radiologists can actually place a tube into the gallbladder with help from their imaging equipment and remove infection or troublesome gallstones from the gallbladder. This procedure can alleviate symptoms in some patients, who may not even require any additional intervention. These practices are not common, however, and they are usually reserved for the very ill patient who might not survive an open operation or is at extremely high risk to develop a certain complication.

Gallstones can migrate out of the gallbladder and cause problems if they lodge in and obstruct the common bile duct. This places the patient at high risk for developing jaundice and infection in the biliary system. The standard method for dealing with this problem continues to be open surgery. In this procedure, the gallbladder is removed through an incision and the common bile duct is also opened. The gallstones are removed through a variety of techniques, and the duct is then closed. A tube is placed in the duct to keep it open, because otherwise it could scar and become narrowed. Many of these patients must be hospitalized for a number of days, making this surgery an expensive one.

Internists who specialize in the diseases of the abdomen have become proficient at performing endoscopic techniques. These techniques came about after the development of fiberoptics, which allow one to see through a tube, even if it is bent at a variety of angles. An endoscope, composed of surgical instruments, a light source, and fiberoptic cables, can be used to examine the lining of the stomach and intestines, allowing the diagnosis of many conditions.

Endoscopy is performed by inserting the endoscope through the mouth and into the patient's stomach and the first part of the intestines. From this location, the area where the common bile duct opens into the intestines can be seen, and this is often where gallstones become lodged. The gallstones can be removed with instruments attached to the scope, thus solving the patient's problem. Unfortunately, this technique does not remove the gallbladder, the source of the gallstones, and the patient is at some risk for a recurrence. This risk can be minimized by enlarging the opening where the duct enters the intestinal tract. This technique, too, is advantageous for patients who are elderly or ill and cannot withstand the trauma of surgery and anesthesia.

There are other options besides surgery or dietary changes for the treatment of patients with gallstones. Medicines are available that can dissolve the gallstones by changing the chemical nature and solubility of bile. Such drugs, however, are not ideal: They work only for certain types of gallstones, are expensive, and may produce side effects. In addition, there may be a recurrence of the gallstones when a patient stops taking these medicines. Such a result indicates that the bile-concentrating action of the gallbladder combines with a given patient's bile composition to create a gallstone-forming environment. Thus, gallstones will continue to form unless the gallbladder is removed or the bile is again altered when the taking of such medicines is resumed. Patients can also have the gallstones broken up into very small pieces, as is often done with kidney stones, by high-frequency sound waves aimed at the gallstones. This procedure, however, known as lithotripsy, has drawbacks: It works in only a small percentage of patients (those with a limited number of small gallstones), and the results have not been uniformly consistent or satisfactory.

PERSPECTIVE AND PROSPECTS

Diseases of the gallbladder and biliary system are common in modern industrialized societies. The exact etiologies are not entirely clear, but they may involve dietary mechanisms or other customs of the Western lifestyle. There is also evidence that genetic factors are important, as gallbladder disease often runs in families. Traditionally, the treatment of non-life-threatening gallbladder disease has been conservative, with dietary discretion being the most important factor. When that failed, or if the condition was more serious, the gallbladder was removed. Open cholecystectomy was long considered the best method for dealing with these problems. This operation has been recently challenged by endoscopic and laparoscopic techniques, which have become widely available and enjoyed great success. These new treatment options will become more important as increasing medical costs promote the refinement of less invasive and better techniques. Nevertheless, open cholecystectomy is sometimes the only option for a patient, and less invasive techniques can have limitations as well as complications.

Basic scientific research is also important in this field. Investigations into the mechanisms of gallstone formation are critical to the understanding of gallbladder diseases, as gallstones are the cause of many of these problems. As with many other diseases, prevention might be the key to eliminating many gallbladder diseases, making biliary colic, cholecystitis, and common bile duct diseases rare.

—*Mark Wengrovitz, M.D.*

See also Abdomen; Abdominal disorders; Cholecystectomy; Cholecystitis; Gastroenterology; Gastroenterology, pediatric; Gastrointestinal disorders; Internal medicine; Jaundice; Kidney stones; Laparoscopy; Liver; Liver cancer; Liver disorders; Liver transplantation; Obesity; Pain; Pancreatitis; Stone removal; Stones; Ultrasonography.

FOR FURTHER INFORMATION:

Blumgart, L. H., ed. *Surgery of the Liver and Biliary Tract*. 3d ed. 2 vols. Edinburgh, Scotland: Churchill Livingstone, 2000. This authoritative text offers a comprehensive, detailed description of the subject.

Cameron, John L., ed. *Current Surgical Therapy*. 6th ed. St. Louis: C. V. Mosby, 1998. An excellent textbook that covers all surgical problems, including those related to gallbladder and gallstone removal.

Krames Communications. *The Gallbladder Surgery Book*. San Bruno, Calif.: Author, 1991. This helpful book provides the general reader with an understanding of the symptoms of gallbladder diseases, their most common causes, and treatment options.

_____. *Laparoscopic Gallbladder Surgery*. San Bruno, Calif.: Author, 1991. This work offers information regarding laparoscopic cholecystectomy to patients who are facing gallbladder surgery.

Maingot, Rodney. *Maingot's Abdominal Operations*. Edited by Michael J. Zinner et al. 10th ed. Stamford, Conn.: Appleton and Lange, 1997. This textbook has long been considered the classic work on all surgical disciplines. Contains an excellent section on gallbladder diseases.

GALLBLADDER REMOVAL. *See* CHOLECYSTECTOMY.

GALLSTONES. *See* GALLBLADDER DISEASES; STONE REMOVAL; STONES.

GANGLION REMOVAL

PROCEDURE

ANATOMY OR SYSTEM AFFECTED: Feet, hands, tendons

SPECIALTIES AND RELATED FIELDS: Dermatology, family practice, general surgery

DEFINITION: The removal of fluid-filled sacs which usually develop on the tendons of the wrists, fingers, or feet.

INDICATIONS AND PROCEDURES

Sacs containing synovial fluid surround tendons to reduce the friction on adjacent tissues during movement. These sacs can form cysts, known as ganglions, that range in size from a pea to a golf ball. Smaller ganglions are more common and often spontaneously disappear. A ganglion is not harmful unless it causes pain or the patient desires its removal for cosmetic reasons. Ganglion formation typically occurs around the tendons of the wrist.

In order to remove a ganglion, the physician will disinfect the skin overlying the cyst and insert a needle attached to a syringe in order to aspirate the fluid from the ganglion. Unfortunately, this procedure usually reduces the ganglion's size only temporarily. Some physicians will make an incision into the skin and remove the whole ganglion. This procedure requires thorough disinfection of the skin using alcohol and/or povidone-iodine and may require a local anesthetic such as lidocaine to be injected under the skin. Surgical instruments are used to dissect the cyst wall from the tendon and surrounding tissues. The total removal of the ganglion usually prevents recurrence.

USES AND COMPLICATIONS

As with any invasive procedure, the physician performing the surgical removal of a ganglion must be cautious so as to prevent infections or damage to surrounding healthy tissues.

The larger the ganglion, the greater are the potential complications. A longer incision must be made, which allows a large site for potential bacterial invasion and infection. The larger ganglion also requires more extensive dissection from surrounding tissues, which increases the possibility of injury to these structures. Although it is rare, tendons, ligaments, and nerves can be permanently damaged in ganglion removal. For example, if the ganglion was located in the wrist and the underlying tendons and nerves were severely damaged, the result may be a limited use or loss of use of the hand.

—*Matthew Berria, Ph.D.,*
and Douglas Reinhart, M.D.

See also Abscess removal; Abscesses; Cyst removal; Cysts; Nervous system; Neurology; Tendon disorders; Tendon repair.

FOR FURTHER INFORMATION:

Breslau, R. C. "Ganglion of the Glenohumeral Joint: An Unusual Axillary Tumor." *Southern Medical Journal* 59, no. 5 (May, 1966): 566.

Kikuchi, Kenji, and Masahiro Saito. "Ganglion-Cell Tumor of the Filum Terminale: Immunohistochemical Characterization." *Tohoku Journal of Experimental Medicine* 188, no. 3 (July, 1999): 245-256.

Lenfant, C., R. Paoletti, and A. Albertini, eds. *Biotechnology of Growth Factors: Vascular and Nervous Systems*. New York: Karger, 1992.

McLendon, Roger E. *Pathology of Tumors of the Central Nervous System: A Guide to Histological Diagnosis*. New York: Oxford University Press, 2000.

GANGLIONS. *See* CYSTS; GANGLION REMOVAL.

GANGRENE
DISEASE/DISORDER
ANATOMY OR SYSTEM AFFECTED: All

SPECIALTIES AND RELATED FIELDS: Bacteriology, internal medicine, microbiology

DEFINITION: Necrosis (death of tissue) resulting from blood loss and bacterial invasion followed by putrefaction; may be initiated by a variety of diseases and conditions, and if left untreated may result in need for amputation or in death.

KEY TERMS:

anaerobic: referring to conditions that favor the growth of an organism in the absence of oxygen

cellulitis: an infection of the skin which, if left untreated, can abscess and kill the affected tissue

collagenase: an enzyme that breaks down the proteins of collagen tissue, a primary component of connective tissue (ligaments and tendons)

debridement: cleansing of a wound by removal of dirt, foreign objects, damaged tissue, and cellular debris, in order to promote healing

exotoxin: a toxic protein, such as an enzyme, excreted by microorganisms into the environment

Gram's stain: a stain used to classify bacteria as either gram-positive (they retain the primary stain of crystal violet when subjected to treatment with a decolorizer) or gram-negative (no coloration)

hemolysis: the premature breakdown of red blood cells

hyaluronidase: an enzyme that breaks down hyaluronic acid, the gel-like matrix of connective tissue

lecithinase: an enzyme that breaks down lecithin, a kind of phospholipid that is a component of human cells (such as red blood cells)

necrosis: localized tissue death that occurs in groups of cells in response to disease or injury

CAUSES AND SYMPTOMS

The term "gangrene" is used when wounded or traumatized tissue has become so badly infected by bacteria that the tissue dies. The infection can be localized, but the threat of the gangrene spreading to other tissue is very serious: It can rapidly become fatal to the patient.

There are approximately thirty different clostridial bacteria species that can cause infection in the human body as they release toxins into the system. Five species of clostridia can cause gangrene. *Clostridium perfringens* is the most common culprit: This species is responsible for about 90 percent of invasive infections in damaged tissue. The other four species are *C. novyi*, *C. septicum*, *C. sordellii*, and *C. histolyticum*.

Gangrene

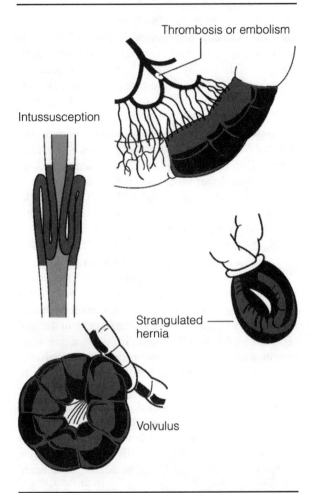

Gangrene may occur as a result of obstruction of the organs through a variety of means: strangulation, thrombosis, embolism, intussusception, volvulus, or other obstruction. The most dangerous form of gangrene, however (not pictured here), is gas gangrene, which results from infection by clostridial bacteria and usually occurs as a result of war wounds or other severe trauma.

Clostridia are bacilli (rod-shaped) bacteria. They are anaerobic and form spores that are heat-resistant. These spores are larger than the cells that produce them, but they are not motile.

C. perfringens is found in all types of soil, including desert sand and marine sediments. The spores produced by these bacteria can survive for years until conditions are right for germination. In addition to the soil, these bacteria are found in the mouth, vaginal tract, and intestinal tract. While these species can

go undetected and be innocuous for a lifetime, they can cause gangrene in the intestinal tract and the adjoining peritoneum in persons with a bowel obstruction. They can also become dangerously active if freed into the abdominal cavity during invasive surgery or postoperatively if some of the intestine is isolated from the blood supply (ischemia). A type of gangrene, anaerobic puerperal sepsis, may result if the uterus is traumatized by surgical procedures such as septic instrumental abortions. This gangrene is especially dangerous, as mortality is high even with immediate treatment.

C. perfringens works anaerobically in tissue that has been deprived of oxygen. This deprivation can result from a decreased blood supply caused by damaged or crushed blood vessels or clots that block the flow of blood; the release of sulfhydryl groups or oxidases (oxygen-consuming enzymes) by traumatized tissue (from a wound, tourniquet, or foreign body); diseases that may damage the circulatory system, such as diabetes or arteriosclerosis; aerobic bacteria that use up the available oxygen in a given area; or chemicals introduced by soil or dirt that kill cells. Without living cells, there is no tissue to receive oxygen from the circulatory system. The anaerobes thrive in this oxygen-poor environment, since they also take advantage of and use the vitamins, amino acids, salts, and carbohydrates of damaged and dying cells. As the bacteria grow and reproduce in this environment, they infect neighboring tissue, including the lymphatic system. More cells are killed, which in turn provides a larger anaerobic environment in which the bacteria can increase in number. This spreading process can be very quick; a whole limb can become affected within a matter of hours. Bacteremia, toxemia, and hemolysis then develop, followed by circulatory failure, renal shutdown, and death.

Types of wounds that have a greater likelihood of developing anaerobic infections are jagged shrapnel wounds in soldiers on the battlefield, accidents (such as those caused by car wrecks) that result in crushed or torn limbs, wounds contaminated by dirty hands or instruments, and wounds resulting from human or animal bites. These wounds can be jeopardized by clostridial spores that are in the soil, or, as in the case of abdominal surgery, perforation of the large intestine may liberate clostridia into the area. The spores only germinate under anaerobic conditions; once they begin reproducing, however, they can maintain their own anaerobic environment.

Gangrenous infections can be divided into three categories: simple contamination, cellulitis, and gas gangrene. Simple contamination is infection with clostridia and/or streptococcal bacteria. Visible signs of simple contamination include a brown discharge of pus with a putrid odor. While this infection may increase in severity, it is possible that healing may result instead.

The second category of gangrenous infection is anaerobic cellulitis. Anaerobic cellulitis may be a worsened condition of simple contamination or may be the initial contamination of clostridia. It can develop within three or four days of exposure. Typically, the bacteria will multiply within connective tissue spaces and release gas. As gas is produced, the resulting pressure keeps the wound open and allows seepage of a foul-smelling discharge. This infection may remain localized or may spread, but little pain is associated with this form.

Gas gangrene, the most dangerous form of this type of infection, is also known as malignant edema. Its incubation period may be a mere four to six hours or may be as long as six weeks. Gas gangrene is not painless; the onset is sudden, with a feeling of increased weight in the affected area. The sufferer will feel critically ill, look pale, sweat, and be delirious, maniacal, or totally apathetic. The patient should be monitored for shock. The wound has not changed in appearance, but there may be an odorless discharge. Gas released is trapped between muscle fibers and can be found by palpitation. If treatment is not begun, toxemia, hemolytic anemia, and renal failure (caused by tubular necrosis) may occur; death then follows.

The seriousness of the invasion is determined by the location of the infection. The least worrisome is an infection of the subcutaneous skin layers that develops slowly, producing little pain with its inflammation. Even so, gas released from the bacteria may be trapped within the affected area and can be palpated (a sensation known as crepitance). This localized infection, referred to as clostridial anaerobic cellulitis, is not particularly dangerous.

Gas gangrene will more likely occur when the affected area is a deep infection of the muscle layers. The muscle cells are abundant in carbohydrates, a rich energy source for the pervasive bacteria. The bacteria release two by-products as they consume cells: hydrogen gas and toxins. The gas collects and puts so much pressure on the sheets of muscles that the fibers begin to separate. In these gaps between fibers, the fluid accumulates and can further decrease the likelihood of the tissue's survival. The toxins emitted by the bacteria move quickly into more muscle cells, causing necrosis. This form of infection causes intense pain, and the rapid spread of the bacteria magnifies the symptoms. Affected muscle becomes pale, then fails to respond to stimuli. Following this stage, the muscle turns deep red and then black as the gangrene progresses. The skin covering the muscle also undergoes discoloration; a bronze tint colors the taut skin, and blisters filled with dark fluid appear. Eventually, even the skin blackens. The area is so inflamed that crepitance is hard to ascertain.

Though usually associated with skin and muscle, gangrene can also involve the lungs, pleural cavity, eye, brain, liver, or uterus.

TREATMENT AND THERAPY

When gas gangrene occurs, it should be considered a medical emergency. Because gas gangrene spreads and infects so rapidly and endangers either a limb or the patient's life, the use of the laboratory in diagnosis is minimal before treatment: If the physician waits two or three days while the bacteria are cultivated and identified, the patient will likely lose a limb or may die.

The surest way to detect the presence of *C. perfringens* to diagnose gas gangrene is to aspirate some of the fluid that is seeping from the wound. Since these bacteria may normally inhabit the human environment, care must be taken not to contaminate the sample. Using needle and syringe aspiration rather than swabs will help keep the sample clean. If a section of tissue is removed to study, it must not be exposed to air; the bacteria would not survive the oxygen bath, and the readings would therefore be inaccurate. To ensure that no oxygen contamination has occurred, the syringe used to collect the fluid should be capped off and the sample should be injected into a transport container that is oxygen-free. This container would be a vial filled with nitrogen gas or carbon dioxide, filled with a reducing agent, or filled with a solution containing thioglycolate or cysteine.

Once the specimen has reached the laboratory, it should first be examined by microscope. In order for the bacteria to be seen in the microscope, a Gram's stain should be done. It is important to pinpoint the genus and species of bacteria so that proper treatment can begin as soon as possible. Since *C. perfringens* is gram-positive, the stain pattern and the bacterial size and shape immediately identify this bacteria as an anaerobe. Identifying characteristics would be a rod shape (either large and blunt-ended or long, skinny, and pointed), irregular staining, or the presence of cocci of different sizes. Not only can shape and size be detected, but an estimate of bacterial number can indicate the extent of the infection as well.

After a preliminary identification of the bacteria has been accomplished with staining and microscopy, cultivation and definitive identification follow. The specimen is inoculated onto several media (such as meat glucose, thioglycolate, and blood agar) and allowed to incubate anaerobically for forty-eight to seventy-two hours at 35 to 37 degrees Celsius. Then the samples are examined to detect colonization and the presence or absence of hemolysis. Final identification is made by compiling information about the results of the Gram's stain, the structure of the colony, biochemical reactions, and a determination of the end products released as glucose is fermented. This determination is made by infusing the colony with a glucose broth and monitoring the end products that are released using gas chromatography. Another test to detect *C. perfringens* measures lecithinase production. There is no value in examining the blood serum in a gangrene patient's blood.

Mortality rates for cases of gas gangrene that do not receive treatment range from 40 to 60 percent. Therefore, if signs indicate the presence of clostridia, immediate surgery is important to examine the affected tissue. The wound (and all tissue showing signs of bacterial invasion) should be thoroughly and aggressively debrided (cleansed) and the infected area removed. Depending on the extent of the infection, amputation of the area may be indicated to prevent further spread of the disease. Antibiotic therapy is also given in an attempt to stop bacterial growth; penicillin is the drug of choice.

If the infection has not progressed to the point that amputation is necessary, hyperbaric oxygen can sometimes be used for successful treatment. This treatment consists of putting the patient in a chamber of pure oxygen for a brief period several times a day. This environment is too rich for the bacteria to survive. The exposure to these conditions does not alter the oxygen-carrying capabilities or saturation of red blood cells. It does result in an important difference in the oxygen tension of the serum (and thereby the lymph in the interstitial tissue). The significance of this variation is that it may interrupt toxin synthesis and bacteria growth. This enhances the body's ability to combat the infection in that it allows normal phagocytic and host defense mechanisms to take control.

Although clostridial infections are not usually transmissible from one person to another, patients diagnosed with gas gangrene should be placed on drainage/secretion precautions. This simply means that those in contact with the patient should wear gowns and gloves and should wash their hands thoroughly after touching the patient or any contaminated articles. Those articles that are contaminated should be disposed of or cleaned thoroughly. Autoclaving of instruments and equipment should ensure adequate sterilization. Boiling and chemical disinfection is not enough to kill resistant spores contaminating other articles. To be rid of the infective organisms completely, dressings should be burned, bed linens autoclaved, and mattresses and pillows sterilized in an ethylene oxide chamber. The relatively small danger of transmission is to other patients with surgical or traumatic wounds.

Antitoxins have been developed for gas gangrene, but they are not reliable and have not come into practical use. Since there is no effective antitoxin against gangrene induced by *C. perfringens*, prevention lies in how the wound is treated. There must be a thorough debridement and an adequate dosage of antibiotics. In addition, final closure of the wound should be delayed for two or three days to allow complete drainage of the area. Any bandage or cast that must be applied should allow adequate circulation of air (an airless environment would encourage growth of *C. perfringens*).

PERSPECTIVE AND PROSPECTS

The first anecdotes describing gangrene were in the seventeenth century. Since the Napoleonic Wars, gas gangrene has caused much death and disfigurement. In World War I, this was especially the case; as many as 10 percent of all wounded soldiers were infected. Many who would have survived their injuries succumbed to gas gangrene. In most of these cases, infection came through contaminated soil that had been fertilized with human and animal waste. The contamination most often was by several clostridial species.

Early surgical procedures carried the same risk; lack of sanitary conditions and poor (or absent) disinfection techniques led to far more deaths than injuries warranted. By the late 1800's, anaerobes were identified as the culprits causing putrefaction and infections associated with tissue necrosis, gas emissions in tissue, and a foul odor. The scientists credited with first isolating *C. perfringens* as the causative bacteria in gas gangrene were George Nuttall and William Welch in 1892. Though these bacteria were extensively studied, it was not until the 1960's that adequate diagnostic technology was available for clinical use. Because of this technology, there was a far smaller impact of gangrene on the battlefields of the Vietnam War. The threat of gangrene is still a reality, however, in the postoperative patient.

C. perfringens is also implicated in another common health hazard: food poisoning. This species is responsible for 3 percent of food poisoning outbreaks and 11 percent of single cases. Such food poisoning usually occurs with ingestion of meat, poultry, and gravies that are contaminated with *C. perfringens*. Most outbreaks are associated with restaurant, dormitory, or bulk food preparation and not with home cooking. Once the bacteria enter the intestinal tract, they make their presence obvious within eight to twenty-four hours. Typically, the disease is mild, producing discomfort in the form of abdominal pain and diarrhea. It usually runs its course in twenty-four hours. Medicinal treatment is unwarranted; the manifestations of this disease are often mild enough that the infection is undiagnosed.

C. perfringens may have the opportunity to multiply before the food is eaten. Contaminated dishes should be thoroughly reheated to prevent illness. Since *C. perfringens* produces endospores that are heat resistant, simply cooking or heating the food may be insufficient. Contamination is reinforced because heating also drives off oxygen, creating an environment in which the bacteria thrive. Therefore, those spores that survive the heating process are encouraged in this oxygen-poor medium to reproduce and grow quickly. Clostridial food poisoning can be avoided by refraining from eating foods that have been sitting out for prolonged periods. When there is a delay between preparation and eating, then food should be kept at very warm or very cool temperatures (above 60 degrees Celsius or below 5 degrees Celsius).

—*Iona C. Baldridge*

See also Amputation; Bacterial infections; Embolism; Food poisoning; Frostbite; Hernia; Hernia repair; Infection; Poisoning; Thrombosis and thrombus; Wounds.

FOR FURTHER INFORMATION:

Jawetz, Ernest, Joseph L. Melnick, and Edward A. Adelberg. *Medical Microbiology*. 19th ed. Norwalk, Conn.: Appleton and Lange, 1991. A comprehensive microbiology text written primarily for medical students but also used by physicians and health science students. Some background is helpful in reading through the sections on microbiological principles, immunology, pathogenesis, and chemotherapy.

Morello, Josephine A., Helen Eckel Mizer, Marion E. Wilson, and Paul A. Granato. *Microbiology in Patient Care*. 6th ed. Dubuque, Iowa: Wm. C. Brown, 1998. This text is addressed to beginning students of health-related fields. It is divided into a section introducing the principles of microbiology and a section relating microbial diseases and their epidemiology. Well written and illustrated.

Pelczar, Michael J., Jr., E. C. S. Chan, and Noel R. Krieg. *Microbiology: Concepts and Applications*. New York: McGraw-Hill, 1993. After the history of microbiology is presented, fundamental concepts of microbiology are balanced with medical microbiology, environmental microbiology, and microbial genetics.

Schaechter, Moselio, Gerald Medoff, and Barry I. Eisenstein, eds. *Mechanisms of Microbial Disease*. 3d ed. Baltimore: Williams & Wilkins, 1999. A readable textbook designed for medical students, graduate students, and advanced undergraduate students. Combines microbiology with the study of infectious diseases, relating both subjects to the major human systems.

GASTRECTOMY
PROCEDURE

ANATOMY OR SYSTEM AFFECTED: Abdomen, gastrointestinal system, stomach

SPECIALTIES AND RELATED FIELDS: Gastroenterology, general surgery, oncology

DEFINITION: The surgical removal of all or part of the stomach.

KEY TERMS:

anesthesia: the use of drugs to inhibit pain and alter consciousness

duodenum: the first part of the small intestine, located just after the stomach and before the jejunum

hemostasis: the control of bleeding

incision: a cut made with a scalpel

The Three Major Kinds of Gastrectomy

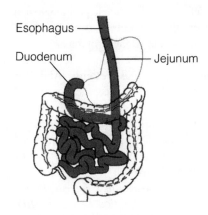

Total gastrectomy
The whole stomach is removed, the esophagus is joined to the jejunum, and the end of the duodenum is sealed.

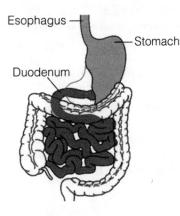

Billroth I (partial) gastrectomy
The remaining part of the stomach is joined to, the duodenum.

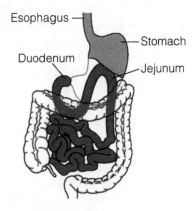

Billroth II (partial) gastrectomy
The remaining part of the stomach is joined to the jejunum, and the end of the duodenum is sealed.

jejunum: a region of the small intestine located after the duodenum

suture: a thread used to unite parts of the body

INDICATIONS AND PROCEDURES

The stomach is an important organ in the gastrointestinal system. It receives the food that has been swallowed from the esophagus and immediately begins to process it. The stomach produces and secretes gastric juices, which include hydrochloric acid and an enzyme called pepsin for digestion. As the stomach collects it, food is churned and mixed with the gastric fluid before it is passed to the first region of the small intestine, the duodenum. Occasionally, the stomach becomes cancerous or has an ulcer that will not heal and thus must be surgically removed.

Complete removal of the stomach, a total gastrectomy, is a relatively rare operation usually performed to treat stomach cancer. Partial gastrectomy, however, in which only the diseased portion of the stomach is removed surgically, is fairly common. A partial gastrectomy is often performed to treat a peptic ulcer that fails to heal after medical treatment. Peptic ulcers, which include gastric and more commonly duodenal ulcers, may not respond to drug therapy and can place the patient at risk for bleeding into the gastrointestinal tract or even complete perforation of the

stomach or duodenal wall. Therefore, the indications for gastrectomy include perforation, obstruction, massive bleeding, and severe abdominal pain.

Gastrectomy requires hospitalization, general anesthesia, and postoperative care. An anesthesiologist will administer a general anesthetic rendering the patient unconscious and insensible to pain during the operation. A nasogastric tube is passed into the stomach via the nose and nasal cavity so that any stomach contents can be removed using suction before an incision is made into the stomach.

During total gastrectomy, the whole stomach is removed and the esophagus is attached to the jejunum. The two most common types of partial gastrectomy surgeries are the Billroth I and Billroth II. A surgeon performing a Billroth I will remove the diseased part of the stomach and attach the remaining healthy stomach to the duodenum. The Billroth I is also known as gastroduodenostomy. This operation preserves most of the digestive functions. Billroth II gastrectomy requires the surgeon to perform a gastrojejunostomy in which the remaining stomach is joined with the jejunum and bypasses the duodenum. Thus the opening of the duodenum must be closed to prevent the digestive contents from escaping into the abdominal cavity.

During the recovery period, the nasogastric tube is left in place to help drain the secretions from the gastrointestinal system until the body is recovered enough to eliminate these secretions normally. Once the normal movement of the digestive tract (peristalsis) is detected, the patient is given very small amounts of fluid. If the intestines can process the ingested fluids, then the nasogastric tube is removed and the amount of fluid ingested is gradually increased. Typically, if there is no pain or nausea and vomiting, the patient can be started on a diet containing small amounts of solid food.

Uses and Complications

The risk of complications is relatively high in a total gastrectomy and lessens if smaller portions of the stomach are removed. The overall rate of complications is approximately 10 percent.

Since the stomach has such an important role in the process of digestion, it is not surprising that complications and adverse effects occur postsurgically. Some of the most common symptoms noted after gastrectomy include a feeling of discomfort and fullness after ingesting a relatively small meal. This feeling is attributable to the fact that the stomach volume has been reduced in a partial gastrectomy or eliminated in a total gastrectomy. New ulcers may also form and necessitate further drug treatment. Gastritis (inflammation of the stomach lining) may also occur after surgery, as well as a condition called dumping syndrome. Patients with dumping syndrome feel weak, nauseated, and light-headed after a meal because the food moves too rapidly out of the stomach. Most of these side effects can be treated effectively with medications and dietary changes.

Long-term complications include malabsorption problems. Occasionally after gastrectomy, the digestive system cannot compensate adequately for the loss of the stomach, leading to poor digestion and absorption of nutrients. The most common malabsorptive disorder following gastrectomy is the inability to absorb vitamin B_{12}. The stomach produces a substance called intrinsic factor which is required for the absorption of this essential vitamin. Without intrinsic factor and the ability to absorb vitamin B_{12}, the patient must receive monthly injections of the vitamin for the rest of his or her life.

Perspective and Prospects

Early detection of stomach cancers and ulcers may help reduce the need for gastrectomies. Endoscopic examinations in which the physician can observe the lining of the stomach through a surgical tube passed into the patient's mouth and down the esophagus may aid in the early detection of stomach problems such as cancer and ulcers that are failing to heal.

Aggressive medical management of gastrointestinal ulcers will likely reduce the chance that an ulcer will perforate and require gastrectomy. Antiulcer medications are available to reduce the amount of stomach acid released, to add to the protective barrier of the stomach, and to eradicate the bacteria known to cause many ulcers. Destroying the bacteria, *Helicobacter pylori*, increases the likelihood of curing the patient of ulcer formation.

—*Matthew Berria, Ph.D.,*
and Douglas Reinhart, M.D.

See also Cancer; Digestion; Gastroenterology; Gastrointestinal disorders; Gastrointestinal system; Ileostomy and colostomy; Oncology; Stomach, intestinal, and pancreatic cancers; Ulcer surgery; Ulcers; Vitamins and minerals.

For Further Information:

Clayman, Charles B., ed. *The American Medical Association Encyclopedia of Medicine*. New York: Random House, 1994. A concise presentation of numerous medical terms and illnesses. A good general reference.

Schwartz, Seymour I., ed. *Principles of Surgery*. 7th ed. New York: McGraw-Hill, 1999. A standard textbook on the topic. Intended for practicing surgeons, but valuable to general readers for its details.

GASTRITIS. *See* ABDOMINAL DISORDERS; GASTROINTESTINAL DISORDERS.

GASTROENTERITIS. *See* ABDOMINAL DISORDERS; GASTROINTESTINAL DISORDERS.

GASTROENTEROLOGY
SPECIALTY

ANATOMY OR SYSTEM AFFECTED: Abdomen, gallbladder, gastrointestinal system, intestines, liver, pancreas, stomach, throat

SPECIALTIES AND RELATED FIELDS: Internal medicine, microbiology, nutrition, oncology

DEFINITION: The subspecialty of internal medicine devoted to the digestive tract and the organs aiding digestion.

KEY TERMS:

biopsy: the use of special needles, forceps, and suction capsules to remove tissue samples for examination

endoscope: a long, maneuverable tube containing fiber optics through which physicians can view the gastrointestinal tract directly

enzyme: any of a large group of cell-produced proteins that act as catalysts for the chemical reactions necessary for digestion

motility: the spontaneous motion of the gastrointestinal tract's organs

peristalsis: the rhythmic waves of muscle contraction that move food through the esophagus, stomach, and intestines

procedure: any medical treatment which involves physical manipulation or invasion of the body

sphincter: a ringlike muscle that acts as a one-way valve to control the flow of fluids and waste

stool: the food wastes, mixed with bile and bacteria, that are eliminated through the anus

stricture: the narrowing of a passageway

SCIENCE AND PROFESSION

The gastrointestinal (GI), or digestive or alimentary, tract is a hose of layered membranes, about seven to nine meters long, that runs from the throat to the anus, allowing matter from the external world to pass through the human body. Along with its allied organs, glands, and nerve networks, the GI passage extracts the nutrients from food that are needed to fuel the body and excretes any substances that are left over. Physicians specializing in the GI system, gastroenterologists, care for everything from the upper esophageal sphincter to the anus; other specialists care for the mouth.

The GI tract has five major sections, each performing a different service: the esophagus, the stomach, the small intestine, the colon, and the anorectum. The esophagus begins where the throat ends, just below the vocal cords. It is a straight tube, about 20 to 22 centimeters long, with a valve at the top (upper esophageal sphincter). When food, formed into a ball and softened by chewing, enters from the mouth, rhythmic waves of muscle contractions (peristalsis) squeeze it smoothly toward the stomach, a trip that lasts about seven seconds. Peristaltic pressure triggers the lower esophageal sphincter to open, dropping the ball of food into the stomach; the sphincter immediately closes so that no stomach acids wash up into the esophagus.

The stomach, an ear-shaped bag that holds one to two liters of material, has three adjoining sections. First, the fundus, just below the lower esophageal sphincter, stores food. Second, the body mixes hydrochloric acid into the food, which breaks down proteins and kills bacteria, as well as a variety of enzymes, most of which also attack protein; a chemical is also introduced that prepares vitamin B_{12} for absorption in the small intestine. Third, the antrum grinds the food and pumps it through a sphincter (the pylorus) into the small intestine. Food usually takes from one to six hours to pass through the stomach.

The small intestine, about 3 meters long, loops and coils in the region from the rib cage to the pelvis. The first major loop, a squared U-shape, is the duodenum. Here bile from the liver and the gallbladder breaks down fats; water may come in from the blood if the food is salty, and enzymes from the pancreas and intestinal membrane glands continue digestion. The next section, the jejunum, absorbs most of the juices mixed with the food during digestion—up to 8 liters—as well as minerals and nutrients. The last section, the ileum, takes out bile salts and vitamin B_{12}. After about three to five hours, the remnants of food, moved by peristalsis, reach another sphincter, the ileocecal valve.

The ileocecal valve admits the remaining contents into the colon, which is wider and has segments like a caterpillar. Also called the large intestine, it rises along the right side of the body in the ascending colon; turns ninety degrees into the transverse colon, which crosses to the left side of the body; and turns another ninety degrees into the descending colon, which drops to the sigmoid (S-shaped) colon—altogether a passage of more than a meter. The colon receives watery matter from the small intestine each day, and colon bacteria, of which there is a great variety, mix with the solids and complete digestion. The colon absorbs most of this remaining water.

The anorectum is the last stop. The rectum stores fecal matter, the waste products of digestion: bile, bacteria, undigested fiber, cells sloughed from intestinal linings, and mucus. When a sufficient mass has built up, about 100 to 200 grams, pressure signals the time for defecation. The puborectalis muscle, which is under conscious control after toilet training, relaxes, tilting the feces into a vertical position. The anal sphincter opens, and the feces exit the body as stool. It normally takes from four to seventy-two hours for wastes to pass through the colon.

Three organs attached to the GI tract participate in digestion: the liver, the gallbladder, and the pancreas. The liver makes bile, an oily green liquid which aids the absorption of fats and fat-soluble vitamins and which stores and processes absorbed nutrients, as well as removing toxic substances from food. Bile travels from the liver through the common bile duct into the duodenum; along the way, the gallbladder, a small pouch, stores the bile until it is needed. In addition to making insulin, the pancreas secretes various enzymes for digestion into the duodenum via the pancreatic duct.

The enteric nervous system (ENS), or "gut brain," regulates peristalsis, secretions, and some immune responses throughout the digestive tract, although its mechanisms are not completely understood. The ENS comprises an intricate network of nerves and ganglia laced through the linings of the gut membranes and muscles, and it senses the presence of food through various hormones and neurotransmitters. The vagus nerve connects the esophagus and stomach to the base of the brain; sacral nerves do the same job for the colon. Other nerves reach from the GI tract to the spinal cord.

Mark Twain advised people to eat whatever they liked and then let the foods fight it out in the stomach. When the GI tract reacts to disagreeable foods, however, the result can be pain; in fact, because of the great number of possible malfunctions (deadly or not), the GI tract is responsible for more discomfort and misery than any other major system.

Gastroenterologists spend the largest percentage of their time treating maladies that cause pain but do no lasting harm. For example, gas, a perennial problem for people of all ages, causes bloating, and its pain is sometimes so severe that it is mistaken for a heart attack. An array of poorly understood functional disorders of the colon, called irritable bowel syndrome (IBS), affects 15 to 20 percent of Americans who have nausea, diarrhea or constipation, and abdominal distress; this condition is popularly known as "nervous stomach." Although not dangerous, it produces a bewildering variety of stomachaches. Likewise, chronic stomach and motility irregularities in the esophagus can affect digestion. Proctalgia fugax is intermittent, intense pain in the rectum.

Many GI diseases, however, are deadly. Various cancers grow in the stomach, esophagus, and, most commonly among Americans, colon. (Cancers rarely begin in the small intestine.) Gastroesophageal reflux disease (GERD) occurs when stomach juices repeatedly sluice into the esophagus, where they irritate and inflame the membrane. Aside from causing a burning sensation, the juices can erode through the membrane, creating ulcers. If the membrane is eaten through entirely, a hole opens into the body cavity around the gut, spilling food, blood, and digestive juices. Emergency surgery is then needed. Ulcers can also occur in the stomach and duodenum as a result of motility disorders, excess acid, or drugs, especially alcohol and aspirin, that irritate the membrane. Colitis and Crohn's disease are serious inflammations of the gut lining, especially in the colon; except for some forms of colitis that are caused by bacteria, the mechanism behind such inflammation remains unknown, but the disorders frequently require surgery to remove damaged and inflamed areas.

Similarly, tears in the gut lining, strictures, passages blocked by chunks of food, exposed veins (varices), infected sacs in the colon (diverticula), and communicable diseases such as dysentery and hepatitis produce potentially deadly symptoms.

DIAGNOSTIC AND TREATMENT TECHNIQUES

An extensive battery of tests, procedures, and medications enable gastroenterologists to cure or palliate many GI diseases. In addition to the traditional physician's tools of the physical examination and the patient's medical history, high-tech instruments let gastroenterologists see inside parts of the gut, produce images of it, remove tissue and stones, stop bleeding, and destroy tumors. Medicines kill bacteria, help regulate motility, speed the healing of damaged tissue, and control diarrhea and constipation. Yet the GI tract is a very intricate system, and at times the gastroenterologist's most effective remedy is sympathy and advice about changing patients' behavior or diet so that they learn to live with their diseases.

Before treatment can begin, the disease must be identified. An interview with the patient and a medical examination constitute the first step in narrowing the range of possible causes of distressing symptoms. Symptoms described by the patient or discovered by the physician are clues to the underlying causes and suggest the kinds of tests that will most likely isolate the actions of a specific disease. Blood tests can reveal abnormal levels of white cells or chemicals and the presence of infection. Samples of digestive juices likewise can show chemical imbalances, infections, and bleeding, as can stool samples. Biopsies of the gut membrane, liver, and tumors allow pathologists to inspect tissue damage and look for viruses or bacteria. For example, a patient with yellowish skin (jaundice) and a tender liver who complains of nausea and chills may lead a physician to suspect hepatitis. The physician will then order a blood serum test, looking for specific proteins typical of hepatitis infection, and a liver biopsy to learn the type of hepatitis.

Some diseases, especially those destroying or inflaming tissue or involving motility problems, require imaging to identify, as do blockages and strictures. To obtain pictures of the gut, physicians use ultrasonography, X rays, magnetic resonance imaging (MRI), and computed tomography (CT) scans. Ultrasonographs transmit sound waves through the body and judge the density of tissues by the intensity and pattern of reflection; they are particularly useful for spotting gallstones. X rays, MRIs, and CT scans pass radiation through the body, which is recorded on film or by sensors that feed data to a computer to construct an image. Plain X rays show the pattern of air and gas distribution in the digestive tract and can detect obstructions; X rays may also be taken after barium, a radioopaque element, has been swallowed or inserted in the colon so that it coats the GI tract's walls and makes them easier to see. Such imaging helps the physician to locate strictures, perforations, cancers, diverticula, blockages, and distended areas.

Few tests are more revealing, however, than a direct look inside the GI tract. Until the 1960's, this could not be done without exploratory surgery. At that time, the endoscope became widely available. Developed by British, American, and Japanese scientists, the endoscope is a long, flexible, maneuverable tube filled with fiber optic strands and a central channel for inserting various instruments. A light source at its tip illuminates the area ahead of the scope; the fiber optics collect the reflected light and pass it directly to the eye of the examining physician at the scope's opposite end, to a television monitor, or to a camera. There are many types of endoscopes, of which three are most common: The meter-long upper gastrointestinal panendoscope (or gastroscope), inserted through the mouth, can be used for seeing well into the duodenum; the 60-centimeter flexible sigmoidoscope is used in the rectum and sigmoid colon; and the lower panendoscope (or colonoscope)—180, 140, 100, or 70 centimeters long—inserted through the anus, can be worked through the entire colon and as

much as 30 centimeters into the ileum. Most of the small intestine cannot be seen by endoscopy.

With endoscopy, gastroenterologists can spot and examine a diseased or damaged area of the gut and perform a biopsy so that tissue can be examined under a microscope. Yet endoscopes can do even more than that. They can push a wad of food obstructing the esophagus into the stomach, stretch open a stricture, or clear a clogged duct with wires inserted through the scope's channel; small balloons can be inflated inside the gut to widen constricted passages. Similarly, endoscopes with wire attachments can open a passage between the surface skin and the stomach, allowing food to be put directly in the stomach for patients incapable of swallowing, a procedure called percutaneous endoscopic gastrostomy (PEG). With looped and electrified wires, they can remove polyps, cut away tissue, and cauterize bleeding vessels and ulcers. One such procedure, endoscopic retrograde-cholangiopancreatography (ERCP), can image the biliary and pancreatic ducts and allow removal of gallstones without surgery. Drugs may also be injected through the endoscope to control bleeding from varicose veins (sclerotherapy), and fiber optics permit the use of lasers to vaporize cancerous tissue.

Gastroenterologists use drugs to sedate patients during procedures and to treat dysfunctions and diseases. Other medications available are too numerous and their administration too complex to describe in detail, but basically they ease pain, check diarrhea and vomiting, decrease acid production to permit ulcers to heal, soften the stool of constipated patients, control motility problems (such as spasms), regulate secretions, speed coagulation at bleeding sites, or kill harmful bacteria and parasites. GI pain, especially from irritable bowel syndrome, is notoriously difficult to treat because of the diversity of contributing causes, including emotional problems. Researchers turn out a steady supply of new drugs each year, but improvements are slow, and new drugs require extensive clinical trials to determine proper dosage and detect harmful side effects. Sometimes, a placebo—that is, a pill with no active ingredient, a "sugar pill"—is enough to make a patient feel better. The interaction between a patient's gut, nervous system, and personality is intricate and sometimes highly idiosyncratic.

Gastroenterologists do not simply react to disease and trauma with treatments; they also try to prevent trouble from starting in the first place. A large part of their job involves educating patients. They discuss diets that can reduce GI pain and warn against the abuse of drugs, especially alcohol and tobacco, that are known to contribute to heartburn and ulcers. They routinely screen patients over the age of fifty for cancer, sometimes by endoscopic examination, especially if there is a family history of cancer.

PERSPECTIVE AND PROSPECTS

Jan Baptista van Helmont, a seventeenth century medical chemist, was the first to describe the diseases and digestive juices of the GI tract scientifically. Gastroenterology can be said to have started with his studies (he also coined the word "gas"). Yet no one directly observed the operations of digestion until 1833, when U.S. Army surgeon William Beaumont cared for a French Canadian with a bullet wound to the stomach. The wound remained open, and Beaumont could watch the action of gastric juices and the stomach's mixing and grinding action. Throughout the nineteenth century, there were advances in the understanding and treatment of the GI tract, including the introduction of enemas and gastric lavage (washing out), X rays, and an early form of endoscopy.

Like most branches of medicine, twentieth century technology greatly expanded gastroenterology's role in diagnosing, preventing, and treating disease. Imaging and endoscopy especially have revolutionized the field. In 1932, Rudolph Schindler developed a flexible gastroscope, and in 1943, Lester Dragstedt performed the first vagotomy (surgically cutting the vagus nerve) to reduce stomach acid secretions. Advances were also made to heal peptic ulcers with a special diet. The second half of the twentieth century saw an escalating number of refinements and innovations in procedures but was most remarkable for the development of drugs.

This progress has meant that far fewer surgical procedures are needed for common GI diseases. Because of new medicines, ulcer disease rarely requires surgery. Gallstones in the common bile duct that once necessitated surgical removal now may be taken out during an ERCP; a stent (perforated tube) can be inserted into a blocked bile duct under a gastroenterologist's guidance to keep bile flowing from the liver. Screenings for colon cancer and the removal of polyps, which can become cancerous, often identify cancerous or precancerous areas early and permit surgeons to remove tumors before the cancer spreads, sometimes making surgery unnecessary. Patients who once might have died because of a blocked or strictured esophagus can now be relieved and quickly released from the hospital. The overall trend has been shorter hospital stays and lower medical costs for common ailments. The sophistication of equipment and the training needed to treat difficult problems, however, has correspondingly inflated costs, as has the tendency to medicate painful ailments that sufferers once had to steel themselves to endure, such as irritable bowel syndrome.

Despite the expansion of gastroenterology's procedures and knowledge, it is far from an independent field. Gastroenterologists typically act as consultants, caring for patients only after they have been screened by family practitioners, emergency room doctors, and internists. Moreover, gastroenterologists rely on pathologists to decipher the information in biopsied tissue samples, radiologists to interpret imaging, neurologists to trace nervous system problems, and surgeons to repair perforated gut walls and remove diseased organs or transplant new ones. Finally, specially trained nurses and technicians must help them with many procedures and ensure that patients follow prescribed dietary and drug regimens.

—*Roger Smith, Ph.D.*

See also Abdomen; Abdominal disorders; Appendectomy; Appendicitis; Bulimia; Bypass surgery; Celiac sprue; Cholecystectomy; Cholecystitis; Cholera; Colic; Colitis; Colon and rectal polyp removal; Colon and rectal surgery; Colon cancer; Colonoscopy; Constipation; Crohn's disease; Diarrhea and dysentery; Digestion; Diverticulitis and diverticulosis; *E. coli* infection; Emergency medicine; Endoscopy; Enemas; Enzymes; Fistula repair; Food biochemistry; Food poisoning; Gallbladder diseases; Gastrectomy; Gastroenterology, pediatric; Gastrointestinal disorders; Gastrointestinal system; Gastrostomy; Glands; Heartburn; Hemorrhoid banding and removal; Hemorrhoids; Hernia; Hernia repair; Hirschsprung's disease; Ileostomy and colostomy; Indigestion; Internal medicine; Intestinal disorders; Intestines; Irritable bowel syndrome (IBS); Lactose intolerance; Liver; Liver cancer; Liver disorders; Liver transplantation; Malabsorption; Malnutrition; Metabolism; Nausea and vomiting; Nutrition; Obstruction; Pancreas; Pancreatitis; Peristalsis; Pinworm; Poisonous plants; Proctology; Pyloric stenosis; Roundworm; Salmonella infection; Shigellosis; Soiling; Stomach, intestinal, and pancreatic cancers; Stone removal; Stones; Tapeworm; Taste; Toilet training; Trichinosis; Ulcer surgery; Ulcers; Vagotomy; Weight loss and gain; Worms.

FOR FURTHER INFORMATION:

Brandt, Lawrence J. *The Clinical Practice of Gastroenterology.* 2 vols. Edinburgh, Scotland: Churchill Livingstone, 1999. Details virtually all of the adult and pediatric gastroenterologic problems encountered in practice. Features a full section on liver disease and synthesizes new advances in molecular immunology and imaging techniques.

Heuman, Douglas M., A. Scott Mills, and Hunter H. McGuire, Jr. *Gastroenterology.* Philadelphia: W. B. Saunders, 1997. This volume in the Saunders text and review series discusses digestive system diseases, the physiology of the digestive system, and the methods employed in the field of gastroenterology. Includes a bibliography and an index.

Janowitz, Henry D. *Indigestion: Living Better with Upper Intestinal Problems from Heartburn to Ulcers and Gallstones.* New York: Oxford University Press, 1994. Janowitz discusses common ailments of the upper GI tract with special attention to degenerative diseases afflicting people as they age. His style is clear and straightforward, aimed at general readers who want to prevent illness or to manage an existing one. Accompanied by charts and illustrations.

Massoni, Margaret. "Nurses' GI Handbook." *Nursing 20.* (November, 1990): 65-80. Intended as a primer on GI problems for nurses, this article contains many illustrations of the gut, surgical techniques, and physical examination methods; lists of symptoms and the disorders they suggest; and tables of biochemical tests.

Morrissey, John F., and Mark Reichelderfer. "Medical Progress: Gastrointestinal Endoscopy." *The New England Journal of Medicine* 325 (October 17 and 24, 1991): 1142-1150, 1214-1223. This two-part review article presumes a sophisticated understanding of medicine; however, it is readable, if difficult, and clearly defines medical standards for using endoscopy in detecting, preventing, and treating most GI disorders.

Peikin, Steven. *Gastrointestinal Health.* Rev. ed. New York: HarperCollins, 1999. Concerned almost wholly with the effect of nutrition on GI maladies, the author offers a self-help guide for the afflicted. After explaining the GI tract's workings and describing common symptoms, Peikin specifies diets that he argues will relieve symptoms.

Steiner-Grossman, Penny, Peter A. Banks, and Daniel H. Present, eds. *People . . . Not Patients: A Source Book for Living with Inflammatory Bowel Disease.* Rev. ed. Dubuque, Iowa: Kendall/Hunt, 1997. This book is for those suffering from ulcerative colitis or Crohn's disease. Easy-to-understand, detailed discussions of the diseases are accompanied by illustrations and photographs.

GASTROENTEROLOGY, PEDIATRIC

SPECIALTY

ANATOMY OR SYSTEM AFFECTED: Abdomen, gallbladder, gastrointestinal system, intestines, liver, pancreas, stomach, throat

SPECIALTIES AND RELATED FIELDS: Internal medicine, neonatology, nutrition, pediatrics

DEFINITION: The diagnosis and treatment of diseases and disorders of the digestive tract in infants and children.

KEY TERMS:

biopsy: a small sample of tissue, such as from the lining of the gastrointestinal tract, which is removed for laboratory study to aid in diagnosis

endoscopy: the use of a small-diameter, flexible tube of optical fibers with an external light source to examine visually the interior of the body, such as the gastrointestinal tract

SCIENCE AND PROFESSION

The pediatric gastroenterologist is a pediatrician who has received extra training in the diagnosis and treatment of gastrointestinal diseases and disorders. The full course of training requires a medical degree followed by three years of pediatric residency, plus an additional three years of solely studying children's gastrointestinal diseases. The six years of postdoctoral training are almost always conducted at a large teaching hospital.

The gastrointestinal tract extends from the mouth to the anus. It is responsible for the ingestion, digestion, and absorption of food and for the elimination of unusable waste from the diet. Its principal parts are the esophagus, the stomach, the small intestine and colon, and the liver, gallbladder, and pancreas.

Children suffer the same wide range of gastrointestinal problems that afflict adults. Each age group, however, has its own special problems. For example, children very rarely have stomach or colon cancer, both relatively common in adults. On the other hand, diarrhea is a very common cause of infant death worldwide but is seldom life-threatening for adults.

Childhood gastrointestinal disease varies widely in its severity, from simple constipation needing only a change in diet to liver disease so severe that the child must undergo a liver transplant in order to survive. Common problems that a pediatric gastroenterologist might treat include gastroenteritis, constipation, chronic diarrhea, gastroesophageal reflux (especially in infants), and infections such as bacterial dysentery or viral hepatitis. Less common disorders are peptic ulcers, inflammatory bowel diseases (IBDs) such as ulcerative colitis and Crohn's disease, and malabsorption disorders involving the ability of the intestines to absorb nutrients from digested food.

The liver, gallbladder, and pancreas are abdominal organs that connect directly with the gastrointestinal tract. They are important in the digestion and absorption of food and in the metabolism of the basic sugars, fats, and proteins that are absorbed by the intestines. The diagnosis and treatment of disorders of these organs is part of gastroenterology.

Anatomical defects of the gastrointestinal tract can occur, such as intestinal malformations, obstructions, imperforate anus, and congenital fistulas between the trachea and esophagus. They are generally treated both by the gastroenterologist and by a general or pediatric surgeon, who performs any necessary surgery.

Since the gastrointestinal tract is critical in the digestion and absorption of food, a pediatric gastroenterologist must know much about nutrition. The physician will often prescribe the proper diet for a particular ailment. Occasionally, this program includes parenteral nutrition, in which a patient is fed intravenously with a complex solution of nutrients.

Most of the gastroenterologist's time is spent in the clinic, examining patients and prescribing medications, or performing procedures such as endoscopy of the stomach or colon. A minority of this specialist's patients require hospitalization, few of whom will be seriously or terminally ill.

A child's intestinal disease, especially if serious, can be very stressful for the patient's parents. The pediatric gastroenterologist must be able to communicate clearly with parents and to support them emotionally during the child's illness.

DIAGNOSTIC AND TREATMENT TECHNIQUES

Much of the pediatric gastroenterologist's work involves obtaining a thorough, detailed history of the ailment from the child and parent. Often, skillful questioning will lead to the proper diagnosis and suggest the best treatment. A careful physical examination of the entire child, not simply the abdomen, is also important.

The pediatric gastroenterologist conducts a wide variety of laboratory tests in evaluating the nature and severity of the illness, such as complete blood counts and liver enzyme measurements. Bowel movement specimens often provide important data, such as the presence of blood or infectious bacteria in the intestines.

The pediatric gastroenterologist performs several diagnostic and therapeutic procedures. Flexible endoscopy is the use of a thin, bendable tube of optic fibers to view the interior of the esophagus, stomach, or colon. The physician can obtain biopsies, small samples of gastric or intestinal tissue, through the endoscope and can remove benign intestinal growths called polyps. The gastroenterologist may place a pH probe, a small electrode on a wire, in the esophagus to test acidity levels for periods as long as twenty-four hours. This probe is used to monitor acid reflux from the stomach into the esophagus. This disease, called gastroesophageal reflux can lead to weight loss, recurrent pneumonia, or a scarred esophagus if left untreated.

Liver transplantation may be necessary when a child suffers irreversible liver failure as a result of severe hepatitis, congenital abnormalities such as biliary atresia (failure of the bile ducts to form properly), or some disorders of the body's metabolism. The pediatric gastroenterologist is an important member of the transplant team.

PERSPECTIVE AND PROSPECTS

Subspecialties of pediatrics began to be recognized in the middle of the twentieth century. The first organization for pediatricians interested in gastroenterology was formed in the early 1970's.

In adult gastroenterology, diagnostic tools such as endoscopy and therapies such as antirejection medications for transplantation procedures improved rapidly in the last quarter of the twentieth century. Taking advantage of this new knowledge, pediatric gastroenterologists were also able to diagnose accurately more disorders in their own patients and to treat them effectively.

—*Thomas C. Jefferson, M.D.*

See also Abdomen; Abdominal disorders; Appendectomy; Appendicitis; Bulimia; Bypass surgery; Celiac sprue; Cholera; Colic; Colitis; Colon and rectal surgery; Constipation; Crohn's disease; Diarrhea and dysentery; Digestion; *E. coli* infection; Emergency medicine; Endoscopy; Enemas; Enzymes; Fistula repair; Food biochemistry; Food poisoning; Gastroenterology; Gastrointestinal disorders; Gastrointestinal system; Glands; Heartburn; Hernia; Hernia repair; Hirschsprung's disease; Ileostomy and colostomy; Indigestion; Internal medicine; Intestinal disorders; Intestines; Lactose intolerance; Liver; Liver disorders; Malabsorption; Malnutrition; Metabolism; Nausea and vomiting; Nutrition; Obstruction; Pancreas; Pancreatitis; Pediatrics; Peristalsis; Pinworm; Poisonous plants; Proctology; Pyloric stenosis; Roundworm; Salmonella infection; Shigellosis; Soiling; Tapeworm; Taste; Toilet training; Trichinosis; Weight loss and gain; Worms.

FOR FURTHER INFORMATION:

Kirschner, Barbara S., and Dennis D. Black. "The Gastrointestinal Tract." In *Nelson Essentials of Pediatrics*, edited by Richard E. Behrman and Robert M. Kliegman. 3d ed. Philadelphia: W. B. Saunders, 2000. A chapter in a great text for medical students rotating through pediatrics. It has thorough explanations of diseases and treatments.

Walker, W. Allan, et al., eds. *Pediatric Gastrointestinal Disease: Pathophysiology, Diagnosis, Management*. 3d ed. St. Louis: C. V. Mosby, 2000. This reference textbook deals extensively with the pathophysiologic basis of gastrointestinal disease in children of all ages. An approach to dealing with the families of children with gastrointestinal diseases augments the in-depth approach to disease manifestations and management. A careful approach to diagnosis follows.

GASTROINTESTINAL DISORDERS
DISEASE/DISORDER

ANATOMY OR SYSTEM AFFECTED: Abdomen, gastrointestinal system, intestines, stomach

SPECIALTIES AND RELATED FIELDS: Gastroenterology, internal medicine, microbiology

DEFINITION: The many problems that can affect the gastrointestinal tract, such as infections, injuries, dysfunctions, tumors, congenital defects, and genetic abnormalities.

KEY TERMS:

gastroenterologist: a medical specialist in diseases of the gut

endoscope: any of several flexible fiber-optic scopes used to examine the inside of the gut; it is equipped with tools to cauterize wounds or remove tissue or gallstones

intestines: the section of the gut between the anus and the stomach, consisting of the rectum, colon, and small bowel (subdivided into the ileus, jejunum, and duodenum)

motility: the spontaneous movements of the gut during swallowing, digestion, and elimination

mucosa: the tissue lining the interior of the gastrointestinal tract, through which nutrients pass into the bloodstream

stool: the waste products excreted from the body upon defecation; feces

tumor: a mass of abnormal cells that can be cancerous

CAUSES AND SYMPTOMS

What and how people eat, their digestion, and their toilet habits affect their health more than any other voluntary daily activity. Breathing, circulation, the brain's control of most bodily functions—these normally take place without conscious thought. The intake of nourishment and elimination of wastes, by contrast, afford a great variety of choices. Accordingly, poor or self-destructive eating and toilet habits lie behind many gastrointestinal (GI) disorders. Yet not all disorders result from an individual's habits. Many arise because of a person's cultural or physical environment, some are hereditary or congenital, and a fair amount have no known cause. All told, more than one hundred disorders may originate in the GI tract and its organs, including infections, cancer, dysfunctions, obstructions, autoimmune diseases, malabsorption of nutrients, and reactions to toxins taken in during eating, drinking, or breathing. Furthermore, diseases in other organs, systemic infections such as lupus, immune suppression such as that caused by acquired immunodeficiency syndrome (AIDS), reactions to altered body conditions as during pregnancy, and psychiatric problems can all reverberate to the gut.

The symptoms of GI disorders range from mildly annoying to life-threatening, although seldom does any single symptom except massive bleeding lead quickly to death. Indigestion, bloating, and gas send more people to gastroenterologists than any other set of symptoms, and they often reflect nothing more than overeating. Pain anywhere along the gut, aversion to food (anorexia), and nausea are general symptoms common to many disorders, although pain in the chest is likely to come from the esophagus while pain in the abdomen points to a stomach or intestinal problem. Red blood in the stool indicates bleeding in the intestines, black (digested) blood suggests bleeding in the upper small bowel or stomach, and vomited blood indicates injury to the stomach or esophagus—all dangerous signs indeed. Chronic diarrhea, fatty stool, constipation, difficulty in swallowing, hiccuping, vomiting, and cramps point to disturbances in the GI tract's orderly, wavelike contractions or absorption of nutrients and fluid. Pruritus (intense itching) can come from something as transient as a mild drug reaction or as serious as cancer. Dysentery (bloody diarrhea) usually comes from severe inflammation or lesions caused by viruses, bacteria, or other parasites. Malnourishment is a sign of badly disordered digestion, and ascites (fluid accumulation in body cavities) can result from serious disease in the liver or pancreas. Likewise, jaundice, the yellowing of the skin or eyes because of excess bile, signals problems in the liver, pancreas, or their ducts.

The large number and complexity of GI disorders do not allow a quick, comprehensive summary. Fortunately, many are uncommon, and the most frequent problems can be described through a tour of the GI tract. The GI tract is basically a tube that moves food from one end to the other, extracting energy and biochemical building blocks for the body along the way. So a disorder that interrupts the flow in one section of the intestines can have secondary effects on other parts of the gut. Disorders seldom affect one area alone.

The esophagus. The GI tract's first section, the esophagus, is simply a passageway from the mouth to the stomach. Although it rarely gets infected, the esophagus is the site of several common problems, usually relatively minor, if painful. Muscle dysfunctions, including slow, weak, or spasmodic muscular movement, can impair motility and make swallowing difficult, as can strictures, which usually occur at the sphincter to the stomach. The mucosal lining of the esophagus is not as hardy as in other parts of the gut. When acid backflushes from the stomach into the esophagus, it inflames tissue there and can cause burning and even bleeding, a condition popularly known as heartburn and technically called gastroesophageal reflux disease (GERD). Retching and vomiting, usually resulting from alcohol abuse or associated with a hiatal hernia, can tear the mucosa. Smokers and drinkers run the risk of esophageal cancer, which can

spread down into the gut early in its development and then becomes deadly; however, it accounts for only about 1 percent of cancers. Most of these conditions can be cured or controlled if diagnosed early enough.

The stomach. In order to store food and prepare it for digestion lower in the gut, the stomach churns it into a homogenous mass and releases it in small portions into the small bowel; meanwhile, the stomach also secretes acid to kill bacteria. Bacteria that are acid-resistant, however, can multiply there. One type, *Helicobacter pylori*, is thought to be involved in the development of ulcers and perhaps cancer. Overuse of aspirins and other nonsteroidal anti-inflammatory drugs (NSAIDs) can also cause stomach ulcers. A variety of substances, including alcohol, can prompt inflammation and even hemorrhaging. Stomach cancer has been shown to strike those who have a diet high in salted, smoked, or pickled foods; the most common cancer in the world, although not in the United States, it has a low survival rate. When stomach muscle function fails, food accumulates until the stomach overstretches and rebounds, causing vomiting. Some foods can coalesce into an indigestible lump, and hair and food fibers can roll into a ball, called a bezoar; such masses can interfere with digestion.

The small intestine. The five to six meters of looped gut between the stomach and colon is called the small intestine. It secretes fluids, hormones, and enzymes into food passing through, breaking it down chemically and absorbing nutrients. Although cancers seldom develop in the small intestine itself, they frequently do so in the organs connected to it, the liver and pancreas. The major problem in the small bowel is the multitude of diseases causing diarrhea, dysentery, or ulceration: They include bacterial, viral, and parasitic disease; motility disorders; and the chronic, progressive inflammatory illness called Crohn's disease, which also ulcerates the bowel wall. Although most diarrhea is temporary, if it persists diarrhea severely weakens patients through dehydration and malnourishment. For this reason, diarrheal diseases caused by toxins in water or food are the leading cause of childhood death worldwide. Furthermore, the small bowel can become paralyzed, twisted, or kinked, thereby obstructing the passage of food. Sometimes its contents rush through too fast, a condition called dumping syndrome. All these disorders reduce digestion, and if they are chronic, then malnutrition, vitamin deficiency, and weight loss ensue.

The large intestine. The small intestine empties into the large intestine, or colon, the last meter of the GI tract; here the water content of digestive waste matter (about a liter a day) is reabsorbed, and the waste becomes increasingly solid along the way to the rectum, forming feces. Unlike the small bowel, which is nearly sterile under normal conditions, the colon hosts a large population of bacteria that ferments the indigestible fiber in waste matter, and some of the by-products are absorbed through the colon's mucosa. Bacteria or parasites gaining access from the outside world can cause diarrhea by interfering with this absorption (a condition called malabsorption) or by irritating the mucosa and speeding up muscle action. For unknown reasons, the colon can also become chronically inflamed, resulting in cramps and bloody diarrhea, an illness known as ulcerative colitis; Crohn's disease also can affect the colon. Probably because it is so often exposed to a variety of toxins, the colon is particularly susceptible to cancer in people over fifty years old: Colorectal cancer accounted for the second highest number of cancer deaths in 1993, with an equal proportion of men and women. As people age, the muscles controlling the colon deteriorate, sometimes forming small pouches in the bowel wall, called diverticula, that can become infected (diverticulitis). In addition, small knobs called polyps can grow, and they may become cancerous. One of the most common lower GI disorders is constipation, which may derive from a poor diet, motility malfunction, or both.

The rectum. The last segment of the colon, the rectum collects and holds feces for defecation through the anus. The rectum is susceptible to many of the diseases affecting the colon, including cancer and chronic inflammation. The powerful anal sphincter muscle, which controls defecation, can be the site of brief but intensely painful spasms called proctalgia fugax, which strikes for unknown reasons. The tissue lining the anal canal contains a dense network of blood vessels; straining to eliminate stool because of constipation or diarrhea or simply sitting too long on a toilet can distend these blood vessels, creating hemorrhoids, which may burn, itch, bleed, and become remarkably annoying. If infected, hemorrhoids or anal fissures may develop painful abscesses (sacs of pus). Extreme straining can cause the rectum to turn inside out through the anus, or prolapse.

The liver. The GI tract's organs figure prominently in many disorders. The liver is a large spongy organ that filters the blood, removing toxins and dumping them with bile into the duodenum. A number of viruses can invade the liver and inflame it, a malady called hepatitis. Acute forms of the disease have flulike symptoms and are self-limited. Some viruses, however, as well as alcohol or drug abuse and worms, cause extensive cirrhosis (the formation of abnormal, scarlike tissue) and chronic hepatitis. Although only recently common in the United States, viral hepatitis has long affected a large percentage of people in Southeast Asia; because hepatitis can trigger the mutation of normal cells, liver cancer is among the most common cancers worldwide. Hepatitis patients often have jaundice, as do those who, as a result of drug reactions, cancer, or stones, have blocked bile flow. Because of congenital or inherited errors of metabolism, excess fat, iron, and copper can build up in the liver, causing upper abdominal pain, skin discolorations, weakness, and behavioral changes; complications can include cirrhosis, diabetes mellitus, and heart disease.

The gallbladder. A small sac that concentrates and stores bile from the liver, the gallbladder is connected to the liver and duodenum by ducts. The concentrate often coalesces into stones, which seldom cause problems if they stay in one place. If they block the opening to the gallbladder or lodge in a duct, however, they can cause pain, fever, and jaundice. Although rare, tumors may also grow in the gallbladder or ducts, perhaps as a result of gallstone obstruction.

The pancreas. Lying just behind the stomach, the pancreas produces enzymes to break down fats and proteins for absorption and insulin to metabolize sugar; a duct joins it to the duodenum. The pancreas can become inflamed, either because of toxins (largely alcohol) or blockage of its duct, usually by gallstones. Either cause precipitates a painful condition, pancreatitis, that may last a few days, with full recovery, or turn into a life-threatening disease. If the source of inflammation is not eliminated, chronic pancreatitis may develop and with it the gradual loss of the pancreas' ability to make enzymes and insulin: Severe abdominal pain, malnutrition, diarrhea, and diabetes may develop. Pancreatic cancer, once rare in the United States, ranked fifth among cancers causing death during 1993. Scientists are unsure of the causes; pancreatitis, gallstones, diabetes, and alcohol have been implicated, but only smoking is well attested to increase the risk of contracting pancreatic cancer, which is very lethal and difficult to treat.

Only about 1 percent of patients live more than a year after diagnosis.

Functional diseases. Finally, some disorders appear to upset several parts of the GI tract at the same time, often with no identifiable cause but with chronic or recurrent symptoms. Gastroenterologists call them functional diseases, and they afflict as much as 30 percent of the population in Western countries. People with irritable bowel syndrome (IBS) complain of abdominal pain, urgency in defecation, and bloating from intestinal gas; they often feel that they cannot empty their rectums completely, even after straining. Functional dyspepsia manifests itself as upper abdominal pain, bloating, early feelings of fullness during a meal, and nausea. Also included in this group are various motility disorders in the esophagus and stomach, whose typical symptom is vomiting, and pseudo-obstruction, a condition in which the small bowel acts as if it is blocked but no lesion can be found. Many gastroenterologists believe that emotional disturbance plays a part in some of these diseases.

TREATMENT AND THERAPY

The majority of GI disorders are transient and pose no short-term or long-term threat to life. The body's natural defenses can combat most bacterial and viral infections in the gut without help. Even potentially dangerous noninfectious conditions, such as pancreatitis, resolve on their own if the irritating agent is eliminated. Many disorders require a gastroenterologist's help, however, and even despite help can make people semi-invalids. Regulation of diet and the use of drugs to combat infections or relieve pain are important treatments. If these fail, as is likely to happen in such serious conditions as chronic inflammatory disease and cancer, cures or palliation is yet possible because of gastroenterological technology, particularly endoscopy, and surgical techniques developed in the twentieth century.

While it is not true that GI disorders would necessarily disappear with improved diet, since genetic disorders would remain, gastroenterologists stress that proper nourishment is the first line of defense against trouble. For example, incidence of stomach cancer plummets in countries where people eat fresh foods and use refrigeration rather than salting and smoking to preserve food. Regions where fiber makes up a high percentage of the diet, such as Africa, have a far lower incidence of inflammatory bowel disease. Last, and certainly not least, groups that do not drink alcohol or smoke (such as Mormons) have far lower incidences of cancer and inflammatory disease throughout the GI tract.

—*Roger Smith, Ph.D.*

See also Abdomen; Abdominal disorders; Appendectomy; Appendicitis; Bacterial infections; Botulism; Bypass surgery; Candidiasis; Celiac sprue; Cholecystitis; Cholera; Cirrhosis; Colic; Colitis; Colon and rectal polyp removal; Colon and rectal surgery; Colon cancer; Colon therapy; Colonoscopy; Constipation; Crohn's disease; Diabetes mellitus; Diarrhea and dysentery; Digestion; Diverticulitis and diverticulosis; Enemas; Fistula repair; Food poisoning; Gallbladder diseases; Gastrectomy; Gastroenterology; Gastroenterology, pediatric; Gastrointestinal system; Gastrostomy; Heartburn; Hemorrhoid banding and removal; Hemorrhoids; Hernia; Hernia repair; Hirschsprung's disease; Ileostomy and colostomy; Incontinence; Indigestion; Internal medicine; Intestinal disorders; Intestines; Irritable bowel syndrome (IBS); Jaundice; Kwashiorkor; Lactose intolerance; Liver; Liver cancer; Liver disorders; Malabsorption; Malnutrition; Metabolism; Nausea and vomiting; Nutrition; Obstruction; Pancreas; Pancreatitis; Peristalsis; Peritonitis; Pinworm; Poisoning; Poisonous plants; Proctology; Protozoan diseases; Pyloric stenosis; Roundworm; Salmonella infection; Shigellosis; Soiling; Stomach, intestinal, and pancreatic cancers; Tapeworm; Toilet training; Trichinosis; Tumor removal; Tumors; Typhoid fever and typhus; Ulcer surgery; Ulcers; Vagotomy; Weight loss and gain; Worms.

FOR FURTHER INFORMATION:

Heuman, Douglas M., A. Scott Mills, and Hunter H. McGuire, Jr. *Gastroenterology*. Philadephia: W. B. Saunders, 1997. A review of digestive system diseases and methods of treating them. Includes a bibliography and an index.

Janowitz, Henry D. *Indigestion: Living Better with Upper Intestinal Problems from Heartburn to Ulcers and Gallstones*. New York: Oxford University Press, 1994. Clear explanations of common ailments, especially those related to aging, to help people prevent or manage GI disorders. With charts and illustrations.

Sachar, David B., Jerome D. Waye, and Blair S. Lewis, eds. *Pocket Guide to Gastroenterology*. Rev. ed. Baltimore: Williams & Wilkins, 1991. In detailed outlines intended for physicians, this handbook contains a wealth of information from which general readers can profit despite the extensive use of medical terminology.

Thompson, W. Grant. *The Angry Gut: Coping with Colitis and Crohn's Disease*. New York: Plenum Press, 1993. In addition to highlighting the significant similarities and differences of these two syndromes and stressing the importance of a correct diagnosis, Thompson broaches more sensitive topics that seem to be ignored by the medical profession.

GASTROINTESTINAL SYSTEM

ANATOMY

ANATOMY OR SYSTEM AFFECTED: Abdomen, gallbladder, intestines, liver, pancreas, stomach, teeth, throat

SPECIALTIES AND RELATED FIELDS: Dentistry, gastroenterology, internal medicine, nutrition, oncology, otorhinolaryngology

DEFINITION: A compartmentalized tube that is equipped to reduce food, both mechanically and chemically, to a state in which it is absorbed and used by the body; this system includes the mouth, esophagus, stomach, small intestine, and colon (large intestine), as well as the salivary glands, pancreas, liver, and gallbladder.

KEY TERMS:

absorption: the movement of digested food from the small intestine into blood vessels and from blood into body cells

bolus: food that has been mixed with saliva and formed into a ball; the bolus passes from the mouth to the stomach through a process called swallowing or deglutition

chyme: the semiliquid state of food as it is found in the stomach and first part of the small intestine

digestion: the mechanical and chemical breakdown of food into physical and molecular units that can be absorbed and used by cells

enzymes: substances that aid in the chemical digestion of food; enzymes are produced and secreted by glands found in digestive organs

peristalsis: a muscular contraction that helps to move food through the digestive tube

sphincter: a circular muscle that controls the opening and closing of an orifice

villus: a fingerlike projection in the small intestine that provides a site for the absorption of digested food into the circulatory and lymph systems

STRUCTURE AND FUNCTIONS

The gastrointestinal system or alimentary canal exists as a tube which runs through the body from mouth to anus. The wall of the tube is composed of four layers of tissue. The outermost layer, the serosa, is part of a large tissue called the peritoneum, which covers internal organs and lines body cavities. Extensions of the peritoneum called mesenteries anchor the organs of digestion to the body wall. Fatty, apronlike structures that hang in front of the abdominal organs are also modifications of the peritoneum. They are called the lesser and the greater omentum. The muscular layer, composed of circular and longitudinal muscles, makes up the bulk of the wall of the tube. The contractions of this layer aid in moving materials through the tube. Nerves, blood vessels, and lymph vessels are found in the third layer, the submucosa. The innermost or mucous layer has glands for secretion and modifications for absorption.

The tube is compartmentalized, and each section is equipped to accomplish some part of the digestive process. The mechanical phase of digestion involves the physical reduction of food to a semiliquid state; this is accomplished by tearing, chewing, and churning the food. Chemical digestion utilizes enzymes to reduce food to simple molecules that can be absorbed and used by the body to provide energy and to build and repair tissue.

The mouth (also called the buccal or oral cavity) marks the beginning of the gastrointestinal system and the digestive process. The mouth is divided into two areas. The vestibule is the space between the lips, cheeks, gums, and teeth. Lips, or labia, are the fleshy folds that surround the opening to the mouth. The skin covers the outside, while the inside is lined with mucous membrane. The colored part of the lips, called the vermilion, is a juncture of these two tissues. Because the tissue at this point is unclouded, underlying blood vessels can be seen. A membrane called the labial frenulum attaches each lip to the gum, or gingivalum.

The oral cavity occupies the space posterior to the teeth and anterior to the fauces or opening to the throat. It is bounded on the sides by cheeks and on the roof by an anterior bony structure called the hard palate and a posterior muscular area, the soft palate. The uvula, a cone-shaped extension of the soft palate, can be seen hanging down in front of the fauces. The floor of the oral cavity is formed by the tongue and associated muscles. Taste buds are found on the surface of the tongue. The bottom of the tongue is anchored posteriorly to the hyoid bone. Anteriorly, the membranous frenulum lingua anchors the tongue to the floor of the mouth. The tongue's movement is controlled by extrinsic muscles that form the floor of the mouth and by intrinsic muscles that are part of the tongue itself. The movements of the tongue assist in speaking, swallowing, and forming food into a bolus.

Teeth, found in gum sockets, are the principal means of mechanical digestion in the mouth. Human teeth appear in two sets. The deciduous or milk teeth are the first to appear. There are usually ten in each jaw, and they are replaced by the second, permanent set during childhood. The permanent set consists of sixteen teeth in each jaw. The four incisors and two canines have sharp chiseled edges, which permit biting and tearing of food. The four premolars and six molars have flat surfaces that are used in grinding the food. Frequently, the third pair of molars or wisdom teeth do not erupt until later in adolescence. The crown of a tooth appears above the gum line while

The Organs of the Gastrointestinal System

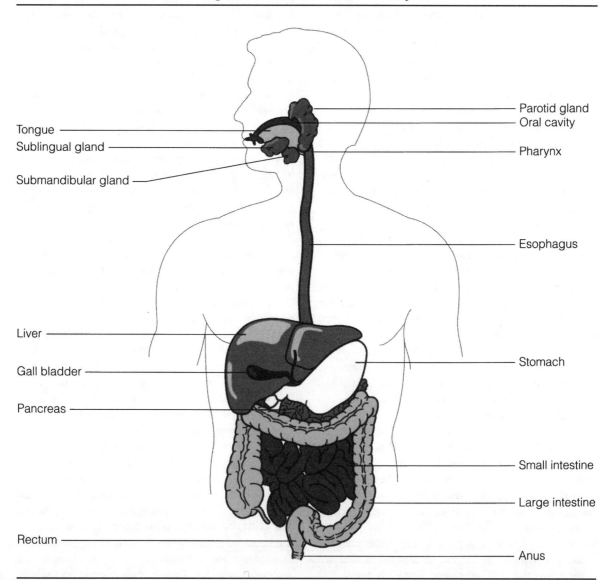

the roots are embedded in the gum socket. The small area between the crown and the root is called the neck. The crown is covered with enamel and the root with cementum. Dentin is beneath the covering in both areas and forms the bulk of the tooth. The central cavity of the tooth is filled with a soft membrane called pulp. Blood vessels and nerves are embedded in the pulp.

At the rear of the mouth, the fauces or opening leads to the pharynx. The pharynx is a common passageway for the movement of air from nasal cavity to trachea and food from mouth to esophagus. The esophagus is a tube approximately 25 centimeters long. Most of the esophagus is located within the thoracic cavity, although the lower end of the tube pierces the diaphragm and connects with the stomach in the abdominal cavity. Both ends of the esophagus are controlled by a circular muscle called a sphincter. The movement of food through the esophagus is assisted by gravity and the contractions of the muscularis layer. No digestion is accomplished in either the pharynx or the esophagus.

The stomach, a J-shaped organ, is divided into four areas: the cardia, fundus, body, and pyloris. The cardia lies just below the sphincter at the juncture of esophagus and stomach, while the fundus is a pouch that pushes upward and to the left of the cardia. The large central area is the body, and the lower end of the stomach is the pyloris. Here another sphincter, the pyloric valve, controls the opening between stomach and intestine. The mucosa of the stomach is arranged in folds called rugae. The rugae permit distension of the organ as it fills. Gastric and mucus glands are present in the mucosa. The gastric glands produce and secrete enzymes that are specific for protein digestion, as well as hydrochloric acid, which creates the proper acid environment for enzyme action. The muscularis of the stomach wall has three layers of muscle with a circular, longitudinal, and oblique arrangement. The muscle arrangement facilitates the churning action that reduces the food to a semiliquid called chyme. The pyloric valve relaxes under neuronal and hormonal influence, and the chyme is moved into the small intestine.

The site for the completion of digestion and the absorption of digested material is the small intestine. This tube, with a 2.5-centimeter diameter and a length of 6.4 meters, is coiled into the mid and lower abdomen. The first 25 centimeters of the small intestine constitute the duodenum. This is followed by the

jejunum, which is 2.5 meters long. The ileum, at 3.6 meters, terminates at the ileocecal valve, which connects the small to the large intestine. The interior of the small intestine is characterized by the presence of fingerlike projections of the mucosa called villi that contain blood and lymph capillaries and circular folds of submucosa (the plicae circularis), both of which provide absorption surface for the digested food. Mucosal glands produce enzymes that contribute to the digestion of carbohydrates, lipids, and proteins. Enzymes from the pancreas and bile from the liver enter the small intestine at the duodenum and aid the chemical digestion.

The final compartment in the gastrointestinal system is the large intestine, sometimes called the bowel or colon. This tube, with a diameter of 6.5 centimeters and a length of 1.5 meters, is divided into the cecum; the ascending, transverse, and descending colon; the rectum; and the anal canal. The cecum is a blind pouch located just below the ileocecal valve. The fingerlike appendix is attached to the cecum. The ascending colon extends from the cecum up the right side of the abdomen to the underside of the liver, where it turns and runs across the body. The colon descends along the left side of the abdomen. The last few centimeters of colon form an S-shaped curve which gives the section its name, sigmoid colon. Three bands of longitudinal muscle called taeniae coli run the length of the colon. Contraction of these bands causes pouches or haustra to form in the colon, giving the tube a puckered appearance. The sigmoid colon leads into the rectum, a 20-centimeter segment which terminates in a short anal canal. The anus is the opening from the anal canal to the exterior of the body.

DISORDERS AND DISEASES

Because the primary function performed in the gastrointestinal system is the physical and chemical preparation of food for cellular absorption and use, any malfunction of the process has implications for the overall metabolism of the body. Structural changes or abnormalities in the anatomy of the system interfere with the proper mechanical and chemical preparation of the food.

Teeth are the principal agents of mechanical digestion or mastication in the mouth. Dental caries or tooth decay involves a demineralization of the enamel through bacterial action. Disrupted enamel provides an entrance for bacteria to underlying tissues, resulting in infection and inflammation of the tissues. The resulting pain and discomfort interfere with the biting, chewing, and grinding of food. Three pairs of salivary glands secrete the water-based, enzyme-containing fluid called saliva. These glands can be the target of the virus that causes mumps. (Although the pain and swelling that are typical of this disease can prevent swallowing, the more important effect of the virus in males is the possible inflammation of the testes and subsequent sterility.)

The gastroesophageal sphincter at the lower end of the esophagus controls the movement of materials from the stomach into the esophagus. Relaxation of this sphincter allows a backflow of food (gastroesophageal reflux) to occur. The acidity of the stomach contents damages the esophageal lining, and a burning sensation is experienced. Substances such as citric fruits, chocolate, tomatoes, alcohol, and nicotine as well as body positions that increase abdominal pressure, such as bending or lying on the side, induce heartburn or indigestion. A hiatal hernia occurs when a defect of the diaphragm allows the lower portion of the esophagus and the upper portion of the stomach to enter the chest cavity; it causes heartburn and difficulty in swallowing.

Pathologies and abnormalities of the stomach and intestines are studied in the medical science called gastroenterology. The stomach is the site of both mechanical and chemical digestion. Although small amounts of digested food begin to pass into the small intestine within minutes following a meal, the chyme usually remains in the stomach for three to five hours. Relaxation of the gastroesophageal sphincter will result in reflux; and stimulation by nerves from the medulla of the brain can cause the forceful emptying of stomach contents through the mouth. This is called vomiting and may be brought about by irritation, overdistension, certain foods, or drugs. Excessive vomiting results in dehydration, which in turn upsets electrolyte and fluid balance.

Chemical digestion in the stomach requires an acidic environment. This is provided by gastric glands, which secrete hydrochloric acid. The tissue lining the stomach protects it from this acidity and prevents self-digestion. Oversecretion of the gastric juices or a breakdown of the stomach lining can cause lesions or peptic ulcers to form in the mucosal lining. Gastritis, the inflammation of the stomach mucosa brought on by the ingestion of irritants such as alcohol and aspirin or an overactive nervous stimu-

lation of the gastric glands, may be the underlying cause of ulcer formation. Ulcers can form in the lower esophagus, stomach, and duodenum because these are the organs that come in contact with gastric juice. The terms "gastric ulcer" and "duodenal ulcer" refer to peptic ulcers located in the stomach and the first portion of the small intestine, respectively.

Gastroenteritis could involve the stomach, the small intestine, or the large intestine. It is a disorder marked by nausea, vomiting, abdominal discomfort, and diarrhea. The condition has various causes and is known by several names. Bacteria are a common cause of the condition known as food poisoning. Amoebas, parasites, and viruses can bring about the symptoms associated with intestinal influenza or travelers' diarrhea. Allergic reactions to food or drugs may cause gastroenteritis.

Although diverticulitis may be found anywhere along the gastrointestinal tract, it is most commonly found in the sigmoid colon. This disorder results from the formation of pouches or diverticula in the wall of the tract. Undigested food and bacteria collect in the diverticula and react to form a hard mass. The mass interferes with the blood supply to the area and ultimately irritates and inflames surrounding tissue. Abscess, obstruction, and hemorrhage may develop. A diet lacking in fiber appears to be the major contributor to this disorder.

Colitis, or inflammation of the bowel, is accompanied by abdominal cramps, diarrhea, and constipation. It may be brought about by psychological stress, as in irritable bowel syndrome, or may be a manifestation of such disorders as chronic ulcerative colitis and Crohn's disease.

A change in the rate of motility through the colon or large intestine results in one of two disorders: diarrhea or constipation. As food passes through the colon, water is reabsorbed by the body. If the food moves too quickly through the colon, then much of the water will remain in the feces and diarrhea results. Severe diarrhea affects electrolyte balance. Viral, bacterial, and parasitic organisms may initiate the rapid motility of substances through the colon. Another condition, called constipation, develops from sluggish motility. When the food remains for too long a time in the bowel, too much water is reabsorbed by the body. The feces then become dry and hard, and defecation is difficult. Lack of fiber in the diet and lack of exercise are the leading causes of constipation.

Hemorrhoids are varicose veins that develop in the rectum or anal canal. Varicose veins are the result of weakened venous valves. Factors such as pressure, lack of muscle tone as a result of aging, straining at defecation, pregnancy, and obesity are among the common contributors. Hemorrhoids become irritated and bleed when hard stools are passed.

Disorders in the accessory organs contribute to the malfunctioning of the gastrointestinal system. Gallstones, cirrhosis of the liver, pancreatitis, and pancreatic cancer are among the major diseases affecting the digestive process. These disorders generally involve the obstruction of tubes or the destruction of glands, so that enzymes do not reach the intended site of digestion.

PERSPECTIVE AND PROSPECTS

The proper functioning of the gastrointestinal system is dependent on the anatomical structure and health of the organs. The organs provide the site for the mechanical and chemical digestion of food, the absorption of food and water, and the elimination of waste material. Two factors play a primary role in causing anatomical abnormalities in digestion: aging and eating disorders.

The aging process gradually changes anatomical structure. In order for food to be chewed properly, teeth must be in good health. Dental caries, periodontal disease, and missing teeth prevent the proper mastication of food. Because of these problems, older people tend to avoid foods that require chewing. This may lead to an unbalanced diet. Another age-related change in the mouth is the atrophy of the salivary glands and other secretory glands, which interferes with chemical digestion and swallowing. A loss of muscle tone in the organ walls impedes mechanical digestion and slows down the movement of food through the system. Often, the elimination of waste material becomes difficult and constipation results.

Eating disorders such as anorexia nervosa and bulimia contribute to digestive malfunctioning. These disorders are most often associated with but are not limited to young women. Anorexia is self-imposed starvation, while bulimia is characterized by a binge-purge cycle which incorporates vomiting and/or an abusive use of laxatives. Both conditions induce nutrient deficiencies and upset water and electrolyte balances. The vomiting of the acid contents of the stomach damages esophageal, pharyngeal, and mouth tissue. It also destroys tooth enamel. In addition to the harm done to the gastrointestinal system, eating disorders affect several other systems, such as the reproductive system.

The field of medical science that studies and diagnoses digestive system disorders is gastroenterology. Gastroenterologists use several investigative techniques. Blood tests and stool examination are used to detect internal bleeding and deficiency disorders. For a time, X rays were the only nonsurgical means of obtaining information on the structure of internal organs. The advent of nuclear medicine in the 1950's led to the use of radioisotopes in body scanning procedures. Instruments capable of a more detailed and direct visualization were developed, such as fiber optics and the fluoroscope. Fiber optics involves the use of long, threadlike fibers of glass or plastic that transmit light into the organ and reflect the image back to the viewer; this method allows the physician to detect ulcers, lesions, neoplasms, and structural abnormalities. The fluoroscope uses X rays to permit continuous observation of motion within the organs.

The 1970's saw the development of more sophisticated scanning and imaging techniques. Computed tomography (CT) scanning uses X-ray techniques to scan very thin slices of tissue and presents a defined, unobstructed view. Magnetic resonance imaging (MRI) can provide detailed information even to the molecular level; energies from powerful magnetic fields are translated into a visual representation of the structure being studied. Another technique, ultrasonography, passes sound waves through a body area, intercepts the echoes that are produced, and translates them into electrical impulses, which are recorded and interpreted by the physician.

—Rosemary Scheirer, Ed.D.

See also Abdomen; Constipation; Diarrhea and dysentery; Digestion; Endoscopy; Enzymes; Food biochemistry; Gastroenterology; Gastroenterology, pediatric; Gastrointestinal disorders; Glands; Hemorrhoids; Hernia; Host-defense mechanisms; Indigestion; Internal medicine; Intestinal disorders; Intestines; Laparoscopy; Lipids; Liver; Malnutrition; Metabolism; Muscles; Nausea and vomiting; Nutrition; Obstruction; Peristalsis; Proctology; Sense organs; Systems and organs; Taste; Teeth.

FOR FURTHER INFORMATION:

McMinn, R. M. H., and R. T. Hutchings. *McMinn's Color Atlas of Human Anatomy.* 4th ed. St. Louis: Mosby Year Book, 1998. Although this atlas is intended for an advanced student of human anatomy, the average reader can profit from the marvelous diagrams and pictures. The pictures are especially helpful in visualizing the organs as they actually appear in the human body.

Moog, Florence. "The Lining of the Small Intestine." *Scientific American* 245 (November, 1981): 154-176. This article incorporates a historical perspective in the detailed explanation of absorption as it occurs in the small intestine. The article requires some scientific literacy but is not beyond the comprehension of a reader with a high school science background.

Tortora, Gerard J., and Sandra R. Grabowski. *Principles of Human Anatomy and Physiology*. 9th ed. New York: John Wiley & Sons, 2000. This highly readable text gives a clear and accurate description of the anatomy and physiology of the gastrointestinal system. The illustrations and diagrams are excellent. The authors include descriptions of major disorders and clinical applications.

GASTROSTOMY
PROCEDURE

ANATOMY OR SYSTEM AFFECTED: Abdomen, gastrointestinal system, stomach

SPECIALTIES AND RELATED FIELDS: Gastroenterology, oncology

DEFINITION: The creation of a hole through the wall of the abdomen into the stomach in order to feed a patient who is unable to swallow.

INDICATIONS AND PROCEDURES

Gastrostomies are carried out during situations in which a patient is unable to swallow food. This condition may result from cancer or strictures of the esophagus; when an esophageal fistula is present, causing the diversion of swallowed food; or when a patient is unconscious. In some cases, the patient is a child who has swallowed a caustic substance, causing damage to the esophagus. Under such circumstances in which a gastrostomy is warranted, an artificial opening is prepared through the abdominal wall into the stomach, and a tube is inserted through the opening.

The gastrostomy tube, which is usually made of plastic or nylon, may be permanently inserted or removed after each feeding. The development of the Barnes-Redo prosthesis has alleviated some of the problems associated with permanent gastrostomies.

The device, which is permanently installed, has a cap placed over the opening between feedings. When it is time to eat, the cap is removed, and a catheter is placed through the tube into the stomach, allowing food or liquids to be fed to the patient. When the meal is finished, the catheter is removed and the cap replaced on the gastrostomy tube.

Food for gastrostomy patients cannot be solid. It is recommended that any food first be thoroughly cooked and then blended into a mushy consistency. Patients should smell and taste the food prior to feeding, both to minimize difficulty in adjustment to the situation and to stimulate gastric secretions, which will aid in digestion.

USES AND COMPLICATIONS

Care must be taken with gastrostomy patients to minimize the chance of infection. Any tubes that will be inserted into the stomach must be sterilized prior to use. In addition, the skin around the gastrostomy tube must be protected from gastric juices such as stomach acid, which could cause irritation. The major adjustment for these patients, however, is often psychological—particularly for those with permanent gastrostomies, since meals are often times for social gatherings.

—*Richard Adler, Ph.D.*

See also Cancer; Catheterization; Critical care; Critical care, pediatric; Gastroenterology; Gastroenterology, pediatric; Gastrointestinal disorders; Gastrointestinal system; Nutrition; Poisoning; Stomach, intestinal, and pancreatic cancers.

FOR FURTHER INFORMATION:

Broadwell, Debra C., and Bettie S. Jackson, eds. *Principles of Ostomy Care*. St. Louis, Mo.: Mosby, 1982.

Gauderer, Michael W. L., and Thomas A. Stellato. *Gastrostomies: Evolution, Techniques, Indications, and Complications*. Chicago, Ill.: Year Book Medical, 1986.

Ponsky, Jeffrey L., ed. *Techniques of Percutaneous Gastrostomy*. New York: Igaku-Shoin, 1988.

GENE THERAPY
PROCEDURE

ANATOMY OR SYSTEM AFFECTED: All

SPECIALTIES AND RELATED FIELDS: Biotechnology, ethics, genetics, oncology, pulmonary medicine

DEFINITION: A procedure that attempts to cure a condition by adding specific genes to cells. The expression of these genes results in the production of specific proteins.

KEY TERMS:

adenovirus: a virus whose genetic material is in the form of deoxyribonucleic acid (DNA); it can be engineered to carry genes for gene therapy

chromosome: a long thread of DNA that includes many genes and is complexed with protein; at cell division, each chromosome duplicates and becomes tightly wound into a compact unit, allowing a complete set of chromosomes to be delivered to each daughter cell

deoxyribonucleic acid (DNA): the genetic material of organisms

gene: a stretch of DNA that codes for a specific protein

genome: a complete set of genetic information for an organism

messenger ribonucleic acid (mRNA): an RNA copy of a gene's coding region that leaves the nucleus and enters the cytoplasm, where it is translated into protein; the product of gene transcription

nonviral vector: a gene delivery system that packages DNA in molecules such as lipids that protect it from degradation

plasmid: a stable loop of DNA from bacteria that can be engineered to carry nonbacterial genes of choice

retrovirus: a virus whose genetic material is in the form of RNA; upon infecting a cell, its RNA is first transcribed into DNA by the enzyme, reverse transcriptase, and this DNA is then inserted randomly into the cell's genome; can be used to carry genes for gene therapy

viral vector: a virus that has been engineered to carry specific genes, allowing the delivery of these genes to cells that the virus infects, a method used in gene therapy

INDICATIONS AND PROCEDURES

Gene therapy is a new technology that holds great promise for treating a variety of illnesses. Still primarily in its experimental stages, its major goal is to transfer genes into cells that will be of therapeutic use. Where defective genes are responsible for causing inherited diseases such as cystic fibrosis, it is hoped that the defective gene can be replaced by a corrected copy of the gene. Where a disease state, such as cancer or acquired immunodeficiency syndrome (AIDS), could be improved by delivering therapeutic substances to specific sites, it is hoped that genes coding for therapeutic products could be transferred to specific cells at specific sites. The cells that are being targeted for gene therapy are somatic cells, body cells other than those that give rise to eggs or sperm. This ensures that the therapy does not affect future generations.

Gene therapy relies on a number of advances in genetics that have increased the understanding of what genes are and how they work. A gene is a stretch of deoxyribonucleic acid (DNA) that functions as a blueprint for a particular protein. Genes are connected together into long strands of DNA called chromosomes contained within each cell's nucleus. When a gene is expressed, an intermediate molecule is made called messenger ribonucleic acid (mRNA), which represents a copy of the blueprint encoded by the gene. Once made, the mRNA leaves the nucleus and enters the cytoplasm, where the protein machinery of the cell decodes the message, translating it into a specific protein. When a gene is defective—that is, when a mutation has caused an alteration in the DNA sequence of the gene—there can be a number of consequences. The mutation may prevent the gene from being expressed, with the result that no protein product is made. The mutation may cause an incorrect mRNA to be made, with the result that a faulty protein product is made. These results can lead to a serious disease condition. Cystic fibrosis, for example, is caused by mutations in the cystic fibrosis gene, CFTR, that result in a faulty CFTR protein being made. This protein is a chloride-ion-channel protein that helps to control the viscosity of cellular secretions. When this protein is defective, cellular secretions become very viscous, which is the basis for the major symptoms of the disease.

Identifying the genetic basis for inherited diseases has been aided considerably by information from the Human Genome Project, which is identifying the position and function of numerous human genes. This effort, coupled with new technologies for copying genes and inserting them into cells, has made it possible to design a number of protocols for gene therapy. Because the control over gene expression is so exquisitely complex, it has been exceedingly difficult to achieve the fine control over the expression of the introduced genes that is necessary for many applications of gene therapy. Experimentally introduced genes, for example, are typically expressed only over short periods of time, such as weeks or months. In addition, it has been difficult to control the amount of product produced by these genes; usually the amount is insufficient for curing the disease. Advances in the field, however, are rapid, and new uses for gene therapy are being suggested that do not require long-term expression of the therapeutic gene.

Inserting copies of genes into cells can be done in a variety of ways, typically using cloning vectors. A vector is anything that will deliver a copy of the gene to the cells. Viruses are often used as vectors because of their ability to bring genetic material into a cell with great efficiency, infecting as many as 100 percent of the cells to which they are exposed. Since viruses are normally pathogens, however, they must first be engineered so that they can no longer multiply or cause disease. This is done by removing certain viral genes before inserting the gene of choice into the virus. Retroviruses and adenoviruses are two types that are often used. A retrovirus inserts its genetic material directly into the host cell's genome, making the inserted genes stable. A retrovirus will infect only dividing cells and, by inserting its genes into the cell's genome, may interfere with normal cell function. An adenovirus infects both dividing and nondividing cells but does not insert its genetic material into the host cell's genome. The advantage of using adenoviruses is that they do not carry the risk of interfering with normal gene function. The genetic material brought into the cell, however, is less stable and can easily be lost.

Nonviral vectors can also be used to deliver genes to their target cells. One of the more successful methods is to use lipids to envelop the gene. Typically, a gene is contained within a stable circular DNA construct called a plasmid. When surrounded by lipids, these plasmids form small lipid spheres called lipoplexes, which can enter cells. Amino acid polymers have also been used to coat DNA for the delivery of genes to specific cell types that bind these amino acids. These nonviral vectors are less efficient than viral vectors, infecting as few as one in every ten thousand cells; however, they do not carry some of the risks involved in using viruses. A more direct method, in which naked DNA is injected directly into a tissue, has yielded results as well, although how the cells take up the DNA is not known.

When gene therapy is being delivered, treatment can be either in vivo, in which the viral or nonviral vector is introduced directly into the patient's body, or ex vivo, in which the target cells are removed from the patient, treated, and then returned to the patient's body. Ex vivo methods allow the selection of cells that have incorporated the therapeutic gene and their growth in culture to increase cell number greatly before returning them to the patient.

USES AND COMPLICATIONS

Gene therapy is being investigated as a tool for treating a number of disorders. As of 1998, however, no patient had been cured of a disease using gene therapy, despite more than one hundred clinical trials involving more than two thousand patients. Nevertheless, there was a report of success in using gene therapy to cause the growth of new blood vessels around blocked blood vessels. This use of gene therapy—in which genes are added to cells not to replace a faulty gene product but to cause the production of a substance such as a growth factor in a selected location—greatly increases the possible applications beyond the correction of inherited genetic disorders.

Initially, it was thought that gene therapy would first be used to cure a number of disorders caused by defects in a single gene. By 1990, candidates for the earliest gene therapies included beta-thalassemias, severe combined immunodeficiency syndrome (SCID), hemophilia types A and B, familial hypercholesterolemia, inherited emphysema, cystic fibrosis, Duchenne muscular dystrophy, and lysosomal storage disease. By 1995, gene therapies for most of these diseases were in clinical trials, but without any clear successes. By then, however, added to this list of disorders in clinical trials were a number in which treatment was aimed not at correcting a single gene but at delivering a gene product to a specific site. Among these were gene therapies for rheumatoid arthritis, AIDS, and cancer. By 1997, about 50 percent of all gene therapy research was focused on cancer, with the next largest group of studies, about 10 percent, focused on AIDS.

The first authorized human gene therapy was performed on a four-year-old girl, Ashanti DeSilva, who had adenosine deaminase (ADA) deficiency. Without treatment, this genetic deficiency leads to a fatal malfunctioning of the immune system. In 1990, a correct version of the ADA gene packaged in a retroviral vector was delivered by injection to the young girl. Several other young patients were treated afterward, but DeSilva was the only patient to show marked improvement in her condition. In all cases, however, the more traditional treatment, in which a synthetic version of ADA is administered in the form of PEG-ADA, was continued, indicating that the gene therapy did not cure the condition completely.

Cystic fibrosis is another disease that has been thought to be potentially curable through gene therapy. Several characteristics make it a promising candidate. Since correcting the gene CFTR in as few as 6 percent of the cells of an affected organ can produce normal function, not all cells would need to incorporate a functional gene. Also, the cells in most critical need of correction are those lining the airways of the lungs, cells that are easily accessible for in vivo treatment. Most trials have involved using an adenovirus as a vector to carry the CFTR gene, since these viruses normally infect human airways—they are the viruses that produce the common cold. The engineered viruses carrying the CFTR gene are delivered through an aerosol spray. Although patients show partially corrected chloride ion transport, the effect is short lived because most of the cells incorporating the corrected gene are short lived. Consequently, the gene therapy must be repeated every few months, but this method soon becomes ineffectual. Because the adenovirus stimulates an immune response, with repeated treatment the patient's immune system soon destroys the viral vector. Therefore, nonviral vectors are being tried in order to avoid an immune response.

A number of gene therapies that have entered clinical trials have been aimed at cancer. Among these are therapies designed to make tumor cells incorporate genes for substances such as interleukin-2 that will stimulate or augment an immune system attack against the cancer. In other approaches, genes dubbed "suicide" genes, which cause cell death, are being incorporated into tumor cells. Other trials have been aimed at trying to correct the genes that have caused the cells to become cancerous. An alternative approach has been to introduce the multidrug resistance (MDR) gene into normal bone marrow cells in order to increase their resistance to the toxic effects of the chemotherapy used to kill cancer cells.

Quite a different use of gene therapy has been to insert genes into highly accessible cells, such as muscle or skin fibroblasts, to turn them into protein factories for particular components that normally would be produced elsewhere—for example, to produce clotting factors, normally produced in the liver, that are missing in hemophiliacs.

PERSPECTIVE AND PROSPECTS

Before clear successes in gene therapy can be anticipated, gene delivery methods must be improved to

In the News: Benefits and Risks of Gene Therapy

Gene therapy trials in the United States have come under scrutiny since 1999, when the Food and Drug Administration terminated a clinical trial after the death of a teenage participant. Some institutions suspended their gene therapy trials while further research of the techniques and discussion of patients' rights was conducted. In contrast to this dire news in the United States, physicians in France announced in 2000 that two babies who underwent gene therapy for severe combined immunodeficiency syndrome (SCID) have have shown no signs of disease for over one year, and a third child has been disease-free for four months following gene therapy. This was the first clear-cut report of any benefit of gene therapy persisting for a significant length of time.

On the basic research front, a common challenge in gene therapy may soon be solved. Viruses are typically used to deliver genes to cells because they integrate their genetic material (and the gene of interest) directly into chromosomes. However, viruses are expensive to prepare and store, they sometimes cause an undesired immune response in a patient, and the most promising gene therapy viruses are not capable of carrying the large genes needed to treat diseases such as cystic fibrosis and muscular dystrophy. Stanford University researchers are using transposons, naturally occurring mobile DNA elements, to package genes and insert them into chromosomes. Studies have shown 5-6 percent of hemophiliac mice greatly improved after gene therapy via the transposon method. While this research is a long way from use in humans, any method that does not use a virus is a welcome innovation to the gene therapy community.

—*Karen E. Kalumuck, Ph.D.*

reach more of the target cells, precise control over expression of the delivered gene must be acquired to ensure adequate amounts of product, and methods for "targeted" gene insertion must be developed, whereby a faulty gene is replaced exactly by a correct copy of the gene. Until this fine control can be achieved, the best candidate genes for gene therapy are those whose products do not need to be tightly controlled.

Although major successes in gene therapy are yet to occur, the field is rapidly expanding, encompassing new areas that bring renewed optimism. One of these areas involves the use of antisense oligonucleotides (antisense RNA and DNA). These molecules, which can be made to bind to specific mRNAs, preventing their translation into protein, are being developed to block the production of certain deleterious proteins. They are being tested in clinical trials against diseases such as cancer and AIDS. Novel approaches such as these show promise in providing new weapons against disease.

—*Mary S. Tyler, Ph.D.*

See also Acquired immunodeficiency syndrome (AIDS); Cancer; Clinical trials; Cloning; Cystic fibrosis; DNA and RNA; Genetic diseases; Genetics and inheritance; Hemophilia; Human Genome Project; Mutation; Viral infections.

FOR FURTHER INFORMATION:

Bank, Arthur. "Human Somatic Cell Gene Therapy." *BioEssays* 18 (December, 1996): 999-1007. A sophisticated discussion of clinical trials in gene therapy, focusing primarily on cancer.

Clark, William R. *The New Healers: The Promise and Problems of Molecular Medicine in the Twenty-first Century.* New York: Oxford University Press, 1999. Clark's background as a teacher of immunology helps him initiate readers into the realm of molecular biology and gene therapy, the likely linchpin in eradicating most of the four thousand genetic disorders within the next fifty years.

Felgner, Philip L. "Nonviral Strategies for Gene Therapy." *Scientific American* 276 (June, 1997): 102-106. Explains how lipoplexes (DNA surrounded by lipids) rather than viruses could be used as a method of delivering genes.

Friedmann, Theodore. "Overcoming the Obstacles to Gene Therapy." *Scientific American* 276 (June, 1997): 96-101. Discusses in vivo and ex vivo methods of gene therapy and the advantages and disadvantages of different gene delivery systems.

Ho, Dora Y., and Robert M. Sapolsky. "Gene Therapy for the Nervous System." *Scientific American* 276 (June, 1997): 116-120. Predicts ways in which gene therapy might be used to combat neurological disorders such as Parkinson's disease and stroke.

Lyon, Jeff, and Peter Gorne. *Altered Fates, Gene Therapy, and the Retooling of Human Life.* New York: W. W. Norton, 1995. The story of gene therapy as told by two journalists who have covered the topic extensively in their work.

Old, R. W., and S. B. Primrose. *Principles of Gene Manipulation: An Introduction to Genetic Engineering.* Oxford, England: Blackwell Scientific, 1994. An in-depth but easy-to-understand explanation of modern techniques for manipulating and cloning genes.

U.S. House of Representatives. Hearing Before the Committee on Science, Space, and Technology. *Gene Therapy: Status, Prospects for the Future, and Government Policy Implications.* No. 168. Washington, D.C.: U.S. Government Printing Office, 1994. An in-depth report from scientists, ethicists, and physicians about gene therapy, as well as testimony concerning Ashanti DeSilva, one of the first recipients of gene therapy.

GENETIC COUNSELING
SPECIALTY

ANATOMY OR SYSTEM AFFECTED: Cells, reproductive system, uterus

SPECIALTIES AND RELATED FIELDS: Cytology, embryology, genetics, obstetrics, preventive medicine, psychology

DEFINITION: The scientific field that uses several biochemical and imaging techniques, as well as family histories, to provide information about genetic conditions or diseases in order to help individuals make medical and reproductive decisions.

KEY TERMS:

chromosomal abnormality: any change to the number, shape, or appearance of the forty-six chromosomes in each human cell; the presence of many such abnormalities will prevent the normal development of an individual and lead to a miscarriage

dominant genetic disease: a disease caused by a mutation in a gene that need be inherited from only one parent in order to exert its effect

genetic screening: a program designed to determine whether individuals are carriers of or are affected by a particular genetic disease

karyotype: a photograph of the chromosomes taken from the cells of an individual; a karyotype can be used to predict the sex of a fetus or the presence of a large chromosomal abnormality

mutation: an alteration in the DNA sequence of a gene that usually leads to the production of a nonfunctional enzyme or protein and, thus, a lack of a normal metabolic function; this defect may cause a medical condition called a genetic disease

recessive genetic disease: a disease caused by a mutation in a gene that must be inherited from both parents in order for an individual to show the symptoms of the disease; such a disease may show up only occasionally in a family history, especially if the mutation is rare

Science and Profession

Genetic counseling is a process of communicating to a couple the medical problems associated with the occurrence of an inherited disorder or birth defect in a family. Included in this process is a discussion of the prognosis and treatment of the problem. Specific reproductive options include abortion of an ongoing pregnancy, birth control or sterilization to prevent additional pregnancies, artificial insemination, the use of surrogate mothers, embryo transplantation, and adoption.

In all cases, the role of the counselor is to provide unbiased information and options to the couple seeking advice. The counselor must not only discuss the medical implications of a condition but also help to alleviate the emotional impact of positive diagnoses and, in particular, to assuage the guilt or denial that a diagnosis may elicit in parents.

The two major categories of medical problems covered by counselors are birth defects and genetic diseases. The first group includes Down syndrome and spina bifida, while the latter includes hemophilia, sickle-cell disease, and Tay-Sachs disease. Although the distinction between these two categories can sometimes blur, the key difference involves the clear pattern of inheritance shown by the genetic diseases.

Humans have between thirty thousand and thirty-five thousand genes. Genes are segments of deoxyribonucleic acid (DNA) that are arranged in linear fashion along the forty-six chromosomes. Most genes contain the information necessary for the cells to produce a specific protein, which often is involved in controlling some critical physiological function. For example, the beta globin gene produces a protein

called beta globin that makes up half of the hemoglobin that carries oxygen in the red blood cells.

A genetic disease can occur when the DNA changes in structure. Such a change is also known as a mutation. A mutation can lead to the production of a defective protein that cannot carry out its normal function, thus causing a physiological defect. In the case of beta globin, changing only one of the 106 molecules that make up this protein leads to a form of hemoglobin that can produce nonfunctional protein aggregates in red blood cells. These aggregates can cause the red blood cells to collapse and take on a sickle shape. Such cells lose their function, and the tissues are starved for oxygen—a condition known as anemia. This defect, which is called sickle-cell diseasea, is a fatal, heritable disease. As with all genetic disease, such mutations are relatively rare. Certain diseases may, however, be more prevalent within certain ethnic groups; for example, African Americans have a high incidence of sickle-cell disease, and Ashkenazic Jews have a high incidence of Tay-Sachs disease.

Humans have two of each kind of chromosome; one set of twenty-three is inherited from the mother, and the other set of twenty-three is inherited from the father. Thus, each person has two copies of each gene, one located on a maternal chromosome, the other on a paternal one. Many types of defects, such as sickle-cell disease, require that both genes have mutations in order for the disease to have an effect. Individuals who have one normal gene and one with a mutation are normal but carry the disease; they can pass the mutation on to the next generation in their eggs and sperm. This type of disease is called a recessive genetic disease. The only way a child can have sickle-cell disease is if both parents are carriers, since it is unlikely that a person affected by the disease will live long enough to have children.

Since it is equally likely for each parent to pass on the normal gene in eggs or sperm as to pass on the mutation, the laws of probability predict that, on the average, one-fourth of such a couple's offspring should have the disease. One of the major tasks of a genetic counselor is to advise couples of these probabilities if the diagnoses and family histories suggest that they are carriers. Since the laws of genetics involve random occurrences, however, it is possible that in a family with three or four children, all the children will be normal, or that in another family, all the children will have the disease. This degree of uncertainty produces stress and anxiety in couples who seek counseling only to hear that they indeed are at risk. Discussing concepts that involve sophisticated genetic or biochemical themes or issues of probable risk with couples untrained in scientific thinking is difficult, especially considering the highly emotional atmosphere of such discussions.

Other diseases, such as Huntington's chorea, also known as Woody Guthrie's disease for the folksinger who was afflicted by it, are caused by a dominant mutation. A mutation is dominant when an individual needs to inherit only one copy of the mutation in order to have the disease. Unlike recessive diseases that can disappear from a family for generations, a dominant mutation can be inherited only from a person who has the disease. In most cases, such a person has one normal gene and one with the mutation, which means that there is a 50 percent chance that the gene will be passed on. Huntington's chorea is a particularly insidious genetic disease, because the symptoms usually begin to show only in middle age, often after child-bearing decisions have been made. Thus, the children of an afflicted parent must decide whether they will marry and have children before they know whether they have inherited the mutation from their parents.

There are no cures for the permanent physiological defects that result from genetic disease. In some cases, the disease symptoms can be controlled by supplementing the protein that is lacking. Some forms of insulin-dependent diabetes and most cases of hemophilia can be treated in this way. In other cases, as with the disease phenylketonuria (PKU), special diets can prevent the severe neurological problems that inevitably lead to childhood death if the disease is left untreated.

DNA technology and genetic engineering offer potential cures for some diseases in which the primary defect caused by the mutation is well understood. Gene therapy is a process by which an additional copy of a normal gene is inserted into the cells of an affected individual or the defective gene is replaced by a normal one. Successful experiments with animals have given scientists confidence that these techniques will provide cures for many genetic diseases. These same DNA technologies are making better diagnosis possible and, as in the case of cystic fibrosis, are helping to extend the lives and enhance the quality of life of individuals afflicted with incurable diseases.

One of the more controversial aspects of genetic counseling is the procedure of screening. In this procedure, individuals suspected to be at risk are tested for the presence of a mutation. Screening can let people know whether they have a disease as well as whether they are carriers of the disease and therefore can pass the disease on to their children. Screening can be extended to all individuals, regardless of family or ethnic history. For example, in the United States, most states require that all newborn infants undergo a PKU test. This simple test involves taking a small sample of blood by pricking the heel of the baby. Although the costs of this screening are not insignificant, the benefit is that those infants found to have the disease can be treated immediately by being placed on a special diet so as to avoid the debilitating effects of the disease.

Other screening procedures are targeted at specific groups. The screening program for Tay-Sachs disease focuses on ethnic Jewish populations. This successful, voluntary program has reduced the incidence of Tay-Sachs disease significantly in the United States. The key to the success of the program was the money spent to educate the targeted group. In addition, key members of the population played a leading role in designing the overall program. Because of the much larger size of the potential group at risk, similar efforts to screen African American populations for sickle-cell disease have been much less successful. Ethical concerns about the motivations behind government-sponsored or government-encouraged screening of minority populations make these programs difficult to implement. In addition, in mandatory programs, concerns about confidentiality and information release become major obstacles.

Diagnostic and Treatment Techniques

Genetic counseling usually begins when a couple or an individual seeks the advice of a family physician or obstetrician regarding the medical risks associated with having a child. Motivating this request may be a previous birth of a child with a defect, a general uneasiness on the part of a couple worried about environmental exposure to potentially harmful agents, a family history of genetic disease, or advanced maternal age (which can be a factor in certain chromosomal abnormalities). Often, the family is referred to a genetic counseling clinic where most of the actual diagnosis and counseling will occur.

Arriving at a proper diagnosis for any obvious condition, as well as giving advice about potential risks, involves obtaining as much family history as possible with respect to the trait, as well as diagnostic information from the couple. If pregnant already, the woman may undergo a prenatal diagnostic procedure that could include ultrasound, blood tests, amniocentesis, and chorionic villus sampling.

Ultrasound is a technique that uses sound waves to visualize the exterior of the developing fetus. This widely used procedure is almost routine in many large urban hospitals. Ultrasound can be used to detect the presence of twins as well as of some profound birth defects such as hydrocephalus (water on the brain) or spina bifida. The latter defect, which involves the failure of the neural tube to close properly during development, leads to weakness, paralysis, and lack of function in lower body areas. The severity of the defect is hard to predict, and, unlike genetic disease, the incidence of recurrence is no higher than normal for subsequent children.

Supplementing ultrasound in the detection of spina bifida is a simple blood test that looks for a protein that the fetus spills into the amniotic fluid in higher quantities if the neural tube fails to close properly. The protein, which is called alpha-fetoprotein, crosses the placenta to circulate in the mother's blood. The amount of this normal protein in the mother's blood correlates with the developmental age of the fetus; therefore, an abnormal level might indicate a problem. Older-than-calculated fetuses and twins can both cause increased levels of alpha-fetoprotein, so care must be taken in this diagnosis. If abnormally high levels of the protein are found, amniocentesis would then be used to measure the protein level in the amniotic fluid, thus increasing the reliability of the diagnosis. In amniocentesis, a few teaspoonfuls of amniotic fluid are removed from the sac that surrounds and protects the developing fetus. Ultrasound is used to visualize the exterior of the fetus to allow the safe removal of this fluid, which contains some fetal cells. Biochemical tests can be performed directly on the fluid and results obtained quickly. Tay-Sachs disease is an example of a genetic disease that can be detected in this fashion, since fetuses with the disease fail to make an enzyme that their normal counterparts do make.

Many techniques, however, require obtaining large numbers of fetal cells and/or DNA. In these cases, the cells must be cultured for one to two weeks in a laboratory in order to get enough material to test. The delay between taking the sample and discussing the results with the clients is a source of stress and anxiety for parents undergoing counseling.

Preparing a karyotype, a photograph showing the numbers and sizes of the chromosomes of the fetus, is a commonly performed procedure following amniocentesis. Normal fetuses contain forty-six chromosomes, and any change in chromosome number, shape, or size can be detected by a skilled clinician. A large percentage of miscarriages involve fetuses with chromosomal abnormalities, so this diagnosis can be critical. A relatively common type of birth defect that can be diagnosed with a karyotype is Down syndrome. Most children born with Down syndrome have forty-seven chromosomes instead of forty-six; thus, this diagnosis is very accurate. In addition, the sex of the fetus can be determined from a karyotype, since male fetuses have an X and a Y chromosome while females have two X chromosomes. This information can be valuable to couples who are at risk for carrying a sex-linked genetic disease such as hemophilia, which could not affect any female offspring. Such information could potentially be used inappropriately for sexual selection of offspring, however, and the counselor must provide this information cautiously.

Amniocentesis is usually performed in the sixteenth week of pregnancy to allow the fetus to grow to a size at which the removal of a small amount of amniotic fluid would not be harmful. Although there is little risk to mother or fetus in this procedure, the delay associated with laboratory culturing means that results are often known in the eighteenth week of pregnancy or even later. At this stage, abortion becomes a more traumatic medical procedure. Chorionic villus sampling, on the other hand, can actually sample small amounts of fetal tissue directly. Since the procedure can safely obtain enough tissue to diagnose most problems and can be performed as early as the ninth or tenth week of pregnancy, abortion becomes a medically less traumatic option.

DNA technology provides the counselor with a battery of new diagnostic procedures that can look directly for the presence of a mutation in the DNA of the fetus. These tests can be performed on parents who are worried about being carriers for a particular disease or can be used on DNA obtained from fetal cells grown in a laboratory. Such tests have very high reliability and can give information about diseases such as sickle-cell disease, Huntington's chorea, muscular dystrophy, and cystic fibrosis.

The counselor's task is to take the diagnostic results and interpret them in the context of the medical history and particular family situation. The counselor must point out the options available, both for further diagnosis to confirm or rebut less-sensitive preliminary tests and to discuss potential medical interventions such as the special diets available for children born with PKU. In cases in which no medical intervention is possible, the severity of the problem should be discussed honestly so that the parents can choose either to continue or to abort the pregnancy. Other options, including adoption, artificial insemination, and embryo transplants, can also be evaluated. Finally, the risk of recurrence of the problem in future pregnancies should be discussed.

Counselors need to realize that their clients are often in emotionally fragile states. They must guard against using bias or interjecting their own personal beliefs or values when counseling their clients. Full disclosure of information, both verbally and in a carefully written report, is usually provided.

Compounding the tasks of the counselor is the fact that, in many cases, exact diagnoses are not yet possible. Sometimes, only the relative risks associated with another pregnancy can be determined. Different couples will perceive risks very differently depending on their own religious and moral backgrounds, as well as on the expected severity of the defect. In the case of a genetic disease such as Tay-Sachs, which is 100 percent fatal and requires extensive hospitalization of the child, a modest risk may be considered unacceptable, while in the case of a birth defect such as Down syndrome, whose severity cannot be predicted, and in which case the child may lead a long and rich life, a modest risk may be considered quite differently.

PERSPECTIVE AND PROSPECTS

The need for centers specializing in genetic counseling arose when it became clear that certain diseases and birth defects had a hereditary component. Many families request the services of counselors from these centers, and the centers are also involved in both voluntary and mandatory screening programs. In the United States, about 4 percent of all newborns suffer from a defect that is recognized either at birth or shortly thereafter. This group includes 0.5 percent who have a chromosomal abnormality that results in an obvious medical problem, 0.5 to 1 percent who have classical genetic diseases, and 2 percent who

suffer from a birth defect that may have a heritable component. Estimates vary, but more than one-third of all children in pediatric hospitals are there because of some association with a genetic disease.

Physicians have always served as counselors to families, but the rapid advances made in genetics and molecular science during the second half of the twentieth century have clearly surpassed the abilities of most physicians to keep current with treatments and diagnoses. The first formal clinic for genetic counseling was established at the University of Michigan in the 1940's. Most clinics specializing in this field were based at large medical centers; first in major metropolitan areas, and later in smaller population centers.

Genetic counseling clinics usually employ a range of specialists, including clinicians, geneticists, laboratory personnel for performing diagnostic testing, and public health and social workers. In 1969, Sarah Lawrence College instituted a master's-level program in genetic counseling to train candidates formally in the scientific, medical, and counseling skills required for this profession. Since that time, many other programs have been established in the United States. Today, most large counseling programs at medical centers use these specially trained personnel. In rural areas, however, family physicians are still a primary source of counseling; thus, genetic training is an important component of basic medical education.

The sophisticated medical diagnostic tools described above allow a counselor to provide abundant information to couples requesting counseling, but the power of DNA technology has expanded and will continue to expand the scope of current practice. Soon, counselors will not have to give advice in terms of probabilities and likelihoods of risk; molecular detection techniques will make possible the absolute identification of not only individuals with a disease but also related carriers.

As these DNA tools become more widely available, counseling will become a more integral part of preventive medicine. A DNA diagnostic procedure for a heritable form of breast cancer is available that allows women who have the mutation to monitor their health closely in order to receive prompt, lifesaving medical intervention. An important ethical issue here is that some women who have been diagnosed as having the mutation are undergoing preventive mastectomies without having developed any growths in order to ensure that they will not develop cancer. This radical therapy carries with it considerable emotional stress and should be undertaken only after consultation with a physician. As DNA-based diagnostic procedures, perhaps coupled with mandatory screening, become more commonplace, concerns about the release of this information to potential employers or health insurers will become more critical.

—*Joseph G. Pelliccia, Ph.D.*

See also Abortion; Amniocentesis; Birth defects; Blood testing; Chorionic villus sampling; DNA and RNA; Down syndrome; Ethics; Gene therapy; Genetic diseases; Genetic engineering; Genetics and inheritance; Hemophilia; Laboratory tests; Mutation; Phenylketonuria (PKU); Screening; Sickle-cell disease; Spina bifida; Tay-Sachs disease; Ultrasonography.

For Further Information:

Filkins, Karen, and Joseph F. Russo, eds. *Human Prenatal Diagnosis*. Rev. 2d ed. New York: Marcel Dekker, 1990. An advanced sourcebook that describes the procedures of prenatal diagnosis in great detail. Contains information on risk, reliability, cost, and so forth.

Harper, Peter S. *Practical Genetic Counselling*. 5th ed. London: Wright, 1998. A good overview of all aspects of genetic counseling, including a discussion of the types of diagnoses, treatments, risks, and emotional strains associated with counseling. Also gives a history of counseling as a discipline.

Mange, Arthur P., and Elaine J. Mange. *Genetics: Human Aspects*. 2d ed. Sunderland, Mass.: Sinauer Associates, 1990. An excellent advanced high school or college text that introduces most of the concepts relevant to genetic counseling, from basic theory to practical applications.

Pierce, Benjamin A. *The Family Genetic Sourcebook*. New York: John Wiley & Sons, 1990. Good background reading on genetics and genetic diseases. The book gives short, clear descriptions of a number of genetic diseases, along with their diagnosis and treatment.

U.S. Congress. Office of Technology Assessment. *Genetic Counseling and Cystic Fibrosis Carrier Screening: Results of a Survey-Background Paper*. Washington, D.C.: Government Printing Office, 1992. Genetic screening is a controversial subject. This source discusses the problems and successes associated with one such effort.

Genetic diseases

Disease/disorder

Anatomy or system affected: All

Specialties and related fields: Embryology, genetics, internal medicine, neonatology, obstetrics, pediatrics

Definition: A variety of disorders transmitted from parent to child through chromosomal material; most people experience disease related to genetics in some form, and research into this area is yielding greater understanding of the relationship between disease and hereditary proclivities toward disease, as well as new strategies for early detection and prevention or therapy.

Key terms:

autosomal recessive disease: a disease which is only expressed when two copies of a defective gene are inherited, one from each parent; present on non-sex-determining chromosomes

chromosomes: rod-shaped structures in each cell which contain genes, the chemical elements that determine traits

deoxyribonucleic acid (DNA): the chemical molecule that transmits hereditary information from generation to generation

dominant gene: a gene which can express its effect when an individual has only one copy of it

gene: the hereditary unit, composed of DNA, that resides on chromosomes

inheritance: the passing down of traits from generation to generation

X-linked: a term used to describe genes or traits that are located on the X chromosome; a male needs only one copy of an X-linked gene for it to be expressed

Causes and Symptoms

Hereditary units called genes determine the majority of the physical and biochemical characteristics of an organism. Genes are composed of a chemical compound called deoxyribonucleic acid (DNA) and are organized into rod-shaped structures called chromosomes that reside in each cell of the body. Each human cell carries forty-six chromosomes organized as twenty-three pairs, each composed of several thousand genes. Twenty-two of the chromosome pairs are homologous pairs; that is, similar genes are located at similar sites on each chromosome. The remaining chromosomes are the sex chromosomes. Human females bear two X chromosomes,

Human Chromosomes

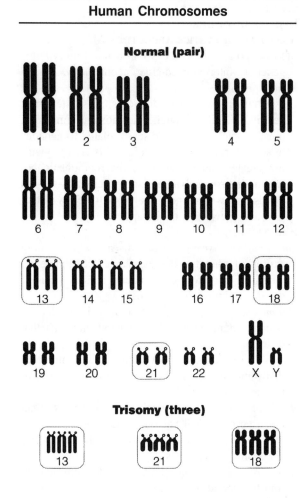

Normal (pair)

Trisomy (three)

Genetic diseases are caused by defects in the number of chromosomes, in their structure, or in the genes on the chromosome (mutation). Shown here is the human complement of chromosomes (23 pairs) and three errors of chromosome number (trisomies) that lead to the genetic disorders Patau's syndrome (trisomy no. 13), Edward's syndrome (trisomy no. 18), and the more common Down syndrome (trisomy no. 21).

and human males possess one X and one Y chromosome.

During the formation of the reproductive cells, the chromosome pairs separate and one copy of each pair is randomly included in the egg or sperm. Each egg will contain twenty-two autosomes (non-sex chromosomes) and one X chromosome. Each sperm will contain twenty-two autosomes and either one X or one Y chromosome. The egg and sperm fuse at fertilization, which restores the proper number of chromosomes, and the genes inherited from the baby's parents will determine its sex and much of its physical appearance and future health and well-being.

Genetic diseases are inherited as a result of the presence of abnormal genes in the reproductive cells of one or both parents of an affected individual. There are two broad classifications of genetic disease: those caused by defects in chromosome number or structure, and those resulting from a much smaller flaw within a gene. Within the latter category, there are four predominant mechanisms by which the disorders can be transmitted from generation to generation: autosomal dominant inheritance, in which the defective gene is inherited from one parent; autosomal recessive inheritance, in which one defective gene is inherited from each parent, who themselves show no signs of the disorder; X-linked chromosomal inheritance (often called sex-linked), in which the flawed gene has been determined to reside on the X chromosome; and multifactorial inheritance, in which genes interact with each other and/or environmental factors.

Errors in chromosome number include extra and missing chromosomes. The most common chromosomal defect observed in humans is Down syndrome, which is caused by the presence of three copies of chromosome 21, instead of the usual two. Down syndrome occurs at a frequency of about one in eight hundred live births, this frequency increasing with increasing maternal age. The symptoms of this disorder include mental retardation, short stature, and numerous other medical problems. The most common form of Down syndrome results from the failure of the two copies of chromosome 21 to separate during reproductive cell formation, which upon fusion with a normal reproductive cell at fertilization produces an embryo containing three copies of chromosome 21.

Gross defects in chromosome structure include duplicated and deleted portions of chromosomes and broken and rearranged chromosome fragments. Prader-Willi syndrome results from a deletion of a small portion of chromosome 15. Children affected with this disorder are mentally retarded, obese, and diabetic. Cri du chat (literally, cat cry) syndrome is associated with a large deletion in chromosome 5. Affected infants exhibit facial abnormalities, are severely retarded, and produce a high-pitched, kitten-like wail.

Genetic diseases caused by defects in individual genes result when defective genes are propagated through many generations or a new genetic flaw develops in a reproductive cell. New genetic defects arise from a variety of causes, including environmental assaults such as radiation, toxins, or drugs. More than four thousand such gene disorders have been identified.

Manifestation of an autosomal dominant disorder requires the inheritance of only one defective gene from one parent who is afflicted with the disease. Inheritance of two dominant defective genes, one from each parent, is possible but generally creates such severe consequences that the child dies while still in the womb or shortly after birth. An individual who bears one copy of the gene has a 50 percent chance of transmitting that gene and the disease to his or her offspring.

Among the most common autosomal dominant diseases are hyperlipidemia and hypercholesterolemia. Elevated levels of lipids and cholesterol in the blood, which contribute to artery and heart disease, are the consequences of these disorders, respectively. Onset of the symptoms is usually in adulthood, frequently after the affected individual has had children and potentially transmitted the faulty gene to them.

Huntington's chorea causes untreatable neurological deterioration and death, and symptoms do not appear until affected individuals are at least in their forties. Children of parents afflicted with Huntington's chorea may have already made reproductive decisions without the knowledge that they might carry the defective gene; they risk a 50 percent chance of transmitting the dread disease to their offspring.

Autosomal recessive genetic diseases require that an affected individual bear two copies of a defective gene, inheriting one from each parent. Usually the parents are simply carriers of the defective gene; their one normal copy masks the effect of the one flawed copy. If two carriers have offspring, 25 percent will receive two copies of the flawed gene and inherit the disease, and 50 percent will be asymptomatic carriers.

Cystic fibrosis is an autosomal recessive disease which occurs at a rate of about one in two thousand live births among Caucasians. The defective gene product causes improper chloride transport in cells and results in thick mucous secretions in lungs and other organs. Sickle-cell disease, another autosomal recessive disorder, is the most common genetic dis-

ease among African Americans in the United States. Abnormality in the protein hemoglobin, the component of red blood cells that carries oxygen to all the body's tissues, leads to deformed blood cells that are fragile and easily destroyed.

X-linked genetic diseases are transmitted by faulty genes located on the X chromosome. Females need two copies of the defective gene to acquire such a disease, and in general women carry only one flawed copy, making them asymptomatic carriers of the disorder. Males, having only a single X chromosome, need only one copy of the defective gene to express an X-linked disease. Males with X-linked disorders inherit the defective gene from their mothers, since fathers must contribute a Y chromosome to male offspring. Half of the male offspring of a carrier female will inherit the defective gene and develop the disease. In the rare case of a female with two defective X-linked genes, 100 percent of her male offspring will inherit the disease gene, and, assuming that the father does not carry the defective gene, 50 percent of her female offspring will be carriers. There are more than 250 X-linked disorders, some of the more common being Duchenne's muscular dystrophy, which results in progressive muscle deterioration and early death; hemophilia; and red-green color blindness, which affects about 8 percent of Caucasian males.

Multifactorial inheritance, which accounts for a number of genetic diseases, is caused by the complex interaction of one or more genes with each other and with environmental factors. This group of diseases includes many disorders which, anecdotally, "run in families." Representative disorders include cleft palate, spina bifida, anencephaly, and some inherited heart abnormalities. Other diseases appear to have a genetic component predisposing an individual to be susceptible to environmental stimuli that trigger the disease. These include cancer, hypertension, diabetes, schizophrenia, alcoholism, depression, and obesity.

DIAGNOSIS AND DETECTION

Most, but not all, genetic diseases manifest their symptoms immediately or soon after the birth of an affected child. Rapid recognition of such a medical condition and its accurate diagnosis are essential for the proper treatment and management of the disease by parents and medical personnel. Medical technology has developed swift and accurate diagnostic methods, in many cases allowing testing of the fetus prior to birth. In addition, tests are available that determine the carrier status of an individual for many autosomal recessive and X-linked diseases. These test results are used in conjunction with genetic counseling of individuals and couples who are at risk of transmitting a genetic disease to their offspring. Thus, such individuals can make informed decisions when planning their reproductive futures.

Errors in chromosome number and structure are detected in an individual by analyzing his or her chromosomes. A small piece of skin or a blood sample is taken, the cells in the sample are grown to a sufficient number, and the chromosomes within each cell are stained with special dyes so that they may be viewed with a microscope. A picture of the chromosomes, called a karyotype, is taken, and the patient's chromosome array is compared with that of a normal individual. Extra or missing chromosomes or alterations in chromosome structure are determined, thus identifying the genetic disease. The analysis of karyotypes is the method used to determine the presence of Down, Prader-Willi, and cri du chat syndromes, among others.

Defects in chromosome number and structure can also be identified in the fetus, prior to birth, using two different sample collecting methods: amniocentesis and chorionic villus sampling. In amniocentesis, a needle is inserted through the pregnant woman's abdomen and uterus, into the fluid-filled sac surrounding the fetus. A sample of this fluid, the amniotic fluid, is withdrawn. The amniotic fluid contains fetal cells sloughed off by the fetus. The cells are grown for several weeks until there are enough to perform chromosome analysis. This procedure is performed only after sixteen weeks' gestation, in order to ensure adequate amniotic fluid for sampling.

Chorionic villus sampling relies on a biopsy of the fetal chorion, a membrane surrounding the fetus which is composed of cells that have the same genetic constitution as the fetus. A catheter is inserted through the pregnant woman's vagina and into the uterus until it is in contact with the chorion. The small sample of this tissue that is removed contains enough cells to perform karyotyping immediately, permitting diagnosis by the next day. Chorionic villus sampling can be performed between the eighth and ninth week of pregnancy. This earlier testing gives the procedure an advantage over amniocentesis, since the earlier determination of whether a fetus is carrying a genetic disease allows safer pregnancy termination if the parents choose this course.

Karyotype analysis is limited to the diagnosis of genetic diseases caused by very large chromosome abnormalities. The majority of hereditary disorders are caused by gene flaws that are too small to see microscopically. For many of these diseases, diagnosis is available through either biochemical testing or DNA analysis.

Many genetic disorders cause a lack of a specific biochemical which is necessary for normal metabolism. These types of disorders are frequently referred to as "inborn errors of metabolism." Many of these errors can be detected by the chemical analysis of fetal tissue. For example, galactosemia is a disease which results from the lack of galactose-1-phosphate uridyl transferase. Infants with this disorder cannot break down galactose, one of the major sugars in milk. If left untreated, galactosemia can lead to mental retardation, cataracts, kidney and liver failure, and death. By analyzing fetal cells obtained from amniocentesis or chorionic villus sampling, the level of this important chemical can be assessed, and, if necessary, the infant can be placed on a galactose-free diet immediately after birth.

DNA analysis can be used to determine whether a genetic disease has been inherited when the chromosomal location of the gene is known, when the chemical sequence of the DNA is known, and/or when particular DNA sequences commonly associated with the gene in question, called markers, are known.

A sequence of four chemical elements of DNA—adenine (A), guanine (G), thymine (T), and cytosine (C)—make up genes. Sometimes the proper DNA sequence of a gene is known, as well as the changes in the sequence that cause disease. Direct analysis of the DNA of the individual suspected of carrying a certain genetic disorder is possible in these cases. For example, in sickle-cell disease, it is known that a change in a single DNA chemical element leads to the disorder. To test for this disease, a tissue sample is obtained from prenatal sources (amniocentesis or chorionic villus sampling). The DNA is isolated from the cells and analyzed with highly specific probes that can detect the presence of the defective gene which will lead to sickle-cell disease. Informed action may be taken regarding the future of the fetus or the care of an affected child.

Occasionally a disease gene itself has not been precisely isolated and its DNA sequence determined, but sequences very near the gene of interest have been analyzed. If specific variations within these neighboring sequences are always present when the gene of interest is flawed, these nearby sequences can then be used as a marker for the presence of the defective gene. When the variant sequences, called restriction fragment length polymorphisms, are present, so is the disease gene. Prenatal testing for cystic fibrosis has been done using restriction fragment length polymorphisms.

Individuals who come from families in which genetic diseases tend to occur can be tested as carriers.

In this way, they will know the risk of passing a certain disease to offspring. For example, individuals whose families have a history of cystic fibrosis, but who themselves are not affected, may be asymptomatic carriers. If they have children with individuals who are also cystic fibrosis carriers, they have a 25 percent chance of passing two copies of the defective gene to their offspring. DNA samples from the potential parents can be analyzed for the presence of one defective gene. If both partners are carriers, their de-

In the News: Finding Genes and Genetic Diseases

The Human Genome Project has had, and will continue to have, a tremendous impact on the study of genetic diseases. New disease genes were being discovered at a dizzying rate during the year 2000, and as data from the Human Genome Project continues to be analyzed, every year should see a quickening of the pace.

Researchers at the Howard Hughes Medical Institute have discovered a genetic defect that causes increased susceptibility to Type II diabetes. Small genetic variations in the gene for a protein-snipping enzyme called calpain-10 are the culprit. Interestingly, the mutations are not found in the actual coding regions of the gene but rather in the noncoding introns.

Genetic defects that cause cancer susceptibility are already well known, and many have been identified that increase the risk of developing breast and colon cancer. Researchers at the Mayo Clinic have added yet one more defect to the list for colon cancer with the discovery of mutations in the AXIN2 gene. Mutations in this gene result in defective mismatch repair, an important DNA repair system, which leads to increased mutation rates in other genes.

Some important advances have also been made in detecting genetic defects. A new technique for early detection of Down syndrome, one of the most common birth defects, has been developed through a collaborative effort by public and private researchers. The technique involves an ultrasound examination and a simple blood test for two chemicals, free Beta hCG and PAPP-A. The results of the tests are submitted to a special mathematical analysis that assigns risk. High-risk cases are of-

fered additional tests, such as chorionic villus sampling or amniocentesis. A study published in the August, 2000, issue of *Obstetrics and Gynecology* found that 91 percent of the women carrying a baby with Down syndrome were in the high-risk group. The new test will be marketed as UltraScreen by GeneCare Medical Genetics Center, Chapel Hill, North Carolina, and NTD Laboratories, Huntington Station, New York.

Two independent groups of researchers have developed new genetic screening tests that greatly improve accuracy, especially in cases where a person is only carrying one copy of the faulty gene, which has been a notoriously tricky screening problem. Bert Vogelstein and his colleagues at The Johns Hopkins University Oncology Center and the Howard Hughes Medical Institute have developed a much more accurate test for defective genes involved in colon cancer. The test involves culturing human cells and fusing them with a special line of mouse cells, thus isolating single human chromosomes. Based on the results from their work, the new test seems to be better than twice as sensitive as currently used methods. Albert de la Chapelle, director of the Human Cancer Genetics Program at Ohio State University's Comprehensive Cancer Center, reported on a very similar approach that holds promise for detecting cancer-causing gene defects. Additional applications of their procedure might hold promise for identifying women who are carriers of a single copy of X-linked genetic disease genes such as hemophilia and Duchenne muscular dystrophy, as well as many other similar genetic diseases.

—Bryan Ness, Ph.D.

cision about whether to have children will be made with knowledge of the possible risk to their offspring. If only one or neither of them is a carrier, their offspring will not be at risk of inheriting cystic fibrosis, an autosomal recessive disease. Carrier testing is possible for many genetic diseases, as well as for disorders which appear late in life, such as Huntington's chorea.

Many of the gene flaws of multifactorial diseases, those that interact with environmental factors to produce disease, have been identified and are testable. Individuals armed with the knowledge of having a gene which puts them at risk for certain disorders can incorporate preventive measures into their lifestyle, thus minimizing the chances of developing the disease. For example, certain cancers, such as colon and breast cancer, have a genetic component. Individuals who test positive for the genes that predispose them to develop cancer can modify their diets to include cancer-fighting foods and receive frequent medical checkups to detect cancer development at its earliest, most treatable stage. Those with genes that contribute to arteriosclerosis and heart disease can modify their diets and increase exercise, and those with a genetic predisposition for alcoholism could avoid the consumption of alcohol.

PERSPECTIVE AND PROSPECTS

The scientific study of human genetics and genetic disease is relatively new, having begun in the early twentieth century. There are many early historical records, however, which recognize that certain traits are hereditarily transmitted. Ancient Greek literature is peppered with references to heredity, and the Jewish book of religious and civil laws, the Talmud, describes in detail the inheritance pattern of hemophilia and its ramifications upon circumcision.

The Augustinian monk Gregor Mendel worked out many of the principles of heredity by manipulating the pollen and eggs of pea plants over many generations. His work was conducted from the 1860's to the 1870's but was unrecognized by the scientific community until 1900.

At about this time, many disorders were being recognized as genetic diseases. Pedigree analysis, a way to trace inheritance patterns through a family tree, was used since the mid-1800's to track the incidence of hemophilia in European royal families. This analysis indicated that the disease was transmitted through females (indeed, hemophilia is an X-linked disorder).

In the early 1900's, Sir Archibald Garrod, a British physician, recognized certain biochemical disorders as genetic diseases and proposed accurate mechanisms for their transmission.

In 1953, Francis Crick and James D. Watson discovered the structure of DNA; thus began studies on the molecular biology of genes. This research resulted in the monumental discovery in 1973 that pieces of DNA from animals and bacteria could be cut and spliced together into a functional molecule. This recombinant DNA technology fostered a revolution in genetic analysis, in which pieces of human DNA could be removed and put into bacteria. The bacteria then replicate millions of copies of the human DNA, permitting detailed analysis. These recombinant molecules also produced the human gene product, thereby facilitating the analysis of normal and aberrant genes.

The recombinant DNA revolution spawned the development of the DNA tests for genetic diseases and carrier status. Knowledge of what a normal gene product is and does is exceptionally helpful in the treatment of genetic diseases. For example, Duchenne's muscular dystrophy is known to be caused by the lack of a protein called dystrophin. This suggests that a possible treatment of the disease is to provide functional dystrophin to the affected individual. Ultimately, medical science seeks to treat genetic diseases by providing a functional copy of the flawed gene to the affected individual. While such gene therapy would not affect the reproductive cells—the introduced gene copy would not be passed down to future generations—the normal gene product would alleviate the genetic disorder.

—Karen E. Kalumuck, Ph.D.

See also Albinos; Alzheimer's disease; Amniocentesis; Attention-deficit disorder (ADD); Autoimmune disorders; Birth defects; Breast cancer; Breast disorders; Cerebral palsy; Chorionic villus sampling; Colon cancer; Color blindness; Congenital heart disease; Cystic fibrosis; Diabetes mellitus; DNA and RNA; Down syndrome; Dwarfism; Embryology; Environmental diseases; Fetal alcohol syndrome; Fragile X syndrome; Gene therapy; Genetic counseling; Genetic engineering; Genetics and inheritance; Gigantism; Hemophilia; Hydrocephalus; Human Genome Project; Immunodeficiency disorders; Klinefelter syndrome; Laboratory tests; Marfan syndrome; Mental retardation; Multiple sclerosis; Muscular dystrophy; Mutation; Neonatology; Neurofibromatosis;

Obstetrics; Oncology; Pediatrics; Phenylketonuria (PKU); Porphyria; Progeria; Screening; Sickle-cell disease; Spina bifida; Tay-Sachs disease; Thalassemia; Turner syndrome.

FOR FURTHER INFORMATION:

Bellenir, Karen, ed. *Genetic Disorders Sourcebook: Basic Information About Heritable Diseases and Disorders Such as Down Syndrome, PKU, Hemophilia, and Von Willebrandt Diseases*. New York: Omnigraphics, 1996. This nontechnical sourcebook offers basic information about lifestyle expectations, disease management techniques, and current research initiatives for the most common types of genetic disorders, including a resource list of three hundred genetic disorders and related topics.

Edlin, Gordon. *Human Genetics*. Boston: Jones and Bartlett, 1990. Presents excellent background on the principles of genetics and molecular biology for the nonscientist. This sound introduction is used to discuss human reproduction, heredity, and genetic disease in a clear, informative, and thorough style.

Gormley, Myra Vanderpool. *Family Diseases: Are You at Risk?* Reprint. Baltimore: Genealogical, 1998. The author, a certified genealogist and syndicated columnist, explores the relationship between family trees and genetic diseases. Written in popular language, this book gives instruction on how to assess a family's genetic risk, information on the latest scientific breakthroughs, and direction for obtaining further information.

Grant Cooper, Necia, ed. *The Human Genome Project: Deciphering the Blueprint of Heredity*. Mill Valley, Calif.: University Science Books, 1994. Written to be accessible to the general reader, this book provides a basic introduction to the ideas underlying classical and molecular genetics before going on to describe the purpose of the Human Genome Project.

Marshall, Elizabeth L. *The Human Genome Project: Cracking the Code Within Us*. New York: Franklin Watts, 1997. Describes the Human Genome Project and its process of gene mapping, including concerns of critics of the project. Suitable for grades eight through twelve. Includes an extensive glossary and a bibliography.

Maxon, Linda, and Charles Daugherty. *Genetics: A Human Perspective*. Dubuque, Iowa: Wm. C. Brown, 1992. This textbook, designed for persons with no science background, thoroughly covers the background information on cells and genetics needed for an informed understanding of human genetic disease.

Millunsky, Aubrey. *Choices, Not Chances*. Boston: Little, Brown, 1989. The author is an outstanding medical geneticist and pediatrician who has written this informative, nontechnical guide for those interested in genetic disease. Includes a broad discussion of particular diseases, genetic counseling, reproductive options, law, and ethics.

_____, ed. *Genetic Disorders of the Fetus: Diagnosis, Prevention, and Treatment*. Baltimore: The Johns Hopkins University Press, 1998. This source treats a number of issues, from fetal cells in the maternal circulation to ethical issues surrounding a misdiagnosis, in chapters written by experts in the field. Recommended for clinicians in training and scientists working on the laboratory side of prenatal genetic testing.

Pierce, Benjamin. *The Family Genetic Sourcebook*. New York: John Wiley & Sons, 1990. Pierce presents an excellent discussion of human inheritance patterns for the nonscientist and a catalog of more than one hundred genetic traits and diseases and their inheritance patterns.

Shaw, Michael, ed. *Everything You Need to Know About Diseases*. Springhouse, Pa.: Springhouse Press, 1996. This well-illustrated consumer reference, compiled by more than one hundred doctors and medical experts, describes five hundred illnesses and conditions, their causes, symptoms, diagnosis, treatment, and prevention. A valuable reference book for everyone interested in health and disease. Of particular interest is chapter 21, "Genetic Disorders."

Tropp, Burton E. *Biochemistry: Concepts and Applications*. Belmont, Calif.: West/Wadsworth, 1997. This book presents the basic concepts of biochemistry, including proteins and their functions, genetic information, and recombinant DNA technology. A good source for basic biochemical information.

Wingerson, Lois. *Mapping Our Genes*. New York: E. P. Dutton, 1990. Using an engaging narrative style and many anecdotal stories as illustrations, Wingerson provides an account of the history of scientific discoveries that have led to the human genome initiative, an effort to map the chromosomal location of all human genes.

GENETIC ENGINEERING

PROCEDURE

ANATOMY OR SYSTEM AFFECTED: Cells

SPECIALTIES AND RELATED FIELDS: Biochemistry, biotechnology, cytology, ethics, genetics, microbiology, pharmacology

DEFINITION: The use of recombinant DNA technology to create DNA carrying specific genes or parts of genes that can be transferred from one organism to another to alter an organism's genetic makeup.

KEY TERMS:

cloning: making many identical copies; the techniques genetic engineers use to recombine molecular fragments of deoxyribonucleic acid (DNA) from different sources and to reproduce those fragments in bacteria or other organisms

Escherichia coli: a common bacterium that inhabits the human intestinal tract; used by genetic engineers to carry and propagate cloned DNA fragments and to produce proteins from the cloned genes

gene: the specific sequence of nucleotides in a DNA molecule; a gene acts as a code to direct the synthesis of a specific protein

genetically modified organism (GMO): organism whose DNA has been modified by the introduction of foreign DNA by genetic engineering

recombinant DNA: the technology of joining or recombining DNA molecular fragments of different types or from different organisms; also, the fragments themselves

restriction endonuclease: an enzyme that responds to a specific, short sequence of nucleotides within a DNA molecule by binding to that sequence and breaking the DNA strands near the sequence

INDICATIONS AND PROCEDURES

The revolutionary potential of the biotechnology industry was first realized in 1973, when Stanley Cohen of Stanford University, Herbert Boyer of the University of California at San Francisco, and their coworkers introduced recombinant deoxyribonucleic

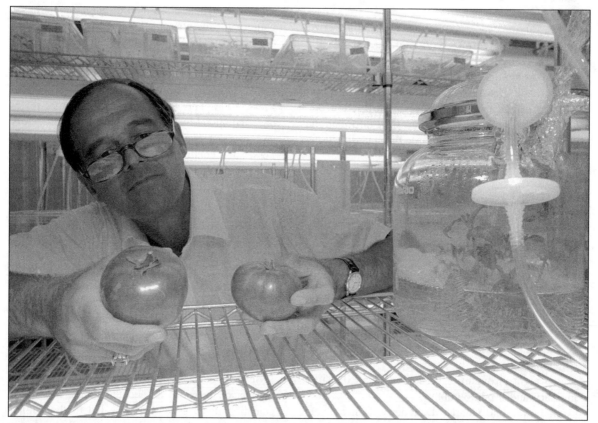

Controversy has surrounded the use of genetic engineering to alter food products. These tomatoes were designed to have a vine-ripened flavor and texture. (AP/Wide World Photos)

acid (DNA) technology to the world. They had isolated separate molecules of DNA, combined them into a single molecule in a test tube, and reinserted the molecule into the common bacterium *Escherichia coli* (*E. coli*). In 1974, Cohen and a coworker wrote in an article published in the *Proceedings of the National Academy of Sciences*:

> . . . the replication and expression of genes in *E. coli* that have been derived from a totally unrelated bacterial species (i.e., *Staphylococcus aureus*) now suggests that interspecies genetic recombination may be generally attainable. Thus, it may be practical to introduce into *E. coli* genes specifying metabolic or synthetic functions (e.g., photosynthesis, antibiotic production) indigenous to other biological classes.

As it turned out, it did become practical to introduce foreign genes into bacteria, and the biotechnology industry began to develop around the techniques of recombinant DNA and genetic engineering. In 1982, the first genetically engineered product was approved for use in humans. The human gene for insulin had been cloned into bacteria, and the bacteria were producing large amounts of the insulin protein, which then could be collected, packaged, and sold. The company producing insulin found an immediate market among diabetics, who had been relying on insulin from cattle and pigs to control their disease.

Genetic engineering relies foremost on the ability of the scientist to cut and rejoin DNA molecules and to increase the ability of bacteria to take up DNA from a culture solution. One type of enzyme that cuts a linear DNA molecule into fragments is called a restriction endonuclease or restriction enzyme. Restriction enzymes cut DNA into predictable, reproducible-sized fragments by cutting at specific nucleotide sequences.

DNA is a long, fibrous molecule composed of two intertwined chains. Each chain is composed of subunits called nucleotides. The four nucleotides—adenine (A), cytosine (C), guanine (G), and thymine (T)—are arranged in different combinations in a linear order much as words and sentences are composed of a specific linear order of the twenty-six subunits known as letters. Each nucleotide in a chain is held firmly to the adjacent nucleotide by covalent chemical bonds. The nucleotide sequence of the second chain is based on that of the first, and the chains are held intertwined together by relatively weak hydrogen chemical bonds. Adenine on one chain always lies across from and creates hydrogen bonds with thymine on the other chain (A-T), and cytosine always lies across from and bonds to guanine (C-G).

The specific sequences at which most restriction enzymes cut are palindromes. A palindrome is a sequence of nucleotides or letters that is the same when read both forward and backward. The palindrome recognized by the first restriction enzyme discovered, called EcoRI, is GAATTC. By itself, this sequence does not look like a palindrome, but consider the sequence of the other strand, following the A-T and C-G bonding rules stated above. The sequence of the opposite strand would be CTTAAG. The first strand reads in the forward direction the same as the second strand reads in the backward direction. This is a palindromic sequence of nucleotides. Other common restriction enzymes recognize sequences such as GGTACC (CCATGG on the other strand) and AAGCTT (TTCGAA).

Besides cutting DNA sequences at predictable locations, restriction enzymes have an additional useful property. The ends of the fragments left by many restriction enzymes are uneven. These uneven ends provide a means by which different fragments can easily be rejoined. For example, when the restriction enzyme EcoRI cuts a DNA molecule into two fragments, the GAATTC sequence on one strand would be left as G on the left fragment and as AATTC on the right fragment, while the other strand would be CTTAA on the left fragment and G on the right fragment. Therefore, any fragment left by EcoRI would have an overhang of AATT on one side and TTAA on the other side. If these overhanging ends from two fragments were to meet, the A-T bonding rule would allow the ends to overlap and bond together by the weak hydrogen bonds. In the parlance of genetic engineering, fragment ends such as these are known as "sticky ends." When sticky ends have met and bound, a second enzyme, ligase, will form the strong covalent bonds of the individual strands.

Recombinant DNA molecules made by combining fragments of DNA from different sources such as bacteria and humans rely on the fact that restriction enzymes leave the same type of ends on every fragment they generate. Therefore, fragments can be rejoined in almost any desirable combination by ligase. The types of DNA fragments that are commonly joined by genetic engineers include a DNA fragment containing a gene of interest, such as the human insu-

The Use of Genetic Engineering

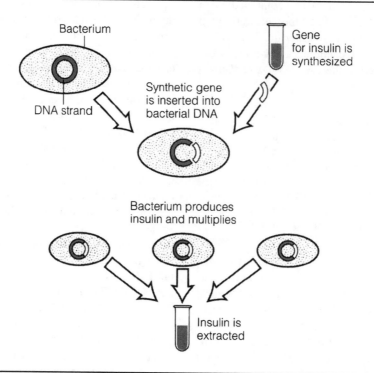

Bacterium

DNA strand

Gene for insulin is synthesized

Synthetic gene is inserted into bacterial DNA

Bacterium produces insulin and multiplies

Insulin is extracted

Genetic engineering, the manipulation of genetic material, can be used to synthesize large quantities of drugs or hormones, such as insulin.

lin gene, and a special DNA fragment which will allow that gene to propagate and be expressed in bacteria. Once the appropriate fragments are combined, the recombinant DNA molecule must be inserted into the bacteria.

Because inserting new genetic information into a bacterium will change or transform the genetic makeup of that bacterium, this procedure is called transformation. First, bacterial cells are grown in a broth and then concentrated into a pellet by centrifugation. The cells are then suspended in a solution containing the salt called calcium chloride. The DNA is also placed in a calcium chloride solution. The salt and DNA aggregate, and the mixture is put with the bacterial cells. By mechanisms that are not well understood, the DNA molecules find their way into the bacterial cells. The bacteria are once again grown in broth, and the inserted DNA is able to replicate. If the proper fragments are joined, then protein such as insulin is made by the bacteria using the genetic information contained within the nucleotide sequence of the inserted human DNA fragments.

The discovery of enzymes to cut, rejoin, and otherwise manipulate DNA has given the genetic engineer important tools to help study the structure and function of genes. Moreover, genetic engineers and biotechnologists have developed techniques using these enzymes to recombine genes contained on DNA molecules from organisms of different species and different kingdoms to manufacture valuable and medically useful products.

USES AND COMPLICATIONS

One of the greatest potential uses of genetic engineering technology is in the diagnosis and treatment of human disease. The first genetically engineered product, approved by the Food and Drug Administration in 1982, was marketed by the Eli Lilly company under the product name of Humulin—a human form of insulin for the treatment of diabetes mellitus.

It is estimated that as many as two hundred million people in the world suffer from diabetes. Diabetes is a disease that results in an overaccumulation of glucose, a sugar, in the blood. In normal individuals, the protein hormone called insulin is produced by the pancreas and used by the body to maintain appropriate blood glucose levels. Patients suffering from diabetes must take injections of insulin daily. The traditional source of this insulin has been beef and pork pancreas acquired from slaughterhouses, but there are problems associated with this source. The methods of extracting insulin can be tedious and costly and provide a relatively small amount of insulin from a large amount of animal tissue. Also, a common problem among diabetics is allergic reactions to impurities in the insulin preparation and resistance to the insulin itself. Genetic engineering has provided a way to obtain pure, human insulin in large quantities.

In normal human cells, an insulin precursor is synthesized as a single protein chain that is then split into two pieces, which remain held together by strong chemical bonds to create the active form of insulin. By using techniques similar to those described above, scientists engineer separate genes into bacteria to produce each of the two pieces that compose insulin. Each segment is purified from the bacteria and then combined chemically to form active insulin. Although the insulin is produced by bacteria, the genetic instructions used by those bacteria are human in origin, and the insulin protein is indistinguishable from insulin actually produced in human cells. While it takes more than 700 kilograms of animal pancreas to yield only 100 grams of insulin, these techniques allow the production of 100 grams of insulin from a single 2,000-liter culture of bacteria. Furthermore, a 2,000-liter culture is relatively small on an industrial scale, which can use huge vats for cultures as large as 100,000 liters.

Insulin is only one of many human proteins that are useful for medical purposes. Another example is a protein called erythropoietin that stimulates the production of red blood cells, or erythrocytes, the oxygen-carrying cells in the blood. A normal function of the kidneys is to help remove toxic substances from the body. Sufferers of kidney disease can undergo a treatment known as dialysis that substitutes for the kidneys' cleansing function. Dialysis is a much safer alternative for most patients than kidney transplantation. Because the kidneys also normally produce erythropoietin, however, patients with diseased kidneys often have a low number of red blood cells and suffer from severe anemia. Anemia can be alleviated with blood transfusions, but transfusions carry the risk of blood-borne diseases such as hepatitis and acquired

immunodeficiency syndrome (AIDS). Fortunately, genetically engineered erythropoietin is available to stimulate red blood cell production in kidney dialysis patients, providing a safe remedy for their anemia.

Transgenic livestock are used to produce biopharmaceuticals. Genes for useful pharmaceutical proteins can be produced in the milk of transgenic livestock. To do this, a cloned gene of a useful pharmaceutical protein is fused to the transcriptional promoter of a gene that is expressed in milk, such as b-lactoglobin. The DNA is then introduced into the animal. The gene is introduced into a fertilized egg by microinjection, and the egg is implanted into a female animal. Female offspring that develop are checked for the presence of the transgene and the expression of the recombinant protein in the milk of the animal. Although sheep and goats have been used, cows may be the preferred animals to use to produce biopharmaceuticals because they produce large quantities of milk (10,000 liters a year). The proteins, generally with the appropriate modifications, are relatively easily isolated from milk. TPA (tissue plasminogen activator), which is administered to heart attack victims to dissolve clots, and clotting factor VIII, the gene needed for efficient clotting of blood that is lacking in patients with hemophilia A, are two examples of biopharmaceutical drugs produced in the milk of transgenic animals.

Another medical use of genetic engineering involves the creation of safe and effective vaccines for viral diseases. The use of recombinant DNA technology has lead to the development of better vaccines. A conventional vaccine uses a killed or disarmed pathogen that is injected into an organism. The organism develops an immune response to the material injected and becomes resistant to the pathogen. Relatively rare side effects of conventional vaccines include an allergic reaction in some individuals receiving the vaccine and the possibility that a disarmed pathogen could become active and cause the disease. Recombinant DNA technology is used to produce vaccines that never contained the live pathogen. In such vaccines, only a protein of the pathogen (for example, the coat protein of a pathogenic virus) is used to stimulate the organism to develop immunity to the pathogen. DNA vaccines, in which only a small piece of the pathogen DNA is used to immunize an organism, are being developed.

In developing nations, millions still die from infectious diseases for which immunizations are nonexistent, unreliable, or too costly. The development of oral vaccines that do not need refrigeration should be a huge help in fighting infectious diseases around the world. Drs. Charles J. Arntzen, from the Boyce Thompson Institute at Cornell University, and William H. R. Langridge, from Loma Linda University, have been involved with the production of edible vaccines in plants. The purpose of a vaccine is to prime the immune system to destroy a specific viral or bacterial pathogen quickly. Food vaccines are genetically engineered to contain antigens (proteins that will induce the immune response) but they do not contain genes to allow the whole pathogen to form. Arntzen and Langridge have shown that tomato or potato plants can make antigens from pathogens such as enterotoxigenic *E. coli*, *Vibro cholerae*, and the hepatitis B virus. Feeding these antigen-containing tubers or fruits to test animals stimulated a mucosal (referring to the mucous membranes of the airway passages) and a systemic immune response that protected the animals from exposure to the pathogens. Some potential concerns about edible vaccines included whether the antigen would be degraded by the gut and whether the antigen would be degraded by cooking, as in cooking the tuber for eating. Antigens delivered in plant foods survive the trip through the stomach well enough to activate the immune system. Cooking of potatoes does not always destroy the anti-

gen, so cooked edible vaccines may be possible. Some tests have also been done in humans, where several volunteers showed a systemic response to a food vaccine containing a hepatitis B antigen. The studies done so far demonstrate that edible vaccines are feasible, but much more work is needed to develop useful vaccines.

Genetic engineering is also being applied to human cells in attempts to treat cancer and genetic diseases. Medical treatments using genetic engineering are called human gene therapies. In gene therapy, genes may be added, deleted, or altered to change the properties of certain cells within the body. Human gene therapy may succeed in providing cures for some of the more than three thousand known genetic diseases. One particularly severe disease is readily amenable to gene therapy. Adenosine deaminase (ADA) deficiency results when an individual's own cells are unable to produce the enzyme ADA. The most harmful effect of this deficiency is the lack of an effective immune system to fight disease. Consequently, the individual must live in an almost entirely sterile environment to avoid potentially harmful bacteria, fungi, and viruses. Bone marrow cells could be extracted from an ADA-deficient person, however, and a new ADA gene could be inserted into the cells. When the bone marrow cells are replaced, they should function normally.

In the News: Gene Switches

Gene switches are controllable, inducible gene expression systems. The expression of an introduced gene is tightly controlled to allow the gene to be expressed at a certain time, in a certain tissue, and to a certain level. Such systems will be important in determining the role a specific protein plays in signaling pathways, in cell development and differentiation, and in the pathogenesis of a disease. Molecular gene switches may also play an important role in the development of controllable human gene therapies for the treatment of genetic diseases. Such systems would allow the expression of a therapeutic protein to be regulated to produce that protein only at a specific time, when needed, and then terminate the expression of the protein. Regulated expression systems would allow crop plants to be used as bioreactors to pro-

duce recombinant proteins. Highly regulated expression of a gene is useful if the gene product is harmful to the cell. Many different types of gene switches have been constructed, including those based on steroid hormone receptors and on tetracycline-controlled activation of transcription (production of messenger RNA). For example, in one type of tetracycline-regulated gene switch, if tetracycline is not present, the TetR repressor protein binds to a region of the introduced gene's promoter and prevents transcription of the gene. The inducer tetracycline, when present, binds the TetR repressor protein, changing its conformation so that it cannot bind the promoter, and transcription of the gene occurs.

—*Susan J. Karcher, Ph.D.*

PERSPECTIVE AND PROSPECTS

Genetic engineering began in the 1970's, a period of heightened public concern about the safety of the citizens and environment and of distrust of established institutions. This fact, along with the nature of the technology—changing nature's or God's design, depending on one's beliefs—placed genetic engineering under great public scrutiny.

Human gene therapy brings up several important ethical questions. First, do humans have the moral and ethical right to alter the genetic makeup of themselves or others? A more critical question is whether one has the right to alter the genetic makeup of future generations. Gene therapy of normal body cells that will die when the individual dies, such as the two examples cited above, is called somatic cell gene therapy. Most people see little ethical problem with such techniques. Yet the potential also exists to alter genetically sperm and egg cells, the germ cells, so that future progeny will all carry the alterations.

Scientists involved in the early development of recombinant DNA methodology saw the danger of reckless experimentation. In fact, in 1974, those scientists called for a worldwide moratorium on genetic engineering until they could discuss the safety concerns. In 1975, the scientists met at Asilomar, California, and developed a set of guidelines under which they would conduct their research. In 1976, the National Institutes of Health (NIH) stepped in and issued formal guidelines based on those recommended at the Asilomar conference. Since the initial NIH guidelines, concern about the potential risks of genetic engineering has subsided. In fact, the NIH guidelines have been relaxed several times. Most experiments are now performed in an open laboratory environment with little containment other than that used for handling normal bacteria or viruses.

In addition to those concerned about the issues of safety, opponents of genetic engineering include those who question the ethics and morality of altering the genetic makeup of organisms, especially humans. Genetic recombination takes place every day in the natural world, but this recombination is usually limited to members of the same species. When organisms reproduce, groups of genes from each parent are recombined to form progeny. It is considered that such events are controlled by the laws of nature or by God. Yet scientists have taken the process one step further, developing the ability to recombine genes from different organisms. Many people, including

some scientists, believe that genetic engineering goes against the laws of nature or is playing God; they call for a halt to genetic engineering. Many others, scientists and laypersons alike, believe that genetic engineering mimics natural events such as viral infections and evolution and that the potential benefits—scientific, social, and medical—are too great to stop genetic engineering.

Although beneficial applications of genetic engineering are in use, there is still a great deal of concern and controversy over the use of genetically modified organisms (GMOs) as human food. One of the earliest developments in the genetic engineering of food was the discovery in 1979 that dairy cows, when injected with a synthetic cow growth hormone, recombinant bovine somatotropin (rBST), increased their milk-producing capacity. In 1990 and 1991, the American Medical Association, the American Pediatric Association, and the National Institutes of Health concluded that milk and meat from cows treated with rBST were as safe as untreated ones. In 1993, the Food and Drug Administration (FDA) approved the use of rBST in dairy cows. In 1990, a genetically engineered form of rennet used in making cheese was approved with little public attention. In 1994, Calgene's Flavr Savr (delayed-ripening) tomato was the first genetically engineered whole food approved for the market by the FDA. By 1999, about twenty genetically modified foods had cleared the premarket approval process in the United States, Canada, Europe, and Japan. Such approved GMOs included herbicide-tolerant soybeans, canola, oilseed rape, and sugar beet; insect-resistant corn and potatoes; and disease-resistant squash and papaya.

In 1999 and 2000, there was a strong public reaction against GMOs in Europe and the United States. In May, 2000, a survey of public perception of biotechnology in Europe, called the "Eurobarometer," indicated that most Europeans consider many applications of biotechnology to be beneficial to society. The survey showed that Europeans regarded the "technological modification of plants used as human food as high risk, but the pharmaceutical applications of biotechnology as useful." Consumer concerns are based on ethical issues (whether scientists should create new life forms) and on safety issues (whether adequate testing has been done to determine the risks). In Britain, in 1994, a cheese and a tomato paste, which were clearly labeled as coming from GMOs, were available to the consumer. The consumers had a choice between the genetically modified and traditional varieties, and there appeared to be little public concern. Later, however, public concern was triggered when soybean products from genetically modified plants were used in about 60 percent of manufactured foods without appropriate labeling.

There are a large number of questions about GMOs. For example, what is the risk of creating a superweed from the escape of engineered genes in crop plants? What is the risk of an allergic reaction to the transgene? GMOs typically contain antibiotic-resistant genes. What might be the risks to the environment or to humans or animals consuming these antibiotic-resistant genes? The patenting of GMOs and the use of "terminator gene" technology to produce sterile seed allow corporations to have a monopoly on the GMOs they produce. What will be the economic consequences of crops with terminator genes for developing countries using traditional farming practices?

Much of the controversy surrounding GMOs might be avoided if the foods were clearly labeled as "genetically modified" so that the consumer is informed and has a choice, but the resolution of this issue is ongoing. In reality, most people place varying emphases on each of these perspectives, and the emphasis often changes depending on what ethical decisions one is trying to make. In the case of an issue such as genetic engineering—which is often technically complex, which touches the very foundations of religious beliefs, and which has such great medical potential—one must carefully evaluate all perspectives and make responsible and informed decisions.

—Gary J. Lindquester, Ph.D.;
updated by Susan J. Karcher, Ph.D.

See also Antibiotics; Bacteriology; Bionics and biotechnology; Cancer; Cells; Chemotherapy; Cloning; Cytology; Diabetes mellitus; DNA and RNA; Enzymes; Ethics; Fetal tissue transplantation; Gene therapy; Genetics and inheritance; Hormone replacement therapy; Hormones; Immunization and vaccination; Mutation; Pharmacology.

FOR FURTHER INFORMATION:

Anderson, W. French, and Elaine G. Diacumakos. "Genetic Engineering in Mammalian Cells." *Scientific American* 254 (July, 1981): 106-121. Describes the difficulties of cloning genes into mammalian cells, a prerequisite to human gene therapy using genetic engineering.

Drlica, Karl. *Understanding DNA and Gene Cloning: A Guide for the Curious*. New York: Wiley, 1997. Provides an introduction to molecular cloning.

Frank-Kamenetskii, Maxim D. *Unraveling DNA—The Most Important Molecule of Life*. Rev. ed. Reading, Mass.: Addison-Wesley, 1997. This very readable book provides an excellent history of the discovery of DNA and genetic engineering.

Gasser, Charles S., and Robert T. Fraley. "Transgenic Crops." *Scientific American* 266 (June, 1992). Describes how to introduce genes into plants.

Gilbert, Walter, and Lydia Villa-Komaroff. "Useful Proteins from Recombinant Bacteria." *Scientific American* 242 (April, 1980): 74-94. Describes the cloning and expression of human insulin and interferon.

Grobstein, Clifford. "The Recombinant-DNA Debate." *Scientific American* 237 (July, 1977): 22-33. Provides an early historical account of the experiments and the regulation of recombinant DNA research.

Langridge, William H. R. "Edible Vaccines." *Scientific American* 283 (September, 2000): 66-71. Describes efforts to create edible vaccines in plants.

McHughen, Alan. *Pandora's Picnic Basket: The Potential and Hazards of Genetically Modified Foods*. New York: Oxford University Press, 2000. McHughen offers a balanced, informed look at the new technology of genetically modified foods. He easily imparts a basic understanding of the molecular genetics required to understand genetic modification and the controversy it sparks.

Nicholl, Desmond. *Introduction to Genetic Engineering*. Cambridge, England: Cambridge University Press, 1994. A valuable textbook for the nonspecialist and anyone interested in genetic engineering. It provides an excellent foundation in molecular biology and builds on that foundation to show how organisms can be genetically engineered.

Rifkin, Jeremy. *The Biotech Century: Harnessing the Gene and Remaking the World*. New York: Jeremy P. Tarcher/Putnam, 1998. Addresses the social aspects of biotechnology.

Shannon, Thomas. *What Are They Saying About Genetic Engineering?* New York: Paulist Press, 1985. Presents both sides of many ethical issues related to genetic engineering—the role of the scientist in society, the dangers of knowledge that can be misused, and the effects of genetic engineering on social structure. Includes examples of the applications of biotechnology.

Velander, William H., et al. "Transgenic Livestock as Drug Factories." *Scientific American* 276 (January, 1997). Provides an overview of biopharmaceutical applications of transgenic animals.

Watson, James, and John Tooze. *The DNA Story.* San Francisco: W. H. Freeman, 1981. A fascinating documentary of the history of gene cloning, from the first cloning in 1973 through the Asilomar conference and public debates on the issue, the government guidelines, and the patenting of the first engineered life-forms. Includes copies of personal letters, newspaper clippings, and editorial cartoons documenting the genetic engineering debate.

Wilmut, Ian, Keith Campbell, and Colin Tudge. *The Second Creation: Dolly and the Age of Biological Control.* New York: Farrar, Straus and Giroux, 2000. Science writer Tudge helps the scientists responsible for cloning the sheep Dolly tell their story. Discusses the groundwork laid by others and the scientific methodology they employed in cloning the first mammal from the cell of an adult of its species.

Yount, Lisa. *Biotechnology and Genetic Engineering.* New York: Facts on File, 2000. Addresses social aspects of genetic engineering. Designed for students in grades six through twelve, this volume is an excellent resource for students, teachers, and library media specialists. Well researched, it includes an extensive chronology, biographical listings, a glossary, and an annotated bibliography.

GENETICS AND INHERITANCE

BIOLOGY

ANATOMY OR SYSTEM AFFECTED: All

SPECIALTIES AND RELATED FIELDS: Embryology, forensic medicine, genetics, pediatrics

DEFINITION: The passage of traits from parents to offspring in discrete units called genes.

KEY TERMS:

allele: a version of a gene; different alleles of a gene have slightly different nucleotide sequences, resulting in differences in the protein encoded in the gene

chromosome: one of the DNA molecules of a nucleus; in humans, chromosomes occur in twenty-three pairs; with each member of a pair having the same genes but possibly having different alleles of the genes

deoxyribonucleic acid (DNA): the hereditary molecule, in which sequences of nucleic acids encode genetic information

dominant allele: the version of a gene that produces a recognizable trait in offspring when present in only one of the two chromosomes of a pair

fertilization: the process by which chromosome pairs, separated in production of egg and sperm cells, are rejoined

gene: a sequence of nucleotides in DNA encoding a protein

meiosis: a division mechanism in which homologous chromosomes are separated and delivered singly to egg or sperm cells; as a part of meiosis, recombination generates new combinations of alleles

nucleotide: a chemical subunit of DNA; different sequences of linked nucleotides spell out instructions for the assembly of proteins

recessive allele: a version of a gene that must be present on both chromosomes of a pair in order to produce a recognizable trait in offspring

recombination: the reciprocal exchange of segments between the two chromosomes of a pair, producing new combinations of alleles

THE RULES OF INHERITANCE

The primary genes of interest to heredity consist of a set of coded directions for making proteins. Each gene codes for a protein; distinct versions of a gene, which encode slightly different versions of the protein, may be carried in the same or different individuals. The distinct versions of a gene, called alleles, are responsible for differences in hereditary traits among individuals. Each individual receives a combination of alleles encoding proteins that directly or indirectly determine traits such as eye, skin, and hair color; height; and, to a degree, characteristics such as personality, behavior, and intelligence.

In molecular terms, genes consist of a sequence of chemical units called nucleotides, linked end to end in long, linear deoxyribonucleic acid (DNA) molecules. There are four kinds of nucleotides in DNA; each gene has its own nucleotide sequence. The alleles of a gene differ slightly in nucleotide sequence—some alleles differ in the substitution of only a single nucleotide. There are many thousands of genes arranged in tandem on the DNA molecules of a human cell; each DNA molecule is known as a chromosome. In humans, the chromosomes occur in twenty-three pairs, for a total of forty-six chromosomes. The two members of a chromosome pair contain the same genes in the same order, but different alleles of a gene may be present in the two members of a pair. One member of a chromosome pair is derived from the female parent of the individual; the other member is derived from the male parent. These are called the maternal and paternal chromosomes of the pair.

Inheritance, and the variation in traits among individuals, depends on two processes that separate and rejoin the chromosome pairs in sexual reproduction. One is a division mechanism, meiosis, which occurs in cell lines leading to egg or sperm cells. Meiosis separates the chromosome pairs and places one member of each pair in an egg or sperm cell. The particular combination of maternal and paternal chromosomes delivered to an egg or sperm cell is random. This random segregation, as it is called, is one source of the variability between offspring in a family. Because there are so many chromosomes, the possibility that two egg or sperm cells produced by the same individual could receive the same combination of maternal and paternal chromosomes is very small—equivalent to one chance in 8.4 million. Another important source of variability comes from a mechanism that occurs before the pairs are separated in meiosis. In this mechanism, called recombination, the two members of a chromosome pair line up side by side and exchange segments perfectly and reciprocally. As a result, alleles are exchanged between the pairs, generating new combinations of alleles. The variability generated by recombination adds to that produced by independent segregation of maternal and paternal chromosomes, so that it is essentially impossible for an individual to produce two egg or sperm cells that are genetically the same.

The second process underlying inheritance is fertilization, in which a sperm and an egg cell fuse, rejoining the twenty-three pairs of chromosomes. Fertilization is another random process, in which any of the millions of sperm cells ejaculated by a male and any of the hundreds of egg cells carried in a female may join. The total variability generated by independent segregation of alleles, recombination, and random union of gametes is such that each human individual, except identical twins, receives a unique combination of alleles. Thus the possibility that any individual has or will ever have a genetic double in the human population, except for an identical twin, is essentially zero. (In the case of identical twins, a single fertilized egg divides to produce two separate, genetically identical cells; instead of remaining together to produce a two-celled embryo, as is normally the case, the cells separate to create two embryos, which develop into genetically identical individuals.)

Because chromosomes occur in pairs, each individual receives two alleles of every gene of the human complement. The two alleles may be the same or different. Some alleles are dominant in their effects, so that one copy of the allele on either chromosome is sufficient to produce the trait encoded in the allele. Other alleles are recessive, so that both chromosomes of the pair must carry the allele for the trait to appear in offspring. In humans, few physical traits are determined by a single gene. Most are the result of complex interactions between several genes, as well as environmental influences. Nonetheless, some traits do tend to follow certain inheritance patterns, but there are exceptions. For example, brown eyes tend to be dominant to blue eyes. If either chromosome carries the brown eye allele, the individual will usually have brown eyes. To have blue eyes, an individual usually carries two genes for blue eyes. Human traits that tend toward dominant inheritance include nearsightedness and farsightedness, astigmatism, dark or curly hair, early balding in males, normal body pigment (as compared to albinism), supernumerary fingers or toes, short fingers or toes, and webbing between fingers and toes. Alleles that tend to be expressed in a recessive fashion include blond hair, straight hair, and congenital deafness.

Although each individual normally carries a maximum of two alleles of any gene, several or many alleles of a gene may exist in the human population as a whole. The major histocompatibility complex (MHC), for example, occurs in hundreds of different alleles throughout the human population—so many that unrelated individuals are unlikely to carry the same combination of MHC alleles. The proteins encoded in these alleles are recognized by the immune system as "self" or "foreign." Unless the same, or a very similar combination of MHC alleles is present, cells are recognized by the immune system as foreign, and the cells are destroyed. Therefore, MHC combinations recognized as foreign are the primary factor in the rejection of tissue or organ transplants among humans. If the transplant does not come from an individual with the same or a very similar MHC combination, rejection is likely unless the immune system is suppressed by drugs such as cyclosporin.

The Inheritance of Genetic Disorders

DOMINANT

One parent affected

50% offspring affected,
regardless of sex

Both parents affected

75% offspring affected,
regardless of sex

RECESSIVE

One parent affected

No offspring affected
All carriers

Both parents carriers

25% offspring affected
50% carriers, regardless of sex

SEX-LINKED RECESSIVE

Mother carrier

50% sons affected
50% daughters carriers

Father affected

All sons normal
All daughters carriers

□ **Male**   ○ **Female**

The best donor for a transplant is a close relative, who is most likely to have a similar MHC combination. Because identical twins have the same MHC combination, tissues and organs can be transplanted between them with no danger of rejection.

Sex is determined by a pair of chromosomes that is different in males and females. Females have two members of the pair, the X chromosomes, which have the same genes in the same order but which may have different alleles of the genes. One member of the XX pair was derived from the female's father, and the other from her mother. Males have only one member of this pair, a single X. In addition, males have a small, single chromosome, the Y, which is not present in females. Thus females are XX, and males are XY. During meiosis in females, the XX pair is separated, so that an egg cell may receive either member of the pair. In males, the X and Y are separated, so that a sperm cell receives either an X or a Y. In fertilization, the X chromosome carried by the egg may be joined with an X-carrying sperm, producing a female (XX), or, the egg may be fertilized by a sperm cell carrying a Y, producing a male (XY). Thus in humans, the sex of the offspring is determined by the type of sperm cell, an X or a Y, fertilizing the egg. Most genes carried on an X chromosome have no counterparts on the Y chromosome. Therefore, traits encoded in genes on the X chromosomes (almost none are carried on the Y) are inherited differently from traits carried on other chromosomes of the set, in a pattern known as sex-linked inheritance.

DISORDERS AND DISEASES

Many human diseases, involving every system in the body, depend on the presence of particular dominant or recessive alleles and are directly inherited. Only the disposition for development of other diseases is inherited—that is, some individuals inherit a combination of alleles that increases the possibility that a genetically based disease will develop during their lifetimes.

The list of diseases contracted through inheritance of a dominant allele is long and impressive. Among the more important of these diseases are achondroplasia, in which individuals are short-statured; familial hypercholesterolemia, in which cholesterol concentration in the blood is abnormally high, leading to vascular disease, particularly of the coronary arteries; Huntington's disease, a disease characterized by dementia, delusion, paranoia, and abnormal movements that begins in persons between twenty and fifty years of age and progresses steadily to death in about fifteen years; Marfan syndrome, a disease of connective tissues involving the skeleton, eyes, and cardiovascular system, characterized by elongated limbs, abnormal position of the eye lens, and structural weakness of blood vessels, particularly of the aorta; neurofibromatosis, characterized by tumors dispersed throughout the body and coffee-colored skin lesions; polycystic kidney disease, in which dilated cysts grow in the kidneys and interfere with kidney function, leading to hypertension and chronic renal failure; spherocytosis, another disease in which blood cells are fragile and easily broken during travel through the circulatory system, producing anemia and jaundice; and thalassemia, a group of diseases most common in persons of Mediterranean descent in which hemoglobin production is faulty, leading to anemias that range from mild to severe.

Diseases caused by recessive genes also appear in the human population. Although many persons are carriers for these diseases, affected persons are rare because both alleles must be present in the recessive form for the disease to develop. Diseases in this category include albinism; sickle-cell disease, common in persons of African descent, in which hemoglobin is faulty, leading to fragility of red blood cells, anemia, blockage of blood vessels, and susceptibility to infection; phenylketonuria (PKU), in which the amino acid phenylalanine accumulates in excess in the bloodstream, leading to nervous system damage including mental retardation; Tay-Sachs disease, most common in persons of Jewish descent, characterized by accumulation of lipid molecules in nerve cells leading to motor incoordination, blindness, and mental deterioration; and glycogen storage diseases, with symptoms ranging from cramps to serious muscular and cardiac disease and convulsions. Sickle-cell disease is recessively inherited. A person with one copy of the sickle-cell gene makes enough normal hemoglobin to have symptoms of the disease only under extreme low oxygen conditions. Cystic fibrosis, one of the most common of genetically determined diseases in Caucasians, is probably also attributable to a recessive allele. In this disease, sweat- and mucus-secreting glands are affected; the most serious effects are caused by the secretion of unusually thick and viscid mucus, leading to blockage of ducts in the lungs, liver, pancreas, and salivary glands. Most critical to survival is blockage of passages in the lungs, producing a chronic cough and persistent pulmonary infections. The average life expectancy of persons with cystic fibrosis is twenty years of age.

A number of diseases are caused by recessive genes carried on the X chromosomes and are inherited in sex-linked patterns. Among these are one form of diabetes (diabetes insipidus) in which glucose uptake by cells is faulty, leading to the accumulation of glucose in the blood; hemophilia, in which the blood-clotting mechanism is deficient, making afflicted persons subject to uncontrolled bleeding; and some forms of muscular dystrophy, characterized by progressive muscular weakness. The Duchenne muscular dystrophy appears early in life, progresses rapidly, and leads to death in most cases by the age of twenty.

Because males receive only one copy of the X chromosome, recessive genes are fully expressed in males—there is no chance for a normal allele to compensate for the effects of the recessive gene. For a sex-linked disease to appear in females, both X chromosomes must carry the recessive allele. For these reasons, sex-linked recessive diseases are much more common in males than in females; for some, appearance of the disease is limited almost exclusively to males.

The molecular basis for some genetically based diseases is known. In familial hypercholesterolemia, for example, receptors for cholesterol on cell surfaces are faulty or not produced, preventing the normal uptake of cholesterol from the bloodstream. As a result, cholesterol accumulates and reaches a dangerously high concentration in the blood. In persons carrying dominant alleles for familial hypercholesterolemia on both chromosomes of the pair, coronary arterial disease advances so rapidly that death from heart attack by the age of twenty is frequent. The disease is among the most common of genetically based defects—about 1 in 500 persons has at least one allele for hypercholesterolemia and develops premature coronary artery disease. In PKU, individuals lack an enzyme normally produced in the liver. The enzyme, phenylalanine hydroxylase, converts excess phenylalanine into another amino acid, tyrosine. Without the enzyme, phenylalanine taken in the diet accumulates to dangerously high levels in the body. Some forms of PKU are treatable by restricting dietary intake of phenylalanine from infancy onward.

Some persons have a genetically determined predisposition to develop certain cancers with greater frequency than the average in the population. About 5 percent of cancers are strongly predisposed—that is, individuals inherit a marked tendency to develop the cancer. Among these are familial retinoblastoma, in which retinal tumors develop; familial adenomatous polyps of the colon; and multiple endocrine neoplasia, in which tumors develop in the thyroid, adrenal medulla, and parathyroid glands. Often underlying these strongly predisposed cancers is the inheritance of a faulty gene (called an oncogene) that promotes uncontrolled cell division, or the opposite—inheri-

tance of a faulty gene that in its normal form suppresses cell division (called a tumor suppressor gene). Typically, oncogenes are inherited as dominant genes, and tumor suppressor genes as recessives. In addition, some cancers, including breast, ovarian, and colon cancers other than familial adenomatous polyps, show a degree of predisposition in family lines.

PERSPECTIVE AND PROSPECTS

The primary features of meiosis and fertilization—random segregation of chromosome pairs in meiosis and random rejoining of pairs in fertilization—makes heredity subject to analysis by mathematical techniques. In fact, mathematical analysis of heredity was carried out successfully before there was any understanding concerning meiosis or DNA. The groundwork for this analysis was laid down in the 1860's by an Austrian monk, Gregor Mendel. Mendel's research approach and his conclusions were so advanced that they were misunderstood and unappreciated during his lifetime.

Mendel chose garden peas for his research because they could be grown easily and they possessed several hereditary traits that were known to breed true—that is, to appear dependably in offspring. Mendel crossed pea plants with different traits in various combinations. On analyzing the results of his crosses, Mendel realized that the numbers of offspring exhibiting different traits could be explained mathematically if he assumed that parents contain a pair of factors governing the inheritance of each trait. Furthermore, he concluded that the factors separate, or segregate, independently as gametes are formed and are reunited randomly at fertilization. He also discovered that some traits are inherited as dominant and some as recessive. Mendel's factors were later called genes.

Until Mendel's time, inheritance was commonly believed to occur through a blending of maternal and paternal characteristics. Mendel's work showed instead that traits are passed on as units; depending on whether a trait is dominant or recessive, it may appear in all offspring or only in a definite, predictable percentage. Some time after Mendel's discoveries, in the early 1900's, meiosis was discovered. At this time, Walter Sutton pointed out that Mendel's genes and chromosomes behave similarly in meiosis and fertilization: Both genes and chromosomes occur in pairs that separate randomly in meiosis and are rejoined at fertilization. Genes were therefore concluded to be carried on the chromosomes. Further genetic research confirmed that Mendel's findings with plant genes also apply to animals, including humans, and worked out many additional features of inheritance, including genetic recombination and sex linkage. Later, in the 1950's, almost one hundred years after Mendel's findings, James D. Watson and Francis Crick discovered the structure of DNA and deduced the fact that hereditary information is encoded in the sequence of nucleotides in DNA.

Research in human genetics differs from genetic investigation in other organisms because, for obvious reasons, it is impossible to set up experimental crosses to test whether particular diseases are inherited. Instead, human family lines are analyzed carefully in pedigrees to trace the appearance of disease over several generations. If a disease is genetically determined, it shows up in definite patterns as dominant, recessive, or sex-linked among parents and offspring in the pedigrees. On this basis, prospective parents can be counseled on the chances that their offspring will develop a hereditary disease.

In June of 2000, Francis Collins, director of the National Human Genome Research Initiative, and J. Craig Venter, of Celera Genomics, announced that they had jointly sequenced the entire human genome and that the first working draft was available. Sequencing the human genome will allow scientists to directly compare healthy DNA to DNA harboring disease genes. Discovering the disease genes and studying them will lead to much more rapid understanding of disease processes, as well as the development of diagnostic procedures and potential therapy and cures, than allowed by the techniques available before the completion of this initiative.

—Stephen L. Wolfe, Ph.D.;
updated by Karen E. Kalumuck, Ph.D.

See also Aging; Albinos; Alzheimer's disease; Amniocentesis; Autoimmune disorders; Biostatistics; Birth defects; Blood testing; Breast cancer; Cancer; Chorionic villus sampling; Cloning; Colon cancer; Color blindness; Cystic fibrosis; Diabetes mellitus; Disease; DNA and RNA; Down syndrome; Dwarfism; Embryology; Enzymes; Gene therapy; Genetic counseling; Genetic diseases; Genetic engineering; Gigantism; Hemophilia; Human Genome Project; Immunodeficiency disorders; In vitro fertilization; Laboratory tests; Mental retardation; Multiple births; Muscular dystrophy; Mutation; Neurofibromatosis; Obstetrics; Oncology; Parkinson's disease; Pathology; Pediatrics; Phenylketonuria (PKU); Porphyria; Pregnancy and gestation; Preventive medicine; Reproductive system; Rh factor; Screening; Sexual differentiation; Sexuality; Sickle-cell disease; Tay-Sachs disease.

FOR FURTHER INFORMATION:

Campbell, Neil A. *Biology: Concepts and Connections.* 5th ed. Redwood City, Calif.: Benjamin/ Cummings, 1999. This classic introductory textbook provides an excellent discussion of essential biological structures and mechanisms. Of particular interest are the chapters entitled "Mendel and the Gene Idea," "The Chromosomal Basis of Inheritance," and "The Molecular Basis of Inheritance."

Edlin, Gordon. *Genetic Principles: Human and Social Consequences.* Boston: Jones and Bartlett, 1984. A readable textbook of general genetics, with an emphasis on human genetics and the medical and social consequences of heredity. Contains many photographs and diagrams that expand on the text.

Goodenough, Ursula. *Genetics.* 3d ed. New York: Holt, Rinehart & Winston, 1984. One of the best available college textbooks of genetics. The book is comprehensive, lucidly written, and contains many informative illustrations. Covers genetics from classical to modern times.

Lewin, Benjamin. *Genes: VII.* New York: Oxford University Press, 2000. A college textbook that discusses the entire field of molecular biology and genetics, with many references to the structure and activity of the cell nucleus. Although written at the college level, it is readable and accessible to a general audience. Many highly informative illustrations and diagrams are included.

Marieb, Elaine N. *Essentials of Human Anatomy and Physiology.* 6th ed. Redwood City, Calif.: Benjamin/ Cummings, 2000. This introductory anatomy and physiology textbook, easily accessible to those with little science background, is richly illustrated with diagrams and photographs, which help to illuminate body systems and processes. In-depth discussions of prevalent diseases and disorders and of current areas of research make this an all-around useful reference work.

Wolfe, Stephen L. *Molecular and Cellular Biology.* Belmont, Calif.: Wadsworth, 1993. Chapter 25, "Meiosis and Genetic Recombination," describes these mechanisms. The book, written at the college level, is highly readable and illustrated with many informative diagrams and photographs.

GENITAL DISORDERS, FEMALE

DISEASE/DISORDER

ANATOMY OR SYSTEM AFFECTED: Genitals, reproductive system, uterus

SPECIALTIES AND RELATED FIELDS: Family practice, gynecology, obstetrics, oncology, urology

DEFINITION: All maladies affecting the reproductive organs of women.

KEY TERMS:

cervix: the narrow portion of the uterus situated at the upper end of the vagina

cyst: a closed sac having a distinct border which develops abnormally within a body space or structure

estrogen: the hormone responsible for female sexual characteristics, produced primarily by the ovaries

Fallopian tubes: tiny tubes that connect the ovaries to the uterus; after ovulation, the egg travels through these tubes, and its fertilization by sperm occurs here

hormone: a chemical compound produced at one site in the body which travels to other parts of the body to exert its effect

hysterectomy: the surgical removal of the uterus; in a total hysterectomy, the uterus, ovaries and Fallopian tubes are removed

laparoscopy: a surgical procedure in which an instrument is inserted into the abdominal cavity through tiny incisions in the abdomen; usually performed without hospitalization

CAUSES AND SYMPTOMS

Diseases and disorders of the female genitals, both internal organs and outward anatomical structures, encompass a huge number of different types of conditions that can range in severity from merely physically annoying to life-threatening. These disorders affect the vulva, vagina, uterus, ovaries, and Fallopian tubes. Many develop from unknown causes, and others have clear-cut origins, such as sexually transmitted diseases. Some have immediately recognizable symptoms, while others are silent until the disease has progressed to a serious stage. Early recognition of symptoms or abnormalities and proper treatment can alleviate pain and save lives.

Endometriosis is a chronic, recurring disease in which the tissue that lines the uterus grows into the abdominal cavity. This tissue normally thickens with blood vessels in preparation for receiving a fertilized egg. In endometriosis, the tissue overgrows the uterus, invades the Fallopian tubes, and reaches the abdominal cavity, where it continues to grow. This abnormally growing tissue will attach to any nearby internal organs, such as the ovaries, bladder, Fallopian tubes, and rectum. The endometrial tissue responds to the same hormonal cues that signal the sloughing off of the uterine lining during menstruation; however, the blood from the endometrial tissue cannot leave the abdominal cavity, leading to inflammation. As the inflammation subsides, it is replaced with scar tissue. This process will repeat with each menstrual cycle, and the scarring can result in infertility, organ malfunction, or adhesions that bind organs together. Some women with endometriosis experience no symptoms, while many experience severe abdominal pain before, during, and after their menstrual periods. Endometrial tissue can be sometimes diagnosed with a pelvic exam, but a definitive diagnosis can be reached only with laparoscopy. The cause of endometriosis is unknown, but some evidence suggests an inherited tendency to develop endometriosis.

Vaginitis is a general term for infections of the vagina. The most common of these is commonly called a yeast infection, caused by the fungus *Candida albicans*. This fungus is usually a harmless organism which lives in nearly everyone's intestinal tract and in the vagina of 20 to 40 percent of American women. Symptoms are caused when the organism grows at an accelerated rate and include severe itching, vaginal discharge, and burning upon urination. Many situations may cause the enhanced growth of the fungus, including use of antibiotics which disturb the acid balance within the vagina, stress, use of oral contraceptives and corticosteroids, and the low estrogen levels that accompany the menopause.

Uterine fibroids are benign tumors made mainly of muscle tissue that can grow inside the uterus or along its outer surface. They grow slowly and are dependent on the hormone estrogen for continued growth. They are usually not problematic, but if they become very large they may cause extremely heavy bleeding during menstruation and can interfere with pregnancy and childbirth. Their cause is unknown, but they will shrink or disappear after the menopause.

Uterine prolapse occurs when the pelvic muscles are no longer able to support the pelvic organs, and the uterus "falls" into the vagina. A feeling of one's "insides falling out" is typical of this disorder, which is often precipitated by one or more difficult births.

Ovarian cysts form when an egg developing inside a follicle within the ovary does not ovulate but instead keeps growing. Small cysts will be painless, but larger ones (up to 7.5 centimeters in diameter) may cause abdominal pain. Most cysts will go away on their own, but some can rupture and cause severe pain.

The hallmark of cancer is uncontrolled cell growth. Cancer may prove fatal by causing destruction of a particular organ at the site of origin or by spreading throughout the body and damaging other organs and systems. All the organs of the female reproductive system can be affected by cancer. Cervical cancer begins in superficial layers of the cervix but may spread rapidly through the vagina and throughout the body. Cervical cancer can be detected in its early, most curable stages by a Pap smear. Endometrial cancer affects the glands which line the uterus. It can occur at any age, but the most common age of onset is sixty. Abnormal bleeding accompanies this disorder, which is diagnosed by examination of a biopsy of uterine tissue. Sarcomas of the uterus are malignant tumors of muscle tissue frequently confused with benign fibroids. This rare cancer is aggressive and difficult to treat. Ovarian cancer constitutes about 25 percent of female reproductive tract cancers, is difficult to detect and cure, and therefore has a high mortality rate. There are no early symptoms, and the cancer seems to occur frequently in those with a family history of the disease. Cancers of the Fallopian tubes and vagina are very rare, but vaginal cancer occurs with greater frequency in women whose mothers were treated with the synthetic estrogen diethylstilbestrol (DES) during the 1940's through the 1960's with the intent of preventing miscarriages. Cancer of the vulva, a form of skin cancer, is relatively easy to treat and has a high cure rate.

Sexually transmitted diseases (STDs) can involve any part of the female genital system. STDs of bacterial origin include gonorrhea and chlamydia, which are major precursors to pelvic inflammatory disease (PID) and syphilis. Untreated, these diseases can lead to serious complications. STDs with a viral cause include genital herpes, genital warts, and acquired immunodeficiency syndrome (AIDS). The causative agent of trichomoniasis is a protozoan. Each STD can be transmitted through direct sexual contact with an infected person, and each has its own set of symptoms and diagnostic criteria.

TREATMENT AND THERAPY

A variety of treatments are available for endometriosis, depending on the severity of the disorder. Over-the-counter or prescription anti-inflammatory drugs may give immediate relief of pain, but the condition itself is frequently treated with hormone therapy. Birth control pills that are high in the hormone progestin and low in estrogen can help shrink endometriosis. Danazol, a synthetic male hormone, suppresses the production of estrogen by the ovaries, thereby helping to eliminate the condition, but it has undesirable side effects. In some cases, surgical removal of the tissue is necessary. In laparoscopy, an instrument is inserted through tiny abdominal incisions and used to remove the tissue. In the most severe cases, a complete hysterectomy (removal of the uterus and ovaries) is performed.

Yeast infections that result in vaginitis must be properly diagnosed by a physician. Two medications for yeast infections are available without a prescrip-

Sites of Common Nonmalignant Female Genital Disorders

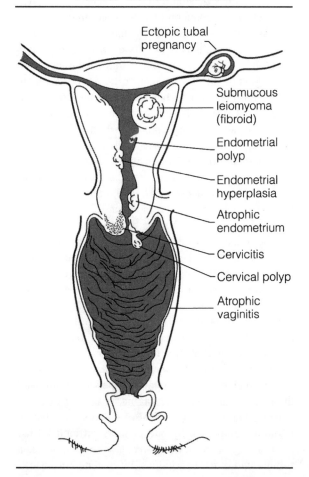

Ectopic tubal pregnancy

Submucous leiomyoma (fibroid)

Endometrial polyp

Endometrial hyperplasia

Atrophic endometrium

Cervicitis

Cervical polyp

Atrophic vaginitis

tion: miconazole and clotrimazole, available under brand names in most pharmacies. If a severe infection does not respond to this treatment, cortisone may be prescribed. Yeast infections have a tendency to recur, and taking precautions to prevent additional episodes is advised. Some ways in which to reduce the chance of reinfection include eating a cup of yogurt daily, avoiding sweets, reducing stress, wearing cotton underwear, avoiding tight-fitting clothing, avoiding feminine hygiene sprays, and using vinegar-and-water or povidone-iodine douches.

If no major discomfort is experienced by the woman when uterine fibroids are first detected, usually no treatment beyond regular observation is necessary. For those experiencing pain or difficulty in conception or pregnancy, the fibroids may be surgically removed in an operation called a myomectomy; in severe cases, a hysterectomy is performed. A laparoscope can be used to remove tumors on the outside of the uterus, or a hysteroscope can be inserted through the cervix, which uses a laser to burn away internal fibroids. Synthetic hormones called gonadotropin-releasing hormone agonists block the ovaries' production of estrogen, which leads to shrinking of the fibroids and the possible avoidance of surgery. Even with surgery, about 25 percent of fibroids grow back within five years.

A prolapsed uterus is frequently treated by hysterectomy, but other therapies are possible. Kegel exercises, designed to strengthen the muscles of the pelvic floor, are effective if done regularly for an extended period of time. A pessary, a ring-shaped device which fits around the cervix and props up the uterus, is another alternative, though an inconvenient one. Major surgery to resuspend the uterus is a surgical option to hysterectomy.

Ovarian cysts will usually be resorbed into the ovary within one to three menstrual cycles. Proper monitoring by a physician is needed to determine if the cysts have cleared. If the cyst does not disappear within three months or if it increases in size, ultrasound and/or laparoscopy will be used to determine if a different type of ovarian tumor is present, which would necessitate surgical removal.

Cancer treatment is highly specialized for the particular variety of the disease, its severity, and consideration of the affected individual. Typical treatments include surgical removal of the tumor and/or affected organ, radiation therapy, chemotherapy, and immunotherapy (the reinforcement of the immune system,

generally administered after radiation or chemotherapy). When diagnosed in premalignant stages, cervical abnormalities may be treated by cryosurgery (freezing and killing the abnormal cells) or laser destruction of the abnormal cells. Advanced cervical cancer is treated by hysterectomy. Endometrial cancer is treated with total hysterectomy, including the uterus, ovaries, and Fallopian tubes, and if the cancer has spread, radiation and/or chemotherapy. The only known cure for uterine sarcoma is total hysterectomy, and removal of both the ovaries and the Fallopian tubes is performed for ovarian cancer. The tumors of vaginal cancer are eliminated surgically or with laser treatment.

Sexually transmitted diseases of bacterial origin are treated successfully with antibiotics. Drug therapy can also eliminate trichomoniasis. There are no cures for the virally transmitted STDs. Certain drugs can reduce the frequency of outbreaks of genital herpes, and genital warts may be removed by freezing, burning, or surgery. No cure exists for AIDS, and only experimental drugs are available to prolong life.

PERSPECTIVE AND PROSPECTS

The diagnosis and treatment of female genital disorders and diseases have evolved from a state of some being considered psychosomatic to a field which spurs the continued development and improvement of diagnostic and treatment technologies. It is also a field which has been a major force in the mass screening of diseases and in public health issues. Many conditions such as endometriosis have historically been misdiagnosed and the associated pain dismissed as nonexistent—to the dismay of the suffering woman. This and other conditions such as prolapsed uterus and fibroids were typically treated with the drastic surgery of hysterectomy. Women have demanded that more research into the causes of these disorders, and options to hysterectomy, be developed. Laparoscopy has replaced hysterectomy in many cases, preserving the uterus and childbearing capacity.

The treatment of all female cancers has benefited from research into the cause and treatment of these disorders. For decades, the Pap smear has been routinely used with American women on an annual basis, and it has been responsible for saving thousands of lives through early detection of abnormal cervical cells that may progress to a cancerous state. Public education about the necessity of early cancer detection has helped to improve the survival chances of individuals with cancer, and sensitive blood tests can detect some cancers at their most treatable stages, long before any symptoms occur. Discovery of the hereditary nature of female genital cancers has established routine monitoring of those at risk for the disease, again resulting in early detection. New, better radiation and chemotherapy treatments, as well as improved immune system support, benefit all cancer patients. The connection between certain "cancer-fighting" foods and good health has led to a revision of Americans' eating habits.

While some sexually transmitted diseases are easily cured with antibiotics if caught early, those of viral origin are not and may have fatal consequences. Information through such diverse means as television and grade-school programs has educated people about this problem and the best ways to protect themselves from becoming victims of an incurable STD. Continuing research into diagnostic methods and treatment regimes in this area will lead to improved health for everyone.

—*Karen E. Kalumuck, Ph.D.*

See also Amenorrhea; Candidiasis; Cervical, ovarian, and uterine cancers; Cervical procedures; Childbirth; Childbirth complications; Chlamydia; Circumcision, female, and genital mutilation; Conception; Contraception; Culdocentesis; Cystitis; Dysmenorrhea; Ectopic pregnancy; Electrocauterization; Endometrial biopsy; Endometriosis; Episiotomy; Gonorrhea; Gynecology; Herpes; Infertility in females; Menopause; Menorrhagia; Menstruation; Miscarriage; Ovarian cysts; Pelvic inflammatory disease (PID); Pregnancy and gestation; Premature birth; Premenstrual syndrome (PMS); Reproductive system; Sexual dysfunction; Sexuality; Sexually transmitted diseases; Sterilization; Stillbirth; Syphilis; Urology; Urology, pediatric; Warts.

FOR FURTHER INFORMATION:

Boston Women's Health Book Collective. *Our Bodies, Ourselves for the New Century.* New York: Simon & Schuster, 1998. Gives expanded and accessible information on a broad range of topics concerning women's health. An excellent reference book for all women. A listing of local, national, and international resources is included.

Carlson, Karen J., Stephanie A. Eisenstat, and Terra Ziporyn. *The Harvard Guide to Women's Health.* Cambridge, Mass.: Harvard University Press, 1996. Some three hundred clearly written, alphabetically arranged entries provide authoritative information for the lay public on both mental and physical diseases, tests, symptoms, and commonly asked questions.

Foley, Denise, and Eileen Nechas. *Women's Encyclopedia of Health and Emotional Healing: Top Women Doctors Share Their Unique Self-Help Advice on Your Body, Your Feelings, and Your Life.* Emmaus, Pa.: Rodale Press, 1993. A very readable and informative book filled with practical information and anecdotal examples covering all aspects of women's physical and emotional health.

Gray, Mary Jane, and Florence Haseltine. *The Woman's Guide to Good Health.* Yonkers, N.Y.: Consumer Reports Books, 1991. This practical and comprehensive guide is written by physicians and gives complete information about the myths, risks, and alternatives regarding female diseases, diagnosis, and treatment. A useful appendix includes a list of societies for support and further information.

Novotny, P. P. *What Women Should Know About Chronic Infections and Sexually Transmitted Diseases.* New York: Dell, 1991. This compact, easy-to-understand book gives complete and accurate information on the transmission, diagnosis, and prevention of all sexually transmitted diseases that affect women. A handy reference guide.

Shaw, Michael, ed. *Everything You Need to Know About Diseases.* Springhouse, Pa.: Springhouse Press, 1996. This well-illustrated consumer reference, compiled by more than one hundred doctors and medical experts, describes five hundred illnesses and conditions, their causes, symptoms, diagnosis, treatment, and prevention. Of particular interest is chapter 9, "Gynecologic Disorders."

GENITAL DISORDERS, MALE
DISEASE/DISORDER

ANATOMY OR SYSTEM AFFECTED: Genitals, reproductive system

SPECIALTIES AND RELATED FIELDS: Family practice, oncology, proctology, urology

DEFINITION: Disorders and diseases of the male reproductive system, including sexual dysfunction, infertility, genital cancer, and sexually transmitted diseases.

KEY TERMS:

autonomic nervous system: the part of the vertebrate nervous system that controls involuntary actions

dysfunction: the disordered or impaired function of a body system or organ

endocrine: relating to the production or action of a hormone

hormone: a substance which creates a specific effect in an organ distant from its site of production

impotence: the inability to have or maintain an erection satisfactory for sexual intercourse

organic: pertaining to, arising from, or affecting a body organ

parasympathetic nervous system: the part of the autonomic nervous system that stimulates digestion, slows the heart, and dilates blood vessels, acting in opposition to sympathetic nerves

psychogenic: originating in the mind or in mental conditions and activities

spermatogonia: cells of the testes that become sperm during spermatogenesis

sphincter: a ringlike muscle which constricts or relaxes to close or open a body orifice or passage, as required by normal body function

sympathetic nervous system: the part of the autonomic nervous system that represses digestion, speeds up the heart, and constricts blood vessels, acting in opposition to parasympathetic nerves

PROCESS AND EFFECTS

Before discussion of male genital disorders and diseases, it is useful to describe the male genital system, which is composed of the scrotum, testes, epididymis, vas deferens, prostate and bulbourethral glands, seminal vesicles, penis, and urethra. The scrotum, composed of skin and underlying muscle, encloses the two testes and protects these sperm-making organs.

Each human testis is an ovoid structure about 5.0 centimeters long and 3.3 centimeters in width. A testis is composed of seminiferous tubules, a structure which surrounds the sperm-producing tubules, and accessory cells (the Leydig cells). The production of sperm, spermatogenesis, is controlled by hormones from the brain's hypothalamus and pituitary glands. It begins with the secretion of testosterone, the main male hormone, by Leydig cells. Brain hormone and testosterone actions cause the metamorphosis of cells called spermatogonia into sperm during a two-month passage through the seminiferous tubules.

The highly coiled seminiferous tubules, tiny in diameter and more than 200 meters long, coalesce into the efferent tubules, which release sperm into the epididymis. In a twelve-day trip through the highly coiled, 4.5-meter-long epididymis, sperm attain the ability to move (motility) and to fertilize a human egg cell, or ovum. Next, they enter the vas deferens, paired structures that connect the epididymis of each testis to its ejaculatory duct and the urethra. The only known vas function is to transport sperm, as a result of the action of nearby nerves and muscles, into the latter structures. The vas are cut in bilateral vasectomy surgery, which is often used for male sterilization.

The prostate, seminal vesicles, and bulbourethral glands produce the secretions that constitute most sperm-containing semen, which is ejaculated during intercourse. The prostate gland is situated immediately below the urinary bladder and surrounds the portion of the urethra closest to the bladder. It is a fibromuscular gland which empties into the male urethra on ejaculation. Prostate secretions contain important enzymes and make up a quarter of the seminal fluid.

The seminal vesicles are 7.5 centimeters long and empty into the ejaculatory ducts. They produce more than half of the liquid portion of semen, contributing fluid rich in fructose, the main nutrition source of sperm. The tiny, paired bulbourethral (or Cowper's) glands are located below the prostate. They secrete lubricants into the male urethra that ease semen passage.

The male urethra passes from the urinary bladder, through the prostate, and then through the penis. At the end of the penis, it reaches the outside of the body, to pass semen and urine. The penis, a cylindrical erectile organ, surrounds most of the male urethra and contains three cavernous regions. One, the corpus spongiosum, is found around the urethra. The others, the paired corpora cavernosa, are erectile tissues that fill with blood to produce an erection upon male sexual arousal. Erection is a complex reflex which involves both the sympathetic and parasympathetic portions of the human nervous system.

At the time of erection, nerve impulses dilate blood vessels that communicate with the corpora cavernosa and allow them to fill with blood. Sphincters then close off the portion of the urethra closest to the urinary bladder. At the same time, sperm, prostate secretions, bulbourethral gland secretions, and seminal vesicle secretions enter the urethra. Next, muscle contractions propel the ejaculate out of the urethra. The blood then leaves the corpora cavernosa, and the penis resumes its unexcited state.

COMPLICATIONS AND DISORDERS

Proper male sexual function involves several closely coordinated hormone, nervous, and chemical processes. After a discussion of the male genital system, it thus becomes clear that many factors can cause male genital problems and diseases. Male infertility, for example, can be attributable to inadequate sperm production; undersecretion by the seminal vesicles, Cowper's glands, and/or prostate; malfunction of other endocrine glands or of the nervous system; and dysfunction or lack of the epididymis. Impotence, the inability to have or maintain a satisfactory erection for intercourse, is another frequent male genital problem. It may be psychogenic or caused by anatomic dysfunction, disease, or medications used to treat health problems.

The male sexual response cycle is mediated by the complex interplay of parasympathetic and sympathetic nerves. For example, penis erection is mostly parasympathetic, while ejaculation is largely attributable to sympathetic enervation. Dysfunction disorders include low sexual desire, impotence (erectile dysfunction), and lost orgiastic control (premature ejaculation). Impotence is the most frequent of these problems.

Erectile dysfunction is said to occur when the failure to complete successful intercourse occurs at least 25 to 30 percent of the time. Most often, it is short term (secondary impotence) and related to individual partners or to temporary damage to male self-esteem. Secondary impotence may also be caused by diseases such as diabetes mellitus, medications such as tranquilizers and amphetamines, alcoholism and other psychoactive drug addictions, and minor genital abnormalities. Aging is not necessarily a cause of impotence, even in octogenarians.

Long-lasting (or primary) impotence that occurs despite corrective medical treatment is generally attributable to severe psychopathology and must be treated by psychotherapy and counseling. Psychogenic impotence is implicated when an erection can be achieved by masturbation. The treatment of impotence caused by organic problems may include testosterone administration, the discontinuation of drug therapy or addictive drugs, or corrective surgery, which may include inflatable penis implants.

Male infertility is a problem found in about a third of all cases in which American couples are unable to have children. The problem is thus estimated to occur in 4 to 5 percent of American men. There are a wide number of causes for male infertility, which is always caused by the failure to deliver adequate numbers of mature sperm into the female reproductive tract as a result of organic problems. Impaired spermatogenesis, a frequent cause of male infertility, may have numerous causes. Examples include severe childhood mumps, brain and/or testicular hormone imbalances, drug abuse, obstruction or anatomic malformation of the seminal tract (especially the seminiferous tubules and epididymis), and a defective prostate gland.

Diagnosis includes careful physical examination by a urologist and evaluation of ejaculated semen to identify the number, activity, and potential for fertilization of its sperm. Blood tests will identify hormone imbalances and other possible causative agents. Many treatments are possible for male infertility, ranging from medications, to corrective surgery, to artificial insemination with sperm collected and frozen until enough are on hand to effect fertilization.

Cancer of the male genital organs may occur in the prostate, urethra, penis, or testis. The most important of these is prostate cancer. Urethral cancer is rare. More common is carcinoma of the penis, which occurs most often in uncircumcised men who practice poor genital hygiene. It is very often located beneath the foreskin and does not spread quickly. Total or partial removal of the penis is often required in advanced cases that have been ignored for long periods. Testicular cancers account for most solid genital malignancies in young men. These cancers appear as painful scrotal masses which increase rapidly in size. Any large, firm mass arising from a testis is suspicious and should be examined immediately by X ray, computed tomography (CT) scan, and tests for various tumor markers seen in the blood. Treatment of these tumors includes surgery, radiation, and chemotherapy. Survival rates vary greatly and depend upon the cancer type. Cancer of the prostate and other male genital organs is not clearly understood and may have hormonal and chemical bases. It is believed that periodic self-examination is the most valuable preventive methodology.

Common disorders of the male genital organs include priapism, hydrocele and spermatocele, testicular torsion, and varicocele. Priapism is persistent, painful erection not accompanied by sexual arousal. It is caused by a poorly understood mechanism and is characterized by both pain and much-thickened blood in the corpora cavernosa. Priapism often occurs after prolonged sexual activity and may accompany prostate problems, genital infections such as syphilis, and addictive drug use. Treatment of priapism includes spinal anesthesia, anticoagulants, and surgery. In the absence of prompt, effective treatment, priapism may end male sexual function permanently.

Hydrocele is a common, noncancerous scrotum lesion most common in men over forty. The problem is caused by fluid accumulation resulting from testis inflammation. Hydrocele is not painful and is removed surgically only if excessive in size. Closely related in appearance is a spermatocele, which contains sperm and occurs adjacent to an epididymis. Both hydroceles and spermatoceles are said to transilluminate: They are both so transparent that a flashlight beam will pass through them. Testicular torsion is a twisting of the vas deferens, which causes pain and swelling; surgery is required to return blood flow to the testis. Varicocele describes varicose veins of the testis, which is common and usually harmless.

Sexually transmitted diseases can also affect the male genitals. These diseases include herpes, gonorrhea, syphilis, chlamydia, and genital warts. For the prevention of sexually transmitted diseases, abstention, the careful choice of sexual partners, and the use of male or female condoms are useful.

PERSPECTIVE AND PROSPECTS

Treatment of the various types of male genital disorders and diseases has evolved greatly. Particularly valuable are the strides made in the treatment of impotence. It has been realized that such sexual dysfunction is often a consequence of organic problems that may be remedied by the cessation of causative medication use or by minor surgery. In addition, the utilization of inflatable penis implants in the cases where insoluble psychogenic or organic problems occur has been a milestone in the treatment of this emotionally devastating male genital problem.

Wide examination of the entire spectrum of male genital problems has led to numerous advantageous treatments and to an understanding that withholding unneeded medical treatments can be beneficial. For example, information regarding spermatoceles, hydroceles, and many related nonacute male genital problems has decreased the incidence of unnecessary male genital surgery, and its related risks, for patients.

Another important concept is that of frequent self-examination of the male genitals. This practice has led to a shortening of the time lag between the ap-

pearance of a suspicious mass in the scrotum, testes, or other male sex organ and medical attention from professionals (such as urologists) trained both to evaluate their seriousness and to treat them. Early detection has diminished the severity of many genital cancers and facilitated their treatment. Moreover, several clinical tests for such lesions have become more available and more widely used by the public.

It is hoped that these avenues and others, as well as further advances in both diagnostic techniques and treatment possibilities, will eventually eradicate male genital diseases and disorders. Two areas in need of advancements are priapism and prostate cancer, which is an effective killer.

—*Sanford S. Singer, Ph.D.*

See also Candidiasis; Chlamydia; Circumcision, male; Gonorrhea; Herpes; Hydrocelectomy; Hypospadias repair and urethroplasty; Infertility in males; Orchitis; Penile implant surgery; Prostate cancer; Prostate gland; Prostate gland removal; Reproductive system; Sexual dysfunction; Sexuality; Sexually transmitted diseases; Sterilization; Stones; Syphilis; Testicles, undescended; Testicular surgery; Testicular torsion; Urology; Urology, pediatric; Vasectomy; Warts.

FOR FURTHER INFORMATION:

American Psychiatric Association. *Diagnostic and Statistical Manual of Mental Disorders: DSM-IV-TR*. Rev. 4th ed. Washington, D.C.: Author, 2000. This compilation includes diagnostic criteria and other useful facts about mental problems associated with male genital diseases. It thus provides insight into the psychogenic aspects of these afflictions.

Berkow, Robert, and Andrew J. Fletcher, eds. *The Merck Manual of Diagnosis and Therapy*. 17th ed. Rahway, N.J.: Merck Sharp & Dohme Research Laboratories, 1999. This book abounds with useful data on the characteristics, etiology, diagnosis, and treatment of male genital disorders and diseases. Written for physicians, it is also quite useful to general readers.

Montague, Drogo K. *Disorders of Male Sexual Function*. Chicago: Year Book Medical, 1988. This medical text is useful to all readers wishing detailed information on aspects of men's health, including male reproductive anatomy and physiology, terminology, clinical evaluation, pharmacology, and the treatment of male sexual diseases.

Sherwood, Lauralee. *Human Physiology: From Cells to Systems*. 4th ed. Belmont, Calif.: Wadsworth, 2001. This college text contains useful information on the male genital system, background endocrinology, spermatogenesis, aspects of sexual dysfunction, and sexually transmitted diseases in men. Also a source of many explanatory illustrations.

Geriatrics and Gerontology

Specialties

Anatomy or system affected: All
Specialties and related fields: All
Definition: Geriatrics refers to the social and health care of the elderly; gerontology is the study of the aging process.

Key terms:

decubitus ulcer: ulceration of the skin and subcutaneous tissues, resulting from protein deficiency and prolonged, unrelieved pressure on bony prominences

dementia: a deterioration or loss of intellectual faculties, reasoning power, memory, and will that is caused by organic brain disease

glaucoma: an eye disease characterized by increased intraocular pressure, which can lead to degeneration of the optic nerve and ultimately blindness if left untreated

Medicare: the popular designation for 1965 amendments to the U.S. Social Security Act, providing hospitalization and certain other benefits to people over the age of sixty-five

polypharmacy: the prescription of many drugs at one time, often resulting in excessive use of medications and adverse drug interactions

prostate: in men, the organ surrounding the neck of the urinary bladder and beginning of the urethra; its secretions make up about 40 percent of semen

The Study of Aging

The field of geriatrics deals with the care of the elderly. The U.S. government's definition of elderly includes persons sixty-five years or older. Geriatricians are physicians with specialized training in geriatric medicine who restrict their practices to caring for persons seventy-five years or older. These patients are most likely to suffer from specific geriatric syndromes, including dementia, delirium, urinary incontinence, malnutrition, osteoporosis, falls and immobility, decubitus ulcers, polypharmacy, and sleep disorders. The majority of older persons in the United States live in family settings with their spouses or children. Approximately 30 percent of older persons live alone, the majority of them being women. The proportion of older persons (those over 65) who live in nursing homes is about 5 percent; this number increases strikingly with age, with 22 percent of Americans aged eighty-five or older residing in a nursing home.

The focus of geriatric medicine is on improving functional disability and treating chronic disease conditions that impair a person's ability to perform such activities of daily living as bathing and dressing, maintaining urinary and bowel continence, and eating. A more objective measure of an older person's ability to live independently is the instrumental activities of daily living scale. This scale measures an individual's ability to use the telephone, obtain transportation, go shopping, prepare meals, do housework and laundry, self-administer medicines, and manage money.

The maximum life span of an organism is the theoretical longest duration of that organism's life, excluding premature, unnatural death. The maximum life span of humans is unknown, although most experts believe it to be approximately 120 years. Most people will die of disease or accident, however, before they reach this biological limit. Attempts to understand why this occurs have led to the development of several theories of aging. The aging process is controlled, in large part, by genetic mechanisms. Aging is a biologic process characterized by a progressive development and maturation leading to senescence and death. There are profound changes in cells, tissues, and organs as well as in physiological, cognitive, and psychological processes. Aging is not the acquisition of disease, although aging and disease can be related. In the absence of disease, normal aging is a slow process. It involves the steady decline of organ reserves and homeostatic control mechanisms, which is often not apparent unless there is maximal exertion or stress on an individual system or on the total organism.

Numerous changes in the body occur as people age. For example, one can expect to lose two inches in height from age forty to age eighty. This shrinkage results from a decrease in vertebral bone mass and in the thickness of intervertebral disks, as well as from postural alterations with increased flexion or bending at the hips and knees. Total body fat increases as one ages, accompanied by decreases in muscle mass and total body water. Such changes in body composition have important implications for drug treatments and nutritional plans. For example, fat-soluble medications exhibit a longer duration of action in the elderly. Older persons also experience a thinning of the dermal layer of the skin, with thinner blood vessels, decreased collagen, and less skin elasticity. Sun damage can accelerate these changes. Graying of the hair reflects a progressive loss of functional melanocytes from the hair bulbs. The number of hair follicles of the scalp decreases, as does the growth rate of remaining follicles. The brain also alters with age: The weight of the brain declines, blood flow to the brain decreases, and there is a loss of neurons in specific areas of the brain. These changes in brain structure are highly variable and do not necessarily affect thinking and behavior.

Many changes occur in the vision of the older person. Loss of elasticity in the lens leads to presbyopia, the most common visual problem associated with aging. Presbyopia is a condition in which the distance that is needed to focus on near objects increases. Cataracts increase in prevalence with age, although unprotected exposure of the eyes to ultraviolet rays has been implicated in the pathogenesis as well. Glaucoma also occurs more often in the elderly.

Older persons often experience hearing loss from degenerative processes, including atrophy of the external auditory canal and thickening of the tympanic membrane. The result is presbycusis, a bilateral hearing loss for pure tones. Higher frequencies are more affected than lower ones, and the condition is more severe in men than in women. Pitch discrimination also declines with age, which may account for an increased difficulty in speech discrimination.

The heart alters with age, although the significance of these changes is unclear in the absence of disease. There are declines in intrinsic contractile function and electrical activity. The resting heart rate and cardiac output do not change, but the maximum heart rate decreases in a linear fashion and may be estimated by subtracting a person's age from 220. There are also modest increases in systolic blood pressure.

Minor changes occur in the gastrointestinal system. The liver and pancreas maintain adequate function throughout life, although the metabolism of specific drugs is prolonged in older people. Kidney function declines with age, with a 30 percent loss in renal mass and a decrease in renal blood flow. A linear decline in the ability of the kidneys to filter blood after the age of forty can lead to a decrease in the clearance of some drugs from the body.

In the endocrine system, the blood glucose level before meals changes minimally after the age of forty, although the level of blood glucose after meals increases. These changes may be related to decreases in muscle mass and a decreased insulin secretion rate. Glucose intolerance with aging must be distinguished from the hyperglycemia that can accompany diabetes mellitus; the latter requires treatment. No clinically significant alterations in the levels of the thyroid hormone occur, although the end organ response to thyroid hormones may be decreased. The hypothalamic-pituitary-adrenal axis remains intact. Plasma basal and stimulated norepinephrine levels are higher in healthy elderly individuals than in the young. The secretion of hormones such as androgens and estrogens falls sharply as a result of the loss of endocrine cells.

DISEASES THAT COMMONLY AFFECT THE ELDERLY

One of the chronic diseases frequently seen in elderly people is osteoporosis. Osteoporosis is defined as a decreased amount of bone per unit of volume; mineralization of the bone remains normal. Many studies have shown that bone mass decreases with age. Vertebral fractures resulting from osteoporosis cause deformity of the spine, loss in height, and pain. The absolute number of vertebral fractures that occur in older persons has been difficult to estimate, as some of these fractures go undiagnosed. The approximately 200,000 hip fractures that the elderly in the United States suffer annually have much more serious consequences. The lifetime risk of hip fracture by the age of eighty is approximately 15 percent for white women and 7 percent for white men. The risk of hip fracture by this age is significantly less in African Americans, with a 6 percent risk for women and a 3 percent risk for men.

One approach to preventing osteoporosis is to maximize the amount of bone that is formed during adolescence. Under normal circumstances, people begin to experience a net bone loss after the age of thirty-five. In women, the onset of menopause accelerates bone loss because of the decline in estrogen levels. Relative calcium deficiency has also been implicated in age-related osteoporosis. By definition, age-related osteoporosis is a diagnosis of exclusion. An older patient who has suffered a fracture first should be evaluated for other causes of osteoporosis, including hyperparathyroidism, hyperthyroidism, diabetes, glucocorticoid excess, or, in men, hypogonadism. Other secondary causes of osteoporosis include malignancy, such as multiple myeloma, leukemia, or lymphoma, and the drug-related effects of alcohol or steroids. Any identifiable causes should be corrected.

People at increased risk for age-related osteoporosis include those with a family history of the disease; light hair, skin, and eyes; and a small body frame. Bone densitometry or quantitative computed tomography (CT) scanning can be performed to provide the most accurate estimates of the risk of an initial fracture. There are a number of prevention and treatment strategies for patients. One should ensure an adequate calcium intake; the current recommendation is a daily intake of 1,200 milligrams of calcium for postmenopausal women. Weight-bearing exercise should be performed throughout the life span. In postmenopausal women, estrogen treatment is often given. While estrogen has not been shown conclusively to increase bone density, it does prevent further bone loss. In patients who cannot take estrogen, an alternative treatment is the hormone calcitonin. Calcitonin works by inhibiting osteoclast function, thereby halting the otherwise normal breakdown of bone.

A disorder that is commonly seen in elderly men is benign prostatic hypertrophy. The incidence of this disease increases in a progressive fashion, with approximately 90 percent of men aged eighty affected by this condition. The pathogenesis of prostatic hypertrophy is hormonal, caused by increased levels of dihydrotestosterone formed from the testosterone within the gland itself. The usual symptoms are those of urinary obstruction, which include hesitancy, straining, and decreased force and dimension of the urinary stream. Screening for benign prostatic hypertrophy includes two parts. The first is a blood test for prostate-specific antigens. The second is a digital rectal exam to inspect the prostate gland. Patients with positive findings will require further evaluation. A significant increase in prostatic tissue may need to be removed surgically. In patients with minimal disease, drug treatment may be used. Finesteride is an inhibitor of the enzyme 5-alpha reductase that is responsible for the conversion of testosterone to dihydrotestosterone. It slows the rate of increase in prostate tissue mass.

Depression is a common problem in both men and women as they get older. The elderly can experience transient mood changes that are the result of an iden-

tifiable stress or loss. In older persons, however, depression may be related to some medical condition, particularly dementia, which is associated with multiple strokes or Parkinson's disease. Major depression is more common in hospital and long-term care settings, where the prevalence is about 13 percent. The symptoms of depression include significant weight change, insomnia or hypersomnia, psychomotor agitation or retardation, decreased energy and easy fatigability, feelings of worthlessness or excessive guilt, decreased ability to think or concentrate, and recurrent thoughts of death or suicide. The diagnosis of major depression can be made if at least five of these symptoms are present for at least two weeks. Depressive symptoms must be taken seriously in the elderly. The rate of suicide in older persons is higher than for other groups, with older white males having the highest rates of any age, racial, or ethnic group.

Another depressive disorder experienced by the elderly is dysthymia. Dysthymic disorders are characterized by less severe symptoms than those associated with major depression and by a duration of at least two years. The symptoms generally include at least two of the following: poor appetite or overeating, insomnia or hypersomnia, low energy and fatigue, low self-esteem, poor concentration or difficulty in making decisions, and feelings of hopelessness. Dysthymia may be primary or secondary to a preexisting chronic psychiatric or medical illness, with accompanying loss of function and debilitation.

Adjustment disorders with depressed mood are also seen in older persons. Such disorders occur within three months of a stressful situation and last up to six months. The prototypical situation is the depressive reaction that follows an acute medical illness. In the elderly, the four most common stressors are physical illness, reactions to the death of family and friends, retirement, and moving to an institutional setting. In dealing with depressive symptoms, however, it is important to consider other diagnoses, such as underlying medical illnesses, drug reactions to prescribed or over-the-counter medicines, hypochondriasis, alcohol abuse, and dementias. In older patients, the disorder most often associated with depression is dementia.

A thorough diagnostic evaluation can help in the diagnosis of a depressive disorder and can rule out other complicating problems. A careful history is elicited from the patient and from a family member or caretaker. A formal mental status examination is conducted to uncover abnormalities in concentration, speech, psychomotor skills, cognitive ability, and memory. Laboratory blood tests often include a complete blood count, chemical analysis, and thyroid function tests. Abbreviated neuropsychological tests can differentiate between patients with dementia and those with depression alone. The treatment of depression includes psychotherapy and pharmacotherapy. Behavioral interventions, such as special weekly activities and assignments, can be helpful. Most often, some kind of antidepressant medication is effective.

PERSPECTIVE AND PROSPECTS

In the United States, there has been increasing interest in the fields of geriatrics and gerontology because of the country's changing demographics. In 1989, thirty-one million Americans were sixty-five years of age and older. This represents about one in eight persons. Because of the very large numbers in the baby-boom age group—that is, people born between 1945 and 1964—it is expected that the number of elderly people will increase dramatically by the year 2030 to about sixty-five million elderly persons. The elderly will compose approximately 22 percent of the total U.S. population.

Another reason for the increase in the size of the older population in the United States is an increase in life expectancy. Life expectancy is defined as the average number of years a person is expected to live, given population mortality rates. It can be calculated for any age category but is usually given as life expectancy from birth. The life expectancy in the United States is much higher than in undeveloped countries and in most other developed countries as well. This figure rose steadily throughout the twentieth century. A child born in 1988 could expect to live seventy-five years, while someone born in 1900 could expect to live only fifty years. Most of this increase in life expectancy is attributable to a decreased death rate for infants and children resulting from improvements in sanitation, active immunization against childhood diseases, and advances in medical treatments. For persons aged sixty-five, there was an increase in life expectancy over that same time period of only five years, probably the result of improved medical therapies.

As Americans live longer, the length of time that older persons will rely on society for their care increases as well. This situation places a greater burden on those persons who are working, as they must support greater numbers of people receiving Social Security and Medicare benefits, and requires a rethinking of the age requirements to be eligible for these programs. In 1997, while older persons represented 13 percent of the population, they accounted for 38 percent of the total costs for health care. Other factors adding to the cost of health care include such new technologies as specialized imaging equipment, complex laboratory procedures, and new therapeutic drugs. The goal of much research in geriatric medicine is to prevent or slow down the effects of aging so that the elderly may live in good health. Further research to understand better the mechanisms involved in human aging will help to design preventive and treatment strategies.

—*RoseMarie Pasmantier, M.D.;*
updated by L. Fleming Fallon, Jr.,
M.D., Ph.D., M.P.H.

See also Aging; Aging: Extended care; Alzheimer's disease; Arthritis; Bed-wetting; Blindness; Bone disorders; Brain disorders; Cataract surgery; Cataracts; Critical care; Death and dying; Dementias; Depression; Domestic violence; Emergency medicine; Endocrinology; Estrogen replacement therapy; Euthanasia; Family practice; Fatigue; Hearing loss; Hip fracture repair; Hormone replacement therapy; Hospitals; Incontinence; Memory loss; Nursing; Nutrition; Ophthalmology; Orthopedics; Osteoporosis; Pain management; Paramedics; Parkinson's disease; Pharmacology; Physician assistants; Psychiatry; Psychiatry, geriatric; Rheumatology; Sleep disorders; Spinal cord disorders; Spine, vertebrae, and disks; Suicide; Visual disorders.

FOR FURTHER INFORMATION:

Coni, Nicholas, and Steven Webster. *Lecture Notes on Geriatrics.* 5th ed. Oxford, England: Blackwell Scientific, 1998. Easy-to-read study notes on geriatric medicine. Discusses the different changes that occur in the patient during the aging process and characterizes the different diseases seen in the elderly.

Coni, Nicholas, William Davison, and Stephen Webster. *Ageing: The Facts.* 2d ed. London: Oxford University Press, 1992. This manageable volume contains a wealth of data and information related to aging. It is written for general readers.

Ferri, Fred F., Marsha Fretwell, and Tom J. Wachtel. *Practical Guide to the Care of the Geriatric Patient.* 2d ed. St. Louis: Mosby Year Book, 1997. An excellent resource. The text is clearly written, and the index is especially useful. Nonprofessional readers will have no trouble understanding this book.

Hampton, Roy, and Charles Russell. *The Encyclopedia of Aging and the Elderly.* New York: Facts on File, 1992. Much well-stated information is presented. The scope is broad—lifestyle, myths and misconceptions, medical and legal concerns, death and dying. Statistical information is presented in charts and tables, appendices list organizations, and the bibliography is useful.

Isaacs, Bernard. *The Challenge of Geriatric Medicine.* London: Oxford Medical, 1992. This volume presents the issues associated with geriatric medicine and the care of older citizens. It is well written and should be of interest to most readers who want additional information on this subject.

Margolis, Simeon, and Hamilton Moses III, eds. *The Johns Hopkins Medical Handbook: The One Hundred Major Medical Disorders of People over the Age of Fifty.* Rev. ed. Garden City, N.Y.: Random House, 1999. This definitive home medical reference for adults offers an in-depth guide to the most common medical problems occurring in adults over fifty. The directory of hospitals and other health care resources, from support groups to treatment centers, is comprehensive.

Stenchever, Morton A. *Health Care for the Older Woman.* New York: Chapman and Hall, 1996. A reference that provides medical practitioners and students with comprehensive, current information specific to the care of middle-aged and advanced-aged women. It covers health maintenance issues, including diet, exercise, safety, psychological and psychosocial problems, social problems, and grief and loss.

GERMAN MEASLES. *See* CHILDHOOD INFECTIOUS DISEASES; RUBELLA.

GESTATION. *See* PREGNANCY AND GESTATION.

GIARDIASIS
DISEASE/DISORDER

ANATOMY OR SYSTEM AFFECTED: Gastrointestinal system

SPECIALTIES AND RELATED FIELDS: Family practice, gastroenterology, pediatrics

DEFINITION: An acute or chronic parasitic infection of the gastrointestinal system.

CAUSES AND SYMPTOMS
The parasite *Giardia lamblia*, which causes giardiasis, is acquired through the ingestion of contaminated food or water. This organism can also be spread by person-to-person contact involving fecal contamination. It is the most frequent parasite acquired by children in day care centers and preschools.

After exposure, the incubation period before the onset of symptoms is one to two weeks. After infection, only 25 to 50 percent of affected individuals become symptomatic. The disease is characterized by abdominal pain, cramps, flatulence, weight loss, and diarrhea, which in many cases may be chronic (of a duration longer than fifteen days).

TREATMENT AND THERAPY
Some cases of giardiasis are self-limited. Symptomatic cases, however, in which the diagnosis has been confirmed by laboratory studies, need to be treated. Furazolidone, metronidazole, and paromomycin are effective drugs in the treatment of giardiasis. Furazolidone and metronidazole are equally efficacious; the first may be more practical in children because of its availability in liquid form.

Giardiasis can be prevented by strict hand-washing, especially in those individuals who are in close contact with patients with diarrhea or children in diapers at day care centers. Another important consideration in the prevention of giardiasis resides in the purification of drinking water, which can be achieved through boiling or chemical decontamination. It has been demonstrated that breast-feeding protects infants against symptomatic infection.

PERSPECTIVE AND PROSPECTS
G. lamblia was first observed by microscopist Antoni van Leeuwenhoek in 1675. It was once considered a harmless organism, but its pathogenic role was clearly established in the 1960's. This parasite is one of the most common protozoans able to infect humans in the United States and other developed countries.

—*Benjamin Estrada, M.D.*

See also Diarrhea and dysentery; Food poisoning; Gastroenterology; Gastroenterology, pediatric; Gastrointestinal system; Parasitic diseases.

FOR FURTHER INFORMATION:
Gracey, Michael, ed. *Diarrhea.* Boca Raton, Fla.: CRC Press, 1991.

Greenberger, Norton J. *Gastrointestinal Disorders: A Pathophysiologic Approach*. 4th ed. Chicago: Year Book Medical, 1989.

Thompson, W. Grant. *Gut Reactions: Understanding Symptoms of the Digestive Tract*. New York: Plenum Press, 1989.

Walker, W. Allan, et al., eds. *Pediatric Gastrointestinal Disease: Pathophysiology, Diagnosis, Management*. 3d ed. St. Louis, Mo.: C. V. Mosby, 2000.

GIGANTISM

DISEASE/DISORDER

ANATOMY OR SYSTEM AFFECTED: Arms, bones, brain, circulatory system, endocrine system, eyes, hands, hair, legs, musculoskeletal system, reproductive system

SPECIALTIES AND RELATED FIELDS: Biochemistry, cardiology, endocrinology, family practice, general surgery, internal medicine, neurology

DEFINITION: A rare congenital disease that begins in children with pituitary gland tumors that make too much growth hormone, which yields pituitary giants who often die at relatively young ages. After adolescence, the disease is manifested as acromegaly, which is quite serious over the long term.

KEY TERMS:

acromegaly: a disease of adults initially characterized by pathological enlargement of bones of the hands, feet, and face; caused by chronic pituitary gland overproduction of growth hormone by tumors

congenital: referring to a condition (such as a health problem) present or occurring at birth

growth hormone: a hormone produced by the pituitary gland that mediates overall growth

pituitary gland: a peanut-sized gland at the base of the vertebrate brain; its hormone secretions control many other hormone-producing (endocrine) glands and hence control growth, gender maturation, and many other life processes

CAUSES AND SYMPTOMS

Gigantism is a rare disease caused by the presence of tumors of the peanut-sized pituitary gland, located at the base of the brain. Such tumors produce an excess of growth hormone, the biomolecule responsible for overall growth. In children or adolescents having these tumors, excess growth hormone results in overgrowth of all parts of the body. Gigantism occurs because the bones of the arms and legs have not yet cal-

cified and can grow much longer than usual. Hence, an afflicted child becomes very large in size and very tall, often reaching a height of more than 6 feet, 6 inches.

A young child afflicted with pituitary gigantism grows in height as much as 6 inches per year. Thus, an important symptom that identifies the problem is that such children are much taller and larger than others of the same age. In many cases, this great size difference may lead to individuals who are more than twice the height of their playmates. Excessive growth of this sort should lead parents to seek the immediate advice of their family physician, who can aid in the selection of a specialist to identify the problem and develop an appropriate treatment.

As gigantism proceeds, pituitary tumors often invade and replace the rest of the pituitary gland. This is unfortunate, because the pituitary gland produces several other hormones—called trophic hormones—which control mental processes, gender maturation, and healthy overall growth. Consequently, prolonged, untreated gigantism may yield a huge individual who is mentally ill, possessed of various psychoses, sexually immature, and quite unhealthy. In addition, the human musculoskeletal system is not designed to accommodate individuals attaining the great heights of many postadolescent pituitary giants. Hence, it is fairly common that the giants have great difficulty standing and walking; some can do so only with the aid of canes. Moreover, the average life expectancy of a full-sized pituitary giant is shorter than that of individuals of normal stature, and many die by the middle of the third decade of their lives.

In cases where pituitary tumors that oversecrete growth hormone occur after calcification of the long bones is complete—after adolescence—gigantism will not occur. Such individuals develop acromegaly. This often-fatal disease, progressive throughout life, thickens bones and causes the overgrowth of all body organs. Hands and feet grow larger, and the lower jaw, brow ridges, nose, and ears enlarge, coarsening the features. More damaging is the development of headaches, high blood pressure that can lead to heart attacks, irritability, and even cancer over the long run. It should be noted that these disabilities are rarely seen in pediatric patients and most often begin in the fourth decade of life. Many medical scientists believe that pituitary gigantism and acromegaly are the basis for the legends about giants and ogres.

TREATMENT AND THERAPY

If a diagnosis of gigantism or acromegaly seems probable, the physician or specialist involved will order a blood test to identify the amount of growth hormone present in the body. Computed tomography (CT) and magnetic resonance imaging (MRI) scans will also be carried out, especially in those suspected of having acromegaly, to identify possible organ changes away from normal size. In cases where growth hormone levels are high and cannot be reduced by chemotherapy—for example, with antigrowth hormone drugs such as somatostatin and bromocriptine—and/or a tumor is identified as being present via CT and MRI, surgery or radiation therapy to destroy the tumor will be attempted.

PERSPECTIVE AND PROSPECTS

It must be recognized that the success of any therapeutic regimens or their combination will prevent additional gigantism or symptoms of acromegaly from occurring. It is not possible, however, to reverse preexisting consequences of the pituitary tumors on young children and adolescent pituitary giants or older giants and acromegalics.

For this reason, it is essential for worried parents or adult patients to visit an appropriate physician as quickly as possible. Such foresight will usually minimize problems associated with either manifestation of pituitary tumors and enable an afflicted individual to have the best possible future life. In addition to extirpating causative tumors, it will then become possible, after additional blood tests plus the thorough examination of CT and MRI data, to identify which body organs need to be treated and to arrest or minimize health complications, such as those associated with the reproductive, cardiovascular, and musculoskeletal systems.

—Sanford S. Singer, Ph.D.

See also Birth defects; Bones and the skeleton; Congenital heart disease; Dwarfism; Endocrine disorders; Endocrine system; Endocrinology; Endocrinology, pediatric; Growth; Hormones; Orthopedics, pediatric.

FOR FURTHER INFORMATION:

Berkow, Robert, and Andrew J. Fletcher, eds. *Merck Manual of Diagnosis and Therapy*. 17th ed. Rahway, N.J.: Merck Sharp & Dohme Research Laboratories, 1999. This book abounds with useful data on the characteristics, etiology, diagnosis, and treatment of gigantism. Written for physicians, it is also quite useful to general readers.

Clayman, Charles B, ed. *American Medical Association Family Medical Guide*. New York: Random House, 1994. An excellent reference for the beginner. The scientific accuracy of the text is not compromised by its accessibility.

Imura, Hiroo, ed. *The Pituitary Gland*. 2d ed. New York: Raven Press, 1994. Discusses such topics as the physiology of the pituitary gland, pituitary hormones, the hypothalmo-hypophyseal system, and the diagnosis of pituitary diseases.

Landau, Elaine. *Standing Tall: Unusually Tall People*. New York: Franklin Watts, 1997. This respectful treatment of a sensitive subject opens with actual, personal stories. It explores the role of unusually sized characters in folklore, then explains the causes and challenges of uncommon growth patterns.

Tierney, Lawrence M., Jr., et al., eds. *Current Medical Diagnosis and Treatment: 2001*. 39th ed. New York: McGraw-Hill, 2000. This text, updated yearly, is the point of reference for physicians and other health care practitioners. It incorporates each year's biomedical research discoveries that have immediate, relevant, and applicable use for the patient.

GINGIVITIS

DISEASE/DISORDER

ANATOMY OR SYSTEM AFFECTED: Gums, mouth, teeth

SPECIALTIES AND RELATED FIELDS: Dentistry

DEFINITION: A superficial inflammation of the gums, gingivitis is associated with a destructive buildup of plaque on the gums and between the teeth. The plaque contains bacterial toxins and enzymes that cause irritation, resulting in red, swollen gums that bleed easily. The infection may progress slowly and almost unnoticeably until pockets form between the teeth and gums. If left untreated, the condition can result in periodontitis, in which the teeth detach from the gums. Good oral hygiene can help prevent plaque formation, but professional scaling of the teeth is necessary to remove the deposits that develop.

—Jason Georges and Tracy Irons-Georges

See also Cavities; Dental diseases; Dentistry; Endodontic disease; Periodontal surgery; Periodontitis; Root canal treatment; Teeth; Tooth extraction; Toothache.

Development of Gingivitis

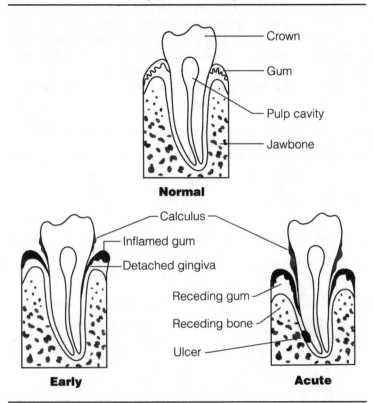

Normal

Crown
Gum
Pulp cavity
Jawbone

Calculus
Inflamed gum
Detached gingiva
Receding gum
Receding bone
Ulcer

Early

Acute

FOR FURTHER INFORMATION:

Smith, Rebecca W. *The Columbia University School of Dental and Oral Surgery's Guide to Family Dental Care*. New York: W. W. Norton, 1997.

Ward, Brian R. *Dental Care*. New York: Franklin Watts, 1986.

Woodall, Irene R., ed. *Comprehensive Dental Hygiene Care*. 4th ed. St. Louis: C. V. Mosby, 1993.

GLANDS

ANATOMY

ANATOMY OR SYSTEM AFFECTED: Breasts, endocrine system, gastrointestinal system, genitals, nervous system, pancreas, reproductive system, skin

SPECIALTIES AND RELATED FIELDS: Biochemistry, dermatology, endocrinology, gastroenterology, gynecology, vascular medicine

DEFINITION: Organs or areas of the body that produce, store, and secrete fluids, exerting a profound effect on growth, energy production, chemical balance, reproduction, and health.

KEY TERMS:

adrenal glands: the endocrine glands on top of the kidneys, which produce a large number of hormones involved in metabolism and in response to stress

endocrine system: the system of glands located throughout the body that produces hormones and secretes them directly into the blood for delivery by the circulatory system

hormone: a product of the endocrine glands transported throughout the bloodstream which controls and regulates other glands or organs by chemical stimulation

pancreas: the gland located under the stomach that produces insulin and glucagon, the hormones responsible for control of the body's blood sugar level

parathyroid glands: four tiny structures on the back of the thyroid, chiefly concerned with the regulation of calcium and phosphorus

pituitary gland: a tiny gland located under the brain which controls the thyroid, adrenal, and sex glands

sex glands: the ovaries in the female and the testes in the male, which secrete hormones involved in reproduction

thyroid gland: an endocrine gland located in the neck, which regulates the rate of energy production throughout the body

STRUCTURE AND FUNCTIONS

A gland is any tissue or organ that produces and releases a fluid. Some, such as digestive or sweat glands, secrete their juices through a duct or tube. These glands are known as exocrine glands, meaning "externally secreting." Other glands pass their secretions directly into the blood that flows through them. Known as endocrine or "internally secreting" glands, these are the ones that produce hormones. This article will focus only on the endocrine glands and their hormones that control, stimulate, and regulate almost every important function in the body.

Although there are hundreds of known or suspected hormones, there are only several major endocrine glands to produce them. They include the pituitary, pineal gland, and hypothalamus in the brain; the thyroid, parathyroid glands, and thymus in the neck; and the adrenal glands and pancreas in the abdomen. In addition, the female ovaries in the pelvic cavity and the male testes in the scrotum contribute their hormones to the widespread work of the endocrine system.

The largest endocrine organ, the thyroid, is quite small, weighing only about an ounce. It is butterfly-shaped and wrapped around the windpipe in the throat. By means of the two iodine-containing hormones that it produces, called thyroxine (T_4) and triiodothyronine (T_3), this gland controls the rate of the body's metabolism; that is, these hormones control the speed at which energy-producing chemical reactions occur in all the cells of the body. They also play a crucial role in oxygen use, protein synthesis,

The Major Glands of the Human Body

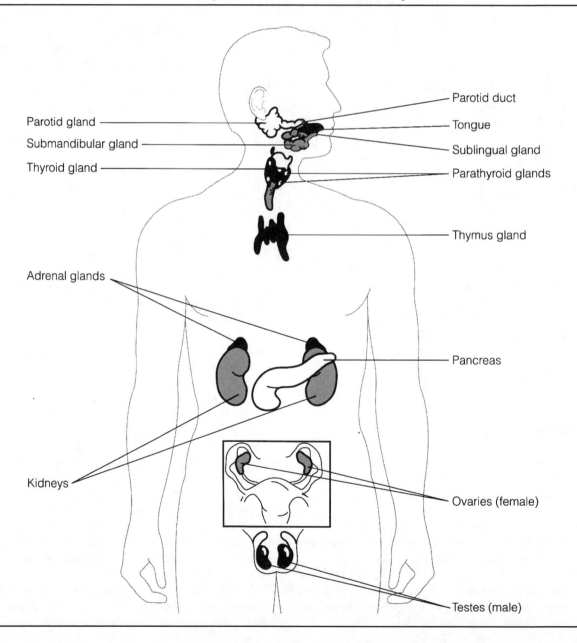

Parotid duct

Parotid gland

Tongue

Submandibular gland

Sublingual gland

Thyroid gland

Parathyroid glands

Thymus gland

Adrenal glands

Pancreas

Kidneys

Ovaries (female)

Testes (male)

and the development of the central nervous system. A third thyroid secretion, calcitonin, has a completely different role. By opposing the work of the parathyroids discussed below, it prevents the existence of too much calcium in the blood.

The four tiny parathyroid glands on the back of the thyroid are each only 0.25-inch wide. They supply parathyroid hormone, which maintains the proper balance of calcium in various parts of the body. It is very important to the bones, nerves, muscles, and blood that each contain the exact amount of calcium needed to function correctly. If there is not enough calcium, parathyroid hormone instructs the intestine to absorb more calcium and the kidneys to retain more. If the blood still has an insufficient level of calcium, parathyroid hormone causes it to be released from storage in the bones.

The pancreas, found behind the stomach, is unusual because it is both an exocrine gland, producing digestive enzymes for the intestine, and an important endocrine gland. Its major hormones, insulin and glucagon, are the major regulators of the blood sugar level. Soon after a meal is digested, insulin is released, enabling all cells in general but liver cells in particular to take excess sugar out of the blood at a rapid rate. The liver's stored sugar is then released steadily into the blood between meals because of the steady glucagon production in the pancreas. The careful balancing of these two hormones enables the body to have just the right sugar content in the blood at all times.

The hormones that bring about the most striking changes in both anatomy and behavior are known as the sex hormones. Because sex hormone levels are high in the fetus, they directly influence the development of its sex organs.

Somewhere around the age of eleven, the level of a girl's estrogens rises sharply, causing female puberty. These hormones, produced in the two ovaries (located in the pelvic cavity), cause breast development, the growth of pubic and underarm hair, and the broadening of hips and thighs. Each month of the woman's life until the menopause, the ovarian estrogen and progesterone levels rise and fall, controlling the release of an egg or ovum from her ovary. These same hormones have prepared the uterus to support and nourish a developing embryo if the egg is fertilized.

The two testes, located in the scrotal sac, by their production of testosterone and other androgens bring about male puberty around the age of thirteen. These hormones are responsible for such male secondary sex characteristics as facial hair, deepening of the voice, and heavier muscles and bones. The testes' secretions seem also to cause the greater aggressiveness of men compared to women. Their prime function, however, is aiding the production of healthy sperm.

The two-inch-long adrenal glands, perched on top of the kidneys, are actually two glands in one. The outer 80 percent is called the cortex, while the inner part is named the medulla. The adrenals produce dozens of hormones, most of which are involved in some way with one's ability to cope with stress. One of the major adrenal cortex hormones is cortisol. It helps maintain blood pressure, regulates fluid levels, directs protein and sugar metabolism, increases or decreases body fat reserves, and affects the immune system. A second area of the cortex secretes aldosterone, which directs the kidney to retain sodium and excrete potassium, controlling their levels in the blood. The third cortex area, surprisingly, produces some testosterone and estrogen in both males and females.

The adrenal medulla responds to sudden stress by pouring epinephrine, formerly called adrenaline, into the blood. Dramatic changes in the working of the heart, lungs, liver, muscles, and many other organs then enable the body to cope with sudden emergencies.

The thymus gland, behind the breastbone, is very unusual because it is quite large in a newborn, grows throughout childhood, but shrinks drastically from puberty onward. It is the source of several important secretions, including thymosin, which activates the T cells and B cells. These lymphocytes, a type of white blood cell, provide immunity to disease by destroying invading organisms.

The tiny pineal gland, less than a quarter of an inch long, is embedded close to the very center of the brain. Although the exact function of this pinecone-shaped structure is a mystery, it appears to be the only gland producing melatonin. Proven to be involved in seasonal reproduction in other mammals, melatonin seems to be related to puberty in humans.

The careful and precise control of most of these glands is the work of the pituitary, causing it to be called "the master gland." This small gland, about 0.5 inch in size, has three distinct parts: the front or anterior pituitary, the back or posterior pituitary, and a tiny middle section.

The anterior pituitary sends thyroid-stimulating hormone (TSH) to the thyroid, causing it to release T_3 and T_4. It also secretes adrenocorticotropic hormone (ACTH), which causes the adrenal cortex to give off its many secretions. In the female, the follicle-stimulating hormone (FSH) that the anterior pituitary sends to the ovary causes an egg to mature, while in the male it fosters sperm development. Luteinizing hormone (LH), from the anterior pituitary, triggers the monthly release of an egg and then coaxes the ovary to produce progesterone. The male's LH causes clusters of cells in the testes, called interstitial cells, to produce testosterone. As if these were not enough important jobs for the anterior pituitary to have, it secretes growth hormone (GH) to stimulate body growth until maturity and secretes prolactin or lactogenic hormone to cause the female breast to produce milk for a nursing baby.

The posterior pituitary secretes only two hormones: oxytocin, which brings about labor and birth, and antidiuretic hormone (ADH), which is also known as vasopressin. ADH causes the kidney to reabsorb the proper amount of water needed by the body, a most important function.

Long after the anterior pituitary was named "the master gland," it was learned that the hypothalamus is the master of the master. This small area of tissue below the brain produces a number of releasing hormones and inhibiting hormones which, in turn, carefully control the anterior pituitary's secretion of FSH, LH, TSH, ACTH, prolactin, and growth hormone. The hypothalamus is also the source of oxytocin and ADH, which is then stored by the posterior pituitary until it is needed by the body.

DISORDERS AND DISEASES

In 1970, only a few dozen hormones from the endocrine glands were known to medical science. By 1990, at least two hundred had been discovered. An understanding of their actions and interactions has generated numerous helpful medical applications.

These complex interactions, involving the concept of feedback, have made possible many treatments for defective glands. Feedback means that healthy glands are self-regulating. For example, more calcium in the blood causes less parathyroid hormone to be released, and then the lowered amount of blood calcium causes more parathyroid hormone production. All glands have these feedback loops, but those involving the hypothalamus, pituitary, and one of its target glands are particularly complicated.

Appropriate medical treatment of thyroid disease, for example, requires careful understanding of its feedback mechanism. An increase in thyroid-stimu-

lating hormone releasing hormones (TRH) from the hypothalamus normally causes the pituitary to give off its thyroid-stimulating hormone. This in turn triggers the production of thyroxine and triiodothyronine.

The type of thyroid disease in which insufficient thyroid hormones are produced is called hypothyroidism. It is quite common, with one in every one thousand men and two in every one hundred women afflicted at some time during life. It is often caused by an inability of the thyroid gland to produce enough hormone, the result of a disease of the pituitary that prevents it from producing TSH or a disease of the hypothalamus that prevents it from producing TRH. Surprisingly, an underactive thyroid is often enlarged but still unable to produce enough T_3 or T_4. This enlargement is called a goiter. In the type called Hashimoto's disease, the hypothyroidism develops because the body mistakenly produces antibodies that destroy the thyroid tissue.

Because of the complexity of the chemical feedback loop involved in thyroid gland control, many cases of hypothyroidism have been caused inadvertently by drugs given for other conditions. Among these medicines are lithium carbonate, used to treat manic depressives; expectorants containing potassium iodide, prescribed for respiratory infections; and a host of other drugs. Physicians prescribing these drugs and patients using them need to watch carefully for the development of symptoms such as intolerance to cold, puffy face and back of hands, weight gain, high blood pressure, yellowed skin, and loss of hair.

Adults afflicted with hypothyroidism, no matter what the cause, also commonly suffer some disturbances to their nervous system, experiencing lethargy, slowness of thought, poor memory, and slowness of reaction to events occurring around them. Even more disastrous are the effects of an underactive thyroid in infants, where it causes mental retardation and stunted physical growth. If diagnosed early enough, the infant can be successfully treated in the same manner as an adult, with lifelong daily doses of TSH, T_3, and T_4 in individually and carefully adjusted amounts.

In addition, like any gland, the thyroid can oversecrete as well as undersecrete. Hypersecretion is also quite common, with three or four out of one thousand people having this disease, the majority being women. The resulting excessive rate of metabolism causes many possible symptoms including intolerance to heat, irritability, excessive perspiration, heart palpitations, rapid weight loss, weakness, shortness of breath, and sore, bulging eyes.

There are two main types of hyperthyroidism. By far the most common is called Graves' disease. It is brought about when the patient's own immune system creates antibodies that cause continuous excess hormone production by the thyroid even though the pituitary is sending the normal amount of TSH. The less common cases of hyperthyroidism involve lumps or nodules that form in the thyroid and oversecrete T_3 and T_4 for no apparent reason. One of three treatments is usually used to cure hyperthyroidism: Radioactive iodine is given to destroy part of the overactive gland, surgery is used to remove part of the gland, or certain drugs are prescribed that prevent the thyroid from producing its hormones.

As common as thyroid disorders are, there is no endocrine disorder as common as diabetes mellitus, which afflicts one out of every one thousand people. When certain cells of the pancreas are destroyed and cannot produce insulin, the person is said to have insulin-dependent diabetes (IDD). This type is most often found in children and young adults. Non-insulin-dependent diabetes (NIDD) occurs more frequently in middle-aged and older people. This condition occurs because the person's tissues become resistant to the insulin; no matter how much the pancreas tries to produce it, sugar is not able to enter the tissues properly. IDD patients are suspected to have been born with genes that make their immune systems destroy their insulin-producing pancreatic cells by mistake, after they have been exposed to certain viruses. NIDD also seems to be inherited, but stress, various illnesses, and obesity rather than viruses trigger the lack of response to insulin as the person ages.

Patients who develop either type of diabetes mellitus usually soon exhibit some if not all of the following symptoms: constant thirst and urination; loss of weight, strength, and energy; frequent hunger pains; and the inability of cuts or bruises to heal. The long-term effects of the very high blood sugar level of diabetics vary from patient to patient. They often include heart disease and high blood pressure, unhealed wounds which become gangrenous, kidney failure, endless infections, nerve damage, and possible coma.

Treatment for diabetes attempts to make the body's cells absorb sugar normally. This can often be achieved through diet, medicines that stimulate insulin production, other drugs that make the tissues more responsive to the work of insulin, and, if necessary, injections of insulin itself. These traditional methods may or may not ever be completely replaced by exciting possibilities explored in the early 1990's: insulin pumps to deliver a steady supply and full or partial pancreas transplants.

Although no one objects to attempts to aid sufferers of thyroid disorders or diabetes mellitus, ethical questions have arisen concerning defects in some endocrine glands. A striking example involves a lack of growth hormone from the pituitary. Doctors, parents, and youngsters often disagree over whether GH therapy should be given to a child who is noticeably shorter than peers at a given age. Because GH, like any hormone, may produce many unwanted side effects, there is much controversy over this particular medical application of endocrine gland research.

PERSPECTIVE AND PROSPECTS

Glands, together with the nervous system, are the body's means of control and coordination. Given this fact, the discovery of each gland's functions had ramifications for medical science as a whole.

Although the ancient Greeks, Romans, and Chinese suspected the importance of some glands, it was only in the seventeenth century that scientists began to acquire useful knowledge of them. At that time, the Englishman Thomas Wharton first recognized the difference between duct and ductless glands. In the 1660's, Théophile Bordeu, a Frenchman regarded by many as the founder of endocrinology, declared that some parts of the body gave off "emanations" that had dramatic effects on other parts of the body. Following Bordeu's lead, the Dutchman Fredrik Ruysch claimed in the 1690's that the thyroid poured important substances into the bloodstream.

Then, in 1775, Percival Platt made an unusual discovery in London while repairing a hernia in a female patient. When he inadvertently removed her ovaries, the woman's menstrual period ceased. This led John Davidge to realize the importance of the ovaries in controlling menstruation. Also in the late 1700's, doctors began to associate a swollen neck, bulging eyes, and a racing pulse with a swollen thyroid gland; they suspected a cause-and-effect relationship.

Thomas Addison, an English physician, found diseased adrenals by autopsy in a group of patients who had exhibited all the same symptoms. He published in 1849 that he definitely suspected another cause-and-effect relationship. That same year, the first experimental proof of the functions of a hormone was found by A. A. Berthold in Germany. Roosters whose testes he had removed lost all usual male characteristics. Testes that had been left free in the abdomens of other birds soon attached themselves, grew blood vessels, and produced the expected rooster characteristics.

Two major breakthroughs occurred in the late 1800's when Paul Langerhans found the actual pancreas cell clusters, called islets, that produce insulin and when Charles-Edouard Brown-Séquard developed a technique to use extracts from glands to determine their function.

The year 1900 brought three major discoveries: William Bayliss and Ernest Starling found that a chemical messenger from the intestine causes the pancreas to excrete digestive juice; Jokichi Takamine discovered that adrenaline increases heart rate and blood pressure; and Alfred Frölich described dwarfed individuals who had suffered previous pituitary damage.

In 1914, in Minnesota, Edward Kendall obtained the chemical he named thyroxine from animal thyroids. Similarly, in 1921, Frederick Banting and Charles Best isolated insulin from the pancreases of animals. By 1948, Kendall and many other workers had isolated two dozen adrenal cortex hormones; Philip Hench made medical news when he first used the one named cortisone to relieve, though not cure, arthritis.

By the mid-1970's, Rosalind Yalow and her colleagues had perfected a technique called radioimmunoassay, which uses radioactive materials to measure minute quantities of hormones. This enables physicians to measure the circulating level of nearly every hormone and diagnose anyone with an excess or deficiency. Many hormones such as insulin, growth hormone, and estrogen can then be given to supplement what the body is underproducing; these have been very expensive and hard to obtain in quantity from animals or deceased humans. By the 1980's, two new techniques called recombinant DNA and the polymerase chain reaction gave promise of unlimited, pure, and readily accessible hormones. For example, human genes transferred to yeast enable them to produce thymosin, while bacteria now produce human insulin.

Future research on the glands will continue to take many directions but is sure to focus on the dozens, if not hundreds, of secretions called prostaglandins. This army of hormonelike substances is believed to play an enormous number of roles in the human body.

—Grace D. Matzen

See also Abscess drainage; Abscesses; Addison's disease; Adrenalectomy; Brain; Breasts, female; Cyst removal; Cysts; Diabetes mellitus; Dwarfism; Endocrine disorders; Endocrinology; Endocrinology, pediatric; Gigantism; Goiter; Hormone replacement therapy; Hormones; Hyperparathyroidism and hypoparathyroidism; Hypoglycemia; Mastectomy and lumpectomy; Mumps; Pancreas; Parathyroidectomy; Prostate gland; Prostate gland removal; Systems and organs; Testicular surgery; Thyroid disorders; Thyroid gland; Thyroidectomy.

FOR FURTHER INFORMATION:

Brook, Charles G. D., and Nicholas J. Marshall. *Essential Endocrinology.* Rev. 3d ed. Cambridge, Mass.: Blackwell Science, 1996. This text addresses the field of endocrinology, describing the physiology of the endocrine glands and the hormones that they produce. Includes an index.

Clark, John, ed. *The Endocrine System: Miraculous Messenger.* New York: Torstar Books, 1985. This beautifully illustrated book presents solid factual information in a lively, highly readable manner. Provides many interesting applications of knowledge about the endocrine glands.

Little, Marjorie. *The Endocrine System.* Rev. ed. New York: Chelsea House, 2000. This volume is intended not only to provide basic knowledge but also to enable the general reader to pursue the subject through its lengthy bibliography. Also includes a helpful glossary and an extensive list of organizations which will provide further information.

Morgan, Brian L. G., and Roberta Morgan. *Hormones: How They Affect Behavior, Metabolism, Growth, Development, and Relationships.* Los Angeles: Price, Stern, Sloan, 1989. Part 1 uses simply written case histories to explain each gland and its effect on the body. Part 2 is an excellent guide to hormonal problems. A useful bibliography is included.

Shaw, Michael, ed. *Everything You Need to Know About Diseases.* Springhouse, Pa.: Springhouse, 1996. This well-illustrated consumer reference, compiled by more than one hundred doctors and medical experts, describes five hundred illnesses and conditions, their causes, symptoms, diagnosis, treatment, and prevention. Of particular interest is chapter 12, "Hormone and Gland Disorders." Rev. ed. New York: Prentice Hall, 1987. An excellent reference for those particularly interested in the pancreas gland and diabetes. Contains an extensive list of sources from which more information may be obtained.

GLAUCOMA

DISEASE/DISORDER

ANATOMY OR SYSTEM AFFECTED: Eyes

SPECIALTIES AND RELATED FIELDS: Ophthalmology, optometry

DEFINITION: A group of eye diseases characterized by an increase in the eye's intraocular pressure; early diagnosis through regular eye examinations can manage the effects of the disease, while late diagnosis may result in impaired vision or blindness.

KEY TERMS:

aqueous humor: the liquid filling the space between the lens and the cornea of the eye, which nourishes and lubricates them

ciliary body: a structure built of muscle and blood vessels which produces the aqueous humor

cornea: the curved, transparent membrane forming the front of the outer coat of the eyeball that serves primarily as protection and focuses light onto the lens

intraocular pressure: the degree of firmness of the eyeball, as controlled by the proper secretion and drainage of the aqueous humor

lens: a transparent, flexible structure, convex on both surfaces and lying directly behind the iris of the eye; it focuses light rays onto the retina

ophthalmic laser: a high-intensity beam of light which permits a surgeon to cut tissue precisely in the treatment of eye diseases

optic disc: the portion of the optic nerve at its point of entrance into the rear of the eye

peripheral vision: side vision, or the visual perception to all sides of the central object being viewed

retina: the thin, delicate, and transparent sheet of nerve tissue that receives visual stimuli and transmits them to the brain through the optic nerve

tonometer: an instrument used to measure the eye's intraocular pressure, thus checking for the presence of glaucoma

CAUSES AND SYMPTOMS

Glaucoma is an eye disease caused by higher-than-normal pressure inside the eye. The intraocular pressure can increase slowly or suddenly for various reasons but always with detrimental results. Of all the possible causes of blindness, glaucoma is among the most common, but it is also the most preventable. If diagnosed early, it can be controlled and the loss of sight avoided. What complicates the problem is that the most common form of glaucoma shows no symptoms until extensive, irreversible damage has occurred.

To understand this disease, it is necessary to know what occurs within the eye when the intraocular pressure increases. The inner surface of the cornea is nourished by the aqueous humor, which is also called the aqueous fluid. This secretion from the ciliary body flows into the space behind the iris and then through the pupil into the space in front of the iris. Where the front of the iris joins the back of the cornea is a point called the venous sinus, at the anterior drainage angle. Here the aqueous humor is reabsorbed and transported to the bloodstream. In a normal eye, this drainage process works correctly and the balance between the amount secreted and the amount reabsorbed maintains a constant intraocular pressure. In glaucoma, the drainage part of the process works inefficiently. For a variety of reasons, some of which are not fully understood, the drainage mechanism is defective. The upset balance in secretion drainage causes the unwanted increase in intraocular pressure in one eye or, more commonly, in both. The iris is pushed forward, further inhibiting drainage of the aqueous fluid.

Even a very small elevation in intraocular pressure will affect the eye adversely, causing damage to its particularly delicate parts. Although the eye as a whole is quite tough, the optic nerve is vulnerable to increased pressure. This vital connection between the eye and the brain is damaged by the stress within the harder eyeball. The delicate nerve fibers and blood vessels of the optic disc, as the beginning of the optic nerve is called, then die. Once they die, they can never be regenerated or replaced, and blindness is the result. The destruction of the optic disc causes a condition called cupping. A normal optic disc is quite level with the retina. Glaucoma causes it to collapse, creating a genuine indentation. Thus, cupping is a definite sign of glaucoma.

The damage that glaucoma inflicts is progressive. The defect in drainage does not necessarily worsen, and the pressure, once elevated, does not necessarily continue to increase. Once begun, however, the killing of the optic nerve cells continues until the resulting loss of vision progresses to total blindness. The first nerve fibers to die are the ones near the outer edge of the optic disc, which originates near the periphery of the retina. The first decrease in vision, therefore, is in one's peripheral vision. Then, as each layer of nerve fibers dies, the visual field narrows and narrows.

This slow, progressive route to blindness is typical of the most common type of glaucoma, called chronic simple glaucoma. It is called "simple" because the rise in intraocular pressure does not result from any known underlying reason. Although individuals with a family history of glaucoma are more prone to the disease, it is not directly hereditary. Moreover, not everyone with a family history of glaucoma will develop the disease. For reasons that are not well understood, people of African ancestry have glaucoma in much greater numbers than those of European ancestry. In the United States, the incidence of glaucoma among African Americans is three times that of Caucasians.

In persons of all races, chronic simple glaucoma usually begins after the age of forty; however, the aging process does not seem to be a direct cause of glaucoma. Unlike the formation of senile cataracts, which result from inevitable eye changes as one grows older, glaucoma's development is not explained by the aging process. It can safely be said that glaucoma seems to occur in persons who have a tendency toward inadequate aqueous fluid drainage. As those persons grow older and their bodies lose their resiliency in general, the drainage problem reaches a point where it begins to raise the intraocular pressure beyond the normal range. Those with untreated chronic simple glaucoma are seldom aware of the disease before considerable damage has been done. The progressive death of nerve fibers is ordinarily very slow because the elevation of pressure is slight and causes no pain or blurriness of sight.

Chronic simple glaucoma makes up about 95 percent of all cases of the disease. Several other rare types together make up the other 5 percent. In chronic secondary glaucoma, the drainage defect is caused by some complication of a different eye problem. The causes of chronic secondary glaucoma include inflammation from an eye infection, an allergic reaction, trauma to the eye, a tumor, or even the presence of a cataract. Medications such as corticosteroids can sometimes cause this type of glaucoma to

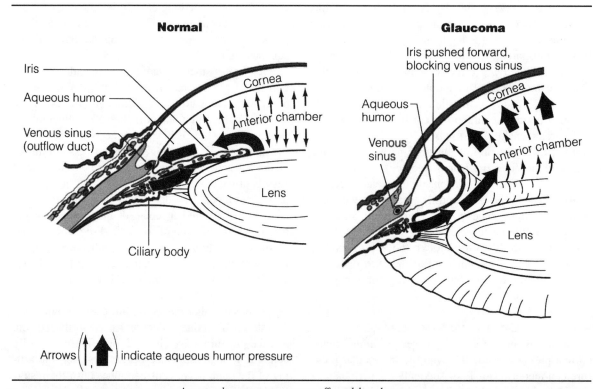

A normal eye versus an eye affected by glaucoma.

develop. Whatever the cause, chronic secondary glaucoma exhibits the same increased pressure, slow nerve destruction, and ultimate loss of vision as chronic simple glaucoma.

A third variety, acute glaucoma, is both rare and dramatic in its onset. The increase in intraocular pressure is many times higher than that in chronic glaucoma. It also occurs very rapidly, sometimes within hours. The anterior drainage angle where drainage is accomplished is almost totally blocked. The eyeball becomes so hard that the elevated pressure can often be felt simply by touching the front of the eye. The great pressure causes terrible pain and immediate damage to the eye. When nausea, vomiting, and severe headaches accompany eye pressure, acute glaucoma should be suspected. Immediate treatment is required to prevent blindness. Acute glaucoma can be either simple or secondary. It is termed simple when a drainage area that has always been abnormally narrow suddenly becomes totally blocked. It is called secondary when it is precipitated by some other eye condition.

The rarest type of glaucoma, congenital glaucoma, is present at birth or develops during early infancy. It results from the incorrect formation of drainage canals while the eye is developing. Because a baby's eyeball is much smaller and softer than an adult's, this glaucoma is often recognized by the bulging of the eyes.

It is quite easy for an eye doctor to detect even the apparently symptomless chronic glaucoma, and the rate of successful treatment is high. It is unfortunate, then, that glaucoma is responsible for innumerable cases of permanent loss of vision. In the vast majority of these patients, the destruction of the eye could have been prevented. If everyone over the age of forty had an annual eye examination, blindness caused by glaucoma could be essentially eliminated.

TREATMENT AND THERAPY

The treatments available for glaucoma include eyedrops, ointments, pills, and surgery, using both scalpels and lasers. In both acute and congenital glaucoma, there is no time for the use of medications. Patients need to be admitted to the hospital and operated on immediately if their eyesight is to be saved.

If diagnosed early, cases of both chronic simple and chronic secondary glaucoma can often be effectively treated by medications. The first drug given in the form of eyedrops was discovered in the nine-

teenth century. Called pilocarpine, it is obtained from the leaves or roots of a South American bush. The drug is classified as a miotic because it constricts the pupil of the eye. Constriction of the pupil draws it away from the drainage angle, automatically increasing the drainage of aqueous fluid and therefore decreasing the pressure. To be effective, it is generally used four times a day. Other glaucoma drugs act to decrease the secretion of the fluid, which also decreases the intraocular pressure. Timolol maleate, the most frequently prescribed drug for glaucoma, works in this fashion. It usually needs to be used twice a day. Some ophthalmologists prefer to use some of both types of drops for the same patient, decreasing pressure by both mechanisms. Others prescribe one medication that produces both effects. Dipivefrin is one such medication.

In either case, to avoid possible unpleasant side effects the most dilute concentration, to be used the fewest times each day, is prescribed first. If this does not control the pressure, more concentrated drops, to be used more times daily, must then be prescribed. The medications in these eyedrops can often be used more easily by elderly patients in the form of a gel, an ointment, or a tiny disc which is placed on the cornea. Although considerably more costly than frequent drops, these methods are less of a nuisance. The gels and ointments need only be used once a day, while the discs are time-released over an entire week.

If drops or gels do not produce the desired reduction in pressure, pills can be used, not to replace the drops but to supplement them. These tablets are essentially diuretics that decrease the production of aqueous humor. Taken once a day, or less frequently in a time-release capsule, acetazolamide is the drug most often prescribed.

There are also several fast-acting drugs that can be injected into a vein to lower pressure by rapidly pulling some aqueous fluid into blood vessels in the eye, bypassing the drainage angle. These are not used in the treatment of chronic glaucoma except as preparation for a planned surgery. They are, however, often used when patients are admitted to the hospital for acute glaucoma to prevent damage until emergency surgery can be performed.

In the great number of patients, chronic glaucoma can be controlled by one of these medications. In those rare cases when it cannot, surgery must be performed. Although initially successful, such surgeries must often be repeated in the future. As with the above medications, glaucoma surgery aims to decrease the intraocular pressure by decreasing secretion or increasing effective drainage.

Although surgery can never reverse the optic nerve damage that has already occurred, it is often effective in preventing further destruction. The first of these surgical procedures was developed in the mid-nineteenth century. Called an iridectomy or iridotomy, it attempts to provide a better access to the patient's drainage angle by removing part of the iris. A second type of surgical procedure, known as a trabeculectomy or filtering operation, attempts to control intraocular pressure by creating a new, wider drainage outlet for the aqueous humor. Until the use of lasers, both of these operations were done completely manually by a surgeon with steady hands using sharp blades on a tiny part of the eye.

To perform an iridectomy, the surgeon must cut a tiny hole into the edge of the iris with surgical scissors, allowing aqueous fluid to flow into the space between the iris and the cornea. Covered by the upper eyelid, this small hole is visible only by close examination and should not let in unwanted extra light or cause any discomfort to the patient.

The filtering operation, or trabeculectomy, can be performed in several different ways, but each involves the eye surgeon's use of a knife called a scalpel to create an artificial canal through the outer wall of the patient's eye. The passageway created, known as a fistula or filtering bleb, permits the aqueous humor to drain properly from the inner eye. By removing a part of the abnormal tissue from the drainage angle, the surgeon unclogs the drainage mechanism.

A different approach to glaucoma control does not involve cutting. It attempts to help the patient by destroying part of the source of the excess fluid, the oversecreting ciliary body. When a cold probe is applied to the ciliary body, the procedure is termed cryotherapy; when a hot probe is used, the method is called cyclodiathermy. No incision is required in either case because the probes are applied externally. A very common side effect of these two procedures, however, is fairly severe inflammation. Even when inflammation does not occur, the desired result may be only partially achieved. Both cryotherapy and cyclodiathermy are less commonly done than either iridectomy or trabeculectomy, and the procedures are usually only performed on older patients.

Many of these manual procedures are being replaced by several types of laser therapy. A laser is a precisely directed beam of high-intensity light that can function as a surgical knife. Laser surgery is generally safer than the older methods because it is less invasive to the body, as no incision is made in the eye. It can be done on an outpatient basis with only a local anesthetic. Recovery time, the likelihood of complications, and postoperative discomfort are all lessened. Patients with acute glaucoma, chronic simple glaucoma, and certain types of secondary glaucoma (depending on the cause) can be successfully treated with lasers.

Both iridotomy and trabeculectomy can be performed by the use of an instrument called the argon laser. This particular laser is relatively low-powered, but it is efficient and very popular with ophthalmologists. After a drop of anesthetic is placed in the eye, the surgeon aims the highly focused argon beam at a precise location within the affected eye. The beam need only be directed into the eye for one-tenth of a second to achieve its effect. In an iridotomy, the laser simply drills a tiny hole in the iris for the fluid to circulate freely, while in a trabeculectomy several laser cuts are made on the clogged drainage angle to open it. A more sophisticated ophthalmic laser is the YAG laser. After a drop of anesthetic is placed on the eye, a weak "aiming beam" of helium-neon laser light is shone directly into the afflicted eye to pinpoint the area to be treated. This is followed by two to five bursts of the YAG laser, which drills a hole for better drainage.

All the above treatments for glaucoma, whether medical or surgical, have the potential for serious side effects and complications. Consequently, research continues to seek therapies with better rates of success and fewer complications.

PERSPECTIVE AND PROSPECTS

The development of ways to diagnose glaucoma has paralleled the general development of the ophthalmologist's tools. These devices in turn reflect the links between the science of those branches of physics that study pressure, lenses, mirrors, and light and the science that studies the normal and abnormal functioning of the eye.

In 1851, the German doctor Hermann von Helmholtz invented the ophthalmoscope, which enables one to study the interior of the eye. His instrument focuses a beam of light into the patient's eye and then magnifies its reflection. If this test reveals early signs of cupping of the optic disc, glaucoma can be diagnosed long before other symptoms have appeared.

Intraocular pressure can be measured with an instrument called a tonometer. The two basic varieties are called Schiötz tonometry and applanation tonometry. Both only became possible after biochemists developed anesthetic drops to put in the eye so that the patient would not feel the device touching the very sensitive cornea. The earlier of the two devices, developed in 1905 by the Norwegian physician Hjalmar Schiötz, is a very simple device that is still the most widely used tonometer in the world. With the patient lying down and looking upward, the physician places the hand-sized instrument directly on the cornea. A simple lever is moved by the pressure within the eye to indicate whether that pressure is within the normal range or dangerously high. The Goldman applanation tonometer is considered even more accurate and is often used to confirm the results of the simpler Schiötz device. An orange dye called fluorescein is added to the anesthetic. The patient, in a sitting position, rests the head against a bar to steady it. The doctor uses a tonometer to touch the cornea while simultaneously peering into it with a well-illuminated microscope.

More specialized glaucoma examination may require gonioscopy, visual field tests, or tonography. The gonioscope has mirrors and facets to provide an illuminated view of the drainage angle, a normally dark corner at a 90 degree angle from the examiner. Excessive narrowing of the angle is a dangerous indication of glaucoma. There are many kinds of visual field tests, but all give a map of the central area where vision is sharp and more acute, versus the peripheral area where it is weaker. Since damage to the optic nerve always causes a narrowing of the visual field, this mapping is very important. The ability to measure the field has grown from oculokinetic perimetry—using an inexpensive test chart, pencil, record sheet, and human examiner— to the expensive and sophisticated automated perimetry, which generates a computer analysis for the physician. Tonography does not measure the visual field but again attacks the problem by measuring the intraocular pressure. Unlike the ordinary use of tonometry, which involves momentary contact with the cornea, tonography uses the tonometer for four minutes to massage the eye. In a normal eye, pressure will drop; in a glaucoma patient, it will not.

All these tests, developed through years of oph-thalmic research, have given medical science invaluable tools to diagnose glaucoma and prevent blindness.

—*Grace D. Matzen*

See also Blindness; Cataract surgery; Cataracts; Eye surgery; Eyes; Laser use in surgery; Ophthalmology; Optometry; Sense organs; Visual disorders.

FOR FURTHER INFORMATION:

Eden, John. *The Physician's Guide to Cataracts, Glaucoma, and Other Eye Problems*. Yonkers, N.Y.: Consumer Reports Books, 1992. This excellent book provides the reader with nontechnical yet truly accurate explanations of the functioning of the normal eye and of the disease conditions glaucoma and cataracts.

Epstein, David L., et al., eds. *Chandler and Grant's Glaucoma*. Rev. 4th ed. Baltimore: Williams & Wilkins, 1997. A standard text on glaucoma. Includes bibliographic references and an index.

Galloway, N. R. *Common Eye Diseases and Their Management*. 2d ed. New York: Springer-Verlag, 1999. While this text may be difficult material for the general reader, it is useful for obtaining more precise medical information. Intended for medical students but accessible to nonscientists because of the author's writing style.

Neal, Helen. *Low Vision*. New York: Simon & Schuster, 1987. Interesting approach to ophthalmology, providing technical material in a light, readable style. Aims to give the reader a solid understanding of how to avoid eye problems. Includes in its lengthy appendix several lists of further resources, organizations, and products for the visually impaired.

Rubman, Robert H., and Howard Rothman. *Future Vision: Space-Age Techniques to Save Your Sight*. New York: Dodd, Mead, 1987. Rubman, a doctor, brings to this volume his extensive knowledge of and skill in practicing ophthalmology. Rothman, an accomplished freelance writer of science materials, makes Rubman's knowledge genuinely accessible to the nonscientist.

Samz, Jane. *The Encyclopedia of Health: Vision*. New York: Chelsea House, 1990. Contains a rather brief treatment of the topic of glaucoma. This volume is more useful for understanding the normal eye, eye tests in general, and a diversity of other eye diseases. Includes lists of helpful organizations and further readings, as well as a brief glossary.

GLOMERULONEPHRITIS

DISEASE/DISORDER

ANATOMY OR SYSTEM AFFECTED: Kidneys, urinary system

SPECIALTIES AND RELATED FIELDS: Bacteriology, internal medicine, nephrology, virology

DEFINITION: The filtering units of the kidneys are known as glomeruli, and inflammation of these structures is called glomerulonephritis. There are two main types: acute and chronic. Acute glomerulonephritis follows an infection, usually by streptococcal bacteria but also by the viruses that cause chickenpox, mumps, syphilis, measles, and malaria. After the underlying infection is cured, the kidney disorder generally disappears without treatment. Chronic glomerulonephritis, however, has no cure and develops slowly and without symptoms. Renal failure often results, and dialysis or kidney transplantation may be required. The chronic form may be caused by other renal disorders or systemic disorders such as lupus erythematosus.

—Jason Georges and Tracy Irons-Georges
See also Bacterial infections; Dialysis; Internal medicine; Kidney disorders; Kidney transplantation; Kidneys; Lupus erythematosus; Nephrectomy; Nephritis; Nephrology; Nephrology, pediatric; Renal failure; Stone removal; Stones; Transplantation; Urinary system; Urology; Urology, pediatric; Viral infections.

FOR FURTHER INFORMATION:

Cameron, Stewart. *Kidney Disease: The Facts.* 2d ed. New York: Oxford University Press, 1986.

Dische, Frederick E. *Concise Renal Pathology.* 2d ed. Oxford, England: Oxford University Press, 1995.

Legrain, Marcel, Jean-Michel Suc Legrain et al. *Nephrology.* Translated by M. Cavaille-Coll. New York: Masson, 1987.

Whitworth, Judith A., and J. R. Lawrence. *Textbook of Renal Disease.* 2d ed. New York: Churchill Livingstone, 1994.

GLYCOLYSIS

BIOLOGY

ANATOMY OR SYSTEM AFFECTED: Cells, muscles, musculoskeletal system

SPECIALTIES AND RELATED FIELDS: Biochemistry, cytology, exercise physiology, pharmacology, sports medicine

DEFINITION: The chemical process of splitting a molecule of glucose in order to obtain energy for other cellular processes; at times of intense activity, glycolysis produces most of the energy used by muscles.

KEY TERMS:

adenosine triphosphate (ATP): an important biological molecule that represents the energy currency of the cell; the energy in a special high-energy bond in ATP is used to drive almost all cellular processes that require energy

aerobic: occurring in the presence of oxygen

anaerobic: occurring in the absence of oxygen

cellular respiration: a complex series of chemical reactions by which chemical energy stored in the bonds of food molecules is released and used to form ATP

chemical energy: the energy locked up in the chemical bonds that hold the atoms of a molecule together; food molecules, such as glucose, contain much energy in their bonds

creatine phosphate: an energy-containing molecule present in significant quantities in muscle tissue; energy is stored in a high-energy bond similar to that of ATP

enzyme: a biological catalyst that speeds up a chemical reaction without itself being used up; enzymes are made of protein, and a single enzyme can usually only catalyze a single chemical reaction

nicotinamide adenine dinucleotide (NAD): a molecule used to hold pairs of electrons when they have been removed from a molecule by some biological process; the empty molecule is denoted by NAD^+, while it is denoted as NADH when it is carrying electrons

STRUCTURE AND FUNCTIONS

Glycolysis is the first step in the process that cells use to extract energy from food molecules. Although energy can be extracted from most types of food molecule, glycolysis is usually considered to begin with glucose. In fact, the term "glycolysis" actually means the splitting (*lysis*) of glucose (*glyco*). This is a good description for the process, since the glucose molecule is split into two halves. The glucose molecule consists of a backbone of six carbon atoms to which are attached, in various ways, twelve hydrogen atoms and six oxygen atoms. The glucose molecule is inherently stable and unlikely to split spontaneously at any appreciable rate.

When the energy is extracted from a glucose molecule, it is stored, for the short term, in a much less stable molecule called adenosine triphosphate (ATP). The ATP molecule consists of a complex organic molecule (adenosine) to which are attached three simple phosphate groups. While the first phosphate is attached by what one could call a "normal" chemical bond, the second and third phosphates are attached by high-energy bonds. These are chemical bonds that require a considerable amount of energy to create. Therefore, the ATP molecule can store much energy. When one of the high-energy bonds of ATP is broken, a large amount of energy is released. Usually, only the bond holding the last phosphate is broken, producing a molecule of adenosine diphosphate (ADP) and a free phosphate group. The phosphate group is only split from ATP at the precise moment when energy is required by some other process in the cell. This breaking of ATP provides the energy to drive cellular processes. The processes include activities such as the synthesis of molecules, the movement of molecules, and the contraction of muscle. The third phosphate can be reattached to ADP using energy released from glycolysis, or by other components of cellular respiration. The production of ATP can be diagrammed as follows:

energy from glycolysis + ADP + phosphate → ATP

Similarly, the breakdown of ATP can be diagrammed as:

ATP → ADP + phosphate + usable energy

With this understanding of how ATP works, one can look at how it is generated in the cell by glycolysis.

The first step in the production of energy from food is really an energy-consuming process. Since glucose is inherently a stable molecule, it must be activated before it will split. It is activated by attaching a phosphate group to each end of the six-carbon backbone. These phosphate groups are supplied by ATP. Therefore, glycolysis begins by using the energy from two ATP molecules. The atoms of the glucose molecule are also rearranged during the activation process so that it is changed into a very similar sugar, fructose. A fructose molecule with a phosphate group on either end is called fructose 1,6-diphosphate. Thus one can summarize the activation process as:

glucose + 2 ATP → fructose 1,6-diphosphate + 2 ADP

Fructose 1,6-diphosphate is a much more reactive molecule and can be readily encouraged to split by the appropriate enzyme. The split produces two identical molecules with the rather cumbersome name of phosphoglyceraldehyde, usually abbreviated to PGAL. Each PGAL consists of a three-carbon backbone with attached oxygen and hydrogen atoms, and a phosphate group at the end. Each PGAL molecule then undergoes several changes, only the important results of which will be mentioned. At one point, the PGAL molecule picks up a free phosphate group at the opposite end from where one is already attached. Various arrangements of the atoms convert the bonds holding the phosphate groups into high-energy bonds. These phosphate groups are then able to be transferred to ADP molecules producing ATP. Since each PGAL produces two ATPs, and two PGALs are produced from each original glucose, four ATP molecules are produced all together. Since two ATPs were used to activate the glucose, the cell has a net gain of two ATP molecules for each glucose molecule used.

The rearrangement of the atoms leaves them in a form called pyruvic acid. Pyruvic acid still contains much energy locked up in its chemical bonds. In most of the cells of the body and most of the time, pyruvic acid will be further broken down and all of its energy released. This further breakdown of pyruvic acid requires oxygen and is beyond the scope of this topic. It should be pointed out, however, that the complete breakdown of two molecules of pyruvic acid can produce more than thirty additional ATP molecules. With the addition of oxygen, the end products are the simple molecules of carbon dioxide and water.

Other products of the rearrangement of PGAL are energy-containing electrons. Electrons are highly energetic and have a negative electrical charge. They cannot be allowed simply to dart around the cell by themselves. Instead, they are picked up and carried by molecules specially designed for this purpose. These energy-carrying molecules have the rather intimidating name of nicotinamide adenine dinucleotide, abbreviated to NAD. Biologists have more or less agreed to a conventional notation for this molecule, to allow the reader to know whether the molecule is carrying electrons or is empty. Since the empty molecule has a net positive charge, it is denoted as NAD^+. When full, it holds a pair of electrons. One electron would neutralize the positive charge, while two result in a negative charge. The negative charge attracts one of the many hydrogen ions (H^+) in the cell. Thus when carrying electrons the molecule is denoted NADH.

These energy-carrying electrons have little significance most of the time in most of the cells of the body. The NADH molecules are able to donate their electrons to systems that generate ATP from them. These systems, however, require the use of oxygen. Although the body has an excellent respiratory system and circulatory system to obtain and deliver oxygen to all parts of the body, there are times when it is inadequate. When a muscle is working very hard, there simply is not enough blood supply to bring all the oxygen that the muscle needs.

The oxidative pathways that completely break down pyruvic acid are limited by the lack of oxygen in very active muscles. The ability to deal with electrons from NADH is also drastically reduced. Glycolysis can continue even in the absence of oxygen, but the electrons produced by glycolysis must be dealt with.

There is a very limited amount of NAD^+ in each cell. NAD^+ is designed to hold electrons briefly, while they are transferred to some other system. In the absence of oxygen, the electrons are transferred to pyruvic acid. Since pyruvic acid cannot be broken down without oxygen, there is an ample supply. Transferring electrons from NADH to pyruvic acid allows the empty NAD^+ to pick up more electrons produced by glycolysis. Therefore, glycolysis can continue producing two ATP molecules from each glucose molecule used. While two ATPs per glucose molecule is a small amount compared to the more than thirty ATPs produced by oxidative metabolism, it is better than none at all.

The process of generating energy (ATPs) in the absence of oxygen is referred to as fermentation. Most people are familiar with the fermentation of grapes to produce wine. Yeast has the enzymes to transfer electrons from NADH to pyruvic acid and to convert the resulting molecule into alcohol and carbon dioxide. No further energy is obtained from this process. Alcohol still contains much of the energy that was in glucose. Humans and other mammals have different enzymes than yeast cells. These enzymes transfer the electrons from NADH to pyruvic acid, producing lactic acid.

THE ROLE OF GLYCOLYSIS IN MUSCLE ACTIVITY

When yeast is respiring anaerobically (without oxygen), it will continue producing alcohol until it poisons itself. Most yeast cannot tolerate more than about 12 percent alcohol, the concentration found in most wine. The lactic acid produced by fermentation in humans is also poisonous. People, however, do not respire completely anaerobically. The two ATPs produced per glucose molecule used are simply not enough to supply the energy needs of most human cells. Muscle cells have to be somewhat of an exception. There are times when one asks the muscle cells to use energy much faster than one can supply them with oxygen. One may consider a muscle working under various levels of physical activity and examine its oxygen requirements and waste products.

At rest, a muscle requires very little ATP energy. For an individual sitting on the couch watching television, energy demands are minimal. The lungs inhale and exhale slowly and take in enough oxygen to keep its concentration in the blood high. A relatively slow heart rate can pump enough of this oxygen-rich blood to the muscles to supply their very minimal needs. As soon as one uses a muscle, however, its ATP consumption increases dramatically. Even if an individual simply walks as far as the refrigerator, large quantities of ATP are required to cause the leg muscles to contract. Muscle cells maintain a constant level of ATP so that, as soon as one asks a muscle to contract, it can do so. The ATP that is broken down is almost instantly regenerated from an additional energy store peculiar to muscle cells. Creatine phosphate is a molecule similar to ATP, in that the phosphate group is attached by a high-energy bond. There is more creatine phosphate in muscle cells than ATP. As soon as ATP is broken down, phosphates, and their high-energy bonds, are transferred from creatine phosphate. Within the first few seconds of activity, the ATP concentration in a muscle cell remains almost constant, but the creatine phosphate level begins to drop.

As soon as the creatine phosphate concentration drops, the aerobic (oxygen-requiring) respiratory processes speed up. These processes break down glucose all the way to carbon dioxide and water and release plenty of ATP. This ATP can then be used for muscle contraction. If the muscle has now stopped contracting, the new ATP produced will be used to rebuild the store of creatine phosphate.

Within the first minute or so of muscle contraction, the use of oxygen can be quite high. The circulatory system has not yet responded to this increased oxygen demand. Muscle tissue, however, has a reserve of oxygen. The red color of most mammalian muscles is attributable to the presence of myoglobin, which is similar to hemoglobin in that it has a strong affinity for oxygen. The myoglobin stores oxygen directly in the muscle, so that the muscle can operate aerobically while the circulatory and respiratory systems adjust to the increased oxygen demand.

At low or moderate muscle activity, the carbon dioxide produced by aerobic respiration in muscles will trigger an increase in the activity of both the circulatory and the respiratory systems. The increased demand for oxygen by the muscles is supplied by an increased blood flow. Jogging around a track or participating in aerobic exercises would be considered low to moderate muscular activity. Respiration rate and pulse rate both increase with jogging. This increase in oxygen supply to the muscles provides all that they need. The level of creatine phosphate will be lower than that in resting muscles, but it will soon be replenished when the activity is stopped. The muscle cells have a good supply of food molecules in the form of glycogen. Glycogen is simply a long string of glucose molecules connected together for convenient storage. At a rate of activity such as that created by jogging, the glycogen supply can last for hours. Even after it is used up, glycogen stored in the liver can be broken down to glucose and carried to the muscles by the blood. An individual will probably want to stop jogging before his or her muscles will want to quit.

High levels of muscular activity pose a different set of problems. After more than about a minute of vigorous exercise, the muscles begin to use ATP faster than oxygen can be supplied to regenerate it. The additional ATP is supplied by lactic acid fermentation. Glucose is only broken down as far as pyruvic acid, then converted to lactic acid by the addition of electrons from NADH. Lactic acid begins to accumulate in the muscle tissue. Since the body is still using large amounts of ATP but not taking in enough oxygen, it is said to enter a state of oxygen debt. When the muscular activity ends, the oxygen debt is repaid.

One can use an example of someone running to catch a bus, sprinting for 50 yards at full speed. That is not enough time for the circulation and lungs to respond to the increased demand for oxygen. The muscles have made up the difference between supply and demand with lactic acid fermentation. The individual now sits down in the bus and pants—to repay his or her oxygen debt.

Some of the oxygen will go to replenish the store in muscle myoglobin. Some of it will be used in oxi-dative metabolism in the muscle to replenish the reserves of creatine phosphate. The rest will be used to deal with the accumulated lactic acid. The lactic acid is not all dealt with in the muscle where it was produced. Being a small molecule, it easily enters the bloodstream. In muscles throughout the body, it can be converted back to pyruvic acid. Pyruvic acid can then reenter the oxidative pathway and be used to generate ATP, with the use of oxygen. The lactic acid, then, is being used as a food molecule to supply the needs of resting muscle. Much of the lactic acid is metabolized in the liver. Some of it will be metabolized with oxygen to produce the energy to convert the rest of it back to glucose. The glucose can then be circulated in the blood or stored in the liver or muscles as glycogen. A minimal amount of lactic acid is excreted in the urine or in sweat.

If the subject of the preceding example kept running at full speed, having missed the bus and run all the way to the office, lactic acid would build up in the muscles and in the blood. If the office was far enough away, the subject would eventually reach the point of exhaustion and stop running. At that point, the level of lactic acid in the leg muscles would be high enough to inhibit the enzymes of glycolysis. Glycolysis would slow down so that lactic acid would not become any more concentrated. The muscles' supply of creatine phosphate would be almost exhausted, but the ATP supply would be only slightly lower than in a resting muscle. The body is protected from damaging itself: Too much lactic acid would lower the pH to dangerous levels, and the absolute lack of ATP causes muscles to lock, as in rigor mortis. The body's self-protection mechanisms force one to stop before either of these conditions exists. Once the subject stops running, and pants long enough, he or she can continue. The additional oxygen taken in by increased respiration will have metabolized a sufficient amount of lactic acid to allow the muscles to start working again.

PERSPECTIVE AND PROSPECTS

Cellular respiration is the process by which organisms harvest usable energy in the form of ATP molecules from food molecules. Lactic acid fermentation is the form of respiration used by human muscles when oxygen is in limited supply. Glycolysis is the energy-producing component of lactic acid fermentation, which is much less efficient than aerobic cellular respiration. Fermentation harvests only two molecules of ATP for every glucose molecule used, while aerobic respiration produces a yield of more than thirty molecules of ATP. Most forms of life will only resort to fermentation when oxygen is absent or in short supply. While higher forms of life such as humans can obtain energy by fermentation for short periods, they incur an oxygen debt which must eventually be repaid. The yield of two molecules of ATP for each glucose molecule used is simply not enough to sustain their high demand for energy.

Nevertheless, lactic acid fermentation is an important source of ATP for humans during strenuous physical exercise. Even though it is an inefficient use of glucose, it can provide enough ATP for a short burst of activity. After the activity is over, the lactic acid produced must be dealt with, which usually requires the use of oxygen.

Most popular exercise programs focus on aerobic activity. Aerobic exercises do not place stress on muscles to the point where the blood cannot supply enough oxygen. These exercises are designed to improve the efficiency of the oxygen delivery system so that there is less need for anaerobic metabolism. Training programs in general attempt to tune the body so that the need for lactic acid fermentation is reduced. They concentrate on improving the delivery of oxygen to the muscles, storing oxygen in the muscles, or increasing the efficiency of muscular contraction.

—*James Waddell, Ph.D.*

See also Cells; Enzymes; Exercise physiology; Food biochemistry; Metabolism; Muscles; Sports medicine.

FOR FURTHER INFORMATION:

Camp, Pamela S., and Karen Arms. *Exploring Biology.* 2d ed. Philadelphia: W. B. Saunders, 1984. A lighter introductory biology text. Chapter 12, "Cellular Respiration," provides an overview of the process and a clear stepwise description of glycolysis. The pronunciation guide in the margin is a unique feature.

Campbell, Neil A. *Biology: Concepts and Connections.* 5th ed. Redwood City, Calif.: Benjamin/Cummings, 1999. A very thorough and complete introductory biology text. Chapter 9, "Cellular Respiration: Harvesting Chemical Energy," covers both aerobic and anaerobic respiration. The author points out the interconnectedness of many processes.

Lehninger, Albert L. *Bioenergetics.* New York: W. A. Benjamin, 1971. Chapter 4, "Generation of ATP in Anaerobic Cells," provides a detailed but very readable account of the anaerobic portion of respiration. The chapter also provides a succinct account of enzyme action in general.

Margaria, Rodolfo. "The Sources of Muscular Energy." *Scientific American* 226 (March, 1972): 12. This article points out the relative amounts of energy from aerobic and anaerobic sources used by active muscle. The discussion leads to tips on developing the most effective training regimen.

Shephard, Roy J. *Biochemistry of Physical Activity.* Springfield, Ill.: Charles C Thomas, 1984. Chapter 3, "Carbohydrates and Phosphagen," provides a detailed description of energy production and use in muscles.

GOITER

DISEASE/DISORDER

ANATOMY OR SYSTEM AFFECTED: Endocrine system, glands, throat

SPECIALTIES AND RELATED FIELDS: Endocrinology, internal medicine

DEFINITION: A goiter is an enlargement of the thyroid, the butterfly-shaped gland found over the trachea and below the larynx in the neck. It may be

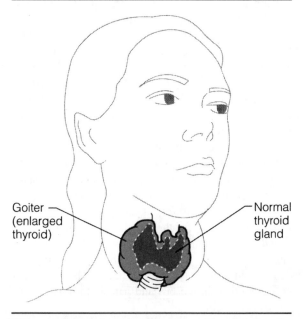

Goiter (enlarged thyroid); dashed lines show relative size of normal thyroid.

attributable to inflammation (as from an autoimmune disorder) or to a benign or malignant tumor, or the condition may be classified as simple goiter. Simple goiter is either endemic, related to such nutritional factors as the iodine deficiency characteristic of malnutrition, or sporadic, following the ingestion of certain foods or drugs. Goiters can also occur as a result of benign nodules that usually strike middle-aged women. Regardless of the cause, the enlarged thyroid gland can reach enormous proportions, resulting in respiratory and circulatory problems. Treatment depends on the cause and may include hormone replacement or surgery.

—*Jason Georges and Tracy Irons-Georges*
See also Autoimmune disorders; Endocrine disorders; Endocrinology; Endocrinology, pediatric; Hyperparathyroidism and Hypoparathyroidism; Malnutrition; Thyroid disorders; Thyroid gland; Thyroidectomy; Tumors.

FOR FURTHER INFORMATION:

Bayliss, R. I., and W. M. Tunbridge. *Thyroid Disease: The Facts.* New York: Oxford University Press, 1991.

Brook, Charles G. D., and Nicholas J. Marshall. *Essential Endocrinology.* Rev. 3d ed. Cambridge, Mass.: Blackwell Science, 1996.

Little, Marjorie. *The Endocrine System.* Rev. ed. New York: Chelsea House, 2000.

Wood, Lawrence C., David S. Cooper, and E. Chester Ridgeway. *Your Thyroid: A Home Reference.* 3d ed. New York: Ballantine Books, 1995.

GONORRHEA

DISEASE/DISORDER

ANATOMY OR SYSTEM AFFECTED: Eyes, genitals, reproductive system

SPECIALTIES AND RELATED FIELDS: Bacteriology, gynecology, obstetrics, public health, urology

DEFINITION: One of the most common and treatable sexually transmitted diseases, gonorrhea is an infection of the urogenital tract. In men, the symptoms may be painful urination and a yellow discharge from the penis; in women, the symptoms may be painful urination, a cloudy discharge and blood from the vagina, and abdominal discomfort. Some people have no symptoms, however, and become lifetime carriers of the disease. Gonorrhea can also be transmitted from mother to baby during childbirth, affecting the eyes and possibly causing blindness. Adults may also contract conjunctivitis associated with gonorrhea. If left untreated, the disease can become serious, resulting in blindness, systemic infection, and pelvic inflammatory disease in women.

—*Jason Georges and Tracy Irons-Georges*
See also Blindness; Conjunctivitis; Eyes; Genital disorders, female; Genital disorders, male; Gynecology; Reproductive system; Sexually transmitted diseases; Urology.

FOR FURTHER INFORMATION:

Brodman, Michael, John Thacker, and Rachael Kranz. *Straight Talk About Sexually Transmitted Diseases.* New York: Facts on File, 1993.

Eng, Thomas Rand, and William T. Butler, eds. *The Hidden Epidemic: Confronting Sexually Transmitted Diseases.* Washington, D.C.: National Academy Press, 1997.

Fish, Raymond M., Elizabeth Trupin Campbell, and Suzanne R. Trupin. *Sexually Transmitted Diseases: Problems in Primary Care.* Los Angeles: Practice Management Information, 1992.

Quetel, Claude. *History of Syphilis.* Baltimore: The John Hopkins University Press, 1990.

GOUT

DISEASE/DISORDER

ANATOMY OR SYSTEM AFFECTED: Feet, joints

SPECIALTIES AND RELATED FIELDS: Internal medicine, podiatry, rheumatology

DEFINITION: A form of arthritis of the peripheral joints, often characterized by painful, recurrent acute attacks and resulting from deposits of uric acid in joint spaces.

KEY TERMS:

acute gout: a very painful gout attack, most common in the left big toe; usually the first indicator of occurrence of the disease

arthritis: any of more than a hundred related diseases, including gout, that are characterized by joint inflammation

cartilage: a tough, white, fibrous connective tissue attached to the bone surfaces that is involved in movement

corticosteroid: a fatlike steroid hormone made by the adrenal glands, or similar synthetic chemicals manufactured by pharmaceutical companies

gene: a piece of the hereditary material deoxyribonucleic acid (DNA) that carries the information needed to produce an inheritable characteristic

genetic engineering: also called recombinant DNA research; a group of scientific techniques that allow scientists to alter genes

hyperuricemia: the presence of abnormally high uric acid levels, which usually leads to gout symptoms

rheumatologist: a physician who studies rheumatoid arthritis and related diseases

secondary gout: gout symptoms caused by other diseases and by therapeutic drugs

synovial fluid: the thick, clear, lubricating fluid that bathes joints and helps them to move smoothly

tophaceous gout: chronic gout that may be characterized by tophi, severe joint degeneration, and/or serious kidney problems

tophi: lumps in the cartilage and joints of chronic gout sufferers, caused by crystals of uric acid

CAUSES AND SYMPTOMS

Gout, once called the affliction of kings, is a hereditary disease that causes inflammation of the peripheral joints. It is also called gouty arthritis because arthritis means joint inflammation and describes more than a hundred related diseases. Gout has afflicted humans since antiquity, and it was first described by Hippocrates in the fifth century B.C.E. It usually first presents itself as an extremely painful swelling of the big toe of the left foot in men over the age of forty. Gout attacks, termed acute gout, are quite rare in premenopausal women. In fact, more than 90 percent of all gout sufferers are men. The prevalence of gout is extremely high in Pacific Islanders, with 10 percent of adult males afflicted. One characteristic portrayal of gout sufferers, which may come from the "affliction of kings" concept, is of obese and obviously affluent individuals. This is partly a misconception because gout is a very democratic disease, found in the poor as often as in the wealthy. Nevertheless, acute gout attacks are often brought on by very rich meals or by drinking sprees, so obesity is accurately portrayed as a contributing factor.

An acute gout attack may occur in almost any joint, with the most common sites after the big toe being the ankles, fingers, feet, wrists, elbows, and knees. Such attacks are not often seen in the shoulders, hips, or spine and, if they do occur, appear only after a gout sufferer has had many previous attacks in other joints. Acute gout of the big toe occurs so often that it has been given its own name, podagra. Common explanations for the very frequent occurrence of podagra are that considerable pressure is placed on the big toe in the process of walking and that most people are right-handed and are therefore "left-footed," putting more pressure on the left foot than on the right one in walking or in sports.

An acute gout attack is preceded by feelings of weakness, nausea, chills, and excessive urination. Then, the area that is affected becomes red to purple, swollen, and so tender that the slightest touch is very painful. This pain is so severe that many sufferers describe it as being crushing, or even excruciating. Acute gout attacks come on suddenly, and many victims report suddenly being jolted awake by pain in the night. Fortunately, such attacks are few and far between and usually last only from a few days to a week. In addition, more than half of those who have one attack of podagra will never have another gout attack.

The problems associated with acute gout are attributable to a chemical called uric acid. Uric acid does not dissolve well in the blood and other biological fluids, such as the synovial fluid in joints. When overproduced by the body or excreted too slowly in urine, undissolved uric acid forms sharp crystals. These crystals and their interactions with other joint components cause the pain felt by gout sufferers. It is interesting to note that gout is caused by the overproduction of uric acid in some individuals and by uric acid underexcretion in others. Many of the foods that seem to cause gout are rich in chemicals called purines, which are converted to uric acid in the course of preparation for excretion by the kidneys.

Much more dangerous to gout victims than the acute attacks is leaving the disease untreated. When this happens, crystals of uric acid produce lumps or masses in the joints throughout the body and in the kidneys. In the joints, the masses, called tophi, lead to inflammation, scarring, and deformity that can produce an irreversible degenerative process. Tophi are most common in the fingers and the cartilage of various parts of the body, and external tophi are found in the cartilage of the ears of gout sufferers. The visible tophi, however, are only representative, and undetected uric acid masses may be widely spread throughout the body. Such untreated gout is called chronic or tophaceous gout.

Tophaceous gout is another disease with a long history. It was first described by the Greek physician Galen in the second century C.E. Another extremely dangerous aspect of tophaceous gout is unseen kidney stones, which will cause great pain on urination,

Gout

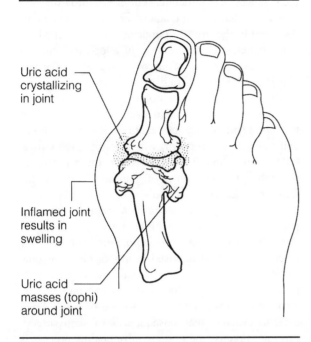

Uric acid crystallizing in joint

Inflamed joint results in swelling

Uric acid masses (tophi) around joint

The big toe is a common site for gout.

produce high blood pressure, and even cause fatalities in 3 to 5 percent of afflicted persons.

The prime indicator of gout is high blood levels of uric acid, called hyperuricemia; however, this condition, without other symptoms, does not always signal existent, symptomatic gout. Therefore, the best indicator of the presence of the disease is a combination of hyperuricemia, acute attacks, and observed uric acid in the synovial fluid of all troublesome, gouty joints.

Some investigators propose that gout sufferers are highly intelligent because such famous individuals as Michelangelo, Leonardo da Vinci, Martin Luther, Charles Darwin, and Benjamin Franklin were afflicted with the disease. This trend, however, may indicate that famous people are usually able to afford a lifestyle that causes the predilection to high uric acid levels (for example, the eating of purine-rich foods and high alcohol consumption). Rheumatologists who have studied gout would argue that alcoholism is a better predictor for the disease because it is very common in heavy drinkers. In fact, studies in which gout patients were given purine-rich diets or purine-rich diets plus alcoholic beverages showed that alcohol increased the number and severity of gout attacks.

Gout is also associated with a number of other diseases, including Down syndrome, lead poisoning, some types of diabetes, psoriasis, and kidney disease. Furthermore, a number of therapeutic drugs used in chemotherapy for cancer, diuretics, and some antibiotics can cause acute gout symptoms. These types of gout are differentiated from the hereditary disease already described—so-called primary gout—by the term "secondary gout." Drug-induced secondary gout goes away quickly when administration of the offending drug is stopped.

Another group of diseases that have symptoms somewhat similar to gout are called pseudogout. They have an entirely different cause (mineral crystals in the joints), occur in men and women with equal frequency, usually begin in extreme old age, and are treated quite differently.

It is also interesting that while premenopausal women are nearly gout-free, the disease becomes fairly common after the menopause. This fact supports a role for female hormones in preventing the disease. Primary gout in women is usually much more severe and destructive than gout in men. In those families in which maternal gout is observed, it is likely that occurrence of the disease in male offspring will occur earlier than is usual, such as near the age of thirty.

TREATMENT AND THERAPY

Once primary gout has been diagnosed, three methods are available for treating it: therapeutic drugs, surgery, and special diets. Most often, gout treatment uses therapeutic drugs, with the drug of choice being colchicine. Colchicine treatment can be traced back for thousands of years, to Egypt in 1500 B.C.E. Originally, it was given as an extract of the meadow saffron plant, *Colchicum autumnale*. In modern times, the pure chemical has been isolated for medicinal use.

Colchicine is reportedly a specific remedy for gout and has no effect on any other type of arthritis. In fact, the reversal of severe joint pain with colchicine is often used as a diagnostic tool that tells physicians that the joint disease being treated is indeed gout. Colchicine can be utilized to treat acute gout attacks or can be taken routinely for long periods of time. Its actions in the handling of acute attacks are quick and profound. In some cases, however, colchicine will have side effects, including severe stomach cramps, nausea, and diarrhea. When these effects occur, colchicine use is discontinued until they disappear and then its reuse is instituted.

Most of the basis for colchicine action is its decrease of the inflammation that causes the pain of gout attacks. This action is believed to be attributable to colchicine's interaction with white blood cells that destroy uric acid crystals and subsequent prevention of the cells from releasing inflammatory factors. Other drugs that work in this way are nonsteroidal anti-inflammatory drugs (NSAIDs) such as aspirin, ibuprofen, indomethacin, naproxin, and phenylbutazone. Colchicine and NSAIDs are usually given by mouth. In some cases, anti-inflammatory steroid hormones called corticosteroids, such as prednisone and prednisolone, are used to treat acute gout. The corticosteroids are given by injection into the gouty joint. Despite the rapid, almost miraculous effects of these steroids, they are best avoided unless absolutely necessary because they can lead to serious medical problems.

Another group of antigout medications consists of the uricosuric drugs. Two favored examples of such drugs are probenecid (Benemid) and sulfinpyrazone (Anturane). The uricosuric drugs prevent the occurrence of hyperuricemia and eventual tophaceous gout by increasing uric acid excretion in the urine, therefore lowering the uric acid levels in the blood. This lowering has two effects: the prevention of the attainment of uric acid levels in the blood and joints that lead to crystal or tophus formation and the eventual dissolution of crystals and tophi as blood levels of uric acid drop.

Uricosuric drugs have no effect, however, on an acute gout attack and can sometimes make such attacks even more painful. For this reason, uricosuric drug therapy is always started after all acute gout attack symptoms have subsided. Aspirin blocks the effects of the uricosuric drugs and should be replaced with acetaminophen (for example, Tylenol) whenever they are utilized for chemotherapeutic purposes. Side effects of excessive doses of uricosuric drugs can include headache, nausea and vomiting, itching, and dizziness. Their use should be discontinued immediately when such symptoms occur. Later reuse of the uricosuric drugs is usually possible.

The third category of antigout drugs is a single chemical, allopurinol (usually, Lopurin or Zyloprim). This drug lowers the body's ability to produce uric acid. It is highly recommended for all gout-afflicted people who have kidney disease that is severe enough for kidney stones to form. It has undesired side effects, however, that include skin rashes, drowsiness, a diminished blood count, and severe allergic reactions. As a result, the use of allopurinol is disqualified for many patients. One advantage of allopurinol chemotherapy over the use of uricosuric agents is the fact that it can be taken along with aspirin.

The end result of a chemotherapeutic regimen with uricosuric drugs and/or allopurinol is the lowering of the blood and urinary uric acid levels so that crystals and tophi do not form or, where formed, redissolve. Often, their combination with colchicine is useful for preventing the occurrence of gout attacks during the initial chemotherapy period.

While surgery is not a common treatment for gout, people who have large tophi that have opened up, become infected, or interfere with joint mobility may elect to have them removed in this fashion. In some cases, severe disability or joint pain caused by the degenerative effects of long-term tophaceous gout is also corrected surgically. Care should be taken, however, to evaluate the consequences of such surgery carefully because the postoperative healing process is often quite slow and many other problems can be encountered.

Media sources often praise special diets in treating gout, without firm proof of their effectiveness. The finding that gout is usually a hereditary disease resulting from metabolic defects that either prevent uric acid excretion or cause its accumulation has pointed out that most dietary factors have a relatively small effect on the disease. Consequently, chemotherapy is much more effective than dietary intervention for diminishing gout symptoms. Nevertheless, there are several incontestable dietary aspects essential to the well-being of persons afflicted with gout.

First, dieting is quite useful, and overweight gout sufferers should lose weight. Such action is best taken slowly and under medical supervision. In fact, excessively fast weight loss can temporarily worsen gout symptoms by elevating blood uric acid levels. In addition, excesses of a number of foods should be avoided by gout sufferers because they are overly rich in the purines that give rise to uric acid when the body processes them. Some examples are the organ meats (liver, kidneys, and sweetbreads), mushrooms, anchovies, sardines, caviar, gravy and meat extracts, shellfish, wine, and beer. Modest intake of these foods is allowable. For example, the daily intake of one can of beer, a glass of wine, or an ounce or two of hard liquor is permissible. The gout sufferer should remember that excessive alcohol intake often brings on acute gout attacks and, even worse, will contribute to worsening tophus and kidney stone formation.

Another adjunct to the prevention or diminution of gout symptoms is the daily intake of at least a half gallon of water or other nonalcoholic beverages. This will help to flush uric acid out of the body, in the urine, and may help to dissipate both tophi and kidney stones. Plain water is best, as it contains no calories that will increase body weight, potentially aggravating gout and leading to other health problems.

PERSPECTIVE AND PROSPECTS

Many sources agree that primary gout is under control in most afflicted people, who can look forward to a normal life without permanent adverse effects of the disease. Those individuals who seek medical treatment at the first appearance of gout symptoms may combine chemotherapy, an appropriate diet regimen, and alcohol avoidance to prevent all but a few acute attacks of the disease. In addition, they will not develop tophi or kidney problems.

Even those afflicted persons who put off treatment until kidney stones or tophi appear can be helped easily. Again, an appropriate diet and the wise choice of chemotherapy agents will prevail. Only the patients who neglect all gout treatment until excessive joint damage and severe kidney disease occur are at serious risk, yet even with these individuals, remission of most severe symptoms is usually possible. The long-term neglect of gout symptoms is unwise, however, because severe tophaceous gout can be both deforming and fatal.

Currently, the eradication of most primary gout, not gout treatment, is seen as the desired goal of research. It is believed that a prime methodology for the eradication of gout will be the use of genetic engineering for gene replacement therapy. Primary gout sufferers are victims of gene lesion diseases: Their bodies lack the ability, because of defective genes, to control either the production or the excretion of uric acid. It is hoped that gene replacement technology will enable medical science to add the missing genes back into their bodies. Other research aspects viewed worthy of exploration in the attempts to vanquish primary gout are the understanding of how to cause white blood cells to destroy uric acid crystals in the joints more effectively and safely and to decode the

basis for the gout-preventing effects of female hormones related to their presence in premenopausal women.

—*Sanford S. Singer, Ph.D.*

See also Alcoholism; Arthritis; Down syndrome; Feet; Foot disorders; Lead poisoning; Obesity; Podiatry; Rheumatology; Urinary disorders.

FOR FURTHER INFORMATION:

Berkow, Robert, and Andrew J. Fletcher, eds. *The Merck Manual of Diagnosis and Therapy.* 17th ed. Rahway, N.J.: Merck Sharp & Dohme Research Laboratories, 1999. Contains a useful exposition of the characteristics, etiology, diagnosis, and treatment of gout and its relationship to other forms of arthritis. Designed for physicians, the material is also useful for less specialized readers. Information on related topics is also included.

Devlin, Thomas E. *Textbook of Biochemistry: With Clinical Correlations.* New York: Wiley-Liss, 1992. This college textbook presents considerable information on gout, hormones, genetic engineering, and related topics. Includes chemical structures, diagrams, and references useful to the reader. All descriptions are simple but scholarly.

Fries, James F. *Arthritis: A Take-Care-of-Yourself Health Guide for Understanding Your Arthritis.* 5th ed. Reading, Mass.: Addison-Wesley, 1999. Covers gout and pseudogout in a chapter on crystal arthritis, discussing the features, prognosis, and treatments of both problems. Crystal arthritis types are very well differentiated and integrated into the consideration of arthritis.

Scriver, Charles R., et al., eds. *The Metabolic Basis of Inherited Disease.* 6th ed. 2 vols. New York: McGraw-Hill, 1989. This classic medical text contains an excellent chapter on gout describing the symptoms, diagnosis, biochemistry, and genetics of the disease in great detail. Aimed at health science professionals, the book contains much important information for the diligent general reader as well. Important pictures, diagrams, and large number of handy references are included.

2000 Physician's Desk Reference Companion Guide. Montvale, N.J.: Medical Economics, 2000. This atlas of prescription drugs includes those used against gout—their manufacturers, useful dose ranges, metabolism and toxicology, and contraindications. This text, found in most public libraries, is useful for both physicians and patients.

GRAFTS AND GRAFTING

PROCEDURE

ANATOMY OR SYSTEM AFFECTED: All

SPECIALTIES AND RELATED FIELDS: Critical care, dermatology, emergency medicine, general surgery, genetics, immunology, neurology, physical therapy, plastic surgery

DEFINITION: The transplantation of tissue from one part of the body to another or from one individual to another in order to treat disease or injury; such surgery requires careful genetic matching in order to avoid a harmful immune response.

KEY TERMS:

allograft: a graft of tissue from one individual to another individual (usually between close relatives)

autograft: a graft of tissue from one part of an individual's body to another

graft-versus-host disease (GVHD): a genetic incompatibility between tissues in which immune system cells from the grafted tissue attacks host tissue

histocompatibility: tissue compatibility, as determined by histocompatibility protein antigens present on the cell membranes of all tissue cells

histology: the study of tissues and their development, roles, and locations within the body

host-versus-graft disease (HVGD): a tissue rejection in which the immune system cells of the graft recipient attack the grafted tissue from a donor individual

immune response: the reaction of an intricate system of cells, which identify, attack, immobilize, and remove foreign tissue from the body through chemical signals

leukocytes: white blood cells, immune system cells which either produce antibodies or phagocytically consume cells and tissues that are genetically foreign in nature

tissue: a specialized region of cells that forms organs within the body; the four principal types are epithelial, connective, nervous, and muscular

totipotence: the capacity for cells of a given tissue type to regenerate and replace killed or damaged cells within a given body region

INDICATIONS AND PROCEDURES

In medicine, a graft is a tissue region which is transferred from one part of the body to another body part (autograft) or from one individual to another individual (allograft). Grafts between individuals of differing species (xenografts) also are possible. The actual transfer of tissue is called a transplant. The identification and matching of appropriate tissue types and the surgical connection of the tissue constitute grafting.

Examples of autografts include the use of leg veins to reconstruct the coronary arteries during heart bypass surgery, skin transplants during reconstructive facial surgery, and thumb/big toe interposable transplants following the loss of a hand or foot digit. Examples of allografts include major organ transplantations (including that of the heart, liver, and kidney), bone marrow transplantation, and blood transfusions between two genetically matched individuals. Xenograft examples include the grafting of animal tissue such as skin or stomach epithelia to the equivalent body parts in humans.

Genetic matching of donor and recipient tissues in grafting and transplantation is critical to the success of the tissue graft. Thus, tissue compatibility, termed histocompatibility, is of primary importance for successful grafting. Autografts are the most successful grafts because they occur on the same individual, and consequently there is no genetic difference between donor and recipient cells. As the genetic difference between donors and graft recipients increases, however, the probability decreases that a graft will be successful.

For example, grafts between identical twins are highly successful because the donor and recipient are genetically identical; hence, the situation is the same as an autograft. Grafts between siblings are likely to succeed. Allografts between people having distinct genetic differences, however, are less likely to succeed. Xenografts are extremely difficult except for basic mammalian tissues, such as epithelial tissue.

Histology is the study of tissues and their development within the human body. The four principal tissue types within the human body and within other mammalian species are epithelial tissue, which lines the surfaces of organs inside and outside throughout the body; connective tissue (such as cartilage, bone, fat, and blood), which provides structure or transport throughout the body; nervous tissue, which conducts electrical impulses as information networks throughout the body; and muscular tissue, which provides contractility and movement for various body parts. All organs consist of a specific pattern of these four tissues: Epithelial tissue provides cover and protection, connective tissue provides support, nervous tissue provides information from the central control regions of the brain, and muscular tissue allows responses to localized change in the organ. In addition, the cells of tissues subspecialize for unique roles within the tissue of which they are a part. For example, nervous system cells may specialize to form receiving sensory neurons or transmitting motor neurons.

Regardless of tissue type, each of the thousand trillion cells in an individual possesses the same basic genes as the others, and therefore many of the same proteins are expressed throughout the body. All cells within an individual have proteins located within the lipid bilayers of their cell membranes. Several of these proteins are located on every single cell of the individual and thus serve as genetic identification markers for the individual's immune system. These cell surface identification proteins are called histocompatibility proteins.

The histocompatibility proteins, of which there are many, are encoded by a battery of human genes called the major histocompatibility complex (MHC). These proteins ensure tissue compatibility for all cells in an individual with respect to that individual's immune system. The cells of the immune system recognize the specific histocompatibility proteins of one's own cells as "self" markers. Foreign cells, which are missing a few or many of the individual's specific set of histocompatibility proteins, are recognized by the immune system as "nonself" and are attacked. This self-versus-nonself reaction is how the immune system distinguishes its own cells from any invading foreign cells and tissues. Therefore, the histocompatibility proteins play a critical role in the successful identification of one's own cells and the destruction of infections, such as those caused by bacterial or fungal cells.

An immune response occurs when immune system cells called leukocytes (white blood cells) cannot locate the specific "self" histocompatibility proteins on a sampled cell. A type of leukocyte called a T lymphocyte will release a protein called immunoglobulin to immobilize the foreign "nonself" cell lacking the correct histocompatibility antigens (the proteins on the cell membranes). Immunoglobulins, also called antibodies, are proteins secreted by T lymphocytes to immobilize foreign antigens.

After the T lymphocyte antibodies have immobilized the antigens on the foreign cells, another type of leukocyte called a B lymphocyte produces antibodies that attack the foreign antigens. Furthermore, the B lymphocytes will multiply themselves, creating millions of copies to produce a clone army of B lymphocytes, all of which make the same antibodies targeted at the same foreign antigens. These specialized clones constitute a memory cell line, which will attack these antigens again if the organism is exposed to them in the future. This reaction is the basis of immunization.

Furthermore, after the T and B lymphocyte antibodies immobilize the foreign antigens, phagocytic leukocytes such as neutrophils and macrophages migrate to the region to ingest and completely destroy the foreign cells. This process will continue until either the foreign cells are vanquished or the immune system is exhausted.

The immune response just described may appear simple, but it is very complicated. In addition to the complex chemical identification of histocompatibility proteins on all of an individual's cells, the production of specific antibodies by T and B lymphocytes involves an extraordinary rearrangement of genes within these immune cells that is still poorly understood.

The immune response directly affects grafts and grafting. For transplants performed between two individuals, most tissues require a close genetic match between the donor and the recipient. They should be as closely related to each other as possible so that

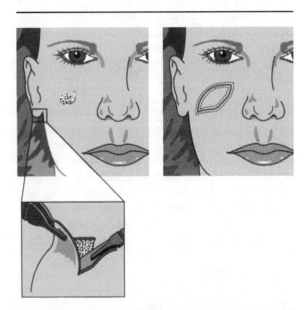

Skin grafting requires the excision of tissue from a less noticeable location, such as behind the ear, and its relocation to an injured or more cosmetically important area, such as the face.

they share a common genetic heritage and, therefore, a high probability that their respective cells have most, if not all, of the same histocompatibility proteins. A close genetic relationship between the graft donor and recipient maximizes the chance that a graft will succeed and that an immune response against nonself tissues will not occur.

USES AND COMPLICATIONS

Grafts, grafting, and transplants between individuals are extremely important in the treatment of maiming or disfiguring accidents and life-threatening diseases. A huge demand exists for grafted tissue, not merely organ transplants, for use in a variety of medical conditions and procedures.

The most common and successful types of grafts are autografts from one part of an individual's body to another part, or from one identical twin to her or his sibling. In autograft cases, there is a perfect match for the histocompatibility proteins on all the cells and tissues. Thus, an immune response will not occur unless the immune system is abnormal in some way, as with such autoimmune diseases as lupus erythematosus and rheumatoid arthritis.

An example of an autograft is the transfer of a vein from the leg to the heart in a patient suffering from coronary artery disease; the grafted vein serves as a replacement coronary artery supplying blood, nutrients, and oxygen to the heart muscle. Another type of autograft is the transfer of skin from the abdomen or pelvic region to the face as part of reconstructive plastic surgery. A severed thumb can be replaced by the big toe, its equivalent digit on the foot.

Allografts, those between different individuals, can be successful if there is careful genetic matching between the donor and recipient tissues. Because of the specificity of matching for certain tissue and cell types, donor-recipient matching may mean an average of any two people out of a thousand or, with more critical tissue lines such as stem cells, two people out of ten million. Often, siblings will serve as tissue donors. Otherwise, the lengthy process of finding possible tissue donors and determining their specific histocompatibility profiles must be conducted before the graft can take place between a recipient and a matched tissue donor.

Grafts are simple between generalized surface tissue such as epithelial and connective tissues. Pig epithelial tissue has been used for skin and stomach tissue grafts on human recipients. Bone marrow transplants for aplastic anemia and leukemia patients, however, require more difficult histocompatibility matching. The use of fetal nervous tissue grafts into the brain tissue of Alzheimer's disease patients has yielded promising results in regenerating brain tissue and slowing the acceleration of this debilitating disease, which generally strikes the elderly.

Grafts are useful for tissue lines lacking totipotence, the ability to regenerate damaged or dead cells. The example cited above of fetal tissue being used to treat Alzheimer's disease is a clear illustration of such tissue-grafting applications. Mature brain tissue in adult humans cannot regenerate. Fetal tissue grafts, however, have facilitated the regenerative capacity of some brain tissue in these patients.

Likewise, stem cell lines such as the red bone marrow of flat bones, where white blood cells (leukocytes) and red blood cells (erythrocytes) are manufactured, are important targets for tissue grafting. In leukemia, a patient's bone marrow is rapidly producing malignant leukocytes. It is clear that the stem cell line producing these cells is aberrant in such patients. Consequently, a small graft of bone marrow tissue from a histocompatible donor's bone marrow may lead to the establishment of a healthy stem cell line in the patient to stop the overproduction of aberrant cells.

In any grafting process, the donor tissue is surgically inserted and secured into the recipient's tissue site. There, the tissue, if successful, can grow and expand into the localized organ region to perform its correct function in the individual's body. In the event that there is not a histocompatible match between the donor tissue within the recipient's body, two possible rejection mechanisms can ensue. In host-versus-graft disease (HVGD), which is the most common type, the recipient's immune system releases antibodies and eventually destroys the donor tissue. In graft-versus-host disease (GVHD), immune system cells transplanted with the donor tissue into the recipient migrate into the recipient's tissues and attack the cells; the recipient will become ill and may die. The grafted tissue has rejected the entire body into which it has been transferred.

PERSPECTIVE AND PROSPECTS

In 1990, the Nobel Prize in Physiology or Medicine was awarded to American medical researchers Joseph E. Murray of the Harvard Medical School and E. Donnall Thomas of Seattle's Fred Hutchinson Cancer Research Center. These two scientists were pioneers in the use of grafts, grafting, and tissue transplants to save people's lives. Murray performed the first successful kidney transplant, between two identical twins, in 1954. Murray teamed with Thomas at Harvard to study methods for preventing host-versus-graft rejections. During the 1960's at the University of Washington, Thomas developed the technique of destroying a potential bone marrow recipient's immune system using radiation, followed by the grafting of donor bone marrow tissue into the patient, thereby increasing the chances that the transplant will succeed before the patient's immune system can become active again. Both scientists also made important discoveries concerning the major histocompatibility proteins.

Grafts and grafting play a vital role in medicine. Grafts can save the lives of people with such diseases as leukemia, anemia, and cancer. Grafts also can be useful in reconstructing damaged organs and skin, especially for burn victims. Still, much research is needed to understand histocompatibility better and to reduce the chance of tissue rejection.

—*David Wason Hollar, Jr., Ph.D.*

See also Alzheimer's disease; Amputation; Bone grafting; Bone marrow transplantation; Breast surgery; Burns and scalds; Cleft lip and palate repair; Corneal transplantation; Critical care; Critical care, pediatric; Dermatology; Dermatopathology; Emergency medicine; Fetal tissue transplantation; Hair transplantation; Heart transplantation; Heart valve replacement; Immune system; Kidney transplantation; Laceration repair; Leukemia; Liver transplantation; Malignant melanoma removal; Pigmentation; Plastic surgery; Skin; Skin lesion removal; Transplantation.

FOR FURTHER INFORMATION:

Alberts, Bruce, et al. *Molecular Biology of the Cell.* 3d ed. New York: Garland, 1994. This comprehensive work by several outstanding molecular biologists is a detailed survey of developmental biology with special emphasis on vertebrate animals, particularly humans. Chapter 17, "The Immune System," is an excellent discussion of the immune system, grafts, rejection, and histocompatibility.

Beck, William S., Karel F. Liem, and George Gaylord Simpson. *Life: An Introduction to Biology.* 3d ed. New York: HarperCollins, 1991. An outstanding introductory textbook for biology majors that is clearly written and beautifully illustrated. Chapter 23, "Immunity," is a good discussion of basic concepts, including descriptions of immune reactions and various types of transplants such as blood type ABO and Rh factor matchups.

Eisen, Herman N. *General Immunology: An Introduction to Molecular and Cellular Principles of the Immune Response.* 3d ed. Philadelphia: J. B. Lippincott, 1990. This incredibly thorough and concise work describes in great detail the various workings of animal immune systems, including types of antibodies, immune system cells, grafts, graft rejection, histocompatibility proteins, and the genetic basis of the immune response.

Memmler, Ruth L., Barbara J. Cohen, and Dena L. Wood. *Memmler's The Human Body in Health and Disease.* 9th ed. Philadelphia: J. B. Lippincott, 2000. This book is a thorough but brief introduction to human anatomy, physiology, and disease that is written specifically for the layperson. Chapter 17, "Body Defenses, Immunity, and Vaccines," describes the immune system, transplants, and graft rejection.

Palca, Joseph. "Overcoming Rejection to Win a Nobel Prize." *Science* 250 (October 19, 1990): 378. Palca's article is an announcement of the 1990 Nobel Prize for Physiology or Medicine awarded to Americans Joseph E. Murray and E. Donnall Thomas, pioneers in grafting and transplant medical research. Palca discusses the careers of these two scientists and the major experiments leading to their momentous discoveries.

GRAM STAINING

PROCEDURE

ANATOMY OR SYSTEM AFFECTED: Cells, immune system

SPECIALTIES AND RELATED FIELDS: Bacteriology, biochemistry, cytology, microbiology

DEFINITION: A staining process used as a means of differentiating microorganisms, which are classified as either gram-positive or gram-negative.

KEY TERMS:

cell wall: a structure outside the cell membrane of most bacteria, composed of varying amounts of carbohydrates, lipids, and amino acids

gram-negative: referring to microorganisms that appear pink following the Gram-staining procedure

gram-positive: referring to microorganisms that appear violet following the Gram-staining procedure

Gram's stain: a method of staining bacteria as a primary means of differentiation and identification

lipopolysaccharide (LPS): a major component of the cell wall of gram-negative bacteria; the toxicity of LPS is associated with illnesses caused by gram-negative organisms

mordant: a chemical that acts to fix a stain within a physical structure; the role played by iodine in Gram's stain

peptidoglycans: repeating units of sugar derivatives that make up a rigid layer of bacterial cell walls; found in both gram-positive and gram-negative cells

INDICATIONS AND PROCEDURES

The observation and identification of bacteria are of obvious primary importance in the study of microorganisms. Even with the use of powerful microscopes, direct observation of unstained bacteria is difficult. The use of stains to increase their contrast with the background allows bacteria to be observed more easily.

As a result of resident acidic groups—polysaccharides or nucleic acids—the surfaces of bacteria tend to be negatively charged. Conversely, the dye portion of common stains such as methylene blue or crystal violet consists of positively charged ions. For staining purposes, a sample of bacteria is placed on a glass slide and allowed to dry. The solution of stain is flooded over the bacterial "smear" for about a minute, and the slide is then rinsed. The main purpose of such simple stains is to allow the cells to be observed.

In contrast with simple stains, differential staining methods do not stain all cells in the same manner. Bacteria grown under different environmental conditions, or bacteria that may differ from one another in their physical structure, will exhibit different staining properties when treated with differential stains. Gram staining (also called Gram's stain) is an example of a differential stain.

Gram staining is a relatively simple procedure and is among the first practices learned by students in microbiology laboratories. The process begins with the preparation of a bacterial smear on the slide. A stain, crystal violet, is allowed to flood the dried smear. The slide is rinsed, and a solution of iodine is dropped over the smear. The iodine functions as a mordant, fixing the crystal violet into a complex insoluble in water. Following another rinse, the smear is covered with either an alcohol or an acetone "destaining" solution for several seconds, rinsed again, and counterstained with the red dye safranin. After a last wash, the bacteria are observed with a mi-

croscope. If they were not destained by the alcohol step, retaining the blue or violet color, they are considered gram-positive; if they have stained pink because of the counterstain safranin, they are considered gram-negative.

The precise means by which Gram staining works is not entirely clear. The cell wall structure of gram-positive bacteria either prevents the alcohol/acetone solution from removing the crystal violet-iodine complex from the cell or prevents the solution from having access to the complex. Though the question remains whether the cell wall structure is the sole determining factor in the differential procedure, there is no doubt that the cell wall features are primary factors in the determination of Gram-staining results. Therefore, the structure of the cell wall in most bacteria reflects the Gram-staining characteristics.

The cell wall structure found in gram-positive bacteria differs significantly from that in gram-negative cells. While both contain a rigid layer called the peptidoglycan, the peptidoglycan layer is much thicker and makes up a significantly larger portion of the cell wall in gram-positive bacteria. In contrast, a significant portion of the cell wall found in gram-negative bacteria is composed of lipid derivatives.

The peptidoglycan portion of the cell is composed of repeating units of two sugar derivatives: N-acetylglucosamine and N-acetylmuramic acid. The peptidoglycan within the wall is in the form of sheets, layered on top of one another. In gram-positive bacteria, approximately 90 percent of the cell wall material consists of peptidoglycan; among gram-negative bacteria, about 10 percent of the wall is represented by this rigid layer.

These cell wall structures are stabilized by short chains of amino acids that cross-link the layers of peptidoglycan. Formation of the cross bridges is an enzymatic process called transpeptidation. The antibiotic penicillin inhibits the enzyme that carries out the formation of such cross-links. The result is a weakening in the cell wall, and possibly cell death. Since the peptidoglycan layer of gram-negative bacteria represents a much smaller proportion of the cell wall, such microorganisms are often more resistant to the action of penicillin than are gram-positive bacteria.

During the Gram-staining procedure, decolorization of the cell is carried out during the wash with alcohol or acetone. The thick peptidoglycan layer found in gram-positive bacteria, however, prevents movement of the crystal violet-iodine complex from the cell. Thus, the cells do not decolorize; they retain their violet appearance.

The peptidoglycan layer is a small proportion of the gram-negative cell wall. Much of the outer wall in these bacteria is a layer of lipopolysaccharide (LPS), which acts as a physical barrier but also contains pharmacological properties. The LPS layer is a complex structure containing a lipid portion (lipid A), a core polysaccharide consisting of a variety of sugars, and an outer layer of branched sugars called the O-region (O-polysaccharide). The LPS layer is anchored to the thin peptidoglycan portion of the cell wall through a lipoprotein complex. The LPS portion of gram-negative cell walls is often termed endotoxin because of its pharmacological activity. Release of LPS as a result of cell death during certain types of infection can result in high fever or shock.

Since the cell wall of gram-negative bacteria contains proportionately little peptidoglycan, the crystal violet-iodine complex is easily removed during the Gram-staining procedure. Following the alcohol step, the cells again appear colorless. Therefore, when they are counterstained with the safranin, the bacteria will appear pink.

An evaluation of Gram-staining characteristics is generally the first step in the identification of newly isolated bacteria. Most bacteria can be classified as either gram-positive or gram-negative, and this step, along with characterization of the shape of the organism, is of immense importance in narrowing down the possible identities of an isolate.

Further means of identification generally involve the use of selective or differential types of media. These processes utilize the biochemical properties of bacteria for their identification. A selective medium is one in which chemical compounds have been added that inhibit the growth of certain forms of bacteria but allow the growth of others. For example, the chemical dye eosin-methylene blue (EMB) inhibits the growth of gram-positive bacteria while allowing gram-negative bacteria to grow. If a mixed culture of bacteria is inoculated onto EMB medium, only the gram-negative microorganisms will grow. A differential medium will allow a variety of bacteria to grow, but different types of bacteria may produce different reactions on the medium. Since EMB agar contains lactose as a carbon source, it is also a differential medium. Bacteria that ferment lactose produce a green metallic color of colony on EMB; bacteria that do not ferment lactose produce a pink colony.

Biochemical tests are more useful for the identification of organisms that are gram-negative than for those that are gram-positive. Biochemical variations among both genera and species of gram-positive bacteria tend to be too variable for effective identification of these organisms. By contrast, such biochemical results among gram-negative bacteria generally do not vary significantly within the species and hence are useful means of further identification.

The biochemical tests used for identification of gram-negative bacteria can be summarized in the form of a flow chart. Such charts represent the series of tests that divide bacteria into smaller and smaller groups. For example, following a determination of morphological and Gram-staining characteristics, differential tests may be carried out to observe the ability of the bacteria to ferment various types of carbohydrates. A series of broths containing such sugars as glucose, lactose, or sucrose are inoculated. Generally, a pH indicator such as the chemical phenol red is included, as is an inverted glass tube (Durham tube) for observation of gas production. If the organism can ferment lactose and produces acid and gas, the broth tube of lactose will appear yellow and there will be a gas bubble in the Durham tube. If the organism does not ferment lactose, no growth or change from the red color of the broth will be observed in that tube.

Further differentiation of either lactose-positive or lactose-negative organisms, to continue with this particular example, can be carried out with other biochemical tests. Certain species of bacteria are capable of removing a molecule of carbon dioxide from amino acids; others are not. In some cases, multiple tests can be run at the same time. For example, a common differential test for gram-negative bacteria utilizes a medium called triple sugar iron (TSI) agar. TSI agar contains a small amount of glucose and larger amounts of lactose and sucrose, hence the designation of triple sugar. Iron is also contained in the medium. The agar is prepared in a test tube and allowed to harden on a slant. Organisms are inoculated onto the surface of the slant and stabbed into the butt of the slant. If glucose alone is fermented, only enough acid is produced to turn the butt yellow. If either lactose or sucrose is fermented, both the slant and butt of the agar will turn yellow. Production of hydrogen sulfide gas is indicated by a black precipitate from iron sulfide; other gas production is indicated by bubble formation in the region of the stab. In this manner, inoculation of a single type of medium can provide multiple tests for identification.

At one time, each of these differential tests had to be carried out individually. Beginning in the 1970's, however, a variety of media kits became available that allow fifteen to twenty tests to be run simultaneously. These kits consist of strips of miniaturized versions of biochemical tests that permit the rapid identification of gram-negative bacteria.

Even though some biochemical tests are less helpful in the identification of gram-positive bacteria, some characteristics of these organisms can be used. These organisms may be round (cocci) or rod-shaped (bacilli). If bacilli, they may be aerobic (they utilize oxygen) or anaerobic (they do not utilize oxygen). By testing for coagulase, an enzyme which will cause the coagulation of plasma, cocci can be further differentiated.

Finally, serological methods can be used in the identification of either gram-positive or gram-negative organisms. In these tests, a fluorescent dye is attached to molecules of antibodies, proteins directed against the surface molecules of specific bacteria. The ability of the antibodies to attach to bacteria is indicative of the species.

USES AND COMPLICATIONS

The use of Gram-staining methodology is arguably the single most important step in the identification of microorganisms; its applications are far-ranging. Most diseases of humans and other animals, as well as of plants, are caused by microorganisms. Isolation and identification of disease-causing bacteria are key aspects in understanding the etiology of such diseases. Many aspects of technology, from the discovery or development of new antibiotics to the development of new strains of microbes, utilize such methodologies as Gram's stain in the identification of fresh isolates.

Clinical methods for the identification of infectious agents follow a series of defined steps. The particular material involved depends on the type and site of infection and can include such fluids as blood, urine, pus, or saliva (sputum). The specific symptoms of the illness may also provide clues as to the particular agents involved.

For example, among the most common infections are those of the urinary tract. These are particularly common nosocomial, or hospital-acquired, infections. Samples are taken with a sterile swab, which is used to inoculate special types of selective or differential media. Generally speaking, such infections are usually associated with gram-negative bacteria. The majority of these infections, about 90 percent, are caused by *Escherichia coli* (*E. coli*), a common intestinal organism. To a lesser extent, such infections may be associated with other genera such as *Klebsiella*, *Pseudomonas*, *Proteus*, or *Streptococcus*. All but *Streptococcus* are gram-negative bacilli.

Confirmation of the Gram morphology follows growth on selective media. The media of choice in this example are those selective for gram-negative bacteria: either eosin-methylene blue or MacConkey agars. Both inhibit the replication of bacteria such as *Staphylococcus*, commonly found on the surface of the skin and a possible contaminant during the swabbing of the site of infection.

The presence of the sugar lactose in either MacConkey or EMB agar allows these media to be differential in addition to being selective. Lactose fermenters such as *Escherichia*, *Klebsiella*, or *Enterobacter* will produce pink colonies on MacConkey agar, while gram-negative organisms such as *Proteus*, *Pseudomonas*, or *Salmonella*, which do not ferment lactose, will produce colorless colonies on this medium. Analogous results can be seen with other differential enteric agars. More detailed types of analysis using other forms of media or utilizing immunological methods may be necessary to fine-tune the diagnosis, or antibiotic susceptibility tests may simply be conducted to determine the treatment of choice.

In some instances, Gram morphology may be sufficient for the identification of a microorganism. For example, the presence of gram-negative cocci in a cervical smear from a patient suspected of having contracted a sexually transmitted disease is indicative of a *Neisseria gonorrhoeae* infection. The identification can be confirmed using immunological methods or through growth on selective media such as Thayer-Martin agar, which contains antibiotics inhibitory to most other gram-negative bacteria.

If the clinical sample consists of blood or cerebrospinal fluid, both of which are normally sterile, either gram-negative or gram-positive organisms may be involved. The initial step toward identification is a Gram's stain of the material. Gram-negative bacteria can be identified using methods already described. Generally speaking, the bacterial content of blood during bacteremia will be too low for ready observation. For this reason, blood samples are inoculated into bottles of nonselective growth media, one of which is grown under aerobic conditions and one under anaerobic conditions. If and when growth becomes apparent, smears are prepared for Gram staining.

Gram-positive cocci will almost always be members of either of two genera: *Staphylococcus* or *Streptococcus*. The two can be differentiated on the basis of catalase production, an enzyme which degrades hydrogen peroxide; staphylococci produce the enzyme, while streptococci do not. A variety of commercial kits are available for rapid identification of species. These contain a battery of tests based on biochemical properties of the organisms, including tolerance of high salt, fermentation of unusual sugars, and growth characteristics on blood agar plates (nutrient agar containing sheep red blood cells).

The identification of gram-positive bacilli is more difficult, given their biochemical variation even within the genus. The major subdivisions of this group are based on their tolerance of oxygen. Obligate gram-positive anaerobes, organisms that cannot tolerate oxygen, include the genus *Clostridium*, members of which cause tetanus, gangrene, and food poisoning. Aerobes and facultative anaerobes, which are oxygen-tolerant, include the genera *Bacillus*, *Corynebacterium*, and *Listeria*. Further identification often requires immunological means.

The gram-negative bacillus *E. coli* is frequently used as a marker for sewage contamination of water supplies. Since it is a common intestinal organism and rarely found in soil, its presence in water samples is indicative of possible fecal contamination of that water. Testing for the presence and level of *E. coli* utilizes the biochemical properties of the microbe. Various quantities of the water sample are placed in tubes of lactose broth; growth is indicative of a lactose fermenter and is presumptive for the presence of *E. coli*. A sample of the lactose culture is then streaked on EMB agar. The development of metallic green-colored colonies of gram-negative bacilli confirms the presence of *E. coli*. The smaller the volume of the water sample that produced growth in lactose, the higher the level of *E. coli* in that sample. In a sense, *E. coli* serves as a surrogate marker in these tests. It may not itself be a pathogen (though some strains of *E. coli* may indeed cause severe intestinal infections), but other gram-negative intestinal pathogens such as *Salmonella*, *Shigella*, or *Vibrio*, even if present in water supplies, may be in a concentration too low for ready detection. Therefore, the presence of *E. coli* suggests possible fecal contamination, al-

lowing for proper sewage treatment. Conversely, the absence of *E. coli* in the water sample indicates that fecal contamination, and therefore the presence of other intestinal pathogens, is unlikely.

PERSPECTIVE AND PROSPECTS

During the latter portion of the nineteenth century, the role of bacteria as etiological agents of disease became apparent. Eventually the experimental observations linking the presence of bacteria with various illnesses coalesced in the so-called germ theory of disease. During the early 1880's, the German physician Robert Koch, along with his colleagues and students, developed an experimental method that could be applied to associate a particular organism with a specific disease. These procedures eventually became known as Koch's postulates. Inherent in Koch's postulates was the necessity to observe the microbial agent, either in tissue or following growth in the laboratory. Staining methods, however, were often crude or imprecise. The best one might hope for was to be able to at least observe the organism.

Hans Christian Gram, a Danish physician working with C. Friedlander in Berlin during the early 1880's, was able to introduce a highly effective method of staining bacteria. Gram's method was a modification of that developed earlier by Paul Ehrlich. The procedure began by first staining the sample with Gentian Violet in aniline water, followed by treatment with iodine in a potassium iodide solution. Gram found that when tissue sections or smears treated in such a manner were washed with dilute alcohol, certain types of bacteria (or schizomycetes, as they were then known) became decolorized (gram-negative), while other forms of bacteria retained their violet appearance (gram-positive). The procedure, published in 1884, was shown to be applicable for most types of bacteria. As a result, a process for differentiation between various types of bacteria became available. In addition, the ability to detect smaller quantities of bacteria in tissue increased significantly.

—*Richard Adler, Ph.D.*

See also Bacterial infections; Bacteriology; Cells; Cytology; *E. coli* infection; Laboratory tests; Microbiology; Salmonella infection; Shigellosis; Staphylococcal infections; Streptococcal infections.

FOR FURTHER INFORMATION:

Alcarno, I. Edward, and Lawrence M. Elson. *Microbiology Coloring Book.* New York: HarperCollins,

1996. This volume is one in a series of "coloring books" that are excellent sources of information. Detailed instructions help the reader navigate the intricacies of the world of microbes through observation and reading. This book is jammed with useful facts about the biology of microorganisms and the methods used to study them.

Goodsell, David. *The Machinery of Life.* New York: Springer-Verlag, 1993. A short book on the biology of the cell for the general reader. The section on *Escherichia coli* as the prototype for bacteria is well written and easy to understand. Especially striking are the large number of computer graphics illustrating molecular structures.

Koneman, Elmer, Stephen Allen, V. R. Dowell, Jr., and Herbert Sommers. *Color Atlas and Textbook of Diagnostic Microbiology.* 5th ed. Philadelphia: J. B. Lippincott, 1997. Presents methods of identification for most organisms likely to appear in a clinical laboratory. Of particular interest are the large number of color photographs illustrating results for major staining methods and biochemical tests.

Madigan, Michael T., John M. Martinko, and Jack Parker. *Brock Biology of Microorganisms.* 9th ed. Upper Saddle River, N.J.: Prentice Hall, 2000. An outstanding microbiology text. The authors provide a thorough description of bacteria and the means by which they are studied. Relevant to this topic are chapters on methods of isolation and characterization.

Singleton, Paul. *Introduction to Bacteria.* 2d ed. New York: John Wiley & Sons, 1992. The author has written a concise description of bacteria and their roles in nature. Included are chapters on bacterial structure and methods of classification and identification. Portions of the book cover molecular aspects of cells.

GRAY HAIR
DISEASE/DISORDER

ANATOMY OR SYSTEM AFFECTED: Hair
SPECIALTIES AND RELATED FIELDS: Dermatology
DEFINITION: The reduction in hair pigmentation that is a natural by-product of aging.

CAUSES AND SYMPTOMS

Hair color is produced by tiny pigment cells in hair follicles called melanocytes. Each melanocyte has long, armlike extensions that carry the pigment granules known as melanin to the hair cells. In the course of a lifetime, the production of pigment-forming enzymes drops, and the activity of the melanocytes in each follicle begins to wane, resulting in gray hair. Each individual's melanocyte clock is different, but in Caucasians the reduction of melanocyte activity usually occurs earlier than in other ethnic groups. On the average, graying starts at age thirty-four in Caucasians, in the late thirties in Asians, and at age forty-four in African Americans.

Pigment loss starts at the root, with some strands of hair gradually fading in color, while others may grow in gray or white. Initial graying can be accelerated by hyperthyroidism, anemia, autoimmune disease, severe stress, or vitamin B_{12} deficiency. Disorders of skin pigmentation, such as vitiligo, can also result in the loss of hair pigmentation.

Once gray hair begins to appear, the rate at which it progresses over the rest of the head depends entirely upon each individual. It does not appear to be a function of the original hair color or texture, ethnic background, or the condition of the scalp. By age fifty, 50 percent of Caucasians are significantly gray. As hair loses its pigment, it often gets drier, resulting in coarser, wirier hair.

TREATMENT AND THERAPY

For some individuals, gray hair is a symbol of maturity, while for others it is an embarrassing sign associated with the aging process. In most cases, graying can be readily masked if so desired. Effective chemical and vegetable rinses and dyes are available.

—*Alvin K. Benson, Ph.D.*

See also Aging; Hair loss and baldness; Hair transplantation; Pigmentation; Skin; Skin disorders.

FOR FURTHER INFORMATION:

Carper, Jean. *Stop Aging Now!* New York: Harper-Collins, 1995.

Feinberg, Herbert S. *All About Hair.* Alpine, N.J.: Wallingford Press, 1978.

Levine, Norman. *Pigmentation and Pigmentary Disorders.* Boca Raton, Fla.: CRC Press, 1993.

Schneider, Edward L., and John W. Rowe. *Handbook of the Biology of Aging.* 4th ed. San Diego: Academic Press, 1996.

GRIEF AND GUILT
DISEASE/DISORDER

ANATOMY OR SYSTEM AFFECTED: Psychic-emotional system

SPECIALTIES AND RELATED FIELDS: Family practice, psychiatry, psychology

DEFINITION: Grief and accompanying guilt are common reactions to the fact or eventuality of serious losses of various kinds, especially death; every person eventually experiences grief, and while grief is normal, its effects can be incapacitating.

KEY TERMS:

abnormal grief: an unhealthy response to a loss, which may include anger, an inability to feel loss, withdrawal, and deterioration in health

grief: a multifaceted physical, emotional, psychological, spiritual, and social reaction to loss

guilt: a cognitive and emotional response often associated with the grief experience in which a person feels a sense of remorse, responsibility, and/or shame regarding the loss

loss: the sudden lack of a previously held possession, physical state, or social position or the death of a loved one

CAUSES AND SYMPTOMS

During life, people unavoidably experience a variety of losses. These may include the loss of loved ones, important possessions or status, health and vitality, and ultimately the loss of self through death. "Grief" is the word commonly used to refer to an individual's or group's shared experience following a loss. The experience of grief is not a momentary or singular phenomenon. Instead, it is a variable, and somewhat predictable, process of life. Also, as with many phenomena within the range of human experience, it is a multidimensional process including biological, psychological, spiritual, and social components.

The biological level of the grief experience includes the neurological and physiological processes that take place in the various organ systems of the body in response to the recognition of loss. These processes, in turn, form the basis for emotional and psychological reactions. Various organs and organ systems interact with one another in response to the cognitive stimulation resulting from this recognition. Human beings are self-reflective creatures with the capacity for experiencing, reflecting upon, and giving meaning to sensations, both physical and emotional. Consequently, the physiological reactions of grief that take place in the body are given meaning by those experiencing them.

The cognitive and emotional meanings attributed to the experience of grief are shaped by and influence interactions within the social dimensions of life. In other words, how someone feels or thinks about grief influences and is influenced by interactions with family, friends, and helping professionals. In addition, the individual's religious or spiritual frame of reference may have a significant influence on the subjective experience and cognitive-emotional meaning attributed to grief.

The grief reactions associated with a loss such as death vary widely. While it is very difficult and perhaps unfair to generalize about such an intensely personal experience, several predictors of the intensity of grief have become evident. The amount of grief experienced seems to depend on the significance of the loss, or the degree to which the individual subjectively experiences a sense of loss. This subjective experience is partially dependent on the meaning attributed to the loss by the survivors and others in the surrounding social context. This meaning is in turn shaped by underlying belief systems, such as religious faith. Clear cognitive, emotional, and/or spiritual frameworks are helpful in guiding people constructively through the grief process.

People in every culture around the world and throughout history have developed expectations about life, and these beliefs influence the grief process. Common questions in many cultures include "Why do people die?" "Is death a part of life, or a sign of weakness or failure?" "Is death always a tragedy, or is it sometimes a welcome relief from suffering?" and "Is there life after death, and if so, what is necessary to attain this afterlife?" The answers to these and other questions help shape people's experience of the grief process. As Elisabeth Kübler-Ross states in *Death: The Final Stage of Growth* (1975), the way in which a society or subculture explains death will have a significant impact on the way in which its members view and experience life.

Another factor that influences the experience of grief is whether a loss was anticipated. Sudden and/or unanticipated losses are more traumatic and more difficult to explain because they tend to violate the meaning systems mentioned above. The cognitive and emotional shock of this violation exacerbates the grief process. For example, it is usually assumed that youngsters will not die before the older members of the family. Therefore, the shock of a child dying in an automobile crash may be more traumatic than the impact of the death of an older person following a long illness.

Death and grief are often distasteful to human beings, at least in Western Judeo-Christian cultures. These negative, fearful reactions are, in part, the result of an individual's difficulty accepting the inevitability of his or her own death. Nevertheless, in cultures which have less difficulty accepting death and loss as normal, people generally experience more complicated grief experiences. The Micronesian society of Truk is a death-affirming society. The members of the Truk society believe that a person is not really grown up until the age of forty. At that point, the individual begins to prepare for death. Similarly, some native Alaskan groups teach their members to approach death intentionally. The person about to die plans for death and makes provisions for the grief process of those left behind.

In every culture, however, the grief-stricken strive to make sense out of their experience of loss. Some attribute death to a malicious intervention from the outside by someone or something else; death becomes frightening. For others, death is in response to divine intervention or is simply the completion of "the circle of life" for that person. Yet for most people in Western societies, even those who come to believe that death is a part of life, grief may be an emotional mixture of loss, shock, shame, sadness, rage, numbness, relief, anger, and/or guilt.

Kübler-Ross points out in her timeless discourse "On the Fear of Dying" (*On Death and Dying*, 1969) that guilt is perhaps the most painful companion of death and grief. The grief process is often complicated by the individual's perception that he or she should have prevented the loss. This feeling of being responsible for the death or other loss is common among those connected to the deceased. For example, parents or health care providers may believe that they should have done something differently in order to detect the eventual cause of death sooner or to prevent it once the disease process was detected.

Guilt associated with grief is often partly or completely irrational. For example, there may be no way that a physician could have detected an aneurysm in her patient's brain prior to a sudden and fatal stroke. Similarly, a parent cannot monitor the minute-by-minute activities of his adolescent children to prevent lethal accidents. Kübler-Ross explains a related phenomenon among children who have lost a parent by pointing out the difficulty in separating wishes from deeds. A child whose wishes are not gratified by a parent may become angry. If the parent subsequently dies, the child may feel guilty, even if the death is some distance in time away from the event in question.

The guilt may also involve remorse over surviving someone else's loss. People who survive an ordeal in which others die often experience "survivor's guilt." Survivors may wonder why they survived and how the deceased person's family members feel about their survival, whether they blame the survivors or wish that they had died instead. As a result, survivors have difficulty integrating the experience with the rest of their lives in order to move on. The feelings of grief and guilt may be exacerbated further if survivors believe that they somehow benefited from someone else's death. A widow who is suddenly the beneficiary of a large sum of money attached to her husband's life insurance policy may feel guilty about doing some of the things that they had always planned but were unable to do precisely because of a lack of money.

Last, guilt may result when people believe that they did not pay enough attention to, care well enough for, or deserve the love of the person who died. These feelings and thoughts are prompted by loss—loss of an ongoing relationship with the one who died, as well as part of the empathetic response to what it might be like to die oneself.

Feelings of guilt are not always present, even if the reaction is extreme. If individuals experience guilt, however, they may "bargain" with themselves or a higher power, review their actions to find what they did wrong, take a moral inventory to see where they could have been more loving or understanding, or even begin to act self-destructively. Attempting to resolve guilt while grieving loss is doubly complicated and may contribute to the development of what is considered an abnormal grief reaction.

The distinctions between normal and abnormal grief processes are not clear-cut and are largely context-dependent; that is, what is normal depends on standards that vary among different social groups and historical periods. In addition, at any particular time the variety of manifestations of grief depend on the individual's personality and temperament; family, social, and cultural contexts; resources for coping with and resolving problems; and experiences with the successful resolution of grief.

Despite this diversity, the symptoms that are manifested by individuals experiencing grief are generally grouped into two different but related diagnostic categories: depression and anxiety. It is normal for the grieving individual to manifest symptoms related to anxiety and/or depression to some degree. For example, a surviving relative or close friend may temporarily have difficulty sleeping, or feel sad or that life has lost its meaning. Relative extremes of these symptoms, however, in either duration or intensity, signal the possibility of an abnormal grief reaction.

In *Families and Health* (1988), family therapist William Doherty and family physician Thomas Campbell identify the signs of abnormal grief reactions as including periods of compulsive overactivity without a sense of loss; identification with the deceased; acquisition of symptoms belonging to the last illness of the deceased; deterioration of health in the survivors; social isolation, withdrawal, or alienation; and severe depression. These signs may also include severe anxiety, abuse of substances, work or school problems, extreme or persistent anger, or an inability to feel loss.

TREATMENT AND THERAPY

There is no set time schedule for the grief process. While various ethnic, cultural, religious, and political groups define the limits of the period of mourning, they cannot prescribe the experience of grief. Yet established norms do influence the grief experience inasmuch as the grieving individuals have internalized these expectations and standards. For example, the typical benefit package of a professional working in the United States offers up to one week of paid "funeral" leave in the event of the death of a significant family member. On the surface, this policy begins to prescribe or define the limits of the grief process.

Such a policy suggests, for example, that a mother or father stricken with grief at the untimely death of a child ought to be able to return to work and function reasonably well once a week has passed. Most individuals will attempt to do so, even if they are harboring unresolved feelings about the child's death. Coworkers, uncomfortable with responding to such a situation and conditioned to believe that people need to "get on with life," may support the lack of expression of grief.

Helpful responses to grief are as multifaceted as is grief itself. Ultimately, several factors ease the grief process. These include validating responses from significant others, socially sanctioned expression of the experience, self-care, social or religious rituals, and possibly professional assistance. Each person responds to grief differently and requires or is able to use different forms of assistance.

Most reactions to loss run a natural, although varied, course. Since grief involves coming to grips with the reality of death, acceptance must eventually be both intellectual and emotional. Therefore, it is important to allow for the complete expression of both thoughts and feelings. Those attempting to assist grief-stricken individuals are more effective if they have come to terms with their own feelings, beliefs, and conflicts about death, and any losses they personally have experienced.

Much of what is helpful in working through grief involves accepting grief as a normal phenomenon. Grief-related feelings should not be judged or overly scrutinized. Supportive conversations include time for ventilation, empathic responses, and sharing of sympathetic experiences. Helpful responses may take the form of "To feel pain and sadness at this time is a normal, healthy response" or "I don't know what it is like to have a child die, but it looks like it really hurts" or "It is understandable if you find yourself thinking that life has lost its purpose." In short, people must be given permission to grieve. When it becomes clear that the person is struggling with an inordinate amount of feelings based on irrational beliefs, these underlying beliefs—not the feelings—may need to be challenged.

People tend to have difficulty concentrating and focusing in the aftermath of a significant loss. The symptoms of anxiety and depression associated with grief may be experienced, and many of the basic functions of life may be interrupted. Consequently, paying attention to healthy eating and sleeping schedules, establishing small goals, and being realistic about how long it may take before "life returns to normal" are important.

While the prescription of medication for the grief-stricken is fairly common, its use is recommended only in extreme situations. Antianxiety agents or antidepressants can interfere with the normal experiences of grief that involve feeling and coming to terms with loss. Sedatives can help bereaved family members and other loved ones feel better over the short term, with less overt distress and crying. Many experts believe, however, that they inhibit the normal grieving process and lead to unresolved grief reactions. In addition, studies suggest that those who start on psychotropic medication during periods of grief stay on them for at least two years.

The grief process is also eased by ritual practices that serve as milestones to mark progress along the way. Some cultures have very clearly defined and well-established rituals associated with grief. In the United States, the rituals practiced continue to be somewhat influenced by family, ethnic, and regional cultures. Very often, however, the rituals are confined to the procedures surrounding the preparation and burial of the body (for example, viewing the body at the mortuary, a memorial service, and interment). As limited as these experiences might be, they are designed to ease people's grief. Yet the grief process is often just beginning with the death and burial of the loved one. Consequently, survivors are often left without useful guidelines to help them on their way.

Another common, although unhelpful, phenomenon associated with the process is for the grief-stricken person initially to receive a considerable amount of empathy and support from family, friends, and possibly professionals (such as a minister or physician) only to have this attention drop off sharply after about a month. The resources available through family and other social support systems diminish with the increasing expectation that the bereaved should stop grieving and "get on with living." If this is the case, or if an individual never did experience a significantly supportive response from members of his or her social system, the role of psychotherapy and/or support groups should be explored. Many public and private agencies offer individual and family therapy. In addition, in many communities there are a variety of self-help support groups devoted to growth and healing in the aftermath of loss.

PERSPECTIVE AND PROSPECTS

The grief process, however it is shaped by particular religious, ethnic, or cultural contexts, is reflective of the human need to form attachments. Grief thus reflects the importance of relationships in one's life, and therefore it is likely that people will always experience grief (including occasional feelings of guilt). Processes such as the grief experience, with its cognitive, emotional, social, and spiritual dimensions, may affect an individual's psychological and physical well-being. Consequently, medical and other health care and human service professionals will probably always be called upon to investigate, interpret, diagnose, counsel, and otherwise respond to grief-stricken individuals and families.

In the effort to be helpful, however, medical sci-

ence has frequently intervened too often and too invasively into death, dying, and the grief process—to the point of attempting to disallow them. For example, hospitals and other institutions such as nursing homes have become the primary place that people die. It is important to remember that it has not always been this way. Even now in some cultures around the world, people die more often in their own homes than in a "foreign" institution.

In the early phases of the development of the field of medicine, hospitals as institutions were primarily devoted to the care of the dying and the indigent. Managing the dying process was a primary focus. More recently, however, technological advances and specialty development have shifted the mission of the hospital to being an institution devoted to healing and curing. The focus on the recovery process has left dying in the shadows. Death has become equated with failure and associated with professional guilt.

It is more difficult for health care professionals to involve themselves or at least constructively support the grief process of individuals and families if it is happening as a result of the health care team's "failure." In a parallel fashion, society has become unduly fixated on avoiding death, or at least prolonging its inevitability to the greatest possible extent. The focus of the larger culture is on being young, staying young, and recoiling from the effects of age. As a result, healthy grief over the loss of youthful looks, stamina, health, and eventually life is not supported.

Medical science can make an important contribution in this area by continuing to define the appropriate limits of technology and intervention. The struggle to balance quantity of life with quality of life (and death) must continue. In addition, medical science professionals need to redouble their efforts toward embracing the patient, not simply the disease; the person, not simply the patient; and the complexities of grief in death and dying, not simply the joy in healing and living.

—Layne A. Prest, Ph.D.

See also Death and dying; Depression; Emotions: Biomedical causes and effects; Midlife crisis; Neurosis; Phobias; Postpartum depression; Psychiatric disorders; Psychiatry; Psychiatry, child and adolescent; Psychiatry, geriatric; Psychoanalysis; Stress; Suicide.

FOR FURTHER INFORMATION:

Doka, Kenneth J., ed. *Living with Grief After Sudden Loss: Suicide, Homicide, Accident, Heart Attack*

Stroke. Washington, D.C.: Taylor & Francis, Hospice Foundation of America, 1997. Provides information that will be useful for individuals dealing with the different kinds of adjustment related to the death of a loved one or the loss of functioning or abilities.

Klass, Dennis, Phyllis R. Silverman, and Steven L. Nickman, eds. *Continuing Bonds: New Understandings of Grief*. Washington, D.C.: Taylor & Francis, 1996. Examines cross-cultural manifestations of bereavement, particularly the psychological aspects. Includes a bibliography and an index.

Kübler-Ross, Elisabeth, ed. *On Death and Dying*. New York: Collier Books, 1970. This book is, and will remain, a classic in the field. Kübler-Ross shares the experience of many years working with dying patients and their families.

Staudacher, Carol. *Beyond Grief: A Guide for Recovering from the Death of a Loved One*. New York: Barnes & Noble Books, 2000. A clear and readable guide to the grief process. The author provides specific examples relevant for some of the most painful grief experiences: those following the death of a spouse, child, or parent at an early age.

GROWTH

BIOLOGY

ANATOMY OR SYSTEM AFFECTED: All

SPECIALTIES AND RELATED FIELDS: Embryology, endocrinology, obstetrics, orthopedics, pediatrics

DEFINITION: The development of the human body from conception to adulthood; growth occurs at different rates for different systems over this period, and varies by sex and individual as well.

KEY TERMS:

accretion: a type of growth in which new, nongrowing material is simply added to the surface

allometric growth: unequal rates of growth of different body parts, or in different directions

developmental biology: broadly, the study of ontogeny; narrowly, the study of how gene action is controlled

embryonic stage: that part of ontogeny during which organs are formed

fetal stage: that part of ontogeny after the organs are formed but before birth takes place

interstitial growth: growth throughout a structure, usually in all directions

isometric growth: equal rates of growth of all parts, or in all directions

ontogeny: the entire developmental sequence, from conception through the various embryonic stages, birth, childhood, maturity, senescence, and death; also, the study of this sequence

ossification: the formation of bone tissue

PROCESS AND EFFECTS

The human body grows from conception until adult size is reached. Adult size is reached in females around the age of eighteen and in males around twenty or twenty-one, but there is considerable variation in either direction. (Nearly all numerical measurements of growth and development are subject to much variation.) On the average, males end up with a somewhat larger body size than females because of these two or three extra years of growth.

Growth begins after conception. The first phase of growth, including approximately the first month after conception, is called embryonic growth, and the growing organism is called an embryo. During embryonic growth, the most important developmental process is differentiation, the formation of the various organs and tissues. After the organs and tissues are formed, the rest of prenatal growth is called fetal growth and the developing organism is called a fetus. Respiratory movements begin around the eighteenth week of gestation, during the fetal stage; limb movements (such as kicking) begin to be felt by the mother around the twenty-fourth week, with a considerable range of variation. At birth, the average infant weighs about 3.4 kilograms (7.5 pounds) and measures about 50 centimeters (20 inches) in length.

Growth continues after birth and throughout childhood and adolescence. From the perspective of developmental biology, childhood is defined as the period from birth to puberty, which generally begins at twelve years of age, and adolescence continues from that point to the cessation of skeletal growth at around the age of eighteen in females and twenty or twenty-one in males. The long period of adulthood that follows is marked by a stable body size, with little or no growth except for the repair and maintenance of the body, including the healing of wounds. After about age sixty, there may be a slight decline in body height and in a few other dimensions.

By one year of age, the average baby is 75 centimeters (30 inches) long and weighs 10 kilograms (22 pounds). (There is actually a slight decline in weight in the first week of postnatal life, but this is usually regained by age three weeks.) For ages one to six, the

Growth from Infancy to Adulthood

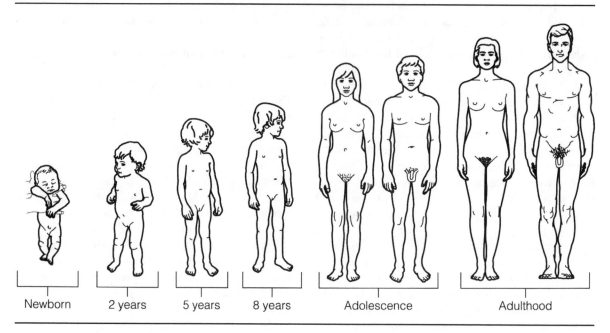

Newborn   2 years   5 years   8 years   Adolescence   Adulthood

average weight (in kilograms) can be approximated by the equation "weight = age × 2 + 8." For ages seven to twelve, growth takes place more rapidly: Average weight (in kilograms) can be approximated by "weight = age × 3.5 − 2.5," while average height (in centimeters) can be approximated for ages two to twelve by the equation "height = age × 6 + 77." Head circumference has a median value of about 34.5 centimeters at birth, 46.3 centimeters at an age of one year, 48.6 centimeters at age two, and 49.9 centimeters at age three. All these figures are about 1 centimeter larger in boys than in girls, with considerable individual variation. Median heights and weights, when differentiated by sex, reveal that boys and girls are generally similar until age fourteen, after which boys continue to gain in both dimensions.

Growth of the teeth takes place episodically. In most children, the first teeth erupt between five and nine months of age, beginning with the central incisors, the lower pair generally preceding the upper pair. The lateral incisors (with the upper pair first), the first premolars, the canines, and the second premolars follow, in that order. All these teeth are deciduous teeth ("baby teeth") that will eventually be shed, to be replaced during late childhood by the permanent teeth. At one year of age, most children have between six and eight teeth.

Growth takes place in several directions. Growth at the same rate in all directions is called isometric growth, which maintains similar proportions throughout the growth process. Isometric growth occurs in nautilus shells and a variety of other invertebrates. Most of human growth, however, is allometric growth, which takes place at different rates in different directions. Allometric growth results in changes in shape as growth proceeds. Moreover, different parts of the body grow at different rates and in different directions. During fetal development, for example, the head develops in advance of the fore and hind limbs, and the fetus at about six months of age has a head which is about half its length. The head of a newborn baby is about one-third of its body length, compared to about one-seventh for an adult. In contrast, the legs make up only a small part of the body length in either the six-month-old fetus or the newborn baby, and their absolute length and proportionate length both increase throughout childhood and adolescence.

Growth of the skeleton sets the pace for growth of the majority of the body, except for the nervous system and reproductive organs. Most parts of the skeleton begin as fast-growing cartilage. The process in which cartilage tissue turns into bone tissue is called ossification, which begins at various centers in the bone. The first center of ossification within each bone is called the diaphysis; in long bones, this ossification usually takes place in the center of the bone, forming the shaft. Secondary centers of ossification form at the ends of long bones and at certain other specified places; each secondary center of ossification is called an epiphysis. In a typical long bone, two epiphyses form, one at either end. Capping the end of the bone, beyond the epiphysis, lies an articular cartilage. Between the epiphysis and the diaphysis, the cartilage that persists is called the epiphyseal cartilage; this becomes the most rapidly growing region of the bone. During most of the growth of a long bone, the increase in width occurs by accretion, a gradual process in which material is added at a slow rate only along a surface. In the case of a bone shaft, increase in width takes place only at the surface, beneath the surrounding membrane known as the periosteum. By contrast, the epiphyseal cartilage grows much more rapidly, and it also grows by interstitial growth, meaning that growth takes place throughout the growing tissue in all directions at once. As the epiphyseal cartilage grows, parts of it slowly become bony, and those bony portions grow more slowly.

During the first seven or eight years of postnatal life, the growth of the epiphyseal cartilage takes place faster than its replacement by bone tissue, causing the size of the epiphyseal cartilage to increase. Starting around age seven, the interstitial growth of the epiphyseal cartilage slows down, while the replacement of cartilage by bone speeds up, so that the epiphyseal cartilage is not growing as fast as it turns into bone tissue; the size of the epiphyseal cartilage therefore starts to decrease. At the time of puberty, the hormonal influences create an adolescent growth spurt during which the individual's bone growth increases for about a one-year period. In girls, the adolescent growth spurt takes place about two years earlier than it does in boys—the average age is around twelve in girls, versus about fifteen in boys—but there are tremendous individual variations both in the extent of the growth spurt and in its timing. At age fourteen, most girls have already experienced most of their adolescent growth spurt, while most boys are barely beginning theirs. Consequently, the average fourteen-year-old girl is a bit taller than the average fourteen-year-old boy.

At around eighteen years of age in females and twenty or twenty-one years of age in males, the replacement of the epiphyseal cartilage by bone is finally complete, and bone growth ceases. The age at which this occurs, and the resulting adult size, both vary considerably from one individual to another. For the rest of adult life, the skeleton remains more or less constant in size, diminishing only slightly in old age.

Most of the other organs of the body grow in harmonious proportion with the growth of the skeleton, reaching a maximum growth rate during the growth spurt of early adolescence and reaching a stable adult size at around age eighteen in women and age twenty or twenty-one in men. The nervous system and reproductive system, however, constitute major exceptions to this rule. The nervous system and brain grow faster at an earlier age, reaching about 90 to 95 percent of their adult size by one year of age. The shape of the head, including the shape of the skull, keeps pace with the development of the brain and nervous system. For this reason, babies and young children have

Median Heights and Weights from Childhood to Adulthood

	Boys		Girls	
Age	Height (cm)	Weight (kg)	Height (cm)	Weight (kg)
2	87	12	87	12
3	95	15	94	14
4	103	17	102	16
5	110	19	108	18
6	117	21	115	20
7	122	23	121	22
8	127	25	127	25
9	132	28	132	28
10	138	31	138	33
11	143	35	145	37
12	150	40	152	42
13	157	45	157	46
14	163	51	160	50
15	169	57	162	54
16	174	62	162	56
17	176	66	163	57
18	177	69	164	57

heads that constitute a larger proportion of their body size than do the heads of adults.

The growth of the reproductive system also follows its own pattern. Most reproductive development is delayed until puberty. The reproductive organs of the embryo form slowly and remain small. The reproductive organs of children, though present, do not reach their mature size until adolescence. These organs, both the internal ones and the external ones, remain small throughout childhood. Their period of most rapid growth marks the time of puberty, which spans ages eleven through thirteen, with a wide range of variation. At this time, the pituitary gland begins secreting increased amounts of the follicle-stimulating hormone (FSH), which stimulates the growth and maturation of the gonads (the ovaries of females and the testes of males). The ovaries or testes then respond by producing increased amounts of the sex hormones testosterone (in males) or estrogen (in females), which stimulate the further development of both primary and secondary sexual characteristics. Primary sexual characteristics are those which are functionally necessary for reproduction, such as the presence of a uterus and ovaries in females or the presence of testes and sperm ducts in males. Secondary sexual characteristics are those which distinguish one sex from another, but which are not functionally necessary for reproduction. Examples of secondary sexual characteristics include the growth of breasts or the widening of the hips in females, the growth of the beard and deepening of the voice in males, and the growth of hair in the armpits and pubic regions of both sexes.

Growth takes place psychologically and socially as well as physically. Newborn babies, though able to respond to changes in their environment, seem to pay attention to such stimuli only on occasion. At a few weeks of age, the baby will respond to social stimuli (such as the sound of the mother's voice) by smiling. Babies usually can grasp objects by five months of age, depending on the size and shape of the object. By six months, most babies will show definite signs of pleasure in response to social stimulation; this may include an open-mouth giggle or laugh. At seven months of age, most babies will respond to adult facial expressions and will show different responses to familiar adults as opposed to strangers. The age at which babies learn to crawl varies greatly, but most infants learn the technique by nine or ten months of age. Social imitation begins late in the first year of life. Also, by this time, children learn object perma-

nence, meaning that they will search for a missing object if they have watched it being hidden. Walking generally develops around eighteen months of age, but the time of development varies greatly.

Jean Piaget (1896-1980) was a pioneer in the study of the social and cognitive development of children. Piaget identified four stages of cognitive and social growth, which he called sensorimotor, preoperational, concrete operational, and formal operational. In the sensorimotor stage, from birth to about two years of age, infants begin with reflexes such as sucking or finger curling (in response to touching their palms). Starting with these reflexes, they gradually learn to understand their senses and apply the resulting information in order to acquire important adaptive motor skills that can be used to manipulate the world (as in picking up things) or to navigate about and explore the world (as in walking). Socially, infants develop ways to make desirable stimuli last by such acts as smiling. In the preoperational stage, which lasts from about two to six years of age, children acquire a functional use of their native language. Their imagination flourishes, and pretending becomes an important and frequent activity. Most of the thinking at the preoperational stage is egocentric, however, which means that the child perceives the world only from his or her own point of view and has difficulty seeing other points of view.

The concrete operational stage spans the years from about seven to eleven years of age. This is the stage at which children learn to apply logic to concrete objects. For example, they realize that liquid does not change volume when poured into a taller glass, and they develop the ability to arrange objects in order (for example, by size) or to classify them into groups (for example, by color or shape). The final stage is called the formal operational stage, beginning around age twelve. This is the stage of adolescence and adulthood, when the person learns to manipulate abstract concepts in such areas as ethical, legal, or mathematical reasoning. This is also the stage at which people develop the ability to construct hypothetical situations and to use them in arguments.

COMPLICATIONS AND DISORDERS

Disorders of growth include dwarfism, gigantism, and several other disorders such as achondroplasia (chondrodystrophy). Dwarfism often results from an insufficiency of the pituitary growth hormone, also called somatostatin or somatotrophic hormone. Some short-statured individuals are normally proportioned, while others have proportions differing from those of most other people. An overabundance of growth hormone causes gigantism, a condition marked by unusually rapid growth, especially during adolescence. In some individuals, the amount of growth hormone remains normal during childhood but increases to excessive amounts during the teenage years; these individuals are marked by acromegaly, a greater than normal growth which affects primarily the hands, feet, and face.

Achondroplasia, also called chondrodystrophy, is a genetically controlled condition caused by a dominant gene. In people having this condition, the epiphyseal cartilages of the body's long bones turn bony too soon, so that growth ceases before it should. Those exhibiting chondrodystrophy therefore have short stature and childlike proportions but rugged faces that look older than they really are.

Inadequate growth can often result from childhood malnutrition, particularly from insufficient amounts of protein. If a child is considerably shorter or skinnier than those of the same age, that child's diet should be examined for the presence of malnutrition. Intentional malnutrition is one of the characteristic features of anorexia nervosa. The opposite problem, overeating, can lead to obesity, although obesity can also result from many other causes, including diabetes and other metabolic problems.

PERSPECTIVE AND PROSPECTS

As a phenomenon, growth of both wild and domestic animals was well known to ancient peoples. Hippocrates (c. 460-c. 370 B.C.E.), considered the father of medicine, wrote a treatise on embryological growth, and Aristotle (384-322 B.C.E.) wrote a longer and more complete work on the subject. During the Renaissance, Galileo Galilei (1564-1642) studied growth mathematically and distinguished between isometric and allometric forms of growth, arguing that the bones of giants would be too weak to support their weight.

The most important era in the study of human embryonic development was ushered in by the Estonian naturalist Karl Ernst von Baer (1792-1876), who discovered the human ovum. From this point on, detailed studies of human embryonic and postnatal development proceeded at a rapid pace, especially in Germany. Much of the modern understanding of growth in more general or mathematical terms de-

rives from the classic studies of the British anatomist D'Arcy Wentworth Thomson (1860-1948). In the twentieth century, Piaget became a leader in the study of childhood social and cognitive growth phases.

—*Eli C. Minkoff, Ph.D.*

See also Aging; Childbirth; Conception; Dwarfism; Embryology; Endocrine disorders; Endocrinology; Endocrinology, pediatric; Failure to thrive; Gigantism; Glands; Hormones; Hypertrophy; Malnutrition; Menopause; Menstruation; Nutrition; Pregnancy and gestation; Puberty and adolescence; Sexuality; Vitamins and minerals; Weight loss and gain.

FOR FURTHER INFORMATION:

Behrman, Richard E., ed. *Nelson Textbook of Pediatrics*. 16th ed. Philadelphia: W. B. Saunders, 2000. Contains a considerable amount of useful information, including graphs and growth charts. Offers advice for the monitoring of growth development in children and adolescents.

Gray, Henry. *Gray's Anatomy*. Edited by Peter L. Williams et al. 38th ed. New York: Churchill Livingstone, 1995. The classic work on anatomy, containing the most thorough descriptions. The excellent color illustrations provide much realistic detail in most cases and well-selected highlights in a few. Developmental stages are covered in detail.

Moore, Keith L., and T. V. N. Persaud. *The Developing Human*. 6th ed. Philadelphia: W. B. Saunders, 1998. Excellent descriptions and illustrations of all developmental stages of human growth are provided in this useful work.

Oski, Frank A., ed. *Oski's Pediatrics: Principles and Practice*. 3d ed. Philadelphia: J. B. Lippincott, 1999. Contains many good descriptions and illustrations of different stages of development, various disorders common in children, and several treatments for these disorders.

Rosse, Cornelius, and Penelope Gaddum-Rosse, eds. *Hollinshead's Textbook of Anatomy*. 5th ed. Philadelphia: Lippincott-Raven, 1997. A very thorough, up-to-date, detailed reference work. Provides helpful descriptions and illustrations, including descriptions of the immature stages of growth.

GUILLAIN-BARRÉ SYNDROME
DISEASE/DISORDER

ANATOMY OR SYSTEM AFFECTED: Immune system, muscles, musculoskeletal system, nerves, nervous system

SPECIALTIES AND RELATED FIELDS: Internal medicine, neurology

DEFINITION: An acute degeneration of peripheral motor and sensory nerves, known to physicians as acute inflammatory demyelinating polyneuropathy, a common cause of acute generalized paralysis.

KEY TERMS:

antibody: a substance produced by plasma cells which usually binds to a foreign particle; in Guillain-Barré syndrome, antibodies bind to myelin protein

antigen: any substance that stimulates white blood cells to mount an immune response

areflexia: loss of reflex

autoimmune disorder: a condition in which the immune system attacks the body's own tissue instead of foreign tissue

B cell: a type of white blood cell that produces antibodies

CSF protein: a protein in the cerebrospinal fluid which is usually very low

demyelination: a loss of the myelin coating of nerves

electromyogram: the external recording of electrical impulses from muscles

macrophage: a white blood cell that engulfs foreign protein; in Guillain-Barré syndrome, it also attacks myelin

motor weakness: muscle weakness resulting from the failure of motor nerves

nerve conduction velocity: the speed at which a nerve impulse travels along a nerve

neurogenic atrophy: shrinkage of muscle caused by a loss of nervous stimulation

neuropathy: a condition in which nerves are diseased, are inflamed, or show abnormal degeneration

phagocytosis: the process of engulfing particles

polyneuropathy: neuropathy found in many areas

CAUSES AND SYMPTOMS

Guillain-Barré syndrome (GBS) is an acute disease of the peripheral nerves, especially those that connect to muscles. It causes weakness, areflexia (loss of reflex), ataxia (difficulty in maintaining balance), and sometimes ophthalmoplegia (eye muscle paralysis). GBS demonstrates a variable, multifocal pattern of inflammation and demyelination of the spinal roots and the cranial nerves, although the brain itself is not obviously affected. By the 1990's, it was the most common cause of generalized paralysis in the United States, averaging two cases per 100,000 people per year. The disease was first described in the early 1900's by Georges Guillain and Jean-Alexander Barré, two French neurologists. Little was known of the cause of GBS or the mechanism for its symptoms, however, until the 1970's. Since then, symposia sponsored by the National Institute of Neurological and Communicative Disorders and Stroke have shed more light on this condition.

Most individuals with GBS have a rapidly progressing muscular weakness in more than one limb and also experience paresthesia (tingling) and numbness in the hands and feet. These sensations have the effect of reducing fine muscle control, balance, and one's awareness of limb location. The prevailing scientific opinion regarding GBS is that it is an autoimmune disorder involving white blood cells, which for some unknown reason attack nerves and/or produce antibodies against myelin, the insulating covering of nerves. The weakness is usually ascending in nature, beginning with numbness in the toes and fingers and progressing to total limb weakness. The demyelination is more prominent in the nerves of the trunk and occurs to a lesser extent in the more distal nerves. The brain and spinal cord are protected from GBS by the blood-brain barrier, although antibodies to myelin have been found in the cerebrospinal fluid of some patients.

With GBS, there is often a precipitating event such as surgery, pregnancy, upper respiratory infection, viral infection (such as cytomegalovirus), or vaccination. Preexisting debilitating illnesses such as systemic lupus erythematosus (SLE) or Hodgkin's disease also seem to predispose a person to GBS. GBS has been diagnosed in patients having heart transplants in spite of the fact that they are receiving immunosuppressive drugs. The increased risk with such surgery may be attributable to the stress associated with the procedure. Most patients who come down with GBS have had some prior condition that placed stress on the immune system prior to the appearance of GBS.

The patient with GBS is frequently incapable of communicating as a result of paralysis of the vocal cords. Typically, motor paralysis will worsen rapidly and then plateau after four weeks, with the patient bedridden and often in need of respiratory support. Autonomic nerves can also be affected, causing gastrointestinal disturbances, adynamic ileus (loss of function in the ileum of the small intestine), and indigestion. Other, less common symptoms include pupillary disturbances, pooling of blood in limbs, heart rhythm disturbances, and a decrease in the heart muscle's strength. These patients are usually hypermetabolic because considerable caloric energy goes into an immune response that is self-destructive and into mechanisms that are attempting to repair the damage.

In addition to the loss of myelin, cell body damage to nerves may result and may be associated with permanent deficits. If the nerve cell itself is not severely damaged, regrowth and remyelination can occur. Antibodies to myelin proteins and to acidic glycolipids are seen in a majority of patients. Blood serum taken from patients with GBS has been shown to block calcium channels in muscle, and experiments in Germany have found that cerebrospinal fluid from GBS patients blocks sodium channels.

Like most autoimmune conditions, GBS is cyclic in nature; the patient will have "good" days and "bad" days because the immune system is sensitive to the levels of steroid hormones in the body, which are known to fluctuate. In addition to paralysis, there is significant pain with GBS. Many of the nerve fibers that register the pain response (nociceptors) are nonmyelinated and therefore are not interrupted in GBS. Pain management can be difficult, requiring the use of such drugs as fentanyl, codeine, morphine, and other narcotics. The course of the disease is variable and is a function of the level of reactivity of the patient's immune system. The autoimmune attack is augmented in those patients experiencing activation of serum complement protein induced by antibodies. Recovery usually takes months, and frequently the patient requires home health care. Complications can lead to death, but most patients recover fully, though some have residual weakness.

The physician must be careful to distinguish GBS from lead poisoning, chemical or toxin exposure, polio, botulism, and hysterical paralysis. Diagnosis can be confirmed using cerebrospinal fluid (CSF) analysis. GBS patients have protein levels greater than 0.55 gram per deciliter of CSF. Macrophages are frequently found in the CSF, as well as some B cells. Nerve conduction velocity will be decreased in these patients to a value that is 50 percent of normal in those nerves that are still functioning. These changes can take several weeks to develop. With GBS, macrophages and T cells have been shown to be in contact with nerves, as evidenced in electron micrographs. T-cell and macrophage activation in these individuals point to an immune response gone awry, possibly precipitated by a virus or exposure to an antigen that is foreign but similar in appearance to one of the proteins in myelin. T cells, upon encountering an unrecognizable antigen, will produce interleukin 2, initiate attack, and recruit macrophages to participate. The use of an anti-T-cell drug theoretically should improve nerve function, but researchers at the University of Western Ontario failed to find any benefit from the infusion of an anti-T-cell monoclonal antibody. Unexpectedly, GBS has been found in patients testing positive for the human immunodeficiency virus (HIV) who are asymptomatic, in spite of the fact that their T cells are under attack from the HIV virus and are diminished in number. Although myelin proteins are thought to be the immunogens, other candidates include gangliosides in the myelin. Antiganglioside antibodies have been seen in a majority of the GBS patients. This trait may distinguish GBS from amyotrophic lateral sclerosis (Lou Gehrig's disease) and multiple sclerosis, which seem to involve different myelin proteins as antigens.

In GBS, the white blood cells attack peripheral motor nerves more often than other types of nerves, implying a biochemical difference between motor and sensory nerves that has yet to be discovered. One possible cause of this disease is a similarity between a protein or glycolipid that is present normally in myelin and coincidentally on an infectious agent, such as a virus. The immune system responds to the agent, resulting in a sensitization of the macrophages and T cells to that component of myelin. B cells are then stimulated to produce antibodies against this antigen, and they unfortunately cross-react with components of the myelin protein. The severity of the disease will depend on the number of macrophages and lymphocytes activated and whether serum complement-binding antibodies are being produced. Serum complement proteins are activated by a particular class of antibodies, resulting in the activation of enzymes in the blood that potentiate tissue destruction and neurogenic atrophy. Serum complement levels can be determined by a serum complement fixation test.

In severe cases of GBS, intercostal muscles are more severely compromised and respiratory function needs to be monitored closely. The immune response will subside when T-suppressor cells have reached their peak levels. Halting the autoimmune response will not reverse the symptoms immediately, since it takes time for antibody levels to decrease and for the nerves to regrow and remyelinate, which occurs at the rate of 1 to 2 millimeters per day. Some nerves will undergo retrograde degeneration and be lost from the neuronal pool. Other nerves will have more closely spaced nodes and conduct impulses at a lower velocity. Nerve sprouting will also occur, which will result in one nerve's being responsible for more muscle fibers or serving a larger sensory area and in decreased fine motor control.

TREATMENT AND THERAPY

In Guillain-Barré syndrome, the amount of muscle and nerve involvement can be assessed by performing an electromyogram, which can reveal the amount of motor nerve interruption and the conduction velocity of the nerves that continue to function. Based upon the assumption that an autoimmune response is in progress, corticosteroids such as prednisolone and methylprednisolone are sometimes administered in high doses. The benefits of such drugs have been shown to be marginal, while the side effects are considerable.

More recently, a procedure known as plasmapheresis has been tried with better results, especially when performed in the first two weeks. This procedure involves removing 250 milliliters (a little more than a pint) of plasma from the blood every other day and replacing this volume with a solution containing albumin, glucose, and appropriate salts. Six treatments are typical and usually result in a faster recovery of muscle control than for those not receiving plasmapheresis. Because relapses may occur if the patient produces new antibodies to myelin, immunosuppressants are given to the patient after plasmapheresis. Another procedure, intravenous immunoglobulin therapy, is in the clinical trial stage and is based on the strategy of blocking the binding of antibodies to nerves.

Cyclosporine, a T-cell inhibitor, is also being tried, with some promising results. Some researchers note, however, that transplant patients, who routinely take cyclosporine, have a higher-than-normal risk of developing GBS. Others emphasize that no one knows what their risk for GBS would be without the administration of cyclosporine. Because of the variability of the body's immune response, the benefits of this drug will depend on whether, in a given individual, it is an antibody response or T-cell response. Cyclosporine will benefit those who have a strong T-cell response. T-cell reactivity can be tested with the mixed lymphocyte assay, and T-cell counts can be done.

Cerebrospinal fluid filtration is also being tried in order to remove reactive white blood cells and antibodies. Serum so filtered loses its nerve-inhibiting ef-

fect, as evidenced by its application to in vitro nerve and muscle cells. GBS has been mimicked in animal models, which show antibody and T-cell reactivity to myelin protein. Guillain-Barré syndrome has many of the characteristics of an autoimmune disease and could serve as a model for an acquired autoimmune condition.

PERSPECTIVE AND PROSPECTS

Guillain-Barré syndrome is an example of a delicate physiological balance gone awry. The immune system has the difficult task of distinguishing between self and enemy, and if it detects the latter it must either inactivate or eliminate the intruder. Mistakes in recognition or communication between immune cells can cause either an unintended attack or the failure to attack when appropriate. GBS probably represents an unnecessary attack on self tissue, in this case myelin, and may be considered a form of hyperimmunity. Many diseases fall into this category. They include rheumatoid arthritis, juvenile diabetes, Crohn's disease, ulcerative colitis, Graves' disease, multiple sclerosis, amyotrophic lateral sclerosis, ankylosing spondylitis (inflammation of the joints between the vertebrae), and systemic lupus erythematosus. The other type of response, hypoimmune, is seen in cancer and immunodeficiency diseases such as acquired immunodeficiency syndrome (AIDS).

Questions that arise with GBS are the same ones that arise in many other diseases. It must be determined why the immune system chose this time to initiate an attack against a self-antigen. The answer could be a mistake in recognition, an error in translating the deoxyribonucleic acid (DNA) code in the bone marrow cells, an alteration of the antigen by some environmental factor, or an alteration of an antigen-detector protein on a white blood cell. Researchers also try to discover if there is a genetic predisposition for GBS. Seeking answers about GBS may shed light on other conditions as well, and treatments beneficial to GBS patients have a high probability of benefiting patients with other immune disorders. GBS is a reminder that physiological stress can translate to immunological stress, and under stress the immune system can make mistakes. Failure to react can result in diseases such as cancer, and unnecessary action can lead to diseases such as GBS.

—*William D. Niemi, Ph.D.*

See also Ataxia; Autoimmune disorders; Immune system; Immunology; Motor neuron diseases; Nervous system; Neuralgia, neuritis, and neuropathy; Neurology; Neurology, pediatric; Numbness and tingling; Paralysis; Stress.

FOR FURTHER INFORMATION:

Barr, Murray L., and John A. Kierman. *The Human Nervous System.* 7th ed. Philadelphia: J. B. Lippincott, 1998. A softbound text designed for a medical school introductory course in the basic sciences. Provides a good foundation for understanding the nervous system, with some discussion of demyelination.

Lechtenberg, Richard. *Synopsis of Neurology.* Philadelphia: Lea & Febiger, 1991. A pocket-sized book with summary descriptions of the most common neurological syndromes. Covers diagnostic techniques and symptoms associated with neurological problems, including Guillain-Barré syndrome.

Merrill, Jean E., Michael C. Graves, and Donald G. Mulder. "Autoimmune Disease and the Nervous System: Biochemical, Molecular, and Clinical Update." *Western Journal of Medicine* 156, no. 6 (1992): 639-646. This review summarizes information published on the immunological aspects of many of the classic autoimmune conditions up to 1992.

Nicholls, John G., A. Robert Martin, and Bruce G. Wallace. *From Neuron to Brain.* 4th ed. Sunderland, Mass.: Sinauer Associates, 2000. An excellent and detailed neurobiology text that can help the reader understand the basis and consequences of demyelinating conditions such as Guillain-Barré syndrome.

Noback, Charles R., Norman L. Strominger, and Robert J. Demarest. *The Human Nervous System.* 4th ed. Philadelphia: Lea & Febiger, 1991. A concise, easy-to-read paperback that offers a good balance of physiology and anatomy. Well illustrated.

Pearlman, Alan L., and Robert C. Collins. *Neurobiology of Disease.* New York: Oxford University Press, 1990. An advanced text that provides detailed descriptions of most neurological abnormalities. Contains a good description of Guillain-Barré syndrome and a chapter devoted to demyelinating disease.

GULF WAR SYNDROME

DISEASE/DISORDER

ANATOMY OR SYSTEM AFFECTED: Blood, brain, cells, chest, eyes, gastrointestinal system, gums, hair, immune system, joints, muscles, psychic-emotional system, skin

SPECIALTIES AND RELATED FIELDS: Biochemistry, environmental health, epidemiology, ethics, occupational health, psychology, public health

DEFINITION: A popular term used to describe collectively a variety of symptoms, not a specific disease, suffered by veterans of the Persian Gulf War.

KEY TERMS:

cytokines: proteins which are used by white blood cells to communicate with similar cells

organophosphates: chemical pesticides

pyridostigmine bromide: a chemical that prevents damage from possible nerve gas exposure

sarin: a nerve gas that can cause convulsions and death

CAUSES AND SYMPTOMS

This condition is characterized by flulike symptoms, which sufferers complain of experiencing simultaneously but which do not indicate any specific known disease. Such physical symptoms include chronic fatigue, fever, muscle and joint pain and weakness, and intense headaches. Some patients report episodes of memory loss, insomnia, nightmares, and limited attention spans as well as neuropsychological disorders, such as depression, anxiety attacks, and mood swings. Respiratory problems, diarrhea and gastrointestinal distress, blurred vision, arthritis, bleeding gums, hair loss, and skin rashes sometimes accompany other symptoms.

Physicians disagree about the causal factors of Gulf War syndrome. While some medical professionals diagnose veterans' symptoms as resulting from exposure to wartime toxins, bacteria, or viruses, other doctors state that the symptoms are psychosomatic and due to posttraumatic stress disorder. Gulf War syndrome has not been attributed to any infectious disease that veterans might have contracted in the Persian Gulf. Significantly, no laboratory abnormality or unique characteristic has been identified for this disorder nor has any organ system been isolated as the primary system affected by this condition. Most medical professionals say that Gulf War syndrome is a condition representing factors of several diseases but is not a separate disease.

Many Persian Gulf War veterans believe their ailments are service related. Approximately eight hundred thousand coalition forces were deployed to the Persian Gulf after Iraq invaded Kuwait in August,

1990. About 10 percent of these veterans have claimed to have Gulf War syndrome (statistics vary according to sources). Soldiers hypothesize that exposure to sarin caused the syndrome. Other possible causes include germ and chemical warfare (although no evidence of either has been verified), antianthrax and botulism vaccines, pyridostigmine bromide (PB) tablets, and exposure to radiation from depleted uranium, fumes from burning oil wells, and organophosphates.

TREATMENT AND THERAPY

Because they do not think their concerns are being seriously addressed, many veterans rely on self-diagnosis based on other veterans' accounts exchanged orally, in the press, or on the Internet. Self-medication with over-the-counter pain relievers is a common treatment on which veterans depend for the soothing of symptoms. Physicians prescribe more potent pharmaceuticals and physical therapy to alleviate symptoms and reinforce patients' immune systems. The American, Canadian, and British governments have established medical programs through publicly funded veterans' administrations and privately endowed medical institutions to research the syndrome's causes, ascertain its etiology, identify derivative presentations of the syndrome, develop effective treatment methods, and offer medical care for veterans exhibiting Gulf War syndrome symptoms.

Physicians recommend that some veterans suffering Gulf War syndrome undergo counseling to address neuropsychological symptoms and assist readjustment to peacetime or civilian life and frustration with enduring chronic sickness. Exercise, a nutritional diet, and support groups are also helpful to many veterans suffering Gulf War syndrome. Genetic testing of veterans and their spouses is also sometimes pursued to determine causation of birth defects in some veterans' children, which are often incorrectly attributed to Gulf War service. Complications associated with treatment of Gulf War syndrome include possible common side effects of pain relievers, such as drowsiness. Patients also risk becoming addicted to pain relievers that they use to numb the ever-present aches associated with chronic illnesses.

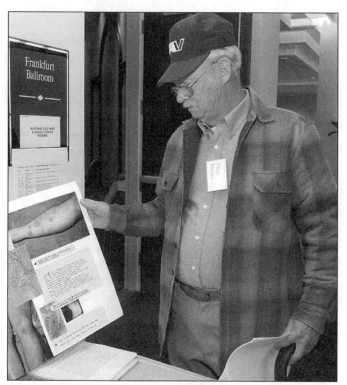

Gulf War veteran Floyd McCain examines a poster at a conference sponsored by the National Gulf War Resource Center. McCain returned from the conflict with headaches, dizziness, night sweats, memory loss, and numerous skin cancers and other lesions. (AP/Wide World Photos)

PERSPECTIVE AND PROSPECTS

Originally identified when some American, British, and Canadian Gulf War veterans complained of various ailments after returning home in 1991, Gulf War syndrome was sensationalized in the press as a mystery illness. Physicians familiar with military medical history recognized similarities with symptoms documented in soldier populations as early as the American Civil War. This awareness suggested that the syndrome was indicative of a common wartime factor rather than a unique occurrence in the Gulf War.

Gulf War syndrome became politicized as government officials and veterans disagreed regarding description of and funding for treatment of the syndrome. After clinical investigations of twenty thousand Gulf War veterans, the Institute of Medicine declared that no Gulf War syndrome existed, although some soldiers did suffer nonchronic illnesses, such as malaria. Five independent panels confirmed the conclusion that no unique case of an illness had been proven.

Physicians and scientists representing the Departments of Defense, Veterans Affairs, and Health and Human Services stated that the rates of incidence of Gulf War veterans' symptoms, hospitalization, and mortality are not greater than those reported for the general population and that many veterans may have already been genetically predisposed to certain physiological conditions. They also questioned why veterans from other countries, especially Arab nations, did not report syndrome symptoms nor were any similar reports issued after World War II soldiers returned from the Persian Gulf.

Determined to understand Gulf War syndrome, some researchers hypothesize how variables possibly affected veterans' immune symptoms to cause physiochemical reponses, such as increased cytokine production and brain cell damage. Others claim that chemical exposure contaminated soldiers' bloodstreams and is to blame for renal failure and cancers. Unless additional research determines a singular illness, Gulf War syndrome will remain a puzzling, vague, controversial condition with no specific cure or prevention for future military forces. A Veterans Administration Persian Gulf Health Registry and Department of Defense Persian Gulf Health Surveillance System were created to monitor veterans' health status and to detect patterns that might possibly provide further insights about the complexities of Gulf War syndrome.

—Elizabeth D. Schafer, Ph.D.

See also Environmental diseases; Environmental health; Epidemiology; Poisoning; Toxicology.

FOR FURTHER INFORMATION:

Blanck, Ronald R., and members of the Persian Gulf Veterans Coordinating Board. "Unexplained Illnesses Among Desert Storm Veterans: A Search for Causes, Treatment, and Cooperation." *Archives of Internal Medicine* 155 (February 13, 1995): 262-268.

Bloom, Saul, et al. *Hidden Casualties: Environmental, Health, and Political Consequences of the Persian Gulf War.* Berkeley, Calif.: Arms Control Research Center, North Atlantic Books, 1994.

Eddington, Patrick G. *Gassed in the Gulf: The Inside Story of the Pentagon-CIA Cover-up of Gulf War Syndrome.* Washington, D.C: Insignia, 1997.

Hersh, Seymour M. *Against All Enemies: Gulf War Syndrome, the War Between America's Ailing Veterans and Their Government.* New York: Ballantine Books, 1998.

National Defense Research Institution. *A Review of the Scientific Literature as It Pertains to Gulf War Illnesses.* 7 vols. Santa Monica, Calif.: Rand, 1998.

GYNECOLOGY
SPECIALTY

ANATOMY OR SYSTEM AFFECTED: Breasts, genitals, reproductive system, uterus

SPECIALTIES AND RELATED FIELDS: Endocrinology, family practice, obstetrics, oncology, psychiatry, psychology

DEFINITION: The branch of medicine concerned with the diseases and disorders that are specific to women, particularly those of the genital tract, as well as women's health, endocrinology, reproductive physiology, family planning, and contraceptive use.

KEY TERMS:

anterior: toward the front of the body or any structure

menarche: the establishment or beginning of the menstrual cycle in a woman

menopause: the permanent cessation of the menstrual cycle, signifying the conclusion of a woman's reproductive life

menstruation: the cyclic bleeding that normally occurs, usually in the absence of pregnancy, during the reproductive period of the human female; typically occurs at twenty-eight-day intervals

posterior: toward the back or rear of the body or any structure

puberty: the physiological sequence of events by which a child is transformed into an adult; the growth of secondary sexual characteristics occurs, reproductive functions begin, and the differences between males and females are accentuated

SCIENCE AND PROFESSION

To understand gynecology, it is first necessary to have a working knowledge of relevant female anatomy and physiology. Broadly, the female reproductive organs are divided into two groups: external and internal organs. The external organs are the vulva and vagina; the internal organs are the uterus, Fallopian tubes, and ovaries. Within each group are many specific components, most of which are analogous to structures in the male because they are derived from the same sources during embryological development.

The vulva is the portion of the female genitals which is externally visible. It is a complex structure, composed of the following parts: the labia major, labia minor, mons pubis, clitoris, vestibule, urethra, entrance to the vagina, hymen, and Bartholin's (or vulvovaginal) glands.

The outermost parts of the female anatomy are the labia major, or outer lips. These raised folds of skin have fatty, or adipose, tissue beneath the surface. Compared to surrounding skin, they are darker in color; this is especially true in women who have dark hair. At birth, the labia major are relatively flat and lie at about the same level as adjacent skin. At puberty, they increase in thickness, one of the secondary sexual characteristics that helps to define puberty. The labia major provide protection for the labia minor and cover the entrance to the vagina. The external surface of the labia major is covered with a heavy growth of hair. This pubic hair is usually curly and darkly colored. Its appearance is another visible characteristic of secondary sexual development. There is some hair on the inside surfaces of the labia major, but this is much more sparse and lightly colored than the externally visible pubic hair. The labia major correspond to the skin of the scrotum in males.

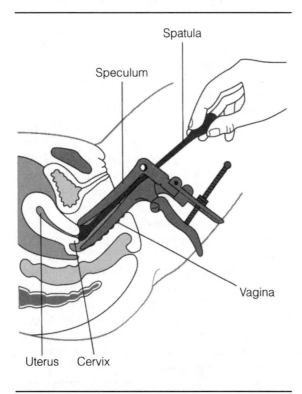

A routine gynecological examination includes a Pap smear, in which a spatula is used to perform a biopsy of the cervix for laboratory analysis.

Immediately anterior to the labia major is a mound of fatty tissue called the mons pubis. This tissue, which is also covered with pubic hair, provides a protective cushion during sexual activities. It extends to the lowermost portion of the abdomen. There is no corresponding structure in the male.

The labia minor are two firm folds of skin that lie immediately underneath the labia major. Anteriorly, they provide a covering of skin for the clitoris called a prepuce. From this origin, they sweep posteriorly to encircle the opening to the vagina. While no hairs are found on the labia minor, there are many small sebaceous glands. These glands secrete a slightly oily liquid that keeps the skin soft and moist. (There are sebaceous glands in most, but not all, areas of the skin throughout the body.) Males have a prepuce that covers the tip of the penis, analogous to the prepuce covering the clitoris. The only analogue to the labia minor in males is a raised ridge of skin between the penis and the scrotum.

The clitoris is a small, cylindrical organ that corresponds to the male penis. It has erectile tissue within it; during sexual excitation, the clitoris increases slightly in size by becoming longer. Normally, the glans of the clitoris is the only portion of the organ that is externally visible. The clitoris is covered by the prepuce, and its body extends anteriorly under the mons pubis.

The vestibule becomes visible when both the labia major and the labia minor are separated. It is an area rather than a particular structure. The vestibule encompasses the opening to the urethra and the entrance to the vagina. The skin of the vestibule extends to form the hymen which partially covers the vaginal entrance in most but not all females. In many cultures, the hymen is a symbol of virginity, although it may be broken and lost prior to the beginning of sexual activity. There are no corresponding structures in the male.

The urethra is a tube that carries urine from the bladder to the surface of the body. The opening in the vestibule is called the urethral meatus. It is anterior to the opening to the vagina. Immediately to the sides of the urethral meatus are tiny glands that secrete mucus, called the lesser glands of the vestibule. Opening into the surface of the vestibule immediately below the urethra are two ducts which lead to Skene's glands. The physiological function of these glands is not known, although they do harbor the bacteria that cause the sexually transmitted disease gonorrhea. In males, the urethra is much longer. It is found on the underside of the penis and exits the body at the tip of the penis.

Immediately to the side of the opening to the vagina are two glands. The function of Bartholin's glands is to secrete mucus that provides lubrication for the portions of the vagina nearest to the opening. In the male, there are two corresponding structures called Cowper's glands, which also produce mucus for lubrication.

The vagina is a tube of muscle that connects the vulva with the uterus. In adult females, it is 9 to 10 centimeters in length. When a woman is standing upright, the vagina extends upward and backward from the opening to the uterus. There is a slight cuplike expansion near the uterus. It is here that the actual connection between the vagina and uterus is made through a muscular structure called the cervix. The muscles of the vagina are normally constricted, thus closing the tube. The vagina can stretch to accommodate a penis during intercourse and a fetus during birth.

The cervix is a ring of muscle; the central opening is called the cervical os. Throughout most of the month, the cervical os forms a tight barrier. When the lining of the uterus is sloughed during a menstrual period, the cervix relaxes slightly. During childbirth, the cervix dilates to 10 centimeters (about 4 inches).

The uterus is a hollow, thick-walled, muscular organ. It normally forms a right angle with the vagina, angling upward and anteriorly. The bladder is immediately below and anterior to the uterus. In a nonpregnant woman, the uterus is pear-shaped. In a woman who has never been pregnant, it is 8 centimeters in length, 6 centimeters wide, and 4 centimeters thick. It increases in size during pregnancy; after birth, it shrinks but does not quite return to its size prior to pregnancy. The lining of the uterus is shed approximately every twenty-eight days during a normal menstrual period. The first menstrual period signals the onset of puberty in a female and the beginning of her reproductive life; this event is called menarche.

The Fallopian tubes are two canals that transport eggs from the ovary to the uterus. They are approximately 11 centimeters in length. The tubes are wide near the ovaries and become narrow toward the uterus. The ovaries are two almond-shaped bodies found in the pelvic cavity, just below the outer portions of the Fallopian tubes. The ovaries are about 3.5

by 2 by 1.5 centimeters in size, although there can be much variation. They are supported by several broad ligaments and attached to the uterus by the ovarian ligament. The ovaries contain eggs, which are released at monthly intervals between puberty and the menopause.

DIAGNOSTIC AND TREATMENT TECHNIQUES

The gynecological examination is an important event for women; it is difficult to overemphasize its importance. All women should have a gynecological examination annually. This process should begin at menarche and continue throughout the remainder of a woman's life. For the examination, a woman lies on her back. For much of the procedure, her knees are raised to allow access to the pelvis and genitalia. Stirrups are commonly provided for support of the feet.

The gynecological exam begins with a visual inspection of the external genitalia. The mons pubis and pubic hair are inspected for abnormalities such as unusual growths and organisms that can spread disease. Next, the labia major, labia minor, vestibule, and clitoris are visually inspected for pathology; the lesions of many sexually transmitted diseases are visible without a microscope. The same areas are then palpated to check for lumps or other abnormalities. Cysts and nontender growths are frequently discovered in this manner.

The next portion is a bimanual examination. The examiner places one hand on the patient's abdomen and gently inserts two fingers of the other hand into the patient's vagina; gloves are worn at all times. The examiner proceeds to feel the uterus and ovaries. The internal hand is used to displace organs and push the uterus toward the skin, where it is manipulated by the external hand. Surface contours can be felt in this manner. Each ovary is then palpated. Because they are small in size, the ovaries may be difficult to feel.

The third portion of the examination is a visual inspection of the interior of the vagina and the surface of the cervix. To accomplish this, a speculum is used to hold the vagina in an open position. The speculum is an instrument made of metal or plastic that has two flat blades that can be moved apart. The speculum is gently inserted into the vagina, and, once it is in place, the instrument is opened. The blades displace the walls of the vagina and allow an examiner direct visual access to its interior. The walls are checked for lesions and other problems. The surface of the cervix is inspected. The cervical os is not usually penetrated.

While the speculum is in an open position, the fourth portion of the gynecological examination is completed: A Pap smear is obtained. A long swab is inserted and moved over the surface of the cervix, picking up mucus from the surface. A second swab is then put up to the cervical os but not inserted. A second sample of mucus is thus obtained. Both are sent to a laboratory for processing. The speculum is closed and removed; the gynecological examination is complete.

The purpose of the Pap smear is to check for cancer of the cervix. The swab picks up mucus that contains cells from the cervix. Cancer is characterized by the growth of abnormal cells. The Pap smear is able to detect these abnormal cells long before a lesion is visually apparent. By detecting abnormal cells early, physicians have more time available for treating the problem, and more time means that more treatment options exist. The end result is that patients have a greater probability of surviving the cancer. The Pap smear is an example of a screening test. The point of both annual examinations and screening tests is to prevent problems from becoming major or life-threatening by detecting them early. Prevention is far easier than attempting a treatment or cure. It is also less costly.

Many sexually transmitted diseases (STDs) are discovered during a gynecological examination. Examples of such diseases are syphilis, gonorrhea, herpesvirus, Papillomavirus, chancroid, granuloma inguinale, lymphogranuloma venereum (chlamydia), and acquired immunodeficiency syndrome (AIDS).

Syphilis is a disease with an early infectious phase that attacks the genitalia and a later, less-specific phase that can involve any organ of the body. Female victims complain of painful sores on their labia major, internal surfaces, labia minor, walls of the vagina, and surface of the cervix. Syphilis can be treated effectively with antibiotics. Gonorrhea is an infectious disease that mainly affects the mucous membranes of the genitalia, the internal surface of the urethra, the cervix, and the rectum. During the birth process, the eyes of newborn babies can be infected if the mother has the disease. Gonorrhea causes inflammation and a foul discharge. It can usually be treated with antibiotics, but a number of drug-resistant strains of the bacteria have emerged. Herpes is a viral disease that can cause great pain and suffering by attacking nerves; there is no discharge. It can be spread to babies during the birth process as well. There is no effective treatment for herpes. Papillomaviruses are thought to be transmitted through intimate sexual contact. They are important clinically because they have been linked to cancer of the cervix; there is no effective cure. Chancroid is an acute, localized infection that produces tender ulcers; it can be treated with antibiotics. In contrast, granuloma inguinale is a mildly contagious, chronic, and progressive disease that involves the skin and lymphatic system but is most commonly found on the genitalia. Lymphogranuloma venereum, or chlamydia, is usually restricted to the genitalia as well. Women can have these diseases and be unaware of their presence. They can be treated relatively effectively. AIDS is also transmitted sexually. The prospects for effective treatment seem remote; the disease has proved uniformly fatal.

Other diseases are of gynecological importance. Pelvic inflammatory disease (PID) usually follows the migration of bacteria into the pelvic area and involves the uterus, Fallopian tubes, ovaries, and adjacent tissues. It is diagnostic for a variety of different organisms, usually bacteria. The Fallopian tubes are probably the most vulnerable organs to be affected. If diagnosed early enough, pelvic inflammatory disease can be effectively treated. If allowed to go untreated, however, it can lead to sterility.

Endometriosis is defined as a condition in which tissue resembling that normally found inside the uterus is found outside the uterus. All organs of the pelvis are potential targets. The study of this disease is growing in importance because endometriosis is a common cause of sterility. Treatment frequently involves the surgical removal of the tissue and sometimes of the organs that it invades.

Ectopic pregnancy is the leading cause of maternal mortality in the United States. Most ectopic pregnancies occur in the Fallopian tubes, although abdominal pregnancies are occasionally reported. The most reliable way to diagnose ectopic pregnancy is by regular gynecologic examination.

Many gynecological problems associated with the female reproductive system are not diagnosed in a timely fashion, leading to needless pain, suffering, and death. A major reason for this finding is that many gynecologic conditions are asymptomatic—that is, they do not cause pain or other problems for the victim. Frequently, however, women deny that they have gynecological diseases. Pain can be ignored; lesions can be overlooked. Admitting to the reality of a sexually transmitted disease can be difficult or impossible for many women. Virtually all the diseases and problems associated with the female reproductive system can be detected through examinations. The key to effective treatment is early detection, with annual gynecological examinations providing the best opportunity to do so.

PERSPECTIVE AND PROSPECTS

Gynecology is a broad field that addresses many topics. Gynecology does not deal with disease states: The events of conception and pregnancy are also a part of this field. There are psychological aspects to gynecology, as seen in the denial exhibited by women with silent or "undesirable" conditions. There are issues of pressing urgency for women, such as cancer of the cervix, infertility, and AIDS.

Gynecology is widely accessible to contemporary women. Information about bodies and gynecology is available from many sources. If all women had regular gynecological examinations, half of the people in any given population would probably be much healthier. The detection and treatment of cancer of the cervix and uterus would become much easier; the number of deaths would probably decline. Similarly, the attack rates for pelvic inflammatory disease and endometriosis would probably also decline; these disorders contribute significantly to infertility in the United States. Issues relating to pregnancy and contraception can frequently be resolved by consultation with a gynecologist. Regular gynecological examinations can assist women as they begin the menopause. Many of the myths surrounding older age in females can be dispelled: There is no need to abandon sexual activity; regular checkups must be continued; and hormone replacement therapy can reduce the effects of physiological aging.

—*L. Fleming Fallon, Jr., M.D., Ph.D., M.P.H.*

See also Abortion; Amenorrhea; Amniocentesis; Biopsy; Breast biopsy; Breast cancer; Breast disorders; Breast-feeding; Breasts, female; Cervical, ovarian, and uterine cancers; Cervical procedures; Cesarean section; Childbirth; Childbirth complications; Chlamydia; Chorionic villus sampling; Circumcision, female, and genital mutilation; Conception; Contraception; Culdocentesis; Cyst removal; Cystectomy; Cystitis; Cysts; Dysmenorrhea; Electrocauterization; Endocrinology; Endometrial biopsy; Endometriosis; Endoscopy; Episiotomy; Genital disorders, female; Glands; Gonorrhea; Herpes; Hormone replacement therapy; Hysterectomy; In vitro fertilization; Incontinence; Infertility in females; Laparoscopy; Mammography; Mastectomy and lumpectomy; Mastitis; Menopause; Menorrhagia; Menstruation; Myomectomy; Nutrition; Obstetrics; Ovarian cysts; Pelvic inflammatory disease (PID); Peritonitis; Postpartum depression; Pregnancy and gestation; Premenstrual syndrome (PMS); Reproductive system; Sex change surgery; Sexual dysfunction; Sexuality; Sexually transmitted diseases; Sterilization; Syphilis; Tubal ligation; Ultrasonography; Urethritis; Urinary disorders; Urology; Warts.

FOR FURTHER INFORMATION:

Boston Women's Health Book Collective. *Our Bodies, Ourselves for the New Century.* New York: Simon & Schuster, 1998. Contains in-depth discussions of topics covered in this article. This book was written by women for women and is one of the best reference works available on this subject for the general reader.

Cunningham, F. Gary, et al., eds. *Williams Obstetrics.* 20th ed. Stamford, Conn.: Appleton and Lange, 1997. This standard textbook in obstetrics would complement a similar text in gynecology. Provides wide coverage of events related to pregnancy and childbirth. A well-written text for the serious reader who wants in-depth information.

Dechnery, William. *Current Obstetric and Gynecological Diagnosis and Treatment.* 7th ed. Norwalk, Conn.: Appleton and Lange, 1991. Discusses the diagnosis and treatment of gynecological disorders in a brief and concise format. The section authors are recognized experts in their fields. Treatment protocols are included.

Jones, Howard W., III, Anne Colston Wentz, and Lonnie S. Burnett. *Novak's Textbook of Gynecology.* 11th ed. Baltimore: Williams & Wilkins, 1988. A standard textbook widely used in medical education throughout the world. Uses medical terminology but is accessible to a general reader who is patient. Excellent pictures accompany the text.

Tyler, Sandra L., and Gail M. Woodall, eds. *Female Health and Gynecology: Across the Lifespan.* Bowie, Md.: R. J. Brady, 1982. The authors have written an excellent text for the general reader. Concepts are clearly presented in language that is readily understood. The book covers most major aspects of gynecology. It is objective in coverage of contemporary and controversial issues and does not champion any particular philosophy or point of view.

GYNECOMASTIA

DISEASE/DISORDER

ANATOMY OR SYSTEM AFFECTED: Breasts, glands

SPECIALTIES AND RELATED FIELDS: Endocrinology, family practice, pediatrics

DEFINITION: Gynecomastia is the term for development of glandular, not fatty, breast tissue in males. Other than embarrassment, the major consequence is a slight increase in the probability of breast cancer, which is otherwise rare in males. The presence of gynecomastia, however, can reflect a hormonal imbalance—such as from a tumor, an extra X chromosome, or exogenous steroids—that may have other, more severe, health consequences. Enlarged breasts in children and adolescents also occur in benign forms. Newborns of both sexes may show mild breast enlargement shortly after birth as a result of maternal hormones. Some boys develop a slight swelling of breast tissue around puberty. Both conditions are temporary.

—Linda Mealey, Ph.D.

See also Breast cancer; Breast disorders; Breasts, female; Endocrine system; Endocrinology; Endocrinology, pediatric; Hormones; Neonatalogy; Pediatrics; Puberty and adolescence.

FOR FURTHER INFORMATION:

Hall, Peter Francis. *Gynaecomastia.* Glebe, Australia: Australasian Medical, 1959.

Masters, William H., Virginia E. Johnson, and Robert C. Kolodny. *Human Sexuality.* 5th ed. New York: HarperCollins College, 1995.

Scheike, Ole. *Male Breast Cancer.* Copenhagen: Munksgaard, 1975.

Hair loss and baldness
Disease/disorder

Anatomy or system affected: Hair, head, skin

Specialties and related fields: Dermatology, endocrinology, plastic surgery

Definition: Symptoms of genetic factors, endocrine disorders, and aging which occur in both men and women, although more frequently in men, affecting more than one-half of the male population.

Key terms:

alopecia: a condition in which all hair falls out, not only that on the scalp but also eyebrows, eyelashes, and even body hair

follicle: a small, saclike cavity for secretion or excretion

hair shaft: the hair itself, consisting of the central part (medulla), the middle part (cortex), and the outer part (cuticle)

psoriasis: a chronic skin disease characterized by scaly, reddish patches

seborrhea: a dermatologic condition characterized by an excessively dry (seborrhea oleosa) or oily skin (seborrhea sicca)

Causes and Symptoms

The major reason that hair on the scalp thrives more lavishly than on other parts of the body is that scalp hairs are produced by the largest follicles found in human skin. Throughout the early years of infancy, these follicles increase in size, shedding their hairs about every two to six years to clear a path for a new hair that grows thicker and longer than the one that it replaced. In the mid-teens, nearly every follicle in an individual's scalp is generating an actively growing hair, and by the late teens scalp hair reaches its adult size, populating the scalp in numbers that will never again be equaled.

For most adults entering their twenties, this situation reverses, and hair loss begins to occur—either permanently or temporarily. At this stage in their development, nearly every man and more than 80 percent of women find their hairlines receding. As the years progress, the shedding continues, and the density of scalp hair continues to diminish. Nearly all the permanent hair loss that affects the human scalp is produced by the natural aging process and/or common baldness.

Common, or male pattern, baldness (baldness is classified into various groups depending on its pattern on the scalp) affects at least 20 million Americans. The term "baldness" is often used when a definite hairline recession, a bald spot on the crown, thinning over the top of the scalp, or a combination of the three is detected. The sides and rear scalp fringe areas are usually spared, except for the inevitable thinning that accompanies age. These regions appear to be capable of generating enough two-to-six-year hair cycles to keep them well covered for most, if not all, of a male's average life span.

The less frequent causes of permanent hair loss can be categorized into three groups. The first involves injury to follicles created by constant tension or pulling of scalp hair. Tight ponytails or chignons, worn over a number of years, often result in permanent bald patches on the sides of the head. In addition, tight rollers and the process of hair weaving kill follicles. The second infrequent cause of permanent hair loss is physical injury, such as a laceration or burn. If hair is ironed as a method of straightening over a period of years, hair follicles will become damaged. The third cause involves various inflammatory skin

---

Patterns of Hair Loss

Male pattern

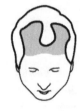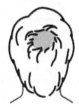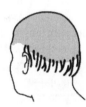

Women (rare, after pregnancy)

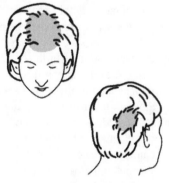

Patchy hair loss
(from infection, disease or stress)

disorders and growths that occasionally affect the scalp. For example, a scalp wen, or cyst, tends to occur in families and requires no treatment unless it appears to be growing. Removal involves a simple office procedure and eliminates the bald spot that results from pressure of the enlarging cyst upon adjacent scalp follicles.

Nearly all humans lose some scalp hair every day. The number of falling hairs, however, often varies considerably from day to day. This daily variation in hair loss is not an indication of abnormality. An average of thirty to sixty hairs may be shed from the scalp each day. While days, weeks, and months may pass with little to no hair loss, large numbers of hairs may be lost over similar time periods. The yearly average, however, remains fairly constant.

This daily variation in hair loss merely reflects the fact that hair follicles act independently of one another. Their three-year growth and three-month rest cycles occur randomly. Aside from the tendency to lose more hair in the autumn, chance dictates the periods when the scalp will contain more resting hairs (hairs having small whitish roots).

Dandruff and its two related conditions of seborrhea and psoriasis, both scaly scalp conditions, may create a significant diffuse hair loss. Because these conditions are so common, they account for most of the shedding that requires medical treatment. In most cases, these problems can be controlled without medical assistance.

Temporary hair loss can result from alopecia areata, pregnancy, severe illness, surgery, certain medications, hormonal disorders, or dieting. Alopecia areata is a condition that usually produces temporary shedding of scalp—and occasionally body—hair. In most cases, the hair regrows spontaneously or after medical therapy has ended. Occasionally, if this problem begins during childhood, all the scalp and body hair may be lost permanently. Extensive shedding may follow pregnancy or the discontinuation of birth control pills. After several months, however, the hair usually begins to regrow. Hair loss may also result from a severe illness associated with high fever (usually influenza) or an extensive surgical procedure. In the case of surgery, the cause is related to changes in body chemistry. Various medications can also create hair loss. The main offenders are the amphetamines, blood thinners, antithyroid drugs, anticancer drugs (as well as radiation treatments), and birth control pills. Hormonal disorders, particularly thyroid dysfunction, can create a thinning problem, but this condition is rarely an isolated symptom. In rare instances, improper nutrition can result in hair loss, such as in the case of dieters who eliminate protein from their daily food intake.

The conditions responsible for temporary shedding usually create a thinning problem quite rapidly. Aside from hair breakage or forcible extraction (hair pulling), the problem is usually one of increased numbers of resting hairs, resulting in massive hair loss. (The two conditions primarily responsible for creating permanent hair loss—aging and common baldness—usually develop slowly, over many years. Thinning occurs simply because the scalp follicles are no longer capable of producing new hairs.)

If something occurs to double the number of resting hairs from their normal 15 to 30 percent, then hundreds of hairs may fall each day. If this lasts for several months, about one-third of the scalp's hair may be lost. A loss of about 30 to 40 percent is required before thinning becomes obvious. After the shedding abates, it may take years for the scalp hair to return to its original density, since the new hairs can grow only about an inch every two months.

TREATMENT AND THERAPY

Scientific research in the area of hair loss has produced a drug that has been relatively effective in some individuals. The drug minoxidil was originally used as an antihypertensive medication; however, 70 percent of patients taking it reported unexpected hair growth, occasionally in such undesirable places as the forehead. A 0.2 percent minoxidil solution for external use was devised by a major drug company in the United States and marketed under the name Rogaine. The Food and Drug Administration approved Rogaine as the only prescription drug that effectively combats baldness.

Although it is uncertain how the drug works, it is believed that minoxidil enables shrunken follicles to grow back to a size capable of producing sturdy, visible hairs. Minoxidil has been shown to have promising, though limited, results. It is best at filling in those patchy gaps that herald the beginnings of baldness. Between one-third and one-half of men in some studies exhibited "significant" or "cosmetically acceptable" hair growth. Minoxidil is not a cure, however, and it requires a lifetime commitment. When the drug is stopped, hair thins out within months.

Another nonsurgical method for achieving permanent hair is hair weaving, a process that originated in the African American culture in the nineteenth century. Weaving hair involves braiding it tightly so that a toupee or smaller weft (section of hair) can be attached permanently. All that is required is a sufficient amount of hair remaining on the scalp to serve as an anchor for a hairpiece.

The braids are usually formed from the thicker hair found on the sides and back of the scalp. A semicircular ridge is created that holds a hairpiece firmly in place. If enough hair is still growing on top of the scalp, it can be twisted into smaller braids to anchor individual wefts. This type of weave permits better aeration and easier cleansing of the scalp.

A hair "fusion," "bonding," or "linking" is exactly like a weave except that the hairpiece or wefts are glued, instead of tied, onto the braided hair. This so-called chemical bond is insoluble in water and quite caustic. Frequent hair breakage has limited the usefulness of this method.

While weaved or fused hair does not grow, it still requires regular care and maintenance to keep it looking acceptable. The scalp hair used to anchor the weave naturally continues to grow. As it grows, the attached hair starts to ride above the scalp. Thus the weave or fusion must be reanchored frequently (as often as every three weeks). In addition, the tension placed on the anchoring scalp hair creates accelerated shedding, and this hair loss is often irreversible.

Hair implants, also known as medical or suture implants, have become the principal method for fixing a hairpiece securely to the scalp. Implants are usually not permanent, are only quasi medical, and are to be distinguished from transplants, with which they share a resemblance in name only. Implants are stitches made from either stainless steel or nylon-type materials that are sewn into the scalp and tied into rings. Like the weave hair braids, the knotted stitches act as anchors, holding a hairpiece or several wefts against the barren scalp. If the implants secure a hairpiece, only two or perhaps six stitches are needed. If the implants anchor many smaller wefts of hair, however, more than a dozen stitches must be sewn into the scalp. A physician must perform this procedure, since only someone with a medical license can inject a local anesthetic and sew stitches into the scalp. The problems generated by sewing and leaving stitches in the scalp, however, are pain, infection, and scarring.

In the 1970's, a surgical procedure known as tunnel grafting was developed. This procedure is not available in implant clinics. A 2.5-by-7.5 centimeter rectangle of skin is removed from behind each ear. The two pieces are immediately grafted to the front and back of the scalp to form two loops that serve as anchors for a hairpiece. While the operation is relatively simple to perform, extreme care must be taken to ensure proper graft acceptance and healing. Although this method avoids the pitfalls of implanted stitches, it still retains two of the problems common to any kind of artificial anchoring device. Since only two loops are available to fix a hairpiece, the hairpiece can still lift off the scalp. In addition, the skin loops are as vulnerable to injury as suture loops. Scalp lacerations resulting from forcible removal of the hairpiece have occurred.

From the discovery of hair transplants in the 1960's to 1978, it has been estimated that approximately one million people—both men and women—underwent such transplants. As with implants, a medical license is mandatory in order to inject a local anesthetic into the scalp and make the surgical incisions required for a hair transplant. Doctors who specialize in hair transplants are usually dermatologists, some are plastic surgeons, and a few acquire the training that enables them to perform this procedure.

Even the baldest scalp contains thousands of transplantable hair follicles. To move them where they are most needed, three surgical methods have been developed, employing scalp grafts known variously as "flaps," "strips," and "plugs." While all three methods are used, most hair transplants are performed with plug grafts because they are simpler and safer to work with and yield the most satisfying results. The transplant candidate need only be bald enough to justify undergoing the procedure and be endowed with enough side and rear fringe scalp hair to make the procedure worthwhile.

To create a flap or "full thickness" graft, a surgeon cuts out three sides of a rectangular patch of scalp from above the ears and swings it over to the bald area to create a new hairline. Thus is a major hospital procedure requiring considerable surgical expertise. Although a fairly large portion of bald scalp can be provided with instant hair density, this method is fraught with problems. To ensure a proper take, or graft survival, the blood vessels feeding the transplant must remain intact while they are moved along with it. Because the vessels are quite fragile, they are frequently damaged, resulting in poor graft survival and catastrophic hair loss.

To alleviate this problem, a variation of this type of transplant, known as a free flap procedure, was developed by a team of Japanese surgeons. The free flap is cut out on all four sides, completely severing the blood supply. After setting the graft into its new location, the surgeons meticulously reestablish its blood supply to the recipient blood vessels using a delicate microsurgical technique.

Even if this technical obstacle is surmounted, however, other aesthetic problems remain. The first problem involves the surgical scar that delineates the border between the forehead and the transplanted hairline. Little can be done to minimize this scar. The other problem concerns the unnatural direction in which the newly transplanted hair grows. A flap graft cannot provide hair that will grow in the direction of the hair that has been lost. Hairs growing from the sides of the scalp exit much closer to the surface than in other areas. When transplanted to the frontal area, these hairs lie much too flat against the scalp. Thus, while a flap may provide a faster way to achieve a high-density transplant, the problems of graft survival and poor aesthetic results have limited its usefulness.

A surgical strip graft is a narrow rectangular patch of scalp, cut out on all four sides, that is usually transplanted to create a hairline. Unlike the larger flap, its blood supply need not be moved along with it or be laboriously reestablished. After the strip is placed into its new location, the adjacent bald scalp sends new blood vessels directly into it. Like a flap graft, however, it must be sewn into place. If it is used to create a hairline, an unsightly scar will mark its border with the forehead as well. While this procedure can be performed in an office rather than at a hospital, extreme care must be taken to avoid damaging this delicate graft. Despite the most painstaking precautions, poor takes result quite often. Areas of nongrowth are common, and not infrequently the entire graft becomes almost completely devoid of hair.

A "hair transplant" usually refers to a procedure in which a small cylinder of hair-bearing scalp, or plug, is taken from the rear or side fringe areas and transferred to either the bald crown or the scalp's frontal region. While this transplant method requires several sessions to approach the density of hair acquired with a flap graft, the ease with which it can be performed, coupled with its superior aesthetic results, make it the logical choice for surgically replacing hair.

The surgeon uses a trephine, or "punch," to remove the cylindrical section of scalp, properly called a do-nor graft rather than a plug. The graft is quite small, measuring about 0.8 centimeter deep by 0.5 centimeter in diameter. The hair follicle is intimately related to all three skin layers. The bulb—or hair-producing portion of the follicle—lies within and is cushioned by the fat, or adipose, layer. The entire follicle is supported by and receives its nourishment from the fibrous portion of skin, or dermis, which is about 0.6 centimeter thick in the scalp. The skin mantle, or epidermis, provides the opening, or "pore," through which the hair exits to the surface of the scalp.

When a donor graft is removed, all three skin layers must be included. The hair is actually superfluous to the procedure: The hair follicle is all that is essential. After removing the hair-bearing donor grafts, the physician next punches out identical sections of bald scalp. The term "plug" actually refers to the hairless cylinder of scalp that is taken from the bald area. The donor graft is placed into the void left by the removal of the bald plug. Light pressure is applied for several seconds to allow the blood to clot and hold the graft in place. Because these grafts are so small and clotting occurs so rapidly, stitches are not required to fix them in place.

Within hours, new blood vessels move into the graft from the surrounding skin to feed the new section. Within several days, as healing continues, the graft and its adjacent host skin become one. Keeping the grafts small facilitates easy penetration by these vital blood vessels. When larger grafts, or strips, are used, the blood supply may not reach all the hair follicles, and they die.

Because of their small size, the rounded edges of the grafts blend into the host skin quite evenly, creating an acceptable hairline. While they might appear obvious on close inspection, they are always less noticeable than the borders left by flaps and strips. Because the grafts are small and are taken from the rear half of the scalp, where the hairs grow out in the same manner as the front and crown hairs, they can be directed to duplicate exactly the original pattern of growth in the bald host areas. This method is a minor office procedure that, in the hands of an experienced physician, is considered safe, with little discomfort experienced by the patient.

PERSPECTIVE AND PROSPECTS

The observation that eunuchs are not subject to gout or baldness was made by Hippocrates in the year 400 B.C.E. and is contained in the *Hippocratic Corpus* as a short medical truth or aphorism. Aristotle, himself balding, was interested in the fact that eunuchs did not become bald and were unable to grow hair on their chests. These observations were either forgotten or overlooked for the next twenty-five centuries, and medical science remained baffled by male pattern baldness until James B. Hamilton, an anatomist, in 1949 again made the observation that eunuchs did not become bald. His suggestion that androgens are a prerequisite and incitant in male pattern baldness and his later classification of the patterns and grades of baldness are landmarks in the study of male pattern baldness. Subsequent investigations of hair loss confirmed the significance of androgens in male pattern baldness, and Hamilton's classification remains in use.

Hamilton demonstrated conclusively that the extent and development of male pattern baldness were dependent on the interaction of three factors: androgens, genetic predisposition, and age. In summary, he found that genetic, endocrine, and aging factors are interdependent. No matter how strong the inherited predisposition, male pattern alopecia will not result if androgens are missing. Neither are the androgens able to induce baldness in individuals not genetically predisposed to baldness. The action of aging is demonstrated by the immediate loss of hair upon exposure to androgens in the sixth decade of life, whereas hair in young men exposed to androgens tends to remain much longer.

Over the centuries, men have tried every imaginable approach to retain hair. They have shampooed their scalps with tar, petroleum, goose dung, and cow urine. They have stuck their heads into rubber caps connected to vacuum pumps to suck recalcitrant hairs to the surface. In the 1960's, hair transplants became the most efficient and aesthetically pleasing method of retaining scalp hair. Research in the area of drug treatment continues.

—Genevieve Slomski, Ph.D.

See also Aging; Dermatology; Gray hair; Hair transplantation; Plastic surgery; Pregnancy and gestation; Psoriasis; Skin; Skin disorders.

FOR FURTHER INFORMATION:

"Bothered by Baldness? Here Are Your Options." *Health News* 18, no. 3 (June/July, 2000): 3. The vast majority of men with thinning hair have "male pattern baldness." Some of the treatments available to men to prevent baldness are discussed, including medication and hair transplants.

Norwood, O'Tar T., and Richard C. Shiell. *Hair Transplant Surgery.* 2d ed. Springfield, Ill.: Charles C Thomas, 1984. The authors discuss the surgical techniques for transplanting hair. Accessible to the general reader. Includes bibliographical references.

Setterberg, Fred. "The Naked Truth About Baldness." *In Health* 3 (September/October, 1989): 112-118. This article summarizes for the general reader the main causes of permanent hair loss and discusses treatment options such as transplants and the drug minoxidil.

Stough, Dow B., and Robert S. Haber, eds. *Hair Replacement: Surgical and Medical.* St. Louis: C. V. Mosby, 1996. This book discusses hair loss and its various treatments, such as stimulants and transplantation.

HAIR TRANSPLANTATION
PROCEDURE
ANATOMY OR SYSTEM AFFECTED: Hair, head, skin
SPECIALTIES AND RELATED FIELDS: Dermatology, general surgery, plastic surgery
DEFINITION: The surgical relocation of healthy hair follicles to a part of the scalp where shrunken follicles are producing short, thin hair or no hair.

INDICATIONS AND PROCEDURES

There are several types of balding that may cause a patient to seek out a hair transplantation procedure. Androgenetic alopecia (common baldness) is a condition that can affect both men and women who are genetically predisposed to it. Usually beginning in late adolescence or early adulthood, androgenetic hormones cause hair follicles gradually to grow smaller and eventually to yield hair that can be detected only by a microscope, or no hair at all.

Different patterns of balding have been observed. Frontal recession is a gradual process during which the frontal hairline retreats from the forehead. In vertex thinning, the hair on the crown of the head gradually disappears, exposing the scalp; the denuded area grows slowly in a concentric pattern. With complete balding, progressive frontal recession combines with vertex balding to create a condition in which hair is present only in a rim at the sides and back of the scalp.

Several surgical styles have been developed to perform hair transplantation, and techniques continue to evolve to improve the appearance of the scalp and hair. In one common procedure, small grafts of scalp

Hair Transplantation

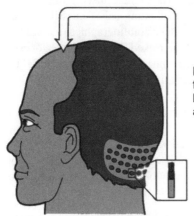

Plugs of hair are taken from the back of the head and transplanted

Before

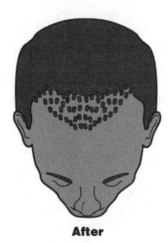

After

In the punch graft method of hair transplantation, tiny plugs of hair are taken from areas of the scalp where hair growth is still abundant and are inserted into areas where growth has stopped, usually the forehead or the crown.

containing one or two healthy hair follicles, called micrografts, are removed surgically and set into the frontal scalp to create a natural-looking hairline. The area behind the frontal hairline is filled in with large grafts, and the gaps between the large grafts are filled in with minigrafts, which contain three or four hairs. This process can involve several sessions over a long time, sometimes as long as ten years, depending on the patient's natural hair thickness and degree of balding. The freshly grafted hair falls out but is replaced with new growth in a few weeks.

More than fifty thousand hair transplantation procedures are performed each year in the United States, and the number is expected to increase as more practitioners are trained and the cost, which often amounts to several thousand dollars, is reduced.

—Russell Williams, M.S.W.

See also Dermatology; Grafts and grafting; Hair loss and baldness; Plastic surgery; Skin; Transplantation.

FOR FURTHER INFORMATION:

Hannapel, Coriene E. "Hair Transplant Advances Add Up to Better Results." *Dermatology Times* 21, no. 6 (June, 2000): 35. Dr. Walter P. Unger, codirector of dermatologic surgery at the University of Toronto, discusses the shift to using only follicular units for transplanting, as opposed to using both follicular units and minigrafts.

Sams, W. Mitchell, Jr., and Peter J. Lynch, eds. *Principles and Practice of Dermatology.* 2d ed. New York: Churchill Livingstone, 1996. This is a new edition of a dermatology reference guide and text emphasizing accurate diagnosis by succinct discussions in eighty-five presentations featuring color photographs. The contributing dermatologists detail all major topics in the field of dermatology.

Segell, Michael. "The Bald Truth About Hair." *Esquire* 121, no. 5 (May 1, 1994): 111-117. A guide to avoiding baldness is offered. Baldness can occur in three ways: vertex baldness (the top of the head), frontal recession, or a combination of both.

HALITOSIS
DISEASE/DISORDER

ANATOMY OR SYSTEM AFFECTED: Gastrointestinal system, mouth, nose, respiratory system, stomach

SPECIALTIES AND RELATED FIELDS: Dentistry, family practice, otorhinolaryngology

DEFINITION: Halitosis, commonly known as bad breath, is usually the result of such habits as drinking alcohol, smoking, and eating pungent foods, including onions and garlic. Over time, the offensive odor may no longer be noticeable to the patient. The odor is eliminated if these habits are stopped. Halitosis may also be attributable to chronic infections of the mouth, throat, and lungs. Poor oral or dental hygiene, sinusitis, tonsillitis, and bronchiectasis (distortion and consequent damage of the bronchi in the lungs) may be responsible for the foul breath; treatment consists in addressing the underlying condition.

—*Jason Georges and Tracy Irons-Georges*

See also Abdominal disorders; Alcoholism; Cavities; Dental diseases; Dentistry; Food biochemistry; Gastroenterology; Gastroenterology, pediatric; Gastrointestinal disorders; Gastrointestinal system; Indigestion; Nasopharyngeal disorders; Otorhinolaryngology; Pharyngitis; Sinusitis; Sore throat; Tonsillitis.

FOR FURTHER INFORMATION:

Ring, Malvin E. *Dentistry: An Illustrated History.* New York: Harry N. Abrams, 1985.

Smith, Rebecca W. *The Columbia University School of Dental and Oral Surgery's Guide to Family Dental Care.* New York: W. W. Norton, 1997.

Ward, Brian R. *Dental Care.* New York: Franklin Watts, 1986.

Woodall, Irene R., ed. *Comprehensive Dental Hygiene Care.* 4th ed. St. Louis, Mo.: C. V. Mosby, 1993.

HALLUCINATIONS
DISEASE/DISORDER

ANATOMY OR SYSTEM AFFECTED: Brain, nervous system, psychic-emotional system

SPECIALTIES AND RELATED FIELDS: Neurology, psychiatry, psychology

DEFINITION: The perception of sensations without relevant external stimuli.

Society often associates hallucinations with psychotic behavior, because schizophrenia and other forms of mental illness frequently involve hallucinations. Another widely publicized example of these symptoms is the use of hallucinogenic drugs, for example, LSD (lysergic acid diethylamide) or marijuana. One must also consider the role of hallucinations in religious experiences and megalomania; such perceptions occur when ordinary people are subjected to extraordinary stimuli.

Medical science has resisted the study of hallucinations and treated them as symptoms of mental illness. Increasing evidence shows, however, that they arise from specific brain and nervous system structures involving specific biological experiences and common reactions to stimuli. Consequently, people suffering from drug abuse, alcoholism, and disorders similar to Alzheimer's disease, in which severe loss of memory can provoke illusions, are subject to hallucinations.

Since a hallucination can be the result of physical causes as well as the traditional mental unbalance of schizophrenia or manic depression, it is difficult to categorize its symptoms. An individual experiencing hallucinations at times other than waking or falling asleep should see his or her doctor. If the incidents are attributable to a serious illness, early detection is possible. If they are an effect of a particular medication, the prescription should be changed immediately.

—*K. Thomas Finley, Ph.D.*

See also Addiction; Alcoholism; Alzheimer's disease; Bipolar disorder; Brain; Brain disorders; Delusions; Dementias; Intoxication; Narcolepsy; Neurology; Neurology, pediatric; Paranoia; Poisonous plants; Psychiatric disorders; Psychiatry; Psychiatry, child and adolescent; Psychiatry, geriatric; Psychosis; Schizophrenia; Sleep disorders; Stress.

FOR FURTHER INFORMATION:

Asaad, Ghazi. *Hallucinations in Clinical Psychiatry: A Guide for Mental Health Professionals.* New York: Brunner/Mazel, 1990. Discusses the diagnosis and treatment of hallucinations. Includes bibliographical references and an index.

Lennox, Belinda R., et al. "Spatial and Temporal Mapping of Neural Activity Associated with Auditory Hallucinations." *The Lancet* 353, no. 9153 (February 20, 1999): 644. Results show the strong association of the right middle temporal gyrus with the experience of auditory hallucination in the patient studied, supporting the hypothesis that auditory hallucinations reflect abnormal activation of auditory cortex.

Siegel, Ronald K. *Fire in the Brain: Clinical Tales of Hallucination.* New York: E. P. Dutton, 1992. This textbook describes clinical case studies of patients suffering from hallucinations. Includes bibliographical references.

Slade, P. D., and R. P. Bentall. *Sensory Deception: A Scientific Analysis of Hallucinations.* Baltimore: The Johns Hopkins University Press, 1988. Discusses the mechanisms of hallucination. Includes bibliographical references and an index.

Stephens, G. Lynn, and George Graham. *When Self-Consciousness Breaks: Alien Voices and Inserted Thoughts.* Cambridge, Mass.: MIT Press, 2000. Utilizes a number of case studies to explain alienated self-consciousness. Includes bibliographical references and an index.

HAMMERTOE CORRECTION
PROCEDURE
ANATOMY OR SYSTEM AFFECTED: Blood vessels, bones, feet, musculoskeletal system, nervous system, tendons

SPECIALTIES AND RELATED FIELDS: General surgery, orthopedics, podiatry

DEFINITION: The surgical removal of ligaments and joining of the middle joints in the toes to correct hammertoe, a deformity in which the toes bend downward abnormally.

INDICATIONS AND PROCEDURES
A hammertoe is a painful deformity which usually affects the second toe. The clawlike appearance of the toe results from malignancy of the joint surface or shortening and weakening of the foot and toe muscle. People with diabetes mellitus are prone to hammertoe development because of the nerve and muscle damage frequently associated with the disease. In other cases, hammertoe results from the wearing of shoes that are too short and do not fit properly. High-heeled shoes, which place pressure on the front of the foot and compress the smaller toes tightly together, can contribute to hammertoe formation. Painful calluses form on the tops of toes when the deformed toe rubs against the top of the shoe. Special orthotics and pads are often used to redistribute pressure and relieve pain. In severe cases, surgery may be required.

Before the operation, blood and urine studies are conducted and X rays are taken of both feet. Hammertoe correction surgery begins with the injection of a local anesthetic. To prevent bleeding in the surgical area, a tourniquet is applied above the ankle. An incision is made through the skin above the affected joint. The tendons that attach to the toes are located and cut free of the connective tissue to the foot bone. The tendons are then divided, enabling the toe to lay straight. To keep the toe from bending, the middle joints are permanently connected together with fine pins and wires. Fine sutures are used to close the skin, and the tourniquet is removed. After the surgery, additional blood studies are taken. Sutures are usually removed seven to ten days after the procedure.

USES AND COMPLICATIONS
The correction of hammertoe usually arises out of a need to correct severe deformity or relieve persistent pain. During recovery, flat, comfortable shoes should be worn. After recovery, shoes should be worn that fit well and do not cramp the toes or put undue stress on the front of the foot. Though full recovery from surgery is expected in four weeks, vigorous exercise should be avoided for six weeks after surgery. Once the time for healing has passed, the affected toe will appear in a normal position, and pain will be relieved. Because of the connecting of joints in the toe, however, movement of the toes will be limited.

Possible complications associated with hammertoe correction include excessive bleeding and surgical wound infection.

—*Jason Georges*

See also Bone disorders; Bones and the skeleton; Feet; Foot disorders; Hammertoes; Lower extremities; Orthopedic surgery; Orthopedics; Podiatry.

FOR FURTHER INFORMATION:
Copeland, Glenn, and Stan Solomon. *The Foot Doctor.* Emmaus, Pa.: Rodale Press, 1986.

Lorimer, Donald L., ed. *Neale's Common Foot Disorders: Diagnosis and Management.* Rev. 4th ed. New York: Churchill Livingstone, 1993.

Shangold, Jules, and Frank Greenberg. *Opportunities in Podiatric Medicine.* Skokie, Ill.: VGM Career Horizons, 1982.

HAMMERTOES
DISEASE/DISORDER
ANATOMY OR SYSTEM AFFECTED: Feet

SPECIALTIES AND RELATED FIELDS: Orthopedics, podiatry

DEFINITION: Toes that are bent permanently at the joint nearest to the foot; the closely related term "clawtoe" denotes a toe that is bent at both joints.

CAUSES AND SYMPTOMS
Hammertoes and clawtoes can occur in one or more of the four smaller toes on each foot, with the second toe being the most common site for these deformities. Hammertoes and clawtoes are thought to be caused by muscle imbalance, contraction of the tendons, and enlargement of the toe joints. Although anyone can develop these conditions, they are felt to be caused primarily by wearing high heels or shoes that are too tight. It is common for people to develop painful corns and calluses in association with these conditions, particularly on the top or on the tip of the toe where it is most likely to rub against the shoe. Furthermore, people with hammertoes or clawtoes may experience considerable pain if the toe gets inflamed

and may also develop skin ulcers from the rubbing of their shoes against the bent toe. These ulcers can become infected and develop abnormal channels to the skin surface called sinus tracts. These conditions may also cause significant problems with walking for the affected individual.

TREATMENT AND THERAPY

Treatment of hammertoes or clawtoes depends on the severity of the condition and whether there are secondary complications such as corns or ulcers. The simplest treatment is to change to shoes with broad toes and soft soles that cushion the foot and to avoid wearing high heels and shoes that pinch the toes. Accompanied by excellent foot care such as callus and corn removal, this may be all that is required to prevent pain and irritation of the toes. In cases that are more advanced, various inserts can be added to the shoes. These include metatarsal bars, orthotics, and other devices. A metatarsal bar supports the ball of the foot, spreading the pressure normally put on this area over a greater part of the foot. Orthotics are specially molded plastic devices that serve much the same purpose. In some cases, podiatrists (foot doctors) or orthopedists recommend toe caps, padded sleeves that help prevent friction between the toe and the shoe. In a few cases, it may be necessary to cut the tendons in the toe or to perform arthroplasty (repair of the joint itself) to provide relief.

—*Rebecca Lovell Scott, Ph.D.*

See also Bone disorders; Bones and the skeleton; Corns and calluses; Foot disorders; Lower extremities; Skin; Skin disorders.

FOR FURTHER INFORMATION:

Copeland, Glenn, and Stan Solomon. *The Foot Doctor.* Emmaus, Pa.: Rodale Press, 1986.

Lorimer, Donald L., ed. *Neale's Common Foot Disorders: Diagnosis and Management.* Rev. 4th ed. New York: Churchill Livingstone, 1993.

Shangold, Jules, and Frank Greenberg. *Opportunities in Podiatric Medicine.* Skokie, Ill.: VGM Career Horizons, 1982.

HAND-FOOT-AND-MOUTH DISEASE
DISEASE/DISORDER

ALSO KNOWN AS: Vesicular stomatitis with exanthem
ANATOMY OR SYSTEM AFFECTED: Mouth, skin
SPECIALTIES AND RELATED FIELDS: Dermatology, family practice, pediatrics

DEFINITION: Hand-foot-and-mouth disease is a generally mild infectious illness caused by the Coxsackie virus. It is characterized by a blistery rash in the mouth and on the extremities. After an incubation period of three to six days, symptoms begin with fever, appetite loss, exhaustion, and a sore mouth. A day later, blisters appear in the mouth and on the hands and feet. Rarely, severe internal complications can occur. The disease peaks in the summer and fall. No treatment exists, but hand-foot-and-mouth disease usually resolves spontaneously in two weeks.

—*Connie Rizzo, M.D.*

See also Childhood infectious diseases; Dermatology, pediatric; Fever; Rashes; Viral infections.

FOR FURTHER INFORMATION:

Clayman, Charles B., ed. *The American Medical Association Family Medical Guide.* 3d rev. ed. New York: Random House, 1994.

Goldsmith, Lowell A., Gerald S. Lazarus, and Michael D. Tharp. *Adult and Pediatric Dermatology: A Color Guide to Diagnosis and Treatment.* Philadelphia: F. A. Davis, 1997.

Schmitt, Barton D. *Your Child's Health: The Parents' Guide to Symptoms, Emergencies, Common Illnesses, Behavior, and School Problems.* Rev. ed. New York: Bantam Books, 1991.

Spock, Benjamin, and Steven J. Parker. *Dr. Spock's Baby and Child Care.* 7th rev. ed. New York: Pocket Books, 1998.

HANTA VIRUS
DISEASE/DISORDER

ANATOMY OR SYSTEM AFFECTED: Kidneys, lungs, respiratory system
SPECIALTIES AND RELATED FIELDS: Critical care, environmental health, epidemiology, internal medicine, pulmonary medicine, public health, virology
DEFINITION: An often-fatal viral infection carried by rodents that causes influenza-like symptoms and respiratory failure.

CAUSES AND SYMPTOMS

Hanta virus, which is distantly related to Ebola virus, is transmitted through contact with the urine and droppings of wild rodents, such as the deer mouse and cotton rat. Contact usually involves the inhalation of contaminated particles in dust. Hanta virus is not transmissible between humans.

Infection takes two major forms. In South America, one strain causes hemorrhagic fever with renal syndrome, involving kidney failure, hemorrhaging, and shock. In the United States, another strain results in hantavirus pulmonary syndrome. Early symptoms mimic influenza; they include fever, chills, muscle aches, nausea and vomiting, malaise, and a dry cough. After initial improvement, increasing shortness of breath follows and may progress to pulmonary edema, internal bleeding, respiratory failure, and death.

TREATMENT AND THERAPY

Diagnosis of hantavirus pulmonary syndrome involves physical examination for hypoxia, hypotension, and adult respiratory distress syndrome. Laboratory tests show an elevated white blood cell count and a decreasing platelet count, and chest X rays may reveal edema. The presence of hanta virus is confirmed through serological testing.

There is no cure for hantavirus pulmonary syndrome; treatment is focused on alleviating the symptoms. This condition must be treated in the intensive care unit (ICU) of a hospital, as careful monitoring of respiratory function and blood gases is essential. In severe cases, the use of an endotracheal tube and a ventilator becomes necessary. Experiments have been performed with intravenous ribavirin therapy; the efficacy of this treatment is being evaluated. Unfortunately, even with aggressive measures, the death rate ranges from 50 to 80 percent.

PERSPECTIVE AND PROSPECTS

The incidence of hantavirus pulmonary syndrome seemed to rise sharply in the 1990's. Epidemiologists were uncertain whether the number of cases increased or more cases were reported following identification of the virus in the United States in 1993.

Because much remains to be learned about the transmission, development, and treatment of hanta virus infection, public health efforts have been in education and prevention. Hikers and campers are thought to be at a greater risk; they are urged to avoid exposure to rodent droppings and questionable water sources. People entering cabins, sheds, or other buildings that have not been used recently should air out the building first and use disinfectant on all surfaces.

—*Tracy Irons-Georges*

See also Edema; Environmental diseases; Environmental health; Epidemiology; Lungs; Pulmonary diseases; Pulmonary medicine; Respiration; Viral infections; Zoonoses.

FOR FURTHER INFORMATION:

Cockrum, E. Lendell. *Rabies, Lyme Disease, Hanta Virus, and Other Animal-Borne Human Diseases in the United States and Canada.* Tucson, Ariz.: Fisher Books, 1997.

Meyer, Andrea S., and David R. Harper. *Of Mice, Men, and Microbes: Hantavirus.* New York: Academic Press, 1999.

Pan American Health Organization. *Hantavirus in the Americas: Guidelines for Diagnosis, Treatment, Prevention, and Control.* Washington, D.C.: Author, 1999.

HARE LIP. *See* CLEFT LIP AND PALATE.

HAY FEVER

DISEASE/DISORDER

ALSO KNOWN AS: Allergic rhinitis

ANATOMY OR SYSTEM AFFECTED: Nose, respiratory system

SPECIALTIES AND RELATED FIELDS: Otorhinolaryngology, virology

DEFINITION: Rhinitis is the inflammation of the mucous membrane that lines the nose. It is caused by a common cold virus or by an allergic reaction to airborne allergens. Allergic rhinitis is commonly called hay fever. Its symptoms include itchy eyes, frequent sneezing, a stuffy nose with a clear discharge, and sometimes wheezing. Allergic rhinitis can be treated by eliminating as many allergens from one's environment as possible. Thoroughly cleaning living spaces and removing allergy-causing elements, such as animals and plants, can help prevent onset. The symptoms can be treated with antihistamines, decongestants, nasal sprays, and eye drops.

—*Jason Georges and Tracy Irons-Georges*

See also Allergies; Common cold; Multiple chemical sensitivity syndrome; Nasopharyngeal disorders; Otorhinolaryngology; Sense organs; Sinusitis; Smell; Sneezing; Viral infections.

FOR FURTHER INFORMATION:

Joneja, Janice M. V., and Leonard Bielory. *Understanding Allergy, Sensitivity, and Immunity.* New Brunswick, N.J.: Rutgers University Press, 1990.

Kuby, Janis. *Immunology.* New York: W. H. Freeman, 2000.

Roitt, Ivan. *Essential Immunology*. 9th ed. Boston: Blackwell Scientific, 1997.

Young, Stuart, Bruce Dobozin, and Margaret Miner. *Allergies*. Rev. ed. New York: Plume, 1999.

HEAD AND NECK DISORDERS
DISEASE/DISORDER

ANATOMY OR SYSTEM AFFECTED: Bones, brain, head, muscles, musculoskeletal system, neck, nervous system, respiratory system, spine, throat

SPECIALTIES AND RELATED FIELDS: Dentistry, emergency medicine, neurology, otolaryngology, sports medicine

DEFINITION: Physical trauma or neurological problems affecting the head and neck, including the spinal cord.

The head and neck region of the human body houses a sophisticated collection of structures including the special sense organs (structures for breathing, speaking, and eating) and the brain, brain stem, and cervical (neck) portion of the spinal cord. A multitude of disorders or injuries can occur in this complex region.

Trauma to the head and neck. Head or neck trauma can result from a harsh blow on the head, as can occur in a fall or with a strike from an object. These injuries are commonly seen in young, basically healthy persons who come to emergency rooms during evenings or weekends as a result of sports accidents, automobile accidents, or domestic or street violence. In the older age group, strokes and aneurysms are more common problems. Some of these accidents or events can cause permanent nerve and brain damage to the injured person.

Concussions and contusions of the head are common results of head trauma, which induces an internal neurological response. A concussion is a loss of consciousness or awareness of one's surroundings that may last a few minutes or days. Sometimes a concussion appears only as a moderately decreased level of awareness and not a total loss of consciousness. There is no evidence of a change in the brain's structure but, oddly, there is a change in the way in which the brain operates so that alertness is altered. Concussion is presumably a temporary change in brain chemistry, and the damage is reversible unless repeated head blows, such as a professional boxer may experience, are endured. Concussions may occur from other trauma, such as loss of blood flow to the brain, but such trauma is more closely associated with the more urgent threat of permanent brain damage. A contusion is popularly referred to as a bruise. The color associated with a fresh bruise is attributable to an aggregation of blood in an area that was damaged, causing many small blood vessels to rupture and release blood into the surrounding tissue. A bruise around the eye, temple, or forehead causes a black eye.

Automobile accidents rank as one of the common causes of head and neck injury. One of the more familiar complaints after a car accident is the condition called whiplash. Whiplash is the lay person's term for hyperextension of the neck, whereby the head is thrust backward (posteriorly) abruptly and beyond the normal range of neck motion. Hyperflexion occurs when the head is abruptly thrust in the forward (anterior) direction—sometimes as a recoil from hyperextension. The pain of whiplash originates from the damage to the anterior longitudinal ligament along the neck region of the spinal cord. This ligament can be overly stretched or even torn as a result of a sudden snap or jerk of the neck. Furthermore, the bony vertebrae may also grind against one another after the trauma, causing additional irritation, swelling, and pain in the neck area.

One of the common troubles of a gun or knife wound to the head and neck region is superficial and

Compression from:

Depressed bone

Internal bleeding

Pressure on brain stem due to swelling

Head trauma may result in compression of the brain, consequent distortions, and severe neurological reactions.

deep lacerations (cuts). If left unsutured, a deep scalp wound can cause death by hemorrhage. Superficial lacerations to the face may also cause considerable bleeding; such wounds generally are not life-threatening, but they often require stitches in order to heal.

Trauma to the head and neck area can arise from spontaneous internal events such as a stroke, an embolus, or an aneurysm. Each of these conditions is serious and potentially life-threatening because of the risk of losing blood flow to the brain and other vital tissues of the head and neck region.

Neurological problems of the head and neck. Although the bony cranium offers some protection to the head, the neck is, in some regards, more vulnerable to intrusion. Breathing can be interrupted by severing the left or right phrenic nerve, each of which innervates its corresponding half of the most important muscle of breathing, the diaphragm.

The left or right vagus nerve may also be severed. The vagus nerves supply the sympathetic system of the thorax and abdomen, and they also innervate the vocal cords. Severance of one of the vagus nerves causes a hoarseness of the voice as a result of the loss of function of one-half of the vocal cords. If both vagus nerves are damaged—a rare event—then the ability to speak is forever lost.

The sympathetic trunk is another nerve at risk in the neck. Severance of this nerve leads to Horner's syndrome, which consists of a group of signs including ptosis (drooping eyelids), constricted pupils, a flushed face as a result of vasodilation, and dry skin on the face and neck because of the inability to sweat.

Transection (the complete severance) of the lower cervical spinal cord causes upper and lower limb paralysis and trouble with urination, and damage to the upper cervical cord can cause death because of loss of innervation to the muscles of respiration. Hemisection (partial severance) of the cervical spinal cord can also cause Horner's syndrome. Damage to the spinal cord can occur from a knife or gun wound or from crushing or snapping the cord by sudden impact, as with an injury from an earthquake or an automobile accident.

—*Mary C. Fields, M.D.*

See also Amnesia; Aneurysmectomy; Aneurysms; Ataxia; Brain; Brain disorders; Cluster headaches; Coma; Computed tomography (CT) scanning; Concussion; Craniosynostosis; Craniotomy; Dementias; Dizziness and fainting; Electroencephalography (EEG); Embolism; Encephalitis; Epilepsy; Hallucinations; Headaches; Hemiplegia; Hydrocephalus; Laryngitis; Memory loss; Meningitis; Migraine headaches; Nasal polyp removal; Nasopharyngeal disorders; Neuralgia, neuritis, and neuropathy; Neurology; Neurology, pediatric; Neurosurgery; Numbness and tingling; Palsy; Paralysis; Paraplegia; Pharyngitis; Quadriplegia; Seizures; Shunts; Sinusitis; Spinal cord disorders; Sports medicine; Strokes; Thrombosis and thrombus; Torticollis; Unconsciousness; Voice and vocal cord disorders.

For Further Information:

Clayman, Charles B., ed. *The American Medical Association Family Medical Guide.* New York: Random House, 1994. The perfect beginner's guide, not only to head and neck medicine but to any common medical topic as well.

Moore, Keith L. *Clinically Oriented Anatomy.* 4th ed. Baltimore: Williams & Wilkins, 1999. Moore addresses the normal human anatomy and offers clinical commentary for the sake of relevance. Enhanced by multicolored, detailed sketches. Expertly written.

Headaches

Disease/disorder

Anatomy or system affected: Brain, head, nervous system, psychic-emotional system

Specialties and related fields: Family practice, internal medicine, neurology

Definition: A general term referring to pain localized in the head and/or neck, which may signal mere tension or serious disorders.

Key terms:

cluster headache: a severe type of headache, characterized by excruciating pain; attacks occur in groups, or clusters

migraine headache: a type of headache characterized by pain on one side of the head, often accompanied by disordered vision and gastrointestinal disturbances

prophylactic treatment: a treatment focusing on preventing disease, illness, or their symptoms from occurring

symptomatic treatment: a treatment focusing on aborting disease, illness, or their symptoms once they have occurred

tension-type headache: a type of headache characterized by bandlike or caplike pain over the head

CAUSES AND SYMPTOMS

In 1988, an ad hoc committee of the International Headache Society developed the current classification system for headaches. This system includes fourteen exhaustive categories of headache with the purpose of developing comparability in the management and study of headaches. Headaches most commonly seen by health care providers can be classified into four main types: migraine, tension-type, cluster, and "other" acute headaches.

Migraine headaches have been estimated to affect approximately 12 percent of the population. The headaches are more common in women, and they tend to run in families; they are usually first noticed in the teen years or young adulthood. For the diagnosis of migraine without aura ("aura" refers to visual disturbances or hallucinations, numbness and tingling on one side of the face, dizziness, or impairment of speech or hearing—symptoms that occur twenty to thirty minutes prior to the onset of the headache), the person must experience at least ten headache attacks, each lasting between four and seventy-two hours with at least two of the following characteristics: The headache is unilateral (occurs on one side), has a pulsating quality, is moderate to severe in intensity, or is aggravated by routine physical activity. Additionally, one of the following symptoms must accompany the headache: nausea and/or vomiting, or sensitivity to light or sounds. The person's medical history, a physical examination, and (where appropriate) diagnostic tests must exclude other organic causes of the headache, such as brain tumor or infection. Migraine with aura is far less common.

Migraines may be triggered or aggravated by physical activity, by menstruation, by relaxation after emotional stress, by ingestion of alcohol (red wine in particular) or certain foods or food additives (chocolate, hard cheeses, nuts, fatty foods, monosodium glutamate, or nitrates used in processed meats), by prescription medications (including birth control pills and hypertension medications), and by changes in the weather. Yet the precise pathophysiology of migraines is unknown. It had been posited that spasms in the blood vessels of the brain, followed by the dilation of these same blood vessels, cause the aura and head pain; however, studies using sophisticated brain and cerebral blood-flow scanning techniques indicate that this is likely not the case and that some type of inflammatory process may be involved related to the permeability of cerebral blood vessels and the resultant release of certain neurochemicals.

Tension-type headaches are the most common type of headache; its prevalence is approximately 79 percent. Tension-type headaches are not hereditary, are found more frequently in females, and are first noticed in the teen years of young adulthood, although they can appear at any time of life. For the diagnosis of tension-type headaches, the person must experience at least ten headache attacks lasting from thirty minutes to seven days each, with at least two of the following characteristics: The headache has a pressing or tightening (nonpulsating) quality, is mild or moderate in intensity (may inhibit but does not prohibit activities), is bilateral or variable in location, and is not aggravated by physical activity. Additionally, nausea, vomiting, and light or sound sensitivity are absent or mild. Furthermore, the patient's medical history and physical or neurological examination exclude other organic causes for the headache apart from the following: oral or jaw dysfunction, muscular stress, or drug overuse. Tension-type headache sufferers describe these headaches as a bandlike or caplike tightness around the head, and/or muscle tension in the back of the head, neck, or shoulders. The pain is described as slow in onset with a dull or steady aching.

Tension-type headaches are believed to be precipitated primarily by emotional factors but can also be stimulated by muscular and spinal disorders, jaw dysfunction, paranasal sinus disease, and traumatic head injuries. The pathophysiology of tension-type headaches is controversial. Historically, tension-type headaches were attributed to sustained muscle contractions of the pericranial muscles. Studies indicate, however, that most patients do not manifest increased pericranial muscle activity and that pericranial muscle blood flow and/or central pain mechanisms might be involved in the pathophysiology of tension-type headaches. It is also believed that muscle contraction and scalp muscle ischemia play some role in tension-type headache pain.

Cluster headaches are the least frequent of the headache types and are thought to be the most severe and painful. Cluster headaches are more common in males, with estimates of 0.4 to 1.0 percent of males being affected. Traditionally, these headaches first appear at about thirty years of age, although they can start later in life. There is no genetic predisposition to these headaches. For the diagnosis of cluster headaches, the person must experience at least ten severely painful headache attacks, typically on one side of the face and lasting from fifteen minutes to three hours. One of the following symptoms must accompany the headache on the painful side of the face: a bloodshot eye, tearing, nasal congestion, nasal discharge, forehead and facial sweating, contraction of the pupils, or drooping eyelids. Physical and neurological examination and imaging must exclude organic causes for the headaches, such as tumor or infection. Cluster headaches often occur once or twice daily, or every other day, but can be as frequent as ten attacks in one day, recurring on the same side of the head during the cluster period. The temporal "clusters" of these headaches give them their descriptive name.

A cluster headache is described as a severe, excruciating, boring, sharp, and burning pain through the eye. The pain is occasionally throbbing but always unilateral. Radiation of the pain to the teeth has been reported. Duration of a headache can range from ten minutes to three hours, with the next headache in the cluster occurring sometime the same day. Cluster headache sufferers are often unable to sit or lie still and are in such pain that they have been known, in desperation, to hit their heads with their fists or to smash their heads against walls or floors.

Cluster headaches can be triggered in susceptible patients by alcohol consumption, subcutaneous injections of histamine, and sublingual use of nitroglycerine. Because these agents all cause the dilation of blood vessels, these attacks are believed to be associated with dilation of the temporal and ophthalmic arteries and other extracranial vessels. There is no evidence that intracranial blood flow is involved. Cluster headaches have been shown to occur more frequently during the weeks before and after the longest and shortest days of the year, lending support for the hypothesis of a link to seasonal changes. Additionally, cluster headaches often occur at about the same time of day in a given sufferer, suggesting a relationship to the circadian rhythms of the body. Vascular changes, hormonal changes, neurochemical excesses or deficits, histamine levels, and autonomic nervous system changes are all being studied for their possible role in the pathophysiology of cluster headaches.

Acute headaches, using the International Headache Society's classification scheme, constitute many of the headaches not mentioned above. Distinct from the other headache types, which are often considered to be chronic in nature, acute headaches often signify underlying disease or a life-threatening medical condition. These headaches can display pain distribution and quality similar to those seen in chronic headaches. The temporal nature of acute headaches, however, often points to their seriousness. Acute headaches of concern are usually the first or worst headache the patient has had or are headaches with recent onset that are persistent or recurrent. Other signs that cause a high index of suspicion include an unremitting headache that steadily increases without relief, accompanying weakness or numbness in the hands or feet, an atypical change in the quality or intensity of the headache, headache upon exertion, recent head trauma, or a family history of cardiovascular problems. Such headaches can point to hemorrhage, meningitis, stroke, tumor, brain abscess, hematoma, and infection, which are all potentially life-threatening conditions. A thorough evaluation is necessary for all patients exhibiting the danger signs of acute headache.

TREATMENT AND THERAPY

Because there are several hundred causes of headaches, the evaluation of headache complaints is crucial. Medical science offers myriad evaluation techniques for headaches. The initial evaluation includes a complete history and physical examination to determine the factors involved in the headache complaint, such as the general physical condition of the patient, neurological functioning, cardiovascular condition, metabolic status, and psychiatric condition. Based on this initial evaluation, the health care professional may elect to perform a number of diagnostic tests to confirm or reject a diagnosis. These tests might include blood studies, X rays, computed tomography (CT) scans, psychological evaluation, electroencephalograms (EEGs), magnetic resonance imaging (MRI), or studies of spinal fluid.

Once a headache diagnosis is made, a treatment plan is developed. In the case of acute headaches, treatment may take varying forms, from surgery to the use of prescription medications. For migraine, tension-type, and cluster headaches, there are several common treatment options. Headache treatment can be categorized into two types: abortive (symptomatic) treatment or prophylactic (preventive) treatment. Treatment is tailored to the type of headache and the type of patient.

A headache is often a highly distressing occurrence for patients, sometimes causing a high level of anxiety, relief-seeking behavior, and a dependency on the health care system. The health care provider must consider not only biological elements of the illness but also possible resultant psychological and sociological elements as well. An open, communicative relationship with the patient is paramount, and treatment routinely begins with soliciting patient collaboration and providing patient education. Patient education takes the form of normalizing (or "decatastrophizing") the headache experience for patients, thereby reducing their fears concerning the etiology of the headache or about being unable to cope with the pain. Supportiveness, understanding, and collaboration are all necessary components of any headache treatment.

There are a number of abortive pharmacological treatments for migraine headaches. Ergotamine tartrate (an alkaloid or salt) is effective in terminating migraine symptoms by either reducing the dilation of extracranial arteries or in some way stimulating certain parts of the brain. Isomethaptine, another effective treatment for migraine, is a combination of chemicals that stimulates the sympathetic nervous system, provides analgesia, and is mildly tranquilizing. Another class of medications for migraines are nonsteroidal anti-inflammatory drugs (NSAIDs); these drugs, as the name implies, work on the principle that inflammation is involved in migraine. Both narcotic and nonnarcotic pain medications are often used for migraines, primarily for their analgesic properties; the concern in prescribing potent narcotic pain medications is the potential for their overuse. Antiemetic medications prevent or arrest vomiting and have been used in the treatment of migraines. Sumatriptan, a vasoactive agent that increases the amount of the neurochemical serotonin in the brain, shows promise in treating migraines that do not respond to other treatments.

Prophylactic treatments for migraines include betablockers, methysergide, and calcium channel blockers, which are believed to interfere with the dilation or contraction of extracranial arteries by acting on the sympathetic nervous system or on the central nervous system itself. Antidepressants, medications used typically for the treatment of depression, have also been found to prevent migraine attacks; there appears to be an analgesic effect from certain antidepressants that is effective for chronic migraines. Antiseizure medications have been found to be useful for some migraine patients, although the mechanism of action is unknown. NSAIDs have also been used as a preventive measure for migraines.

There are several nonpharmacological treatment options for migraine headaches. These include stress management, relaxation training, biofeedback (a variant of relaxation training), psychotherapy (both individual and family), and the modification of headacheprecipitating factors (such as avoiding certain dietary precipitants). Each of these treatments has been found to be effective for certain patients, particularly those with chronic migraine complaints. For some patients, they can be as effective as pharmacological treatments. The exact mechanism of action for their effect on migraines has not been established. Other self-management techniques include lying quietly in a dark room, applying pressure to the side of the head or face on which the pain is experienced, and applying cold compresses to the head.

The abortive treatment options for tension-type headaches include narcotic and nonnarcotic analgesics, because of their pain-reducing properties. More often with tension-type headaches, the milder over-the-counter pain medications (such as aspirin or acetaminophen) are used. NSAIDs, simple muscle relaxants, or antianxiety drugs can also be used. Muscle relaxants and antianxiety drugs are believed to relax smooth muscles, reducing scalp muscle ischemia and therefore head pain.

Prophylactic treatments for tension-type headaches include antidepressants, narcotic and nonnarcotic analgesics, muscle relaxants, and antianxiety drugs. Occasionally, "trigger-point injections" are used to relieve tension-type headaches. Trigger points are areas within muscles, primarily in the upper back and neck, that are hypersensitive; when stimulated, they can cause headaches. These trigger points can be injected with a local anesthetic or steroid to decrease their sensitivity or to eliminate possible inflammation in the area.

Nonpharmacological treatment of tension-type headaches is similar to that for migraines and includes stress management, relaxation training, biofeedback, and psychotherapy. Psychotherapy has been found to be a very important adjunct to any treatment of tension-type headaches because the illness, particularly when chronic, can lead to a pain syndrome characterized by family dysfunction, medication overuse, and vocational disruptions. Other self-management techniques include taking a hot shower or bath, placing a hot water bottle or ice pack on the head or back of the neck, exercising, and sleeping.

For cluster headaches, one of the most excruciating types of headache, the most common abortive treatment is administering pure oxygen to the patient for ten minutes. The exact mechanism of action is unknown, but it might be related to the constriction of dilated cerebral arteries. Ergotamine tartrate or similar alkaloids given orally, intramuscularly, or intravenously can also abort the attack in some patients. Nasal drops of a local anesthetic (lidocaine hydrochloride) or cocaine have been used to interrupt the activity of the trigeminal nerve that is believed to be involved in cluster attacks. The efficacy of these treatments is inconclusive.

Prophylactic treatment of this headache type is crucial. Ergotamine, methysergide, calcium channel blockers, antiseizure medications, and steroidal anti-inflammatory medications have been used with some success in the prevention of cluster attacks. The mechanism of action for these medications is unknown. Lithium carbonate, a drug commonly prescribed for bipolar disorder, has been found to be effective for some cluster patients. This medication is believed to affect certain regions of the brain, possibly the hypothalamus.

While no nonpharmacological treatment strategies are routinely offered to cluster headache patients, surgery is an option in severe cases, particularly if the headaches are resistant to all other available treatments. Percutaneous radio frequency thermocoagulation of the trigeminal ganglion is a surgical procedure that destroys the trigeminal nerve pathway, the chief nerve pathway to the face. Modest successes have been found with this extreme treatment option.

PERSPECTIVE AND PROSPECTS

Headaches are among the most common complaints to physicians and quite likely have been a problem since the beginning of humankind. Accounts of headaches can be found in the clinical notes of Arateus of Cappadocia, a first century physician. Descriptions of specific headache subtypes can be traced to the second century in the writings of the Greek physician Galen. Headaches are a prevalent health problem that affects all ages and sexes and those from various cultural, social, and educational backgrounds.

The lifetime prevalence estimates of headaches is 93 percent for males and 99 percent of females. Studies in the United States estimate that 65 to 85 percent of the population will experience a headache within a year. Data from cross-cultural studies echo the significance of this public health problem: Frequent, severe headaches are reported by 10.4 percent of men and 35.3 percent of women in Thailand; 17.6 percent of men and 20.2 percent of women in urban Africa report a history of recurrent headaches; 57 percent of men and 73 percent of women in Finland report at least one headache in the previous year; and 39 percent of men and 60 percent of women in New Zealand also report an annual headache frequency.

As these data indicate, the prevalence of headaches is greater in women, although the reason is unknown. Age seems to be a mediating factor as well, with significantly fewer people sixty-five years of age or older reporting headache problems. There are no socioeconomic differences in prevalence rates, with persons in high-income and low-income brackets having similar rates. There are data to suggest that people with college educations or higher report headaches more often than those with only some high school education. The only vocational area that has been tied to increased rates of headaches are people who work at computer terminals.

The total economic costs of headaches are staggering. Headaches constitute approximately 1.7 percent of all visits to physician offices. Of visits to hospital emergency rooms, 2.5 percent are for headaches. The expenses associated with advances in assessment techniques and routine health care have risen rapidly. The cost in lost workdays adds to this economic picture. Thirty-six percent of headache sufferers in one study reported missing one or more days of work in the previous year because of headaches. The scientific study of headaches is necessary to understand this prevalent illness. Efforts, such as those by the International Headache Society, to develop accepted definitions of headaches will greatly assist efforts to identify and treat headaches.

—Oliver Oyama, Ph.D.

See also Anxiety; Brain; Brain disorders; Cluster headaches; Head and neck disorders; Migraine headaches; Multiple chemical sensitivity syndrome; Neuralgia, neuritis, and neuropathy; Neurology; Neurology, pediatric; Sinusitis; Stress; Stress reduction; Tumor removal; Tumors.

FOR FURTHER INFORMATION:

Blanchard, Edward B., and Frank Andrasik. *Management of Chronic Headaches: A Psychological Approach.* New York: Pergamon Press, 1985. The authors review the evaluation and treatment of headaches from a psychological perspective. Alternative, nonpharmacological treatments for headaches are described in detail.

Diamond, Seymour. "Migraine Headaches." *The Medical Clinics of North America* 75, no. 3 (May 1, 1991): 545-566. Diamond is one of the world's authorities on headaches. His article is well organized and comprehensively addresses the subject of migraines in a readable and interesting format. A practical guide to treating the headache patient.

Rapoport, Alan M., and Fred D. Sheftell. *Headache Relief.* New York: Simon & Schuster, 1991. The book takes the often-complicated theory, evaluation, and treatment of headaches and explains each area in very understandable terms for the layperson. The authors describe a "how-to" approach to treating headaches.

Raskin, Neil H. *Headache.* 2d ed. New York: Churchill Livingstone, 1988. A review of headaches from a technical perspective. The reader looking for a thorough resource study of headaches will find this text useful. The review of common headache types is comprehensive and reflects the research on headaches in the mid-1980's.

Saper, Joel R., et al., eds. *Handbook of Headache Management: A Practical Guide to Diagnosis and Treatment of Head, Neck, and Facial Pain.* 2d ed. Baltimore: Williams & Wilkins, 1999. A manual for doctors with patients complaining of headache pain.

HEALING
BIOLOGY

ANATOMY OR SYSTEM AFFECTED: All

SPECIALTIES AND RELATED FIELDS: Alternative medicine, cytology, dermatology, family practice, hematology, histology, immunology, plastic surgery, vascular medicine

DEFINITION: The process of mending damaged tissue by which an organism restores itself to health.

KEY TERMS:

collagen: a white fibrous protein produced by the body to fill in areas destroyed by injury; the healing component more commonly thought of as scar tissue

delayed primary closure: a procedure in which the wound is left open four to six days and then sewn closed; used for infected or contaminated wounds

healing by primary intention: the most desirable healing in the least amount of time, with minimal scar tissue formation; the edges of the wound close together

healing by secondary intention: less desirable healing of a wound, with replacement of damaged area by granulation tissue; delayed healing and excessive scar formation occur

regeneration: the renewal, regrowth, or restoration of destroyed or missing tissue; the production of new tissue

tensile strength: the greatest stress that can be placed on a tissue without tearing it apart; relative to the strength of a tissue

wounds: injuries classified as open or closed depending on whether the skin is broken; types of open wounds include abrasions, lacerations, avulsions, punctures, and incisions

THE HEALING PROCESS

The human body is not able to reproduce injured parts during the healing process. Most injured tissue in the body is replaced with collagen, a white protein known as scar tissue. Body areas capable of reproducing, or regenerating, include the outer layer of skin and the inner layers of the intestines.

The human body is involved in a continuous process of self-healing every day. The outer layer of the skin is constantly rubbed off, yet the body is able to replace (regenerate) new skin to take its place. Another body area capable of regeneration is the innermost layer of the intestine. All other types of tissue, however, such as muscle, fat, blood vessels, or even bones, must rely on other ways to heal when injured. How quickly the body heals depends on many factors, but the process is a predictable one. The healing process includes three phases: the acute inflammatory phase, the repair or regeneration phase, and the remodeling phase.

The first phase of healing, the immediate inflammatory phase, includes the first three or four days after the injury. This process, carried out by vascular, chemical, and cellular events, leads to the repair of tissue, to regeneration, or to scar tissue formation. If the hand is sliced open by a piece of broken glass, the first healing response would be a temporary decrease in blood flow, known as vasoconstriction, that lasts from a few seconds up to several minutes. This narrowing of the blood vessel occurs because of a decrease in the diameter of the blood vessels at the injury site and prevents the person from bleeding to death. With extensive vessel damage, however, the

The Healing Process

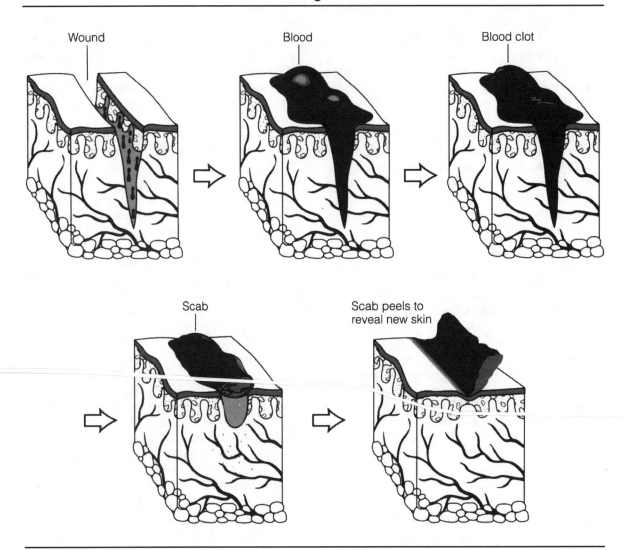

Wound

Blood

Blood clot

Scab

Scab peels to reveal new skin

body is unable to close off enough vessels, and life-threatening hemorrhaging may occur.

When only a small amount of tissue is cut, the blood begins to seal the broken vessels by coagulation, also known as blood clot formation. The next step is activation of the chemicals needed in the healing process, which is possible only after the blood vessel diameter increases in a process called vasodilation. During vasodilation, the blood flow is slowed and the blood becomes thicker, resulting in swelling. At this point, a buildup or accumulation of fluid results from the seeping of plasma, the fluid portion of the blood, through the vessel walls. This seeping or leakage results from the difference in pressure within the vessel and outside its walls. The amount of swelling at the injury site depends on the amount of seeping, which in turn depends on how much tissue damage has occurred.

Because the blood flow is slower, the concentration of red blood cells and white blood cells is increased. The white blood cells line up and adhere to the inside walls of small blood vessels, known as venules. These white blood cells then pass through the venule walls and are chemically attracted to the injury site over the next several hours. A specialized connective tissue cell, known as a mast cell, is also sent to the injury site. Mast cells contain heparin and histamine. Heparin prolongs the clotting time of blood by temporarily preventing coagulation, while histamine causes dilation of the capillaries. During this earliest phase, both heparin and histamine are important factors, since their actions allow other specialized cells to move into the injured area. The amount of bleeding and fluid buildup at the injury site depends on the extent of damage and how easily materials can cross the walls of intact vessels. Both of these conditions influence the healing process.

The second phase of healing can be called the repair or regeneration phase. For tissue capable of regeneration, this phase involves the restoration of destroyed or missing tissue. For other types of tissue, this second phase would entail the repair process. The healing of a deep cut in the hand would not be considered regeneration, since the body is not able to remake all the different layers of skin and muscle injured. This healing phase would extend forward from the previously described inflammatory phase. During this phase, the cut is naturally cleaned through the body's ability to remove cellular waste, the help of the red blood cells, and the formation of a blood clot.

Two types of healing can occur. Primary healing, or healing by primary intention, could take place in the hand laceration example, since the edges are even and close together. If this injury resulted in a large piece of tissue being removed, then the body would fill the gap with scar tissue. The replacement of tissue with scar tissue is an example of secondary healing, or healing by secondary intention. A torn muscle would be an example of secondary healing if it is allowed to heal on its own by the formation of scar tissue within the muscle.

No matter which type of healing occurs, several factors regulate how quickly and how completely this process takes place. Because blood vessels and cells are deprived of oxygen and die from the injury, this new cellular waste or debris must be cleaned from the area before repair or regeneration can take place. This tissue death promotes the formation of new capillary buds on the walls of the intact vessels. As these mature, the injury site is newly supplied with oxygenated blood and the healing process continues into the third phase.

The third phase of healing, known as the remodeling phase, includes the laying down of young scar tissue that increases in strength over the next year. Although the healing process has no distinct time frame, it is believed that three to six weeks is needed for the production of scar tissue. There must be a balance between the toughness and the elasticity of the scar. The amount of stress placed on a newly formed scar will determine the tensile strength of the collagen content. If stress or strain is placed on this forming scar tissue too early, the healing process will take longer. A desirable outcome would be a scar of adequate collagen content through the development of sufficient mature collagen fibers of proper tensile strength. Adequate tensile strength is also affected by how long inflammation is present.

If an injury site has inflammation that lasts up to one month, it is considered a subacute inflammation. When it lasts for months or years, it is then called chronic inflammation. Chronic inflammation is a condition where small traumas happen repeatedly; it is often seen in overuse injuries. Because this type of injury lasts longer, different types of chemicals try to initiate complete healing. The role of some of these special chemicals is not completely understood.

The healing of a broken bone, similar in many ways to the healing of the skin, is somewhat easier to understand. The first phase shows the same acute inflammation that lasts about four days, involving clotting blood, dead bone cells, and soft tissue damage around the injury site. The second phase, the repair and regeneration phase, differs slightly when a bone is broken, since the blood clot (hematoma) becomes granulated and builds between the two bone ends. The bone produces a specialized cell that turns into a soft or hard fibrous callus, matures into cartilage, and finally becomes bone with a firmly woven network of cells.

The beginning soft callus is a network of unorganized bone that forms at the two broken edges and is later absorbed and replaced by a hard callus. With appropriate care, a broken bone will develop a new network in the center and eventually become primary bone. The amount of oxygen available in the area determines this development. It is important to keep in mind that when the injury is severe enough to break a bone, then the blood supply is interrupted, lowering the amount of oxygen that is available. Low oxygen could result in the formation of only fibrous tissue or cartilage. Strong, healthy bone results when oxygen and the correct amount of compression are available. The third phase, the remodeling phase, describes the time when the callus has been reabsorbed and special intersecting bone fibers cover the broken area. It may take many years for this entire process to be completed, until the bone has regained its normal shape and ability to withstand stresses.

DISORDERS AND TREATMENT

Any of the three stages of healing can be delayed or prevented. The three main causes for failed healing are poor blood supply, poor immobilization, or infection.

The healing process within the body can be seriously hampered if the blood supply is poor, since the delivery of nutrients, chemicals, hormones, and specialized building materials to the injury site is hampered. It is extremely important that oxygen levels are adequate for proper healing. If the blood supply is not sufficient, then the tissue may die, especially in broken bone fragments. Fortunately, most tissues of the body have a good blood supply, as demonstrated by the amount of bleeding that takes place when the skin and underlying tissues are injured.

The second condition that interferes with healing is excessive movement because the body part was not immobilized. In order for the scar tissue or even new bone to become well organized, the two edges of the injured tissue must be kept close together.

The third reason for poor healing is infection. Although the body has many defenses against infection, foreign material can slow healing. If this infectious material invades the space between the two bone ends of a fracture, the necessary building materials may not reach the site. Infection invading the hand tissue cut by the glass could prevent the edges from healing together because of pus, scab formation, or the interference of germs.

There are many different types of injuries, and several steps must be taken in caring for each type. Soft tissues, the first line of defense against injuries, can be used to describe all tissues other than bone. Soft tissue injuries are classified as either closed or open. In a closed wound, the damage lies below the surface of the skin and the skin remains intact. A sprained ankle or a bruised knee are classified as closed wounds. In an open wound, the skin or mucous membranes such as the lining of the mouth are broken or torn.

There are four types of open soft tissue injuries; each has specific characteristics and heals differently. The first type is an abrasion, in which part of the outer layer of the skin and some underlying tissue is rubbed or scraped off. A common injury of this type is a scraped knee resulting from a fall on the sidewalk. The second type, the laceration, results from a sharp object cutting the skin, such as the previous example of a piece of glass cutting the skin either superficially or very deeply. The third type, an avulsion, results when a piece of skin or even an entire fingertip is torn off or left loosely hanging by a small flap of skin. It is important that this flap not be removed since a physician can sometimes reattach the part. The last type of soft tissue injury is the puncture wound, which results when a sharp object penetrates the skin and into a body part. Such an injury could be a stab from a knife or an ice pick, a splinter stuck in the foot, or even a bullet shot into the leg. The initial management is the same for all four types of injury.

Management of open wounds must include control of bleeding, infection prevention, and immobilization. Two of the above injuries, an avulsion and a puncture wound, require additional special care. In the case of an avulsed body part, the amputated part should be saved; wrapped in a dry, sterile piece of gauze; and placed in a plastic bag. If this bag is kept in something cool, such as a bucket of ice, the possibility of reattachment is increased. An impaled object remaining in a puncture wound should never be removed but held in place and all movement restricted until medical care can be given.

Several medical treatments can aid in promoting the healing process, as can commonsense first aid measures taken immediately after an injury occurs. For example, with a glass cut to the hand one should immediately stop the bleeding by placing a sterile piece of gauze, or a very clean cloth, directly over the laceration. By adding direct pressure over the gauze, the circulation is reduced. If the cut is deep, if the bleeding cannot be controlled, or if a piece of glass remains in the wound, then it is advisable to seek medical attention. A physician would then thoroughly clean the injury site and stitch the two edges together. Immobilizing the two flaps of skin together by sewing them will allow the first two phases of healing to progress. By having the wound inspected and cleaned by medical personnel, the risk of infection is reduced. A small injury can be cared for at home, but infection must be prevented through proper cleansing. Even soap and water, along with a bandage or dressing, will help to ward off infections.

PERSPECTIVE AND PROSPECTS

Many strategies to improve the healing of human tissue have evolved over time—from ancient times, when healers packed mud on the top of sores to draw out the infection, to modern alternative medicines. Every person, at one time or another, receives a cut, scrape, bump, or bruise. Therefore, there is much interest in speeding up the healing process.

Renewed interests in nontraditional approaches to medicine explore the healing powers locked within the human body. The use of homeopathy, acupuncture, and acupressure are examples of alternatives to antibiotics and standard first aid measures to help an injury heal. Holistic health care, hypnosis, and osteopathic medicine offer other areas of exploration. The practice of Chinese medicine includes the use of herbs, crystals, massage, and meditation to allow healing to proceed quickly but through natural means. Even the use of aromatherapy—treatment through the inhalation of specific smells—has gained a foothold in the medical world. The manipulations done by chiropractic doctors offer other possibilities. Some seek cures in nature, from sources below the sea or deep in the forest. Yet, many untapped resources remain. The continuing research in genetics offers vast possibilities, and the link between mental attitude and the immune system presents a rich area for further exploration. Even innovations as simple as a special glue, used to replace sutures or staples for closing wounds, would have an important influence on the future of the healing process.

—Maxine M. Urton, Ph.D.

See also Antibiotics; Aromatherapy; Bleeding; Blood and blood disorders; Chiropractic; Circulation; Dermatology; Grafts and grafting; Histology; Host-defense mechanisms; Immune system; Immunology; Infection; Inflammation; Laceration repair; Meditation; Skin; Surgery, general; Vascular system; Wounds.

FOR FURTHER INFORMATION:

Crosby, Lynn A., and David G. Lewallen, eds. *Emergency Care and Transportation of the Sick and Injured.* Rev. 6th ed. Rosemont, Ill.: American Academy of Orthopaedic Surgeons, 1997. One chapter deals with soft tissue injuries. Offers graphic photographs of actual injuries and discusses care and management. This text is often used in the training of emergency medical technicians, yet chapters are easily understood by nonmedical laypersons.

Eisenberg, David. *Encounters with Qi.* New York: W. W. Norton, 1995. Extensive explanations of the Chinese principles in medicine are covered, from ancient practices through current uses. Examines the uses of herbs, acupuncture, and psychic healing to restore the body's inner balance.

Gach, Michael R. *Acupressure's Potent Points: A Guide to Self-Care for Common Ailments.* New York: Bantam Books, 1990. An extensively illustrated book showing the self-use of acupressure to relieve physical problems by activating the body's natural self-healing processes.

Goldberg, Linn, and Diane L. Elliot. *The Healing Power of Exercise: Your Guide to Preventing and Treating Diabetes, Depression, Heart Disease, High Blood Pressure, Arthritis, and More.* New York: Wiley, 2000. This book explains how exercise can reduce your risk of certain diseases as well as alleviate symptoms.

Handal, Kathleen A. *The American Red Cross First Aid and Safety Handbook.* Boston: Little, Brown, 1992. A comprehensive, fully illustrated guide outlining basic first aid and emergency care steps to be taken until medical assistance can be obtained. Updated materials can also be obtained directly from local Red Cross Association chapters listed in telephone books.

Woodham, Anne, and David Peters. *The Encyclopedia of Healing Therapies.* New York: Dorling Kindersley, 1997. This book explains holistic and complementary medicine and offers a guide to well-being. Also contains information on finding practitioners, a directory of associations, a glossary, and a bibliography.

HEALTH MAINTENANCE ORGANIZATIONS (HMOs)

ORGANIZATION

DEFINITION: A business competitor within a free market economy that provides health care insurance and services to group and individual clients for an established, prepaid monthly premium and that generally attempts to provide care at a lower cost than traditional fee-for-service insurance programs by transferring financial risk to physicians through capitation and other incentives.

KEY TERMS:

disability insurance: a health coverage policy that protects against loss of income resulting from sickness or accident, whereby benefits are structured to pay approximately 40 to 60 percent of earnings up to a maximum total amount

group model HMO: an HMO organized by physicians whereby a private professional corporation is established which then individually contracts with an HMO to provide services exclusively for its subscribers

independent practice association model HMO: a flexible arrangement whereby several office physicians in a community form a networked professional corporation that seeks group contracts among local employers and provides all medical care for a capitated rate per client per month to subscribers, who often choose a personal primary care physician

managed care: the techniques by which an HMO, a health insurance carrier, or a self-insuring employer makes certain that the health care services it is endorsing are cost-effective and of a high quality

point-of-service model HMO: also called an open-ended HMO; a model that includes an option which allows subscribers to seek medical care outside the established network and receive partial reimbursement, with all remaining expenses paid out-of-pocket

preferred providers: physicians and other health care providers and hospitals who choose to provide health care at a reduced cost for subscribers to an HMO

staff model HMO: an HMO that is directly controlled at its headquarters, with all physicians and other health care workers being full-time, salaried employees

ROLE IN THE HEALTH CARE INDUSTRY

A health maintenance organization (HMO) in a free market economy functions in a dual role as both a health insurance company and a provider of health services, roles that were previously separated within the U.S. health care system. HMOs—also known as competitive medical plans, managed care plans, or alternative delivery systems—are generally organized by an employer, physician group, union, consumer group, insurance company, or for-profit health care agency. They were originally formed from one, or a mixture, of the following models: point of service, staff, group, and independent practice association.

The role of an HMO as an insurer is to seek group contracts with employers and individual clients and to negotiate premiums to be prepaid in exchange for covering preagreed benefits. Its role in service delivery is to affiliate with or hire directly physicians to provide the expected volume of care that is required for all subscribers under contract. An HMO owns or contracts with one or more health centers for ambulatory care and with hospitals for inpatient care. Within its private health center or in contracts with free-standing providers, an HMO will furnish services from other health care providers such as physical and occupational therapy, pharmacy, and mental health care, which are rapidly increasing in their level of responsibility.

HMOs are attractive to employers because the annual medical bill for the average subscriber-patient consistently has proved to be approximately 30 percent less than that of conventional insurers. One advantage of HMO membership is that all medical expenses, from routine and emergency care to hospitalization, are covered within a single, fixed monthly premium. In addition, presenting an HMO membership card at time of services with a small copayment means no forms to fill out, no deductibles to pay, and no bills to submit. Disadvantages include that new subscribers often cannot keep a trusted physician they have had for years, providers become extremely busy when they are assigned hundreds of patients in exchange for a fixed fee, and subscribers often must accept fewer choices in treatment options.

PRACTICES AND PROCEDURES

The term "managed care" describes the techniques by which an HMO, a health insurance carrier, or a self-insuring employer makes certain that the health care services that it endorses are high in quality and cost-effective. This system was once used in many countries. Workers joined a mutual aid association and paid premiums, and the association was responsible for hiring enough quality full-time or part-time physicians to provide the required services. These restrictive arrangements could not survive within a country that has a national health insurance law because every covered citizen would then have the right to choose any provider and subsequently bill the system. Managed care is only able to survive in the United States because a compulsory national health insurance law has not been enacted, as has been done in other industrialized countries.

The headquarters of an HMO competitively markets its services to employer groups and individuals and administers the revenue and payments. An HMO generally contracts or directly hires a limited number of physicians in addition to building, staffing, and equipping the necessary number of health centers and hospitals. Its marketing claim is to provide good quality care within the employer's group premium, without seeking further supplements from the employer. Because an HMO and its providers are at personal financial risk, the organization directly imposes financial discipline upon its physicians, hospitals, and other health care providers. The HMO retains a percentage of the premiums paid from employers for its administrative and facility costs and pays a monthly "capitated rate" per client to the providers. HMOs have historically had persistent difficulty in recruiting and retaining physicians, and patients have consistently informed the HMOs that they prefer private offices to health centers.

Managed care procedures generally involve the HMO establishing a network of physicians with superior reputations in each region, with these physicians agreeing to bill the carriers according to limited reimbursement rules. Each client is assigned to a "primary care gatekeeper" who is expected to provide most care in his or her private office for limited fees. When a referral to a specialist, laboratory, or hospital is necessary, authorization is required from the headquarters of the managed care organization. Hospitals contract with these organizations to limit their charges and follow established rules about economical care and prompt discharge. The managed care organization reviews utilization by physicians and hospitals, attempts to correct wasteful practices, and subsequently drops health care providers with expensive and/or poor practice styles.

In contrast to more traditional HMOs, point-of-service plans have more recently emerged. These plans enable clients to have freedom of choice with respect to providers and some treatment options but requires them personally to pay the balance for their chosen higher-priced services. If the patient goes to physicians, hospitals, and other providers within the network and follows rules about utilization and authorization, the out-of-pocket financial costs are minimal. The patient retains the option to go to an out-of-plan provider, pay the bill in full, and then be reimbursed for the limited amount established in the individual plan. The employer's group contract with the managed care organization provides for limited and predictable premiums. The considerable costs of out-of-plan services thus are shifted from the group contract to the individual patient.

Managed care plans will continue to monitor closely the treatment patterns of physicians and encourage them to prescribe cheaper medications, to develop standards that physicians are expected to follow in treatment of various diseases, and to hold utilization review panels that review patient records and decide which treatments a patient's health plan will cover and which it will not. Because of the numerous consumer complaints that arose from actions resulting from the decisions of case managers, who often do not have any medical training, nineteen states had passed comprehensive managed care laws by 1997. In the year 1997 alone, states passed a record 182 laws related to managed care, up from 100 in 1996. Legislation has and undoubtedly will continue to focus on issues such as adopting measures to ban physician gag clauses, to establish consumer grievance procedures, to require disclosure of financial incentives for physicians to withhold care, to hold external reviews of internal decisions to deny care, and to ensure the ability to sue an HMO for malpractice.

Perspective and Prospects

The first HMOs in the United States were established in the 1930's with the pioneering efforts of the Ross-Loos Medical Group in California, but most experienced only minimal growth until the 1970's. Beginning in the early 1970's, HMOs proliferated rapidly, primarily as a result of escalating costs for health care services and increasing competition among a growing number of physicians. The Health Maintenance Organizations Act of 1973 provided federal grants and loans for the establishment of HMOs and required many employers to offer HMO membership to employees as a health insurance alternative. The federal government began to promote the HMO concept as a means by which to control costs by discouraging physicians from performing unnecessary and costly procedures, to meet the increased demand for health insurance particularly in underserved areas, and to foster preventive medicine. Money incentives, which are strongly supported by numerous politicians, are in theory the major forces behind personal freedom of choice, containment of costs, and assurance of quality. Innovated by the Kaiser Foundation Health Plan in California, the Health Insurance Plan of Greater New York, and the Group Health Cooperative of Puget Sound, greater numbers of preferred provider organizations began to appear in the 1980's and 1990's as a more flexible alternative to standard HMOs. Many major health insurers such as Blue Cross and Blue Shield then began exerting control over the daily operations of both HMOs and preferred provider organizations. Managed care was spread rapidly across the United States by the large health insurance companies, largely stimulated by the ongoing difficulties experienced by national policy in containing medical costs. In 1970, there were approximately thirty different managed care plans; by 1997, this number had grown to more than fifteen hundred. In 1997, more than 80 percent of HMOs were for-profit organizations. The significance of this figure is that an increasing amount of money that could be spent on medical care is now being spent on marketing costs and stockholder dividends.

The largest looming question regarding the future of HMOs is whether physicians and other health care workers, as well as client subscribers, will continue to enroll in and thus support the system. Managed care necessarily adds substantial administrative overhead, with the ongoing question of whether the final result is greater efficiency for the entire system or simply for subscribing employers. Another controversial topic of discussion involves the responsibility of an HMO to provide disability insurance, which becomes necessary when a client incurs loss of income resulting from sickness or an accident that is not covered by workers' compensation. An organization that will exert considerable influence in future HMO developments is the American Association of Retired Persons (AARP), a large, nonprofit advocacy group for Americans over the age of fifty with more than 30 million members. It has begun giving endorsements to HMOs that meet its standards of quality and price.

In other industrialized nations, both the services covered and the extent of coverage equal or exceed the coverage of a standard HMO within the United States. Several countries have universal health care insurance coverage, although in many industrialized nations certain categories of residents may be exempt. Notable examples include Germany, which requires the purchase of private health insurance by law; Canada and Sweden, which have public insurance coverage for essentially any citizen; and Great Britain, which has a majority of medical services located within the public sector.

—Daniel G. Graetzer, Ph.D.

See also Allied health; Ethics; Law and medicine; Malpractice.

FOR FURTHER INFORMATION:

Borowsky, Steven J., Margaret K. Davis, Christine Goertz, and Nicole Lurie. "Are All Health Plans Created Equal? The Physician's View." *Journal of the American Medical Association* 278, no. 11 (1997): 917-921. This article contains physician ratings of health plan practices with respect to what promoted or impeded delivery of quality care.

Brink, Susan, and Nancy Shute. "Are HMOs the Right Prescription?" *U.S. News and World Report* 123, no. 4 (October 13, 1997): 60-65. Covered in this well-researched article is the growing dissatisfaction of subscribers with the quality of health care received with a rating of the best HMOs in the United States.

Freeborn, D. K., and C. R. Pope. *The Promise and Performance of Managed Care: The Prepaid Practice Model.* Rev. ed. Baltimore: The Johns Hopkins University Press, 1999. This excellent text highlights the evolution of several common promises of HMOs that employ the prepaid practice model and evaluates their performance based on relevant criteria.

Gold, M. "Health Maintenance Organizations: Structure, Performance, and Current Issues for Employee Health Benefits Design." *Journal of Occupational Medicine* 33, no. 3 (1991): 288-296. From an occupational medicine viewpoint, this article reviews numerous health benefit plans designed for employees of large and small companies by examining consumer satisfaction, quality of health care, and cost-benefit ratio.

Gross, P. "Managed Care: The Perfect Package." *Health Services Journal* 27 (1995): 20-23. This article evaluates what subscribing clients desire in a managed care package and their opportunities for getting it.

Johnsson, Julie. "HMOs Dominate, Shape the Market." *American Medical News* 39, no. 4 (1996): 1-3. A well-written article that outlines the competition among HMOs and how they attempt to obtain lower prices from providers as premiums continue to drop.

Lairson, D. R., et al. "Managed Care and Community-Oriented Care: Conflict or Complement?" *Journal of Health Care for the Poor and Underserved* 8, no. 1 (1997): 36-55. This informative article evaluates models for community health planning and health care reform designed for the medically indigent, including programs that receive support from the U.S. government and programs that do not.

Luft, H. *Health Maintenance Organizations: Dimensions of Performance.* New Brunswick, N.J.:

Transactions, 1987. An excellent review of the infrastructure of health maintenance organizations to the mid-1980's.

Miller, R. H., and H. S. Luft. "Managed Care Plans: Characteristics, Growth, and Premium Performance." *Annual Review of Public Health* 15 (1994): 437-459. An excellent review of managed health care plans that accurately fulfills its title.

Zelman, W. A. *The Changing Health Care Market Place.* San Francisco: Jossey-Bass, 1996. An excellent evaluation of past trends in HMOs and predictions of what the future might hold.

HEARING AIDS

PROCEDURE

ANATOMY OR SYSTEM AFFECTED: Ears, nervous system

SPECIALTIES AND RELATED FIELDS: Audiology, geriatrics and gerontology, neurology, occupational health, otorhinolaryngology

DEFINITION: Devices that enable many people who exhibit hearing loss to show dramatic improvements in their hearing capabilities.

TYPES OF HEARING LOSS

There are three general types of hearing loss, classified according to what structures of the ear may be involved. All types of hearing loss are not equally amenable to improvements with the use of hearing aids. In conductive hearing loss, changes have occurred in the outer and middle ear. Sensorineural hearing loss involves the inner ear. In the third type, damage involves both conductive and sensorineural aspects, resulting in a mixed loss. It is not unusual to find the mixed type of hearing loss among the elderly.

The causes of the different types of hearing loss are varied. In some cases of conductive damage, the loss may be caused by an infection and may be effectively treated by medication. Surgery may be recommended in those cases where the hearing loss is a result of a problem in the middle ear. In the condition known as otosclerosis, a bony growth forms at the base of the stapes and prevents the proper movement of the small, bony ossicles in the middle ear so that normal transmission of the sound wave cannot occur. Otosclerosis is the most common cause of conductive deafness in adults. The condition can usually be corrected by surgically removing the stapes and replacing it with a plastic or metal device.

Hearing aids may be of considerable benefit to most people who have sensorineural hearing loss. However, people with severe sensorineural hearing loss (commonly known as nerve deafness) who do not gain any benefit from hearing aids may use cochlear implants, which allow the auditory nerve to be directly stimulated.

Presbycusis, or age-related deafness, is the most common cause of sensorineural hearing loss among those individuals sixty-five years of age and older. By the age of sixty-five, nearly 20 percent of the population suffers from presbycusis, which results from changes in the inner ear and in the auditory nerve. The inner ear contains hair cells that are, in fact, nerve cells that respond to stimuli, including sound vibrations.

At birth, there are twenty thousand to thirty thousand hair cells in the ear; as they gradually wear out and die during the course of a lifetime, people experience a loss of their ability to hear high-pitched sounds. A person might have difficulty hearing all the words produced by some women and children. Since individuals suffering from presbycusis have trouble hearing only certain things from certain people, they may not be aware of the deterioration in hearing and may not realize that the situation might be improved through use of a hearing aid. The loss of hearing also may affect a person's ears unequally. If the imbalance is severe enough, a person may experience difficulty in localizing sound, which may lead to disorientation.

This condition tends to get progressively worse with age, and certain families are at higher risk than others. Factors that contribute to presbycusis are many, and it is difficult to determine how these factors interact with those "normal" changes that accompany aging. Without a doubt, occupational noise and other everyday noises are major contributors to presbycusis. There is wide variation in the rate of decline in hearing among individuals as they age.

TYPES OF HEARING AIDS

Hearing aids fall into four general types: those worn on the body, those that are part of an eyeglass frame, those worn behind the ear, and those worn in the ear. Some types are effective only for mild hearing loss, whereas other models may be required for more severe hearing impairments. Continued advances in technology have increased the ability of hearing aids to help improve even severe hearing loss. The different types of hearing aids are not used in equal numbers. Relatively few people use the body-worn type or the eyeglass unit. Used somewhat more frequently is the behind-the-ear aid. However, the majority of hearing-impaired people use some form of the in-the-ear type. Like any product, the useful life of a hearing aid will vary, but they should last, on the average, four to five years.

All hearing aids function in a similar manner. A battery furnishes the operational power source. The size of the battery depends on the size of the aid and the amount of power required to carry out its specific function. The life of a battery is related to the length of time the aid is used and the power needs of the hearing aid. Zinc-air batteries usually maintain performance until they go completely dead, whereas other types, such as mercury batteries, tend to weaken before they are entirely drained. Batteries may last three weeks or less, and it is prudent to always have a supply on hand.

Hearing aids work by picking up sound waves with a microphone and converting them into electrical energy. An amplifier unit controls the volume by increasing the strength of the electrical energy. The receiver then converts the electrical signal back into sound waves. One final, but critical, component of the behind-the-ear hearing aid, the body aid, and the eyeglass aid is the earmold, which connects the hearing aid to the ear. Earmolds must be fitted or molded to individual ears. Since the earmold governs the amount and quality of the sound that passes from the aid into the ear, it not only must match the physical characteristics of each ear but also must be chosen on the basis of the type of hearing loss. Once a person begins to wear a hearing aid, it is essential that hearing and the hearing aid be checked regularly. The checkup usually includes an examination of the earmold, since the shape and size of the ear may change over time. A hearing aid is an extremely sensitive instrument that must be carefully adjusted for the individual who is using it.

PERSPECTIVE AND PROSPECTS

In the United States, about 10 percent of the population have some degree of hearing loss. Hearing loss tends to worsen with aging, and, as the proportion of people living past sixty-five years of age increases, so will the percentage of those who develop hearing loss.

The magnitude of the change can be seen in the statistics of aging in the United States. In 1950, there were more than twelve million people over sixty-five years of age (8.1 percent of the population); this number (and percentage) increased dramatically during the second half of the twentieth century and is predicted to reach more than fifty million (17 percent) by the year 2020. This striking change in population structure has profound implications for the treatment of health conditions—including hearing loss—among the elderly. The causes of hearing loss are many and must be pinpointed in individual cases before any treatment can be initiated.

Although the nature and cause of an individual's hearing loss may have been determined and a proper hearing aid may have been decided upon, it does not necessarily mean that a person's hearing problem has been solved. Hearing loss is often referred to as the "invisible handicap." Many people are slow to recognize that their hearing is deteriorating, others are slow to do anything about it, and many go into a period of denial. Individuals may have problems adjusting to wearing hearing aids because they feel embarrassed or do not want to "stand out." Learning to hear with hearing aids also requires a period of adjustment. However, once a hearing-impaired person has overcome these obstacles, a return to a near-normal life, with all its personal and social benefits, follows.

—*Donald J. Nash, Ph.D.*

See also Aging; Audiology; Hearing loss; Hearing tests; Sense organs.

FOR FURTHER INFORMATION:

Carmen, Richard. *The Consumer Handbook on Hearing Loss and Hearing Aids: A Bridge to Healing.* Sedona, Ariz.: Auricle Ink, 1998. Clinical audiologist Carmen, who has been writing books on the topic of hearing loss since 1977, has gathered materials written by various audiologists that discuss hearing loss and how to manage it.

Dugan, Marcia P. *Keys to Living with Hearing Loss.* New York: Barron's Educational Service, 1997. This book is written so anyone can understand the issues associated with a hearing loss. The book would be helpful for an individual to understand his or her own social and emotional problems related to hearing loss or the problems of a loved one.

Pope, Anne. *Hear: Solutions, Skills, and Sources for People with Hearing Loss.* New York: Dorling Kindersley, 1997. Endorsed by the national organization Self Help for Hard of Hearing People, this book explains the principles of sound, how the ear works, and what can go wrong, accompanied by full-color illustrations. Valuable advice is given on choosing a hearing aid, as well as information about other assistive listening devices, and skills such as speech-reading and auditory training.

Wayner, Donna A. *Hear What You've Been Missing: How to Cope with Hearing Loss*. Minneapolis: Chronimed, 1998. Many things can be done to remedy the frustration and confusion brought on by hearing loss. In this book, audiologist Wayner takes readers step-by-step through recognition of a problem, diagnosis, possible solutions, even early prevention and protection. Those who are experiencing hearing loss themselves or suspect family members are will find this book filled with the information they need.

HEARING LOSS
DISEASE/DISORDER

ANATOMY OR SYSTEM AFFECTED: Ears, nervous system

SPECIALTIES AND RELATED FIELDS: Audiology, geriatrics and gerontology, neurology, occupational health, otorhinolaryngology

DEFINITION: Loss of sensitivity to sound pressure changes as a result of congenital factors, disease, traumatic injury, noise exposure, or aging.

KEY TERMS:

aging process: the process in which physiological, neurological, and biological changes affect behavior and function

auditory: referring to the ear and to the sense of hearing

auditory cortex: that portion of the temporal lobe in the human brain where the ascending auditory pathway terminates

auditory nerve: the cochlear branch of the eighth cranial nerve

neural hearing loss: hearing impairment caused by a loss of the neural tissue that constitutes the ascending pathway of the auditory system

ossicles: three small bones located in the middle ear that convey sound pressure changes from the tympanic membrane (eardrum) to the oval window of the cochlea; the bones are commonly referred to as the hammer (malleus), anvil (incus), and stirrup (stapes)

phonology: the study of the sounds that make up any verbal language system

sensory hearing loss: hearing impairment caused by a loss of sensory cells (nerve cells) in the cochlea

THE PHYSIOLOGY OF THE EAR

The normal, young ear is capable of detecting frequencies (tones) from as low as 20 hertz to as high as 20,000 hertz. (Hertz is the current notation for cycles per second.) Actually, in terms of frequency, humans can hear as low as 2 hertz, but about 20 hertz is required for a perception of "tonality." This is an amazing range. At the very low end of the frequency scale, one is not certain whether a tone is being "heard" or whether the sensation is a "tactile" one. (There is some neuroanatomical speculation that the organ of hearing is a very specialized tactile sensor.) At the very high end of the frequency scale, one can detect the highest strings of the violin, the rustle of leaves as they are disturbed by the wind, and the distinctive cry of birds and animals. A host of other sounds in between the lowest and highest frequencies can also be perceived. The subjective, psychological correlate of frequency is pitch. In general, the higher the frequency of a sound, the higher is the perceived pitch.

The ear performs an amazing feat in dealing with the broad range of intensities. Intensity is directly proportional to the magnitude of sound pressure change. The ear is so sensitive to small changes in sound pressure that the normal ear is capable of detecting pressure changes no greater than the diameter of a hydrogen molecule. At the other end of this continuum, the human ear can withstand great amplitude changes in sound pressure without damage. In terms of sound pressure units, the range from the weakest sound detected to the loudest sound tolerated represents a ratio of 10,000,000:1. In other words, the most intense sound pressure that is bearable is on the order of 10,000,000 times as great as the softest one that is perceptible under optimum listening conditions.

Intensity is expressed in decibels. Essentially, the higher the decibel value, the more intense or louder the sound. The ear is sensitive to a range of intensities from about 0 decibels to about 135 decibels. At the very extreme of this range, pain is experienced and permanent damage can occur if the sound intensity is prolonged. The psychological correlate of intensity is loudness. Under ideal conditions, if the intensity is increased by 9 decibels, the signal is perceived as being twice as loud.

The ability to process acoustic information correctly depends on the critical relationship between frequency and intensity. The critical frequency range needed to understand the English phonological system extends from about 300 hertz to 4,000 hertz. Theoretically, if one heard no other sounds above 4,000 hertz and below 300 hertz, one would experience no difficulty in understanding the intended message. Relative to intensity, a listener would have no difficulty in information processing if speech were presented at 65 decibels at a distance of one meter. In addition to the listener's distance from the speech source, speech understanding is also influenced by ambient background noise. For adequate processing to occur, speech must be louder than the ambient noise.

Sound is produced by a generating source such as a musical instrument, sounds of nature, or the vibrations of the human vocal cords that create a voice. The resulting series of sound pressure changes represent all the frequency and intensity characteristics generated at the source. These sound pressure changes travel through the atmosphere at a constant speed (approximately 335 meters per second at sea level). They are channeled through the external ear canal and strike the eardrum (tympanic membrane). The eardrum is sensitive to negative and positive changes in sound pressure and moves in concert with these changes. The greater the sound pressure, the greater is the magnitude of movement. Similarly, the higher the frequency, the more rapid are the movements of the eardrum. In the middle ear of the hearing system are three small bones, called ossicles. The first of these, the hammer (malleus), is attached to the eardrum. The second, the anvil (incus), is attached by ligaments to the malleus and to the third ossicle, the stirrup (stapes), which in turn attaches to the oval window membrane of the cochlea. As the eardrum is displaced in a negative or positive direction by sound pressure changes in the external ear canal, there is an absolute and corresponding movement of the ossicles.

In the cochlea, there are three anatomical divisions: the scala vestibuli, the scala tympani, and the scala media. Each of these spaces is filled with a fluid. The fluid of the scala media is chemically dif-

Anatomy of the Inner Ear

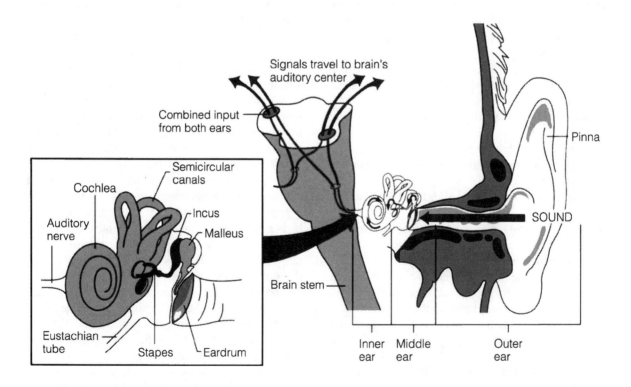

Causes of Hearing Loss

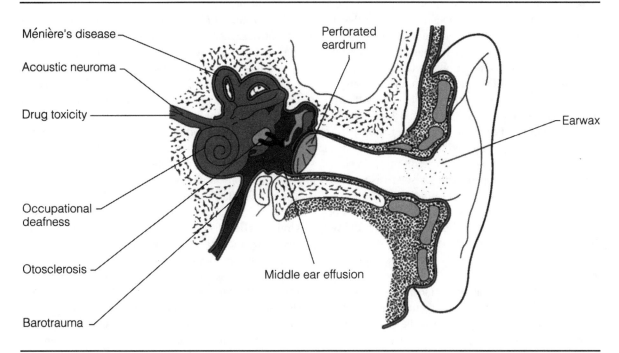

Ménière's disease

Acoustic neuroma

Drug toxicity

Occupational deafness

Otosclerosis

Barotrauma

Perforated eardrum

Earwax

Middle ear effusion

ferent from the fluid in the other two spaces. Housed in the scala media are all the specialized nervous tissues that respond to the movement of the fluid. These specialized nerve cells are situated on top of an anatomical structure called the basilar membrane. The wave forms generated within the fluid are caused by the movement of the stapes bones, as the oval window membrane communicates directly with the fluid of the cochlear space. The rate at which the stapes moves will cause the basilar membrane to be displaced at a site-specific location along its length. High-frequency sounds generate amplitude changes of the membrane at the apical portion. The movement of the membrane causes the small nerve cells (hair cells) to "fire," creating a neural discharge that travels from the cochlea to the temporal cortex of the brain. The neural events generated by sound pressure changes are interpreted by the brain.

CAUSES, SYMPTOMS, AND TREATMENTS
In the truest sense, hearing loss is any reduction in threshold sensitivity for any frequency, including those below or above the range for the normal hearing of speech. The real issue, however, is whether minor changes in sensitivity create significant problems

in understanding speech and other information-bearing acoustic signals. For example, it is known that loss of threshold sensitivity below 300 hertz and above 4,000 hertz has a minimal effect on understanding speech information. It is when hearing loss exists within this critical frequency range that an individual may experience appreciable difficulty in understanding intended messages. The question becomes, then, "What conditions may cause a permanent or temporary loss of hearing, and how is such a loss managed by medical, surgical, or rehabilitative intervention?"

Conductive Hearing Loss. Any barrier or impedance that keeps sound from reaching the cochlea of the human auditory system at its intended loudness is termed "conductive hearing loss." A very common cause of conduction loss is a buildup of earwax (cerumen) in the external ear canal. The production of earwax in the ear canal is essential. It prevents the skin of the ear canal from drying and sloughing off, and it may serve to trap minute foreign particles and keep them from causing damage to the external canal. Normally, earwax will migrate out of the ear and create no conduction problem. It is when the earwax accumulates to an amount sufficient to block sound from entering the ear that something needs to be done. In most cases, earwax can be removed by irrigation. A physician washes out the earwax using a special liquid solution that does not damage the tissue of the ear canal or the eardrum itself.

Another cause of conductive hearing loss is a hole (perforation) in the eardrum, which can be created by a number of conditions, including injury. Depending on the size and location of the hole, surgery (tympanoplasty) is often successful in restoring normal hearing function. For some persons, otosclerosis (a disease causing hardening and fixing of the three small bones in the middle-ear space) results in significant conductive hearing impairment. Otosclerosis prevents these tiny bones from moving efficiently as the eardrum moves, and hearing sensitivity is reduced. Fortunately, advances in surgical procedures have allowed the surgeon to replace the stapes bone with a suitable prosthesis, reinstating relatively normal activity of the ossicles and greatly improving hearing ability.

Congenital malformation of the pinna or the ear canal, known as atresia, is an infrequent cause of conductive hearing loss. Often, when the pinna is malformed, there is no opening into the ear canal. In some cases, the ear canal has failed to develop. Depending on the severity of the malformation, of either the pinna or the ear canal, surgery may be successful in restoring function. Other causes of conductive hearing loss include Eustachian tube malfunction, disruption of the ossicular chain (the three tiny bones in the middle ear), and swelling (edema) of the external ear canal.

A frequently occurring cause of conductive pathology is otitis media. Otitis media may refer to inflammation involving the middle-ear space or to a disorder in which the middle ear is filled with a watery fluid. In some cases, the fluid may harbor bacteria, creating significant medical problems if this condition is not treated early. Such middle-ear effusions are more common in children than in adults. If fluid is present in the middle ear, its mass will restrict the movement of the ossicles and create hearing impairment. Generally, patients with otitis media can be successfully treated through medical or surgical intervention.

It must be noted that conductive pathology does not affect the behavior of inner-ear structures; that is, the inner ear is capable of normal auditory performance. If the conductive pathology is eliminated by appropriate treatment, normal hearing will be restored. Severity of the condition may prevent the restoration of hearing, however, even if an aggressive treatment program is followed.

Sensorineural Hearing Loss. As a major classification of hearing loss, this term is somewhat misleading. Actually, there are two types of hearing loss within this classification. One is a sensory loss which involves the destruction of nerve cells (hair cells) in the cochlea. The other is a neural loss which involves neural cells in the ascending auditory pathway from the cochlea to the brain. It is possible to experience one type of loss without the other. Some examples of sensory loss include the following: loss of nerve cells resulting from traumatic injury to the cochlea, such as from whiplash, sharp blows to the head, or sudden, brief, and intense noises; loss of sensory cells from viral infections such as measles; loss of sensory cells caused by ototoxic drugs such as those in the mycin group (such as streptomycin or kanamycin); congenital problems associated with a lack of embryonic development; and exposure to loud and continuous (long-term) noise, a very common cause of hearing loss in adults. This last type of impairment is different from traumatic injury resulting from sudden, intense noise because it may take months or years for hearing loss caused by long-term noise to manifest itself. Research has also established a clear correlation between the normal aging process and sensory hearing impairment.

When sensory hearing impairment occurs, it is permanent. At the moment, there is no way of regenerating sensory tissue after the cell body has died. The only exception to this rule is found in those patients suffering from Ménière's disease. This disorder is often characterized by vertigo, dizziness, vomiting, and hearing loss. In the initial stages, however, the loss of sensitivity to sound is the result of changes in cellular physiology rather than of necrosis (death) of the nerve cells.

Examples of neural hearing loss are found among those hearing-impaired individuals with tumors, acoustic neuromas (benign tumors), cysts, and other anomalous conditions affecting the transmission of nerve impulses from the cochlea to the brain. Depending on the magnitude of the disorder, neural hearing loss has a much more devastating effect on speech understanding and signal processing than does sensory loss. As with sensory hearing impairment, neural hearing loss is a rather frequent occurrence associated with the aging process. For a sizable portion of those who experience hearing impairment, components of both sensory and neural loss are present. If the cause of the hearing deficit is entirely neural in nature, then the impairment is referred to as a retrocochlear loss.

For some types of neural pathology, medical or surgical intervention can be undertaken successfully. Acoustic neuromas are often removed after they have been confirmed by audiologic, otologic, radiologic, and other diagnostic modalities. The size and location of the neuroma or tumorous growth will often dictate whether hearing can be preserved following surgery.

For those millions suffering from hearing impairment, it is the loss of speech discrimination ability that is of greatest concern. Thousands of studies have been undertaken to investigate the correlation between the magnitude, type, and length of hearing loss and the degree of speech recognition difficulty. One of the essential findings of these studies indicates that, in general, hearing loss is more pronounced for the high frequencies (above 1,000 hertz), whether the loss is caused by disease, drugs, noise, or the aging process. Another major finding is that one's ability to identify vowel and consonant information is frequency-dependent. Vowel identification is dependent on frequencies from about 200 hertz to 1,000 hertz, while consonant identification is dependent on frequencies above 1,000 hertz. A listener understands about 68 percent of speech sounds if nothing above 1,500 hertz is heard and about 68 percent of speech if nothing below 1,500 hertz is heard.

PERSPECTIVE AND PROSPECTS

Hearing loss is quite common and affects some twenty million Americans, ranging from infants to the elderly. The primary reason for preserving hearing is to maintain social adequacy in communication skills. Hearing conservation programs have been instituted by public and private schools, industry, military installations, construction organizations, and more recently, the U.S. government. In 1970, the Occupational Safety and Health Act (OSHA) was passed, making it mandatory for employers to provide safe work areas for workers exposed to noise levels exceeding government standards.

For the hearing impaired, understanding of speech is related to the degree of loss and the type of impairment. Because medical or surgical care cannot always ameliorate the loss, rehabilitation programs may take the form of speech or lipreading to improve communication skills. These rehabilitative programs constituted the treatment of choice until the introduction of wearable electric hearing aids.

Before the advent of electric hearing aids, however, the early ear trumpets were very effective for

In the News: The Vibrant Soundbridge

A September 24, 2000, news story entitled "The Vibrant Soundbridge Provides an Effective Alternative to Hearing Aids," by Kenneth Satterfield, reported that the Vibrant Soundbridge, an implanted device designed to treat moderate-to-severe sensorineural hearing loss (that caused by damage to hair cells or nerves in the inner ear), has received Food and Drug Administration (FDA) approval. The release summarizes the findings of a study involving twenty-nine people who desired an alternative to their hearing aids and had healthy middle ears. Researchers concluded that, relative to hearing aids, all patients preferred the implant and were satisfied with functional hearing and sound quality improvement, and 70 percent claimed improvement with regard to background noise.

An Associated Press release of September 1, 2000, "FDA Approves Implanted Hearing Device,"

by Lauran Neergaard, reported that the FDA, based on a study of eighty-one patients, said that overall hearing gain with the Vibrant Soundbridge was the same as that with an amplifying hearing aid, calling the new device "equally effective but not superior." The device requires the surgical implantation of both a receiver behind the ear and an electromagnet in the middle ear (to vibrate the middle ear bones) and the external placement of a microprocessor containing a battery and microphone behind the ear. Dr. Thomas Balkans, who assisted with the clinical studies, while cautioning against surgery that he deemed unnecessary for most hearing aid users, stated that the 10 percent of patients who have sound clarity and other problems with hearing aids will benefit from these implants.

—*Jack Carter, Ph.D.*

some in restoring speech recognition ability. Through ingenious design, some of the ear trumpets were "acoustically tuned" to provide more amplification in the higher frequencies than in the lower, but the volume of sound was determined by the person talking—often a major problem for the hearing impaired.

With the development of the vacuum tube in the early part of the twentieth century, electric hearing aids became the treatment of choice when medical or surgical intervention was not indicated in resolving the hearing loss. It was possible not only to control the loudness of the hearing aid sound (volume) but also to shape the frequency response of the instrument to match the acoustic needs of the patient. In the second half of the twentieth century, there were significant advances in hearing aid technology. Transistor technology makes it possible to reduce the size of the hearing aid device without sacrificing performance. Computer science has also been used in the design of hearing aids. With digital technology, it is now possible to program electroacoustic characteristics into the hearing aid, which extends its utility.

Recently, major emphasis has been given to hearing conservation. Such continuing efforts have been instrumental in conserving the hearing of tens of thousands who might otherwise suffer from hearing losses sufficient to create problems in speech understanding. Although such programs are too late for millions of hearing-impaired individuals, advances in rehabilitative practices and the scientific application and use of hearing aids have provided them with a quality of life that was not possible only a generation ago.

—*Robert Sandlin, Ph.D.*

See also Aging; Audiology; Ear infections and disorders; Ear surgery; Ears; Hearing aids; Hearing tests; Ménière's disease; Nasopharyngeal disorders; Neuralgia, neuritis, and neuropathy; Otorhinolaryngology; Sense organs; Speech disorders.

FOR FURTHER INFORMATION:

Gerber, Sanford. *Introductory Hearing Science*. Philadelphia: W. B. Saunders, 1974. Somewhat more than a basic text, but one that clearly outlines the various aspects of hearing science, from the measurement of sound and hearing to the use and description of hearing aid devices for the acoustically impaired.

Pascoe, David. *Hearing Aids: Who Needs Them?* St. Louis: Big Bend Books, 1991. This easy-to-read text presents an abundance of data relative to hearing, hearing aid devices, and their use. Answers many questions that may arise concerning hearing aid use in direct and simple terms. One of the most significant aspects of this book is that it explains, in reasonable detail, how to use and evaluate hearing aids.

Yost, William. *Fundamentals of Hearing*. 4th ed. San Diego, Calif.: Academic Press, 2000. This text describes, in easy-to-understand terms, the organ of hearing and its contribution to an individual's behavior. Simple auditory theory is examined, as is the nature of the ear's response to acoustic energy.

HEARING TESTS

PROCEDURE

ANATOMY OR SYSTEM AFFECTED: Ears, nervous system

SPECIALTIES AND RELATED FIELDS: Audiology, neurology, otorhinolaryngology, speech pathology

DEFINITION: Evaluation techniques for determining the type and severity of hearing loss in children.

KEY TERMS:

auditory brainstem response: measurement of the nervous discharge produced by the central auditory system as a response to sound stimulation; also known as brainstem auditory evoked response (BAER) or auditory brainstem potentials (ABR)

auditory nerve: the nerve that conducts sound stimuli to the brain for interpretation

behavioral audiometry: a technique that the audiologist employs to evaluate hearing in infants, toddlers, or uncooperative patients (both children and adults) with developmental deficits

cochlea: the organ localized in the inner portion of the auditory system that detects sound

mastoid: referring to the bone behind the ear

middle ear: the part of the auditory system, consisting of the ossicular chain and the auditory tube, that serves as a conductor of and transducer of sound

otoacoustic emissions: sound produced in the middle ear as a response to the vibration produced by the cochlea when it is stimulated by external sounds

INDICATIONS AND PROCEDURES

Hearing tests are done to establish the presence, type, and severity of hearing impairment in children and adults. Such tests are conducted by an audiologist, although screening tests can also be done by a technician under the supervision of an audiologist. The severity of hearing loss is classified as mild, moderate, moderately severe, severe, and profound. It is also classified according to the anatomic region affected: conductive, sensorineural, or mixed hearing loss.

The selection of tests to evaluate hearing will depend on the patient's age and ability to follow directions and the ability of the audiologist to elicit responses from the patient. When a patient cannot follow instructions such as lifting a hand or pressing a button, a test that does not require the patient's cooperation is used. Two tests that do not require the patient's cooperation are the auditory brainstem potential (ABR) test and the evoked otoacoustic emissions (EOAE) test. Both tests require only that the patient be quiet. For this purpose, the patient may need sedation if normal sleep cannot be induced.

The ABR test requires the placement of four electrodes in the child's head: in both mastoid regions and in the mid forehead and upper center of the head. A stimulus is sent through a small microphone placed in the patient's external ear canal or via headphones. The instrument records the average of the electrical discharges generated by the auditory nerve in response to sound stimuli and produces a tracing of waves that correspond to the different electrical potentials generated in response to the stimuli. Analysis of the waves can determine the presence of hearing loss and measure its severity. The ABR test may be used for screening, to determine whether the subject can hear, or for the clinical evaluation of hearing loss. It can be done at any age. An automated method of ABR testing is available for screening newborn infants for hearing loss; it automatically determines if the patient has passed or failed. The clinical ABR test requires specially trained personnel and takes from forty-five to fifty minutes to perform. The automated method can be applied by a technician.

The EOAE test involves recording the sound produced by hair cells within the cochlea by way of a microphone placed in the outer ear canal. Normally when sound enters the cochlea, the hair cells produce a sound that bounces backward and can be recorded. This sound correlates with the sound sent to the auditory nerve. If there is damage to the hair cells in the cochlea, then no sound is elicited. The EOAE test can be performed without sedation if the patient cooperates by staying quiet. It can be done by a technician and takes approximately ten minutes or less. The EOAE test is used for universal screening of newborn infants. It can be done at all ages to help determine the integrity of the cochlea and thus whether an observed hearing defect is within the cochlea.

Behavioral techniques are the most practical, cost-effective, and time-efficient methods for the accurate assessment of hearing. They give more complete information on the child's hearing as well as functional information about how the child uses his or her hearing. The most simple test is behavioral observation audiometry, in which the audiologist records the behavioral response to an applied sound stimuli of a known frequency. This test can be done with infants up to six months of age, toddlers, and uncooperative patients, such as children or adults with developmental delays. Visual reinforcement audiometry is done with infants and toddlers from six months to twenty-four months of age. It is also used with uncooperative patients. In this test, the patient is submitted to sounds of different intensity and trained to respond to the sound stimuli by means of an attractive stimuli. Every time that the sound appears, the stimuli illuminates. When the patient hears the sound, he or she will look for the reinforcement. Play audiometry is a test that can be used in children over two years of age. The child is taught to move a block or place a puzzle piece every time he or she hears a sound.

PERSPECTIVE AND PROSPECTS

Early detection of hearing loss has become a priority among intervention services because it has devastating effects on language development and consequently on social adaptation. It has been found that the mean age at which deafness is diagnosed is around three, which is after speech development should have occurred. Thus, children with hearing loss are placed at a disadvantage with their peers.

In 1993, the National Institutes of Health (NIH) developed a consensus statement by which all newborn infants in the United States were to be screened for hearing loss. The aim was that by the year 2000, all newborns would have been screened before being discharged from the hospital.

The role of otitis media (middle-ear infections) in producing hearing impairment is an area of great concern and controversy. Special attention to the hearing evaluation of children with recurrent and chronic otitis media is indicated.

—Gloria Reyes Báez, M.D.,
and Hilda Velez Rodriguez, M.S.

See also Ear infections and disorders; Ears; Hearing loss; Neonatology; Physical examination; Screening; Sense organs.

FOR FURTHER INFORMATION:

Elder, Nina. "Now Hear This–Check Your Baby's Hearing." *Better Homes and Gardens* 78, no. 5 (May, 2000): 264. One out of every three hundred U.S. babies is born with a hearing problem, yet only 25 percent of newborns get hearing tests. If a hearing problem is detected within the first six months of life, a child has a good chance of catching up with his or her peers.

Glaser, Gabrielle. "Pediatricians Urge Hearing Tests at Birth." *The New York Times*, April 6, 1999, p. 7. Hearing impairment in infants can cause delays in speech, language, and cognitive development, according to Dr. Philip Ziring. Often, hearing loss is not diagnosed in children until they are two or three years old and are not speaking properly.

Hall, James A. *Handbook of Auditory Evoked Response.* Boston: Allyn & Bacon, 1992. An exhaustive study of auditory evoked response aimed at the medical professional. Includes bibliographical references and an index.

McCormick, Barry, ed. *The Medical Practitioner's Guide to Paediatric Audiology.* Cambridge, Mass.: Cambridge University Press, 1995. A handbook of hearing disorders in infancy and childhood. Includes discussion of the various hearing tests and aids available.

Northern, Jerry L., and Marion P. Downs. *Hearing in Children.* 4th ed. Baltimore: Williams & Wilkins, 1991. Topics covered include hearing and hearing loss, auditory mechanics, medical aspects of hearing loss, deviation of auditory behavior, and amplification.

HEART

ANATOMY

ANATOMY OR SYSTEM AFFECTED: Blood, blood vessels, chest, circulatory system

SPECIALTIES AND RELATED FIELDS: Cardiology, exercise physiology

DEFINITION: The muscle that pumps blood through the body by means of rhythmic contractions.

KEY TERMS:

arteries: vessels that take blood away from the heart and toward the tissues

atria: the upper receiving chambers of the heart that lie above the ventricles

atrioventricular (A-V) node: a small region of specialized heart muscle cells that receives the electrical impulse from the atria and begins its transmission to the ventricles

coronary arteries: the arteries that supply blood to the heart muscle

diastole: the period of relaxation of the heart between beats

sinoatrial (S-A) node: a small region of specialized heart muscle cells that spontaneously generates and sends an electrical signal which gives the heart an automatic rhythm for contraction

systole: the period of contraction of the heart when blood moves out of the heart chambers and into the arteries

veins: vessels that take blood to the heart and from the tissues

ventricles: the lower pumping chambers of the heart located below the atria; they force blood into the arteries

STRUCTURE AND FUNCTIONS

All the cells in the human body are dependent on the blood in the cardiovascular system (the heart and blood vessels) for the transport of gases, nutrients, hormones, and other factors. Likewise, the tissues must have a way to dispose of waste products so that they do not build to harmful levels. All these substances are dissolved in the blood, but something must provide the force to transport the blood to all parts of the body at all times—the heart. This organ must beat continuously from early in development to death. It beats without conscious control and can vary how quickly it moves blood throughout the body depending on the needs and activities of the tissues.

In humans, an individual's heart is about the size of his or her fist and is enclosed in the center of the chest cavity between the lungs. The heart contains specialized muscle cells known as cardiac muscle. These cardiac cells make up most of the thickness of the walls of the heart; they are responsible for moving blood out of the heart and are also involved in maintaining the rhythm of the heartbeat. This heavily muscled layer is referred to as the myocardium. The inner lining of the heart is called the endocardium; it is continuous with the lining of all the blood vessels in the body. The outermost layer of the heart is the epicardium, which covers the myocardium. The heart

The Flow of Blood Through the Heart

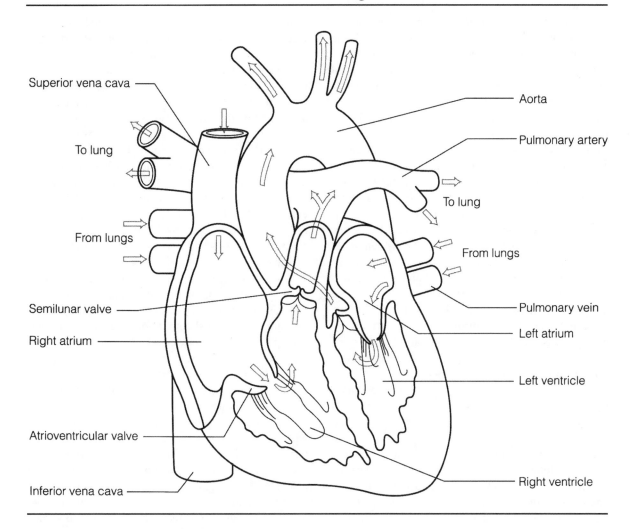

moves as it beats and is contained within a fluid-filled bag called the pericardial sac. The rhythmically beating heart has the potential to rub against adjacent structures (such as the lungs), harming itself and those structures. Therefore, it is important that the heart be encased in the pericardial sac, with its lubricating fluid.

The human heart has four separate chambers. These internal cavities can be identified by their location and function. The upper pair of smaller chambers are known as atria, and the lower larger chambers are called ventricles. Because the atria and ventricles have a muscular wall which separates them into right and left halves, one can refer to the individual chambers as the right atrium and left atrium, and

the right ventricle and left ventricle. The wall that separates the right and left halves of the heart is called the septum. The septum prevents any mixing of blood from the right and left sides of the heart. The atria and ventricles on the same side, however, must allow blood to pass between them in a single direction. This action is accomplished by one-way valves between the atria and ventricles. The valve that allows blood to pass from the right atrium to the right ventricle is called the tricuspid valve because it is made of three flaps. On the left side of the heart is the bicuspid valve (with two flaps), which is also known as the mitral valve. The bicuspid valve allows blood from the left atrium to flow only into the left ventricle. This rather complex anatomy is necessary because the heart must pump blood in one direction and into two separate systems.

The anatomy of the heart often makes more sense if one understands its function or physiology. As an example, one may consider an active cell in the body, perhaps a muscle cell which moves the foot. This cell utilizes oxygen to help metabolize food for energy. During this process, carbon dioxide is produced as a waste product, and high levels of carbon dioxide can be harmful to cells. Therefore, one of the jobs of the cardiovascular system is to deliver oxygen and take away carbon dioxide. Once the carbon dioxide is picked up by the blood, it travels back to the heart via veins and enters the right atrium. From the right atrium, the blood passes the tricuspid valve and enters the right ventricle. The right ventricle then sends the blood past a one-way valve called the semilunar valve into blood vessels that transport it to the lungs. At the lungs, the blood loses carbon dioxide and picks up oxygen. This oxygenated blood must now be delivered to the tissues. First, the blood returns to the heart and enters the left atrium. From the left atrium, blood is pushed past the bicuspid valve into the left ventricle. The blood is then pumped from the powerful left ventricle through another set of semilunar valves into the blood vessels that will carry the blood to all the tissues of the body, including the heart itself. The blood vessels that feed the heart directly are known as coronary vessels.

The orderly pattern by which blood flows through the heart, lungs, and body requires the chambers of the heart to work in a coordinated fashion. The atria contract together to help send blood into the ventricles. The ventricles then contract together so that blood flows through the lungs from the right ventricle and through the tissues of the body from the left ventricle. The tricuspid and bicuspid valves prevent a backflow of blood into the atria when the ventricles contract, and the semilunar valves prevent blood from returning to the ventricles after they have contracted.

Something must coordinate the contraction of the heart so that the atria contract together before the ventricles do so. Highly specialized cells of the myocardium have the ability to conduct electrical impulses rapidly and to discharge spontaneously at a certain rate. These properties allow the heart to be stimulated in a synchronous way and for it to generate its own rate and rhythm. One region of the right atrium is known as the sinoatrial (S-A) node; it functions as the heart's pacemaker. The S-A node has the ability to generate spontaneously an electrical signal with a relatively rapid rhythm. Therefore, it serves to "pace" the heart rate. When the S-A node sends its electrical impulse throughout the atria, the atria contract. There is a slight delay before the impulse reaches the ventricles, which allows the atria to contract fully before the ventricles. The atrioventricular (A-V) node will then pick up the electrical signal and send it through both ventricles via specialized conductive heart muscle fibers known as Purkinje's fibers. Purkinje's fibers transmit the electrical signal ensuring that all the ventricular muscle cells contract at nearly the same time. The ventricles contract in such a way that the bottom tip of the heart (apex) contracts slightly before the region of the ventricles next to the atria (base). Additionally, the ventricles contract in a somewhat twisting motion that causes the heart to "wring out" the blood.

This rather complex system allows the heart to contract at its own rate and in a highly synchronous fashion. Nevertheless, one's heart rate varies depending on one's physical activity or emotional state. For example, during exercise or when an individual is under stress, the heart rate goes up. When one is relaxed, the heart does not beat as rapidly. Therefore, the body must have a way to regulate the rate at which the S-A node signals the heart to contract.

The autonomic nervous system, which functions without one's conscious control, regulates the heart rate. It is divided into two systems: parasympathetic and sympathetic. The parasympathetic nervous system is active during periods of rest and has the ability to slow the heart. During periods of physical or emotional stress, the sympathetic nervous system stimulates the heart to contract more forcefully and at a more rapid rate. The parasympathetic and sympathetic systems communicate with the heart via chemical messengers known as neurotransmitters. The parasympathetic nervous system uses the neurotransmitter acetylcholine to slow the heart, while norepinephrine and epinephrine are the chemicals used by the sympathetic nervous system to increase the heart rate.

DISORDERS AND DISEASES

Even though the heart seems to be adaptable to a variety of situations throughout one's life, it can malfunction. In fact, diseases of the heart and blood vessels are the number one killer in the United States. One common disease that affects the heart directly is coronary artery disease, which can lead to life-threatening heart attacks. Although medical researchers are still investigating the causes of coronary artery disease, most of the evidence points to hypertension (high blood pressure) and atherosclerosis (a buildup of fatty plaque in the walls of arteries).

Hypertension is usually defined as a blood pressure greater than 140/90 millimeters of mercury (mmHg) at rest. A typical blood pressure for a young, healthy adult is 120/80 mmHg. The top number measures the force of blood against an artery wall during the contraction of the heart; this is referred to as the systolic pressure. The bottom number, the diastolic pressure, is a measurement of force when the heart is relaxed. If either systolic or diastolic pressures exceed 140/90 mmHg, the patient is considered hypertensive. The cause of hypertension has not been determined, but it is known that with hypertension the heart must work harder to push the blood through the arteries, including the coronary arteries. Physicians treat hypertension by prescribing drugs that block the effect of the sympathetic nervous system on the heart, such as metoprolol (Lopressor). They may also prescribe drugs such as prazosin (Minipress) that prevent the arteries from becoming too narrow.

Hypertension is also seen in patients who have atherosclerosis. This buildup of fatty materials such as cholesterol under the lining of the artery causes the plaque to protrude, narrowing the diameter of the vessel. This can lead to blood clot formation on artery walls which are irregular. This clot, also known as a thrombus, may dislodge and travel in the bloodstream. Eventually, it may block a small artery, thereby preventing the flow of blood to the tissue. If this happens in a coronary artery, a myocardial infarction (heart attack) will result.

A heart attack occurs when a portion of the heart dies because of a lack of oxygen or a buildup of waste products. Heart muscle has no way of repairing itself, and the resulting damage is permanent. If the patient is transported to the hospital immediately, the emergency room physician may give drugs to prevent further blood clot formation (aspirin and heparin) and to help dissolve the already formed clot (streptokinase and tissue plasminogen activator, or TPA). If the coronary artery is only partially blocked, the patient may suffer from angina pectoris, a chest pain which radiates down the left arm. These patients usually take drugs such as nitroglycerin which help dilate (widen) blood vessels, reestablishing adequate flow to the heart.

Another devastating disease of the heart is congestive heart failure, a condition in which the heart fails to pump enough blood to meet the demands of the body's tissues. The heart becomes enlarged because of the resulting excessive increase in blood volume. There are several causes of heart failure, most of which stem from the fact that the heart loses its ability to pump efficiently. For example, a patient who has had a heart attack may have lost significant function as a result of heart damage. Even without a heart attack, some individuals may have malfunctioning heart valves or other problems that cause an inefficient ejection of blood and thus heart failure.

The cardiovascular system attempts to compensate for heart failure in several ways. The sympathetic nervous system increases the heart rate, and the kidneys retain more fluid to increase blood volume. These compensatory mechanisms help to reestablish adequate blood flow for a while. Because of the increase in blood volume, however, more blood enters the chambers of the heart and causes them to stretch. At some point, the ventricles can no longer force out the increased amount of blood entering them, and they enlarge. This increase in the size of the heart chamber further enlarges the heart and strains the heart muscle. The heart will continue to weaken, unable to keep up with the body's demands. Compensatory mechanisms attempt to meet the body's need for continuous blood flow but in doing so further overload the heart. This vicious circle may lead to complete heart failure and death.

Congestive heart failure may involve only one side of the heart, perhaps because of a heart attack which affected that side. If the heart failure occurs on the left side, the right ventricle is pumping blood to the lungs in an efficient manner but the left ventricle cannot pump all the blood returning from the lungs. Therefore, blood backs up and pools in the lung tissues. Similarly, if the right ventricle begins to fail and the left ventricle is normal, blood begins to pool throughout the body since the right side of the heart cannot keep up in its pumping.

Physicians are able to slow the progression of congestive heart failure by prescribing drugs such as digoxin that increase the force of heart muscle contraction and thereby the amount of blood ejected with each beat. Therapeutic agents such as captopril (Capoten) help to reduce the fluid retention in the kidneys.

Coronary artery disease and heart failure are related to the inability of the heart to contract. In addition, the specialized heart muscle cells that provide the heart's rhythm and conduct the electrical signals necessary for a coordinated heartbeat may be affected by disease. In the resting adult, the heart normally beats about seventy to eighty times per minute. Several conditions exist whereby the heart loses control of its normal rate and rhythm, a serious condition.

For example, if the heart begins to beat too rapidly, the ventricles do not have enough time to fill and the movement of blood to the heart muscle and the rest of the body is impaired. The atria or ventricles may contract at a high rate and lose their coordinated sequence of contraction; this is referred to as atrial or ventricular fibrillation. If immediate action is not taken to reestablish the normal rate and conduction sequence, the patient will die. Emergency measures such as electrical defibrillation may shock the heart into reestablishing its normal rhythm and conduction pathways. It is easy to understand how these abnormal patterns of heart activity occur if one imagines more than one pacemaker attempting to control heart function. The cause of these and other, less severe heart rhythms may be heart damage affecting the conductive pathway, drugs, or even psychological distress.

Heart disease is a major cause of death, but most experts agree that many heart problems are preventable. High blood pressure and high blood levels of fat and cholesterol are associated with an increased incidence of coronary artery disease. Cigarette smoking and excessive weight are also correlated with heart disease. Additionally, exercise seems to be critical in maintaining a healthy heart, as sedentary individuals have a twofold increase in their risk of heart disease when compared to active people.

It is likely that individuals who are at risk can lessen the probability of having heart problems by adopting a more healthful lifestyle, including eating a low-fat diet, stopping smoking, reducing excessive weight and mental stress, and engaging in enjoyable physical activities (with their physicians' permission).

PERSPECTIVE AND PROSPECTS

The role of the heart in the functioning of the human body was questioned by the ancient Egyptians, who attributed breathing to the heart. It was the Chinese who first documented that the heart is responsible for the pulse and movement of blood. They also believed that the heart was the seat of happiness. The ancient Greeks had a different idea about the function of the heart, believing that it was the region where thinking originated.

It was not until William Harvey (1578-1657), an English physiologist, published his experiments on the heart and circulation that scientists believed blood was pumped continuously by the heart. He observed that both ventricles of the heart contracted and expanded at the same time. Harvey also noted that when the heart was removed from an animal, it continued to contract and relax; that is, it had an automatic rhythm.

More than one hundred years after Harvey published his work, Stephen Hales made the first blood pressure measurements. He did so by inserting a tube into the neck artery of a horse and watching the blood rise 3 meters above the animal. Then early in the twentieth century Willem Einthoven invented an instrument to measure electrical currents. This instrument was used by Thomas Lewis to measure the electrical activity in the heart, the first electrocardiograph (ECG).

By the mid-nineteenth century, heart surgeries were being performed to correct heart defects. These early surgeries had to be done with the heart still beating. In 1953, the heart-lung machine was used to take over the pumping function of the heart during surgery so that the surgeon could stop the heart. In 1967, Christiaan Barnard performed the first heart transplantation in a human. Heart transplants were performed during the next ten years with no long-term survivors, usually because of tissue rejection. In 1982, a completely artificial heart was implanted into a patient. This patient died in the spring of 1983.

Heart transplants have become much more successful, however, mainly because of the use of immunosuppressive drugs which help to prevent rejection of the transplanted heart. Similarly, newer drugs and procedures such as coronary bypass surgery, angioplasty, and atherectomy are becoming more effective in treating heart disease. Nevertheless, perhaps the best approach to maintaining a healthy heart is to practice preventive medicine. Scientists are making comparable strides in finding ways to prevent heart disease as they are in treating already existing conditions.

—*Matthew Berria, Ph.D.*

See also Anatomy; Aneurysmectomy; Aneurysms; Angina; Angiography; Angioplasty; Anxiety; Arrhythmias; Arteriosclerosis; Biofeedback; Blue baby syndrome; Bypass surgery; Cardiac rehabilitation; Cardiology; Cardiology, pediatric; Catheterization; Circulation; Congenital heart disease; Electrical shock; Electrocardiography (ECG or EKG); Embolism; Endocarditis; Exercise physiology; Heart attack; Heart disease; Heart failure; Heart transplantation; Heart valve replacement; Hypertension; Internal medicine; Mitral valve prolapse; Pacemaker implantation; Palpitations; Resuscitation; Reye's syndrome; Rheumatic fever; Shock; Sports medicine; Strokes; Systems and organs; Thoracic surgery; Thrombolytic therapy and TPA; Thrombosis and thrombus; Transplantation; Vascular medicine; Vascular system.

FOR FURTHER INFORMATION:

Fox, Stuart I. *Perspectives on Human Biology*. Dubuque, Iowa: Wm. C. Brown, 1991. Chapter 12 of this book provides the nonscientist with a basic understanding of the heart and a few brief descriptions of common heart problems. Presents the material in an easy-to-understand way.

Hales, Dianne. *An Invitation to Health*. 9th ed. Belmont, Calif.: Wadsworth Thomson Learning, 1992. This text should be read by anyone who wishes an overview of health topics. Several chapters deal with the function of the heart and how lifestyle influences its health.

The Incredible Machine. Washington, D.C.: National Geographic Society, 1994. A colorful book which describes in layperson's terms how the body works and how one alters one's own health. The chapter on the cardiovascular system is well written and contains exciting photographs and drawings of the heart.

McGoon, M. *The Mayo Clinic Heart Book*. New York: William Morrow, 1993. One of the most respected texts for laypeople on heart disease. Covers all aspects of anatomy, physiology, diagnosis, treatment, and prevention.

Mackenna, B. R., and R. Callander. *Illustrated Physiology*. 5th ed. New York: Churchill Livingstone, 1990. Provides the reader with a visual explanation of physiology on a basic level. Chapter 5 contains many excellent diagrams, illustrations, and explanations of cardiovascular anatomy and physiology.

HEART ATTACK

DISEASE/DISORDER

ANATOMY OR SYSTEM AFFECTED: Circulatory system, heart

SPECIALTIES AND RELATED FIELDS: Cardiology, critical care, emergency medicine, internal medicine

DEFINITION: Myocardial infarction; the sudden death of heart muscle characterized by intense chest pain, sweating, shortness of breath, or sometimes none of these symptoms.

KEY TERMS:

atherosclerosis: narrowing of the internal passageways of essential arteries caused by the buildup of fatty deposits

atria: the chambers in the right and left top portions of the heart that receive blood from the veins and pump it to the ventricles

fibrillation: wild beating of the heart, which may occur when the regular rate of the heartbeat is interrupted

myocardium: the muscle tissue that forms the walls of the heart, varying in thickness in the upper and lower regions

sinoatrial node: the section of the right atrium that determines the appropriate rate of the heartbeat

ventricles: the chambers in the right and left bottom portions of the heart that receive blood from the atria and pump it to the arteries

CAUSES AND SYMPTOMS

Although varied in origin and effect on the body, heart attacks (or myocardial infarctions) occur when there are interruptions in the delicately synchronized system either supplying blood to the heart or pumping blood from the heart to other vital organs. The heart is a highly specialized muscle whose function is to pump life-sustaining blood to all parts of the body. The heart's action involves the development of pressure to propel blood through arriving and departing channels—veins and arteries—that must maintain that pressure within their walls at critical levels throughout the system.

The highest level of pressure in the total cardiovascular system is to be found closest to the two "pumping" chambers on the right and left lower sections of the heart, called ventricles. Dark, bluish-colored blood, emptied of its oxygen content and laden with carbon dioxide waste instead of the oxygen in fresh blood, flows into the upper portion of the heart via the superior and inferior venae cavae. It then passes from the right atrium chamber into the right ventricle. Once in the ventricle, this blood cannot flow back because of one-way valves separating the "receiving" from the "pumping" sections of the total heart organ.

After this valve closes following a vitally synchronized timing system, constriction of the right ventricle by the myocardium muscle in the surrounding walls of the heart forces the blood from the heart, propelling it toward the oxygen-filled tissue of the lungs. Following reoxygenation, bright red blood that is still under pressure from the thrust of the right ventricle flows into the left atrium. Once channeled into the left ventricle, the pumping process that began in the right ventricle is then repeated on the left by muscular constriction, and oxygenated blood flows out of the aortic valve under pressure throughout the cardiovascular system to nourish the body's cells. Because the force needed to supply blood under pressure from the left ventricle for the entire body is greater than the first-phase pumping force needed to move blood into the lungs, the myocardium surrounding the left ventricle constitutes the thickest muscular layer in the heart's wall.

Pain Associated with Heart Attack

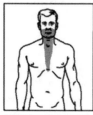

Pain radiating up into jaw and through to back.

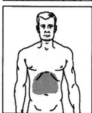

Pain felt in upper abdomen.

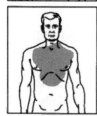

Pressure in the central chest area from mild to severe.

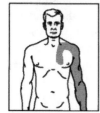

Pain radiating down left arm; may cause sensation of weakness in the arm.

The efficiency of this process, as well as the origins of problems of fatigue in the heart that can lead to heart attacks and eventual heart failure, is tied to the maintenance of a reasonably constant level of blood pressure. If pulmonary problems (blockage caused by the effects of smoking or environmental pollution, for example) make it harder for the right ventricle to push blood through the lungs, the heart must expend more energy in the first stage of the cardiovascular process. Similarly, and often in addition to the added work for the heart because of pulmonary complications, the efficiency of the left ventricle in handling blood flow may be reduced by the presence of excessive fat in the body, causing this ventricle to expend more energy to propel oxygenated blood into vital tissues.

Although factors such as these may be responsible for overworking the heart and thus contributing to eventual heart failure, other causes of heart attacks are to be found much closer to the working apparatus of the heart, particularly in the coronary arteries. The coronary arteries begin at the top of the heart and fan out along its sides. They are responsible for providing large quantities of blood to the myocardium muscle, which needs continual nourishment to carry out the pumping that forces blood forward from the ventricles. The passageways inside these and other key arteries are vulnerable to the process known as atherosclerosis, which can affect the blood supply to other organs as well as to the heart. In the heart, atherosclerosis involves the accumulation, inside the coronary arteries, of fatty deposits called atheromas. If these deposits continue to collect, less blood can flow through the arteries. A narrowed artery also increases the possibility of a variant form of heart attack, in which a sudden and total blockage of blood flow follows the lodging of a blood clot in one of these vital passageways.

A symptomatic condition called angina pectoris, characterized by intermittent chest pains, may develop if atherosclerosis reduces blood (and therefore oxygen) supply to the heart. These danger signs can continue over a number of years. If diagnosis reveals a problem that might be resolved by preventive medication, exercise, or recommendations for heart surgery, then this condition, known as myocardial ischemia, may not necessarily end in a full heart attack.

A full heart attack occurs when, for one of several possible reasons including a vascular spasm suddenly constricting an already clogged artery or a blockage caused by a clot, the heart suddenly ceases to receive the necessary supply of blood. This brings almost immediate deterioration in some of the heart's tissue and causes the organ's consequent inability to perform its vital functions effectively.

Another form of attack and disruption of the heart's ability to deliver blood can come either independently of or in conjunction with an arterially induced heart attack. This form of attack involves a sustained interruption in the rate of heartbeats. The necessary pace or rate of myocardial contractions, which can vary depending on the organism's rate of physical exertion or age, is regulated in the sinoatrial node in the right atrium, which generates its own electrical impulses. The ultimate sources for the commands to the sinoatrial node are to be found in the network of nerves coming directly from the brain. There are, however, other so-called local pacemakers located in the atria and ventricles. If these sources of electrical charges begin giving commands to the myocardium that are not in rhythm with those coming from the sinoatrial node, then dysrhythmic or premature beats may confuse the heart muscle, causing it to beat wildly. In fact, the concentrated pattern of muscle contractions will not be coordinated and instead will be dispersed in different areas of the heart. The result is fibrillation, a series of uncoordinated contractions that cannot combine to propel blood out of the ventricles. This condition may occur either as the aftershock of an arterially induced heart attack or suddenly and on its own, caused by the deterioration of the electrical impulse system commanding the heart rate. In patients whose potential vulnerability to this form of heart attack has been diagnosed in advance, a heart physician may decide to surgically implant a mechanical pacemaker to ensure coordination of the necessary electrical commands to the myocardium.

TREATMENT AND THERAPY

Extraordinary medical advances have helped reduce the high death rates formerly associated with heart attacks. Many of these advances have been in the field of preventive medicine. The most widely recognized medical findings are related to diet, smoking, and exercise. Although controversy remains, there is general agreement that cholesterol absorbed by the body from the ingestion of animal fats plays a key role in the dangerous buildup of platelets inside arterial passageways. It has been accepted that regular, although not necessarily strenuous, exercise is an essential long-term preventive strategy that can reduce the risk of heart attacks. Exercise also plays a role in therapy after a heart attack. In both preventive and postattack contexts, it has been medically proven that the entire cardiovascular system profits from the natural muscle-strengthening process (in the heart's case) and general cleansing effects (in the case of oxygen intake and stimulated blood flow) that result from controlled regular exercise.

The actual application of medical scientific knowledge to assist in the campaign against the deadly effects of heart disease involves multiple fields of specialization. These may range from the sophisticated use of electrocardiograms (ECGs) to monitor the regularity of heartbeats, to specialized drug therapies aimed at preventing heart attacks in people who have been diagnosed as high-risk cases, to coronary bypass surgery or even heart transplants. In the 1980's, highly specialized surgeons at several university and private hospitals began performing operations to implant artificial hearts in human patients.

In the case of ECGs, it has become possible, thanks to the use of portable units that record the heartbeat patterns of persons over an extended period of time, to gain a much more accurate impression of the actual functioning of the heart. Previous dependence on electrocardiographic data gathered during an appointed and limited examination provided only minimal information to doctors.

The domains of preventive surgery and specialized drug treatment to prevent dangerous blood clotting are vast. Statistically, the most important and widely practiced operations that were developed in the later decades of the twentieth century were replacement of the aortic valve, the coronary bypass operation, and with greater or lesser degrees of success, the actual transplantation of voluntary donors' hearts in the place of those belonging to heart disease patients. Coronary bypass operations involve the attachment to the myocardium of healthy arteries to carry the blood that can no longer pass through the patient's clogged arterial passageways; these healthy arteries are taken by the heart surgeon from other areas of the patient's own body.

Another sphere of medical technology, that of balloon angioplasty, held out a major nonsurgical promise of preventing deterioration of the arteries leading to the heart. This sophisticated form of treatment involves the careful, temporary introduction of inflat-

In the News: Heart Attack Risk Predictors and Reducers

At the present time, the calculation of risk for heart attack is determined primarily by evaluation of the level of certain blood lipids such as cholesterol. However, scientists at Brigham and Women's Hospital, in Boston, have found that measuring the level of C-reactive protein, a serum protein normally associated with response to infection, may provide a better means of predicting such risk. The level of C-reactive protein appears to increase as a result of inflammation of the arteries, which is believed to be associated with some heart attacks. Diagnosis of risk in women is particularly important, since it is widely believed that symptoms of angina may result from other causes. Frequently the diagnosis of heart disease is missed in such women when they are brought to the emergency room suffering from chest discomfort.

Risk of either a first or second heart attack may be reduced through the use of so-called superaspirins. Two such drugs, Lamifiban and Aggrastat, appear to relieve angina and reduce the risk of a heart attack by interfering with formation of clots around plaque that has built up in arterial walls. In conjunction with the blood thinner heparin and standard aspirin, superaspirins have been found to decrease the number of episodes of angina, even in patients who do not respond to aspirin alone. The vaccination of elderly or at-risk patients with influenza vaccine has also been found to reduce the risk of heart attack. While the mechanism of protection is unknown, it may reflect the greater incidence of heart attacks resulting from respiratory distress.

—*Richard Adler, Ph.D.*

able devices inside clogged arteries, which are then stretched to increase the space within the arterial passageway for blood to flow. By the 1990's, however, doctors recognized one disadvantage of balloon angioplasty. By stretching the essential blood vessels being treated, this procedure either stretches the plaque with the artery or breaks loose debris that remains behind, creating a danger of renewed clogging. Thus another technique, called atherectomy, was developed to clear certain coronary arteries, as well as arteries elsewhere in the body.

Atherectomy involves a motorized catheter device resembling a miniature drill that is inserted into clogged arteries. As the drill turns, material that is literally shaved off the interior walls of arteries is retrieved through a tiny collection receptacle. Early experimentation, especially to treat the large anterior descending coronary artery on the left side of the heart, showed that atherectomy was 87 percent effective, whereas, on the average, angioplasty removed only 63 percent of the blockage. In addition, similar efforts to provide internal, nonsurgical treatment of clogged arteries using laser beams were being made by the early 1990's.

PERSPECTIVE AND PROSPECTS

The modern conception of cardiology dates from William Harvey's seventeenth century discovery of the relationship between the heart's function as a pump and the circulatory "restoration" of blood. Harvey's much more scientific views replaced centuries-old conceptions of the heart as a blood-warming device only.

Although substantial anatomical advances were made over the next two centuries that helped explain most of the vital functions of the heart, it was not until the early decades of the twentieth century that science developed therapeutic methods to deal with problems that frequently cause heart attacks. Drugs that affect the liver's production of substances necessary for normal coagulation of blood, for example, were discovered in the 1930's. A large variety of such anticoagulants have since been developed to help thin the blood of patients vulnerable to blood clotting. Other drugs, including certain antibiotics, are used to treat persons whose susceptiblitity to infection is known to be high. In these cases, the simple action of dislodging bacteria from the teeth when brushing can cause an invasion of the vital parts of the heart by an infection. This bacterial endocarditis, the result of the actual destruction of heart tissue or the sudden release of clots of infectious residue, could lead to a heart attack in such individuals although they have no other symptoms of identifiable heart disease.

The most spectacular advance in the scientific treatment of potential heart attack victims, however, has been in the field of cardiac surgery. Many advances in open heart surgery date from the late 1950's, when the development of heart and lung replacement machines made it safe enough to substitute electronic monitors for some of the organism's normal body functions. Before the 1950's, operations had been limited to surgical treatment of the major blood vessels surrounding the heart.

Various technical methods have also been developed that help identify problems early enough for drug therapy to be attempted before the decision to perform surgery is made. The use of catheters, which are threaded into the coronary organ using the same vessels that transport blood, became the most effective way of locating problematic areas. The process known as angiography, which uses X rays to trace the course of radio-opaque dyes injected through a catheter into local heart areas under study, can actually tell doctors if drug therapy is having the desired effects. In cases where such tests show that preventive drug therapy is not effective, an early decision to perform surgery can be made, preventing the source of coronary trouble from multiplying the patient's chances of suffering a heart attack.

—Byron D. Cannon, Ph.D.

See also Angina; Arrhythmias; Arteriosclerosis; Bypass surgery; Cardiac rehabilitation; Cardiology; Cardiology, pediatric; Cholesterol; Circulation; Electrocardiography (ECG or EKG); Embolism; Heart; Heart disease; Heart failure; Heart transplantation; Heart valve replacement; Hypercholesterolemia; Hyperlipidemia; Hypertension; Ischemia; Mitral valve prolapse; Pacemaker implantation; Palpitations; Phlebitis; Resuscitation; Thrombolytic therapy and TPA; Thrombosis and thrombus.

FOR FURTHER INFORMATION:

Baum, Seth J. *The Total Guide to a Healthy Heart: Integrative Strategies for Preventing and Reversing Heart Disease*. New York: Kensington, 2000. This book brings together the practices of both conventional and alternative approaches to reversing heart disease and maintaining heart health. Offers great insight into why the integrative approach to maintaining a healthy heart will be the medicine of the new millennium.

Gillis, Jack. *The Heart Attack Prevention and Recovery Handbook*. Point Roberts, Wash.: Hartley & Marks, 1995. Using simple, brief explanations, Gillis's text covers essential information that heart attack victims and families need immediately for reassurance and recovery. Presents excellent discussions of emotional effects on patients, medications, and treatments.

McGoon, M. *The Mayo Clinic Heart Book*. New York: William Morrow, 1993. One of the most respected texts for laypeople on heart disease. Covers all aspects of anatomy, physiology, diagnosis, treatment, and prevention.

Yannios, Thomas A. *The Heart Disease Breakthrough: What Even Your Doctor Doesn't Know About Preventing a Heart Attack*. New York: Wiley, 1999. Yannios, associate director of critical care and nutritional support at Ellis Hospital in Schenectady, New York, describes the smallest components of cholesterol, which can do more damage to the heart than the overall LDL levels that concern so many people.

Zaret, Barry L., Marvin Moser, and Lawrence S. Cohen, eds. *Yale University School of Medicine Heart Book*. New York: William Morrow, 1992. Discusses the prevention and control of heart disease. Illustrated, with a bibliography and an index.

HEART DISEASE
DISEASE/DISORDER

ANATOMY OR SYSTEM AFFECTED: Blood vessels, circulatory system, heart

SPECIALTIES AND RELATED FIELDS: Cardiology, family practice, internal medicine

DEFINITION: One of the leading causes of death in many industrialized nations; heart diseases include atherosclerotic disease, coronary artery disease, cardiac arrhythmias, and stenosis, among others.

KEY TERMS:

cardiac arrhythmia: a disturbance in the heartbeat

coronary arteries: blood vessels surrounding the heart that provide nourishment and oxygen to heart tissue

nodes: areas of electrochemical transmission within the heart that regulate the heartbeat

plaque: an accumulation of matter within artery walls that can impede blood flow

CAUSES AND SYMPTOMS

The heart is a fist-sized organ located in the upper left quarter of the chest. It consists of four chambers: the right and left atria on top and the right and left ventricles at the bottom. The chambers are enclosed in three layers of tissue: the outer layer (epicardium), the middle layer (myocardium), and the inner layer (endocardium). Surrounding the entire organ is the pericardium, a thin layer of tissue that forms a protective covering for the heart. The heart also contains various nodes that transmit electrochemical signals, causing heart muscle tissue to contract and relax in the pumping action that carries blood to organs and cells throughout the body.

Signals from the brain cause the heart to contract rhythmically in a sequence of motions that move the blood from the right atrium down through the tricuspid valve into the right ventricle. From here, blood is pushed through the pulmonary valve into the lungs, where it fulfills one of its major functions: to pick up oxygen in exchange for carbon dioxide. From the lungs, the blood is pumped back into the heart, entering the left atrium from which it is pumped down through the mitral valve into the left ventricle. Blood is then pushed through the aortic valve into the main artery of the body, the aorta, from which it starts its journey to the organs and cells. As it passes through the arteries of the gastrointestinal system, the blood picks up nutrients which, along with the oxygen that it has taken from the lungs, are brought to the cells and exchanged for waste products and carbon dioxide. The blood then enters the veins, through which it is eventually returned to the heart. The heart nourishes and supplies itself with oxygen through the coronary arteries, so called because they sit on top of the heart like a crown and extend down the sides.

The heart diseases collectively include all the disorders that can befall every part of the heart muscle: the pericardium, epicardium, myocardium, endocardium, atria, ventricles, valves, coronary arteries, and nodes. The most significant sites of heart diseases are the coronary arteries and the nodes; their malfunction can cause coronary artery disease and cardiac arrhythmias, respectively. These two disorders are responsible for the majority of heart disease cases.

Coronary artery disease occurs when matter such as cholesterol and fibrous material collects and stiffens on the inner walls of the coronary arteries. This plaque that forms may narrow the passage through which blood flows, reducing the amount of blood delivered to the heart, or may build up and clog the artery entirely, shutting off the flow of blood to the heart. In the former case, when the coronary artery is narrowed, the condition is called ischemic heart disease. Because the most common cause of ischemia is narrowing of the coronary arteries to the myocardium, another designation of the condition is myocardial ischemia, referring to the fact that blood flow to the myocardium is impeded. Accumulation of plaque within the coronary arteries is referred to as coronary atherosclerosis.

As the coronary arteries become clogged and then narrow, they can fail to deliver the required oxygen to the heart muscle, particularly during stress or physical effort. The heart's need for oxygen exceeds the arteries' ability to supply it. The patient usually feels a sharp, choking pain, called angina pectoris. Not all people who have coronary ischemia, however, experience anginal pain; these people are said to have silent ischemia.

The danger in coronary artery disease is that the accumulation of plaque will progress to the point where the coronary artery is clogged completely and no blood is delivered to the part of the heart serviced by that artery. The result is a myocardial infarction (commonly called a heart attack), in which some myocardial cells die when they fail to receive blood. The rough, uneven texture of the plaque instead may cause the formation of a blood clot, or thrombus, which closes the artery in a condition called coronary thrombosis.

Although coronary ischemia is usually thought of as a disease of middle and old age, in fact it starts much earlier. Autopsies of accident victims in their teens and twenties, as well as young soldiers killed in battle, show that coronary atherosclerosis is often well advanced in young persons. Some reasons for these findings and for why the rates of coronary artery disease and death began to rise in the twentieth century have been proposed. While antibiotics and vaccines reduced the mortality of some bacterial and some viral infections, Western societies underwent significant changes in lifestyle and eating habits that contributed to the rise of coronary heart disease: high-fat diets, obesity, and the stressful pace of life in a modern industrial society. Further, cigarette smoking, once almost a universal habit, has been shown to be highly pathogenic (disease-causing), contributing significantly to the development of heart disease, as well as lung cancer, emphysema, bronchitis, and other disorders. In the early and middle decades of the twentieth century, coronary heart disease was considered primarily an ailment of middle-aged and older men. As women began smoking, however, the incidence shifted so that coronary artery disease became almost equally prevalent, and equally lethal, among men and women.

Other conditions such as hypertension or diabetes mellitus are considered precursors of coronary artery disease. Hypertension, or high blood pressure, is an extremely common condition that, if unchecked, can contribute to both the development and the progression of coronary artery disease. Over the years, high blood pressure subjects arterial walls to constant stress. In response, the walls thicken and stiffen. This "hardening" of the arteries encourages the accumulation of fatty and fibrous plaque on inner artery walls. In patients with diabetes mellitus, blood sugar (glucose) levels rise either because the patient is deficient in insulin or because the insulin that the patient produces is inefficient at removing glucose from the blood. High glucose levels favor high fat levels in the blood, which can cause atherosclerosis.

Cardiac arrhythmias are the next major cause of morbidity and mortality among the heart diseases. Inside the heart, an electrochemical network regulates the contractions and relaxations that form the heartbeat. In the excitation or contraction phase, a chain of electrochemical impulses starts in the upper part of the right atrium in the heart's pacemaker, the sinoatrial or sinus node. The impulses travel through internodal tracts (pathways from one node to another) to an area between the atrium and the right ventricle called the atrioventricular node. The impulses then enter the bundle of His, which carries them to the left atrium and left ventricle. After the series of contractions is complete, the heart relaxes for a brief moment before another cycle is begun. On the average, the process is repeated sixty to eighty times a minute.

This is normal rhythm, the regular, healthy heartbeat. Dysfunction at any point along the electrochemical pathway, however, can cause an arrhythmia. Arrhythmias range greatly in their effects and their potential for bodily damage. They can be completely unnoticeable, merely annoying, debilitating, or frightening. They can cause blood clots to form in the heart, and they can cause sudden death.

The arrhythmic heart can beat too quickly (tachycardia) or too slowly (bradycardia). The contractions of the various chambers can become unsynchronized, or out of step with one another. For example, in atrial flutter or atrial fibrillation, the upper chambers of the heart beat faster, out of synchronization with the ventricles. In ventricular tachycardia, ventricular contrac-

tions increase, out of synchronization with the atria. In ventricular fibrillation, ventricular contractions lose all rhythmicity and become uncoordinated to the point at which the heart is no longer able to pump blood. Cardiac death can then occur unless the patient receives immediate treatment.

An arrhythmic disorder called heart block occurs when the impulse from the pacemaker is "blocked." Its progress through the atrioventricular node and the bundle of His may be slow or irregular, or the impulse may fail to reach its target tissues. The disorder is rated in three degrees. First-degree heart block is detectable only on an electrocardiogram (ECG), in which the movement of the impulse from the atria to the ventricles is seen to be slowed. In second-degree heart block, only some of the impulses generated reach from the atria to the ventricles; the pulse becomes irregular. Third-degree heart block is the most serious manifestation of this disorder: No impulses from the atria reach the ventricles. The heart rate may slow dramatically, and the blood flow to the brain can be reduced, causing dizziness or loss of consciousness.

Disorders that affect the heart valves usually involve stenosis (narrowing), which reduces the size of the valve opening; physical malfunction of the valve; or both. These disorders can be attributable to infection (such as rheumatic fever) or to tissue damage, or they can be congenital. If a valve has narrowed, the passage of blood from one heart chamber to another is impeded. In the case of mitral stenosis, the mitral valve between the left atrium and the left ventricle is narrowed. Blood flow to the left ventricle is reduced, and blood is retained in the left atrium, causing the atrium to enlarge as pressure builds in the chamber. This pressure forces blood back into the lungs, creating a condition called pulmonary edema in which fluid collects in the air sacs of the lungs. Similarly, malfunctions of the heart valves that cause them to open and close inefficiently can interfere with the flow of blood into the heart, through it, and out of it. This impairment may cause structural changes in the heart that can be life-threatening.

Heart failure may be a consequence of many disease conditions. It occurs primarily in the elderly. In this condition, the heart becomes inefficient at pumping blood. If the failure is on the right side of the heart, blood is forced back into the body, causing edema in the lower legs. If the failure is on the left side of the heart, blood is forced back into the lungs, causing pulmonary edema. There are many manifestations of heart failure, including shortness of breath, fatigue, and weakness.

Numerous diseases afflict the tissues of the heart wall—the epicardium, myocardium, and endocardium, as well as the pericardium. They are often caused by bacterial or viral infection, but they may also result from tissue trauma or a variety of toxic agents.

TREATMENT AND THERAPY

The main tools for diagnosing heart disease are the stethoscope, the electrocardiograph (ECG), and the X ray. With the stethoscope the doctor listens to heart sounds, which provides information about many heart functions such as rhythm and the status of the valves. The doctor can determine whether the heart is functioning normally in pumping blood from one chamber into the other, into the lungs, and into the aorta. The ECG gives the doctor a graph representation of heart function. Twelve to fifteen electrodes are placed on various parts of the body, including the head, chest, legs, and arms. The activities of the heart are printed on a strip of paper as waves or tracings. The doctor analyzes the printout for evidence of heart abnormalities, changes in heart function, signs of a heart attack, or other problems. Generally, the electrocardiographic examination is conducted with the patient at rest. In some situations, however, the doctor wishes to view heart action during physical stress. In this case, the electrodes are attached to the patient and the patient is required to exercise on a treadmill or stationary bicycle. The physician can see what changes in heart function occur when the cardiac workload is increased. The X ray gives the doctor a visual picture of the heart. Any enlargements or abnormalities can be seen, as well as the status of the aorta, pulmonary arteries, and other structures.

Another standard diagnostic tool is the echocardiograph. High-frequency sound waves are pointed at the heart from outside the body. The sound waves bounce against heart tissue and are shown on a monitor. The general configuration of the heart can be seen, as well as the shape and thickness of the chamber walls, the valves, and the large blood vessels leading to and from the heart. Velocity and direction of blood flow through the valves can be determined.

Various procedures can help the doctor assess the degree of ischemia within the heart. In one test, a radioactive isotope is injected into a vein and its dispersion in the heart is read by a scanner. This procedure can show which parts of the heart are being deprived of oxygen. In another test using a radioactive isotope, the reading is made while the patient exercises, in order to detect any changes in expansion and contraction of the heart wall that would indicate impaired circulation. The coronary angiogram gives a picture of the blockage within the coronary arteries. A thin tube called a catheter is threaded into a coronary artery and a dye that is opaque to X rays is released. The X-ray picture will reveal narrowings in the artery resulting from plaque buildup.

The main goals of therapy in treating heart diseases are to cure the condition, if possible, and otherwise help the patient live a normal life and prevent the condition from becoming worse. In coronary artery disease, the physician seeks to maintain blood flow to the heart and to prevent heart attack. Hundreds of medications are available for this purpose, including vasodilators (agents that relax blood vessel walls and increase their capacity to carry blood). Chief among the coronary vasodilators are nitroglycerin and other drugs in the nitrate family. Also, calcium channel blockers are often used to dilate blood vessels. Beta-blocking agents are used because they reduce the heart's need for oxygen and alleviate the symptoms of angina. In addition, various support measures are recommended by physicians to stop plaque buildup and halt the progress of the disease. These include losing weight, reducing fats in the diet, and stopping smoking. The physician also treats concomitant illnesses that can contribute to the progress of coronary artery disease, such as hypertension and diabetes.

Sometimes medications and diet are not fully successful, and the ischemia continues. In a relatively new procedure, the cardiologist can unblock a clogged artery by a procedure called angioplasty. The physician threads a catheter containing a tiny balloon to the point of the blockage. The balloon is inflated to widen the inner diameter of the artery, and blood flow is increased. This procedure is often successful, although it may have to be repeated. When it is not successful, coronary bypass surgery may be indicated. In this procedure, clogged coronary arteries are replaced with healthy blood vessels from other parts of the body.

When coronary artery disease progresses to a heart attack, the patient should be treated in the hospital or similar facility. The possibility of sudden death is high during the attack and remains high until the patient is stabilized. Emergency measures are undertaken to minimize the extent of heart damage, reduce heart work, keep oxygen flowing to all parts of the body, and regulate blood pressure and heartbeat.

Cardiac arrhythmias can be managed by a variety of medications and procedures. Digitalis, guanidine, procainamide, tocanamide, and atropine are widely used to restore normal heart rhythm. In acute situations, the patient's heart rhythm can be restored by electrical cardioversion, in which an electrical stimulus is applied from outside the body to regulate the heartbeat. When a slowed heartbeat cannot be controlled by medication, a pacemaker may be implanted to regulate heart rhythm.

Treatment of heart valve disorders and disorders of the heart wall is directed at alleviating the individual condition. Antibiotics and/or valve replacement surgery may be required. In many cases, valve disorders can be completely corrected. Cardiac transplantation remains a possible treatment for some heart patients. This is an option for comparatively few patients because there are ten times as many candidates for heart transplants as there are available donor hearts.

PERSPECTIVE AND PROSPECTS

Heart disease became a major killer in the United States in the twentieth century. In the early decades, the best that the medical community could do was to treat symptoms. Since then, the emphasis has shifted to prevention. Hundreds of investigative studies have been undertaken to determine the causes of the most prevalent heart dysfunction, coronary artery disease. Many of these studies have involved tens of thousands of subjects, and they point to a general consensus that coronary artery disease is a multifactorial disorder, the primary elements of which are cholesterol and other fatty substances circulating in the bloodstream, smoking, diabetes, high blood pressure, stress, and obesity.

The reasons that mortality from heart disease is declining include improved medications and treatment modalities, and much credit has to be given to the success of preventive measures. Millions of Americans have stopped smoking and have begun watching their diets. Entire industries are devoted to helping Americans eat more intelligently. While fast-food outlets continued to offer high-fat standards, such as hotdogs and hamburgers, they have also added salads and leaner selections.

Perhaps most important, medical and sociological authorities have turned their attention to children. Because advanced atherosclerosis has been detected in young men and women, cholesterol-watching has become a major preoccupation with parents and school dieticians. In addition, national programs have been instituted to discourage smoking among the young. Whether the rates of coronary heart disease will be lower in these individuals than in their parents remains to be seen, but the success of these measures in the older populations indicates that the prognosis is good.

The prognosis is also good for other heart diseases. New drugs continue to be licensed for the treatment of arrhythmias, and more versatile and reliable pacemakers increase the prospects of a normal life for many patients. Improvements in heart surgery have been particularly impressive, especially those for managing congenital heart defects in neonates and infants. Heart transplants have been successfully performed on these patients, and numerous other procedures promise significant improvement in the prospects of young people with heart disease.

Rheumatic fever, however, one of the major causes of heart disease in children, remains a threat. No vaccine is available for immunization against the streptococcus strains that cause rheumatic fever, but fortunately there are effective antibiotics to control infection in these patients. Rheumatic fever usually develops subsequent to a throat infection. Careful monitoring of the child with a sore throat can avoid progression of the infection to rheumatic fever.

—*C. Richard Falcon*

See also Aneurysms; Angina; Arrhythmias; Arteriosclerosis; Blue baby syndrome; Bypass surgery; Cardiac rehabilitation; Cardiology; Cardiology, pediatric; Cholesterol; Circulation; Claudication; Congenital heart disease; Diabetes mellitus; Eclampsia; Electrocardiography (ECG or EKG); Embolism; Endocarditis; Heart; Heart attack; Heart failure; Heart transplantation; Heart valve replacement; Hypercholesterolemia; Hyperlipidemia; Hypertension; Ischemia; Mitral valve prolapse; Obesity; Pacemaker implantation; Palpitations; Phlebitis; Thrombolytic therapy and TPA; Thrombosis and thrombus; Varicose veins; Venous insufficiency.

FOR FURTHER INFORMATION:

Baum, Seth J. *The Total Guide to a Healthy Heart: Integrative Strategies for Preventing and Reversing Heart Disease.* New York: Kensington, 2000. This book brings together the practices of both conventional and alternative approaches to reversing heart disease and maintaining heart health. Offers great insight into why the integrative approach to maintaining a healthy heart will be the medicine of the new millennium.

Dranov, Paula. *Heart Disease*. New York: Random House, 1990. Devoted to helping the reader become knowledgeable about heart disease and how it is being treated.

Editors of the University of California, Berkeley, Wellness Letter. *The New Wellness Encyclopedia*. Boston: Houghton Mifflin, 1995. A good general medical text with exemplary coverage of the heart diseases, preventive measures, and current therapeutic modalities.

Kowalski, Robert E. *Eight Steps to a Healthy Heart*. New York: Warner Books, 1992. In addition to outlining how to avoid heart disease, this book advises patients with heart disease about how to get the most benefit from their therapy.

Larson, David G., ed. *Mayo Clinic Family Health Book*. 2d ed. New York: William Morrow, 1996. This large reference work was written for the layperson. The sections on the heart diseases are exemplary for clarity and thoroughness.

McGoon, M. *The Mayo Clinic Heart Book*. New York: William Morrow, 1993. One of the most respected texts for laypeople on heart disease. Covers all aspects of anatomy, physiology, diagnosis, treatment, and prevention.

Taylor, George J. *Primary Care Management of Heart Disease*. St. Louis: Mosby, 2000. A resource on the therapy and diagnosis of heart disease. Includes bibliographical references and an index.

Yannios, Thomas A. *The Heart Disease Breakthrough: What Even Your Doctor Doesn't Know About Preventing a Heart Attack*. New York: Wiley, 1999. Yannios, associate director of critical care and nutritional support at Ellis Hospital in Schenectady, New York, describes the smallest components of cholesterol, which can do more damage to the heart than the overall LDL levels that concern so many people.

Zaret, Barry L., Marvin Moser, and Lawrence S. Cohen, eds. *Yale University School of Medicine Heart Book*. New York: William Morrow, 1992. This text will give the reader a clear understanding of the various heart diseases, as well as of current methods of treating and preventing them.

HEART FAILURE
DISEASE/DISORDER

ANATOMY OR SYSTEM AFFECTED: Circulatory system, heart

SPECIALTIES AND RELATED FIELDS: Cardiology, internal medicine, vascular medicine

DEFINITION: A condition in which the heart cannot pump enough blood to meet the needs of the body because its ability to contract is impaired.

KEY TERMS:

congestive heart failure: the stage of heart failure that occurs when a backup of pressure results in accumulation of fluid in the veins and tissues

coronary arteries: the arteries that supply blood to the heart muscle

diuretic: a drug that stimulates the kidneys to eliminate more salt and water from the body

edema: the accumulation of fluid around the cells in tissue

ejection fraction: the ratio of the stroke volume to the residual volume, expressed as a percentage

hormone: a chemical messenger released by a gland which is carried by the blood to its target

inotropic agent: a drug that improves the ability of the heart muscle to contract

optimal length: the length of a heart muscle cell at which stimulation can elicit the maximum possible force development

residual volume: the blood volume left in the heart chamber at the end of a heartbeat

stroke volume: the blood volume leaving either the right or the left side of the heart with each beat; each side usually ejects the same volume per beat

vasodilator: a drug that relaxes blood vessels

CAUSES AND SYMPTOMS

The circulation of the blood has many functions. It is essential for the delivery of oxygen, nutrients, and elements of the immune system to tissues. It also contributes to regulation and communication between different parts of the body by moving chemical messengers from where they are produced to where they have a biological effect. The delivery of warm blood to the surface of the skin is one essential element in temperature control. The blood pressure determines how much water can move across the exchange surfaces in the kidneys, thus affecting water balance in the body. The movement of blood through the kidneys, the lungs, and all tissues is important for waste removal.

All these functions depend on the ability of the heart to contract and eject blood. Blood is pumped, in two serial circuits, from the right heart through the lungs into the left heart and from the left heart around the body back to the right heart. In each circuit, the blood travels through large arteries, then to smaller arterioles, to capillaries (where exchange takes place), and back via small venules and veins to the heart. Heart failure describes the situation in which heart function is reduced. While still able to beat, the heart is unable to meet the circulatory needs of the body. That is, the heart muscle is unable to contract enough to pump the blood adequately.

The severity of the heart failure can be gauged by the ejection fraction, a measure of the pumping capacity of the heart. It is the percentage calculated from the stroke volume (the volume of blood leaving a heart chamber with each beat) divided by the residual volume (the volume left in the heart chamber at the end of a heartbeat). Thus the ejection fraction measures how much blood in the heart chamber can actually leave when the heartbeat occurs. In normal, healthy hearts, this value is 100 percent: The amount that stays in the heart is approximately equal to the amount that leaves it. In mild or moderate heart failure, it ranges approximately between 15 and 40 percent: Less blood leaves the heart with each beat, and more blood remains behind.

The pressure inside the heart at the end of a heartbeat is another index of heart performance. If the heart is failing and more blood is left behind in the heart at the end of a beat, the pressure inside the heart at the end of the beat will be increased. In cases of severe failure, the pressure in the arteries outside the heart will fall.

In failure, the heart cannot supply enough blood for all the functions of the circulation. This fact accounts for the variety of symptoms that accompany heart failure: labored breathing; light-headedness; generalized weakness; cold, pale, or even bluish skin tone; and accumulation of fluid in the extremities and/or lungs. Possible other symptoms include distended neck veins, accumulation of fluid in the abdomen, abnormal heart rate and rhythm, and chest pain.

The specific symptoms of the condition depend on the type of failure, its severity, its underlying causes, and the ways in which the body attempts to compensate. There are several ways to categorize types of heart failure: acute or chronic, forward or backward, and right-sided or left-sided.

Acute heart failure refers to a sudden decrease in heart function. It can be caused by toxic quantities of drugs, anesthetics, or metals or by certain disease states, such as infections. Most often, however, it is caused by a sudden blockage of the coronary arteries supplying the heart muscle. A sudden blockage caused by a blood clot can induce a heart attack and subsequent heart failure, causing chest pain and often abnormal heart rate or rhythm. These effects are sometimes so rapid that there is little time for the body to attempt compensation.

Chronic heart failure is a progressive reduction in heart function that develops over time. It can be caused by inherited or acquired diseases, allergic reactions, connective tissue or metabolic abnormalities, high blood pressure, and anatomical defects. The most common cause, however, is coronary artery disease. This disease narrows blood vessels and leads to a reduction in the amount of blood reaching the heart muscle. It causes reduced oxygen availability and, eventually, a reduction in the ability of the heart muscle to contract.

In the early stages of chronic failure, the hormone and nervous systems promote compensation in the heart, blood vessels, and kidneys to help the heart continue to pump enough blood. These systems stimulate the heart muscle directly to make it beat harder. They also take advantage of the fact that modest stretching of the heart muscle increases its ability to contract. By stimulating the blood vessels to contract, more blood moves back toward the heart, causing a cold, pale, or even bluish skin tone. Stimulation of the kidney to retain water and sodium results in an increase in blood volume, which also moves more blood back to the heart. In each case, the heart muscle is stretched by these increases and, therefore, can contract harder.

Yet these reactions do not constitute a long-term solution. The heart muscle can become fatigued from overwork and can become overstretched. A resulting accumulation of fluid in the heart reduces its ability to contract. Compensation fails, and the additional fluid in the blood starts to back up in the circulation. This condition is called backward heart failure. At the same time, the heart is unable to pump hard enough to move the blood forward against the higher resistance caused by the contraction of the blood vessels. This condition is termed forward heart failure. Congestive heart failure is the stage that occurs when the backup of pressure is worsened by fluid retention and blood vessel contraction. The congestion, or accumulation of fluid, occurs in the veins and tissues.

Left-sided or right-sided heart failure can occur alone or together. The right side of the heart pumps blood to the lungs to be oxygenated, and the left side of the heart pumps oxygenated blood to the organs of the body. Normally, these two sides are well matched so that the same volume moves through each side. When the right heart cannot contract properly, however, blood accumulates upstream in the veins and somewhat less blood reaches the lungs to pick up oxygen, resulting in distended veins and shortness of breath. It is primarily a backward heart failure. Fluid can back up in the veins and increase pressure in the capillaries so that it starts to leak out of the circulation into the surrounding tissues. This leads to an accumulation of fluid (called edema), especially in the liver and lower extremities. In isolated right-sided heart failure, this pressure rarely backs up to such an extent that it causes problems through the rest of the circulation to the left side of the heart.

In contrast, when the left side of the heart cannot contract properly, it can back up pressure so badly that it creates a pressure overload against which the right side of the heart must pump. This increase in the workload on the right side of the heart frequently leads to two-sided heart failure. This outcome is especially common since the disease conditions that exist in the left side are likely to exist on the right as well. In left-sided heart failure, blood accumulates upstream in the lungs, increasing pressure enough to cause a leakage of fluid into the lungs (pulmonary edema). This leakage interferes with oxygen uptake and therefore causes shortness of breath. It also results in inadequate blood flow to the body's tissues, including the muscles and brain, resulting in generalized weakness and light-headedness. Left-sided heart failure is thus both a backward and a forward failure.

TREATMENT AND THERAPY

Treatments for cardiac failure, like its symptoms, depend on a variety of factors. The first goal of treatment is to avoid any obvious precipitating causes of the failure, such as alcohol, drugs, the cessation of necessary essential medications, acute stress, a salt-loaded diet, overexercise, infection, illness, or surgery. The next approach is to take the simplest measures to reduce distension of the heart by controlling salt and water retention and to decrease the workload of the heart by altering the circulatory needs of the

tissues. The former can be achieved by dietary salt restriction, restriction of fluid consumption, or mechanical removal of fluid accumulating around the lungs or abdomen. The latter can be accomplished with bed rest and weight loss.

Typically, drug therapy is also required in order to treat heart failure. No single agent meets all the requirements for optimal treatment, which includes rapid relief of labored breathing and edema, enhanced heart performance, reduced mortality, reduced progression of the underlying disease, safety, and minimal side effects. Therefore, drugs are used in combination to achieve control over sodium and water retention, improve heart contraction, reduce heart work, and protect against blood clots.

The purpose of therapy with diuretic drugs (drugs that increase salt and water loss through the kidneys) is threefold: to reduce the pooling of fluid that can take place in the lungs, abdomen, and lower extremities; to minimize the buildup of back pressure from the accumulation of blood in the veins; and to reduce the circulating blood volume. All these things will lessen the overstretch of the heart muscle and bring it to a level of stretch that is closer to its optimum. Care must be taken, however, not to reduce severely the water content of the blood, which could reduce the stretch on the heart muscle to below the optimum and consequently impair heart contraction. One way to monitor how much water is lost or retained is for patients to empty their bladders and then weigh themselves each day before breakfast. If weight changes steadily or suddenly, then sodium and water loss may be too great or too little. In either case, an adjustment is in order. Some generic diuretic drugs used to treat heart failure include furosemide, ethacrynic acid, the thiazides, and spironolactone.

The purpose of therapy with inotropic drugs (drugs that increase the contractile ability of heart muscle) is to improve the pumping action of the heart. This effect causes an increase in stroke volume (more blood moves out of the heart per beat) and helps compensate for forward failure. The increased output also reduces the backup of blood returning to the heart and thus also compensates for backward failure.

Digitalis, a derivative of the foxglove plant which originated as a Welsh folk remedy, is still the most frequently used inotropic drug for the treatment of chronic heart failure. Because it improves heart muscle contraction, it reverses to some extent all the symptoms of heart failure. Digitalis exerts its effects by increasing the accumulation of calcium inside the heart muscle cells. Calcium interacts with the structure of the shortening apparatus inside the cell to make more contractile interactions within the cell possible. Its disadvantages are that it becomes toxic in high doses and that it can severely damage performance of an already healthy heart.

Other inotropic agents also act to improve contraction by increasing calcium levels within the heart muscle cells. Some of them mimic the naturally produced hormones and neurotransmitters that are released and depleted in early stages of heart failure. These are called the sympathomimetic drugs. They include drugs such as dopamine, terbutaline, and levodopa. While these drugs improve heart performance, they can have serious side effects: increased heart rate, palpitations, and nervousness. One group of inotropic agents improves cardiac contraction while relaxing blood vessels. These drugs, called phosphodiesterase inhibitors, stop the breakdown of an essential cellular messenger molecule which helps to manage calcium levels and other events inside both heart cells and blood vessel cells. Examples of these drugs include amrinone and milrinone. Their use is not common because they can cause stomach upset and fatigue and because they are not clearly superior to other treatments.

The purpose of therapy with vasodilator drugs (drugs that relax the blood vessels) is to decrease the work of the heart. The resulting expansion of the blood vessels makes it easier for blood to be pumped through them. It also leaves room for pooling some of the blood in the veins, decreasing the amount of blood returning to the heart and so reducing overstretching as well. Some of the vasodilators, such as hydralazine, pinacidil, dipyridamole, and the nitrates, act directly on the blood vessels. Other vasodilators, such as angiotensin-converting enzyme (ACE) inhibitors and adrenergic inhibitors, inhibit the release of naturally produced substances that would make the blood vessels contract. Sometimes it is hard to predict the effects of vasodilators because they may act differently in different blood vessels and the body may attempt to offset the effects of the drug by releasing substances that contract blood vessels. Vasodilator drug therapy is usually added to other treatments when the symptoms of heart failure persist after digitalis and diuretic therapy are used.

The purpose of therapy with antithrombotics (blood clot inhibitors) is to prevent any further ob-

struction of the circulation with blood clots. Because heart failure changes the mechanics of blood flow and is the result of damaged heart muscle, it can increase the formation of blood clots. When blood clots form an obstruction in the large blood vessels of the lungs, it is often fatal. Clots can also lodge in the heart to cause further damage to heart muscle or in the brain, where they could cause a stroke. Both the short-acting clot inhibitor heparin and oral agents such as aspirin are used to prevent these effects.

The combination of all these drug therapies, while unable to reverse the permanent damage of heart failure, makes it possible to treat the condition. Individuals treated for heart failure can lead comfortable, productive lives.

If the heart failure progresses to acutely life-threatening proportions and the patient is in all other ways healthy, the next alternative is surgical replacement of the heart. Artificial hearts are sometimes used as a transition to heart transplant while a donor is sought. Yet transplantation is not a perfect solution. Transplanted hearts do not have the nervous system input of a normal heart and so their control from moment to moment is different. They are also subject to rejection. Nevertheless, they provide an enormous improvement in quality of life for severe heart failure patients.

PERSPECTIVE AND PROSPECTS

The vital significance of the pulse and heartbeat have been part of human knowledge since long before recorded history. Pulse taking and herbal treatments for poor heartbeat have been recorded in ancient Chinese, Egyptian, and Greek histories. Digitalis has been used in treatment for at least two hundred years. It was first formally introduced to the medical community in 1785 by the English botanist and physician William Withering. He learned of it from a female folk healer named Hutton, who used it with other extracts to treat more than one kind of swelling. Withering identified the foxglove plant as the source of its active ingredient and characterized it as having effects on the pulse as well as on fluid retention. The plant is indigenous to both the United Kingdom and Europe and may well have been employed as a folk remedy for far longer. It is still the most widely used agent for the treatment of heart failure.

The developments in physiology and medicine during the nineteenth century set the stage for greater understanding and further treatments of heart failure.

It was then that the stethoscope and blood pressure cuff were created for diagnostic purposes. In basic science, cell theory, hormone theory, and kidney physiology led to a better understanding of how heart muscle contraction and fluid balance might be coordinated in the body. The concepts and techniques required to keep organs and tissues alive outside the body with an artificial circulation system were conceived and introduced. Anesthesia and sterile techniques essential for cardiac surgery were developed.

These ideas and accomplishments contributed to important discoveries in the early twentieth century that greatly enhanced the understanding of the early compensatory responses to heart failure. For example, it was found that when heart muscle is stretched, it will contract with greater force on the next beat and that heart muscle usually operates at a muscle length that is less than optimal. Thus, when the amount of blood returning to the heart increases and stretches the muscle in the walls of the heart, the heart will contract with greater force, ejecting a greater volume of blood. This phenomenon, called the Frank-Starling mechanism, was first demonstrated in isolated heart muscle by the German physiologist Otto Frank and in functional hearts by the British physiologist Ernest Henry Starling in 1914.

Subsequent developments in the second half of the twentieth century, such as more specific vasodilator and diuretic drugs as well as the heart-lung machine, have led to the options of more complete drug therapy, artificial hearts (first introduced to replace a human heart by William DeVries in 1982), and heart transplant (first performed by Christiaan Barnard in 1967) as options for the treatment of heart failure.

—Laura Gray Malloy, Ph.D.

See also Arrhythmias; Arteriosclerosis; Cardiology; Cardiology, pediatric; Cholesterol; Circulation; Congenital heart disease; Edema; Endocarditis; Heart; Heart attack; Heart disease; Heart transplantation; Hypercholesterolemia; Hyperlipidemia; Hypertension; Ischemia; Mitral valve prolapse; Obesity; Palpitations; Vascular medicine; Vascular system.

FOR FURTHER INFORMATION:

Campbell, Neil A. *Biology: Concepts and Connections*. 5th ed. Redwood City, Calif.: Benjamin/ Cummings, 1999. An accessible general textbook with an excellent treatment of cardiovascular function and disease in chapter 38. Contains outstanding illustrations and a glossary. A college-level text that is suitable for the high school student as well.

Dox, Ida G., B. John Melloni, and Gilbert M. Eisner. *The HarperCollins Illustrated Medical Dictionary.* New York: HarperCollins, 1993. A home medical dictionary with more than 26,000 medical terms and 2,500 illustrations, including all those of most concern to cardiovascular patients. Defines relevant anatomical structures, functional terminology, and some widely used chemical compounds and drugs under generic names. An excellent resource for high school or college students.

Sherwood, Lauralee. *Human Physiology: From Cells to Systems*. 4th ed. Belmont, Calif.: Wadsworth, 2001. A basic physiology textbook oriented toward an understanding of human function and disease. Superbly well written and offers excellent illustrations. Chapters 9 through 11 address cardiovascular function, with specific reference to heart failure and the cardiovascular abnormalities that precipitate it.

HEART TRANSPLANTATION

PROCEDURE

ANATOMY OR SYSTEM AFFECTED: Chest, circulatory system, heart, lungs, nervous system, respiratory system

SPECIALTIES AND RELATED FIELDS: Cardiology, critical care, emergency medicine, general surgery

DEFINITION: The removal of a diseased heart and its replacement with a healthy donor heart.

KEY TERMS:

cardiomyopathy: a serious acute or chronic disease in which the heart becomes inflamed; it may result from multiple causes, including viral infection

congenital: present at birth

congestive heart failure: abnormal heart function characterized by circulatory congestion caused by cardiac disorders, especially myocardial infarction of the ventricles

coronary atherosclerosis: the accumulation of cholesterol, lipids, and other cellular debris in the coronary arteries, thereby limiting circulation in the heart

immunity: a defense function of the body that produces antibodies to destroy invading antigens and other disease-causing organisms

leukocytes: white blood cells that are important in the development of immunity

primary cardiomyopathy: cardiomyopathy that cannot be attributed to a specific cause *secondary cardiomyopathy:* cardiomyopathy that is attributable to a specific cause (such as hypertension) and that is often associated with diseases involving other organs

INDICATIONS AND PROCEDURES

Heart transplantation is performed when congestive heart failure or heart injury cannot be treated by other conventional medical or surgical means. It is reserved for patients with a high risk of dying within two years. The procedure involves removal of a diseased heart and its replacement with a healthy human heart or possibly an animal heart. In special cases, the surgeon may place the donor heart next to the diseased heart without removing it; this is called a piggy-back transplant.

Patients who are candidates for heart transplantation include those with valvular disease, congenital heart disease, or rare conditions such as tumors. The selection of recipients is based on which patients are likely to exhibit the most pronounced improvement, functional capacity, and life expectancy after surgery. In the United States, the limited availability of donor hearts has necessitated the creation of a national organ procurement and distribution network called the United Network for Organ Sharing (UNOS), which distributes organs based on severity of illness, waiting time, donor and recipient blood types, and body size match.

A heart is about to be removed during a transplantation procedure. (PhotoDisc)

USES AND COMPLICATIONS

The first human heart transplantation was performed on December 3, 1967, by Christiaan Barnard in Capetown, Africa. The heart transplantation procedures that were tried soon afterward usually had a low success rate because the patient's body often rejected the new heart when leukocytes and other cells of the immune system recognized the new heart as foreign material and attacked it. With an improved understanding of immune system functioning and drug intervention, however, survival rates have gradually improved. Currently in the United States, approximately two thousand patients undergo heart transplantation annually in more than 230 heart transplantation centers. The one-year survival rate is 80 percent, the five-year survival rate is 70 percent, the ten-year survival rate is nearly 50 percent, and some patients have lived longer than twenty years, according to statistics from the American Heart Association. About fifteen thousand Americans aged fifty-five or younger (and forty thousand aged sixty-five or younger) would benefit from heart transplantation. Transplantation has been conducted with newborn babies, and adult patients have run marathons and even played professional sports. The average age at which the procedure is performed is forty-seven years for men and thirty-nine years for women.

The complications immediately following this type of surgery include irreversible damage to the heart, because of coronary atherosclerosis or multiple heart attacks, and primary or secondary cardiomyopathy, because the cardiac muscle cells cannot contract normally. Heart transplant recipients must take immunosuppressive (antirejection) medications for the remainder of their lives to prevent rejection; thus they must also cope with the numerous side effects of these drugs. For at least one year after transplantation, the heart is denervated (cut away from the body's nervous system), causing a resting pulse rate of up to 130 beats per minute, as compared to 60 to 80 beats per minute in a normal heart. The chances for longterm success depend in part on the amount of damage or disease in other organs as a result of stroke, chronic obstructive lung disease, and liver or kidney disease. Transplant recipients must also deal with the psychological and emotional strain of the operation and its aftermath. Patients with a history of alcohol and drug abuse or mental illness, and those who lack a social support network of family and friends, are not considered good candidates for heart transplantation.

Perspective and Prospects

The rapid increase in the number of heart transplantations performed worldwide is attributable to specialized medical care and to numerous advances in knowledge regarding surgery, tissue preservation, immunology, and infectious disease. The extraordinary degree of success since the 1970's has enabled many patients who have undergone heart transplantation to live longer and more independent lives. Tremendous strides have been made in diagnosing rejection and developing immunosuppressive medications, and the development of several new antirejection drugs is anticipated soon. New techniques for diagnosing rejection candidates without the performance of a heart biopsy will be a major focus of future research, as will increasing access to donor organs. A better understanding of the immune system may give doctors greater success in transplanting organs from other species (a procedure called a xenograft) instead of human organs. Ongoing research will continue to focus on identifying risk factors for heart disease—such as high blood cholesterol and abnormal lipid subfractions, high blood pressure, diabetes mellitus, family history, and cigarette smoking—as early as possible in order to delay reaching the point at which heart transplantation is necessary.

—*Daniel G. Graetzer, Ph.D.*

See also Cardiac rehabilitation; Cardiology; Cardiology, pediatric; Circulation; Electrocardiography (ECG or EKG); Grafts and grafting; Heart; Heart disease; Heart failure; Heart valve replacement; Immune system; Immunology; Transplantation.

For Further Information:

American College of Sports Medicine. *ACSM's Guidelines for Exercise Testing and Prescription.* 6th ed. Baltimore: Williams & Wilkins, 2000. Covers the standards of exercise testing and therapy, including instruction for patients suffering from heart disease.

American Heart Association. *Heart and Stroke Facts.* Dallas, Tex.: Author, 1994. Contains information for the layperson on cardiovascular and cerebrovascular disease. Includes an index.

Deng, Mario C., et al. "Effect of Receiving a Heart Transplant: Analysis of a National Cohort Entered on to a Waiting List, Stratified by Heart Failure Severity." *British Medical Journal* 321, no. 7260 (September 2, 2000): 540-545. A study of cardiac transplantation in Germany reveals that patients with a predicted low or medium risk of mortality have no reduction in mortality risk as a result of transplantation.

Ewert, Ralf, et al. "Relationship Between Impaired Pulmonary Diffusion and Cardiopulmonary Exercise Capacity After Heart Transplantation." *Chest* 117, no. 4 (April, 2000): 968. Diffusion impairment and reduced performance in cardiopulmonary exercise testing have been found in patients after heart transplantation.

Krau, Stephen D., ed. *Heart Transplantation.* Philadelphia: W. B. Saunders, 2000. Discusses organ procurement, evaluation criteria for the pretransplant patient, and the long-term management of heart transplantation patients, including immunosuppression, complications, and psychological adjustments.

Heart valve replacement

Procedure

Anatomy or system affected: Chest, circulatory system, heart

Specialties and related fields: Cardiology, general surgery

Definition: A surgical procedure that involves removing a defective heart valve and replacing it with another tissue valve or with a mechanical valve.

Key terms:

anticoagulants: a class of drugs that slow the clotting time of blood

bacterial endocarditis: bacterial infection of the heart, which may scar or destroy a valve

Heart Valve Replacement

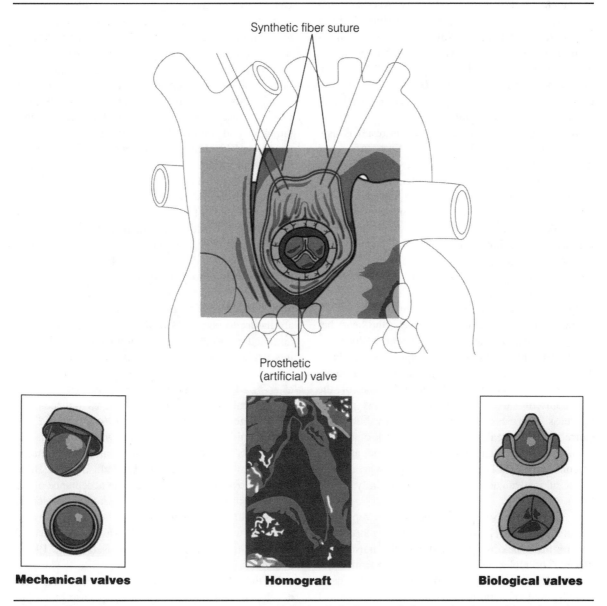

Synthetic fiber suture

Prosthetic
(artificial) valve

Mechanical valves   **Homograft**   **Biological valves**

When heart valves fail, they can be replaced by mechanical valves, which are made from artificial materials such as plastic, metal, and carbon fibers; by homografts, which are taken from cadavers; or by biological valves, which are either taken from pigs or constructed from the tissues of the patient or of a cow.

murmur: the sound made by blood flowing backward through a heart valve

regurgitation: the leakage of blood backward through a valve

stenosis: a condition in which valve tissue has hardened and thickened, interfering with blood flow through the valve

INDICATIONS AND PROCEDURES

Valve replacement surgery is a procedure used when a heart valve no longer functions properly. There are several reasons that a heart valve may fail. Sometimes, a major defect present at birth must be repaired immediately. Minor defects present at birth may go undetected for years. When and if these minor defects become worse as a result of aging, valve replacement surgery may be necessary. Another cause of heart valve damage is infection. Rheumatic fever can cause the scarring of a valve. These scars can become more of a problem with age, and surgery may eventually be necessary. Bacterial endocarditis is another type of infection that can damage the heart very quickly. Valve replacement surgery is often needed as a result of this type of infection.

When a heart valve is damaged, the result is usually stenosis or regurgitation. Stenosis occurs when the valve becomes thick and hard. As a result, normal blood flow through the valve is obstructed. A valve that becomes stretched or weak may not close properly, resulting in blood flowing backward through the valve; this is called regurgitation. When the blood flows backward through the valve, a sound is made. This sound, called a murmur, generally can be heard with a stethoscope.

When a heart valve fails to function properly, the ability of the heart to do work is impaired. In an attempt to maintain normal work levels, the heart begins to enlarge, or experience hypertrophy. When further hypertrophy is no longer possible, the heart fails. This condition will result in permanent damage to the heart muscle and eventually death. Some of the symptoms of valve problems include chest pain or tightness, shortness of breath, temporary blindness, slurred speech, weakness, numbness, lack of coordination, unusually rapid weight gain, fatigue, and loss of consciousness. These symptoms are typically the result of inadequate blood flow, particularly to the brain.

In some cases, surgery can be used to repair the valve. Many times, however, the damage is too extensive for this type of surgery, and the valve must be replaced. The replacement valve may come from a deceased person's heart or from an animal's heart (usually that of a pig), or it may be a mechanical (prosthetic) valve. Prosthetic valves are made from metal, plastic, or carbon ceramic.

During valve replacement surgery, the chest is opened to expose the heart. Blood flow through the heart is diverted through an oxygenator and a pump that maintains the flow of oxygenated blood throughout the body. The surgeon removes the damaged valve and sutures a replacement valve to the heart. Upon completion of the surgery, if the replaced valve functions effectively, normal blood flow is restored through the heart.

USES AND COMPLICATIONS

Heart valve replacement is a very reliable procedure. Although problems with the new valve are possible, the majority of these surgeries are 100 percent effective. Nevertheless, there are two long-term concerns for the patient. Blood thinners or anticoagulants—drugs that slow the clotting process and may prevent blood clots—are usually required with prosthetic valves. These drugs help prevent blood from coagulating in and around the new valve. Some patients must also take antibiotics to prevent additional infections in the heart. Antibiotics are needed especially when patients visit the dentist, when bleeding is likely. If bleeding occurs, bacteria may enter the blood and become lodged in the replacement valve. The ensuing infection can cause further damage to the heart.

When one compares the use of tissue versus mechanical (prosthetic) valves for replacement, some differences emerge. In general, tissue valves work better. In addition, they are less likely to require drugs to increase blood-clotting time. On the other hand, they are harder to obtain. With more people acting as donors and with better preservation techniques becoming available, tissue replacements are preferred.

PERSPECTIVE AND PROSPECTS

Mechanical valves were first used as replacements for damaged valves in the early 1960's. In 1962, the initial clinical use of tissue valves was described. Tissue valve replacements were conducted simultaneously by Donald Ross in England and Sir Brian Barratt-Boyes in New Zealand. The acceptance of tissue valve use was slow because the number of donors was small and the methods for preserving valves for later use were poor. The result was shorter survival times for the replacement valves used in the 1960's and early 1970's.

By the 1980's, better preservation techniques were developed, which allowed surgeons to use living human tissue. These replacements have been found to be superior to nonliving tissues and mechanical valves. In the future, both mechanical and tissue replacements will continue to be used, based on availability and the specific needs of the patient.

—*Bradley R. A. Wilson, Ph.D.*

See also Angiography; Angioplasty; Bleeding; Blood and blood disorders; Bypass surgery; Cardiac rehabilitation; Cardiology; Cardiology, pediatric; Circulation; Electrocardiography (ECG or EKG); Endocarditis; Heart; Heart attack; Heart disease; Heart failure; Heart transplantation; Pacemaker implantation; Rheumatic fever; Thrombolytic therapy and TPA.

FOR FURTHER INFORMATION:

Bonhoeffer, Philipp, et al. "Percutaneous Replacement of Pulmonary Valve in a Right-Ventricle to Pulmonary-Artery Prosthetic Conduit with Valve Dysfunction." *The Lancet* 356, no. 9239 (October 21, 2000): 1403-1405. The authors show that percutaneous valve replacement in the pulmonary position is possible. With further technical improvements, this new technique might be used for valve replacement in other cardiac and non-cardiac positions.

Mitka, Mike. "Final Report on Mechanical vs. Bioprosthetic Heart Valves." *The Journal of the American Medical Association* 283, no. 15 (April 19, 2000): 1947-1948. A long-term follow-up study presented at the annual meeting of the American College of Cardiology has given surgeons a clear answer to the question of whether to perform heart valve replacement with a mechanical or a bioprosthetic device.

Nauer, Kathleen A., Barbara Schouchoff, and Kathleen Demitras. "Minimally Invasive Aortic Valve Surgery." *Critical Care Nursing Quarterly* 23, no. 1 (May, 2000): 66-71. Heart surgery has seen the emergence of minimally invasive techniques in the quest for less traumatic and less painful surgery. This procedure can be provided without the increased cost of endoscopic instrumentation by use of standard instrumentation, cannulation, and prostheses.

Otto, Catherine M. "Timing of Aortic Valve Surgery." *Heart* 84, no. 2 (August, 2000): 211. The timing of aortic valve surgery is described for patients complaining of two conditions: aortic stenosis and chronic aortic regurgitation.

Rahimtoola, Shahbudin H., ed. *Valvular Heart Disease.* 3d ed. Philadelphia: Lippincott, Williams & Wilkins, 2000. Discusses diseases of the heart valve and their treatments. Includes bibliographical references and an index.

HEARTBURN

DISEASE/DISORDER

ANATOMY OR SYSTEM AFFECTED: Chest, gastrointestinal system, stomach

SPECIALTIES AND RELATED FIELDS: Family practice, gastroenterology, internal medicine

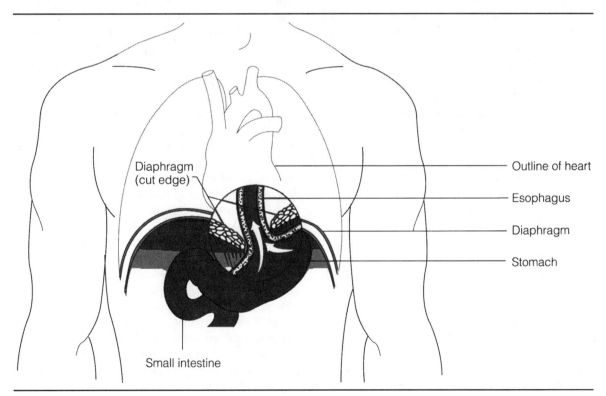

Heartburn is caused by a reflux of stomach acid into the esophagus shortly after eating.

DEFINITION: Also known as acid indigestion, heartburn is characterized by a burning sensation in the middle of the chest that may radiate upward to the throat; the term "heartburn" derives from its similarities to the pain of heart disease. It is caused by a reflux of stomach acids into the esophagus shortly after eating. Overeating, drinking alcohol, and consuming spicy or rich foods may precipitate an attack, as can lying down following a meal. Contributing factors include obesity, pregnancy, stress, emotional upset, the excessive swallowing of air, intestinal gas, congenital defects, and hiatal hernia. Antacids may be used to treat heartburn, and factors that trigger it should be avoided.

—Jason Georges and Tracy Irons-Georges
See also Gastroenterology; Gastroenterology, pediatric; Gastrointestinal disorders; Gastrointestinal system; Hernia; Hernia repair; Indigestion; Nausea and vomiting; Obesity; Pain; Stress; Stress reduction; Ulcer surgery; Ulcers; Vagotomy.

FOR FURTHER INFORMATION:

Janowitz, Henry D. *Indigestion: Living Better with Upper Intestinal Problems.* New York: Oxford University Press, 1992.

_____. *Your Gut Feelings: A Complete Guide to Living Better with Intestinal Problems.* Rev. ed. New York: Oxford University Press, 1994.

Peikin, Steven R., M.D. *Gastrointestinal Health: A Self-Help Nutritional Program to Prevent, Cure, or Alleviate Irritable Bowel Syndrome, Ulcers, Heartburn, Gas, Constipation, and Many Other Digestive Disorders.* Rev. ed. New York: HarperCollins, 1999.

Wolfe, M. Michael, and Sidney Cohen. *Therapy of Digestive Disorders: A Companion to Sleisenger and Fordtran's Gastrointestinal and Liver Disease.* Philadelphia: Saunders, 2000.

HEAT EXHAUSTION AND HEAT STROKE
DISEASE/DISORDER

ANATOMY OR SYSTEM AFFECTED: Blood vessels, circulatory system, skin
SPECIALTIES AND RELATED FIELDS: Critical care, emergency medicine, environmental health, family practice, internal medicine, sports medicine
DEFINITION: Heat-related illnesses in which the body temperature rises to dangerous levels and cannot be controlled through normal mechanisms, such as sweating.

CAUSES AND SYMPTOMS

The human body is well equipped to maintain a nearly constant internal body temperature. In fact, the body temperature of human beings is usually controlled so closely that it rarely leaves a very narrow range of 36.1 to 37.8 degrees Celsius (97 to 100 degrees Fahrenheit) regardless of how much heat the body is producing or what the environmental temperature may be. Humans maintain a constant temperature so that the millions of biochemical reactions in the body remain at an optimal rate. An increase in body temperature of only 1 degree Celsius will cause these reactions to move about 10 percent faster. As internal temperatures rise, however, brain function becomes slower because important proteins and enzymes lose their ability to operate effectively. Most adults will go into convulsions when their temperature reaches 41 degrees Celsius (106 degrees Fahrenheit), and 43 degrees Celsius (110 degrees Fahrenheit) is usually fatal.

A special region of the brain known as the hypothalamus regulates body temperature. The hypothalamus detects the temperature of the blood much like a thermostat detects room temperature. When the body (and hence the blood) becomes too warm, the hypothalamus activates heat-loss mechanisms. Most excess heat is lost through the skin by the radiation of heat and the evaporation of sweat. To promote this heat loss, blood vessels in the skin dilate (open up) to carry more blood to the skin. Heat from the warm blood is then lost to the cooler air. If the increase in blood flow to the skin is not enough, then sweat glands are stimulated to produce and secrete large amounts of sweat. The process, called perspiration, is an efficient means of ridding the body of excess heat as long as the humidity is not too high. In fact, at 60 percent humidity, evaporation of sweat from the skin stops. When the body cannot dissipate enough heat, heat exhaustion and heat stroke may occur.

Heat exhaustion is the most prevalent heat-related illness. It commonly occurs in individuals who have exercised or worked in high temperatures for long periods of time. These people have usually not ingested adequate amounts of fluid. Over time, the patient loses fluid through sweating and respiration, which decreases the amount of fluid in the blood. Because the body is trying to reduce its temperature, blood has been shunted to the skin and away from vital internal organs. This reaction, in combination with a reduced blood volume, causes the patient to go into mild shock. Common signs and symptoms of heat exhaustion include cool, moist skin that may appear either red or pale; headache; nausea; dizziness; and exhaustion. If heat exhaustion is not recognized and treated, it can lead to life-threatening heat stroke.

Heat stroke occurs when the body is unable to eradicate the excess heat as rapidly as it develops. Thus, body temperature begins to rise. Sweating stops because the water content of the blood decreases. The loss of evaporative cooling causes the body temperature to continue rising rapidly, soon reaching a level that can cause organ damage. In particular, the brain, heart, and kidneys may begin to fail until the patient experiences convulsions, coma, and even death. Therefore, heat stroke is a serious medical emergency which must be recognized and treated immediately. The signs and symptoms of heat stroke include high body temperature (41 degrees Celsius or 106 degrees Fahrenheit); loss of consciousness; hot, dry skin; rapid pulse; and quick, shallow breathing.

TREATMENT AND THERAPY

As with most illnesses, prevention is the best medicine for heat exhaustion and heat stroke. When exercising in hot weather, people should wear loose-fitting, lightweight clothing and drink plenty of fluids. When individuals are not prepared to avoid heat-related illness, however, rapid treatment may save their lives. When emergency medical personnel detect signs and symptoms of sudden heat-induced illness, they attempt to do three major things: cool the body, replace body fluids, and minimize shock.

For heat exhaustion, the initial treatment should be to place the patient in a cool place, such as a bathtub filled with cool (not cold) water. The conscious patient is given water or fruit drinks, sometimes containing salt, to replace body fluids. Occasionally, intravenous fluids must be given to return blood volume to normal in a more direct way. Hospitalization of the patient may be necessary to be sure that the body is able to regulate body heat appropriately. Almost all patients treated quickly and effectively will not advance to heat stroke. The activity that placed the patient in danger should be discontinued until one is sure all symptoms have disappeared and steps have been taken to prevent a future episode of heat exhaustion.

Heat stroke requires urgent medical attention, or the high body temperature will cause irreparable damage and often death. Body temperature must be reduced rapidly. With the patient in a cool environment, the clothing is removed and the skin sprinkled with water and cooled by fanning. Contrary to popular belief, rubbing alcohol should not be used, as it can cause closure of the skin's pores. Ice packs are often placed behind the neck and under the armpits and groin. At these sites, large blood vessels come close to the skin and are capable of carrying cooled blood to the internal organs. Body fluid must be replaced quickly by intravenous administration because the patient is usually unable to drink as a result of convulsions or confusion and may even be unconscious. Once the body temperature has been brought back to normal, the patient is usually hospitalized and watched for complications. With early diagnosis and treatment, 80 to 90 percent of previously healthy people will survive.

—Matthew Berria, Ph.D.

See also Critical care; Critical care, pediatric; Dehydration; Emergency medicine; Fever; Hyperthermia and hypothermia; Resuscitation; Shock; Unconsciousness.

FOR FURTHER INFORMATION:

Clayman, Charles B., ed. *The American Medical Association Encyclopedia of Medicine.* New York: Random House, 1994. A concise presentation of numerous medical terms and illnesses. A good general reference.

Hales, Dianne. *An Invitation to Health.* 9th ed. Belmont, Calif.: Wadsworth Thomson Learning, 2000. This text should be read by anyone who wishes an overview of health topics.

Marieb, Elaine N. *Human Anatomy and Physiology.* 5th ed. Redwood City, Calif.: Benjamin/Cummings, 2000. Nonscientists at the advanced high school level or above will be able to understand this fine textbook. It includes a complete glossary, index, pronunciation guide, and other helpful features.

HEEL SPUR REMOVAL

PROCEDURE

ANATOMY OR SYSTEM AFFECTED: Bones, feet, musculoskeletal system

SPECIALTIES AND RELATED FIELDS: General surgery, orthopedics, podiatry

DEFINITION: The surgical removal of a heel spur, a hard, bony growth on the heel.

INDICATIONS AND PROCEDURES

Heel spurs, also known as calcaneal spurs, are hard, bony growths on the heel bone. Pain and tenderness in the sole of the foot under the heel bone are common first indicators of this condition. Painful heel spurs can cause difficulty in walking and standing. Running, jogging, and prolonged standing often contribute to their development, especially when unpadded shoes are worn. When efforts to alleviate pain, such as activity modification and the use of shoes with cushioned heels, have been exhausted, it may be necessary for the spur to be surgically removed.

Most heel spur removal operations are performed at outpatient surgical facilities. Before the operation, blood and urine studies are conducted, and X rays are taken of both feet. Local or spinal anesthetics are administered. The surgeon, orthopedist, or podiatrist conducting the operation will choose a convenient site to make an incision, usually over the spur. Using special instruments, the heel spur is carved free and removed. The opening in the skin is closed with sutures. Barring complications, the sutures can be removed ten to fourteen days later. After the surgery, additional blood studies are taken, and laboratory examination of the removed tissue is performed.

USES AND COMPLICATIONS

Heel spurs form as a result of hard pounding or prolonged stress on the heel of the foot. Shock-absorbing soles in shoes and orthopedic inserts that cushion hard blows to the heel during vigorous exercise can help prevent and aid in recovery from heel spur operations. Following a removal operation, vigorous exercise can be resumed in approximately three months.

Clean cloths or tissues can be pressed against the wound for ten minutes if bleeding occurs within the first twenty-four hours after the surgery. The scar from the incision will recede gradually. Although it is important to keep the foot clean, the wound must be kept dry between baths. For the first two or three days after surgery, the wound should be covered with a dry bandage. Complications associated with heel spur removal surgery can include excessive bleeding and surgical wound infection, which should be examined by a doctor.

—*Jason Georges*

See also Bone disorders; Bones and the skeleton; Feet; Foot disorders; Lower extremities; Orthopedic surgery; Orthopedics; Podiatry.

FOR FURTHER INFORMATION:

Copeland, Glenn, and Stan Solomon. *The Foot Doctor.* Emmaus, Pa.: Rodale Press, 1986.

Lorimer, Donald L., ed. *Neale's Common Foot Disorders: Diagnosis and Management.* Rev. 4th ed. New York: Churchill Livingstone, 1993.

Shangold, Jules, and Frank Greenberg. *Opportunities in Podiatric Medicine.* Skokie, Ill.: VGM Career Horizons, 1982.

HEMATOLOGY

SPECIALTY

ANATOMY OR SYSTEM AFFECTED: Blood, bones, circulatory system, immune system, liver, musculoskeletal system, spleen

SPECIALTIES AND RELATED FIELDS: Cardiology, cytology, forensic medicine, genetics, immunology, oncology, pathology, serology, vascular medicine

DEFINITION: The study of the blood, including its normal constituents, and such blood disorders as anemia, leukemia, and hemophilia.

KEY TERMS:

anemia: a condition characterized by a deficiency of red blood cells or hemoglobin

bone marrow: the soft substance that fills the cavities within bones and that is the site of blood cell production

clotting factors: chemicals circulating in the blood which are necessary for the process of blood clotting

hematologist: one who specializes in the study of blood, its components and disorders

hemoglobin: the iron-containing molecule within red blood cells responsible for oxygen and carbon dioxide transport

leukemia: a condition characterized by the presence of numerous immature white blood cells in the circulating blood

plasma: the fluid portion of blood, containing water, proteins, minerals, nutrients, hormones, and wastes

platelets: specialized cell fragments that initiate blood clotting

red blood cell: a flexible, biconcave blood cell that contains hemoglobin

white blood cell: one of several types of colorless, large blood cells that work together to combat infections

SCIENCE AND PROFESSION

Most branches of medical science study a particular organ that is made of specific tissues and is located in a definite part of the body. Hematology is unique because its subject, the blood, is a liquid tissue constantly in motion and therefore in constant contact with every other tissue and organ of the body.

It has been estimated that blood travels about 16 kilometers (10 miles) an hour. It takes six seconds for blood to travel from the heart to the lungs, about eight seconds from the heart to the brain, and only fourteen seconds from the heart all the way to the toes. Hematologists studying these shifting currents of the blood are able to detect patterns that allow the early discovery of many disorders of the blood itself and of the organs that it supplies.

Blood is a complex material composed of approximately 55 percent plasma and 45 percent cells, which are also called formed elements. The plasma, or liquid portion of the blood, is about 90 percent water and 10 percent substances dissolved or suspended in that water. Part of that 10 percent consists of a remarkable array of substances, including nutrients, gases, salts, wastes, and hormones being transported around the body. The other, larger part of the 10 percent is another remarkable array—plasma proteins such as fibrinogen, albumin, and globulins with a great diversity of functions to accomplish. The modern hematologist's ability to measure and monitor all these plasma components precisely has greatly aided physicians in the treatment of innumerable diseases.

Beyond an analysis of the ingredients of the plasma, hematologists focus on the normal and abnormal conditions of the blood's cells. An individual has 25 trillion red blood cells; 10 million of these cells die or are destroyed each second, and 200 billion new ones need to be made each day. Hematologists discovered that these tiny, biconcave discs packed with hemoglobin transport the vast majority of the oxygen needed constantly by every cell of every organ for energy production.

Before each red blood cell is released from the bone marrow where it is produced, the bulk of its living nucleus is expelled. A small amount of nuclear material remains, as a fine network, in these young cells called reticulocytes. The number of reticulocytes released into the blood is an indication of the activity of the bone marrow. Hematologists use this number in both the diagnosis and the assessment of the response to treatment, in conditions such as the various forms of anemia.

Not only the total number and maturity but also the shape, diameter, and flexibility of red blood cells can give the hematologist important information. For years, such information was gathered by laborious manual methods. Electronic counters can now obtain this information with great speed and even greater accuracy.

Hematologists can also gauge the effectiveness of red blood cells by seeing how much hemoglobin they contain. The amount of this red pigment present—and therefore functioning—was once estimated by being matched against progressively darker-colored glass "standards." Now this figure too is accurately perceived using a precise, photoelectric technique.

Another useful test is called the packed cell volume (PCV) test. It not only reveals the proportion of the red blood cells to the plasma but also allows the calculation of their average size and their hemoglobin content.

An equally common blood investigation is the erythrocyte sedimentation rate (ESR). The erythrocytes, the term that hematologists use to describe red blood cells, normally fall slowly down through the plasma in a standard tube. A very rapid sedimentation rate demonstrates a disturbance in the plasma proteins that may be very dangerous. Usually, the faster they settle out, the sicker the patient, with a wide variety of inflammations as possible causes.

Beginning in the middle of the twentieth century, an increasing number of radioactive tests were developed by which hematologists can assess more accurately total blood volume and the survival time of red blood cells or platelets in circulation. Assessing total volume is important. A loss of more than 1 liter (2 pints) is quite dangerous because it can cause a total collapse of the blood vessels.

This reaction gives a clue about the importance of a second kind of blood cell, the platelet, and its work in stopping bleeding. When a blood vessel is first cut, platelets (or thrombocytes) rush to the site. They swell into irregular shapes, become sticky, clog the cut, and create a plug. The smallest blood vessels rupture hundreds of times a day, and platelets alone are able to make the necessary repairs. If the cut is too large, platelets—which are like sponges filled with diverse and biologically active compounds—disintegrate. Their ingredients react with numerous clotting factors in the plasma to initiate clot formation.

Hematologists check blood samples carefully to ascertain whether their patients possess the normal number of platelets—more than a trillion for the average adult. Since platelets only live about ten days, it is necessary to monitor those patients who exhibit significantly low amounts of these cells. If their bone marrow is not constantly replacing these platelets, these patients might bleed to death from a small cut. On the other hand, doctors must monitor any tendency toward the formation of too many platelets because of the danger of thrombophlebitis, the blockage of a vein by a blood clot.

As with red blood cells, the widespread use of electronic counters has made the measurement of the numbers of platelets and of white blood cells (the third type of blood cell) rapid, efficient, and extremely accurate.

White blood cells are hardest to count because they are the least numerous, making up only 0.1 percent of the total blood. Their number also varies dramatically from 4,000 to 11,000 per cubic centimeter of blood, according to the individual, the time of day, the outside temperature, and many other ordinary factors.

Hematologists can deduce the degree of maturity of circulating white blood cells from the appearance of their nuclei. There are five kinds of white blood cells (or leukocytes), whose normal proportions in the blood are quite specific and change drastically if an infection is present. The number of monocytes, for example, is normally 5 percent. If typhus, tuberculosis, or Rocky Mountain spotted fever organisms are present, the number will rise to 20 or 30 percent. The normal 60 percentage of neutrophils will increase to 75 percent or more in the presence of pneumonia or appendicitis.

DIAGNOSTIC AND TREATMENT TECHNIQUES

Blood to be tested by a hematologist is withdrawn from a vein. A thin smear or film of the blood is placed on a glass slide and stained to bring out identifying features more prominently. The microscope then reveals the proportion of different cell types and any variation from the normally expected amount. This examination alone may give an immediate diagnosis of a particular blood disorder. For example, a red blood cell count that is less than 4 million or more than 6 million per cubic centimeter of blood is considered unusual and is probably an indication of disease.

It often becomes necessary to study not only the circulating blood cells but also the original cells within the bone marrow which produce the erythrocytes, thrombocytes, and leukocytes. The hematologist must then use a long, thin needle to remove a sample of the marrow from within the tibia (shinbone) of a child or the pelvis (hipbone) or sternum (breastbone) of an adult. This test can provide a reliable diagnosis of a specific blood disorder.

The blood disorders that hematologists are routinely called on to diagnose and treat include diseases of the red blood cells, white blood cells, platelets, and clotting factors and failures of correct blood formation.

The disorders involving a deficiency of red blood cells or their hemoglobin are called anemias. There are many types of anemia which are named, distinguished, and treated according to their causes. Some anemias exist because of a lack of the materials needed to build red blood cells: iron, vitamin B_{12}, and folic acid. Other anemias are caused by a shortening of the life span of red blood cells or by inherited abnormalities in hemoglobin. Still others are attributable to chronic infections or cancer.

Iron-deficiency anemia is by far the most common; it is particularly prevalent in women of childbearing age and in children. In young children who are growing rapidly, constant increase in muscle mass and blood volume will cause anemia unless a high enough level of iron is present in the diet. All women between puberty and the menopause lose iron with the menstrual flow of blood and, therefore, are always prone to iron-deficiency anemia. A pregnant woman is even more likely to develop this condition; iron is literally removed from her body and transferred through the placenta to the developing fetus.

The symptoms of iron-deficiency anemia may include a reduced capacity for physical work, paleness, breathlessness, increased pulse and, possibly, a sore tongue. The hematologist witnessing small, misshapen red blood cells deficient in hemoglobin will recommend an increase in iron in the diet. The hematologist will also send this patient for various gastrointestinal tests because of the possibility of internal bleeding or failure of the intestine to absorb iron properly.

Another class of anemias involves a lack of vitamin B_{12} or of folic acid. Without the help of these two substances, the bone marrow cannot build red blood cells correctly. These anemias are diagnosed when the hematologist finds bizarre cells called megaloblasts in the patient's bone marrow. Both vitamin B_{12} and folic acid can be added to the diet or given by injection. The problem may stem, however, not from an insufficient amount of vitamin B_{12} in the diet but from the inability of the stomach lining to produce a substance called intrinsic factor. In this case, the patient will never be able to absorb this vitamin properly and is said to suffer from pernicious anemia.

Those anemias characterized by the early and too frequent destruction of red blood cells are grouped together as hemolytic anemias. Some of these disorders are acquired, while others are inherited. In both types, hemoglobin from the destroyed red blood cells can be detected by the hematologist in the plasma, the urine, or the skin, where it causes the yellowing called jaundice.

Because the many types of anemia are so common, hematologists find that the diagnosis and treatment of these diseases form a large part of their everyday practice. All types of leukemia, on the other hand, are quite rare. They are caused by a change in one kind of primitive blood cell in the bone marrow. The result is uncontrolled growth of these cells, which do not mature but which invade the blood as badly functioning cells. Leukemia is often thought of as cancer of the blood.

Although it is not known what causes leukemia in a particular person, the disease seems to be associated with certain factors, including injury by chemicals or radiation, viruses, and genetic predisposition. Many cases of acute leukemia occur either in children who are under fourteen or in adults who are between fifty-five and seventy-five years of age. In children, it is almost always a disorder in the bone marrow cells that produce the white blood cells, called lymphocytes. This disorder is called acute lymphoblastic leukemia, or ALL. Adult leukemia usually occurs in the bone marrow that forms some other type of white blood cell and is called acute nonlymphoblastic leukemia, or ANLL.

Hematologists diagnose both conditions by their shared symptoms: abnormal bone marrow tissue and a lack of normal white blood cells and platelets in the circulating blood. The patient will often have been referred to the hematologist because of an uncontrollable infection (from a lack of normal white blood cells) or uncontrollable bleeding (from a lack of normal platelets). In both children and adults, anemia usually accompanies acute leukemia because defective bone marrow is not able to produce red blood cells properly either.

Less rare than acute leukemia are the various chronic types. One called chronic granulocytic leukemia (CGL) occurs most often after the age of fifty. Unfortunately, its early symptoms are few and vague, so that the disease may have progressed greatly before its presence would even be suspected. By such time, an enormous enlargement of the spleen, along with elevations in both white blood cell and platelet counts, can be noted.

Two stages are usually seen in chronic granulocytic leukemia. Early treatment can relieve all symptoms, shrink the spleen, and return all blood cells to normal values. Eventually, however, the leukemic condition recurs, and the patient usually lives an average of only three years. Bone marrow transplantation from a suitable donor or a more recent process by which one's own marrow is removed, irradiated, and returned to the bones have become the increasingly common recommendations of the hematologist confronted with this condition.

A second type of chronic leukemia is known as chronic lymphatic leukemia (CLL). Unlike most of the other leukemias, CLL has no known cause, but it is most often found in male patients over the age of forty. Often quite symptomless, it is only discovered by chance. The hematologist is able to diagnose CLL by an increased proportion of abnormal white blood cells present in the blood. Surprisingly, this form of leukemia can vary from a case that remains symptomless, with the patient surviving twenty years or more, to a rapidly progressing case with increasing anemia and constant infections.

The third major class of disorders diagnosed and treated by hematologists consists of those involving abnormal bleeding. The diagnosis is quite simple. The hematologist notes whether bleeding from a tiny puncture in the ear lobe stops within three minutes, as it should. If the bleeding does not stop, the determination of the cause may be difficult: It may involve too few platelets or abnormal or missing clotting factors.

Very precise tests of an increasingly sophisticated nature are now used by hematologists to determine whether a bleeding disorder is attributable to inheritance (as with hemophilia), a vitamin K deficiency, or a side effect of medication or is secondary to a type of leukemia.

PERSPECTIVE AND PROSPECTS

That blood and the vessels that carry it are important to life and health was evident even to ancient peoples. Around 500 B.C.E., Alcmaeon, a Greek, was the first to discover that arteries and veins are different types of vessels. A century later, Hippocrates observed that blood, left to stand, settles into three distinct layers. The top or largest layer is a clear, straw-colored liquid that is now called plasma. The middle layer is a narrow white band that is now known to contain white blood cells. The bottom, quite large layer, he observed to be red; it contains the cells that are now called red blood cells.

Very little else of value seems to have been learned about the blood until the seventeenth century, which witnessed many discoveries in medical science. In 1628, William Harvey, an English doctor, demonstrated scientific evidence of circulation. He found proof of a circular route and of the purpose of circulation. By 1661, the Italian scientist Marcello Malpighi reported seeing the tiny vessels called capillaries in the lungs of the frog.

Another giant step toward modern hematology occurred in the 1660's because of the efforts of Richard Lower of England and Jean-Baptiste Denis of France. Almost simultaneously, they accomplished blood transfusions from dog to dog and, soon after, from animal to human. Some transfusions were very successful; others were fatal to the patient. Almost 250 years would pass before the reason for success or failure would be learned.

In 1688, the Dutch scientist Antoni van Leeuwenhoek was able to describe and measure red blood cells accurately. He also observed that they changed shape to squeeze through tiny blood vessels. It was almost a hundred years later, in the 1770's, that Joseph Priestley, in England, found that the oxygen in the air changed dark blood from the veins into a bright red color. Only in the 1850's did the German researcher Otto Funke find within those red blood cells the compound hemoglobin, which is affected by the presence or absence of oxygen.

Although the first research on blood clotting, by William Hewson, occurred in 1768, the disease called hemophilia, or the failure of the blood to clot, was not described until 1803, by John Otto.

In the United States in the early 1900's, Karl Landsteiner discovered why certain blood can be safely transfused: the existence of the ABO blood types. This renowned hematologist was still advancing his science forty years later when he discovered the Rh system of blood types.

Another renowned hematologist, Max Perutz, worked steadily from 1939 to 1978 to understand fully the structure and function of the hemoglobin molecule. The 1940's had seen another breakthrough when Edwin Cohn, another American, discovered how to separate and purify the various plasma proteins. His work gave fellow hematologists the tools to study individual plasma components in order to learn the exact role of each in the blood. Since that time, scores of hematologists have so advanced this medical science that blood seems to have yielded most of its secrets. The ability of hematologists to treat so many types of anemia, leukemia, and other blood disorders successfully is the fruit of their tireless work.

—Grace D. Matzen

See also Acquired immunodeficiency syndrome (AIDS); Anemia; Bleeding; Blood and blood disorders; Blood testing; Bone marrow transplantation; Cholesterol; Circulation; Cytology; Cytopathology; Dialysis; Fluids and electrolytes; Forensic pathology; Hematology, pediatric; Hemolytic disease of the newborn; Hemophilia; Histology; Hodgkin's disease; Host-defense mechanisms; Hypercholesterolemia; Hyperlipidemia; Immune system; Immunology; Infection; Ischemia; Jaundice; Kidney disorders; Kidneys; Laboratory tests; Leukemia; Liver; Lymphadenopathy and lymphoma; Lymphatic system; Nephrology; Nephrology, pediatric; Rh factor; Septicemia; Serology; Sickle-cell disease; Thalassemia; Thrombolytic therapy and TPA; Thrombosis and thrombus; Toxemia; Transfusion; Vascular medicine; Vascular system.

FOR FURTHER INFORMATION:

Avraham, Regina. *The Circulatory System*. Philadelphia: Chelsea House, 2000. Contains a brief but excellent description of the blood: its many components and their diverse functions. Includes a useful glossary and a lengthy appendix listing other sources of information about blood and circulatory disorders.

Hackett, Earle. *Blood: The Biology, Pathology, and Mythology of the Body's Most Important Fluid.* New York: Saturday Review Press, 1973. This old but classic and, therefore, still relevant volume contains an entertaining but nevertheless factual history of the study of blood from the viewpoint of many peoples in many cultures, from ancient to modern times.

Parker, Steve. *The Heart and Blood*. New York: Franklin Watts, 1989. A very brief but exceptionally well-illustrated volume, using beautiful photography and diagrams most effectively. Written in a clear and concise fashion for a high school audience.

Tortora, Gerard J. *Introduction to the Human Body: The Essentials of Anatomy and Physiology*. 5th ed. New York: Wiley, 2000. A general textbook of anatomy and physiology. Contains one hundred pages of information about the blood, the vessels in which it travels, the heart that pumps it, and the relationship of blood to immunity.

HEMATOLOGY, PEDIATRIC

SPECIALTY

ANATOMY OR SYSTEM AFFECTED: Blood, bones, circulatory system, immune system, liver, musculoskeletal system, spleen

SPECIALTIES AND RELATED FIELDS: Cytology, genetics, immunology, neonatology, pathology, pediatrics, perinatology, serology, vascular medicine

DEFINITION: The diagnosis and treatment of blood disorders in infants and children.

KEY TERMS:

anemia: a red blood cell deficiency caused by a decrease in hemoglobin or red cell production, an increase in cell destruction, or blood loss

erythrocytes: red blood cells

hematology: the scientific, medical study of blood and blood-forming tissues

hematopoiesis: the production of red and white cells and platelets, which occurs mainly in bone marrow

hemorrhage: the loss of a large amount of blood in a short period of time

leukemia: the presence of an increased number of leukocytes in the blood, with the specific disorder classified according to the predominant proliferating cells, the clinical course, and the duration of the disease

leukocytes: white blood cells

leukopenia: an abnormal decrease in white blood cells

neonate: a newborn infant

pediatric: pertaining to neonates, infants, and children up to the age of twelve

polycythemia: an abnormal increase in red blood cells

thrombocytes: platelets

venipuncture: a method of obtaining blood from a vein using a tourniquet, needle, and syringe

SCIENCE AND PROFESSION

Blood, the body's life-sustaining fluid, is composed of red and white cells and platelets floating in plasma. Blood transports oxygen from the lungs to the tissues; removes waste products such as carbon dioxide, urea, and lactic acid; transports hormones and nutrients; removes body heat from central to peripheral parts of the body; clots in order to seal hemorrhages; transports leukocytes and antibodies to fight injury and infection; and stores and circulates elements such as calcium and iron. The diagnosis of hematologic disorders requires the comparison of blood and bone marrow values to established reference ranges. These ranges can vary considerably during a child's growing years, with such important changes as polycythemia in the neonatal period followed by physiologic anemia of infancy, which is maximal at two and a half to three months.

Pediatric hematology involves the ongoing assessment of an infant's or child's blood and bone marrow. This specialty requires such skills as the identification of problems, the setting of goals, the use of appropriate interventions (including diet, teaching, and medication), and an evaluation of the outcome of this care. Routine blood screening involves the removal of blood by a medical laboratory phlebotomist using venipuncture in children and heel or finger stick in infants to assess the following: a complete coronary risk profile with lipid fractionation, a complete blood count (CBC), a chemistry 27 profile, an iron-deficiency profile, and diabetes mellitus screening.

A complete coronary risk profile with lipid fractionation is an assessment of total serum cholesterol, high-density lipoprotein cholesterol, low-density lipoprotein cholesterol, very-low-density lipoprotein cholesterol, total cholesterol/high-density lipoprotein cholesterol ratio, triglycerides, chylomicrons, and possibly apolipoproteins. A CBC involves an analysis of hemoglobin, hematocrit, and red and white blood cell counts with white blood cell differential, including granulocytes (neutrophils, eosinophils, and basophils) and agranulocytes (lymphocytes and monocytes). A chemistry 27 profile assesses important blood constituents such as iron and protein storage, uric acid, several electrolytes, and enzymes. An iron-deficiency profile includes measurements of total iron-binding capacity, percentage of transferrin saturation, and serum ferritin. Diabetes mellitus screening, an assessment of glucose and protein-bound glucose (indicative of the previous seven to fifteen days), is important because only an estimated one-half of all diabetics are diagnosed.

Some of the major manifestations of hematologic disease in infants and children are disorders in the function of red blood cells, white blood cells, or hemostasis. Red blood cell disorders include anemia caused by the inadequate production of erythrocytes and/or hemoglobin as a result of genetic disease or iron deficiency, anemia caused by excessive loss of erythrocytes as a result of hemorrhage or hemolytic problems, polycythemia, erythrocytosis, erythremia, and blood transfusion. Disorders of white blood cells include leukopenia, agranulocytosis, periodic neutropenia, Chediak-Higashi syndrome, and leukemias. Blood diseases associated with defects in hemostasis include disturbances in the mechanism for clotting, such as hemophilia, Von Willebrand's syndrome, deficiencies in factor II (prothrombin), factor XII deficiency, and disorders involving fibrinogen and fibrin; and defects in hemostasis in small vessels, such as thrombocytopenia, Aldrich's syndrome, and thrombopoetin deficiency.

DIAGNOSTIC AND TREATMENT TECHNIQUES

The diagnosis of pediatric hematological disorders begins with a routine blood chemistry analysis, leading to more specific tests and a medical history of the infant or child and family members to determine if the problem is congenital or acquired, chronic or episodic, and static or progressive. Iron deficiency (also called anemia) is probably the most common nutritional problem in the world today. Anemia decreases work capacity by restricting oxygen and carbon dioxide transport and reducing aerobic energy production via the inhibition of iron-dependent muscle enzymes. Therapy for anemia generally involves diet manipulation and medication but is highly variable and depends on the specific causative factors. Since the prevalence of anemia correlates strongly with socioeconomic status, screening intervals and therapy must be planned individually for each child. Up to 20 percent of children from poor homes may be anemic at one year of age, while only 4 percent of children from higher-income homes will be anemic. Anemia becomes less common between three and five years of age, thus diminishing the need for regular screening.

PERSPECTIVE AND PROSPECTS

Future research in pediatric hematology will probably include further investigation of reticulocytes, immature red blood cells that are larger than mature erythrocytes yet nonnucleated, that circulate in the blood for one to two days while maturing. Research into the causes of and prevention techniques for the development of anemia will continue to be a major focus.

Public health authorities have recently recommended routine screening of the entire newborn population for a variety of hereditary diseases, including acquired immunodeficiency syndrome (AIDS). This recommendation is likely to generate considerable controversy. Many states have recently required screening for phenylketonuria (PKU), a condition which can be toxic to brain tissue, even though it occurs in fewer than 1 in 16,000 neonates.

—*Daniel G. Graetzer, Ph.D.*

See also Acquired immunodeficiency syndrome (AIDS); Anemia; Bleeding; Blood and blood disorders; Blood testing; Bone marrow transplantation; Circulation; Cytology; Cytopathology; Dialysis; Fluids and electrolytes; Hematology; Hemolytic disease of the newborn; Hemophilia; Histology; Host-defense mechanisms; Immune system; Immunology; Infection; Ischemia; Jaundice; Kidney disorders; Kidneys; Laboratory tests; Leukemia; Liver; Lymphadenopathy and lymphoma; Lymphatic system; Nephrology, pediatric; Pediatrics; Rh factor; Septicemia; Serology; Sickle-cell disease; Thalassemia; Toxemia; Transfusion; Vascular medicine; Vascular system.

FOR FURTHER INFORMATION:

Nathan, David G., and Stuart H. Orkin, eds. *Nathan and Oski's Hematology of Infancy and Childhood*. Rev. 5th ed. Philadelphia: W. B. Saunders, 1998. This textbook will undoubtedly be useful to many readers not directly involved in clinical or research pediatric hematology. First, it provides basic scientists with a clinical perspective. Second, pediatric and adult subspecialists will occasionally need it to read about rare conditions, and it should be included in the reference collection of every library on adult hematology or general pediatrics.

Smith, C. H. *Smith's Blood Diseases of Infancy and Childhood*. Edited by Denis R. Miller et al. St. Louis: C. V. Mosby, 1978. A thorough text on all aspects of pediatric hematology. Includes bibliographical references and an index.

Wintrobe, M. M., et al. *Wintrobe's Clinical Hematol-*

ogy. 10th ed. Philadelphia: Lea & Febiger, 1999. This edition adds 15 new chapters (for a total of 103), including a new segment on laboratory hematology, with emphasis on interpretation. This section includes new chapters on immunodiagnosis, flow cytometry, clusters of differentiation, cytogenetics, and molecular genetics.

HEMIPLEGIA
DISEASE/DISORDER

ANATOMY OR SYSTEM AFFECTED: Arms, legs, muscles, musculoskeletal system, nerves, nervous system

SPECIALTIES AND RELATED FIELDS: Neurology, physical therapy

DEFINITION: Hemiplegia is paralysis or weakness on one side of the body; it may affect the arm, leg, trunk, or face, or a combination of these. Spastic hemiplegia is characterized by stiff muscles, while flaccid hemiplegia is characterized by wasted, limp muscles. Unlike paraplegia (paralysis from the waist downward) or quadriplegia (paralysis from the neck downward), hemiplegia is attributable to brain injuries and diseases, rather than to spinal cord damage. Hemiplegia can result from a stroke, encephalitis, multiple sclerosis, meningitis, or hemorrhages or tumors in the brain. Physical therapy is used to aid in mobility, and treatment consists of addressing the underlying cause.

—*Jason Georges and Tracy Irons-Georges*

See also Brain; Brain disorders; Cerebral palsy; Encephalitis; Meningitis; Multiple sclerosis; Nervous system; Neurology; Neurology, pediatric; Paralysis; Paraplegia; Physical rehabilitation; Quadriplegia; Strokes.

FOR FURTHER INFORMATION:

Andreoli, Thomas E., et al. *Cecil Essentials of Medicine*. 5th ed. Philadelphia: W. B. Saunders, 2001.

Goroll, Allan H., Lawrence A. May, and Albert G. Mulley, Jr. *Primary Care Medicine*. Rev. 4th ed. Philadelphia: J. B. Lippincott, 2000.

Spence, Alexander P., and Elliott B. Mason. *Human Anatomy and Physiology*. 4th ed. St. Paul, Minn.: West, 1992.

HEMOLYTIC DISEASE OF THE NEWBORN
DISEASE/DISORDER

ALSO KNOWN AS: Erythroblastosis fetalis, Rh incompatibility, ABO incompatibility

ANATOMY OR SYSTEM AFFECTED: Blood, brain, liver, skin

SPECIALTIES AND RELATED FIELDS: Hematology, neonatology, neurology

DEFINITION: The destruction of red blood cells in a fetus by antibodies transferred from the mother.

KEY TERMS:

antibodies: proteins produced by the immune system to destroy invading organisms or those perceived as foreign to the body

bilirubin: a pigment derived from the breakdown of red blood cells

Coombs' test: a test used to determine whether sensitization has occurred

exchange transfusion: the exchange of all or most of a patient's blood for donor blood; in a baby with hemolytic disease, usually performed through the umbilical vein

hemolysis: the rapid destruction of red blood cells

jaundice: yellow pigmentation resulting from the deposition of bilirubin in the skin

kernicterus: brain damage produced by the deposition of bilirubin in the brain

Rhogam: a protein that destroys Rh-positive cells

sensitization: the development of antibodies to a substance

CAUSES AND SYMPTOMS

Hemolytic disease of the newborn is a disorder in which maternal antibodies induce hemolysis of the red blood cells of the fetus or newborn, producing jaundice. The most common causes are ABO or Rh incompatibilities. ABO incompatibility occurs when the mother's blood is type O and baby's blood is either type A or type B. The newborn develops jaundice within the first forty-eight hours of birth as a result of increasing bilirubin levels in the blood. Rh incompatibility can arise when an Rh-negative woman is carrying a second Rh-positive fetus. During the delivery of the first Rh-positive baby, blood from the newborn may pass into the mother's circulation. If no treatment is given, the woman may develop anti-Rh antibodies, which will remain in her circulation. If the fetus in her next pregnancy is also Rh-positive, the anti-Rh antibodies will cross over into the baby's blood, causing hemolysis of the red blood cells. In severe cases, the hemolysis starts in utero and the fetus will develop anemia, progressing to generalized edema with heart failure (hydrops fetalis) and death if the anemia is not corrected.

During the pregnancy, a positive Coombs' test indicates that the woman has been exposed and thus sensitized to Rh factor. A woman who is Rh-negative can become sensitized in three ways: by having delivered an Rh-positive baby following a previous pregnancy and not having received the protein Rhogam; by receiving an erroneous infusion of Rh-positive blood; and by having a spontaneous or induced abortion of an Rh-positive embryo or fetus. A rising concentration of antibodies during the course of the pregnancy indicates that hemolysis is occurring in the fetus. A small amount of amniotic fluid is obtained through a needle inserted through the mother's abdomen to determine the severity of the disease in the fetus. At birth, the baby may have pale skin and an enlarged liver and spleen. Progressive jaundice and anemia develop within the first twenty-four hours. High levels may cause the bilirubin to enter the brain and produce kernicterus. The baby with kernicterus shows little activity (hypoactivity), refuses to suck milk, and experiences seizures that can progress to permanent neurologic damage or to coma and death. Deafness may be a consequence of high bilirubin levels during the newborn period.

TREATMENT AND THERAPY

There is no preventive treatment for ABO incompatibility. Phototherapy, or light therapy, is used to decrease the level of bilirubin. Phototherapy acts on the bilirubin deposited in the skin and makes it water soluble, so that the pigment can be excreted through the gastrointestinal tract. An exchange transfusion may be required to decrease the concentration of bilirubin if it rises to dangerous levels. These levels will depend on the baby's maturation and clinical condition.

Preventive treatment for Rh incompatibility consists of giving Rhogam to all Rh-negative pregnant women at twenty-eight weeks of gestation and within the first seventy-two hours after the delivery of an Rh-positive baby. All Rh-negative women who have experienced an abortion or who have erroneously received a transfusion of Rh-positive blood should also receive Rhogam.

An Rh-negative pregnant woman with a positive Coombs' test needs to have periodic Coombs titers, or antibody concentration measurements, to determine what type of intervention, if any, is required. This test should first be done between sixteen and eighteen weeks of gestation. Rising Coombs titers indicate that hemolysis is occurring in the fetus. Prenatal interventions may include correcting fetal anemia by giving red blood cells directly to the fetus, either into the abdomen or into the umbilical vein. The fetus must be observed with sonography for the development of fetal edema, an ominous sign. At birth, the baby may have severe anemia requiring immediate correction. Phototherapy and an exchange transfusion may be needed if bilirubin rises above acceptable levels. Other modes of therapy such as phenobarbital, agar gel, and rectal suppositories are of limited value in reducing bilirubin in infants with hemolytic disease.

Before discharge from the hospital nursery, a hearing test must be done for all infants who have had jaundice during the neonatal period. Anemia may develop during the first six weeks of life as a result of the persistence of antibodies in the baby's blood. Close follow-up of hemoglobin levels must be done after discharge from the hospital. Blood transfusions may be indicated, as well as iron and folic acid supplementation.

PERSPECTIVE AND PROSPECTS

The incidence of Rh incompatibility has decreased remarkably since the advent of Rhogam. Nevertheless, it still occurs, particularly when unidentified miscarriages have occurred. Rh-negative fetuses can be identified early using special techniques available only in large medical centers. Therapy for hydrops fetalis has improved with the use of cordocentesis. This therapy, which consists of obtaining and transfusing blood directly into the umbilical cord while the fetus is in utero, is available in specialized medical centers and has helped many sensitized babies to survive. Immunoglobulin has been used to block hemolysis, but it cannot be used for treatment. Agents that can metabolize bilirubin are currently under investigation.

—*Gloria Reyes Báez, M.D.*

See also Anemia; Blood and blood disorders; Critical care, pediatric; Emergency medicine, pediatric; Hearing loss; Immune system; Jaundice; Neonatology; Umbilical cord.

FOR FURTHER INFORMATION:

Gruslin-Giroux, Andrée, and Thomas R. Moore. "Erythroblastosis Fetalis." In *Neonatal-Perinatal Medicine: Diseases of the Fetus and Infant*, edited by Avroy A. Fanaroff and Richard J. Martin. 6th ed. St. Louis: C. V. Mosby, 1997. A chapter in an exhaustive resource covering all the major diseases of the infant and fetus. Includes bibliographical references and an index.

Levy, Joseph. "Newborn Jaundice." *Parents Magazine* 69, no. 7 (July, 1994): 59-60. Jaundice is a fairly common condition in newborns because many do not have mature enough livers to process and excrete bilirubin, which causes the yellow color of jaundiced babies. The different types of jaundice, symptoms, and treatments for the disease are discussed.

Segel, George B. "Blood Disorder." In *Nelson Textbook of Pediatrics*, edited by Richard Behrman, Robert M. Kliegman, and Ann M. Arvin. 16th ed. Philadelphia: W. B. Saunders, 2000. A chapter in a standard textbook in the field. Offers detailed information intended mainly for pediatricians.

HEMOPHILIA

DISEASE/DISORDER

ANATOMY OR SYSTEM AFFECTED: Blood

SPECIALTIES AND RELATED FIELDS: Genetics, hematology, serology

DEFINITION: A genetic disorder characterized by the blood's inability to form clots as a result of the lack or alteration of certain trace plasma proteins.

KEY TERMS:

clotting factors: substances present in plasma that are needed for the coagulation of blood

hemophilia A: a genetic blood disease characterized by a deficiency of clotting factor VIII

hemophilia B: a genetic blood disease characterized by a deficiency of clotting factor IX

hemostasis: the process of stopping the flow of blood at an injury site

von Willebrand's disease: a genetic blood disease characterized by a deficiency of the von Willebrand clotting factor

CAUSES AND SYMPTOMS

The circulatory system must be self-healing; otherwise, continued blood loss from even the smallest injury would be life-threatening. Normally, all except the most catastrophic bleeding is rapidly stopped in a process known as hemostasis. Hemostasis takes place through several sequential steps or processes. First, an injury stimulates platelets (unpigmented blood cells) to adhere to the damaged blood vessels and then to one another, forming a plug that can stop minor bleeding. This association is mediated by what is called the von Willebrand factor, a protein that binds to the platelets. As the platelets aggregate, they release several substances that stimulate vasoconstriction, or a reduction in size of the blood vessels. This reduces the blood flow at the injury site. Finally, the aggregating platelets and damaged tissue initiate blood clotting, or coagulation. Once bleeding has stopped, the firmly adhering clot slowly contracts, drawing the edge of the wounds together so that tough scar tissue can form a permanent repair on the site.

Formation of a blood clot involves the participation of nearly twenty different substances, most of which are proteins synthesized by plasma. All but two of these substances, or factors, are designated by a roman numeral and a common name. A blood clot will be defective if one of the clotting factors is absent or deficient in the blood, and clotting time will be longer. The clotting factors, with some of their alternative names, are factor I (fibrinogen), factor II (prothrombin), factor III (tissue factor or thromboplastin), factor IV (calcium), factor V (proaccelerin), factor VII (proconvertin), factor VIII (antihemophilic factor), factor IX (Christmas factor), factor X (Stuart factor), factor XI (plasma thromboplastin antecedent), factor XII (Hageman factor), and factor XIII (fibrin stabilizing factor).

Several of the clotting factors have been discovered by the diagnosis of their deficiencies in various clotting disorders. The inherited coagulation disorders are uncommon conditions with an overall incidence of probably no more than 10 to 20 per 100,000 of the population. Hemophilia A, the most common or classic type of coagulation disorder, is caused by factor VIII deficiency. Hemophilia B (or Christmas disease) is the result of factor IX deficiency. It is quite common for severe hemophilia to manifest itself during the first year of life. Hazardous bleeding occurs in areas such as the central nervous system, the retropharyngeal area, and the retroperitoneal area. Bleeding in these areas requires admission to the hospital for observation and therapy. Joint lesions are very common in hemophilia because of acute spontaneous hemorrhage in the area, specially in weight-bearing joints such as ankles and knees. Urinary bleeding is often present at some time. The appearance of pseudotumors, caused by swelling involving muscle and bone produced by recurrent bleeding, is also common.

Hemophilia is transmitted entirely by unaffected

females (carriers) to their sons in a sex-linked inheritance deficiency. Congenital deficiencies of the other coagulation factors are well recognized, even though bleeding episodes in these cases are uncommon. Deficiency of more than one factor is also possible, although documentation of such cases is very rare, perhaps because only patients with milder variations of the disease survive.

Von Willebrand's disease, unlike the hemophilias that mainly involve bleeding in joints and muscles, involves mainly bleeding of mucocutaneous tissues or skin. It affects both men and women. This disease shares clinical characteristics with hemophilia A, or classic hemophilia, including decreased levels of clotting factor VIII. This similarity made the differentiation between the two diseases very difficult for a long time. It has now been established that there are two different factors involved in von Willebrand's disease, each with a different function. The von Willebrand factor is involved in the adhesion of platelets to the injured blood vessel wall and to one another, and together with factor VIII, circulates in plasma as a complex held by electrostatic and hydrophobic forces. The von Willebrand factor is a very large molecule, consisting of a series of possible multimeric structures. The bigger and heavier the multimer, the better it works against bleeding. Von Willebrand's disease is one of the least understood clotting disorders. Three types have been identified, with at least twenty-seven variations. With type I, all the multimers needed for successful clotting are present in the blood, but in lesser amounts than in healthy individuals. In type II, the larger multimers, which are more active in hemostasis, are lacking, and type III patients exhibit a severe lack of all multimers.

TREATMENT AND THERAPY

The normal body is continually producing clotting factors in order to keep up with natural loss. Sometimes the production is stepped up to cover a real or anticipated increase in the need for these factors, such as in childbirth. Hemophiliacs, lacking some of these clotting factors, may lose large amounts of blood from even the smallest injury and sometimes hemorrhage without any apparent cause. The symptoms of their diseases may be alleviated by the intravenous administration of the deficient clotting factor. How this is done depends on the specific factor deficiency and the magnitude of the bleeding episode, the age and size of the patient, convenience, acceptabil-

ity, cost of product, and method and place of delivery of care.

There are many sources for clotting factors. Fresh frozen plasma contains all the clotting factors, but since the concentration of the factors in plasma is relatively low, a large volume is required for treatment. Therefore, it can be used only when small amounts of clotting factor must be delivered. Its use is the only therapy for deficiencies of factors V, XI, and XII. Plasma is commonly harvested from single donor units to minimize the risk of infection by the hepatitis virus or human immunodeficiency virus (HIV), thus eliminating the risk involved in using pooled concentrates from many donors. Cryoprecipitates are the proteins that precipitate in fresh frozen plasma thawed at 4 degrees Celsius. The precipitate is rich in factors VIII and XIII and in fibrinogen, and carries less chance of infection with hepatitis. Its standardization is difficult, however, and is not required by the Food and Drug Administration. As a result, dosage calculation can be a problem. In addition, there is no method for the control of viral contamination. Therefore, cryoprecipitates are not commonly used unless harvested from a special known and tested donor pool. Clotting factor concentrates present many advantages. They are made from pooled plasma obtained from plasmapheresis or a program of total donor unit fractionation and are widely available. Factors VIII and IX can also be produced from plasma using monoclonal methods. Porcine factor VIII presents an alternative to patients with a naturally occurring antibody to human factor VIII.

Other substances can replace missing clotting factors as well. The synthetic hormone desmopressin acetate (also known by the letters DDAVP) has been used to stimulate the release of factor VIII and von Willebrand factor from the endothelial cells lining blood vessels. It is commonly used for patients with mild hemophilia and von Willebrand's disease. DDAVP has no effect on the concentration of the other factors, and aside from the common side effect of water retention, it is a safe drug. Antifibrinolytic drugs prevent the natural breakdown of blood clots that have already been formed. Although such drugs are not useful for the primary care of hemophiliacs, they are useful for use after dental extractions and in the treatment of other open wounds, after a clot has formed.

Between 10 and 15 percent of the patients affected with severe hemophilia develop factor VIII inhibitors (antibodies), which prevents their treatment with the usual methods. Newer therapeutic approaches have provided additional options for the management and control of bleeding episodes. The use of prothrombin complex concentrates or porcine factor VIII concentrates is indicated for low responders (those with a low amount of antibodies present in their system). An option for high responders is to try to eradicate the inhibitor present in their systems. One way to do this is with a regimen of immunosuppressive drugs. These are very limited in value, however, and cannot be used with HIV-positive hemophiliacs. The drugs used in this approach include substances such as cyclophosphamide, vincristine, azathioprine, and corticosteroids. Another approach utilizes intravenous doses of gamma globulin to suppress, but not eradicate, the inhibitors. Yet another strategy is an immune tolerance regimen, in which factor VIII is administered daily in small amounts. This method causes the inhibitors to decrease and, in some cases, disappear. The regimen can also involve the prophylactic use of factor VIII (or factor VIII in combination with immunosuppressive drugs).

The introduction of plasma clotting factor concentrates has changed the treatment of patients with clotting factor deficiencies. It has brought about a remarkable change in the longevity of these patients and their quality of life. The availability of cryoprecipitates and concentrates of factors II, VII, VIII, IX, X, and XIII has made outpatient treatment for bleeding episodes routine and home infusion or self-infusion a possibility for many patients. Hospitalization for inpatient treatment is rare, and early outpatient therapy of bleeding episodes has decreased the severity of joint deformities.

Nevertheless, other problems are apparent in hemophiliac patients. Viral contamination of the factor concentrates has allowed the development of chronic illnesses, infection with HIV, immunologic diseases, liver and renal diseases, joint disorders, and cardiovascular diseases. While the use of heat for virus inactivation, beginning in 1983, resulted in a reduction in HIV infections, the majority of patients exposed to the virus had already been infected. The strategies to prevent contraction of hepatitis from these concentrates include vaccination against the contaminating viruses and the elimination of viruses from the factor replacement product. The non-A, non-B hepatitis virus is very difficult to remove, however, and the use of monoclonal factors seems to be the only solution

to this problem. In general, difficulties associated with treatment have been largely eliminated through the production of the required clotting factors using recombinant DNA techniques, a process performed independent of human blood.

Treatment of von Willebrand's disease also includes pressure dressing, suturing, and oral contraceptives. A pasteurized antihemophiliac concentrate that contains substantial amounts of von Willebrand factor is used in severe cases.

Hematomas, or hemorrhages under the skin and within muscles, can frequently be controlled by application of elastic bandage pressure and ice. The ones that cannot be controlled easily within a few hours may cause muscle contraction and require factor replacement therapy. Exercise is recommended for joints after bleeding, as it helps protect joints by increasing muscle bulk and power and can also help relieve stress. Devices to protect joints, such as elastic bandages and splints, are commonly used. In extreme cases, orthopedic surgical procedures are readily available.

Analgesics, or painkillers, play an important part in the alleviation of chronic pain. Because patients cannot use products with aspirin and/or antihistamines, which inhibit platelet aggregation and prolong bleeding time, substances such as acetaminophen, codeine, and morphine are used. Chronic joint inflammation is reduced by the use of anti-inflammatory agents such as ibuprofen and of drugs used in rheumatoid arthritis patients.

The need for so many specialties and disciplines in the management of hemophilia has led to the development of multidisciplinary hemophilia centers. Genetic education (information on how the disease is transmitted), genetic counseling (the discussion of an individual's genetic risks and reproductive options), and genetic testing have provided great help to patients and affected families. Early and prenatal diagnosis and carrier detection have provided options for family planning.

PERSPECTIVE AND PROSPECTS

Descriptions of hemophilia are among the oldest known accounts of genetic disease. References to a bleeding condition highly suggestive of hemophilia go back to the fifth century, in the Babylonian Talmud. The first significant report in medical literature appeared in 1803 when John C. Otto, a Philadelphia physician, described several bleeder families with only males affected and with transmission through the mothers. The literature of the nineteenth century contains many descriptions of the disease, particularly the clinical characteristics of the hemorrhages and family histories. The disease was originally called haemorrhaphilia, or "tendency toward hemorrhages," but the name was later contracted through usage to hemophilia ("tendency toward blood"), the accepted name since around 1828.

Transfusion therapy was proposed as early as 1832, and the first successful transfusion for the treatment of a hemophiliac patient was reported in 1840 by Samuel Armstrong Lane. The use of blood from cows and pigs in the transfusions was explored but abandoned because of the numerous side effects. It was not until the beginning of the twentieth century that serious studies on clotting in hemophilia were started. Attention was directed to the use of normal human serum for treatment of bleeding episodes. Some of the patients responded well, while others did not. This result is probably attributable to the fact that some had hemophilia A—these patients did not respond because factor VIII, in which they are deficient, is not present in serum—while some others had hemophilia B, for which the therapy worked. In 1923, harvested blood plasma was used in transfusion, and it was shown to work as well as whole blood. With blood banking becoming a reality in the 1930's, transfusions were performed more frequently as a treatment for hemophilia.

The history of the fractionation of plasma began around 1911 with Dr. Addis, who prepared a very crude fraction by acidification of plasma. In 1937, Drs. Patek and Taylor produced a crude fraction which, on injection, lowered the blood-clotting time in hemophiliacs. In the period from 1945 to 1960, a number of plasma fractions with antihemophiliac activity were developed. The use of fresh frozen plasma increased as a result of advances in the purification of the fractions. Some milestones can be identified in the production of the plasma fractions: the development of quantitative assays for antihemophiliac factors, the discovery of cryoprecipitation, and the development of glycine and polyethylene precipitation.

In 1952, four significant and independent publications indicated that there is a plasma-clotting activity separate from that concerned with classic hemophilia—in other words, that there are two types of hemophilia. One (hemophilia A) is characterized by a deficiency in factor VIII, while the other (hemophilia B) is characterized by deficiency in factor IX. Carriers of hemophilia A can have a mean factor VIII level that is 50 percent lower than that of normal females, while carriers of hemophilia B show levels of factor IX that are 60 percent below normal. The two diseases have the same pattern of inheritance, are similar in clinical appearance, and can be distinguished only by laboratory tests.

Hemophilias are caused by a disordered and complex biological mechanism that continues to be explored. Recombinant DNA techniques have now revealed the molecular defect in factor VIII or factor IX deficiencies in some families, demonstrating that a variety of gene defects can produce the classic phenotype of hemophilia. These techniques have also provided new tools for carrier detection and prenatal diagnosis.

Current treatment of hemophilia has converted the hemophiliac from an in-hospital patient to an individual with more independent status. Crucial in this development has been the creation of comprehensive care centers and of the National Hemophilia Foundation, which provide comprehensive treatment for the hemophilia patient. With the advancement of recombinant DNA technology, the future looks brighter for the sufferers of this disease.

—*Maria Pacheco, Ph.D.*

See also Acquired immunodeficiency syndrome (AIDS); Bleeding; Blood and blood disorders; Genetic diseases; Genetics and inheritance; Transfusion.

For Further Information:

Bloom, Arthur L., ed. *The Hemophilias*. Methods in Hematology 5. New York: Churchill Livingstone, 1982. The series presents accounts of methods for the study of blood and its disorders. This book concentrates on hemophilia, presenting a description of available assay methods, purification methods, and prenatal diagnosis.

Hilgartner, Margaret W., and Carl Pochedly, eds. *Hemophilia in the Child and Adult*. 3d ed. New York: Raven Press, 1989. A compilation of the thoughts and experiences of clinicians who deal with hemophilia, as well as some practical approaches to patient care. A well-organized and informative book.

Jones, Peter. *Living with Haemophilia*. 4th ed. New York: Oxford University Press, 1995. An excellent book for the layperson, it was written specifically for patients and their families. In an easy-to-read, understandable format, explains the transmission of bleeding disorders through families, their manifestations, and their management.

Voet, Donald, and Judith G. Voet. *Biochemistry.* 2d ed. New York: John Wiley & Sons, 1998. A comprehensive biochemistry textbook with an excellent section on blood and blood-clotting mechanisms.

HEMORRHOID BANDING AND REMOVAL
PROCEDURE

ANATOMY OR SYSTEM AFFECTED: Anus, blood vessels, circulatory system, gastrointestinal system, intestines

SPECIALTIES AND RELATED FIELDS: Family practice, gastroenterology, general surgery, proctology

DEFINITION: The surgical ligation and removal of protruding veins from the lower rectum.

INDICATIONS AND PROCEDURES

Hemorrhoids, or piles, result from the protrusion or varicosity of veins found within the mucous membranes of the rectum. Hemorrhoids may develop either inside or outside the rectum, and they are among the more common of human afflictions.

Hemorrhoids generally develop as a result of increased pressure placed on veins within the rectum. The pressure may be attributable to straining as a result of constipation or to prolonged sitting. In women, they often develop during pregnancy and following childbirth. Treatment depends on the severity of discomfort and location of the hemorrhoid.

External hemorrhoids are often not painful, and they may respond to the application of cool compresses or over-the-counter astringent creams. Creams and suppositories containing steroids may be prescribed by a physician. Internal hemorrhoids may not be noticeable unless a vein ruptures, causing some bleeding, pain, and itching. Since bacteria regularly pass through the rectal area, infection may increase the itching and pain, eventually requiring treatment. If discomfort continues and is not relieved through simple medication, the hemorrhoids may require surgical removal. Several methods exist for removal. Often, the vein is stretched and cut off at its base. Local anesthetics may be necessary, and there may be bleeding and discomfort. Internal hemorrhoids may also be eliminated through cryosurgery, the application of subfreezing temperatures to eliminate tissue. The complete surgical removal of the hemorrhoid, hemorrhoidectomy, may be warranted under certain circumstances.

The Removal of Hemorrhoids

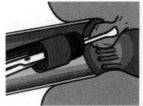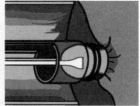

A proctoscope applying
a band to a hemorrhoid

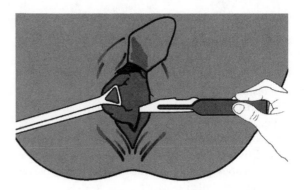

A hemorrhoid being withdrawn
by a clamp and cut off with a scalpel

Severe and distended hemorrhoids may be removed in one of two ways: through the placement of a rubber band around the base of the hemorrhoid, which constricts its blood supply and causes it to wither and drop off; or through surgical excision.

Hemorrhoid banding, also referred to as rubber band ligation and Barron ligation, involves the placement of a tight rubber band at the base of the hemorrhoid. Over the next few days, the vein will degenerate and slough off. The procedure is relatively simple and can be performed on an outpatient basis. Aside from some discomfort for several days, there are few side effects associated with the banding procedure. Warm sitz baths and local astringents may be helpful in reducing any swelling or pain, and the patient should eat a diet conducive to a soft stool.

—*Richard Adler, Ph.D.*

See also Colon and rectal surgery; Colonoscopy; Constipation; Cryotherapy and cryosurgery; Hemorrhoids; Pregnancy and gestation; Proctology; Varicose veins; Vascular medicine; Vascular system.

FOR FURTHER INFORMATION:

Becker, Barbara. *Relief from Chronic Hemorrhoids.* New York: Dell, 1992.

The Hemorrhoid Book: A Look at Hemorrhoids— How They're Treated and How You Can Prevent Them from Coming Back. San Bruno, Calif.: Krames Communications, 1991.

Sachar, David B., Jerome D. Waye, and Blair S. Lewis, eds. *Pocket Guide to Gastroenterology.* Rev. ed. Baltimore: Williams & Wilkins, 1991.

Wanderman, Sidney E., with Betty Rothbart. *Hemorrhoids.* Yonkers, N.Y.: Consumer Reports Books, 1991.

HEMORRHOIDS
DISEASE/DISORDER

ANATOMY OR SYSTEM AFFECTED: Anus, blood vessels, circulatory system, gastrointestinal system, intestines

SPECIALTIES AND RELATED FIELDS: Family practice, gastroenterology, proctology

DEFINITION: Blood-swollen enlargements of specialized tissues that help close the anus, as a result of intravenous pressure in the hemorrhoidal plexus; sometimes called piles.

KEY TERMS:

anus: the valve at the end of the rectum that prevents waste matter from leaking out until a person is ready to defecate

cauterize: to sear tissue with heat or a corrosive substance

dentate line: the junction in the anus where the external skin meets the internal mucosa

gastroenterologist: a physician who specializes in the gastrointestinal tract and related organs

mucosa: the mucus-secreting membrane that lines the surface of internal organs directly exposed to elements from outside the body, such as the lungs and intestines

proctologist: a physician who specializes in diseases of the rectum

rectum: the storage compartment at the end of the colon where wastes collect before defecation

stool: the excreted waste products of digestion

thrombosis: the condition of having a clot in a blood vessel

CAUSES AND SYMPTOMS

Hemorrhoids, some physiologists suggest, are one of the prices that humans pay for walking upright. The vascular system—the veins and arteries that circulate blood—evolved in an animal that walked on all fours. Now that humans spend most of their time standing, gravity puts awkward pressure on the system, and at the bottom of major parts of the system, as in the tissue around the anus, the column of blood above weighs heavily on the network of small blood vessels there. It does not take much additional pressure to cause a vessel's wall to balloon out. When it does, the result is a hemorrhoid, a little pouch protruding on the surface of the anus, similar to a hernia or varicose vein. Most Americans have hemorrhoids, even if they do not realize it, and the major symptoms are rarely dangerous, although they can be extremely annoying. Sometimes, however, hemorrhoids develop into or mask life-threatening diseases.

The term "hemorrhoid" derives from Greek words meaning "blood flowing," an apt description of the circulatory activity in the anal walls and an inadvertently apt warning of what most alarms people— hemorrhoids occasionally bleed. (The alternative, and now obsolescent, term "piles" comes from Latin *pila*, a ball, apparently a metaphor for the appearance of hemorrhoids.) Specifically, the "blood flowing" refers to the supple blood vessels of the internal rectal plexus, a series of pouches that act as cushions to help seal the anus shut. When these pouches become enlarged, they turn into hemorrhoids, which jut from the anus wall and swell up to 3 centimeters in length.

Because of the sphincter that controls defecation, not all hemorrhoids are visible without the aid of special instruments. The anus, an oval opening about three centimeters in front of the spine, is the valve ending the digestive tract. Like the mouth's lips, which begin the tract, the anus can purse shut, a state made possible by two concentric, circular sphincter muscles which act like drawstrings on a cloth bag. When sensors in the rectum signal the time to defecate, these muscles relax to pass stool and then immediately contract to close the anus again. As in the mouth, external skin meets the internal mucosal membrane in the anus; the meeting place is a corrugated joint called the dentate line (or, alternatively, the anorectal juncture or pectinase line). It is in this area—between the skin covering the external (or lower) sphincter and the mucosa over the internal (or upper) sphincter—that hemorrhoids form. Those that bulge out from the dentate line or above are hidden from sight by the closed anus and are called internal hemorrhoids; those that protrude below the closed anus, and so can be seen or felt, are called external hemorrhoids.

External hemorrhoids are the ones famed for vexing people. When the skin is stretched over swelled hemorrhoids, its sense receptors are activated, making the hemorrhoids burn and itch, sometimes so intolerably that the urge to scratch them is uncontrollable. Scratching, especially with abrasive materials such as toilet paper, often scrapes and tears the tissue. The bright red blood from these lesions is easily noticeable on the toilet paper and may even drip into the toilet bowl or onto underclothes. Likewise, the passage of a hard, dry stool often abrades hemorrhoids to the point of bleeding.

Internal hemorrhoids do not itch or burn and rarely cause pain because the mucosal tissue over them has no nerve endings, but they can also bleed when a passing stool damages them. (Pain may be "referred," however, from a damaged internal hemorrhoid to the sciatic nerve, bladder, lower back, or genitals; that is, a person feels little or no pain in the anorectal area, but suddenly pain flares in one of these other areas.) An especially elongated internal hemorrhoid at times can protrude through the anus, a condition called prolapse. Usually, it spontaneously recedes or can be pushed back inside with a finger, but upon rare occasion a group of internal hemorrhoids prolapse, swelling and sending the internal sphincter into painful spasms. A doctor's help may then be required to reduce the pain and fit the hemorrhoids inside.

The blood vessels in the internal rectal plexus swell so easily because they lack valves. Without valves to regulate the local flow of blood, the walls are vulnerable to any sudden increase in pressure. Even a small, transient increase above the normal pressure of blood circulation can cause the vessels to bulge. Often, these bulges disappear when the excess pressure disappears or remain swollen only briefly afterward. If the increased pressure is high enough, however, a permanent protrusion results, drooping from the anal wall like lumps of melted wax on a candle. Even then, if the hemorrhoid is internal, the patient may feel no discomfort and may not realize that a hemorrhoid has formed.

Some people are more susceptible to chronic hemorrhoids than others because of a hereditary lack of elasticity in the blood vessels. In such people, standing for long periods of time can add enough pressure to make hemorrhoids swell. Nevertheless, anyone can get hemorrhoids; all that is needed is enough pressure in the lower abdomen. Straining on the toilet to pass stool is the most common cause. People strain when they are constipated or have diarrhea, and since a poor diet can lead to these conditions, hemorrhoids can be a secondary effect of poor eating habits. Those who like to sit on the toilet a long time, reading or watching television while waiting for a bowel movement, also increase pressure on the anus because of the posture and the compressing effect of the toilet ring; they are likely to develop hemorrhoids. People who regularly lift heavy weights as part of their jobs or for recreation are especially susceptible if they hold their breath while lifting: This action pushes the diaphragm downward on organs below it, including the anus, putting pressure on them. Similarly, during pregnancy women can develop hemorrhoids as the expanding womb crowds and increases pressure on nearby organs; these hemorrhoids are exacerbated by delivery, but they usually go away afterward. Psychologists add to these causes the guilt that some people feel about eat-

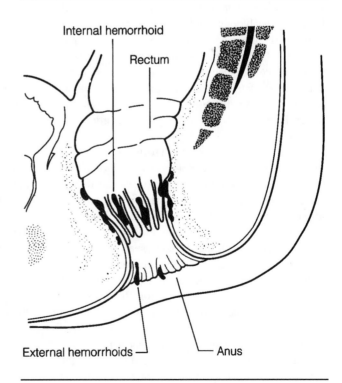

Hemorrhoids

Internal hemorrhoid

Rectum

External hemorrhoids

Anus

ing and excreting, guilt spawned by overindulgence in food or bad toilet training; they bear down on their bowels to defecate as quickly as possible and by doing so stress the hemorrhoidal vessels. Finally, hemorrhoids occasionally develop because of some serious diseases, such as heart failure and cirrhosis of the liver, which elevate pressure in the veins, and rectal cancer, which can create a false sense of fullness so that the person strains to pass a stool that is not really there.

Although they seldom do more than itch, external hemorrhoids can thrombose—develop clots of coagulated blood from a burst or swollen vessel under the skin—and grow as large as a grape. A doctor can relieve the pain by slicing open the hemorrhoid and squeezing out the clot. Left alone, a thrombosed hemorrhoid may rupture, causing a painful and bloody mess that is ripe for infection. Yet the greatest threat of hemorrhoids lies not in the symptoms themselves but in how they might be confused with those of other, deadly diseases. Colorectal cancer, inflammatory bowel disease, and sexually transmitted diseases such as syphilis, gonorrhea, and herpes can lead to discharges of blood, as can anal fissures (cracks in the anal canal), fistulas (tunnel-like passages between an infected gland and mucosa or skin), and abscesses (pus-filled sacs under the mucosa). A person who dismisses the bloody discharge as simply a flare-up of hemorrhoids may be delaying treatment for the real cause. In the case of colorectal cancer, one of the most common cancers in the United States, such a delay can be fatal. Only a doctor has the tools and vantage point to distinguish between the relatively benign hemorrhoids and a dangerous disorder.

TREATMENT AND THERAPY

Since hemorrhoid-like symptoms can be produced by deadly diseases, a thorough checkup at the doctor's office includes an examination of the anus and rectum, especially if the patient has noticed bleeding. In addition to the visual inspection and "digital" examination, during which the doctor inserts a finger and feels around for enlarged hemorrhoids or other masses, patients provide clues by describing the color, amount, and time of bleeding. If the blood is bright red and occurs in small quantities during or just after defecation, hemorrhoids are most likely to blame. If dark red blood or clots appear in the stool or seep out randomly, however, the doctor will look for other causes, inspecting the anus, rectum, and

colon with various types of endoscopes, fiber-optic-filled flexible tubes that can also collect tissue samples. Once the doctor rules out other diseases, the patient has three basic choices: change habits, rely on therapy, or have the hemorrhoids removed.

If a person's hemorrhoids do not cause severe discomfort, the doctor will likely recommend a diet with high fiber and water intake. Fiber and water together make stools bulky and soft. They pass more easily during defecation than small, hard, dry stools. The patient does not have to strain, and so no further pressure is put on existing hemorrhoids. Furthermore, soft stools do not scrape hemorrhoids and cause them to bleed. The doctor will also suggest regular exercise, since this helps the bowels work more efficiently and reduces the chance of constipation. Finally, the patient may receive instructions on the proper way to breathe during heavy exertion so as to lessen the stress on the hemorrhoids. With a better diet, more exercise, and less physical straining, patients may find that hemorrhoids have disappeared completely.

Until hemorrhoids shrink, they plague the patient, and to reduce the itching and burning a number of therapies prove effective, if only temporarily. An ice compress eases the discomfort, as does a sitz bath (sitting for at least fifteen minutes in shallow warm water), which also cleanses the site of potentially infecting wastes and promotes healing in damaged tissue. Should these relatively simple and cheap measures be impracticable, a variety of ointments, creams, medicated pads, and suppositories, either prescription or nonprescription, may provide relief. Some are inert, such as petroleum jelly, and coat and lubricate the hemorrhoids, protecting them from irritation. Some have an astringent effect, tightening and sealing tissue and thereby protecting it. Others have anesthetic ingredients, numbing the tissue, or anti-inflammatory effects, decreasing swelling. None of these medications has a proven capacity to make swelling go away entirely, and those with active ingredients may cause an allergic response. For patients with constipation, doctors may prescribe stool softeners to eliminate straining during defecation. Laxatives are usually to be avoided because the chemicals in them irritate hemorrhoids, and the resulting diarrhea often causes urgency and pressure in the rectal area.

When hemorrhoids become chronically and unusually swollen or the patient can no longer endure the discomfort, removing them is the last resort. This cure is certain, although not necessarily permanent, but it has its cost in pain and recovery time. There are seven basic methods, six that cause the target hemorrhoid to shrivel, to drop off on its own, or both, and one, surgery, that removes it directly.

The surgical removal of hemorrhoids, called hemorrhoidectomy, is a relatively simple operation; nevertheless, it is usually reserved for those patients who for one reason or another cannot undergo one of the other methods. The patient is given a local anesthetic to deaden the tissue in the anus, although some patients are rendered unconscious with a general anesthetic; the surgeon cuts off the hemorrhoid at its base and then sews the wound closed with absorbable sutures. The recovery period may require hospitalization for up to a week, during which pain medication, stool softeners, and anal pads are necessary until the tissues heal. Bed rest after hospitalization and sitz baths may also be necessary. Because of this recovery time—as much as a month all together—hemorrhoidectomies are not widely popular among patients or physicians. Moreover, urine retention, infection, and hemorrhaging after the operation are possible complications.

The remaining methods avoid the trauma of cutting, and the first of them, ligation, is the oldest of all the methods, referred to in the writings of Hippocrates (c. 460-c. 370 B.C.E.). Ancient Greek physicians tied a thread around a hemorrhoid to strangle its blood supply; modern gastroenterologists or proctologists use special rubber bands. The effect is the same: The hemorrhoid dries up, shrivels, and falls off. Little pain accompanies the procedure, which is done in the doctor's office. Ligation, however, can only be used for internal hemorrhoids.

Likewise, sclerotherapy, cryosurgery, and infrared coagulation are only for internal hemorrhoids because the pain would be too intense on external hemorrhoids. In sclerotherapy, the doctor injects a liquid—usually phenol in oil or quinine in urea—that seals closed the blood vessels at the base of the hemorrhoid. With no blood in them, the vessels eventually shrink to normal dimensions and, if stressing pressure on them is not resumed, the hemorrhoid disappears. In cryosurgery, super cold liquid nitrogen or nitrous oxide is applied to the hemorrhoid, freezing it and killing the tissue. The hemorrhoid slowly melts and, as it does, shrinks and finally sloughs off. Popular in the 1970's and early 1980's, cryosurgery lost favor because of the messy and extended recovery

time. Useful for mild, small hemorrhoids, infrared coagulation involves a beam of infrared light that, aimed at the hemorrhoid, shrinks it by cauterizing the tissue. The heat of the beam can cause pain in other parts of the anus during the procedure.

The remaining methods, laser surgery and electric current coagulation, can be used on external hemorrhoids. Like infrared coagulation, laser surgery trains a beam of light—in this case intense visible light—that burns and shrinks the hemorrhoid to a stub. Since the laser cauterizes as it destroys tissue and therefore seals off blood vessels, its main advantage over regular surgery lies in reduced bleeding. Recovery time is shorter, about a week, and hospitalization is usually not necessary. This procedure is much more expensive than a hemorrhoidectomy or ligation, however, because of the cost of laser technology. In electric current coagulation, electrodes pass either direct or alternating current through the hemorrhoids. Because tissue is a poor conductor, the resistance to the current creates heat, which cooks the hemorrhoid, coagulating and shrinking it.

Which method the surgeon, gastroenterologist, or proctologist uses depends partly upon the physician's and patient's preferences and partly upon the size and location of the hemorrhoid. Ligation remains the most frequently used method because it is relatively cheap and fast.

PERSPECTIVE AND PROSPECTS

According to Napoleon's personal physician, piles cost the emperor the Battle of Waterloo, which ended his reign. His hemorrhoids were so inflamed and painful on the morning of the battle that he could not get out of bed, much less sit on his horse. Without his personal direction, the French lost. Popular writers often cite this dramatic example, sometimes with humorous overtones, to demonstrate how seriously hemorrhoids can interfere with the lives of even the great.

Certainly, hemorrhoids are no laughing matter. Yet the long-standing taboo in the United States about excretion and the anus has prompted many Americans either to laugh nervously about their hemorrhoids or to keep silent, preferring to suffer stoically rather than to risk becoming the target of jokes. For this reason, it is nearly impossible to say how many sufferers there are in the United States. Estimates vary from several million people to the entire population over the age of thirty.

Whatever the exact statistic, clearly many people share a problem that embarrasses them too much to discuss openly or that they believe is too trivial for medical attention. If they need relief from the itching and pain, they treat themselves. A large industry in home remedies and over-the-counter medications serves them: Rectal medications alone earned drug companies $178 million in 1999, according to the Consumer Healthcare Products Association. The benefits of such medications are difficult to assess, and some authorities claim that petroleum jelly eases the itching and burning as much as any preparation specifically intended for hemorrhoids. Folk remedies, such as suppositories made of tobacco or compresses soaked in papaya juice, can damage tissue outright, making the problem worse. Moreover, throughout the United States specialized clinics offer surgical cures for hemorrhoids, promising patients quick relief on an outpatient basis and using expensive methods, particularly laser surgery.

Therefore, many people spend a considerable amount of money and time, often wasting both, to tend a chronic discomfort that can as readily be prevented or palliated by a change in habits, doctors claim. Like colon cancer and many other intestinal ailments, hemorrhoids are most common in populations whose diet includes a high number of processed foods, which are low in fiber. While fiber is no panacea, people in cultures whose diet contains significant fiber have larger stools and fewer intestinal complaints in general.

Because hemorrhoids are in most cases preventable or controllable without treatment, they have been cited, along with deadly maladies such as colon cancer and inflammatory bowel disease, in criticisms of both the American diet and Americans' eagerness to rely on medical intervention to save them from their own unhealthy habits. In the case of hemorrhoids— while they are not exclusively a malady of Western civilization—the fast pace and pressures of life, the attitudes about defecation, and the eating habits of industrial cultures help give them a distracting prominence.

—*Roger Smith, Ph.D.*

See also Colon and rectal polyp removal; Colon and rectal surgery; Colon cancer; Colon therapy; Colonoscopy; Cryotherapy and cryosurgery; Endoscopy; Hemorrhoid banding and removal; Intestinal disorders; Intestines; Pregnancy and gestation; Thrombosis and thrombus.

FOR FURTHER INFORMATION:

Becker, Barbara. *Relief from Chronic Hemorrhoids.* New York: Dell, 1992. An excellent book for general readers, it gives advice on every aspect of diagnosis, treatment, removal procedures, and alternative therapies. Special attention is given to improving the patient's diet, and extensive, very specific tables on proper foods accompany the argument for this self-help approach.

"Help for Hemorrhoids Includes Fiber, Fluids, and Fitness." *Environmental Nutrition* 23, no. 4 (April, 2000): 7. Hemorrhoids are a common medical problem, especially for people over age fifty. The best way to prevent hemorrhoids is to avoid constipation by combining a high-fiber diet with plenty of fluids and regular physical activity.

The Hemorrhoid Book: A Look at Hemorrhoids— How They're Treated and How You Can Prevent Them from Coming Back. San Bruno, Calif.: Krames Communications, 1991. Available through doctors' offices, this pamphlet is well worth the trouble to find it. It is fully illustrated, and each illustration is captioned, thereby making the major anatomical features of hemorrhoids clear and memorable, as are the aspects of medical examinations and surgical treatment.

Minkin, Mary Jane. "Prevent Hemorrhoids." *Prevention* 50, no. 6 (June, 1998): 76. Pushing or straining too hard due to constipation is a major reason hemorrhoids develop. Tips on how to prevent constipation are offered.

Okie, Susan. "Colon Susceptible to Other Woes Besides Cancer; The Basics on Everything from Crohn's Disease to Hemorrhoids." *The Washington Post*, February 10, 1998, p. Z19. Between 10 and 20 percent of American adults suffer from irritable bowel syndrome, a set of symptoms that can be painful, inconvenient, and at times disabling.

Sachar, David B., Jerome D. Waye, and Blair S. Lewis, eds. *Pocket Guide to Gastroenterology.* Rev. ed. Baltimore: Williams & Wilkins, 1991. This diagnosis-oriented handbook gives information on all gastroenterological ailments in outline form, making it valuable for quick studies on major problems. The section on hemorrhoids, though superficial, lays out the basic symptoms and treatments.

Wanderman, Sidney E., with Betty Rothbart. *Hemorrhoids.* Yonkers, N.Y.: Consumer Reports Books, 1991. Providing a simple but thorough overview of anatomical problems, causes, medications, therapies, and removal methods, this short book also discusses related complaints, such as fissures and fistulas, and dangerous diseases whose symptoms can be mistaken for those of hemorrhoids.

HEPATITIS

DISEASE/DISORDER

ANATOMY OR SYSTEM AFFECTED: Liver

SPECIALTIES AND RELATED FIELDS: Epidemiology, internal medicine, toxicology, virology

DEFINITION: An inflammatory condition of the liver, characterized by discomfort, jaundice, and enlargement of the organ and bacterial, viral, or immunological in origin; may also result from use of alcohol and other toxic drugs.

KEY TERMS:

alanine aminotransferase: a liver enzyme associated with the metabolism of the amino acid alanine; elevated levels are an indication of liver damage

aspartate aminotransferase: a liver enzyme associated with metabolism of the amino acid aspartate; elevated levels are an indication of liver damage

cirrhosis: chronic degeneration of the liver, in which normal tissue is replaced with fibroid tissue and fat; commonly associated with alcohol abuse but can also result from hepatitis

hepatitis A virus: the virus associated with certain forms of hepatitis; generally contracted through fecal contamination of food and water

hepatitis B virus: the agent associated with severe forms of viral hepatitis; contracted through contaminated blood or hypodermic needles or through contaminated body fluids, and sometimes found in association with hepatitis D virus

hepatitis C virus: formerly referred to as the etiological agent for non-A, non-B viral hepatitis; most often passed in contaminated blood

hepato: a prefix denoting anything associated with the liver—for example, a hepatocyte is a liver cell

jaundice: a symptom of a variety of liver disorders which manifests as yellowish discoloration of the skin, the whites of the eyes, and other tissues; hepatocellular jaundice results from hepatitis

CAUSES AND SYMPTOMS

Hepatitis, a pathology referring to inflammation of the liver, may result from any of a variety of causes but commonly follows bacterial or viral infection. Hepatitis may be associated with an autoimmune phenomenon in which the body produces antibodies against liver tissue. Liver inflammation may also be an aftereffect of the use of alcohol or various hepatotoxic chemicals, either through the taking of illegal drugs or as a side effect of the legal use of pharmacological agents. Among the pharmaceuticals that can cause liver damage are antibiotics such as isoniazid and rifampin and the painkiller acetaminophen.

Symptoms associated with hepatitis are a reflection of the function of the liver. The liver is arguably the most complex organ in the body. More than five hundred different functions have been associated with the organ, including the production of bile for emulsification of fats and the secretion of glucose, proteins, or vitamins for use elsewhere in the body. The liver plays a major role in the detoxification of the blood, removing alcohol, nicotine, and other potentially poisonous substances. The Kupffer cells in the liver function in the removal of infectious agents or foreign material from the blood. More than 10 percent of the blood supply in the body is found within the liver at any time.

Among the functions of the liver is the removal of hemoglobin in the blood, released as a result of the lysis (disintegration) of red blood cells. A breakdown product of hemoglobin is the yellowish compound bilirubin. It is the buildup of bilirubin in blood that results in the appearance of jaundice in cases of inadequate liver function, such as during hepatitis.

Although hepatitis may develop from a variety of causes, it most commonly results from infection of the liver. Nearly any infectious agent may potentially damage the liver, but generally these involve one of several types of viruses, bacteria, fungi, or amoebas. Liver disease may also be significantly exacerbated by alcohol abuse, as is seen in patients with cirrhosis. Regardless of the specific cause, symptoms of liver disease remain similar in most cases. The liver is often enlarged and tender to physical examination. The person may feel tired and run a low-grade fever. It is not unusual for the person to feel nauseous and lose weight. Jaundice is common in most patients; the concentrations of the enzymes alanine aminotransferase (ALT) and aspartate aminotransferase (AST) may rise. Levels of these enzymes, however, are not necessarily indications of the severity of liver disease; in any event, their levels often fall over the course of the disease.

Three particular viruses have been associated with most forms of viral hepatitis (types A, B, and C),

Hepatitis

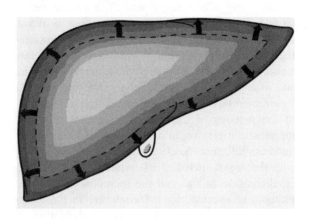

In hepatitis, the liver is enlarged and congested.

while a fourth (type D) appears as a passenger during some cases of hepatitis B. Several additional viruses, designated hepatitis E (HEV) through hepatitis G (HGV), have also been linked to forms of the disease. Hepatitis A results from infection with hepatitis A virus (HAV), a virus classified in the same group as the poliovirus and rhinoviruses (cold viruses). The disease is transmitted through a fecal-to-oral method and is self-limited (running a definite and limited course). Often the disease is subclinical (undetectable), particularly as seen in children. Replication of the virus occurs in hepatocytes (liver cells); the virus then passes into the intestine and is eliminated with the feces. A long incubation period following ingestion may occur, sometimes as long as a month, and during much of this period the person is capable of transmitting the disease. In otherwise healthy individuals, recovery is complete and occurs over several weeks. Anti-HAV antibodies are present in the blood of about 30 to 40 percent of the general population, reflecting the widespread nature of the disease.

Hepatitis B (HBV), formerly called serum hepatitis, is a potentially much more severe form of the disease. The disease in young children is frequently asymptomatic, with appearance of symptoms in older individuals being more common. In general, however, the most frequent result of primary infection with HBV is a mild or subclinical course of infection. The disease is most commonly seen in the fifteen-to-thirty-five age group, in part reflecting its method of transmission (through blood or body fluids).

Persistent infection with HBV, occurring in approximately 1 to 3 percent of patients, can be associated with either an asymptomatic carrier state or chronic hepatitis. The chronic state may be severe, with progression to cirrhosis and cellular degeneration or inflammation. In fact, it is the immune response to the presence of HBV that may contribute to liver degeneration. HBV infection results in the expression of viral antigens, which stimulate an immune response, on the surface of liver cells. Among the inflammatory cells present at the sites of infection are a large proportion of lymphocytes. These include cytotoxic T cells, lymphocytes associated with the killing of virally infected cells. Because immunologically impaired individuals infected with HBV often suffer a mild form of the disease, the possibility exists that it is the immune response itself that contributes to the ensuing liver damage.

Hepatitis B transmission occurs through blood or bodily fluids, including semen and vaginal secretions. Because HBV is also found in saliva, the disease may be transmitted among family members through nonsexual contact. Maternal-neonatal transmission may occur, occasionally while the fetus is in the uterus but more likely during the labor or birth process. There is, however, no evidence for transmission through food or water or by an airborne means.

Clinical features of HBV infections are similar to those associated with other forms of hepatitis. In the asymptomatic form of type B disease, AST or ALT levels may be elevated, but jaundice is absent. Adults with symptomatic hepatitis B may suffer jaundice (icteric hepatitis), or they may not (nonicteric hepatitis). There is generally a mild fever, fatigue, and weakness.

Accompanying an indeterminant number of HBV infections is a second virus, designated the hepatitis D virus (HDV). HDV is a defective virus, capable of replication only in the presence of HBV. Not surprisingly, its geographic distribution and mode of transmission are similar to those of HBV. The prevalence of HDV has been found to be as high as 70 percent in some outbreaks of HBV and nonexistent in others. In most cases, HDV infection results in subclinical or mild hepatitis. In about 15 percent of cases, the disease may progress to a more severe form. HDV may itself be cytopathic (causing pathological changes) for hepatocytes, but this remains to be established firmly.

Based on the exclusion of other types of etiologic agents, including HAV, HBV, Epstein-Barr virus, and cytomegalovirus, non-A, non-B (NANB) hepatitis was considered a clinical entity. During the late 1980's, NANB hepatitis was determined to be caused by a newly isolated infectious agent, designated hepatitis C virus (HCV). The study of HCV was hampered by the inability to grow the virus in cell culture. Ironically, the virus was cloned and characterized before it was even physically observed, allowing for the development of a screening assay used for the detection of contaminated serum. In the United States, approximately 25 percent of hepatitis is associated with HCV. HCV is still recognized as the major complication of blood transfusions or transfusions of blood products, with nearly all cases associated with such transfusions. About 70 percent of cases are asymptomatic, based on measurements of AST or ALT levels. Most cases are mild, with a temporary carrier state established in a large proportion of infected individuals.

Outbreaks of an enterically transmitted NANB hepatitis (NANB hepatitis transmitted through the intestines), designated hepatitis E, have also been found in some parts of the world. Though hepatitis E has been around at least since 1955 (and no doubt earlier, but undocumented), it was only in the late 1980's that it was determined to be a unique form of the disease. Transmission occurs through eating or drinking contaminated food or water, though there is evidence that household contact with infected persons may also transmit the disease. Hepatitis E is most common in the poor countries of Asia, with sporadic outbreaks elsewhere. The few cases found in the United States have involved travelers to these areas.

Acute hepatitis is less commonly associated with infection by other viruses. These include the herpes family of viruses, such as herpes simplex, cytomegalovirus, and Epstein-Barr virus. Because the prevalence of these viruses is quite high, immunosuppressed or immunodeficient patients may be at particular risk.

Certain forms of hepatitis are associated with an autoimmune response. In these cases, the cause is not an infectious agent but rather a form of rejection by the body of its own liver tissue. Autoimmune hepatitis is suspected in individuals in which the disease persists for at least six months with no evidence of exposure to an infectious agent or hepatotoxin. In nearly one-third of these individuals, other immunological diseases such as lupus or arthritis may be present. The clinical manifestations of autoimmune hepatitis are similar to those of other forms of the dis-

ease. Most patients exhibit jaundice, a mild fever, weakness, and weight loss. The liver is often enlarged and tender. Unlike other forms of hepatitis, found equally in men and women, autoimmune hepatitis is most commonly found in women. Prognosis of the disease is unclear, as an unknown percentage of cases are subclinical. Severe forms have a high fatality rate.

TREATMENT AND THERAPY
No specific treatments exist for the various forms of viral hepatitis; hence, treatment is for the most part symptomatic and supportive. Hospitalization may be required in severe cases, but, in general, any restriction of activity is left up to the patient. This is particularly convenient, since recovery often involves a long convalescence. As long as a healthy diet is maintained, no special dietary requirements exist, but a high-calorie diet is often preferable. Drugs or chemicals that are potentially damaging to the liver, including alcohol and certain antibiotics or painkillers, should be avoided.

Hepatitis induced by other forms of infectious agents such as bacteria or fungi may be treated using an appropriate course of antibiotic therapy. In cases of drug-induced disease, avoidance of the chemical is a key to recovery. Bacterial infections of the liver are often associated with patients who are malnourished, such as the elderly or alcoholics, or who may be immunosuppressed. These problems must also be addressed during the course of treatment.

Prevention of the disease is preferable, however, and because the means of viral spread has been well established in most cases, appropriate measures can often be taken. For the most part, the viruses associated with hepatitis have little in common with one another aside from their predilection for hepatocytes. Thus, preventing their spread involves different strategies.

HAV is almost always spread through a fecal-oral means of transmission. Often the source is an infected person involved in the preparation of uncooked foods. Common sense dictates that the person should wash after every use of a toilet, but this is often not the case. Not surprisingly, children attending day care centers frequently become infected. Contaminated groundwater is also a potential source of outbreaks in areas in which proper sewage treatment does not take place. Less commonly, HAV is spread directly from person to person through sexual contact. A method called immunoprophylaxis can prevent the development of symptoms in individuals exposed to hepatitis A by utilizing a form of passive immunity. Developed during World War II, the procedure involves the pooling of serum from immune individuals. Inoculation of the serum into exposed persons is effective in prevention of the disease in most cases.

In 1994, SmithKline Beecham Pharmaceuticals developed and received Food and Drug Administration (FDA) approval for the first vaccine shown to be safe and effective in preventing HAV infection. Manufactured under the trade name Havrix, the vaccine consists of a formalin-inactivated strain of HAV, to be administered in three doses to children. In 1996, a similar vaccine was developed by Merck and Co., to be sold under the trade name Vagta.

The transmission of HBV generally involves passage via contaminated blood or body secretions. In the period prior to the screening of blood, transfusions were the most common means of spreading the disease—hence the designation "serum hepatitis." Since the 1980's, the most common means of documented spread has been through either sexual contact or the sharing of contaminated hypodermic needles. Semen, vaginal secretions, and saliva from infected individuals all contain the active virus, and limiting exchange of these fluids is key to prevention of transmission. Even so, the means of infection in nearly one-third of symptomatic cases remains unknown.

An effective vaccine for prevention of HBV infection was first developed during the 1970's and early 1980's. The vaccination procedure was subsequently modified to create an effective combined active-passive vaccine. Passive immunization utilizes antibodies purified from the blood of donors who have recovered from HBV infection. This hepatitis B immune globulin (HBIG) is combined with a recombinant yeast vaccine that contains hepatitis virus proteins but lacks the genetic material necessary for the virus to replicate. Because HBIG already contains a high level of anti-HBV antibody, it is effective as a postexposure preventive for an individual who has come in contact with the disease. For example, a person exposed to the virus through an accidental needle stick, such as an unimmunized health care worker, may not have time to proceed through the regimen of treatment. The use of HBIG provides a short-term means of protection. The combined vaccine is used as a method of pre-exposure immunization. In the early 1990's, vaccination was recommended to only those persons at high risk for exposure to HBV. This group is composed of homosexual or bisexual men, health care workers (including physicians and dentists), and persons dealing with individuals in whom the disease is commonly found.

Because hepatitis D virus is defective in replication, requiring the presence of HBV, no specific measures of prevention are necessary. Immunization against HBV is sufficient to prevent the spread of HDV.

Treatment of NANB hepatitis consists primarily of allowing the disease to run its course. Because this form of hepatitis is almost exclusively blood-borne and no vaccine exists, prevention requires the exclusion of blood of contaminated individuals from the blood pool available for transfusions. Routine screening of blood for anti-HCV antibodies was begun in 1990. The use of surrogate markers has also proven helpful. For example, elevated levels of ALT and anti-HBV antibodies in the serum of blood donors have been shown to predispose the recipient to NANB hepatitis; hence the exclusion of such blood has been particularly useful in limiting the transmission of the disease. Sharing of contaminated needles is also a means of transmission, requiring increased individual responsibility in order to prevent the spread of the virus. The use of immunoprophylaxis, so helpful in the prevention of transmission of HBV, has not proven effective in the case of HCV.

The transmission of the hepatitis E virus is also through a fecal-oral route. The drinking of water contaminated by sewage has been the most common source of transmission. Because no active means of prevention has been developed, prevention of exposure requires that the individual avoid any food or water potentially contaminated with sewage. This is particularly true in areas of the world in which hepatitis E is found. Though the precaution may seem obvious, the safety of the water, as well as any object washed in the water, is not always readily apparent.

Autoimmune hepatitis results from an aberrant immune system rather than from an infectious agent. Treatment generally involves the use of immunosuppressive drugs to limit the immune response. Corticosteroids such as prednisone, sometimes in combination with azathioprine, have proven effective in the therapy of many patients. Still, in some cases the disease progresses to cirrhosis and results in death. Treatment generally is carried out over a long period of time, at least a year, and relapses are common. Often, the patient requires lifetime therapy. The immunosuppressive activity of the therapy may also leave the patient more susceptible to infection. In some cases, liver transplantation has proven effective, at least in the short term. Because the liver rejection was caused by an autoimmune response in the first place, the transplant may also be subject to the same phenomenon.

PERSPECTIVE AND PROSPECTS

Inflammation of the liver resulting in hepatitis can develop from a variety of mechanisms. Most often, these mechanisms are associated with either a chemical injury or infection by a microbiological agent.

Infections of the liver generally involve one of several viral agents. The association of liver disease, or at least jaundice, with an infectious agent was suspected as early as the time of Hippocrates (the fifth century B.C.E.). Hippocrates described a syndrome which was undoubtedly viral hepatitis. The disease was also described in the Babylonian Talmud about eight hundred years later. Epidemics of the disease have been reported since the Middle Ages; these most likely involved outbreaks of hepatitis A. The spread of this disease through personal contact was confirmed in the 1930's.

Type B, or serum hepatitis, was described as a clinical entity by A. Lurman in 1855. Lurman observed that 15 percent of shipyard workers in Bremen, Germany, who received a smallpox vaccine containing human lymph developed jaundice within the following six months. In the early years of the twentieth century, jaundice frequently developed among patients who received vaccines prepared from convalescent serums or who underwent procedures such as venipuncture using instruments which had not been properly sterilized. By 1926, the blood-borne nature of the disease had been confirmed. In 1942, more than twenty-eight thousand American soldiers developed jaundice after vaccination with a yellow fever vaccine prepared from pooled human serums. By then it had become obvious that at least two forms of infectious agents were associated with viral hepatitis.

The isolation of HBV occurred as a result of studies initiated by Baruch Blumberg in 1963. Blumberg was actually attempting to correlate the development of diseases such as cancer with particular patterns of proteins found in the serum of individuals. His approach was to collect blood from persons in various parts of the world and then analyze their serum proteins. Blumberg found an antigen, a protein, in the blood of Australian aborigines which reacted with antibodies in the blood of an American hemophiliac. Blumberg called the protein the Australia (Au) antigen. It later became apparent that the Au antigen could be isolated from the blood of patients with serum hepatitis. By 1970, it was established that what Blumberg had referred to as the Au antigen was in fact the HBV particle.

HBV is associated with more than simply viral hepatitis. Chronic hepatitis associated with HBV can often develop into hepatocellular carcinoma, or cancer of the liver. The precise reason is unclear; the cancer may result from the chronic damage to liver tissue associated with long-term infection by HBV.

An effective vaccine for the prevention of HBV infection was licensed in 1982. By the late 1990's, the effectiveness of a worldwide vaccination program, under the auspices of the World Health Organization, had led to the possibility that hepatitis resulting from HBV infection, as well as hepatocelluar carcinoma, could be controlled within another decade.

The epidemiological patterns of HCV transmission remained incompletely understood. Between three thousand and four thousand cases of non-A, non-B viral hepatitis were reported annually in the United States, a number that stabilized during the 1990's. The majority of these cases were associated with HCV and account for approximately 25 percent of total cases of viral hepatitis. Nearly all cases are associated with transmission through blood or blood products. With improved methods of screening, the numbers of cases should decrease rapidly.

—*Richard Adler, Ph.D.*

See also Addiction; Alcoholism; Autoimmune disorders; Cirrhosis; Immunization and vaccination; Jaundice; Liver; Liver cancer; Liver disorders; Liver transplantation; Viral infections.

FOR FURTHER INFORMATION:

Gorbach, Sherwood L., John G. Bartlett, and Neil R. Blacklow, eds. *Infectious Diseases*. 2d ed. Philadelphia: W. B. Saunders, 1997. A thorough discussion of infectious diseases. Included is a brief history, an account of the mechanisms of disease and immunity, and a concise discussion of a broad range of infectious agents. The section on hepatitis viruses is well written and not particularly detailed.

Kelley, William, et al., eds. *Textbook of Internal Medicine*. 3d ed. New York: Lippincott-Raven, 1997. A medical textbook on the subject. The book contains an extensive section on liver diseases, including a concise description of viral hepatitis. The discussion of hepatitis viruses is thorough, clear, but not overly detailed.

Levine, Arnold. *Viruses*. New York: W. H. Freeman, 1992. A well-written outline of viruses and their history. Some basic knowledge of biology is helpful in certain areas of the book, but overall the format and style should reach nearly all general readers. The book is profusely and colorfully illustrated. Several sections deal specifically with viral hepatitis.

Palmer, Melissa. *Dr. Melissa Palmer's Guide to Hepatitis and Liver Disease*. Garden City Park, N.Y.: Avery, 2000. Palmer, a nationally recognized hepatologist, provides plainly written medical information explaining how the liver is integral to every aspect of daily functioning and well-being. Includes "The Basics," "Understanding and Treating Viral Hepatitis," "Understanding and Treating Other Liver Diseases," and "Treatment Options and Lifestyle Changes."

Shaw, Michael, ed. *Everything You Need to Know About Diseases*. Springhouse, Pa.: Springhouse Press, 1996. This well-illustrated consumer reference, compiled by more than one hundred doctors and medical experts, describes five hundred illnesses and conditions, their causes, symptoms, diagnosis, treatment, and prevention. Of particular interest is chapter 6, "Liver and Gallbladder."

Spector, Steven. *Viral Hepatitis: Diagnosis, Therapy, and Prevention*. Totowa, N.J.: Humana Press, 1999. This clearly written and readable review of viral hepatitis provides useful information for family physicians interested in this protean disorder. Each chapter is divided into sections, allowing the reader to quickly access desired information.

Zakim, David, and Thomas Boyer, eds. *Hepatology: A Textbook of Liver Disease*. 3d ed. Philadelphia: W. B. Saunders, 1996. A thorough compendium on most aspects of liver disease. The section on hepatitis contains a complete clinical description of the disease and of the biology of the hepatitis viruses.

HERBAL MEDICINE
TREATMENT

ALSO KNOWN AS: Botanical medicine, phytomedicine

ANATOMY OR SYSTEM AFFECTED: All

SPECIALTIES AND RELATED FIELDS: Alternative medicine, nutrition, pharmacology, preventive medicine

DEFINITION: The use of leaves, flowers, stems, seeds, fruits, bark, berries, and roots of plants to prevent, relieve, and treat acute and chronic illnesses and to maintain health.

KEY TERMS:

dietary supplement: a product (other than tobacco) intended to supplement the diet and containing one or more of the following: a vitamin, a mineral, an herb or other botanical, or an amino acid

Dietary Supplement Health and Education Act (DSHEA): a 1994 law that officially created a category of dietary supplements and allowed for the provision of information that is not misleading to consumers regarding a product's benefits and potential side effects

INDICATIONS AND PROCEDURES

According to the American Botanical Council, one-third of adults in the United States use herbal or botanical products in the hope of finding a cheaper, gentler, natural alternative to mainstream medicinal treatments. Herbal medicines are big business, with billions of dollars spent on them each year. Herbal or botanical remedies are no longer confined to the realm of folklore. For example, a female patient may take kava to help calm job stress, echinacea when she feels a cold coming on, and black cohosh for hot flashes.

Herbs and botanicals have active properties similar to regulated drugs. Their prepared compounds are available in different forms, each having its own particular characteristics.

There are tinctures and extracts. If the label is marked "tincture," the preparation contains alcohol or liquid glycerin to allow the active property of the herb to become extracted and concentrated. Extracts use less alcohol or glycerin and water as the essence of the herb is leached out. Tinctures and extracts are a concentrated and cost-effective way of administering herbal compounds. However, the full taste of the herb comes through strongly in a tincture or extract and is sometimes unpleasant. For instance, a tincture of goldenseal, a root used to treat infection, tastes bitter. Using glycerin adds a sweeter taste but in large doses can have a laxative effect.

Another option is capsules and tablets. Ground or powdered forms of raw herbs and botanicals can be found in capsule or tablet form. Generally, there seems to be little difference between the two in terms of clinical results; however, further study is required.

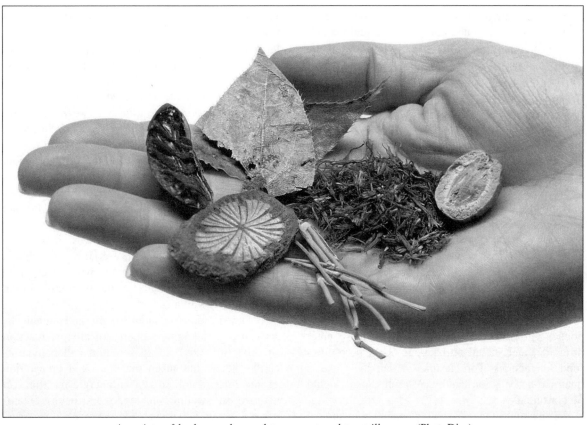

A variety of herbs can be used to prevent and treat illnesses. (PhotoDisc)

The consumer needs to read the label of the preparation to make sure that fresh herbs have been used to make the product.

Finely milled herbs degrade quickly so it is important that herbs be freshly ground and then promptly encapsulated or formed into tablets. With the exception of certain herbal concentrates in capsule form, both capsules and tablets tend to be much weaker than tinctures and extracts.

Other herbal medicines include teas. There are many blends of herbal teas. Some herbs are loose and ready for steeping and others are prepackaged. Herbal teas are also another way of administering liquids. Herbal lozenges are nutrient-rich and naturally sweetened and contain cold-fighting formulas, natural cough suppressants, and decongestant properties. Many lozenges are made without refined sugar and contain vitamin C.

There are also ointments, salves, and rubs in large numbers on the market. Consumer selection depends upon the condition that is being treated. The ointments, salves, and rubs range from calendula oint-

ment (for broken skin and wounds) to goldenseal (for infections, rashes, and skin irritations) to aloe vera gel (to cool and speed the healing of minor burns, including sunburn) to heat-producing herbs (for muscle aches and strains). Herbal and botanical supplements are fast becoming a part of a healthy lifestyle as consumers seek control over their lives and medical problems.

USES AND COMPLICATIONS

When using herbal and botanical treatments, knowledge is the key. Just because a product is considered "natural" does not mean that it is healthful for consumption. The federal government classifies herbal remedies as dietary supplements as defined under the Dietary Supplement Health and Education Act (DSHEA); they are regulated by the Food and Drug Administration (FDA). These preparations do not undergo the rigorous testing demanded by the FDA for other prescription and over-the-counter drugs. Manufacturers are not required to provide detailed information about their products' contents, side effects, safety, or efficacy. They need only to provide reasonable assurance that their products contain no harmful ingredients. Additionally, they are subject to few controls on quality and purity. They cannot make medical claims for the product unless they have FDA approval, but they can make claims about the product's benefits without supporting evidence. For example, a preparation made with ginkgo may be sold to enhance memory but not to treat dementia; echinacea can be labeled an immune-system booster but not a cold remedy.

Consumers need to read about a product they wish to use before taking it. They should be aware that the only required information on herbal/botanical labels is the product's name, the quantity of product being sold (for which no standards now exist), and any appropriate warnings. Very young or very old consumers, those whose metabolism may be compromised due to disease, and those with allergies can have dramatic responses to such preparations. All users need to be aware that herbs/botanicals contain active compounds, just as prescription and over-the-counter drugs do, and should be cautious about herb-drug-food interactions. For questions about their use, a qualified herbalist or health care professional should be consulted.

For example, the following popular medicinal herbs and botanicals can be useful, but they can also cause complications. Flax, which is used to sooth the digestive tract and relieve constipation, can cause agitation, excitement, and rapid breathing. Echinacea, which is used to boost the immune system and treat some infections and insect bites and stings, may complicate autoimmune diseases, such as lupus or multiple sclerosis, and lead to liver damage. Garlic, which is used to lower blood cholesterol and treat infections as an antibiotic and antiseptic, may lead to lowered blood pressure, blood thinning, and diarrhea or stomach upset. Ginsing, which is used to relieve fatigue or debilitation after an illness, may cause headache, insomnia, anxiety, diarrhea, heart palpitations, and increased blood pressure. Black cohosh, which is used to treat hot flashes, may cause dizziness, headache, and nausea. Ginger, which is used to sooth aching muscles, aid digestion, and relieve congestion and fever, may cause diarrhea or upset stomach. Aloe, which is used as a laxative, may cause severe diarrhea or cramps and electrolyte imbalances, and it may alter the absorption of other medications. Ginkgo, which is used to treat memory deficits and increase blood flow, can cause blood thinning, headaches,

restlessness, and irritability. Skullcap, which is used as a sedative and nerve tonic, can lead to severe liver damage. Ephedra (ma huang), which is used as a decongestant and an appetite suppressant, can increase blood pressure and heart rate and lead to heart palpitations, and, in some cases, death. Saw palmetto, which is used to increase urinary flow, reduce residual urine, and decrease urinary frequency in males, has no known serious side effects. St. John's wort, which is used to treat mild to moderate depression, may cause stomach upset and diarrhea. Licorice, which is used to sooth the respiratory tract and increase energy, may cause high blood pressure and dizziness. Valerian root, which is used as a sedative and to reduce nervousness and stress, may cause headache, nausea, and blurred vision. Kava, which is used as a relaxant for stress relief, may cause hypersedation in older individuals or those on prescription drugs such as Valium.

Any medication, including herbs and botanicals, can cause an allergic reaction. An allergic reaction can occur after the first exposure to the allergen or after the patient has taken the medicinal preparation several times. Symptoms of an allergic reaction can include rash, swelling, itching, and difficulty breathing. If a patient believes an allergic reaction is occurring, he or she should call a health care provider, go to the nearest emergency room, or call an emergency medical service provider for help.

PERSPECTIVE AND PROSPECTS

Herbal medicine has a long and respected history. Many medications in wide use today were developed from ancient healing traditions that treated health problems with specific plants. For example, salicylic acid (aspirin) was originally derived from the white willow bark and the meadowsweet plant. Vincristine, used to treat certain types of cancer, comes from the periwinkle plant.

There are more than 750,000 plants on earth. Almost all current research validating herbal medicine has been done in other countries. Pharmaceutical and herbal companies in the United States are just beginning to work together to standardize industry practices and achieve greater consistency in product quality. Consumers of herbals and botanicals need to be smart and be aware that while these preparations can help, they can also cause harm.

—*Linda L. Pierce, Ph.D, R.N., and Julie L. Smith, M.S., R.D./L.D.*

See also Alternative medicine; Antioxidants; Food biochemistry; Homeopathy; Nutrition; Pharmacology; Pharmacy; Self-medication; Supplements; Toxicology.

FOR FURTHER INFORMATION:

Blumenthal, M., ed. *The Complete German Commission E Monographs: Therapeutic Guide to Herbal Medicines*. Austin, Tex.: American Botanical Council, 1998.

Fetrow, C., and R. Avila. *The Complete Guide to Herbal Medicines*. Springhouse, Pa.: Springhouse, 2000.

Foster, S., and V. Tyler. *Tyler's Honest Herbal: A Sensible Guide to the Use of Herbs and Related Remedies*. 4th ed. Binghamtom, N.Y.: Haworth Herbal Press, 1999.

Hoffman, D. *The Complete Illustrated Holistic Herbal: A Safe and Practical Guide to Making and Using Herbal Remedies*. Rockport, Mass.: Element Books, 1996.

Robbers, J., and V. Tyler. *Tyler's Herbs of Choice: The Therapeutic Use of Phytomedicinals*. Binghamtom, N.Y.: Haworth Herbal Press, 1999.

HERMAPHRODITISM AND PSEUDOHERMAPHRODITISM

DISEASE/DISORDER

ANATOMY OR SYSTEM AFFECTED: Genitals, reproductive system, urinary system

SPECIALTIES AND RELATED FIELDS: Embryology, endocrinology, genetics, gynecology, urology

DEFINITION: Abnormal primary sexual characteristics caused by developmental defects.

CAUSES AND SYMPTOMS

Hermaphroditism is a condition in which testicular and ovarian tissues are found in the same person and their urogenital development is ambiguous. A baby with an enlarged clitoris resembling a penis and fused labial-scrotal folds is often designated a male, whereas a baby with a normal clitoris and open labial folds might be considered a female. Generally, inappropriate levels of male and female hormones during fetal development are responsible for ambiguous genitals at birth.

Pseudohermaphroditism is a condition in which either testicular tissues or ovarian tissues, but not both, are found in an individual with ambiguous urogenital development. XY pseudohermaphrodites develop internal testes, but their external genitals and appearance at birth are female. They lack ovaries, Fallopian tubes, and a uterus, but they have a blind (dead-end) vagina. There are two types of XY pseudohermaphrodites, those with testicular feminization syndrome (TFS) and those with *huevodoce* (or *guevedoces*) syndrome (HDS).

As individuals with TFS enter puberty, they begin to grow genital hair and breasts and have the appearance of normal females because they are unable to respond to any form of testosterone. When individuals with HDS begin puberty, the clitoris enlarges into a penislike structure without a urethra. The urethral opening is at the base of the enlarged clitoris. One or both of the internal testes descend into scrotal sacs, and the teenager begins to develop masculine body and facial hair, but there is no breast development. In some cases, the voice deepens, and muscle mass and body shape become more masculine. Individuals with *huevodoce* syndrome develop as they do because they are unable to convert testosterone to 5-alpha-dihydrotestosterone (DHT), the inducer necessary for the early development of male tissues. At puberty, the testes produce very large amounts of testosterone, which is able to make up for the lack of DHT and to stimulate some tissues to develop further.

TREATMENT AND THERAPY

Hormone therapy or even operations to remove vestigial testes at birth might be of value in promoting the development of normal external genitals in hermaphroditic babies. In children with HDS, hormone therapy helps to resolve the ambiguous development of external genitalia at puberty. There are no treatments or therapies for individuals with TFS because these individuals are not responsive to testosterone.

PERSPECTIVE AND PROSPECTS

In general, persons with TFS think of themselves as females. They are sexually attracted to men and usually marry. No treatment should be considered for these individuals. Many individuals with HDS remain in a female role, but some take on the male role as they change at puberty. Hormone therapy might be of value in helping to establish the roles they desire in their culture.

—Jaime S. Colomé, Ph.D.

See also Genetic diseases; Genetics and inheritance; Puberty and adolescence; Reproductive system; Sexual differentiation.

FOR FURTHER INFORMATION:

Fausto-Sterling, Anne. *Sexing the Body: Gender Politics and the Construction of Sexuality.* New York: Basic Books, 2000.

Hellinga, Gerhardus. *Clinical Andrology: A Systematic Approach, with a Chapter on Intersexuality.* London: Heinemann, 1976.

Hunter, R. H. F. *Sex Determination, Differentiation, and Intersexuality in Placental Mammals.* New York: Cambridge University Press, 1995.

Kessler, Suzanne. *Lessons from the Intersexed.* New Brunswick, N.J.: Rutgers University Press, 1998.

HERNIA

DISEASE/DISORDER

ANATOMY OR SYSTEM AFFECTED: Abdomen, gastrointestinal system, intestines, reproductive system, stomach

SPECIALTIES AND RELATED FIELDS: Gastrointestinal system, internal medicine

DEFINITION: A pouchlike mass consisting of visceral material encased in properitoneal tissue (the hernial sac) protruding through an aperture in the abdomen—a result of a weakening in the abdominal wall.

KEY TERMS:

Bassini technique: the most widely accepted surgical method for treating hernias; named after the Italian surgeon Edoardo Bassini

hernioplasty: the surgery performed to treat hernia patients

incarceration: an advanced and dangerous hernial stage which occurs when the hernial sac protrudes well beyond the abdominal aperture and is constricted at the neck

inguinal hernia: the most common form of hernia, in which the hernial sac protrudes into the lower groin area

reducible hernia: a hernia that has not advanced significantly beyond the weakened aperture in the abdomen; such hernias were formerly treated by means of the externally applied pressure of a truss

CAUSES AND SYMPTOMS

A hernia condition exists when either tissues from, or actual portions of, vital internal organs protrude beyond the enclosure of the abdomen as a result of an abnormal opening in several possible areas of the abdominal wall. In most hernias, the protruding material remains encased in the tissue of the peritoneum.

This saclike extension forces itself into whatever space can be ceded by neighboring tissues outside the abdomen. Because of the swelling effect produced, the hernia is usually visible as a lump on the surface of the body. As there are several types of hernias that may occur in different areas of the abdomen, the place of noticeable swelling and the internal organs affected may vary. With the single exception of the pancreas, hernia cases have been recorded involving all other organs contained in the abdomen. The most common hernial protrusions, however, involve the small intestine and/or the omenta, folds of the peritoneum. Another category of hernia, referred to as hernia adipose, consists of a protrusion of peritoneal fat beyond the abdominal wall.

Generally speaking, the cause of hernial conditions involves not only an internal pressure pushing portions of the viscera against the abdominal wall (hence the danger of bringing on a hernia through heavy physical exertion in work or athletics) but also a point of weakness in the abdominal wall itself. Two such points of potential weakness exist in all normal, healthy individuals: the original umbilical ring, which should normally "heal" over after the umbilical cord is severed; and the groin tissues in the lower portion of the abdomen—the region where the most common hernia, the inguinal hernia, occurs. Another possible source of vulnerability to hernia protrusions is connected to the individual's prior surgical history: Scar tissue may prove to be the weakest point of resistance to pressures originating anywhere in the abdominal region.

It should be noted that, because the abdominal tissues of infants and young children are particularly delicate, there is a proportionately higher occurrence of hernial conditions among babies and toddlers. If the hernia is diagnosed and treated early enough, complete healing is almost certain in such cases, most of which do not develop beyond the preliminary, or reducible, stage.

The several stages, or degrees, of hernial development usually begin with what doctors call a reducible hernia condition. At this stage, a patient suffering from hernia, sensing the onset of the disorder, may be able to obtain temporary relief from a developing protrusion by changing posture angle when upright or by lying down. Until the late twentieth century, some physicians preferred to treat reducible hernias by means of an externally attached pressure device, or truss, rather than resorting to surgical intervention.

This form of treatment was gradually dropped in favor of increasingly effective hernioplasty operations.

When a hernial condition enters what is called the stage of incarceration, the advanced protrusion of the sac containing portions of viscera through the opening, or ring, in the abdominal wall can cause very severe complications. If, as is frequently the case, the protruding hernia sac passes through the ring as a fingerlike tube and then assumes a globular form outside the abdominal wall, a state of incarceration exists. As this state advances, the patient runs the risk of hernial strangulation. The constricting pressure of the ring's edges on the hernial sac interferes with circulatory functions in the herniated organ, causing destruction of tissues and, unless surgical intervention occurs, rapid spread of gangrene throughout the affected organ. It was the sixteenth century French surgeon Pierre Franco who carried out the first operation to release a strangulated hernia by inserting a thin instrument between the incarcerated bowel and the herniated sac, then incising the latter without touching the extruded vital organ.

A surprisingly wide range of hernial conditions have been noted and studied. These include hernias in the umbilical, epigastric (upper abdominal), spigelian (transversus abdominal muscle), interparietal, and groin regions. Hernias in the groin can be either femoral or inguinal. Inguinal hernias affecting the groin area have always been by far the most common, accounting for more than three-quarters of hernial cases, particularly among males.

Inguinal hernias share a number of common characteristics with one another and with the other closely associated form of groin hernia, the femoral hernia. Inguinal hernias are all caused by the abnormal introduction of a hernial sac into one of the 4 centimeter-long inguinal canals located on the sides of the abdomen. These canals originate in the lower portion of the abdomen at an aperture called the inguinal ring. They have an external exit point in the rectus abdominal tissue. Located inside each inguinal canal are the ilioinguinal nerve, the genital branch of the genitofemoral nerve, and the spermatic cord. A comparable passageway from the abdomen into the groin area is found at the femoral ring, through which both the femoral artery and the femoral vein pass.

It may take a long period, sometimes years, for the sac to engage itself fully in the inguinal or femoral ring. Once the ring is passed, however, pressures from inside the abdomen help it descend through the

Hiatal Hernia

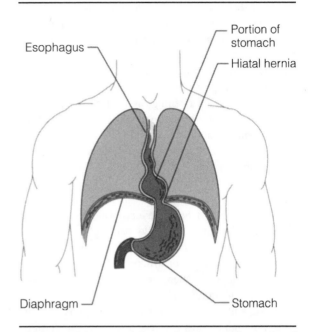

A portion of the stomach has pushed through the weakened abdominal wall.

canal rather quickly. If the external inguinal ring is firm in structure, and particularly if the narrow passageway is largely filled with the thickness of the spermatic cord, the inguinal hernia may be partially arrested at this point. In men, once it passes beyond the external inguinal ring, however, it quickly descends into the scrotum. In women, the inguinal canal contains the round ligament, which may also temporarily impede the further descent of the hernial sac beyond the external inguinal opening.

TREATMENT AND THERAPY

Given the widespread occurrence of hernia conditions at all age levels in most societies, physicians receive extensive training in the diagnosis and, among those with surgical training, the treatment of hernia patients. Near-total consensus among doctors now demands surgery (external trusses having been largely abandoned), but different schools support different surgical methods. With the exception of operations involving the insertion of prosthetic devices to block the extension of hernia damage, most recent inguinal hernioplasty methods derive from the model finalized by the Italian Edoardo Bassini in the late nineteenth century.

Bassini believed that the surgical methods of his time fell short of the goal of complete hernial repair, since most postoperational patients were required to wear a truss to guard against recurring problems. In the simplest of surgical terms, his solution involved the physiological reconstruction of the inguinal canal. The operation provided for a new internal passageway to an external opening, as well as strengthened anterior and posterior inguinal walls. After initial incisions and ligation of the hernial sac, Bassini's method involved a separation of tissues between the internal inguinal ring and the pubis. A tissue section referred to as the "triple layer" (containing the internal oblique, the transversus abdominal, and the transversalis fascia tissue layers) was then attached by a line of sutures to the Poupart ligament, with a lowermost suture at the edge of the rectus abdominal muscle. Such local reconstruction of the inguinal canal proved to strengthen the entire zone against the recurrence of ruptures.

Physicians operating on indirect, as opposed to direct, inguinal hernias confront a relatively uncomplicated set of procedures. In the former case, a high ligation of the peritoneal sac (a circular incision of the peritoneum at a point well inside the abdominal inguinal ring) usually makes it possible to remove the sac entirely. Complications can occur if the patient is obese, since a large mass of peritoneal fatty material may be joined to the sac, obstructing access to the inguinal ring. For normal indirect inguinal hernias, the next basic step, after ensuring that no damage has occurred to the viscera either during formation of the hernia or in the process of relocating the contents of the hernial sac inside the abdomen, is to use one of several surgical methods to reduce the opening of the inguinal ring to its normal size. The physician must also ensure that no damage to the posterior inguinal wall has occurred and that its essential attachment to Cooper's ligament does not require additional surgical attention.

One must contrast the relative simplicity of indirect inguinal hernia surgery to treatment of direct inguinal hernias. In these cases, the hernia does not protrude through the existing inguinal aperture, but, as a result of a weakening of local tissues, passes directly through the posterior inguinal wall. The direct inguinal hernia is usually characterized by a broad base at the point of protrusion and a relatively short hernial sac. When a physician recommends surgical treatment of such hernias, the surgeon must be prepared for the extensive task of surgical reconstruction of the posterior inguinal wall as part of the operation.

Two additional reasons tend to discourage an immediate decision to operate on direct inguinal hernias. First, this form of hernia rarely strangulates the affected viscera, since the aperture stretches to allow protrusion of the hernial sac. Second, once physicians find obvious symptoms of a direct inguinal hernia (a ceding of the weakened posterior inguinal wall to pressures originating in the abdomen), they may decide to examine the patient more thoroughly to determine whether the cause behind the symptoms demands an entirely different prognosis. Such causes of abdominal pressures may range from the effects of a chronic cough to much more serious problems, including inflammation of the prostate gland or other forms of obstruction in the colon itself.

PERSPECTIVE AND PROSPECTS

Because the phenomenon of hernias has been the subject of scientific observation since the onset of formal medical writing itself, a stage-by-stage development of prognoses has been associated with this condition. A main dividing line appears between the mid-eighteenth and mid-nineteenth centuries, however, between the extremely rudimentary surgical treatments of the late Middle Ages and Renaissance and what can be called modern prognoses.

Without doubt the surgical contribution of the sixteenth century Frenchman Pierre Franco, who performed the first operation to release an incarcerated hernia, must be considered a landmark. The major general cause for advancement in knowledge of hernias, however, is tied to the birth of a new era in medical science, characterized by the use, from about 1750 onward, of anatomical dissection to investigate the essential characteristics of a number of common diseases.

Before the relatively long line of contributions that led to general adoption of the Bassini technique of operating on hernias, surgeons tended to follow the so-called Langenbeck method, named after the German physician who pioneered modern hernioplasty. This method held that simple removal of a hernial sac at the point of its protrusion from the abdomen and closing the external aperture would lead to a closing of the sac by "adhesive inflammation." Such spontaneous closing occurs when a severed artery "recedes" to the first branching-off point.

It took contributions by at least two lesser-known late nineteenth century forerunners to Edoardo Bassini to convince the surgical world that hernia operations must involve a high incision of the hernial sac. Both the American H. O. Marcy (1837-1924) and the Frenchman Just Marie Marcellin Lucas-Championnière (1843-1913) have been recognized for their insistence on the necessity of high-incision operations. Their hernia operations, by incising the external oblique fascia, were the first to penetrate well beyond the external ring to expose the entire hernial sac. Following removal of the sac, it was then possible for surgeons to close the transversalis fascia and to repair the higher interior tissues that might have been damaged by the swollen hernia.

Following initial acceptance of the technique of high-incision hernial operations, a number of physicians recommended a variety of methods that might be used to repair internal tissue damage. These methods ranged from simple ligation of the sac at the internal ring, without more extensive surgery involving either the abdominal wall or the spermatic cord, to the much more extensive method practiced by Bassini. Even after the Bassini method succeeded in gaining almost universal recognition, other adaptations (but nothing that represented a full innovation) would be added during the middle decades of the twentieth century. One such method, which borrowed from the German physician Georg Lotheissen's use of Cooper's ligament to serve as a foundation for suturing damaged layers of lower abdominal tissues, earned its proponent, the American Chester McVay, the honor of having the operation named after him.

Finally, one should note that, although few significant changes have occurred in most doctors' view of what must be done surgically to treat hernia patients, surgical use of laser beams in the 1990's began to affect the techniques of hernioplasty, particularly in terms of recovery time.

—*Byron D. Cannon, Ph.D.*

See also Abdomen; Abdominal disorders; Gastroenterology; Gastroenterology, pediatric; Gastrointestinal disorders; Gastrointestinal system; Hemorrhoids; Hernia repair; Intestinal disorders; Intestines.

FOR FURTHER INFORMATION:

Kurzer, Martin, Allan E. Kark, and George W. Wantz. *Surgical Management of Abdominal Wall Hernias.* London: Martin Dunitz, 1999. Although surgeons generally agree that hernias should be treated surgically, which surgical approach is the most appropriate for hernia repair is a much-debated issue. This book examines the various approaches.

Nyhus, Lloyd M., and Robert E. Condon, eds. *Hernia.* 4th ed. Philadelphia: J. B. Lippincott, 1995. Widely recognized and updated joint contribution by a large number of specialized physicians.

Ponka, Joseph L. *Hernias of the Abdominal Wall.* Philadelphia: W. B. Saunders, 1980. A general medical textbook containing excellent illustrative plates.

HERNIA REPAIR

PROCEDURE

ANATOMY OR SYSTEM AFFECTED: Abdomen, gastrointestinal system, intestines, stomach

SPECIALTIES AND RELATED FIELDS: Gastroenterology, general surgery

DEFINITION: Surgery to correct organ or tissue protrusions.

KEY TERMS:

congenital: referring to a disorder which is present at birth

diaphragm: the muscular partition that separates the abdominal and thoracic cavities

esophagus: the muscular tube through which food passes from the throat to the stomach

gangrene: death and decay of a body part as a result of injury, disease, or inadequate blood supply

peritonitis: potentially fatal abdominal inflammation and infection

INDICATIONS AND PROCEDURES

A hernia is an abnormal protrusion of an organ or organ part from its normal body cavity, most often tissue protruding through the abdominal wall. Abdominal hernias may occur in the groin (inguinal hernia), upper thigh (femoral hernia), navel (umbilical hernia), and diaphragm (hiatal hernia). They may be congenital or acquired in later life. Herniated tissue is most often part of the small or large intestine. It can also be part of the bladder or the stomach in femoral and hiatal hernias, respectively. Most hernias occur as a result of strain to the abdominal wall or its injury. For example, they are often caused by athletic overexertion or hard labor. Consequently, men are more subject to acquired hernias than women.

Congenital inguinal hernias in male infants can occur when the testicles of a developing fetus work their way down the inguinal canal to the scrotum. If the tissue sac accompanying them does not close off correctly, congenital hernia occurs. In men, acquired inguinal hernias occur when excess abdominal strain ruptures the intestinal wall and releases a loop of intestine. Inguinal hernias are less common in women and are associated with the canal that holds the round ligament of the uterus. Femoral hernias in both sexes lie on the inner sides of the blood vessels of the thighs and are always acquired, often by overexertion. Umbilical hernias, which may be congenital or acquired, protrude from the navel.

Incisional hernia is caused by the incomplete healing of surgical wounds of the abdomen. A fifth hernia type is hiatal hernia, which occurs at the opening where the esophagus passes through the diaphragm (the hiatus). Such hernias, in which part or all of the stomach passes through the diaphragm, may cause no external symptoms and be diagnosed only when chest X rays are taken for other reasons. If symptoms do occur, they usually include heartburn and chest pain.

Hernias are classified according to severity. Reducible hernias are those which can be resolved by pushing herniated tissue back into its proper position. Irreducible hernias are more serious. They cannot be pushed back manually because of their position, or because of the presence of adhesions that bind them in place. Such hernias can only be corrected with surgery. Strangulated hernias are those whose size and location pinch herniated tissue, cutting off blood flow. They require immediate surgical treatment to prevent the development of gangrene or peritonitis, both of which can be fatal.

Surgical repair is the suggested treatment for most hernias. If the patient is temporarily too ill for surgery, a truss may be used to diminish pain and swelling for inguinal, femoral, umbilical, and incisional hernias. Trusses, however, provide only temporary, symptomatic relief, except perhaps in umbilical hernias of very young children. Extreme caution is necessary: Reducible hernias treated with trusses can become irreducible or strangulated.

Standard hernia surgery can be accomplished in several ways. For the correction of inguinal or umbilical hernias, first the muscle wall is opened. Then, after the herniated loop is moved into an appropriate position, the muscle wall is closed as normally as possible. In more severe types of hernia, repair involving visible protrusions, the abdominal wall is opened, adhesions are cut away, and the tissue is returned to a normal position. Then, the muscle wall is

closed to restore normal muscle layers. When strangulation occurs, damaged tissue is cut away, normal sections are joined together, and viable tissue is returned to the abdomen, followed by abdominal clo-

Hernia Repair

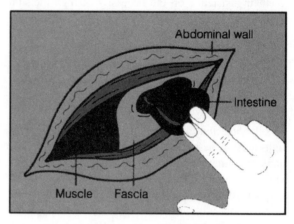

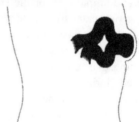

Abdominal wall hernia

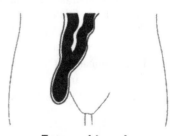

Femoral hernia

A hernia is the protrusion of a tissue or organ (usually a loop of intestine) into another area of the body. With abdominal wall hernias, which include inguinal and umbilical hernias, the intestine protrudes through a weakness in the abdomen; with femoral hernias, the intestine passes down the canal containing the major blood vessels to the thigh and appears as a bulge in the groin area. When a hernia presents a danger to the patient, the intestine must be surgically returned to its proper position.

sure. Incisional hernias are treated similarly, in a fashion dependent on the extent of the external damage and the degree of herniation.

Hiatal hernias are treated medically, whenever possible, because they tend to recur after surgery. Medical treatment includes restriction of activity, weight loss, and diet modification. Surgery is carried out when these efforts fail or if severe adhesions and/or strangulation occurs. The goal of this surgery is to strengthen the closure at the junction between the diaphragm and the esophagus.

USES AND COMPLICATIONS

The surgeries to correct inguinal, femoral, umbilical, and incisional hernias are straightforward. In all cases, but especially in strangulation, patients are checked before release to ensure that normal bowel movement occurs, that incisions have not become infected, and that fever has not developed. At this time, patients are also shown how to protect their incisions before coughing, are advised to maintain a high fluid intake to engender normal bowel function, are warned against overexertion, and are made aware of signs of incision infection. Furthermore, they are advised to resume work or physical activity only after consulting the physician involved.

Patients who have undergone surgery to correct a hiatal hernia are given much the same advice. Their surgery, however, is more extensive and prone to more complications. Therefore, they are provided with recommendations concerning which foods and activities to avoid. Furthermore, they are advised of the extended time period required before they can return to normal function and are told that without careful compliance, the problem will recur.

PERSPECTIVE AND PROSPECTS

Major advances in the treatment of hernias have included better diagnosis of their extent and the necessary means of their correction. Computed tomography (CT) scanning and other imaging techniques can make possible very accurate diagnoses. Progress in the surgical techniques used in hernia repair includes laparoscopy, in which a fiber-optic tube is used to visualize the chest cavity and thus to minimize incision size in the correction of hiatal hernias. All these methodologies are expected to improve in the future.

—*Sanford S. Singer, Ph.D.*

See also Abdomen; Abdominal disorders; Gangrene; Gastroenterology; Gastroenterology, pediatric; Gastrointestinal disorders; Gastrointestinal system; Hernia; Internal medicine; Intestinal disorders; Intestines; Pediatrics; Peritonitis.

FOR FURTHER INFORMATION:
Berkow, Robert, and Andrew J. Fletcher, eds. *The Merck Manual of Diagnosis and Therapy.* 17th ed. Rahway, N.J.: Merck Sharp & Dohme Research Laboratories, 1999. Contains a useful exposition of the characteristics, etiology, diagnosis, and treatment of hernia. Designed for physicians, the material is also useful for less specialized readers. Information on related topics is also included.

Maingot, Rodney. *Maingot's Abdominal Operations.* Edited by Michael J. Zinner et al. 10th ed. Stamford, Conn.: Appleton and Lange, 1997. This textbook has long been considered the classic work on all surgical disciplines.

Tierney, Lawrence M., Jr., et al., eds. *Current Medical Diagnosis and Treatment: 2001.* 39th ed. New York: McGraw-Hill, 2000. This text, updated yearly, is the point of reference for physicians and other health care practitioners. It incorporates each year's biomedical research discoveries that have immediate, relevant, and applicable use for the patient.

HERNIATED DISK. *See* SLIPPED DISK.

HERPES
DISEASE/DISORDER
ANATOMY OR SYSTEM AFFECTED: Genitals, mouth, reproductive system

SPECIALTIES AND RELATED FIELDS: Family practice, gynecology, internal medicine, virology

DEFINITION: A family of viruses that cause several diseases, including infectious mononucleosis, cold sores, genital herpes, and chickenpox; for most individuals, these widespread diseases are mild and of brief duration, but they may be fatal to those with impaired immune systems.

KEY TERMS:
antibody: a protein found in the blood and produced by the immune system in response to bodily contact with a foreign substance, such as a virus

congenital disease: a disease resulting from heredity or acquired while in the womb

disseminated: spread throughout the body

immune system: the body system that is responsible for fighting off infectious disease *immunocompromised:* a condition in which the immune system is impaired in some way, such as being not fully developed, deficient, or suppressed

latent: lying hidden or concealed

primary infection: a person's first infection with a particular virus

recurrent infection: an infection caused by the reactivation of a latent virus

vaccine: a substance given in order to prevent or ameliorate the effect of some disease

virus: the simplest entity that can reproduce; viruses are essentially made of some genetic material in a protective coating; viruses can reproduce only inside a living cell

TYPES OF HERPESVIRUS

Herpesviruses that affect humans include herpes simplex virus types 1 and 2, Epstein-Barr virus, varicella-zoster virus, and cytomegalovirus. Herpesviruses cause three types of infections: primary, latent, and recurrent. Most first-time, or primary, infections with herpesviruses cause few or no symptoms in the victim. Following the primary infection, herpesviruses have the unique ability to become latent, or hidden, in the body. Latent infections may persist for the life of the individual with no further symptoms, or the virus may reactivate (come out of hiding) and cause a recurrent infection. Although herpesvirus infections are often mild in healthy persons, they can cause potentially fatal infections in immunocompromised patients. Persons in this group include infants, whose immune systems are not fully developed; immunodeficient persons, whose immune systems are lacking some important component; and immunosuppressed patients, such as cancer or transplant patients, whose immune systems are being suppressed by immunosuppressive drugs or radiation. Herpesviruses have also been implicated in causing certain types of cancer.

Herpes simplex viruses exist in two forms: type 1 (HSV1) and type 2 (HSV2). HSV1 and HSV2 infections cause the formation of painful or itchy vesicular (blisterlike) lesions, which ulcerate, crust over, and heal within a few weeks. The virus is transmitted from one person to another by direct contact with infected lesions, and the virus enters the recipient through broken skin or mucous membranes. HSV1 usually causes infections above the waist—for example, in the mouth, throat, eye, skin, and brain. Gingivostomatitis, the most common form of primary HSV1 infection, is seen mostly in small children and is characterized by ulcerative lesions inside the mouth. Herpes labialis, or cold sores, the most common recurrent disease caused by HSV1, are characterized by blisters on the outer portion of the lips. HSV1 can also cause infection in any area of the skin where trauma (for example, a burn, scrape, or eczema) gives the virus an opening to get in. HSV1 infection of the eye can lead to scarring and blindness, and HSV1 infection of the brain can lead to death. Genital herpes, a disease transmitted by sexual contact, is most often caused by HSV2. The virus infects the penis in males and the cervix, vulva, vagina, or perineum in females. Two to seven days after infection, painful blisters appear in the genital area; they ulcerate, crust over, and disappear in a few weeks. Fever, stress, sunlight, or local trauma may trigger the virus to come out of hiding and cause a recurrent infection, and about 88 percent of persons with an HSV2 genital infection will have recurrences at a frequency of up to five to eight times per year. A severe form of HSV2 infection, neonatal herpes, occurs when a mother suffering from genital herpes passes the virus to her baby as it travels through the birth canal during delivery. This type of infection is usually disseminated, its death rate is high, and its survivors suffer from severe neurological damage.

Varicella-zoster virus (VZV) causes two diseases: chickenpox (varicella) and shingles (zoster). Chickenpox is a highly contagious common childhood disease caused by a primary infection with VZV. The virus is transmitted during close personal contact with an infected patient via airborne droplets that enter the respiratory tract or via direct contact with skin lesions. Once inside a person, the virus travels from the respiratory tract to the blood, and then to the skin. Ten to twenty-one days after infection, a typical rash appears on the skin and mucous membranes. On skin, the rash begins as red spots that develop into clear, fluid-filled vesicles that become cloudy, ulcerate, scab over, and fall off in a few days. Mucous membrane lesions in the mouth, eyelid, rectum, and vagina rupture easily and appear as ulcers. Fever, headache, tiredness, and itching may accompany the rash. Recovery from chickenpox confers lifelong immunity to reinfection but not latency. Reye's syndrome, an occasional severe complication of chickenpox, is associated with the use of aspirin. A few days after the initial infection has receded, the patient persistently vomits and exhibits signs of brain dysfunction. Coma

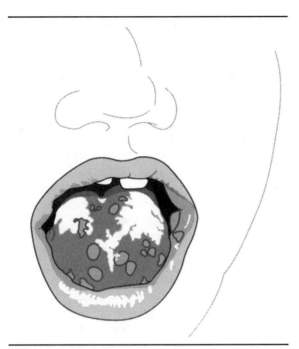

The herpesvirus is responsible for the common cold sore.

and death can follow if the syndrome is not treated. Chickenpox infection in adults is often more severe than in children, and adults run the risk of developing a fatal lung or brain infection.

Individuals with prior varicella infection may later develop shingles, which is caused by the reactivation of latent VZV. More than 65 percent of cases of shingles appear in adults older than forty-five years of age. The mechanism of reactivation is unknown, but recurrence is often associated with physical and emotional stress or a suppressed immune system. Shingles is usually localized to one area of the skin; it begins with pain in the nerves, and then a chickenpox-like rash appears on the skin over the nerves. The pain may be severe for one to four weeks, and recovery occurs in two to five weeks, with pain persisting longer in some elderly patients.

Epstein-Barr virus (EBV) causes infectious mononucleosis, an infection of the lymphatic system. In infected persons, the virus is present in saliva and blood, and thus it is transmitted by intimate oral contact (for example, kissing), sharing food or drinks, or by blood transfusions. Primary infection early in life usually causes no symptoms of disease, whereas primary infection later in life usually causes symptoms of infectious mononucleosis. In countries where sanitation is poor, most people have been infected by the age of five, without symptoms. In contrast, in countries where sanitation is good, primary infection is delayed until adolescence or young adulthood, and thus more than half the people in this age group develop symptoms. Once the infection begins, the virus grows in the throat and spreads to blood and lymph, invading white blood cells called B lymphocytes. The typical symptoms of infectious mononucleosis are extreme exhaustion, sore throat, fever, swollen lymph nodes, and sometimes an enlarged liver and spleen. The disease is self-limiting, and recovery takes place in four to eight weeks. The virus remains latent in the blood, lymphoid tissue, and throat and can continue to be transmitted to others even when no signs of active infection are present. EBV infection has also been associated with chronic fatigue syndrome and several types of cancer.

The widespread cytomegalovirus (CMV) is responsible for a broad spectrum of diseases. As is the case with EBV infection, primary infection by CMV early in life usually results in no symptoms, while primary infection as an adult yields mononucleosis-like symptoms. CMV also causes congenital cytomegalic inclusion disease and is a significant danger to bone marrow transplant patients. The virus is found in body secretions such as saliva, urine, semen, cervical secretions, and breast milk. Babies may acquire the virus from infected mothers congenitally, during birth while passing through the birth canal, or through breast milk. Children in day care may acquire CMV from other children who orally excrete the virus, and parents may get it from their children. CMV may be acquired through sexual transmission and blood transfusions. Patients undergoing transplants, especially bone marrow transplants, are at higher risk for CMV infection, since the virus may be present in the transplanted organs. The mononucleosis-like disease caused by CMV has the same symptoms as EBV-induced mononucleosis except the sore throat, swollen lymph nodes, and enlarged spleen. Congenital cytomegalic inclusion disease causes severe neurological damage, mental retardation, and death in infants; it is a result of primary CMV infection of the mother during pregnancy.

CAUSES, SYMPTOMS, AND TREATMENTS

A physician can often tell whether a person has an HSV infection based on the presence of the characteristic lesions and a history of exposure or previous lesions. For more severe HSV infections, the virus can be isolated and identified from infected tissue to confirm HSV as the causative agent. The major treatment procedure for most mild HSV infections is supportive care. These measures, such as bed rest and medication to relieve itching or pain, treat the symptoms but not the infection. For most infections, the symptoms eventually go away by themselves. For more severe HSV infections, several antiviral drugs have been used. Idoxuridine and trifluridine have been used to treat eye infections. Vidarabine and acyclovir are used to treat encephalitis and disseminated disease; both reduce the severity of the infection but do not reverse any neurological damage or prevent recurrent infections. Acyclovir has also been useful in reducing the duration of primary genital herpes, but not recurrent infection. The use of oral acyclovir to suppress recurrent infection may cause more severe and more frequent infections once the therapy has stopped. The best way to prevent infection with HSV is to avoid contact with a person with active lesions. Victims of genital herpes should avoid all sexual contact during episodes of lesions, to avoid transmitting the virus to someone else. Using condoms may be somewhat helpful in preventing the sexual transmission of HSV2. Newborns, children with eczema or other skin problems, burn patients, and immunocompromised patients should avoid persons with active HSV lesions. Pregnant females with active genital lesions must be delivered by cesarean section, in order to prevent the infection of their infants.

A diagnosis of chickenpox or shingles is based mainly on the symptoms of the patient, since they are so characteristic. It is possible to grow the virus from tissue samples or test the person for antibodies to VZV if necessary. Chickenpox takes care of itself and disappears after a few weeks; therefore, the only treatment needed is supportive care for the patient during that time. Often, drying lotions such as calamine help relieve the itching. It is important to cut the fingernails of especially young children so that they cannot scratch hard enough to break through the skin and leave themselves susceptible to secondary bacterial infection. It is extremely important not to give a child aspirin for the fever, because of the association between the use of aspirin during chickenpox and the development of Reye's syndrome. A child may be given acetaminophen if necessary. Zoster is treated mostly with pain medication to control the pain. Steroids given early in the infection help reduce the severity of the infection, and acyclovir increases the

rate of recovery. Antiviral drugs such as acyclovir, interferon, and vidarabine have been used in the treatment of immunocompromised patients with chickenpox to help reduce the potential severe complications of the disease. For most healthy persons, it is not necessary to prevent chickenpox, since it is a mild disease. It is important for newborns and immunocompromised patients to avoid exposure to persons with chickenpox because of threats such as pneumonia, encephalitis, and death. Since 1981, varicella-zoster immune globin (VZIG) has been available for the prevention and treatment of chickenpox in these patients. VZIG provides a short time of immunity, can lessen symptoms, and is recommended for immunocompromised children exposed to chickenpox, but it has no value once chickenpox has started. A VZV vaccine has been developed and shown to provide temporary protection from severe infection in immunocompromised children.

Unlike diagnoses of most VZV or HSV infections, the diagnosis of an EBV infection cannot be made based on the symptoms alone, because the virus causes a wide range of symptoms that could be caused by many other disease-causing agents. The diagnosis of EBV infection is made, therefore, based on laboratory tests. One test is a blood test in which technicians count the number of and kinds of white blood cells present in a patient. Persons with infectious mononucleosis have an abnormally large number of lymphocytes (one type of white blood cell) in their blood, and many of these lymphocytes have an odd appearance. A second test involves mixing the patients' blood serum (the fluid portion from their blood) with the red blood cells of sheep. The serum from 90 percent of persons with infectious mononucleosis will cause the sheep cells to clump. It is unknown why serum from infectious mononucleosis patients has this odd property (referred to as heterophil-positive). Persons suspected of having EBV but who give a heterophil-negative test are tested more rigorously for antibodies in their blood that are specific for EBV. The isolation of EBV from patients is not routinely performed to confirm a diagnosis of EBV infection, because the techniques needed are too complex for most laboratories. Infectious mononucleosis is a self-limiting disease, which means that it will eventually run its course and go away. Therefore, treatment involves mostly supportive care, such as bed rest and aspirin or acetaminophen for the fever and sore throat. It is also recommended that mononucleosis patients avoid contact sports, to prevent possible rupture of an enlarged spleen. In some severe cases, steroids are administered, and antiviral drugs are in the process of being tested to determine whether they are of any therapeutic value. The best way to prevent an EBV infection is to avoid intimate contact (for example, kissing) with an infected individual. Unfortunately, many persons shed the virus in their saliva without exhibiting any symptoms, so one cannot always tell who is infected and who is not.

Like EBV infection, CMV infection causes vague symptoms, and therefore diagnosis depends on laboratory tests. The virus can be grown from tissue samples, tissue can be examined to look for typical infected cells or the presence of virus, or the blood can be tested to look for antibodies to CMV. Mild cases of CMV need no treatment except supportive measures. Antiviral drugs such as interferon, vidarabine, idoxuridine, and cytosine arabinoside as well as CMV immune globin have all been tested for their benefit in severe cases of CMV infections, but none has been successful. The drug ganciclovir has been shown to have some therapeutic value. Most preventive measures have been aimed at developing a vaccine to prevent congenital CMV and CMV infection in immunosuppressed patients. A CMV vaccine has been developed, but further work is needed. Until better measures are available, it is important to try to avoid infection in immunocompromised patients, especially transplant recipients. The screening of organ donors for the presence of CMV may be helpful in accomplishing this goal. In addition, to prevent congenital CMV, pregnant females need to avoid primary CMV infection during their pregnancies. All pregnant females should be tested for CMV antibodies to determine whether they have already been infected; if not, they should avoid contact with small children who might carry CMV.

PERSPECTIVE AND PROSPECTS

Between 20 and 40 percent of the people in the United States suffer from cold sores, and more than 20 million persons suffer from genital herpes. In addition, HSV1 infection of the eye is the most common cause of corneal blindness in the United States, and HSV2 infection is associated with an increased risk of cervical cancer, which strikes some 15,000 women each year. Two hundred babies in the United States die each year, and 200 more suffer physical or mental impairment caused by HSV infection.

Chickenpox is the second most reported disease in the United States, with more than 200,000 cases per year. This number is probably too low, since many cases go unreported. About 100 deaths per year are attributed to chickenpox.

EBV infection is worldwide, and EBV antibodies can be found in more than 90 percent of most adult populations. EBV infection has been shown to be an important factor in the development of Burkitt's lymphoma (a cancer of the jaw) in Africa and nasopharyngeal carcinoma (a fatal cancer of the nose) in China. EBV has also been linked to chronic fatigue syndrome, but the relationship is not conclusive.

CMV infection is worldwide, with 40 to 100 percent of a population possessing antibodies to CMV. Almost all kidney transplant recipients and half of bone marrow recipients get CMV infection. Congenital CMV infection is the cause of severe neurological damage in more than 5,000 children born each year in the United States.

It is clear from these facts that infections with herpesviruses are a very important public health problem. The infections are widespread, and they cause a significant amount of distress, sickness, and death. The development of vaccines and other drugs to treat these diseases is important for infants and other immunocompromised persons whose lives can be threatened by acquiring a herpesvirus infection. The viruses' ability to become latent and the lack of drugs to destroy the latent viruses, however, make it virtually impossible to eradicate these diseases from the human population. Persons are infected for life, and they may continue to transmit the infection to other persons. Many other viral diseases, such as smallpox, measles, and polio, have been controlled by the use of vaccines that prevent a person from getting the disease, but the development of vaccines for herpesviruses is a complex problem. First, most of the diseases they cause are mild and self-limiting, so there is no pressing need to develop a vaccine quickly. Second, the association of the viruses with cancer causes scientists to proceed with caution in the development of a vaccine. Third, even if a vaccine does become available, it will be a long time before the viruses will be gone from the human population. Since herpesviruses can remain hidden in a person and stay there for life, they will not disappear until all currently infected persons die.

—*Vicki J. Isola, Ph.D.*

See also Cervical, ovarian, and uterine cancers; Chickenpox; Chronic fatigue syndrome; Genital disorders, female; Genital disorders, male; Gynecology; Mononucleosis; Reye's syndrome; Sexually transmitted diseases; Shingles; Viral infections; Warts.

FOR FURTHER INFORMATION:

Biddle, Wayne. *Field Guide to Germs*. New York: Henry Holt, 1995. This comprehensive book is easily accessible to the nonspecialist and includes a discussion of nearly every virus, bacterium, and fungus known to cause human and nonhuman animal disease. The history of the microbe and the treatment of diseases are included.

Ebel, Charles. *Managing Herpes: How to Live and Love with a Chronic STD*. Research Triangle Park, N.C.: American Social Health, 1998. With 20 percent of the American population now carrying the virus that causes genital herpes, the revised edition of this book, first published in 1994 by a nonprofit organization dedicated to stopping sexually transmitted diseases, is timely and welcome.

Langston, D. P. *Living with Herpes*. Garden City, N.Y.: Doubleday, 1983. Written to help patients suffering from herpesvirus infections to understand the disease better. Discusses all types of herpesvirus infections, with a particular emphasis on genital herpes.

Nourse, A. E. *Herpes*. New York: Franklin Watts, 1985. A well-written, informative, and easy-to-read book. Focuses mostly on genital herpes but also includes information on other sexually transmitted diseases and the other herpesvirus infections.

Radetsky, Peter. *The Invisible Invaders: The Story of the Emerging Age of Viruses*. Boston: Little, Brown, 1991. Discusses viruses in general, how they were discovered, and the diseases they cause. Chapter 10 gives an interesting account of the discovery of the links between EBV infection and chronic fatigue syndrome, infectious mononucleosis, and Burkitt's lymphoma.

Regush, Nicholas. *The Virus Within: A Coming Epidemic*. New York: Dutton, 2000. A virus called HHV-6 (a form of the human herpes virus) is at the heart of a controversy brewing in the scientific community. Scientists are uncovering evidence that it may play a role in serious illnesses such as AIDS and multiple sclerosis. Regush makes a strong case for further research.

Zinsser, Hans. *Zinsser Microbiology*. Edited by Wolfgang K. Joklik et al. 20th ed. Norwalk, Conn.: Appleton and Lange, 1992. The information presented in this textbook is thorough, logical, and supplemented by interesting diagrams, photographs, and charts. Chapter 66, "Herpesviruses," gives a complete description of infections with HSV, VZV, EBV, and CMV.

HICCUPS

DISEASE/DISORDER

ALSO KNOWN AS: Hiccoughs

ANATOMY OR SYSTEM AFFECTED: Chest, lungs, muscles, respiratory system, throat

SPECIALTIES AND RELATED FIELDS: Family practice, gastroenterology, neurology

DEFINITION: Involuntary, spasmodic contractions of the diaphragm and the simultaneous closure of the glottis.

CAUSES AND SYMPTOMS

A hiccup is caused by an involuntary, spasmodic contraction of the diaphragm, the large partition of muscles and tendons that separates the chest from the abdomen. The diaphragm draws air into the lungs through rhythmic contractions. When it contracts suddenly, an opening located toward the top of the trachea (windpipe) between the vocal cords in the larynx (voice box) called the glottis snaps shut abruptly. The combination of air being forced through the vocal cords in the larynx and the abrupt closure of the glottis causes the sound associated with hiccups.

There are a number of causes of hiccups, the most common being overdistension of the stomach. Other causes include gastric irritation from spicy or rich foods and nerve spasms. There is some indication that hiccups are controlled by the central nervous system.

Hiccups generally last for a very short time, usually stopping within minutes. People who suffer from hiccups for more than twenty-four hours or who have repetitive attacks are said to suffer from chronic hiccups. This condition is very rare.

People of all ages can suffer from hiccups. Pregnant women report that fetuses sometimes have hiccups in the womb.

TREATMENT AND THERAPY

An attack of hiccups is not serious and is generally self-limiting. A number of techniques to stop are practiced, including holding one's breath, drinking a glass of water, breathing deeply, or breathing into a paper bag.

Babies often suffer from hiccups, particularly during nursing. Some mothers report that feeding the baby a quarter of a teaspoon of sugar mixed in 4 ounces of water calms the hiccups. Doctors suggest that hiccup-prone babies be fed before they are overly hungry and when they are calm.

—*Diane Andrews Henningfeld, Ph.D.*

See also Abdomen; Breast-feeding; Coughing; Respiration.

FOR FURTHER INFORMATION:

Gluck, Michael, and Charles E. Pope II. "Hiccups and Gastrointestinal Reflux Disease: The Acid Perfusion Test as a Provocative Maneuver." *Annals of Internal Medicine* 105 (1996): 219-220.

Heuman, Douglas M., A. Scott Mills, and Hunter H. McGuire, Jr. *Gastroenterology.* Philadephia: W. B. Saunders, 1997.

Launois, J. L., W. A. Bizec, J. C. Whitelaw et al. "Hiccup in Adults: An Overview." *European Respiratory Journal* 6 (1993): 563-575.

Shay, Steven D. S., Robert L. Myers, and Lawrence F. Johnson. "Hiccups Associated with Reflux Esophagitis." *Gastroenterology* 87 (1984): 204-207.

HIP FRACTURE REPAIR

PROCEDURE

ANATOMY OR SYSTEM AFFECTED: Bones, hips, joints, legs, musculoskeletal system

SPECIALTIES AND RELATED FIELDS: Geriatrics and gerontology, orthopedics

DEFINITION: The repair or replacement of a broken hip joint.

KEY TERMS:

arthroplasty: joint replacement

osteoporosis: a loss of bone mass accompanied by increasing fragility and brittleness

INDICATIONS AND PROCEDURES

Hip fracture repair constitutes one of the most common procedures performed by orthopedic surgeons. The human hip consists of two bones, the hipbone and the thighbone (femur), and their point of intersection, a cup-shaped cavity called the acetabulum. This hip joint forms a ball-and-socket mechanism that allows the leg to move in different directions. As a major weight-bearing joint, the hip is vulnerable both to sudden trauma, such as sports injuries, and to degenerative disorders of aging, such as osteoporosis.

If the loss of bone mass associated with osteoporosis is sufficiently advanced, a simple fall from a standing position can shatter the hip joint. The most common fracture involves the femur snapping or cracking just below the rounded end that fits into the acetabulum.

PERSPECTIVE AND PROSPECTS

The repair of hip fractures involves the realignment of the bone fragments and the insertion of a long nail into the bone to hold them together. A plate is attached to the nail and to the healthy bone surrounding the fracture in order to give support.

Because broken bones heal slowly in the elderly, in the past a broken hip almost inevitably resulted in these patients becoming permanent invalids restricted to wheelchairs or, at best, forced to rely on walkers and enjoying only limited mobility. This bleak prognosis changed in the 1960's when orthopedic specialists working with biomedical engineers developed artificial hip joints. The combination of prosthetic devices and surgical techniques known as total hip arthroplasty (THA) allows physicians to return patients to active, independent lives. In THA, the weakened end of the femur is removed and an artificial replacement installed. The replacement can consist of any of a variety of materials, but typically it is constructed of a chromium steel alloy coated with a ceramic polymer that helps resist corrosion as well as providing a surface with which the patient's bone can bond. The end of the prothesis and the surface of the acetabulum are coated with plastic polymers to reduce friction. Research indicates that artificial hip joints last fifteen years or longer before wear and tear on the lining of the ball-and-socket joint creates problems.

—*Nancy Farm Mannikko, Ph.D.*

See also Aging: Extended care; Arthroplasty; Arthroscopy; Bone disorders; Bone grafting; Bones and the skeleton; Emergency medicine; Fracture and dislocation; Fracture repair; Geriatrics and gerontology; Hip replacement; Orthopedic surgery; Orthopedics; Osteoporosis; Physical rehabilitation.

FOR FURTHER INFORMATION:

Sabiston, David C., Jr., ed. *Textbook of Surgery.* 16th ed. Philadelphia: W. B. Saunders, 2001.

Schwartz, Seymour I., ed. *Principles of Surgery.* 7th ed. New York: McGraw-Hill, 1999.

Way, Lawrence W., ed. *Current Surgical Diagnosis and Treatment.* 11th ed. Norwalk, Conn.: Appleton & Lange, 1998.

Wilmore, Douglas W., et al., eds. *Care of the Surgical Patient*. New York: Scientific American, 1992.

HIP REPLACEMENT
PROCEDURE

ANATOMY OR SYSTEM AFFECTED: Bones, hips
SPECIALTIES AND RELATED FIELDS: Orthopedics, rheumatology
DEFINITION: The removal of diseased bone tissue in the hip and its replacement with an artificial device.

INDICATIONS AND PROCEDURES

The most common reason for hip replacement surgery is the decline in efficiency of the hip joint that often results from osteoarthritis. Osteoarthritis is a common form of arthritis that causes joint and bone deterioration, which may lead to the wearing down of cartilage and cause the underlying bones to rub against each other. This may result in severe pain and stiffness in the affected areas. Other conditions that may lead to the need for hip replacement include rheumatoid arthritis (a chronic inflammation of the joints), avascular necrosis (loss of bone caused by insufficient blood supply), and injury.

Generally, physicians may be more inclined to choose less invasive techniques such as physical therapy, medication, or walking aids before resorting to surgery. In some cases, exercise programs may help reduce hip pain. In addition, if preliminary treatment does not improve the patient's condition, doctors may use corrective surgery that is not as invasive as hip replacement. However, when these efforts do not reduce pain or increase mobility, hip replacement may be the best option. In addition, the age of the patient may be an important factor in the decision to replace the hip. The majority of hip replacements are performed on individuals over the age of sixty-five. One of the reasons for this is that the activity level of older adults is lower than that of younger adults, therefore reducing the concern that the new hip will wear out or fail. However, technological advances have improved the quality of the artificial hip, making hip replacement surgery a more likely intervention for younger adults as well.

Generally, a candidate for total hip replacement surgery (THR) possesses a hip that has worn out from arthritis, falls, or other conditions. The hip consists of a ball-and-socket joint where the head of the femur (thigh bone) fits into the hip socket, or acetabulum. In a normal hip, this arrangement provides for a relatively wide range of motion. For some older adults, however, deterioration caused by arthritis and other conditions reduces the effectiveness of this arrangement, compromising the integrity of the hip socket or the femoral head. This state can lead to extreme discomfort.

Total hip replacement may provide the best long-term relief for these symptoms. Total hip replacement involves the removal of diseased bone tissue and the replacement of that tissue with prostheses (artificial devices used to replace missing body parts). Usually, both the femoral head and hip socket are replaced. The femoral head is replaced with a metal ball that is attached to a metal stem and placed into the hollow marrow space of the femur. The hip socket is lined with a plastic socket. Other materials have been used effectively as hip replacements.

In some cases, the surgeon will use cement to bond the artificial parts of the new hip to the bone tissue. This approach has been the traditional method of ensuring that the artificial parts hold. One problem with this method is that over time, cemented hip replacements may lose their bond with the bone tissue. This may result in the need for an additional surgery. However, a cementless hip replacement has been developed. This approach includes a prosthesis that is porous so that bone tissue may grow into the metal pores and keep the prosthesis in place.

Both procedures have strengths and weaknesses. In general, recovery time may be shorter with cemented prostheses since one does not have to wait for bone growth to attach to the artificial prostheses. However, the potential for long-term deterioration of the replaced hip must be considered. A cemented hip generally lasts about fifteen years. With this in mind, physicians may be more likely to use a cemented prosthesis for patients over the age of seventy. Cementless hip replacement may be more advisable for younger and more active patients. Some physicians have used a combination of approaches, known as a "hybrid" or "mixed" hip. This combination relies on an uncemented socket and a cemented femoral head.

USES AND COMPLICATIONS

Total hip replacements are generally quite successful, with about 96 percent of surgeries proceeding without complications. In rare instances, however, complications occur, including blood clots and infections during surgery, and hip dislocation or bone fracture after surgery. In addition, in some cases, bone grafts may be used to assist in the restoration of bone defects. In these instances, bone may be obtained from the pelvis or the discarded head of the femur. Other postoperative complications may include some pain and stiffness.

Patients recovering from total hip replacement usually remain in the hospital up to ten days if there are no complications. However, physical therapists may initiate therapy as soon as the day after surgery. Physical therapy involves the use of exercises that will improve recovery. Many patients are able to sit on the edge of their bed, stand, and even walk with assistance as early as two days after surgery. Patients must remember that their artificial hip may not provide the same full range of motion as an undiseased hip. Physical therapists teach patients how to perform daily activities without placing an undue burden on their new hips. This may require learning a new method of sitting, standing, and performing other activities.

While many factors may affect recovery time, full recovery from surgery may take up to six months. At that point, many patients enjoy such activities as walking and swimming. Doctors and physical therapists may discourage patients from participating in such high-impact activities as jogging or playing tennis, which may burden the new hip. Despite these restrictions, many patients are able to perform normal activities without pain and discomfort. Nonetheless, people who have undergone hip replacement surgery are advised to consult with their doctor about proper exercise and activity levels.

PERSPECTIVE AND PROSPECTS

Total hip replacement is one of the most common surgical interventions that older adults face. The American Academy of Orthopedic Surgeons estimates that more than 120,000 hip replacement surgeries are performed in the United States each year. The average age of the patient who undergoes hip replacement surgery is sixty-seven years, while 67 percent of total hip replacements are performed on individuals age sixty-five or older. Approximately 60 percent of hip replacement surgeries are performed on women.

—*H. David Smith, Ph.D.*

See also Arthritis; Bone disorders; Bones and the skeleton; Hip fracture repair; Orthopedics.

FOR FURTHER INFORMATION:

Baron, John A., Jane Barrett, Jeffrey Katz, and Matthew H. Liang. "Total Hip Arthroplasty: Use and Select Complications in the U.S. Medicare Population." *The American Journal of Public Health* 86, no. 1 (January, 1996). Use and outcomes of primary total hip arthroplasty among U.S. Medicare recipients more than sixty-five years of age were examined by means of physician and hospital claims for a 5 percent random sample during 1986 through 1989.

Bucholz, Robert, and Joseph A. Buckwalter. "Orthopedic Surgery." *The Journal of the American Medical Association* 275, no. 23 (June 19, 1996). The research focus of orthopedic surgery is discussed, including research on the use of recombinant growth factors to induce bone repair and the regeneration of cartilaginous surfaces.

Callaghan, John J. "A Seventy-Six-Year-Old Woman Considering Total Hip Replacement." *The Journal of the American Medical Association* 276, no. 6 (August 14, 1996). A seventy-six-year-old woman complained of many of the signs and symptoms of degenerative joint disease or osteoarthritis of the hip and was at a point where she suffered from a loss of motion.

Duffey, Timothy P., Elliott Hershman, Richard A. Sanders, and Lori D. Talarico. "Investigating the Subtle and Obvious Causes of Hip Pain." *Patient Care* 31, no. 18 (November 15, 1997). A delay in diagnosing the cause of a patient's acute hip pain could lead to significant impairment of the hip. Talarico explains how to maximize one's investigative effort and make the most of treatment.

Dunkin, Mary Anne. "Hip Replacement Surgery." *Arthritis Today* 12, no. 2 (March/April, 1998). Two types of joint prostheses are discussed. Illustrations by Kevin A. Somerville show the difference between a healthy hip joint and cartilage that is damaged.

Finerman, Gerald A. M. *Total Hip Arthroplasty Outcomes*. New York: Churchill Livingstone, 1998. Discusses topics such as the anatomic medullary looking prosthesis, the porous-coated anatomic prosthesis, the anatomic porous replacement system, long-term results of hybrid prostheses, and the hybrid total hip replacement.

Horosko, Marian. "Connected to the Hip Bone." *Dance Magazine*, February, 1999, 89. This article includes a description of metal-metal hip replacement surgery.

MacWilliam, Cynthia H., Marianne U. Yood, James J. Verner, Bruce D. McCarthy, and Richard E.

Ward. "Patient-Related Risk Factors That Predict Poor Outcome After Total Hip Replacement." *Health Services Research* 31, no. 5 (December, 1996). A study identifies factors associated with poor outcome after total hip replacement (THR) surgery. It is the first to present results from the American Medical Group Association (AMGA) THR consortium.

Trahair, Richard C. S. *All About Hip Replacement: A Patient's Guide*. Oxford, England: Oxford University Press, 1999. Includes bibliographical references and an index.

HIPPOCRATIC OATH

ETHICS

DEFINITION: A document, written in the fifth century B.C.E., to offer guidelines for the emerging medical profession, which continues to be the subject of debate in modern practice because of the ethical issues that it addresses.

KEY TERMS:

euthanasia: the practice (particularly in cases involving patients of advanced age) of withholding medical treatments that might sustain life that would otherwise expire "naturally"; in a more controversial form, it is associated with the administration of drugs by physicians in order to avert prolonged suffering

living will: a legally binding document instructing a physician not to prolong life by externally administered life support systems if the patient is unable to express his or her decision concerning forms of medical treatment recommended by a physician

malpractice insurance: insurance policies held by physicians in order to protect them financially in the event of a patient-initiated lawsuit alleging incidents of improper medical decisions or incompetence

MEDICAL CODES OF ETHICS

Western civilization has long held the writings of the fifth century B.C.E. Greek physician Hippocrates, and in particular the Hippocratic oath, as a model of ethical values to be followed in the medical profession. As the nature of Western civilization itself has changed over the centuries, interpretations of the ethical values behind the Hippocratic oath have also changed. The circumstances of modern medical practice and ethical values, however, have ironically made certain elements of the classical Hippocratic tradition even more relevant than they may have appeared in previous eras.

In fact, the Hippocratic oath is only the introductory section of the *Corpus Hippocraticum* (Hippocratic Collection) traditionally attributed to Hippocrates. (There is debate about whether he is the author of all the books or only some.) The actual medical observations of Hippocrates were studied and applied for many centuries, until scientific research rendered many of them recognizably obsolete. A number of sections of the corpus, however, reflect the Greek physician's recurring concern for rules to guide the medical profession. Hippocrates' chapters on "The Art," "Decorum," and "The Law" complement the more famous ethical precepts contained in the oath.

The first part of the oath itself covers the physician's lifelong commitment to his or her teachers. This commitment extends not only to the symbolic bonds of respect but also to obligation to share one's medical practice and even to provide financial assistance to one's teachers, if requested. Additionally, the physician is committed to train, free of charge, the families of his or her teachers in the art of medicine.

The second part of the Hippocratic oath contains the more general pledges that would contribute to its value as an ethical guide for the medical profession. The physician is bound, in a very general way, to help the sick according to his or her ability and judgment in a manner that can never be interpreted as involving injury or wrongdoing. The physician is bound both to confidentiality concerning direct experiences in the patient-doctor relationship and to extreme discretion to avoid the circulation of professional knowledge that is not appropriate for publication abroad.

In addition to these general precepts, all of which have an ethical timelessness that would survive the centuries, there were two points in the oath that refer to specific issues that cannot be separated from the modern debate over medical ethics. Addressing the questions of euthanasia ("mercy killing") and abortion, Hippocrates stated: "I will give no deadly drug to any, though it be asked of me, nor will I counsel such, and especially I will not aid a woman to procure abortion."

Anyone searching for wider guidelines can glean many items of timeless wisdom from other sections of Hippocrates' writings. In the pieces entitled "The Physician" and "Decorum," for example, the personal behavior of doctors is discussed. In all cases, Hippocrates exhorted physicians to maintain even levels of dignity and patience, to practice exemplary personal hygiene, and to avoid excesses in living habits that could introduce an element of distance between themselves and the patients who depend on them. Many centuries later, as in the eighteenth century English essay by Samuel Bard entitled "A Discourse upon the Duties of a Physician," one can see similar concerns for behavioral propriety toward the defenseless: for example, "Never affect to despise a man for the want of a regular education, and treat even harmless ignorance with delicacy and compassion" and protect against the effects of "foolhardiness and presumption." These admonitions are indicative of the defining boundaries of the views of Hippocrates and those of the later, Christian era on the practice of medicine. The main attention of commentators on the Hippocratic corpus in recent generations has been directed to two broad divisions in the main ethical issues that he formulated: the physician's role in abortion and in the decision to end life by either withholding or administering certain treatments. It took many centuries, however, for degrees of emphasis in analyzing the Hippocratic oath to take form. In the interim, and after a delay that separated the classical world from the late medieval world, different interpretations of the Hippocratic oath would appear, each reflecting the cultural environment to which it was meant to apply.

Several factors may explain why centuries passed before systematic attention was given to the rules of medicine first broached in the classical Greek and Roman worlds. The first of these was the general decline of political and economic conditions after the fall of Rome (fifth century C.E.), which had repercussions in a variety of cultural areas. Medical practices tended to revert to quite crude levels until the rediscovery of early medical texts, including those of Hippocrates, sparked interest in improving conditions of medical treatment in the late Middle Ages.

One can say that, in addition to editing elements of Hippocratic teachings to Christianize the pagan references that they contained, a second important redirection occurred in setting down medieval rules for the practice of medicine. It was Holy Roman Emperor Frederick II, around 1241, who specified for the first

The Hippocratic Oath

I will look upon him who shall have taught me this Art even as one of my parents. I will share my substance with him, and I will supply his necessities, if he be in need. I will regard his offspring even as my own brethren, and I will teach them this Art, if they would learn it, without fee or covenant. I will impart this Art by precept, by lecture and by every mode of teaching, not only to my own sons but to the sons of him who has taught me, and to disciples bound by covenant and oath, according to the Law of Medicine.

The regimen I adopt shall be for the benefit of my patients according to my ability and judgment, and not for their hurt or for any wrong. I will give no deadly drug to any, though it be asked of me, nor will I counsel such, and especially I will not aid a woman to procure abortion. Whatsoever house I enter, there will I go for the benefit of the sick, refraining from all wrongdoing or corruption, and especially from any act of seduction, of male or female, of bond or free. Whatsoever things I see or hear concerning the life of men, in my attendance on the sick or even apart therefrom, which ought not to be noised abroad, I will keep silence thereon, counting such things as sacred secrets.

time that the higher authority of the state alone should define institutional procedures for certifying physicians. This was to be done through formal training and examinations in the universities of Naples or Salerno, and later in universities throughout the Western world.

In addition to rules leading to physicians' certification, Frederick II stipulated that doctors must take an oath binding them to obligations that, in comparison to the Hippocratic oath or modern codes of medical ethics, covered very specific issues. One of these was an obligation to report any irregularities in an apothecary's preparation of drugs that were to be dispensed to patients. Another enjoined doctors to provide free medical services to the poor.

If one looks at more modern standards for the regulation of relations between physician and patient, it is possible to suggest that—until some very major changes took place in society's views on delicate questions previously reserved for ecclesiastical law—similar operatives continued to govern the guidelines for medical ethics. In the "Code of Medical Ethics"

(1846-1847) by the American Medical Association (AMA), for example, primary focus is still visibly on the physician's obligation to place the patient's interest before his or her own, particularly in terms of prospects for material or other forms of personal gain. Defense of the public's interest against quackery or the distribution of drugs that are either dangerous or illegally prepared follows, as well as avoidance of "crude hypotheses" or "magnification of the importance of services" sought, merely for the purpose of "temporary effect and popularity." Although there are enormous time spans between the classical Hippocratic model, the medieval variant offered by Frederick II, and the mid-nineteenth century AMA code, all are comparable in their focus on what, in the terminology of the 1847 code, would be called "Duties for Support of Professional Character" (part 1, article 1) or "Duties of the Profession to the Public" (part 2, article 1).

A hundred years later, however, different societal attitudes toward medical ethics would establish themselves in most Western nations, including the United States. Generally stated, the basic changes reflected in ethical debates emphasized (or questioned the rising emphasis on) the protection of individual rights and privacy in matters relating to human life and the intervention of physicians. On the one hand, changing directions in the expression of ethical orientations stemmed from advances made in key areas of medical science in the twentieth century, such as technologies for combatting terminal disease, saving the lives of severely preterm infants, and prolonging life in old age. On the other hand, and in an even broader context, extraordinary scientific discoveries concerning the genetic keys behind life itself introduced an entirely different dimension to medical ethics, that of responsibility for monitoring or "engineering" life that has not yet been conceived.

MODERN APPLICATIONS OF THE HIPPOCRATIC OATH

Although neither the original nor edited versions of the Hippocratic oath are applied today as a condition for becoming a doctor, the medical profession in the United States has definitely formalized publication of what it considers to be a necessary code of medical ethics. Evolving versions of this "Code of Medical Ethics" date from the original (1847) text of the AMA as revised by specific decisions in 1903, 1912, and 1947.

When the AMA adopted a statement under the title "Guide to Responsible Professional Behavior" in 1980, it assigned to a formal body within its organization, the Council on Ethical and Judicial Affairs, the task of publishing, on a yearly basis, updated paragraphs that reflect ethical guidelines for the profession as a whole. These evolving guidelines are organized under such subheadings as "Social Policy Issues," "Interprofessional Relations," "Hospital Relations," "Confidentiality," and "Fees and Charges."

Thus, in the absence of a specific professional oath with detailed provisions, modern physicians are bound to respect the ethical guidelines provided to them by their professional association. Failure to respect these guidelines is tantamount to breaking one's binding ethical obligations and can lead to expulsion from the medical profession.

Several major changes, both in levels of medical technology and in social attitudes toward issues relating to medical practice, have played key roles in several spheres of an ongoing debate concerning medical ethics. In two cases, those of abortion and euthanasia, debate has focused on the ethics of deciding to end life; in the third, referred to generally as genetic engineering, the central question involves both the living and those yet to be born. In all these spheres, the legal and ethical debates have revolved around potential conflicts between physicians and patients but also in the context of wider social values.

Movement from the historical domain of idealized codes or oaths to the more practical and contemporary realm of changing societal reactions to what constitutes injury or breach of professional ethics in several areas of modern medicine is facilitated by reference to landmark legal decisions that have given a modern and quite different meaning to Hippocratic concepts.

Probably the most widely recognized issue reflecting such ethical conflicts, and one that received specific attention in the Hippocratic oath itself, involves abortion. In the United States, the climate of public opinion toward doctor-assisted pregnancy terminations was altered considerably by the landmark 1973 Supreme Court decision *Roe v. Wade*. In this decision, the Court judged that state laws defining abortion as a criminal offense were unconstitutional. The main thrust of the argument in *Roe v. Wade* was that, although the Constitution does not provide a specific guarantee of a civil right of privacy that could be applied to questions of life and death in medical care, parallels exist in Supreme Court decisions on other matters of individual rights with respect to procreation. These rights tend to fall under the Fourteenth Amendment's concept of personal liberty and restrictions on state action. These rights, in the Court's words, are "broad enough to encompass a woman's decision whether or not to terminate her pregnancy."

Reference to the fundamental right of "personal privacy" in *Roe v. Wade* granted individual women and their physicians recourse against specific state laws criminalizing abortion. It did not, however, consider the right to have an abortion to be unqualified. Nor did it extend beyond the domain of pregnancy termination to cover a general assumption that constitutional protection of the right of privacy included the individual's right to "do with one's body as one pleases." In fact, there was an explicit suggestion that the legal definition of protection of an individual's right to privacy where critical medical decisions affecting vital life processes are concerned is "not unqualified and must be considered against important state interests in regulation."

As time passed in the evolving debate over abortion, definitions of what this could mean became colored by the inevitable introduction of religious conceptions of defense of the unborn individual—the fetus—as a possessor of life separate from that of the pregnant woman. This was a precursor to the "right to life" versus "right to choice" debate that would place physicians between two poles of opinion as to where their final obligations should lie.

What seemed most important in the beginnings of the abortion debate (and then, a few years later, the euthanasia debate) was the Supreme Court's inclusion of commentary on Hippocratic ethical precepts as part of its argument justifying recognition of individual rights to final responsibility for the disposition of someone else's "future" life or the disposition of one's own life. The *Roe v. Wade* brief actually argued that the strict Hippocratic injunction against abortion must be recognized as a reflection of only one segment of opinion and values (specifically Pythagorean) at a particular time in history. By underlining the fact that other views and practices were known to be current throughout antiquity, and that later Christian ethics chose to ignore diversity of interpretations of medical ethics in such matters, *Roe v. Wade* implied that diversity of ethical opinion within a social environment must be recognized in order to avoid too narrow a definition of what standards should be followed by physicians in dealing with their patients.

The implications of these two directions in interpreting the ethical bonds between patient and physician—the right to privacy in reaching individual decisions and recognition of a degree of social relativity in defining guidelines for medical ethics—are equally visible in the debate concerning the ultimate source of authority for deciding when to terminate life and the presumed authority of the Hippocratic oath in this process.

Two issues, one involving the ethics of sustaining life by means of advanced medical technology and the other involving the "engineering" of lives according to genetic predictions, fall under the provisions of the Hippocratic oath. As one approaches more contemporary statements of professional obligations of medical doctors, such as the "Principles of Medical Ethics" (1957) of the American Medical Association, one finds that, as certain areas of specificity in classical Hippocratic or Christian medical ethics (the illegality of abortions or the administration of deadly potions) tend to decline in visibility, another area begins to come to the forefront—namely, striving continually to improve medical knowledge and skills to be made available to patients and colleagues.

This more modern concern for the application of advancements in medical knowledge, especially in the technology of medical lifesaving therapy, has introduced a new focus for ethical debate: not "lifesaving" but "life-sustaining" techniques, particularly in cases judged to be otherwise terminal or hopeless. As with the issue of abortion, the question of a doctor's responsibility to use every means within his or her reach to sustain life, even when there is no hope of a meaningful future for the patient, reflects a dilemma regarding Hippocratic injunctions. This debate is more important now than in any earlier era because advanced medical technology has made it possible either to extend the lives of aged patients who would die without life-sustaining machines or—in the case of younger persons afflicted by brain damage, for example—to sustain life although the patient remains in a comatose state.

A prototype in the latter case was a 1976 Supreme Court decision that allowed the parents of New Jersey car accident victim Karen Quinlan to instruct her physician to remove life support systems so that their comatose daughter would die. At issue in this complicated case, which also rested on legal discussions of the constitutional right of privacy, was the question of who should decide that inevitable natural death is preferable to prolongation of life by externally administered means. When the Court took this decision away from an appointed court guardian and gave it to those closest to the patient, the question became whose privacy was being protected. This dilemma is not unlike that inherent in the abortion debate, where the privacy of the pregnant woman is weighed against that of the as-yet-unconscious, unborn child. To whom does the physician's oath to avoid doing injury actually apply?

Legal solutions to subareas of the euthanasia debate were attained in stages, especially in cases of the very aged or patients afflicted with known terminal diseases. A living will, for example, allows individuals to instruct their physicians not to sustain their lives by artificial means if, beyond a certain point, they are unable to express their own will to die. In some cases, this discretion is assigned to the next of kin. In both cases, the objective is to remove ultimate responsibility for inevitable natural death from the physician's shoulders and to place it as closely as possible to within the private sphere of the patient.

A final area of contemporary debate over medical ethics illustrates how far conceptions of ultimate responsibility for the protection of life have gone beyond frames of reference that might have been familiar not only in Hippocrates' time but also as recently as the generation of doctors trained before the 1980's. Impressive advances in the research field of human genetics by the mid-1980's began to make it possible to predict, through analysis of deoxyribonucleic acid (DNA) structures, the likelihood that certain genetic traits (specifically debilitating chronic diseases) might be transmitted to the offspring of couples under study. Inherent in the rising debate over the ethics of such studies, which range from the prediction of reproductive combinations (genetic counseling) through actual attempts to detach and splice DNA chains (genetic engineering), was the delicate question of who, if anyone, should hold the responsibility of determining if individuals have ultimate control over their genes. In the most extreme hypothetical argument, a notion of scientific exclusion of certain gene combinations, or planning of desirable gene pools in future generations, began to appear in the 1980's and 1990's. These notions represent potential problems for medical ethics that, because of exponential changes in technological possibilities, surpass the entire realm of Hippocratic principles.

PERSPECTIVE AND PROSPECTS

Despite the introduction of certain legal precedents that tried to protect both physicians and their patients against dilemmas stemming from the assumed immutable ethical principles of the Hippocratic oath, society continues to witness practical shortcomings in modern understanding of who needs to be protected and how such protection should be institutionalized.

Malpractice insurance offers legal protection to physicians against personal damage claims levied by aggrieved patients or those surviving deceased patients; by the late twentieth century in the United States, these rates had soared. The larger debate regarding whether what physicians have done in individual cases was right or wrong rests on the assumption that his or her judgment can be put to the test by private parties defending their rights against professional incompetence. Therefore, the issue, as well as the institutional and/or legal devices pursued to resolve it, lies beyond the strict realm of a patient's privacy vis-à-vis a physician's responsibilities.

More characteristic examples of the contemporary social-ethical dilemma of whether doctors are fulfilling their appropriate professional responsibilities in recognizing patients' rights to certain types of treatment continue to fall into legally unresolved categories. The most obvious appears to be the ongoing debate concerning the legality of physician-assisted abortions. The considerations that have been introduced clearly go beyond the black-or-white principles that simple comparison with the content of the Hippocratic oath might involve. Courts and legislators involved in the ethics of abortion have had to devote extensive attention to the considerations of how pregnancies were induced (with attention to the anomalies of incest or rape, for example) or to questions of whether tax-appropriated funds gathered from an ethically divided public body can be dispensed to pay for medically approved abortions.

Still other dimensions of contemporary physician-patient relationships reveal that new forms of legislation will be needed before debates over the applicability of Hippocratic principles to modern society will recede from front-page prominence. With living wills having more or less resolved the question of individuals' right to instruct physicians or families to make decisions for them when personal capacities decline to incoherence, signs of new legal dilemmas began to emerge in the 1990's concerning fully coherent, terminally ill patients. Despairing of future suffering that can come well before any question of life support devices arises, some patients contracted their physicians—initially one physician in particular, Jack Kevorkian of Detroit, Michigan—to perform "mercy killing" by the administration of lethal poisons. Thus, one of the specific negative injunctions of the original Hippocratic oath returned the question of individual physicians' ethical and legal obligations to the forefront of public attention and court proceedings more than two millennia after its initial statement.

—*Byron D. Cannon, Ph.D.*

See also Abortion; American Medical Association; Cloning; Education, medical; Ethics; Euthanasia; Genetic engineering; Law and medicine; Malpractice.

FOR FURTHER INFORMATION:

Casarett, David J., Frona Daskal, and John Lantos. "Experts in Ethics? The Authority of the Clinical Ethicist." *The Hastings Center Report* 28, no. 6 (November/December, 1998): 6-11. This article examines the work of Jurgen Habermas, which provides a basis for a model of clinical ethics consultation in which consensus, grounded in moral theory, assumes a central theoretical role.

Fletcher, John C., et al., eds. *Introduction to Clinical Ethics.* 2d ed. Frederick, Md.: University, 1997. This group of essays by contributing authors addresses the topic of ethics in contemporary medicine. Includes a bibliography.

Harron, Frank, John Burnside, and Tom Beauchamp. *Biomedical-Ethical Issues.* New Haven, Conn.: Yale University Press, 1983. A collection of key contemporary documents, including court decisions, state and federal laws, and policy statements by a number of professional associations regarding the most-debated ethical issues in medicine.

Jonsen, Albert R., Mark Siegler, and William J. Winslade. *Clinical Ethics: A Practical Approach to Ethical Decisions in Clinical Medicine.* 4th ed. New York: McGraw-Hill, 1998. Discusses the whole range of medical ethics, including legal issues, confidentiality, care of the dying patient, and euthanasia and assisted suicide.

HIRSCHSPRUNG'S DISEASE
DISEASE/DISORDER

ALSO KNOWN AS: Congenital megacolon

ANATOMY OR SYSTEM AFFECTED: Anus, gastrointestinal system, intestines

SPECIALTIES AND RELATED FIELDS: Cytology, family practice, gastroenterology, pediatrics, proctology

DEFINITION: Hirschsprung's disease occurs when the lower part of the large intestine, including the rectum, has no nerve cells to control the muscles that produce the contractions necessary for a bowel movement. The affected part of the intestine becomes grossly distended, and the baby suffers severe constipation. Diagnosis of the disease is confirmed by an X ray and a biopsy of rectal tissue. An operation removes the affected area of the intestine, and the remaining ends are rejoined.

—*Alvin K. Benson, Ph.D.*

See also Constipation; Gastroenterology, pediatric; Gastrointestinal system; Genetic diseases; Neonatology; Surgery, pediatric.

FOR FURTHER INFORMATION:

Ehrenpreis, Theodor. *Hirschsprung's Disease.* Chicago: Year Book Medical, 1970.

Hadziselimovic, F., and B. Herzog, eds. *Inflammatory Bowel Diseases and Morbus Hirschsprung: Proceedings of the Sixty-fifth Falk Symposium.* Boston: Kluwer Academic, 1992.

Nixon, H. Homewood. *Color Atlas of Surgery for Hirschsprung's Disease.* Oradell, N.J.: Medical Economics, 1985.

HISTOLOGY
SPECIALTY

ANATOMY OR SYSTEM AFFECTED: All

SPECIALTIES AND RELATED FIELDS: Biochemistry, cytology, dermatology, hematology, internal medicine, oncology, pathology, vascular medicine

DEFINITION: The study of the body's tissues—epithelial, connective, muscle, and nerve tissues—to find the changes in structure that can be induced by disease.

KEY TERMS:

collagen: a fibrous protein occurring in many types of connective tissue

connective tissues: tissues containing large amounts of matrix outside the cells

epithelia: tissues that originate in broad, flat surfaces

matrix: organic or inorganic material occurring in connective tissues but located outside the cells

muscle tissues: tissues specialized in such a manner that they respond to stimulation by contracting along their long axes

nerve tissues: tissues specialized in such a manner that they respond to stimulation by conducting nerve impulses along their surfaces

tissues: groups of similar cells that are closely interrelated in function and organized together spatially

TYPES OF TISSUES

Histology is the study of tissues, which are groups of similar cells that are closely interrelated in their function and are organized together by location and structure. The four major types of tissues are epithelial tissue, connective tissue, muscle tissue, and nervous tissue.

Epithelial tissue (or epithelia) includes those tissues that originate in broad, flat surfaces. Their functions include protection, absorption, and secretion. Epithelia can be one-layered (simple) or multilayered (stratified). Their cells can be flat (squamous), tall and thin (columnar), or equal in height and width (cuboidal). Some simple epithelia have nuclei at two different levels, giving the false appearance of different layers; these tissues are called pseudostratified. Some simple squamous epithelia have special names: The inner lining of most blood vessels is called an endothelium, while the lining of a body cavity is called a mesothelium. Kidney tubules and most small ducts are also lined with simple squamous epithelia. The pigmented layer of the retina and the front surface of the lens of the eye are examples of simple cuboidal epithelia. Simple columnar epithelia form the inner lining of most digestive organs and the linings of the small bronchi and gallbladder. The epithelia lining the Fallopian tube, nasal cavity, and bronchi are ciliated, meaning that the cells have small hairlike extensions called cilia.

The outer layer of skin is a stratified squamous epithelium; other stratified squamous epithelia line the inside of the mouth, esophagus, and vagina. Sweat glands and other glands in the skin are lined with stratified cuboidal epithelia. Most of the urinary tract is lined with a special kind of stratified cuboidal epithelium called a transitional epithelium, which allows a large amount of stretching. Parts of the pharynx, larynx, urethra, and the ducts of the mammary glands are lined with stratified columnar epithelia.

Glands are composed of epithelial tissues that are highly modified for secretion. They may be either exocrine glands (in which the secretions exit by ducts that lead to targets nearby) or endocrine glands (in which the secretions are carried by the bloodstream to targets some distance away). The salivary glands in the mouth, the glandular lining of the stomach, and the sebaceous glands of the skin are exocrine glands. The thyroid gland, the adrenal gland, and the pituitary gland are endocrine glands. The pancreas has both exocrine and endocrine portions; the exocrine parts secrete digestive enzymes, while the endocrine parts, called the islets of Langerhans, secrete the hormones insulin and glucagon.

Connective tissues are tissues containing large amounts of a material called extracellular matrix, located outside the cells. The matrix may be a liquid (such as blood plasma), a solid containing fibers of collagen and related proteins, or an inorganic solid containing calcium salts (as in bone).

Blood and lymph are connective tissues with a liquid matrix (plasma) that can solidify when the blood clots. In addition to plasma, blood contains red cells (erythrocytes), white cells (leukocytes), and the tiny platelets that help to form clots. The many kinds of leukocytes include the so-called granular types (basophils, neutrophils, and eosinophils, all named according to the staining properties of their granules), the monocytes, and the several types of lymphocytes. Lymph contains lymphocytes and plasma only.

Most connective tissues have a solid matrix that includes fibrous proteins such as collagen and also elastic fibers, in some cases. If all the fibers are arranged in the same direction, as in ligaments and tendons, the tissue is called regular connective tissue. The dermis of the skin, however, is an example of an irregular connective tissue in which the fibers are arranged in all directions. Loose connective tissue and adipose (fat) tissue both have very few fibers. The simplest type of loose connective tissue, with the fewest fibers, is sometimes called areolar connective tissue. Adipose tissue is a connective tissue in which the cells are filled with fat deposits. Hemopoietic (blood-forming) tissue, which occurs in the bone marrow and the thymus, contains the immature cell types that develop into most connective tissue cells, including blood cells. Cartilage tissue matrix contains a shock-resistant complex of protein and sugarlike (polysaccharide) molecules. Cartilage cells usually become trapped in this matrix and eventually die, except for those closest to the surface. Bone tissue gains its supporting ability and strength from a matrix containing calcium salts. Its typical cells, called osteocytes, contain many long strands by means of which they exchange nutrients and waste products with other osteocytes, and ultimately with the bloodstream. Bone also contains osteoclasts, large cells responsible for bone resorption and the release of calcium into the bloodstream.

Mesenchyme is an embryonic connective tissue made of wandering amoebalike cells. During embryological development, the mesenchyme cells develop into many different cell types, including hemocytoblasts, which give rise to most blood cells, and fibroblasts, which secrete protein fibers and then usually differentiate into other cell types.

Muscle tissues are tissues that are specially modified for contraction. When a nerve impulse is received, the overlapping fibers of the proteins actin and myosin slide against one another to produce the contraction. The three types of muscle tissue are smooth muscle, cardiac muscle, and skeletal muscle.

Smooth muscle contains cells that have tapering ends and centrally located nuclei. Muscular contractions are smooth, rhythmic, and involuntary, and they are usually not subject to fatigue. The cells are not cross-banded. Smooth muscle occurs in many digestive organs, reproductive organs, skin, and many other organs.

The term "striated muscle" is sometimes used to refer to cardiac and skeletal muscle, both of which have cylindrical fibers marked by cross-bands, which are also called cross-striations. The striations are caused by the lining up of the contractile proteins actin and myosin.

Cardiac muscle occurs only in the heart. Its cross-striated fibers branch and come together repeatedly. Contractions of these fibers are involuntary and rhythmic, and they occur without fatigue. Nuclei are located in the center of each cell; the cell boundaries are marked by dark-staining structures called intercalated disks.

Skeletal muscle occurs in the voluntary muscles of the body. Its cylindrical, cross-striated fibers contain many nuclei but no internal cell boundaries; a multinucleated fiber of this type is called a syncytium. Skeletal muscle is capable of producing rapid, forceful contractions, but it fatigues easily. Skeletal muscle tissue always attaches to connective tissue structures.

Nervous tissues contain specialized nerve cells (neurons) that respond rapidly to stimulation by conducting nerve impulses. All neurons contain RNA-rich granules, called Nissl granules, in the cytoplasm. Neurons with a single long extension of the cell body

are called unipolar, those with two long extensions are called bipolar, and those with more than two long extensions are called multipolar. There are two types of extensions: Dendrites conduct impulses toward the cell body, while axons generally conduct impulses away from the cell body. Many axons are surrounded by a multilayered fatty substance called the myelin sheath, which is actually made of many layers of cell membrane wrapped around the axon.

Nervous tissues also contain several types of neuroglia, which are cells that hold nervous tissue together. Many neuroglia have processes (projections) that wrap around the neurons and help nourish them. Among the many types of neuroglia are the tiny microglia and the larger protoplasmic astrocytes, fibrous astrocytes, and oligodendroglia.

Two major tissue types make up most of the brain and spinal cord, or central nervous system. The first type, gray matter, contains the cell bodies of many neurons, along with smaller amounts of axons, dendrites, and neuroglia cells. The second type, white matter, contains mostly the axons, and sometimes also the dendrites, of neurons whose cell bodies lie elsewhere, along with the myelin sheaths that surround many of the axons. Clumps of cell bodies are called nuclei within the brain and ganglia elsewhere. Bundles of axons are called tracts within the central nervous system and nerves in the peripheral nervous system.

HISTOLOGY AS A DIAGNOSTIC TOOL

Many diseases produce changes in one or more body tissues; these changes are so characteristic that the diagnosis of a disease often depends on the microscopic observation of changes in tissues. In order for such a diagnosis to be made, the tissue must be sliced very thin on a machine called a microtome. Some tissues are sliced while frozen; others must be hardened (or "fixed") in chemical solutions. After being sliced, the tissue is usually stained with chemical dyes that make viewing easier. Some tissues are viewed under the light microscope; others are sliced even thinner for viewing by electron microscopy.

Most hospitals have a pathology department that is responsible for these operations. After the tissues are sliced and examined, the pathologist makes a report that usually includes a diagnosis of the disease shown by the tissue samples.

Many diseases result in marked changes in the tissue at the microscopic level. Adaptively altered changes, which are usually reversible, include an increase in cell size (hypertrophy), increase in cell numbers (hyperplasia), a change from one cell or tissue type to another (metaplasia), and a decrease in size by withering (atrophy). Prolonged or repeated insults to the tissue may result in altered or atypical growth patterns (dysplasia). Overwhelming or sustained injury results in irreversible changes such as tissue degeneration or death. Tissue degeneration often includes the accumulation of abnormal amounts of fatty, fibrous, or pigmented tissue. Tissue death in a body that goes on living is called necrosis, and it may be of several types. If tissue death exceeds a certain limit, then the death of the organism results. Once this occurs, the tissues usually release protein-digesting enzymes that digest their own cell contents, a process known as autolysis.

Changes to cellular organelles can often be seen with an electron microscope before they become apparent at the light microscope level. Disturbances of the cell membrane may alter the flow of fluids (especially water) and cause changes to occur in the fluid composition of the cytoplasm. Too much fluid may result in swelling and eventually in bursting of the cells; too little fluid results either in shrinkage or in the coagulation of proteins. Swelling may also be induced by the lack of oxygen flow to the mitochondria, which can also result in the deposition of fats or calcium. The increase in the water content of the cells can also cause swelling in the endoplasmic reticulum and the detachment of ribosomes from the surfaces of the rough endoplasmic reticulum. Most damaging of all are the disturbances of the lysosomes, which can release their protein-digesting enzymes and cause autolysis.

At the light microscope level, other changes that may result from disease processes include the coalescence of numerous dropletlike vacuoles into a single, large, fluid-filled space. Other changes that may indicate disease are abnormal cell shapes, changes in the proportion of blood cells, and the rupture of cell membranes or other structures. Substances that may accumulate in diseased cells include glycogen (a sugar storage product), fibrous deposits of collagen and other proteins, and mineral deposits such as calcium salts. Abnormalities of the nucleus may include nuclear fragmentation, loss of the staining properties of the nucleus, or pyknosis, a shrinkage of the nucleus that also includes the clumping of its chromosomal material.

Edema, or tissue swelling, is a condition that can easily be confirmed by microscopic examination of histological sections. The swelling is marked by an increase in the amount of extracellular fluid. In the case of pulmonary edema, the fluid stains pink and fills the usually empty lung spaces (alveoli).

A different type of change is seen in Barrett's esophagus, a condition caused by the repeated backflow (or reflux) of gastric fluids into the esophagus. The inner lining of the esophagus is usually a stratified squamous epithelium, but in Barrett's esophagus the surface cells become taller, and the lining is changed into a columnar epithelium resembling that of the stomach.

Most cancers are recognized by abnormalities of the affected tissues, usually including more cells in the process of cell division (mitosis). The most dangerous cancers are marked by large tumors with ill-defined, irregular margins. If the cancer tumor is well-defined, small, and has a smooth, circular margin, the cancer is much less of a threat.

In juvenile diabetes, histological examination of the pancreas reveals a greatly reduced number of pancreatic islets, and those that remain are smaller and more fibrous. Herpes simplex infection causes the epidermal cells of the skin to undergo a buildup of fluid and a consequent balloonlike swelling. Warts of the skin are marked by a thickening of the outermost layer (stratum corneum) of the epidermis. Pernicious anemia, or vitamin B_{12} deficiency, results in a deterioration of the glands in the stomach lining. Crohn's disease produces swelling of the affected parts of the intestine, deposition of fat and lymphoid tissue, and ultimately tissue loss and deposition of fibrous scar tissue; the affected parts typically alternate with healthy regions. Cirrhosis of the liver, which is most commonly the result of chronic alcohol abuse, proceeds through a fatty stage (marked by deposition of fatty tissue), a fibrotic stage (marked by small nodules and scars), and an end stage marked by abnormal shrinkage (atrophy) of liver tissue, scars, and larger nodules up to 1 centimeter in diameter. Emphysema, a lung disease found in many smokers, is recognizable histologically by an enlargement of the air spaces and by the presence of black, tarlike deposits within the lung tissue. Fibrocystic changes of the breast may be marked by the deposition of fibrous tissue, by increasing cell numbers, and by the enlargement of the glandular ducts.

Lupus erythematosus, a connective tissue disease,

often produces red skin lesions marked by degeneration and flattening of the lower layers of the epidermis, drying and flaking of the outermost layer, dilation of the blood vessels under the skin, and the leakage of red blood cells out of these vessels, adding to the red color. (The word "erythematosus" means "red.")

Muscular dystrophy has several forms; the most common form is marked in its advanced stages by enlarged muscles in which the muscle tissue is replaced by a fatty substance. Another muscular disease, myasthenia gravis, is often marked by overall enlargement of the thymus and an increase in the number of thymus cells. Myocardial infarction (heart attack), a form of heart disease marked by damage to the heart muscle, is indicated in histological section by dead, fibrous scar tissue replacing the muscle tissue in the heart wall. In patients with arteriosclerosis, the usually elastic walls of the arteries become thicker and more fibrous and rigid. Many of the same patients also suffer from atherosclerosis, a buildup of deposits on the inside of the blood vessels that partially or completely blocks the flow of blood.

In nervous tissue, damage to peripheral nerves often results in a process called chromatolysis in the cell bodies of the neurons from which these axons arise. The nuclei of these cells enlarge and are displaced to one side, while the Nissl granules disperse and the cell body as a whole undergoes swelling. Increased deposits of fibrous tissue characterize multiple sclerosis and certain other disorders of the nervous system. Some of these diseases are also marked by a degeneration of the myelin sheath around nerve fibers. In the case of a cerebrovascular stroke, impaired blood supply to the brain causes degeneration of the neuroglia, followed by general tissue death and the replacement of the neuroglia by fibrous tissue. Cranial hematoma (abnormal bleeding in any of several possible locations) results in the presence of blood clots (complete with blood cells and connective tissue fibers) in abnormal locations. Alzheimer's disease is marked by granules of a proteinlike substance called amyloid, often containing aluminum, surrounded by additional concentric layers of similar composition. Advanced stages of alcoholism are marked in brain tissue by the destruction of certain neurons and neuroglia. Poliomyelitis, or polio, is marked by the destruction of nervous tissue in the anterior horn of the spinal cord.

PERSPECTIVE AND PROSPECTS

The microscopic study of tissues began historically with Robert Hooke's *Micrographia* (1665) and the studies of Marcello Malpighi (1628-1694), but early microscopes were low in quality by today's standards. As microscopes improved, so did their use in studying tissues. During the 1830's, the Scottish botanist Robert Brown (1773-1858) discovered the cell nucleus. Soon, German biologists Matthias Jakob Schleiden (1804-1881) and Theodor Schwann (1810-1882) developed the so-called cell theory, a theory which proclaimed that all living things are constructed of cells and that all biological processes are rooted in processes occurring at the level of cells and tissues. The greatest advances in microscopic optics were made between 1870 and 1900, mostly in Germany, and the study of histology benefited greatly.

The great pathologist Rudolph Virchow (1821-1902) was the first to emphasize the structural changes in cells caused by the disease process; he showed that many diseases could be detected at the cellular level under the microscope. This claim, coupled with the enthusiasm for the cell theory, aroused great interest in the study of cells throughout Europe and later in America. Advances in tissue-staining techniques in microanatomy were made in various countries over a long period; the Czech histologist and physiologist Jan Evangelista Purkinje (1787-1869) was one of the leaders of this early period. Early in the twentieth century, histologists Santiago Ramón y Cajal (1852-1934) of Spain and Camillo Golgi (1844-1926) of Italy shared the 1906 Nobel Prize in Physiology or Medicine for their detailed work on the tissue structure of the nervous system. In the decades after World War II, the electron microscope became a standard instrument for the ultrafine study of tissue details at and even below the cellular level. Today, pathology laboratories routinely use the microscopic examination of tissues as an important tool in diagnosis.

—Eli C. Minkoff, Ph.D.

See also Alzheimer's disease; Arteriosclerosis; Biopsy; Bleeding; Blood and blood disorders; Bones and the skeleton; Cells; Cirrhosis; Crohn's disease; Cytology; Dermatology; Emphysema; Glands; Herpes; Lupus erythematosus; Lymphatic system; Multiple sclerosis; Muscles; Muscular dystrophy; Nervous system; Neurology; Orthopedics; Pathology; Poliomyelitis; Skin; Strokes.

FOR FURTHER INFORMATION:

Fawcett, D. W. *A Textbook of Histology.* 12th ed. New York: Chapman & Hall, 1994. A classic standard, well illustrated with a variety of light micrographs (often in color) and electron micrographs. Most thorough in its descriptions of physiological functions.

Ham, Arthur W., and David H. Cormack. *Histology.* 9th ed. Philadelphia: J. B. Lippincott, 1987. A very thorough textbook that is especially good for bone and other hard tissues. The illustrations (including several in color) are a very good combination of drawings, light micrographs, and electron micrographs.

Kerr, Jeffrey B. *Atlas of Functional Histology.* St. Louis: Mosby, 1999. This volume includes discussion of histology as it applies to the major biological systems, such as the endocrine, respiratory, reproductive, gastrointestinal, nervous, and circulatory systems.

Kessel, Richard G. *Basic Medical Histology.* Oxford, England: Oxford University Press, 1998. This textbook is derived from Kessel's notes, figures, and references accumulated over thirty-five years of teaching histology at the University of Iowa. Suitable for advanced undergraduate students in biology or possibly first-year medical students.

Leeson, C. R., T. S. Leeson, and A. A. Paparo. *Textbook of Histology.* 5th ed. Philadelphia: W. B. Saunders, 1985. Similar to the book by Ham and Cormack but less detailed.

HIV. *See* HUMAN IMMUNODEFICIENCY VIRUS (HIV).

HIVES
DISEASE/DISORDER

ALSO KNOWN AS: Urticaria

ANATOMY OR SYSTEM AFFECTED: Immune system, skin

SPECIALTIES AND RELATED FIELDS: Dermatology, family practice, immunology, internal medicine, pediatrics

DEFINITION: Pink swellings called wheals that may occur in groups on any part of the skin.

CAUSES AND SYMPTOMS

Hives are produced by blood plasma leaking through tiny gaps between the cells lining small vessels in the skin. A natural chemical called histamine is released from mast cells, which lie along the blood vessels in the skin. Allergic reactions, foods, drugs, or other chemicals can cause histamine release.

Hives can vary in size from as small as a pencil eraser to as large as a dinner plate, and they may join together to form larger swellings. When hives are forming, they are usually very itchy; they may also burn or sting. Nearly 20 percent of the general population will have at least one episode of hives in their lifetime. Acute hives may last for a few days to weeks. If they last for more than six weeks, they are called chronic hives.

The most common causes of acute hives are foods, drugs, infections, insect bites, and internal diseases. Other causes are physical stimuli, including pressure, cold, and sunlight.

TREATMENT AND THERAPY

The best treatment for hives is to find the cause and then eliminate it. Unfortunately, this is not always an easy task. Even if a cause cannot be found, antihistamines are usually prescribed to provide some relief. Antihistamines work best if taken on a regular schedule. It may be necessary to try more than one or use different combinations of antihistamines to find out what works best. In severe cases of hives, an injection of epinephrine (adrenalin) or a cortisone preparation can bring dramatic relief.

PERSPECTIVE AND PROSPECTS

In 1927, Sir Thomas Lewis reported the association between wheals and small blood vessel dilation, which later confirmed the importance of histamine as a cause of hives. Years of research showed that apart from allergy, nonimmunological stimuli can cause hives as well. A recent report that some patients with chronic hives may have formed antibodies against the immunoglobulin IgE receptor suggests that the cause of hives could be multifactorial.

—*Shih-Wen Huang, M.D.*

See also Allergies; Bites and stings; Dermatology, pediatric; Immune system; Itching; Rashes; Skin; Skin disorders.

FOR FURTHER INFORMATION:

Joneja, Janice M. V., and Leonard Bielory. *Understanding Allergy, Sensitivity, and Immunity.* New Brunswick, N.J.: Rutgers University Press, 1990.

Kuby, Janis. *Immunology.* New York: W. H. Freeman, 2000.

Roitt, Ivan. *Essential Immunology*. 9th ed. Boston: Blackwell Scientific, 1997.

Young, Stuart, Bruce Dobozin, and Margaret Miner. *Allergies*. Rev. ed. New York: Plume, 1999.

HODGKIN'S DISEASE
DISEASE/DISORDER

ANATOMY OR SYSTEM AFFECTED: Lymphatic system

SPECIALTIES AND RELATED FIELDS: Hematology, internal medicine, oncology, serology

DEFINITION: A neoplastic disorder originating in the tissues of the lymphatic system, recognized by distinctive histologic changes and defined by the presence of Reed-Sternberg cells.

KEY TERMS:

chemotherapy: a modality of cancer treatment consisting of the administration of cytotoxic drugs

combination chemotherapy: the use of multiple chemical agents in the treatment of cancer, each in a lower dosage so that the overall toxicity, but not the effectiveness, is reduced

neoplastic: pertaining to cancerous growths

prognosis: a prediction of the outcome of treatment for a disease on the basis of clinical and pathologic parameters, such as pathology, clinical stage, and presence or absence of symptoms such as fever, night sweats, and unexplained weight loss

radiotherapy: the use of radiation to kill cancer cells or shrink cancerous growth; when high and full doses of radiation (measured in units called rads) are used, the patient is said to be given a "megavoltage"

CAUSES AND SYMPTOMS

Malignant lymphomas are neoplasms of lymphoid tissues and are of two general categories: those related to Hodgkin's disease and others that are collectively called non-Hodgkin's lymphomas. The lymphoid tissues represent the structural expressions of the immune system, which defends the body against microbes. This system is widely spread throughout the body, is highly complex, and interacts closely with other physiologic systems of the body—especially the mucosa that lines the airways and digestive tract, where there is direct exposure to environmental microbes and other foreign substances. The components of this system are aggregations of lymphocytes in the mucosal linings (such as tonsils and adenoids), lymph nodes, and the spleen. The components of the

lymphatic system connect with one another via small lymphatic vessels. The lymph nodes, which are situated in anatomical regions all over the body, interconnect and drain centrally toward the great veins of the body. The cellular components of the immune system are the lymphocytes, also called immunocytes. These account for about 20 percent of blood cells; lymphocytes make up the bulk of the lymphoid tissue that makes up the lymphatic system. The blood cells have a finite life and are disposed of in the spleen, which is the largest lymphoid organ in the body.

There are two major functional immunologic classes of lymphocytes and several other subclasses. Nevertheless, all share similar morphologic appearance, being small round cells almost completely occupied by a round nucleus. The B lymphocyte (the B refers to its bone marrow derivation) can, under proper antigenic stimulation, transform and mature into a plasma cell, which is the cell in charge of producing antibodies. Antibodies are the protein products of the immune system that act by capturing and removing foreign substances, called antigens. The other major class of lymphocytes is the T lymphocyte (the T refers to its thymus derivation). T lymphocytes are of at least two major functional subclasses, which either help or suppress the B lymphocytes in their transformation into plasma cells; thus they are termed helper and suppressor T cells, respectively. Other cellular components of the immune system, cellular monocytes and macrophages, play an important role in carrying and transferring specific immunologic information between the various cellular components of the immune-lymphatic system. This, then, is a highly organized and complex system, with positive and negative biofeedback that maintains optimal, balanced proportions of all the cellular components that make up the system.

Hodgkin's disease is a neoplasm of the lymphoid tissues that usually arises in lymph nodes, often in the neck, and has a varied histologic appearance characterized by the presence of Reed-Sternberg cells. The Reed-Sternberg cell is a giant cell having two nuclei that are situated in a mirror-image fashion. Treatment and prognosis in Hodgkin's disease are determined by two parameters: the histopathologic classification, whereby the morphologic appearance is evaluated by the pathologist, and the clinical staging classification, whereby the extent of spread of the disease and its localization are determined by clinical studies. The pathology is studied by reviewing thinly cut sections of diseased lymph nodes removed from the patient. This study is most important for establishing a diagnosis of Hodgkin's disease and ruling out other conditions that may closely simulate its clinical and/or pathologic features. At times, peer consultations are used to confirm the diagnosis.

Reed-Sternberg cells have a characteristic appearance and must be identified to make a diagnosis of Hodgkin's disease. The pathologic classification of this disease, based on microscopic study, recognizes four different types, each with its own clinical implications regarding survival and prognosis. The classification is based on the relative dominance of lymphocytes when compared to the number of the neoplastic

Staging of Hodgkin's Disease

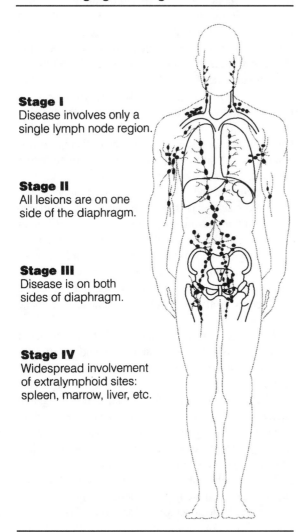

Stage I
Disease involves only a single lymph node region.

Stage II
All lesions are on one side of the diaphragm.

Stage III
Disease is on both sides of diaphragm.

Stage IV
Widespread involvement of extralymphoid sites: spleen, marrow, liver, etc.

Reed-Sternberg cells. In the most favorable type, the lymphocytes predominate and Reed-Sternberg cells are sparse; this type is called lymphocyte predominance. In the worst type, the lymphocytes are very sparse and there are many more Reed-Sternberg cells and their variants; this type is called lymphocyte depletion. In between these two extremes are the mixed-cellularity type, in which there is an even mixture of lymphocytes and Reed-Sternberg cells, and nodular sclerosis, which forms nodules of fibrous scar tissue that surround the mixture of lymphocytes and Reed-Sternberg cells.

This classification has important prognostic implications. It correctly presumes that the neoplastic cells are the Reed-Sternberg cells and their variants, and that the lymphocytes are induced by the immune system to multiply and to fight the spread of the neoplastic cells. It follows that the more the process is successful, the better is the prognosis. Hence lymphocyte predominance carries a more favorable outlook than lymphocyte depletion, with mixed-cellularity types somewhere in between. Nodular sclerosis also carries a good prognosis. Other inflammatory cells are invariably mixed with the lymphocytes and Reed-Sternberg cells; these cells are also part of the body's immune response against cancer cells.

The clinical staging classification of Hodgkin's disease was formulated by a group of experts who met at a workshop in Ann Arbor, Michigan, in 1971. It is based on the proposition that the disease begins in a single group of lymph nodes (usually in the neck) and then spreads to the next adjacent group of lymph nodes, on the same side, before it crosses over to the other side of the body. The disease then advances further across the diaphragm muscle, which separates the thorax from the abdominal cavity, and finally disseminates into the blood to involve the bone marrow and other distant sites. In this schema, stage I represents early stage, with involvement of only a single lymph node region, and stage II is the condition in which two or more such regions are involved on the same side of the diaphragm (that is, either above or below the diaphragm).

In the United States, Hodgkin's disease is an uncommon neoplasm accounting for 7,900 cases, or fewer than 1 percent of all new cases of cancer, and 1,500 deaths, according to 1993 American Cancer Society statistics. This represents an incidence in the United States of 3.2 per 100,000 population overall, with slightly higher incidence in males than females, and in whites than blacks. Incidence trends show a mild rise for the nodular sclerosis type in young adults and a mild decrease of Hodgkin's disease over the age of forty.

Hodgkin's disease can occur at any age, although the highest peak incidence occurs in adolescents and young adults, and smaller peaks occur in the fifth and sixth decades of life. Most patients come to clinical attention because of painless, nontender, enlarged lymph nodes in the neck or armpits (above the diaphragm) or, less commonly, in the groin. In the young adult or adolescent, a mass in the chest may press against the airways to produce a dry, hacking cough and shortness of breath, which may be the patient's first symptoms. Some patients may have anemia or severe itching. At times, especially when the disease is aggressive and extensive, the patient may have a fever, which may run for a few days and then disappear, only to recur after a week or two; there can also be night sweats and weight loss. These symptoms—fever, night sweats, and weight loss—indicate a less favorable prognosis. Younger patients and those with lymphocyte predominance and nodular sclerosis histologic types (favorable histologic types) tend to have limited disease—that is, stages I and II—found primarily above the diaphragm. Older patients and those with mixed-cellularity or lymphocyte depletion types are more likely to have extensive disease involving lymph nodes on both sides of the diaphragm (stage III) or even involving the liver, spleen, and bone marrow (Stage IV).

When a patient with persistent lymph node enlargement seeks medical attention, a lymph node biopsy is usually made to make sure of the diagnosis. Other cancers that may simulate Hodgkin's disease must be excluded, as well as a long list of benign conditions such as infectious mononucleosis and tuberculosis. A series of blood tests, X-ray and other imaging studies, and a bone marrow biopsy are done in order to evaluate the spread of disease and to assign the proper clinical stage. At times, even surgical exploration of the abdomen, with biopsies of abdominal lymph nodes, the liver, and the spleen, is done to assign an accurate stage of Hodgkin's disease; this procedure is called staging laparotomy.

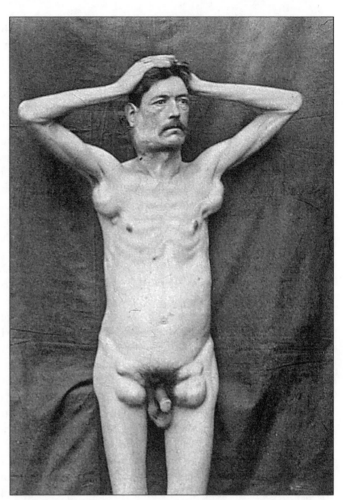

A man with Hodgkin's disease is shown in the Atlas of Clinical Medicine *(1892).* (National Library of Medicine)

TREATMENT AND THERAPY

Modern cancer therapy has achieved its greatest triumph in the treatment of Hodgkin's disease. The advent of a generally acceptable histopathologic classification, accurate staging, improved radiotherapy, effective chemotherapy, and supportive care, such as antibiotics and the transfusion of platelets, have contributed to the impressive 75 percent overall cure rate. The therapy is enhanced by an effective teamwork of medical experts in oncology, radiation therapy, surgery, pathology, and diagnostic radiology.

Because Hodgkin's disease spreads in an orderly fashion through adjacent lymph node groups, effective high-dose radiation can be directed at affected lymph nodes and at their neighboring, uninvolved nodes. Irradiation, with a full dose of 3,500 to 4,000 rads in three to four weeks, can eradicate Hodgkin's disease in involved nodes within the treatment field more than 95 percent of the time. In addition, extended-field irradiation of the adjacent uninvolved nodes is a standard practice used to eradicate minimal or early disease in these lymph nodes.

Stages I and II can be treated with radiotherapy alone by an extended field to include all areas above the diaphragm bearing lymph nodes (the axilla, neck, and chest), and in most cases the lymph nodes in the abdomen. Such treatment cures about 90 percent of patients. For patients in which the disease is found extensively in the chest, chemotherapy is added to the radiotherapy and results in prolonged, relapse-free survival in 85 percent of patients.

A variety of cytotoxic drugs (those that kill cells) are available to treat Hodgkin's disease. Such drugs are similar to nitrogen mustard (which was once used in war) and are toxic to the body. It has been found that when more than one drug is used, each in a smaller dose, the toxicity can be reduced without diminishing effectiveness. Thus combination chemotherapy has evolved. There are many effective regimens of combination chemotherapy that are called by the initials of the individual components; the most widely used is MOPP (mechlorethamine, Oncovin, procarbazine, and prednisone). In stage III, chemotherapy with or without radiotherapy is used, depending upon specific variations within the stage, with cure rates achieved in 75 to 80 percent of patients. Even in stage IV disease, combination chemotherapy (particularly with MOPP) has produced a complete remission in about 75 percent of patients, with a cure rate of more than 50 percent.

Bone marrow transplantation, which is the intravenous infusion of normal marrow cells into the patient shortly after treatment in order to protect the patient from toxicity, has permitted the use of much higher doses of certain drugs. It allows the therapist to irradiate all the patient's bone marrow, eradicating both "good" and "bad" cells, with the hope that the normal marrow cells that are infused will populate the bone marrow and grow there. Bone marrow transplantation has been successfully used mainly in young patients who were resistent to conventional chemotherapy.

PERSPECTIVE AND PROSPECTS

Thomas Hodgkin of Guy's Hospital in London was the first to recognize the disease that would bear his name. In 1832, he described the gross autopsy findings and clinical features of seven patients who had simultaneous enlargement of grossly diseased lymph nodes and spleens, and he considered the condition to be a primary affection of these organs. This condition, he himself records, was vaguely outlined by Marcello Malpighi in 1665. Four years earlier than Hodgkin, David Craige had described the autopsy findings of a similar case. Subsequent histologic examination of tissues from Hodgkin's original cases confirmed the disease in three of them. In 1865, Sir Samuel Wilks elaborated on the autopsy studies of similar cases and published the findings on fifteen patients, calling the condition Hodgkin's disease.

Important histopathologic observations were contributed by William Greenfield in 1878 and E. Goldman in 1892. George Sternberg described the giant cells but believed the condition to be a peculiar form of tuberculosis. The recognition that these cells were an integral part of the disease awaited the careful pathologic observation of Dorothy Reed of The Johns Hopkins Hospital in Baltimore. These cells, appropriately named Reed-Sternberg cells, are the hallmark of Hodgkin's disease.

Controversy as to the nature of this disease led early investigators to study infectious agents as possible etiologic causes, especially the tuberculosis bacillus, but to no avail. More recent studies have examined the roles of other viral infectious agents, especially the agent of infectious mononucleosis, but with no consistent results. At present, the condition is accepted as neoplastic, probably triggered by some unknown environmental agent or agents.

Between 1930 and 1950, major advances included the recognition of meaningful histologic subtypes of Hodgkin's disease correlating with prognosis, and the development by Vera Peters of a clinical staging system. Impressive responses to X-ray therapy were reported at the beginning of the twentieth century, and treatment with megavoltage therapy was further developed. By World War II, it became realistic to speak of curing some patients with early Hodgkin's disease. The potential for a cure meant that accurate histologic diagnosis and estimation of the extent and localization of disease was imperative in planning treatment; a multidisciplinary approach to the diagnosis and treatment was developed. Modern concepts of histologic classification became codified at a conference held in Rye, New York, in 1965, and the clinical staging system was refined into its present form at a workshop held at Ann Arbor, Michigan, in 1971.

Modern effective chemotherapy was developed concurrently with these advances in classification, staging, and radiotherapy. The alkylating agents, created as an outgrowth of studies on nitrogen mustard gas during World War II, provided the first drugs to produce impressive shrinkage of the tumor and significant palliation of the disease. The subsequent developments in modern pharmacology and therapeutics enabled Vince DeVita and his coworkers, in 1970, to design the first effective combination chemotherapy regimen, MOPP.

Today, many more such regimens are being tested; the possibility for cure has become a realistic hope for every patient with Hodgkin's disease. This is the case because of the refinement of ancillary therapies with antibiotics (for infections that may occur during the necessary phases of suppression of the immune system by these powerful toxic drugs) and platelet transfusion technology. Bone marrow transplantation technology also offers strong hope of curing patients with advanced cases who are resistant. The bone marrow is harvested and then reintroduced into a patient whose marrow has been effectively disabled. Immunotherapy is also being investigated. It can boost the patient's ability to combat disease by modulating the body's responses. The drawback to aggressive combinations of chemotherapy and radiotherapy, however, is the emergence of therapy-related leukemia and leukemia-like malignancies several years after the completion of successful therapy for Hodgkin's disease.

—*Victor H. Nassar, M.D.*

See also Bone marrow transplantation; Cancer; Chemotherapy; Lymphadenopathy and lymphoma; Lymphatic system; Malignancy and metastasis; Oncology; Radiation therapy.

FOR FURTHER INFORMATION:

CA: A Cancer Journal for Clinicians 43, no. 1. January/February, 1993. A journal published by the American Cancer Society. This special issue is devoted to a discussion of cancer statistics, including those regarding Hodgkin's disease.

Lacher, Mortimer J., and John R. Redman, eds. *Hodgkin's Disease: The Consequences of Survival.* Philadelphia: Lea & Febiger, 1990. Discusses the treatment of and the complications associated with this disease. Therapy options are analyzed, including chemotherapy, radiotherapy, and the adverse effects of both methods of treatment. Bibliographies and an index are provided.

Lee, G. Richard, et al., eds. *Wintrobe's Clinical Hematology.* 10th ed. Philadelphia: Lea & Febiger, 1999. A textbook of hematologic disorders, with an excellent review of Hodgkin's disease. Written for clinicians and students of medicine.

Williams, Stephanie F., Ramez Farah, and Harvey M. Golomb, eds. *Hodgkin's Disease.* Philadelphia: W. B. Saunders, 1989. A volume in the series Hematology/Oncology Clinics of North America. A thorough review of this disease—its diagnosis, pathology, and treatment. Includes bibliographical references and an index.

Williams, W. J., E. Beuter, A. J. Erslev, and M. A. Lichtman, eds. *Williams Hematology.* 6th ed. New York: McGraw-Hill, 2000. An up-to-date textbook that offers an authoritative review of all aspects of Hodgkin's disease.

HOLISTIC MEDICINE

SPECIALTY

ANATOMY OR SYSTEM AFFECTED: All

SPECIALTIES AND RELATED FIELDS: Alternative medicine, environmental health, nursing, osteopathic medicine, preventive medicine, psychology

DEFINITION: The practice of medicine to maintain both physical and psychological health as a natural deterrent to disease and as a way of realizing one's highest potential.

KEY TERMS:

hospice care: an alternative to hospitalization for the terminally ill or aged that allows for the dignified acceptance of impending death

stress management: the alleviation of stress, a form of preventive medicine borrowed from holistic approaches to common emotional disorders

SCIENCE AND PROFESSION

Although the phenomenon of holistic medicine gained increased attention in the latter half of the twentieth century, most of the principles associated with it have appeared in various forms and in various cultures over the centuries. Ironically, it may have been the progress of medical science generally and the widespread use by doctors of new drugs to treat disease that sparked what some would call holistic medicine's call for a return to basics. For example, some proponents of holism oppose automatic reliance on surgical methods of treating some ailments for not recognizing either their causes or more beneficial modes of treatment. In addition, holists oppose a reliance on drugs not only because they hold certain maladies to be curable (or indeed totally avoidable) without them but also because of possible negative side effects.

A number of quite sophisticated principles could fall under the presumed "basics" of the holistic approach to health. Primary among these is a conviction that—short of obvious conditions involving attacks by virus, bacteria, or chronic debilitation of certain organs of the body, including the nervous system—increased awareness of the nature of bodily functions can help maintain a healthy level of balance within the total organism. Essential to the principle of balance is recognition of the importance of the mind in influencing one's reactions, both psychological and physical, to circumstances in the surrounding environment. Some holists adhere to the Abraham Maslow school of psychology, which places strong emphasis on questions of drive toward "need fulfillment" in both the physical and psychological domains. Certain bodily states can easily be linked to biologically stimulated drives, including hunger and sexuality. Less apparent psychological drives, however, may also trigger physical reactions. Imbalances in fulfilling the natural drives for love or success are held responsible for many forms of physical disorder that could be averted, such as anorexia nervosa, ulcers, and stress.

Several approaches to holistic medicine consider the end goal of good physical health to be not only the avoidance of disease but also the realization of a positive, life-enhancing experience. In some cases, the inspiration for such theories comes from long traditions in Asian philosophies and religions that assume close links between the psychic and the physical realms of life. An assumption that may or may not be shared between such philosophies and holists is that a "true" state of health leads to superior levels of awareness in both spheres.

Physicians interested in holistic medicine need not, however, be tied solely to disease-specific or "consciousness-heightening" aspects of what can be a very general field. Some specialists in geriatrics, for example, adopt holistic approaches to counseling the elderly about natural stages of aging, preparing them to accept, with a minimum of anxiety, the gradual decline that accompanies the end of life. Growing emphasis on hospice care for the terminally ill or aged, as opposed to hospitalization, is connected with this aspect of holistic medicine.

DIAGNOSTIC AND TREATMENT TECHNIQUES

Although individual physicians may espouse holistic approaches, many persons without formal medical training choose to practice it themselves to maintain their bodies and minds in the healthiest state possible. Such practices may be individual and personal, ranging from exercise and dietary habits to meditation. They may also involve group associations supported by the participation of trained physicians or laypersons. It has become possible to find method-specific holistic centers specializing in a range of techniques. These range from, for example, very general holistic health and nutrition institutes to highly specialized centers that strive to treat those suffering from chronic pain through localized electrical nerve stimulation.

Essential to almost all holistic approaches to treatment is an emphasis on the physician's role as a facilitator—someone who is able to help the patient recognize what he or she should do to adopt various attitudes and actions that can alleviate all or part of the observed disorder. In this connection, a number of general practitioners maintain auxiliary personnel to provide various therapies (massages, controlled breathing, and so on) to supplement, or sometimes to replace, such standard treatments as drug prescriptions or minor surgery.

PERSPECTIVE AND PROSPECTS

It was the South African political figure Jan Smuts who, in 1926, first used the specific word "holism" to describe, not holistic medicine per se, but the philosophical principle which holds that whole systems (and therefore whole organisms) involve entities that are greater than, and different from, the sum of their component parts. In medicine, the idea that external factors intervene to affect the way that an organism functions is almost as old as medicine itself. Hippocrates, for example, is known to have been concerned about environmental causes for certain disorders and to have included emotional and nutritional considerations in diagnosing patients.

Two aspects of holistic approaches to health and daily life in the postindustrial world are likely to increase in importance in coming generations: concern over improving dietary habits and exercise patterns. The discovery of the possible long-term harm that can come from poorly balanced diets (particularly those with a high fat content or excessive chemical additives) has made such specialized practices of holists as vegetarianism and fasting more familiar and at least partly attractive to the wider public. Likewise, the holistic emphasis on regular physical exercise for people of all ages has increasingly become part of many general practitioners' standard advice to their patients.

—*Byron D. Cannon, Ph.D.*

See also Aging; Aging: Extended care; Alternative medicine; Death and dying; Environmental diseases; Environmental health; Exercise physiology; Family practice; Meditation; Nutrition; Osteopathic medicine; Preventive medicine; Psychiatry; Psychiatry, child and adolescent; Psychiatry, geriatric; Terminally ill: Extended care.

FOR FURTHER INFORMATION:

Nordenfelt, Lennart. *On the Nature of Health.* Rev. 2d ed. Boston: Kluwer, 1995. Deals with the relationship between good health and the welfare of individuals and society as they interact.

Pelletier, Kenneth R. *Holistic Medicine.* New York: Delacorte Press, 1979. A general text that seeks to strengthen the public image of holistic medicine, both for the prevention and for the treatment of disease, while discounting some popular myths.

Salmon, J. Warren, ed. *Alternative Medicines.* New York: Tavistock, 1984. Offers comparative views of Western and Chinese approaches to holistic medicine but also includes other, less widely recognized alternatives, ranging from chiropractic to psychic healing.

Woodham, Anne, and David Peters. *The Encyclopedia of Healing Therapies.* New York: Dorling Kindersley, 1997. This book explains holistic and complementary medicine and offers a guide to well-being. Also contains information on finding practitioners, a directory of associations, a glossary, and a bibliography.

HOMEOPATHY
SPECIALTY
ANATOMY OR SYSTEM AFFECTED: All

SPECIALTIES AND RELATED FIELDS: Immunology, pathology, pharmacology

DEFINITION: A system of medicine based on the principle that an ill patient can be provided effective and nontoxic treatment through the use of weak or very small doses of a substance that would cause similar symptoms in a healthy individual.

KEY TERMS:

antidote: anything that counteracts the effect of a substance, such as a homeopathic remedy

Materia Medica: the homeopathic pharmacopoeia, a list of remedies with their associated symptoms and uses

potency: the strength of a homeopathic remedy, according to the number of times it has been diluted and succussed

proving: the testing of a substance or remedy on healthy volunteers (provers), who take repeated doses and record in detail any symptoms produced by it

Repertory: an index of symptoms, each heading listing the drugs known to cause the symptom

succussion: violent shaking at each stage of dilution in the preparation of a remedy

tincture: a remedy in liquid form, normally with alcohol and water as a solvent; the most concentrated form is called the mother tincture, from which all dilutions are made

SCIENCE AND PROFESSION

In conventional medicine, diseases, or changes from the normal physiological state, are diagnosed on the basis of symptoms and physical signs. This enables the physician to find a cause for which there is a specific treatment, or to treat the patient's symptoms. There are few treatments, however, that cure the patient as a whole. Sometimes, symptoms are assumed to be the disease, and the method of action is to try to fix the symptoms and not the disease. Suppressing or removing symptoms does not necessarily constitute a cure. Curing patients means restoring them to a sense of well-being that is physical, emotional, and mental. Homeopathic medicine is a form of treatment that studies the person as a whole, with particular interest in the patient as an individual. Homeopathy is a therapeutic method that consists of prescribing for a patient weak or infinitesimal doses of a substance which, when administered to a healthy person, causes symptoms similar to those exhibited by the ill patient. Homeopathic remedies stimulate the defense mechanisms of the body, causing them to work more effectively and making them capable of curing the individual. While controversial and not accepted by most physicians, homeopathy is not intended to substitute for conventional medicine. Rather, it is a system of therapeutics which is meant to enlarge and broaden the physician's outlook, and in some cases,

Homeopathy

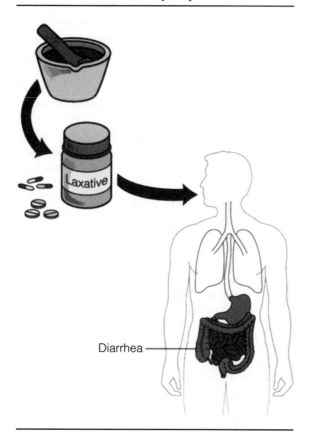

Diarrhea

The principle underlying homeopathy is that taking small amounts of a substance that normally produces a certain symptom will stimulate the immune system to counteract that very symptom. For example, a patient suffering from diarrhea may be given an infinitesimally small dose of a laxative which has been ground into a fine powder with a mortar and pestle.

it might bring about a cure not possible with the usual drugs.

The word "homeopathy" is derived from the Greek words *homoios*, meaning "like" or "similar," and *pathos*, meaning "suffering." A symptom is defined as the changes felt by the patient or observed by another individual that may be associated with a particular disease. When a homeopathic drug or remedy is administered in repeated doses to a group of healthy persons, certain symptoms and signs of toxicity are produced. These symptoms are carefully annotated in what is called the proving of a remedy. In some cases, there are accidental provings—cases in which the symptoms produced by a drug in a healthy person

are observed because of an accident, such as being bitten by a snake. Other sources for the proving of a remedy are the cases in which, after a remedy has been successfully prescribed, symptoms cured by it that were not present in the provings are noted. Some of these symptoms are common to many drugs, and a few are characteristic of particular ones. It is then possible to build a symptom-complex picture which is unique to each drug or remedy. In many cases, when the symptom-complex presented by the patient is compared to the symptom-complex produced by a certain remedy, there will be a resemblance—often a close one—between the patient's symptom picture and the effects of a given drug on healthy persons.

The first and fundamental principle of homeopathy is the selection and use of the similar remedy, based on the patient's symptoms and characteristics and the drug's toxicology and provings. A second principle is the use of remedies in extremely small quantities. The most successful remedy for any given occasion will be the one whose symptomatology presents the clearest and closest resemblance to the symptom-complex of the sick person in question. This concept is formally presented as the Law of Similars, which expresses the similarity between the toxicological action of a substance and its therapeutic action; in other words, the same things that cause the disease can cure it. For example, the effects of peeling an onion are very similar to the symptoms of acute coryza (the common cold). The remedy prepared from *Allium cepa* (red onion) is used to treat the type of cold in which the symptoms resemble those caused by peeling onions. In the same way, the herb white hellebore, which toxicologically produces cholera-like diarrhea, is used to treat cholera.

The homeopathic principle is being applied whenever a sick person is treated using a method or drug that can cause similar symptoms in healthy persons. For example, conventional medicine uses radiation therapy, which causes cancer, to treat this disease. Orthodox medicine, however, does not follow other fundamental principles of homeopathy, such as the use of infinitesimal doses.

Homeopathy stimulates the defense mechanism to make it work more effectively and works on the concept of healing instead of simply treating a disease, combating illness, or suppressing symptoms. Individualization plays a crucial role in homeopathic treatment. Even when two individuals have the same ailment, their symptoms can be different. Remedies are therefore selected on an individual basis, depending on the specific, complete symptom picture of the individual. Homeopathic physicians must develop a different approach to their patients, which involves a diagnosis as well as a study of the whole individual. The way in which some homeopathic remedies work is still unknown, but the persistence of homeopathy since the mid-nineteenth century would seem to suggest its effectiveness in helping sick people.

Some conditions do not respond well to homeopathy, such as those requiring surgery, immediately life-threatening situations such as severe asthma attacks, or situations for which an improvement requires a change in diet (such as iron deficiency) or reduced exposure to environmental stress (a change in lifestyle). Nevertheless, homeopathy appears to help in these cases. For example, it can be useful for faster, complete healing after surgery or after the necessary change in lifestyle has been made. In the United States, both the Food and Drug Administration (FDA) and traditional homeopaths have been concerned about the use of homeopathic remedies to treat serious problems, such as cancer, and their use by unlicensed practitioners. In some cases, the ability to prescribe homeopathic remedies has been restricted to osteopaths, naturopaths, and medical doctors. In some cases, homeopathy does not work; the reason is unknown.

Individuals who have benefited from these remedies may not care whether homeopathy can be scientifically explained or whether research has proven its effectiveness. Nevertheless, some facts suggest that homeopathic medicines are not placebos and that the infinitesimal doses produce true biological action. For example, homeopathic medicines work on animals and are also commonly and successfully used on infants; it is doubtful that psychological suggestion can explain their success in these cases. Moreover, homeopathic microdoses have the capacity to cause symptoms in healthy individuals, and the experience of what is called a healing crisis—temporary exacerbation of symptoms that is sometimes observed during the healing process—cannot be produced by placebos or psychological suggestion. The major drawback to most homeopathic research, however, is that it is rarely published in respected scientific journals, and whatever little has been published has been received with much skepticism from the medical community.

The action of homeopathic medicines supports the theory that each organism expresses symptoms in an effort to heal itself. This homeopathic action can augment, complement, and sometimes replace present medical technologies. For example, abuse of strong medications can lead to resistance to the drugs themselves, allergies, and other unpleasant side effects. In homeopathy, small drug doses have been shown to be more effective than larger ones, which in itself can reduce the undesired side effects associated with the use of common medications.

DIAGNOSTIC AND TREATMENT TECHNIQUES

The first step in treating an illness using homeopathy is taking the case history or symptom picture (the detailed account of what is wrong with the patient as

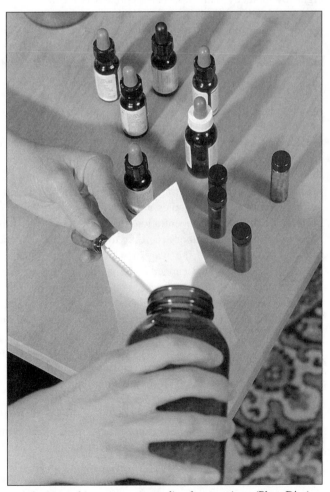

A homeopathist prepares remedies for a patient. (PhotoDisc)

a whole). This is carried out in a similar way by classical doctors and homeopathic practitioners, since most homeopaths are doctors or have some conventional medical training. The symptoms are divided into three categories: general, mental/emotional, and physical.

The homeopath then consults the *Materia Medica* (the encyclopedia of drug effects) and/or the *Repertory* (an index of symptoms from the *Materia Medica* listed in alphabetical order, used as a cross-reference between symptoms and remedies) to decide on the remedy to be used. The professional homeopath works with a number of *Materia Medica* texts compiled by different homeopaths.

The classical homeopath will give only one remedy at a time in order to gauge its effect more efficiently. The best-known unconventional usage of homeopathic medicines is of combination medicines or complexes, normally a mixture of between three and eight low-potency remedies. This approach is useful when the correct remedy is not available or when the practitioner is unsure as to which one to use. These mixtures are commonly sold in health food stores and are named for the disease or symptom that they are supposed to cure. Another unconventional use is what is called pluralism, which is the application of two or more medicines at a time, each of which is taken at a different time of day. This approach is most commonly used in Europe.

Homeopathy is a natural pharmaceutical system that utilizes microdoses of substances to arouse a healing response by stimulating the patient's immune system. Homeopathic remedies are always nontoxic because of the small concentrations used. They do not act chemically but rather according to a particular physical state linked to the way in which they are prepared. They have the capacity of making the ill subject react to his or her disease, and in this way they are considered specific stimulants.

Homeopathic remedies come from the plant, mineral, and animal kingdoms. Plants are the source of more than half of the remedies. They are harvested in their natural state according to strict norms by qualified specialists and are used fresh after thorough botanical inspection. Mineral remedies include natural salts and metals, always in their purest state. Animal remedies may contain venoms, poisonous insects, hormones, or physiological secretions such as musk or squid ink.

In all cases, the starting remedy is made from a mixture of the substance itself, which has been steeped in alcohol for a period of time and then strained. This starting liquid is called a tincture or mother tincture. In the decimal scale, a mixture of one-tenth tincture and nine-tenths alcohol is shaken vigorously, a process known as succussion; this first dilution is called a 1X. (The number in the remedy reveals the number of times that it has been diluted and succussed; thus, 6X means diluted and succussed six times.) In the centesimal scale, the remedy is diluted using one part tincture in a hundred, and the letter *C* is used after the number. The number indicates the degree of the dilution, while the letter indicates the technique of preparation (decimal or centesimal). Insoluble substances are diluted by grinding them in a mortar with lactose to the desired dilution. The greater the dilution of a remedy, the greater its potency, the longer it acts, the deeper it heals, and the fewer doses are needed.

A medicine is chosen for its similarity to the person's symptoms, so that the person's bioenergetic processes are hypersensitive to the substance. One theory used to explain the success of homeopathic remedies, even when they are used in such small concentrations, is that they work through some kind of resonance within the individual's system. There are other examples of high sensitivity to small amounts of substances in the animal kingdom, such as in the case of pheromones, sex attractants that affect only animals of the same species in very small amounts and at a very long distance.

Constantine Hering (1800-1880), the founder of American homeopathy, was the first to make note of the specific features of the healing process to create a holistic assessment tool that can be used to evaluate a patient's progress. His observations are summarized in Hering's Law of Cure: First, the human body seeks to externalize disease, to dislodge it from more serious, internal levels to more superficial ones; for example, in the healing of asthma the patient may exhibit an external skin rash before complete cure is achieved. Second, the healing progresses from the top of the body to the bottom; someone with arthritis will feel better in the upper part of the body earlier than in the lower part. Third, the healing proceeds in the reverse order of the appearance of the symptoms; that is, the more recent symptoms will heal first, and old symptoms may reappear before complete healing.

Homeopathic remedies are most commonly available in tablet form, combined with sugar from cow's milk. The tablets can be soft (so that they dissolve easily under the tongue and are easy to crush) or hard (so that they must be chewed and held in the mouth for a few seconds before being swallowed), or they can be prepared as globules (tiny round pills). The liquid remedies are dissolved in alcohol. Also available are powders that are wrapped individually in small squares of paper (convenient if the remedy is needed for only a few doses or is to be sent by mail), wafers, suppositories, and liniments. Homeopathic tablets will keep their strength for years without deteriorating, but they must be stored in a cool, dark, and dry place with their bottle tops screwed on tightly, away from strong-smelling substances.

The prescribed quantities are the same for babies, children, adults, and older people. The size of a dose is immaterial; it is how often it is taken that counts. The strength (potency) that is needed changes with the circumstances. The greater the similarity between the symptoms and the remedy, the greater the potency to be used (that is, the more dilute the remedy).

The following substances all counteract the effects of a homeopathic remedy to some extent (and as such are considered antidotes): camphor, coffee, menthol/eucalyptus, peppermint, recreational drugs, and any strong-smelling or strong-acting substance.

As with all treatments, there are some dangers associated with homeopathic cures, such as unintentional provings. These take place when, after an initial improvement, the symptoms characteristic of the remedy appear, creating a worse situation for the patient. Sometimes, this reaction takes place because the individual has been taking the remedy for too long, and it can be stopped by discontinuing the remedy or by using an antidote. In other cases, there is a confused symptom picture, the effect being that the remedy is working in a limited way or curing a restricted number of symptoms.

Homeopathy is important in the treatment of bacterial infections (where resistance to antibiotics can develop) and viral conditions. Homeopathic remedies stimulate the person's resistance to infection without the side effects of antibiotics, and they help the body without suppressing the organism's self-protective responses. The remedies used are safer than regular medicines because they exhibit minimal side effects and counterreactions between medicines can be prevented.

Homeopathic remedies are exempt from federal review in the United States. In 1938, any drug listed in the *Homeopathic Pharmacopoeia of the United States* was accepted by the FDA. Consequently, prescribed homeopathics do not have to undergo the rigorous safety and effectiveness testing the regulating agency requires of drugs used in orthodox medicine. Nonprescription homeopathics are also exempt and can be purchased in pharmacies, greengroceries, and health food stores throughout the country. The FDA requires that, as with any over-the-counter drug, a remedy be sold only for a self-limiting condition (such as headaches, menstrual cramps, or insomnia) and that the indications be printed on the label. The ingredients and their dilution must also be listed. Nonhomeopathic active ingredients cannot be included in the preparation.

PERSPECTIVE AND PROSPECTS

The Law of Similars was observed twenty-five centuries ago by Hippocrates and was utilized by people of many cultures, including the Mayans, Chinese, Greeks, and American Indians. In the following centuries, other doctors made similar observations, but they did not come to any practical conclusions. It was not until the end of the eighteenth century that a German physician, Christian Friedrich Samuel Hahnemann, studied the matter further, developed it, and gave it a scientific basis.

Hahnemann recruited a group of healthy subjects to take the remedies and report in a diary the symptoms that they caused, a process called proving the substance. He and his subjects proved more than a hundred remedies and produced a very accurate collection for use by other homeopathy practitioners. He also found that the remedies worked better in very small doses. Homeopathy was initially rejected by the medical profession, but its methods became more accepted when Hahnemann obtained astonishing results with his patients. In 1810, he published a book called *Organon der rationellen Heilkunde* (*The Organon of Homœopathic Medicine*, 1836), in which he presented the philosophy of homeopathy. He also published *Materia Medica pura* in six volumes between 1811 and 1821. These volumes contain the compilations of his provings. As new remedies are discovered, they are added to the compilation. By the time of Hahnemann's death in 1843, homeopathy was established around the world.

In the 1820's, homeopathy arrived in the United States at a time when the state of orthodox medicine was worse than in Europe. Many ordinary people consulted herbalists and bone-setters, so homeopathy was easily accepted and soon flourished. In 1844, the

American Institute of Homeopathy was founded. In 1846, however, the American Medical Association (AMA) was founded, and it adopted a code of ethics which forbade its members to consult homeopaths. Nevertheless, public demand continued. The 1860's through the 1880's saw the heyday of homeopathy in the United States, with the institution of training programs, hospitals, and asylums and the training of thousands of homeopaths in the country.

Developments in orthodox medicine around the end of the nineteenth century strengthened this camp, however, while the homeopathic establishment was weakened by internal division. In 1911, the AMA moved to close many homeopathic teaching institutions because they were considered to provide a poor standard of education. By 1950, all the homeopathic colleges in the United States were either closed or no longer teaching homeopathy. By the 1990's, it was roughly estimated that only five hundred to one thousand medical doctors used homeopathics in their practices, though the number of homeopaths and osteopaths prescribing them had probably increased. Although the AMA has no official statement on homeopathy, it is no longer part of the medical school curriculum.

Homeopathy has exhibited a renaissance, and it is popular throughout the world, especially in France. Perhaps the reasons for this revived popularity include both skepticism surrounding conventional medicine and a need for alternatives in the face of challenging health problems: Homeopathy offers a safe alternative as it seeks to improve the general level of health of the whole person, emotionally as well as physically. It must not be forgotten, however, that this brand of medicine has a long way to go before its curative powers are proven.

—*Maria Pacheco, Ph.D.*

See also Alternative medicine; Disease; Herbal medicine; Immune system; Immunology; Pathology; Pharmacology; Toxicology.

For Further Information:

Aubin, Michel, and Philippe Picard. *Homœopathy: A Different Way of Treating Common Ailments*. Translated by Pat Campbell and Robin Campbell. Bath, England: Ashgrove Press, 1989. An easy-to-read book which includes a critical analysis of orthodox medicine from the perspective of an orthodox doctor turned homeopath, a description of homeopathy, and a section on self-treatment with homeopathy.

Castro, Miranda. *The Complete Homeopathy Handbook: A Guide to Everyday Health Care*. New York: St. Martin's Press, 1991. Examines the principles underlying the theory of homeopathy, as well as how to prescribe and learn the best use of homeopathic medicines that are available over the counter.

McCabe, Vinton. *Practical Homeopathy: A Beginner's Guide*. New York: St. Martin's Press, 2000. McCabe, president of the Connecticut Homeopathic Association and a member of the faculty and board of the Hudson Valley School of Classical Homeopathy, joins philosophy and pharmacy in a practical way in this resource. Includes homeopathic remedies.

Ullman, Dana. *Discovering Homeopathy: Medicine for the Twenty-first Century*. Rev. ed. Berkeley, Calif.: North Atlantic Books, 1991. Includes sections on the history and research methods of homeopathy and an excellent section on sources (books, computer programs, tapes) and general information on homeopathy. Lists pharmacies, organizations, schools, and training programs in the United States.

HORMONE REPLACEMENT THERAPY

PROCEDURE

ANATOMY OR SYSTEM AFFECTED: Endocrine system, glands, psychic-emotional system, reproductive system

SPECIALTIES AND RELATED FIELDS: Endocrinology, gynecology, psychology

DEFINITION: The use of oral or injectable forms of hormones to replace inadequate gland secretions.

INDICATIONS AND PROCEDURES

Hormones are critical substances released by glands, the organs of the endocrine system. Hormone replacement therapy is needed when insufficient amounts of hormones are being produced. Glands can slow or cease secretion because of destruction by tumors, infections, poor nutrition, environmental toxins, normal aging, heredity, and trauma. The most common problems exist with the thyroid (hypothyroidism), pancreas (diabetes mellitus), and ovaries (the menopause). Both thyroid and pancreatic insulin hormone replacement are lifesaving therapies.

After careful testing reveals a hormone deficiency, hormones are administered as either pills or injections. While symptoms, simple blood tests, and X rays may

In the News: Treating Symptoms of the Menopause

Hormone replacement therapy (HRT) involves the administration of hormones to treat individuals with naturally occurring hormonal deficiencies. While endocrinologists are treating large numbers of patients suffering from a wide range of hormonal deficiencies, research into the risks and benefits involved in such treatment is increasingly controversial.

One of the most controversial treatments involves HRT for postmenopausal women who lack estrogen and progesterone. Initially used to treat the unpleasant symptoms associated with the menopause (including hot flashes, irritability, and vaginal dryness), HRT is now considered to have important health benefits for many postmenopausal women. Research has indicated that long-term HRT is related to reduced risk of cardiovascular disease, decreased incidence and severity of osteoporosis, and a slowing of the progression of Alzheimer's disease and cognitive dysfunction in middle-aged and older women. Some recent research now leads to questions about the effectiveness of these protective mechanisms of estrogen-progesterone replacement therapy. Additionally, a great deal of research indicates that postmenopausal hormone replacement leads to an increased risk of breast cancer, ovarian cancer, uterine cancer, thromboembolic (blood-clotting) disease, and gallbladder disease.

Considering the contradictory and controversial research concerning postmenopausal HRT, it is not surprising that many alternative treatments are now being considered. These treatments range from nutritional supplements (like vitamin E and soy products) through nonhormonal drug treatments (like gabapentin) and the use of relaxation techniques (like yoga and Tai Chi Chuan). Clearly, medical treatment of postmenopausal women needs to be individualized. Informed decisions need to be made based on the patient's symptoms, needs, and family history.

—*Robin Kamienny Montvilo, R.N., Ph.D.*

point to a diagnosis, more sophisticated tests are often needed. A sensitive blood test called a radioimmunoassay can determine exact hormone levels. Nuclear scans, using injected radioactive materials, provide vivid images of the affected gland. Biopsies, which are samples of tissue taken from the gland through a needle or incision, can be viewed directly.

USES AND COMPLICATIONS

Hormone replacement therapy reverses the symptoms of hormone deficiency diseases. Without treatment, the diabetic patient, lacking the insulin that regulates blood sugar levels, will suffer coma and death. The patient who lacks sufficient thyroid hormone to regulate the rate of metabolism will also have a fatal outcome if this condition is left untreated. Postmenopausal women, whose ovaries have ceased the production of estrogen and progesterone because of normal aging, may have uncomfortable and sometimes disabling symptoms which can be relieved by hormone replacement.

Definite risks are associated with hormone use because it is very difficult to imitate the precision with which the body normally maintains the blood concentrations of internally produced hormones. Excess dosages can have devastating consequences: Excess amounts of thyroid or insulin hormones can lead to death. Considerable controversy surrounds postmenopausal hormone replacement because of its association with breast and uterine cancer, liver disease, and blood clots. As with all drugs, the benefits and risks of hormones must be weighed and blood levels carefully monitored.

—*Connie Rizzo, M.D.*

See also Diabetes mellitus; Endocrinology; Endocrinology, pediatric; Genetic engineering; Geriatrics and gerontology; Glands; Gynecology; Hormones; Hysterectomy; Menopause; Metabolism; Pancreas; Pediatrics; Pharmacology; Thyroid disorders.

FOR FURTHER INFORMATION:

Goldstein, Steven R. *The Estrogen Alternative.* New York: Putnam, 1998. The work of gynecologist and researcher Goldstein showed that raloxifene, a menopause drug sold under the name Evista, is not harmful, expediting FDA approval. This book, based on case histories and medical reports, enthusiastically promotes raloxifene.

Isselbacher, Kurt J., et al., eds. *Harrison's Principles of Internal Medicine*. 14th ed. New York: McGraw-Hill, 1998. A standard text on internal medicine. Includes bibliographical references and an index.

Jacobwitz, Ruth S. *The Estrogen Answer Book: 150 Most-Asked Questions About Hormone Replacement Therapy*. Boston: Little, Brown, 1999. Jacobwitz has gone through menopause herself and has lectured widely on it, obtaining from the latter experience knowledge of the kinds of questions that women want answered. Includes a list of Web sites for readers seeking further information.

Love, Susan M. *Dr. Susan Love's Hormone Book: Making Informed Choices About Menopause*. New York: Random House, 1997. Chapter by chapter, Love reviews the scientific evidence for the promised benefits of hormone therapy (protection from osteoporosis and heart disease) and for the potential risks (increased chance of breast and endometrial cancer).

Stolar, Mark. *Estrogen: Answers to All Your Questions About Hormone Replacement Therapy and Natural Alternatives*. New York: Avon Books, 1997. An endocrinologist provides, in a question-and-answer format, a comprehensive guide to such topics as estrogen, hormone replacement therapy, and natural remedies, explaining how women can make informed decisions.

HORMONES

BIOLOGY

ANATOMY OR SYSTEM AFFECTED: Circulatory system, endocrine system, glands, psychic-emotional system

SPECIALTIES AND RELATED FIELDS: Biochemistry, endocrinology, pediatrics, pharmacology

DEFINITION: Chemical substances that are secreted by endocrine glands or specialized secretory cells into the blood or surrounding tissues and that serve as the principal regulators of the body's metabolism.

KEY TERMS:

deoxyribonucleic acid (DNA): the basic building block of life, which bears encoded genetic information; it is found mainly in chromosomes and can reproduce

kinase: an enzyme that catalyzes the transfer of phosphate from adenosine triphosphate to another molecule

messenger ribonucleic acid (mRNA): a single-stranded ribonucleic acid that arises from and is complementary to double-stranded deoxyribonucleic acid; it passes from the nucleus to the cytoplasm, where its information is translated into proteins

prohormone: a hormone that must be cut or modified in a specific way in order to achieve full activity

radioimmunoassay: the quantitative measurement of a hormone using an unlabeled hormone to inhibit the binding of a radiolabeled hormone to an antibody

receptor: a molecular structure at the cell surface or inside the cell that is capable of combining with hormones and causing a change in cell metabolism

second messenger: an internal signal produced by a hormone binding to its receptor that transmits further information inside the cell

STRUCTURE AND FUNCTIONS

The definition of the term "hormone" has continued to change over the years. The classic definition is that of an endocrine hormone—that is, one secreted by ductless glands directly into the blood and acting at a distant site. The definition can be expanded to include any chemical substance secreted by any cell of the body that has a specific effect on another cell. A hormone can affect a nearby cell (paracrine action) or the cell that secretes it (autocrine action). Certain hormones are produced by the brain and kidneys, which are not thought of as classic endocrine glands. In fact, the largest producer of hormones is the gastrointestinal tract, which is not usually thought of as an endocrine gland.

Hormones fall into two major categories. There are peptide hormones, which are derived from amino acids, and steroid hormones, which are derived from cholesterol. The different classes of hormones have different mechanisms of action.

Peptide hormones work by interacting with a specific receptor that is located in the plasma membrane of the target cell. These receptors are high-affinity proteins that span the plasma membrane. Receptors have different regions, or domains, that perform specialized functions. One part of the receptor has a specific three-dimensional structure that is similar to a keyhole into which a certain hormone can fit. This allows a very specific action of a hormone in spite of the fact that the hormone is often circulating in very minute quantities in the bloodstream along with myriad other hormones.

There are different classes of plasma membrane receptors. One class is that of the receptor kinases. The insulin receptor is an example. In this case, the part of the receptor molecule that faces the cytoplasm, or inside of the cell, is itself a tyrosine kinase. When insulin interacts with its receptor, a tyrosine molecule on the receptor is phosphorylated. This phosphorylated, or active, kinase can then phosphorylate another protein or enzyme. By using a cascade of phosphorylations and dephosphorylations, the cell can control and amplify a variety of signals to lead to the ultimate effect of the hormone. Another class of membrane receptors includes the G-protein coupled receptor. An example is the beta-2 adrenergic receptor. Epinephrine interacts with this receptor, causing the activation of a signal transducer or G protein. This activated G protein then leads to the activation of adenylate cyclase. This enzyme converts adenosine triphosphate to cyclic adenosine monophosphate (cyclic AMP). Cyclic AMP, which is a prototypical second messenger, activates cyclic AMP-dependent protein kinase (also known as protein kinase A) by binding to its regulatory domain, thereby freeing the catalytic subunit. The catalytic subunit can then phosphorylate other proteins and enzymes, either activating or deactivating them. This is another example of an amplification mechanism.

Steroid hormones exert their effects by means of a mechanism different from that of peptide hormones. All steroids and thyroid hormones have a similar mechanism of action and therefore belong to the steroid/thyroid hormone receptor superfamily. For example, glucocorticoids exert their effects by entering the cell and binding to specific glucocorticoid receptors in the cell nucleus. The glucocorticoid-receptor complex is able to bind specific regulatory DNA sequences, called glucocorticoid response elements. This binding is able to activate gene transcription. This causes an increase in mRNA and, ultimately, the translation of the mRNA to deliver a newly secreted protein. The protein can then act to change the cell's metabolism in some way.

The most common method of hormone measurement is radioimmunoassay, a very powerful technique developed by Solomon A. Berson and Rosalyn S. Yalow in the early 1960's. This technique enables scientists to measure very small amounts of hormones in a variety of body fluids. The concept of radioimmunoassay is that a small amount of a radiolabeled hormone, or tracer, will compete with a native hormone for binding sites on specific antibody molecules. One must separate the antibody bound to the tracer and free the tracer. This is most commonly done by adding a second antibody directed against the antibody-tracer complex.

Most hormones that circulate in the blood are bound to binding proteins. The general binding proteins are albumin and transthyreitin. These two proteins bind many different hormones. There are also specific binding proteins, such as thyroid binding globulin, which binds thyroid hormone, and insulin-like growth factor binding proteins, which bind to the family of insulin-like growth factors. The bound hormone is considered the inactive hormone, and the free hormone is the active hormone. Therefore, binding proteins make it possible to control an active hormone precisely, without having to synthesize a new hormone.

Hormones can be secreted in a variety of time frames. Some hormones, such as testosterone, are secreted in a pulsatile fashion that changes over minutes or hours. To get an accurate hormone level in this case, one can obtain three blood specimens at twenty-minute intervals and pool the samples. Other hormones, such as cortisol, are secreted in a diurnal pattern, with levels varying depending on the time of day. Cortisol levels are highest at about 8 A.M. and fall throughout the day, with the lowest levels occurring between midnight and 2 A.M. The menstrual cycle is an example of the weekly variation of hormone production. The exact control mechanisms that determine the rhythmicity of hormone production are unknown.

The ability to study and utilize hormones has been revolutionized by molecular biology. The first hormone to be made for clinical use based on these techniques was insulin. The need for a secure and steady supply of insulin prompted scientists to look for alternative sources of insulin in the 1970's. At that time, insulin was isolated and purified from animal pancreas glands, mostly those of cows and pigs. It was suspected, however, that insulin could be made in the laboratory via genetic engineering.

In a type of genetic engineering called recombination, DNA molecules from one cell can be cut by restriction enzymes and recombined into the DNA of another cell. In this way, a hybrid molecule is made that will express the foreign DNA contained within it. In the case of insulin, the gene for human insulin was synthesized by isolating purified human insulin and deducing its DNA structure. The human insulin gene then had to be inserted into a cell that would reproduce readily and make the insulin gene product. The bacteria *Escherichia coli* (*E. coli*) K12 strain was chosen as the host cell. The plasmid DNA of the bacteria was removed and cut open by means of endonuclease cleavage, the DNA sequence for the protein to be synthesized was inserted, and the plasmid DNA was reinserted into the bacteria.

Native insulin is produced from a prohormone proinsulin that itself is produced from a pre-prohormone. Proinsulin exists as a single-chain polypeptide of eighty-six amino acids. The insulin molecule exists in a specific three-dimensional structure that is made up of two chains—the alpha chain with twenty-one amino acids, and the beta chain with thirty amino acids—connected by two disulfide bridges. The proinsulin molecule is processed inside the cell, where enzymes cut the single chain in two places after it is folded in such a way as to yield both active insulin and a connecting sequence known as C peptide. When insulin was first produced commercially, the genes for the alpha and beta chains were made separately and then the protein products were combined to make the active hormone. The way in which recombinant DNA human insulin is currently made is by encoding for the proinsulin molecule and then using proteolytic enzymes to cut the molecule in the proper places, yielding insulin and C peptide. This process, which is very similar to the process that the body uses to produce insulin, produces high yields of active hormone.

Modern molecular biology techniques were used to identify a hormone and receptor involved in weight regulation. Genetically obese mice were originally used to identify the *obese* (*ob*) gene product as the hormone leptin. Leptin is a protein hormone produced in adipose cells. The cells secrete leptin into the bloodstream, where it travels to the hypothalamus of the brain. The amount of leptin produced is directly proportional to the amount of adipose tissue present. Leptin signals the hypothalamus to adjust appetite, and to increase the metabolic level accordingly, in order to maintain an ideal weight. *Ob* mice were found to synthesize faulty leptin, so that their brains never received the leptin signal and therefore never gave off the satiety factor. Thus, the mice continued to eat and became obese. *Ob* mice injected with normal leptin lost weight and returned to a normal weight level.

A comparable *ob* gene was identified in humans; however, obese humans were found to produce functional leptin. Subsequently, the receptors for the leptin hormone were identified in both mice and humans. Some fat mice that produced normal leptin were found to have defective leptin receptors in the hypothalamus. The same is believed to happen in humans. If the leptin signal does not reach the brain as the result of a faulty receptor, the brain will not produce the satiety signal. Appetite will remain high, and the number of calories burned will remain low. Thus, either nonfunctional leptin or a defective receptor in the brain may contribute to obesity in humans.

The functioning of leptin may also be responsible for cycles of weight loss and gain in dieters. As obese individuals lose adipose tissue, less leptin is synthesized and the brain may not send out sufficient signals to indicate satiety, thus increasing appetite and food consumption. The leptin-obesity connection is under intensive study.

THE MEDICAL USE OF HORMONES

Hormones that are produced by the body are normally made in small amounts on the order of micrograms or milligrams. These are the physiologic levels of the hormone. Early methods for isolating hormones required extracting very small amounts of hormone from very large amounts of endocrine tissue. This was a tedious process that often yielded insufficient amounts of hormone for clinical use. Medical science has, in recent years, taken advantage of recombinant DNA technology to produce large amounts of native hormones for use in medicine. With large amounts of hormones available to give to people in milligram to gram quantities, one can study the physiologic and pharmacologic effects of these hormones.

One example of the use of large amounts of a hormone produced by genetic engineering is erythropoietin. Erythropoietin is a protein that consists of 166 amino acids plus carbohydrate. In adult humans, the main source of erythropoietin is the kidney. Erythropoietin exerts a major stimulatory effect on hemoglobin synthesis by increasing the number of red blood cells that make hemoglobin. Erythropoietin circulates in the blood in the concentration of about 0.1 to 1 nanomole. Its concentration can be increased fifty to one hundred times in patients with severe anemia. Erythropoietin is essential for the differentiation and development of stem cells from the bone marrow.

Pluripotent stem cells have the ability under different hormonal stimuli to differentiate into lymphoid, megakaryocytic, or erythroid cells. Under the influence of erythropoietin, these cells differentiate into red blood cells.

Most patients who develop kidney failure also suffer from severe anemia because the ability to synthesize erythropoietin is lost as the kidney is destroyed by disease. Giving this hormone to a patient with kidney disease can lead to the restoration of that patient's red blood cell mass. Correcting the anemia that accompanies chronic renal disease can improve the exercise tolerance and overall quality of life of kidney patients. The hormone must be given by injection several times per week. It has been made available to all of the almost 50,000 Americans who have chronic renal failure that requires dialysis. Erythropoietin can also be given to renal failure patients who do not yet require dialysis but who do have anemia. It is also under study for use in the anemia that accompanies the use of drugs to treat acquired immunodeficiency syndrome (AIDS) and cancers. The use of erythropoietin is an important example of the application of pharmacologic amounts of a native hormone.

Calcitonin is a polypeptide hormone with thirty-two amino acids, secreted by specialized C cells of the thyroid gland (also called parafollicular cells). The parafollicular cells make up about 0.1 percent of the total mass of the thyroid gland, and the cells are dispersed within the thyroid follicles. Calcitonin is made from a gene that also produces calcitonin gene related peptide (CGRP) in the central nervous system. The pre-mRNA transcript is cleaved and spliced in different ways to yield the two different peptides. CGRP has been noted to have pharmacological effects on the cardiovascular and central nervous systems, but its physiological role has not been clearly noted. Calcitonin has been isolated from several different animal species, including the salmon, eel, rat, pig, sheep, and chick. There is some structural homology between the different species, and human calcitonin is most similar to rat calcitonin. The fish and chicken molecules are similar and are the most potent. Lowering the serum calcium level is the main physiologic function of the hormone. It does this by inhibiting calcium resorption from bone. Calcitonin acts via the second messenger cyclic AMP. The effect of calcitonin on cultured bone cells in the laboratory can be mimicked by using long-acting analogues of cyclic AMP. Doctors use calcitonin to treat patients with Paget's disease. Paget's disease is a disorder that results in abnormal bone remodeling. This can lead to abnormal areas of bone with symptoms of deformities, bone pain, neurological problems, and bony fractures. The first and most commonly used form of the hormone in the United States is salmon calcitonin. This form is a more potent inhibitor of bone resorption than the human form. A small number of patients given the drug will develop a resistance to it. The etiology of this resistance can be the development of antibodies to the salmon calcitonin. Now that synthetic human calcitonin is available via recombinant DNA technology, patients who have developed a resistance to salmon calcitonin can be switched to the human form. Although the human form is somewhat less potent, the fact that its amino acid structure is identical to that of the native hormone makes it much less immunogenic than salmon calcitonin.

The hormone vasopressin (also known as antidiuretic hormone) is important for water conservation. An increase in plasma osmolality or a decrease in circulating blood volume will normally cause its release. Central diabetes insipidus, a disorder in which there is an absence of vasopressin, is characterized by an inappropriately dilute urine along with a strong stimulus for the release of vasopressin that responds to the exogenous administration of vasopressin. Central diabetes insipidus can be caused by a variety of factors, including trauma, neurosurgery, brain tumors, familial brain infections, and autoimmune disorder. Patients with this disorder do not make measurable levels of vasopressin. Normal levels of vasopressin depend on the plasma osmolality, with the body tightly controlling the plasma osmolality within a very small range. The clinical symptoms of the disease are polyuria and polydipsia. The patient may put out up to 18 liters of urine per day. If such large volume deficits are not remedied, more serious symptoms will ensue. These include hypotension and coma. The acute treatment of any patient with central diabetes insipidus involves the replacement of body water with intravenous fluids. The chronic therapy involves replacement of the hormone vasopressin. There are several different forms of the hormone that may be used, depending on the clinical situation. Aqueous vasopressin is useful for diagnostic testing and for acute management following trauma or neurosurgery. For diagnostic testing, it is often given subcutaneously at the end of the water deprivation test to see whether the patient will respond to the hormone with a decrease in urine output and an increase in urine osmolality greater than 50 percent. After surgery, it can be given either intramuscularly, with a duration of action of about four to six hours, or it can be given by continuous intravenous infusion to ensure a steady level of the hormone. Vasopressin tannate in oil is a long-term preparation that is administered intramuscularly every one to three days. The first long-acting preparation used, it must be mixed carefully and can cause abdominal cramps. The current preferred form of vasopressin is desmopressin (also known as 1-desamino-8-d-arginine vasopressin), which is given intranasally. Native vasopressin is a cyclic polypeptide with nine amino acids. Desmopressin is a vasopressin analogue that is modified in the amino acid 1 and 8 positions. These modifications increase the antidiuretic to pressure-elevating potency ratio by a factor of two thousand and increase the duration of action from six to twenty hours. This is an example of the way in which biochemists can modify a native molecule and change its properties to more desirable ones.

PERSPECTIVE AND PROSPECTS

The study of hormones has been instrumental in understanding how human beings adapt to and live in their environment. Hormones are involved in the regulation of body homeostasis and all critical aspects of the life cycle. The study of hormones has expanded as scientists have produced large amounts of synthetic hormones in the laboratory for use in research.

The history of hormone research is exemplified by the history of insulin. In 1889, Joseph von Mering and Oskar Minkowski demonstrated that pancreatectomized dogs exhibited abnormalities in glucose metabolism that were similar to those seen in human diabetes mellitus patients. This fact suggested that some factor made by the pancreas lowered the blood glucose. The search for this factor led to the discovery of insulin in 1921 by Frederick C. Banting and Charles H. Best. They were able to extract the active principle from the pancreas and to demonstrate its therapeutic effects in dogs and humans. The chemistry of insulin progressed with the establishment of the amino acid sequence and three-dimensional structure in the 1960's. Insulin was the first hormone to be measured by radioimmunoassay, in 1960. Prior to that time, insulin was detected by means of a bioassay that involved the ability of an isolated rat diaphragm muscle to take up glucose from plasma and the comparison

to known amounts of insulin standards. With advances in laboratory techniques in the 1970's, insulin became the first hormone to be commercially available via recombinant DNA technology. This ensured the availability of pure hormone without the need for animal sources. With the discovery of leptin and its receptor and their role in the regulation of weight, drug therapy may help to compensate for defective leptin or the inability to recognize it. Leptin therapy may help obese people who have lost weight keep it off by supplementing their own leptin and causing the brain to secrete the satiety signal.

The ability to synthesize hormones and their receptors has increased greatly. In fact, scientists now can clone genes, or parts of genes, and synthesize the associated protein, so that they have made hormones that are coded for by the body but are of uncertain physiologic function. This method involves amplifying small amounts of DNA isolated from the cell using the technique of polymerase chain reaction (PCR). This allows large amounts of the same piece of DNA to be made in a matter of hours, which can then be transcribed into RNA and translated to yield the hormone. These powerful techniques, developed in the research laboratory, have been applied on a commercial basis and have provided enormous benefits to people. The use of recombinant DNA technology to make hormones that circulate in the body in amounts too small to be used on a commercial basis has enabled doctors to develop new treatments that would not have been possible otherwise. These are very encouraging developments. New techniques are being developed all the time, expanding the knowledge of the human genome. The total human genome includes approximately one billion base pairs of DNA. The Human Genome Project will attempt to clone all the genes encoded for in the human DNA. Even after cloning all the genes, it will be necessary to find a function for each gene product and learn how to control its expression. This opens up exciting possibilities for treating and curing many diseases that are believed to be of a genetic nature.

—RoseMarie Pasmantier, M.D.;
updated by Karen E. Kalumuck, Ph.D.

See also Addison's disease; Cushing's syndrome; Diabetes mellitus; Dwarfism; Endocrine disorders; Endocrinology; Endocrinology, pediatric; Estrogen replacement therapy; Genetic engineering; Gigantism; Glands; Goiter; Growth; Hormone replacement therapy; Hyperparathyroidism and hypoparathyroidism; Hypoglycemia; Insulin resistance syndrome; Melatonin; Menopause; Metabolism; Obesity; Paget's disease; Pancreas; Pancreatitis; Pregnancy and gestation; Puberty and adolescence; Steroid abuse; Steroids; Thyroid disorders; Weight loss and gain.

FOR FURTHER INFORMATION:

Barinaga, Marcia. "Obesity: Leptin Receptor Weighs In." *Science* 271 (January 5, 1996): 29. This article presents a summary of leptin receptor research accessible to the nonspecialist, as well as a discussion of the prospects for obesity drug research.

Bliss, Michael. *The Discovery of Insulin.* Edinburgh: Paul Harris, 1987. Very stimulating reading that recreates the excitement surrounding the discovery of insulin. This novel gives the reader a feeling for the circumstances leading up to that momentous event.

Cooke, Brian A., et al. *Hormones and Their Actions.* Part 2. Amsterdam: Elsevier, 1988. Nice description of second messengers and their role in hormone action. Detailed mechanisms of action for a variety of different hormones are laid out for the reader.

Marieb, Elaine N. *Essentials of Human Anatomy and Physiology.* 6th ed. Redwood City, Calif.: Benjamin/Cummings, 2000. This introductory anatomy and physiology textbook, easily accessible to those with little science background, is richly illustrated with diagrams and photographs, which help to illuminate body systems and processes.

Norman, Anthony W., and Gerald Litwack. *Hormones.* Orlando, Fla.: Academic Press, 1987. A good general discussion of hormones, hormone receptors, and their interactions, as well as the way in which such interactions affect hormone function. The book then describes different hormones based on their anatomic locations and functions.

Rink, Timothy J. "In Search of a Satiety Factor." *Nature* 372 (December 1, 1994): 372-373. A history of the research into weight regulation and how leptin supports prior theories is presented in a general news format. References are provided for further reading.

Wilson, Jean D., and Daniel W. Foster, eds. *Williams Textbook of Endocrinology.* 9th ed. Philadelphia: W. B. Saunders, 1998. This extensive book on endocrinology covers all the different aspects of the field. It is written by recognized experts in endocrinology in a very readable style.

HOSPICE

HEALTH CARE SYSTEM

DEFINITION: Hospice care is a holistic approach to caring for the dying and their families by addressing their physical, emotional, and spiritual needs.

Hospice is a philosophy of care directed toward persons who are dying. Hospice care uses a family-oriented holistic approach to assist these individuals in making the transition from life to death in a manner that preserves their dignity and comfort. This approach, as Elisabeth Kübler-Ross would say, allows dying patients "to live until they die." Hospice care encourages patients to participate fully in determining the type of care that is most appropriate for their comfort. By creating a secure and caring community sensitive to the needs of the dying and their families and by providing palliative care that relieves patients of the distressing symptoms of their disease, hospice care can aid the dying in preparing mentally as well as spiritually for their impending death.

Unlike traditional health care, where the patient is viewed as the client, hospice care, with its holistic emphasis, treats the family unit as the client. There are usually specific areas of stress for the families of the dying. In addition to the stress of caring for the physical needs of the dying, family members often feel tremendous pressure maintaining their own roles and responsibilities within the family itself. The conflict of caring for their own nuclear families while caring for dying relatives places a huge strain on everyone involved and can be a source of anxiety and guilt for the patient as well. Another area of stress experienced by family members involves concern for themselves, that is, having to put their own lives on hold, keeping from getting physically run down, dealing with their newly acquired time constraints, and viewing themselves as isolated from friends and family. Compounding this is the guilt that many caregivers feel over not caring for the dying relative as well or as patiently as they might, or secretly wishing for the caregiving experience to reach an end.

Due to the holistic nature of the care provided, the hospice team is actually an interdisciplinary team composed of physicians, nurses, psychological and social workers, pastoral counselors, and trained volunteers. This medically supervised team meets weekly to decide on how best to provide physical, emotional, and spiritual support for dying patients and to assist the surviving family members in the subsequent grieving process.

This type of care can be administered in three different ways. It can be home-health-agency based, delivered in the patient's own home. It can be dispensed in an institution devoted solely to hospice care. It can even be administered in traditional medical facilities (such as hospitals) that allot a certain amount of space (perhaps a wing or floor, or even a certain number of beds) to this type of care. Fewer than 20 percent of hospices are totally independent and unaffiliated with any hospitals.

PRINCIPLES

Hospice care attempts to enhance the quality of dying patients' final days by providing them with as much comfort as possible. It is predicated on the belief that death is a natural process with which humans should not interfere. The principles of hospice care, therefore, revolve around alleviating the anxieties and physical suffering that can be associated with the dying process, and not prolonging the dying process by using invasive medical techniques. Hospice care is also based on the assertion that dying patients have certain rights that must be respected. These rights include a right to absent themselves from social responsibilities and commitments, a right to be cared for, and the right to continued respect and status. The following seven principles are basic components of hospice care.

The first principle is highly personalized and holistic care of the dying, which includes treating dying patients emotionally and spiritually as well as physically. This interpersonal support, known as bonding, helps patients in their final days to live as fully and as comfortably as possible, while retaining their dignity, autonomy, and individual self-worth in a safe and secure environment. This one-on-one attention involves what can be called therapeutic communication. Knowing that someone has heard, that someone understands and is concerned, can be profoundly healing.

Another principle is treating pain aggressively. To this end, hospice care advocates the use of narcotics at dosages that will alleviate suffering while, at the same time, enabling patients to maintain a desired level of alertness. Efforts are made to employ the least invasive routes to administer these drugs (usually orally, if possible). In addition, pain medication is administered before the pain begins, thus alleviat-

ing the anxiety of patients waiting for pain to return. Since it has been shown that fear of pain often increases the pain itself, this type of aggressive pain management gives dying patients more time and energy to respond to family members and friends and to work through the emotional and spiritual stages of dying. This dispensation of pain medication before the pain actually occurs, however, has proven to be perhaps the most controversial element in hospice care, with some critics charging that the dying are being turned into drug addicts.

A third principle is the participation of families in caring for the dying. Family members are trained by hospice nurses to care for the dying patients and even to dispense pain medication. The aim is to prevent the patients from suffering isolation or feeling as if they are surrounded by strangers. Participation in care also helps to sustain the patients' and the families' sense of autonomy.

The fourth principle is familiarity of surroundings. Whenever possible, it is the goal of hospice care to keep dying patients at home. This eliminates the necessity of the dying to spend their final days in an institutionalized setting, isolated from family and friends when they need them the most. It is estimated that close to 90 percent of all hospice care days are spent in patients' own homes. When this is not possible and patients must enter institutional settings, rules are relaxed so that their rooms can be decorated or arranged in such a way as to replicate the patients' home surroundings. Visiting rules are suspended when possible, and visits by family members, children, and sometimes even pets are encouraged.

The fifth principle is emotional and spiritual support for the family caregivers. Hospice volunteers are specially trained to use listening and communicative techniques with family members and to provide them with emotional support both during and after the patient's death. In addition, because the care is holistic, the caregivers' physical needs are attended to (for example, respite is provided for exhausted caregivers), as are their emotional and spiritual needs. This spiritual support applies to people of all faith backgrounds, as impending death tends to put faith into a perspective where particular creeds and denominational structures assume less significance. In attending to this spiritual dimension, the hospice team is respectful of all religious traditions while realizing that death and bereavement have the ability to both strengthen and weaken faith.

The sixth principle is having hospice services available twenty-four hours a day, seven days a week. Because of its reliance on the assistance of trained volunteers, round-the-clock support is available to patients and their families.

The seventh principle is bereavement counseling for the survivors. At the time of death, the hospice team is available to help families take care of tasks such as planning the funeral and probating the will. In the weeks after the death, hospice volunteers offer their support to surviving family members in dealing with their loss and grief and the various phases of the bereavement process, always aware of the fact that not all bereaved need or want formal interventions.

HISTORY

The term "hospice" comes from the Latin *hospitia*, meaning "places of welcome." The earliest documented example of hospice care dates to the fourth century, when a Roman woman named Fabiola apparently used her own wealth to care for the sick and dying. In medieval times, the Catholic Church established inns for poor wayfarers and pilgrims traveling to religious shrines in search of miraculous cures for their illnesses. Such "rest homes," usually run by religious orders, provided both lodging and nursing care, since the medieval view was that the sick, dying, and needy were all travelers on a journey. This attitude also reflects the medieval notion that true hospitality included care of the mind and spirit as well as of the body. During the Protestant Reformation, when monasteries were forcibly closed, the concepts of hospice and hospital became distinct. Care of the sick and dying was now considered a public duty rather than a religious or private one, and many former hospices were turned into state-run hospitals.

The first in-patient hospice establishment of modern times (specifically called "hospice") was founded by Mary Aitkenhead and the Irish Sisters of Charity under her leadership in the 1870's in Dublin, Ireland. Cicely Saunders, a physician at St. Joseph's Hospice in London, which was founded by the English Sisters of Charity in 1908, began to adapt the ancient concept of hospice to modern palliative techniques. While there, Saunders became extremely close to a Holocaust survivor who was dying of cancer. She found that she shared his dream of establishing a place that would meet the needs of the dying. Using the money he bequeathed her at his death as a starting point, Saunders raised additional funds and opened St. Christopher's Hospice in Sydenham, outside London, in 1967. Originally it housed only cancer patients, but with the financial support of contracts with the National Health Service in England and private donations, it later expanded to meet the needs of all the dying. In fact, no patient has ever been refused because of inability to pay. St. Christopher's has served as a model for the hospices to be built later in other parts of the world.

Even though hospice care did not originate with Cicely Saunders, she is usually credited with founding the first modern hospice, since she introduced the concept of dispensing narcotics at regular intervals in order to preempt the pain of the dying. She was also the first to identify the need to address other, non-physical sources of pain for dying patients.

Two years after St. Christopher's Hospice was opened, Kübler-Ross wrote *On Death and Dying*, which validated the hospice movement by relating stories of the dying and their wishes as to how they would be treated. In 1974, the United States opened its first hospice, Hospice, Inc. (later called the Connecticut Hospice), in New Haven, Connecticut. Within the next twenty-five years, over three thousand hospice programs would be implemented in the United States. In Canada, the first "palliative care" unit (as hospices are referred to in Canada) was opened in 1975 by Dr. Balfour M. Mount at the Royal Victoria Hospital in Montreal. This is considered to be the first hospital-based hospice in North America.

COST

Because of hospice care's reliance on heavily trained volunteers and contributions, and because death is seen as a natural process that should not be prolonged by invasive and expensive medical techniques, hospice care is much less costly than traditional acute care facilities. Because hospice care is a philosophy of care rather than a specific facility, though, legislation to provide monetary support for hospice patients took a great deal of time to be approved. In 1982, the U.S. Congress finally added hospice care as a Medicare benefit. In 1986, it was made a permanent benefit. Medicare requires, however, that there be a prognosis of six months or less for the patient to live. Hospice care is also reimbursable by many private insurance companies.

The National Hospice Organization (NHO) originated in 1977 in the United States as a resource for the many groups across the country who needed assistance in establishing hospice programs in their own communities. The purpose of this organization is to provide information about hospice care to the public, to establish conduits so that information may be exchanged between hospice groups, and to maintain agreed-upon standards for developing hospices around the country. The NHO publishes *Guide to the Nation's Hospices* on an annual basis.

—*Mara Kelly-Zukowski, Ph.D.*

See also Death and dying; Euthanasia; Grief and guilt; Hospitals; Medicare; Terminally ill: Extended care.

FOR FURTHER INFORMATION:

Buckingham, Robert W. *The Handbook of Hospice Care.* New York: Prometheus Books, 1996. Covers the history and philosophy of hospice care while providing practical information as to its cost, how to find hospice programs in your own community, and how to manage grief. Focuses on two target populations for hospice care: children and AIDS victims.

Byock, Ira. *Dying Well: The Prospect for Growth at the End of Life.* New York: Riverhead Books, 1997. President of the American Academy of Hospice and Palliative Medicine at the time he wrote this book, Dr. Byock uses the personal stories of his patients to show the best ways to die. Provides information for the families of the dying who wish to make their loved ones' final days as comfortable and meaningful as possible.

Connor, Stephen R. *Hospice: Practice, Pitfalls, and Promise.* Washington, D.C.: Taylor & Francis, 1998. This book provides a useful outline of the history, structure, and function of hospice programs in the United States, with understandably less emphasis on medical issues. There is clear evidence of wide experience and consideration of the real world of hospice care, not second-hand distillation from the literature.

Lattanzi-Licht, Marcia, John J. Mahoney, and Galen W. Miller. *The Hospice Choice: In Pursuit of a Peaceful Death.* New York: Simon & Schuster, 1998. Definitive resource from the National Hospice Organization. Provides practical information such as range of hospice services, methods of payment, and so on. Intersperses stories of families who have received hospice care with a thorough explanation of its history, principles, and benefits.

Sendor, Virginia F., and Patrice M. O'Connor. *Hospice and Palliative Care: Questions and Answers.* Lanham, Md.: Scarecrow, 1997. The user-friendly question-and-answer style of this volume allows for use as a quick reference. The purpose is to address the questions often asked by individuals faced with a terminal illness and those involved in the care of the terminally ill.

HOSPITALS

HEALTH CARE SYSTEM

DEFINITION: Institutions focused on the management, prevention, and treatment of illness; utilizing a staff of medical and allied health professionals, hospitals provide medical, surgical, and psychiatric treatment along with emergency care and evaluation.

KEY TERMS:

emergency room: a place where rapid evaluation and treatment of sudden illnesses, accidents, and traumas occur

intensive care: continuous medical treatment involving vigilant monitoring of the vital signs of patients with grave physical conditions

outpatient care: evaluation and treatment services not requiring an overnight stay

triage: a process in which patient needs are evaluated by a healthcare team and preliminary treatment plans are made

ORGANIZATION AND FUNCTIONS

Hospitals are run both privately and under public auspices, such as a local, state, or federal government. In general, they can be classified in three ways: nonprofit versus for-profit, general versus specialty, and short-term versus long-term care. Typically, they are organized in a hierarchical fashion: A governing body, such as a board of directors and its committees, oversees an administrator who, in turn, oversees a variety of departmental managers. While the governing body is responsible for defining and fostering the hospital's mission, the administrator guides the implementation of the mission, and the managers enact it. As such, hospitals have feedback mechanisms from the departments and chief administrator back to the board to ensure quality and progress.

STAFF AND SERVICES

Most hospitals have five primary departments for service management: financial, support, nursing, medical, and ancillary. The first two, financial and support, provide nonmedical services, while the remainder provide direct and indirect medical services. The financial department relies on office personnel and manages business functions, such as admissions, data management, accounting, and collections. In contrast, the support department manages administrative functions (such as volunteer services, medical records, purchasing, personnel), environmental concerns (such as maintenance and housekeeping), and nonmedical patient services (such as dietary needs and social services). This department hosts a diverse service staff, ranging from janitors to dietitians to social workers.

As patients, individuals typically enter hospitals through admissions, the emergency room, or a hospital clinic, or via referral from a private doctor. Thus, depending on a patient's route of admission, his or her interaction with different departmental service staff may vary considerably. In any hospital, however, the nursing service has perhaps the greatest visibility, as it fulfills functions in the emergency and operating rooms, outpatient clinics, and inpatient units. In fact, nurses may perform any of the following duties, de-

pending on their level of training and where they work within a hospital: triage, charting, medical room preparation, medication administration, vital signs monitoring, assistance of patients with meals and hygiene, and staff training. In addition, the nursing service typically dominates short-term special care units, such as intensive care and the emergency room, and nonacute care units, such as renal dialysis centers, psychiatric and substance abuse units, and long-term care centers for chronic illnesses.

Equally well known is the medical service, consisting of physicians, osteopathic physicians, podiatrists, dentists, and psychologists. Typically, this service manages the delivery of care for general medicine, surgery, obstetrics and gynecology, pediatrics, and psychiatry. While the nursing service historically has dominated the emergency room, more recently medical staff are leading in this service area. Many different classes of emergency rooms exist, however, ranging from highly staffed physicians and specialists (twenty-four-hours on site) to minimally staffed (an on-call emergency nurse or technician who transfers

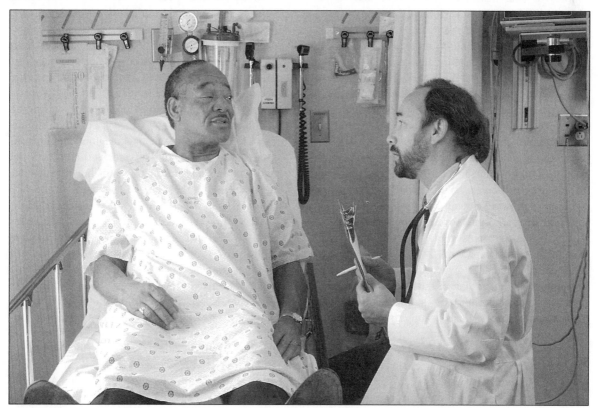

Older adults may find themselves hospitalized for acute illnesses, chronic illnesses, or injuries—all of which present higher risks for the elderly than for younger adults. (Digital Stock)

patients to hospitals with life support equipment). Consequently, this balance between nursing and medical services may vary considerably among hospital emergency rooms.

Finally, ancillary service professionals assist the medical service staff in rendering diagnoses and treating patients. These staff members are highly trained and commonly use sophisticated equipment and methods. Subdepartments composing this service include the laboratory, pharmacy, anesthesiology, physical therapy, electrocardiography (ECG or EKG), electroencephalography (EEG), magnetic resonance imaging (MRI), and inhalation therapy departments. Radiology is also included and has three divisions: diagnostic radiology, therapeutic radiology, and nuclear medicine.

PERSPECTIVE AND PROSPECTS

The word "hospital" was derived from the Greek word *hospitum*, meaning a place for the reception of pilgrims, and the Latin word *hospes*, meaning "guest" or "host." Originally, hospitals existed as temples or churches in ancient Greece and Rome, where priest-physicians performed healing miracles on the mind, body, and spirit. Later, hospitals were run by Christians and church bishops in Europe and served primarily as places of refuge and service for travelers. It was not until 600 C.E. that European hospitals specifically began caring for the sick. Similarly, in America, hospitals were not established until the eighteenth century—and then, only in larger cities. At that time, they primarily functioned as places where the urban poor could receive care and where individuals with contagious diseases could be confined during epidemics. With the advent of modern medicine and developments such as anesthesia and antibiotic drugs, hospitals were seen less as places to be sick and more as places to get well. As a result, they began to take in patients from all sectors of society and with a broader diversity of medical needs.

Today, hospitals are large, financially driven institutions that focus not only on the provision of emergency medical services and healing the very sick but also on the prevention of illness. Increasingly, specialty hospitals are addressing specific groups of patients, such as children, women, elders, and individuals with particular illnesses, such as cancer. In addition, specialty hospitals are taking on identities as centers for research and teaching as they improve treatment methods and strategies. With improved drug therapies and medical procedures, there is also a trend in general hospitals toward outpatient and day care for chronic illnesses replacing a long history of inpatient services. In the future, these trends toward service specialization and outpatient service are expected to continue, with hospitals increasing their use of illness prevention strategies, as well as continuing to improve their delivery of critical care and emergency services for diverse groups of patients.

—*Nancy A. Piotrowski, Ph.D.*

See also Anesthesiology; Critical care; Critical care, pediatric; Emergency care; Geriatrics and gerontology; Malpractice; Nursing; Obstetrics; Oncology; Paramedics; Pediatrics; Physician assistants; Psychiatry; Psychiatry, child and adolescent; Psychiatry, geriatric; Surgery, general; Surgery, pediatric; Terminally ill: Extended care.

FOR FURTHER INFORMATION:

Christman, Luther, and Michael A. Counte. *Hospital Organization and Healthcare Delivery*. Boulder, Colo.: Westview Press, 1981. Details guidelines and rationale for health care risk management, looking beyond conventional hospital-based, clinical initiatives to encompass a variety of health care settings.

Clifford, Joyce C. *Restructuring: The Impact of Hospital Organization on Nursing Leadership*. Chicago: AHA Press, 1998. An examination of the evolution of the role of the chief nursing officer in hospitals responding to a dramatically changing health care environment. Clifford examines the impact of change on the management and administration of clinical nursing services and considers the opportunities and ramifications of how present actions can affect the future of nursing.

Melnick, Glenn, Emmett Keeler, and Jack Zwanziger. "Market Power and Hospital Pricing: Are Nonprofits Different?" *Health Affairs* 18, no. 3 (June, 1999): 167-173. This study shows that nonprofit and government hospitals have steadily become more willing to raise prices to exploit market power and discusses the implications for antitrust regulators and agencies that must approve nonprofit conversions.

Sloane, Robert M., and Beverly LeBov Sloane. *A Guide to Health Facilities: Personnel and Management*. 3d ed. Ann Arbor, Mich.: Health Administration Press, 1992. Offers an overview of health facilities, with a look at hospital administration. Includes bibliographical references and an index.

HOST-DEFENSE MECHANISMS

BIOLOGY

ANATOMY OR SYSTEM AFFECTED: Blood, cells, gastrointestinal system, immune system, skin, urinary system

SPECIALTIES AND RELATED FIELDS: Hematology, immunology, preventive medicine, serology

DEFINITION: Immunological methods that the body uses to protect against external infectious agents and to maintain internal homeostasis, such as those rooted in the skin, sweat, urine, tears, phagocytes, and "helpful" bacteria.

KEY TERMS:

antibodies: proteins produced by immune cells called lymphocytes; antibodies bind to targets called antigens in a highly specific manner

antigen: any substance that causes the formation of a specific antibody; generally a protein

complement: a series of serum proteins that, when activated, carry out a variety of immune functions; the most notable complement function is the lysis of a target

granulocyte: a white blood cell characterized by large numbers of cytoplasmic granules, including neutrophils, eosinophils, and basophils

innate immunity: nonspecific immunity in the sense that prior contact with an infectious agent is not required for proper innate immune response

interferons: a family of proteins; some of these proteins induce an antiviral state within a cell, while others serve to regulate aspects of the immune response

lymphocyte: either of two kinds of small white blood cells; B lymphocytes function to secrete antibodies, while T lymphocytes function to destroy virus-infected cells

macrophage: any of several forms of either circulating or fixed phagocytic cells of the immune system

neutrophil: a circulating white blood cell that serves as one of the principal phagocytes for the immune system

phagocyte: any cell capable of surrounding, ingesting, and digesting microbes or cell debris; in a certain sense, phagocytes function as scavengers

STRUCTURE AND FUNCTIONS

Humans exist in an environment that contains a wide variety of potentially infectious agents. These agents range in size from microscopic viruses—such as rhinoviruses, which cause the common cold—to a wide variety of bacteria and even macroscopic agents such as parasitic worms. In the absence of a functioning immune system, as is observed in persons with acquired immunodeficiency syndrome (AIDS) or congenital immune deficiencies, a person will eventually succumb to overwhelming infections.

Host-defense mechanisms consist of two major components: an innate system that is not dependent on prior exposure to an infectious agent and an acquired immunity that is stimulated by exposure to an agent. In general, the innate system functions in a nonspecific manner, while the acquired immune responses are highly specific.

The first major lines of host defense are the physical barriers to infection. These include the intact skin and the mechanical or physical barriers that serve to protect body openings. Few infectious agents are capable of penetrating intact skin. Numerous sweat glands and follicles are also associated with skin, and their secretion of fatty acids or lactic acid serves to produce an acid environment that inhibits the growth of bacteria. In addition, the high salt content found on the surface of the body also serves to inhibit growth. Bacteria that can resist the high levels of salt and acid, such as *Staphylococcus* or *Streptococcus*, tend to cause skin-related problems such as acne or boils.

Openings of the body, such as the mouth, anus, and vagina, exhibit both the physical barrier of skin and a variety of other defense strategies. Secreted mucus serves to trap foreign particles, which can then be expelled, depending on the tissue, by the ciliary action of the cells, coughing or sneezing, or the washing action of saliva, urine, or tears. Many of these secretions also contain antibacterial or antiviral agents. Gastric juices contain hydrochloric acid, while the enzyme lysozyme, found in tears and saliva, serves to cause the breakdown of certain bacteria.

The normal flora of organisms found within the body also plays an important role in defense. Bacteria in the mouth and gut serve to suppress any external agents that may find their way to those regions. Removal of the innate flora with antibiotics may result in yeast infections of the mouth or vaginal tract, or ulceration by "opportunistic" organisms of the gut.

Penetration of the host by infectious agents initially brings into action other aspects of the innate immune system. This can take the form of a series of "professional" phagocytes, cells that literally eat foreign particles such as bacteria; also included are chemical agents found in tissue and blood.

Two major forms of phagocytes are found in blood and tissues: neutrophils and monocytes/macrophages. Neutrophils represent the most numerous white cells in blood, approximately 60 to 70 percent of the total. They can be recognized by their multilobed nuclei,

The Host-Defense Mechanisms of the Body

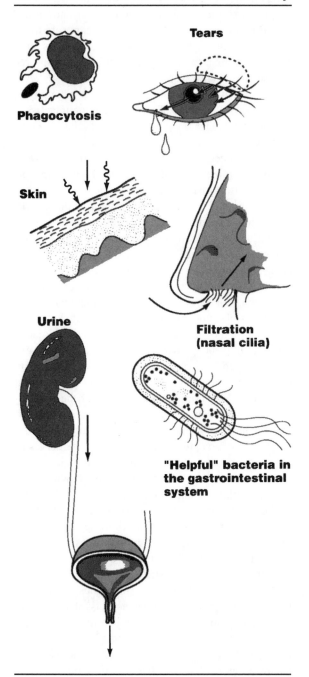

Phagocytosis

Tears

Skin

Filtration
(nasal cilia)

Urine

"Helpful" bacteria in
the gastrointestinal
system

which confer the ability to pass between the endothelial cells of capillaries into sites of tissue infections. When neutrophils locate a target, such as an infectious agent or a dead cell, they surround that target with membranous arms called pseudopods and ingest it. Once the particle is incorporated within this "phagosome," it is ready for killing and digestion.

The killing of ingested organisms such as bacteria involves a series of complicated reactions, the major products of which are highly reactive oxidizing agents such as peroxides or metabolic by-products such as acid. At the same time, digestive organelles within the phagocyte, called lysosomes, fuse with the phagosome. Lysosomes contain numerous digestive enzymes, and these function to digest the engulfed particle. In effect, the particle now ceases to exist.

Monocytes, which are most often observed in their differentiated macrophage stage, function in a similar manner. Unlike circulating cells such as neutrophils, however, macrophages constitute the mononuclear phagocytic system that is associated with many tissues in the body. Examples of tissue-associated macrophages are the Kupffer cells of the liver, the microglia of the brain, and certain alveolar cells of the lungs. In addition to serving a nonspecific phagocytic function, macrophages serve as antigen-presenting cells (APCs) for specific immune responses.

A variety of blood chemicals also can be associated with innate immunity. Complement represents a series of some twenty blood proteins, activated in a cascade fashion, which exhibit a variety of pharmacologic activities. The complement pathway can be initiated upon exposure to certain bacteria. Components of the pathway can serve as chemoattractants for neutrophils. They can increase the efficiency of phagocytosis (opsonization), and they can form a membrane attack complex on the surface of a target, resulting in lysis.

Another type of blood cell may play a role in certain types of parasitic infections: the eosinophil. Granulocytes like the neutrophils, eosinophils contain within their granules digestive enzymes capable of being released against targets such as parasitic worms. The binding of these enzymes on the surface of a target damages the parasite's membrane, resulting ultimately in death of the parasite.

Acquired host defenses, while involving mechanisms similar to those of the innate systems, differ in one important way: They require prior exposure to the antigen. Acquired immunity consists of two major arms: humoral immunity, which represents substances soluble in the blood; and cellular immunity, which utilizes cells targeted against agents in a specific manner.

Humoral immunity centers primarily on proteins called antibodies. Exposure to foreign antigens triggers a series of reactions among three separate types of blood cells: antigen-presenting cells, T lymphocytes, and B lymphocytes. It is the B cell that actually secretes the antibodies.

The process starts when an APC encounters and phagocytizes an antigen. The antigen is digested, and pieces, or determinants, of the antigen are expressed on the surface of the cell. The most common APC is the macrophage, but antigen presentation can also be carried out by dendritic cells found in the dermis of the skin. This portion of the process is analogous to the series of events associated with innate immunity. At this point, however, the determinant is "presented" to appropriate T and B lymphocytes. Only those lymphocytes that possess specific receptors for that antigenic determinant can interact with the APC; it is this aspect that represents the specificity of the reaction. In association with a subclass of T lymphocytes called T helper cells (also known as CD4+ cells), the B cell is stimulated to begin the secretion of large quantities of antibodies. The antibodies recognize and bind only those antigens against which they were produced.

The formation of antigen-antibody complexes is the key to the humoral response. The result of the reaction depends upon the form taken by the antigen. The binding of antibodies to a bacterium or virus results in opsonization, a significantly enhanced ability of phagocytes to engulf the target. Antibody binding to a virus may also inhibit the agent's binding to a target cell, rendering the virus inactive. If the antigen is a toxin, antibody binding will neutralize the molecule.

The other arm of acquired immunity directly utilizes cellular defenses. The key cell here is the T lymphocyte. T lymphocytes mature in an organ called the thymus, which is located in humans near the thyroid in the neck and which provides the basis for the cells' name. T cells are often referred to as "killer cells" (or CD8+ cells), because of their function. They possess receptors on their surfaces that bind to specific target cells, which are generally cells infected with viruses, though T cells are also associated with rejection of foreign grafts. Once the T cell binds to the target,

pharmacologically active granules are released that bind to and disrupt the membrane of the target. Thus, the humoral response is directed primarily against extracellular agents such as bacteria, while the cellular response is directed primarily against internal parasites.

DISORDERS AND DISEASES

In their most obvious form, the mechanisms of host defense protect against disease. Humans exist in an environment that is a sea of microorganisms. Most infections, while often uncomfortable, are not life threatening. It is only when the immune system fails to function properly or is overwhelmed that illness results in the death of the individual. Ironically, the study of these circumstances has provided much knowledge of the functioning of the immune system.

Throughout history, diseases have periodically plagued humanity. Epidemics of viral diseases such as polio and bacterial infections such as bubonic plague or cholera have killed untold millions of persons. Among the most important advances in medicine since the eighteenth century has been the development of vaccination as a means of preventing disease. In the case of passive immunity, host defenses are temporarily augmented, while active immunity, mimicking an actual infection, often provides lifelong protection.

Passive immunity involves the acquisition of preformed antibodies by an individual. Since colostrum, or milk from a nursing mother, contains a form of antibody, this is the most common form of passive immunization. Preformed antibodies may also be given to a person exposed to potentially lethal toxins under circumstances in which there may be insufficient time for a proper immune response. These can include persons exposed to snake venom or tetanus toxin. While temporarily providing protection, passively acquired antibodies survive in the individual only for a short period.

More commonly, vaccines are utilized to provide active immunization by stimulating the acquired host defenses. These vaccines generally utilize inactivated or attenuated parasites that stimulate specific cellular or humoral responses. The prototypes of active immunization are the polio vaccines developed by Jonas Salk and Albert Sabin in the 1950's. Salk's vaccine utilizes a formalin-inactivated poliovirus, while Sabin's consists of attenuated virus. While controversy exists regarding which is superior, both vaccines act in basically the same manner. Exposure to either vaccine results in the production of protective antibodies in the circulation of the individual. In the event of actual infection by poliovirus, the agent would be neutralized before it could reach its target in the central nervous system. Analogous vaccines have been developed against previously common viral diseases such as smallpox, measles, and mumps, and against bacterial diseases such as pertussis (whooping cough) and diphtheria.

The process by which the acquired immune process functions is in part defined by the nature of the antigen. It is also important to remember that the humoral and cellular defense systems are not self-exclusive; each functions in conjunction with the other. If the antigen in question is a bacterium, it is primarily the role of the humoral system to deal with the infection. This can take several forms. The antibody may bind to the surface of the cell, inactivating the cell wall or membrane enzymes, resulting in the death of the cell. The antibody-antigen (bacterium) complex may also activate the complement pathway, resulting in either opsonization or the formation of a membrane attack complex by complement components. Indeed, antibody binding by itself may result in opsonization.

If the antigen is a virus-infected cell, the cellular portion of the response comes into play. Cytotoxic T cells can bind to the target through specific receptors, causing the death of the virus-infected cell. If an antibody binds to viral receptors on the infected cell, cytotoxic cells with receptors for the antibody may show increased affinity for the target in a process called antibody-dependent cell-mediated cytotoxicity (ADCC). The result is the death of the target. The antibody may also serve to neutralize a cell-free virus before the particle can even infect the target cell. Certain bacteria, however, such as the mycobacteria associated with tuberculosis and leprosy, are actually found as intracellular parasites. In such cases, it is the cellular immune system that plays a major role in defense. In this manner, the humoral and cellular defense mechanisms complement each other.

Failure of the immune system to function is clearly illustrated in persons infected with the human immunodeficiency virus (HIV), the virus that causes AIDS. HIV infects the subclass of T lymphocytes called T helper cells. The eventual result is the death and depletion of this subclass of cells. As briefly described earlier, T helper cells are central to the function of both the humoral and the cellular arms of acquired immunity. The interaction of these cells with B lymphocytes is necessary for both antibody production by these cells and their proliferation. The T helper cell is also required for activation and proliferation of the CD8+ cytotoxic T cells.

As AIDS progresses in the individual, the T-helper subclass becomes increasingly depleted. As a result, both the cellular and humoral immune systems become progressively less functional. The person becomes more susceptible to opportunistic organisms in the environment and eventually succumbs to any of a wide variety of diseases.

In rare congenital cases, only certain aspects of the immune system are nonfunctional. These often tragic examples serve to illustrate the role of various cells within the host defense. For example, children with B-cell deficiencies suffer from repeated bacterial infections, while yeast and viral infections rarely result in problems. Children in whom the thymus fails to develop (Di George or Nezelof syndromes), however, suffer from repeated viral infections but rarely from bacterial infections.

Severe combined immunodeficiency syndrome (SCID) affects approximately one out of every 150,000 live births. This genetic disorder is the result of a lack of the enzyme adenosine deaminase (ADA), which ultimately causes a lack of functioning T cells. For years, patients with this disorder had been doomed to living in sterile bubble environments and would die at a young age because of their inability to fight even the mildest infection. Bone marrow transplants for patients with compatible donors can sometimes strengthen the immune system; however, this option is not available for everyone.

In 1990, two unrelated girls with SCID, four and nine years old, were the subject of the first clinical trial of gene therapy. T cells in their blood were isolated and cultured, and normal copies of the ADA gene were introduced into the cells. The genetically engineered T cells were then infused back into the patients over a period of approximately two years. Both girls showed remarkable improvement, with near normal levels of ADA and functioning immune systems, and were thereafter able to lead normal lives. These positive results remained several years after cessation of the actual gene therapy, indicating that this first clinical trial of gene therapy was a success. The door is now open for using gene therapy on other disorders, including those of the immune system.

Host defenses are also utilized within the homeostatic process, which can be defined as maintaining the status quo. An example of such a process is the role of the immune system in protecting humans against various forms of cancer. Although immunosuppressed individuals appear to be at no greater risk for most cancers than normal persons, certain types of skin cancers, as well as certain types of B-cell lymphomas, arise more frequently in these persons. Thus, it is likely that the immune system plays at least some role in protecting the individual from certain forms of cancer. Artificial stimulation of the immune system has, however, been utilized in an attempt to treat sundry forms of advanced cancers. The process involves the removal of immune cells from the patient and the incubation of those cells with a form of interferon generally secreted by T helper cells during their regulation of the immune response. The cells are then returned to the patient. The theory is that, by nonspecifically stimulating cytotoxic cells, some of those cells may serve to destroy the cancer. In some instances, patients have shown improvement.

Clearly, the immune system functions by means of a complex process of cellular interactions. The initial encounter with a foreign infectious agent utilizes an innate system that serves as a first line of defense. Then, through a type of learning process, a specific immune response is generated that provides a more rapid, more efficient means of generating protection.

PERSPECTIVE AND PROSPECTS

Manipulating the host's immune system in order to protect against disease dates back more than a thousand years. In order to protect themselves against smallpox, the Chinese carried out a practice called variolation, in which dried crusts obtained from the pocks of mild cases were inhaled. The practice was copied by early Arabic physicians and eventually made its way to eighteenth century Europe. In the late eighteenth century, an English country physician, Edward Jenner, observed that dairy maids who had recovered from a mild disease called cowpox rarely exhibited the scars associated with smallpox. Jenner reasoned that a person who had been exposed to the cowpox agent would be protected against smallpox. Jenner tested his theory and was proved correct. Smallpox became the first disease that could be prevented by vaccination.

Competition between French and German scientists during the late nineteenth century resulted in much of the existing basic knowledge of host defenses. A Russian, Élie Metchnikoff, working with Louis Pasteur in Paris during the 1880's, developed the views of cellular immunity that are still current. In that same period, the work of Emil von Behring and Paul Ehrlich in Berlin established the role of humoral immunity in protecting against disease.

Active immunization remains the primary method by which an individual may be protected from disease, but the process lends itself to a variety of problems. Not all antigenic determinants of the bacterium or parasite in question are equally important. A response to some antigens may actually hinder the immune response to more important determinants. Furthermore, some individuals react inappropriately to some vaccines, resulting in severe allergic reactions.

For these reasons, much research involves the attempt to isolate only the desired antigen for the vaccine. This has taken several approaches. Purified components, rather than the entire organism, have been used in some vaccines. In some cases, the gene that encodes the desired antigen has been isolated and spliced into the genetic material of a harmless organism. Such an approach has been used to produce a modified hepatitis-B vaccine. The gene encoding the surface antigen of the virus has been spliced into the genome of vaccinia, long used for vaccination against smallpox. When the individual is vaccinated, the hepatitis gene is expressed (though no virus can be made), and the person becomes immune to the disease. In theory, whole cocktails of vaccines can be prepared in a similar manner.

New illnesses and other environmental hazards that affect host defenses continue to arise. AIDS may be unusually lethal, but as a previously unknown disease, it is by no means unique. Nevertheless, the ability of the host immune system to respond to new infectious agents remains a bulwark for maintaining the health of an individual.

—Richard Adler, Ph.D.;
updated by Karen E. Kalumuck, Ph.D.

See also Bacterial infections; Bacteriology; Blood and blood disorders; Cells; Glands; Immune system; Immunization and vaccination; Immunology; Immunopathology; Infection; Skin; Urinary system; Viral infections.

FOR FURTHER INFORMATION:

Bibel, Debra. *Milestones in Immunology.* Madison, Wis.: Science Tech, 1988. A compendium of historic articles related to the development of immunology. In association with each original article is an outline explaining the significance of the material. The book presents the evolution of thought in the field in a clear manner, illustrating how knowledge builds upon previous information.

Life, Death, and the Immune System. New York: W. H. Freeman, 1994. This collection of offprints from *Scientific American* gives detailed information on a host of topics pertaining to the immune system, including AIDS, autoimmune disorders, allergies, and a general description of the physiology of the immune system.

Paul, William E. *Immunology: Recognition and Response.* New York: W. H. Freeman, 1991. Paul has assembled a collection of readings from *Scientific American* that deal with the indicated subject. Most of the articles are written at a level that can be understood by persons with a background in basic science.

Playfair, J. H. L. *Immunology at a Glance.* 7th ed. Boston: Blackwell Scientific, 2000. A collection of short chapters dealing with various aspects of host defense. The material, which is abbreviated, clearly defines the described subjects. The book is written in an introductory manner, though its coverage is extensive.

Roitt, Ivan. *Roitt's Essential Immunology.* 9th ed. Boston: Blackwell Scientific, 1997. A textbook written by a leading authority in the field. Though the chapters explaining the technical aspects of the subject become quite detailed, the introductory material dealing with basic host defense is clear and concise. Numerous photographs are included.

HUMAN GENOME PROJECT

PROCEDURE

ANATOMY OR SYSTEM AFFECTED: All

SPECIALTIES AND RELATED FIELDS: Biochemistry, biotechnology, ethics, forensic medicine, genetics

DEFINITION: A major research initiative to determine the deoxyribonucleic acid (DNA) sequence of all the genetic material within a human being and localize its estimated fifty thousand to one hundred thousand genes.

KEY TERMS:

amino acids: the individual chemical subunits that make up a protein

base: one of the four molecules that make up DNA (guanine, adenine, thymine, and cytosine, abbreviated G, A, T, and C)

chromosome: a long threadlike structure composed of DNA and protein

deoxyribonucleic acid (DNA): the chemical that constitutes genetic material; it consists of four different chemical bases, G, A, T, and C

gene: a discrete unit of hereditary material made of DNA

genome: all the genetic material of an individual organism

organism: any living individual

protein: one of the chemical compounds considered "the building blocks of life"

THE STRUCTURE AND FUNCTION OF DNA

The human genome, like the genomes of all living things, is all the genetic material that makes up an organism. Genetic material is inherited by offspring from parent organisms. The genetic material is deoxyribonucleic acid, or DNA. DNA is a chemical compound that consists of four different bases, or subunits, that are connected to one another via a backbone of sugar and phosphate molecules. There are four different bases, guanine (G), adenine (A), thymine (T), and cytosine (C). Each base in a strand is paired with a complementary base, always A with T and G with C, forming a ladderlike structure with the bases forming the rungs and the sugar-phosphate backbone forming the sides of the ladder. The ladder is twisted into a spiral shape, and this shape is referred to as a double helix.

The sequence of DNA bases contains information that specifies the formation of many different proteins that determine or strongly influence the traits of an organism, including physical traits and the biochemical processes involved in growth, metabolism, and reproduction. In human beings and other complex organisms, DNA and proteins form rod-shaped structures known as chromosomes. Humans have twenty-three pairs of chromosomes.

Discrete units of DNA that specify one heritable trait are referred to as genes. It has been estimated that the human genome consists of about three billion base pairs, divided into between fifty thousand and one hundred thousand genes. Of the entire three billion base pairs of DNA, only about 3 percent are contained in genes. The rest are involved in regulating the production of gene products, maintaining the structure of chromosomes, and other still-unknown functions. Damaged genes or damage to the mechanisms that control protein production by certain genes can directly cause or strongly influence many diseases in humans.

The information stored in the DNA sequence of a gene is converted into a protein by a complex and elegant series of chemical processes. First, the DNA sequence is converted into an intermediary sequence called messenger ribonucleic acid (mRNA). Messenger RNA consists of bases that are complementary to the DNA molecule in a fashion similar to the way in which two DNA strands of a double helix are complementary. The strand of mRNA is then "read" and translated into a protein. Three bases in sequence stand for one of twenty different protein subunits, called amino acids. As the mRNA is read, successive amino acids specified by the DNA sequence of the gene are linked together, ultimately forming a functional protein.

Changes in the DNA sequence, called mutations, may result in a change in the amino acid sequence of the specified protein. These changes may cause the protein to function improperly, or the protein might not be produced at all; in either case, some mutations may cause disease, depending on the gene that was affected by the mutation. Mutations can be caused by chemicals, radiation, or mistakes made when the DNA was copied and reproduced during cell division. If the mutation occurs in egg or sperm cells, it could be passed on to offspring.

Because DNA controls the fundamental processes of life—how adult organisms, with a complex array of tissues and organs, develop from a single egg fertilized by a single sperm—isolating and studying all of the genes involved in these developmental processes would provide an incomparable opportunity to expand human understanding of all life's processes. In addition, understanding normal development would help scientists to understand what has gone wrong when development does not proceed as it should and perhaps lead to ways to prevent or treat birth defects. Many diseases that afflict children and adults, from cancer to blood and neurological disorders, have a strong genetic component. Isolating and studying normal as well as defective genes associated with a specific disease could lead to improved diagnosis and treatment and, possibly, a cure for the disease.

MAPPING GENES

Deciphering the entire DNA sequence of humans is the first step in isolating and studying genes that are involved in human growth, development, health, and disease. As soon as the technology became available, in the late 1980's and early 1990's, an international initiative, the Human Genome Project, was begun to sequence the entire human genome. At the time the initiative was begun, only the genome of a relatively simple bacterium had been sequenced. The human genome, being three thousand times larger, presented a far more complex, monumental task but one with the potential to pave the way for great benefits for humankind.

To facilitate the understanding of how a particular gene works, genes similar to human genes are sought in simpler organisms. The genomes of several commonly used research organisms have been sequenced, including the common fruit fly, *Drosophila melanogaster*, and the round worm, *Caenorhabditis elegans*. Genes tend to be similar in all animals, and if a gene similar to a particular human gene can be identified in a simpler organism, studying the gene in the simpler organism will be much quicker and less expensive and could lead to insights into the functioning of that gene in humans, perhaps ultimately leading to a diagnostic tool or a cure.

For example, when the fly genome sequence was completed in 2000, scientists found that 177 human genes associated with diseases as diverse as cancer, Alzheimer's disease, and the neurological degenerative disorder Tay-Sachs disease had comparable genes in flies. Studying the fly genes could improve the study of these diseases in humans.

By comparing the sequences of the "normal" human genome, as determined by the Human Genome Project, with that of patients with a particular disease, scientists will be able to pinpoint the gene or genes involved in the disease. Pinpointing the gene will facilitate the study of what the normal gene product does and perhaps lead to a cure. However, in most cases it would take years of research to reach that point. For example, the gene that causes Huntington's disease, a rare neurodegenerative disorder that strikes in midlife and is always fatal, was discovered in 1993, and a diagnostic test has been available for it since the late 1980's. Nevertheless, scientists do not understand the cause of the disease, and a cure has not yet been discovered.

Localizing disease genes or genes that predispose individuals to certain disorders, such as heart disease, will more directly lead to diagnostic tests to discover whether one has the genetic makeup that could lead to a particular disorder. Tests to determine whether someone might pass along selected genetic diseases, such as cystic fibrosis, Tay-Sachs disease, and sickle-cell disease, to offspring are already in existence. Potential parents can use the information in planning their families. In cases in which the presence of certain genes may predispose but not directly cause someone to develop a disease (such as heart disease or certain forms of cancer), preventive measures and regular monitoring could be suggested to limit the chance of developing the disease.

A device called a gene chip is being developed that would enable scientists to understand human development and disease at the cellular level. Small pieces of DNA of interest are programmed into the chip, and it is introduced into selected tissues and used to detect which genes are producing which protein products at a particular time and in which tissue. This type of specificity will enable comparison of the healthy and diseased state at the level of the fundamental unit of life, the cell, thus aiding in understanding and curing disease.

Pharmacogenomics is a new field that has sprung up in the wake of the Human Genome Project. In pharmacogenomics, researchers use information about the genetic makeup of individuals to determine how they will respond to particular therapeutic drugs. Initially, drug design for the human population in general will benefit from mapping the human genome. Ultimately, scientists hope that drug treatments will be tailored to individuals, assigning each patient the most effective treatment for his or her individual genetic makeup.

PERSPECTIVE AND PROSPECTS

The first evidence of the role of DNA in genetic makeup was discovered in 1944 by Oswald Avery, Maclyn McCarty, and Colin MacLeod, who discovered that nonpathogenic bacteria could become pathogenic by mixing them with DNA from pathogenic bacteria. Martha Chase and Alfred Hershey, in 1952, provided supporting evidence for DNA's role when they discovered that DNA was the genetic material in bacterial viruses. The three-dimensional structure of DNA was determined in 1953 by Francis Crick and James Watson, with assistance from Rosalind Franklin and Maurice Wilkins. Knowing the three-dimensional structure paved the way for scientists to decipher the processes inherent in DNA's role as the genetic material, including its self-replication,

DNA's genetic code, and the mechanisms that transform that code into proteins. In the mid-1970's, techniques were developed to "clone" or make many copies of selected DNA, cutting DNA from an organism of interest and placing it into rapidly multiplying bacteria. In 1977, two DNA sequencing methods were developed, one by Allan Maxam and Walter Gilbert, and another by Fred Sanger, which is the basic method used to sequence the human genome. A revolutionary advance that helped to set the stage for sequencing the human genome came in the mid-1980's when Kary Mullis developed a technique called the polymerase chain reaction (PCR). PCR allows the rapid production of enormous numbers of copies of specific DNA sequences, thus facilitating their study.

Scientists began discussing the possibilities of sequencing the entire human genome in the mid-1980's. The National Human Genome Research Institute (NHGRI), founded in 1989 as the National Center for Human Genome Research (NCHGR), is funded by the National Institutes of Health and the Department of Energy, along with the British Wellcome Trust. Its task, the Human Genome Project, has been an international effort that has included seventeen genome centers in the United States and five international genome centers, all sharing data and working cooperatively. The original goal was to have the human genome sequenced in fifteen years, by 2005, at a cost of $3 billion, or about $1 for each of the estimated 3 billion human genome base pairs.

The research laboratories followed an orderly process of breaking the genome into large pieces, localizing them to particular sites on chromosomes and then breaking the large pieces into smaller pieces and using automated sequencers to establish their DNA sequence. Development of the automated process was possible thanks to the work of Leroy Hood, who in the 1980's developed a means to tag the DNA with four different dyes, one for each of the DNA bases. The order in which the colors in a mixture of DNA travel through the machine is the order of the DNA bases. The short sequences are then arranged so that they overlap, using computer programs to facilitate the process. As a final step, researchers known as "annotators" locate and identify genes, again aided by computer programs. All the information is posted daily on the centers' Internet site and is accessible to scientists worldwide.

In March, 1998, more than seven years and halfway into the project, only 3 percent of the genome had been sequenced. On May 9 of that year, maverick scientist J. Craig Venter made an announcement that rocked the scientific community: He was forming a new company called Celera Genomics, and this company would sequence the entire human genome in three years, for between $200 million and $300 million.

Celera Genomics used a different sequencing technique than the NHGRI, one called "whole genome shotgun sequencing," which shatters the genome into thousands of short fragments. The ends of these fragments are sequenced, and powerful computers are used to do trillions of computations to overlap the fragments and reconstruct the entire genome. Many scientists believed that this technique could result in great inaccuracies in the sequence.

An unprecedented level of cooperation occurred between the publicly funded NHGRI and privately funded Celera Genomics. On June 23, 2000, in a joint news conference with U.S. president Bill Clinton, Venter and Francis Collins, the director of NHGRI, announced that each group had sequenced the entire genome, five years ahead of the original schedule.

At that time, an estimated 99.9 percent of the human genome sequence had been completed, but significant gaps and inaccuracies exist that both groups are working to resolve. Now researchers are intent on understanding what the sequence means, locating genes, and determining how they affect human health and development. The information contained in the human genome is expected to help doctors understand, diagnose, and treat most, if not all, diseases. Treatments may be tailored to the individual, based on his or her own unique genetic makeup. However, there are real ethical concerns about the power of the data contained in the genome. Concerns exist about the use of the information for screening for insurance purposes or employment and the potential for discrimination based on DNA sequences. In addition, scientists will be able to identify genetic disease or the potential for genetic disease long before treatments are available. The Human Genome Project has provided profound new knowledge that holds much promise for worldwide health but also has the potential for becoming a Pandora's box of difficult ethical challenges.

—Karen E. Kalumuck, Ph.D.

See also DNA and RNA; Ethics; Genetic counseling; Genetic diseases; Genetic engineering; Genetics and inheritance.

FOR FURTHER INFORMATION:

Ridley, Matt. *Genome: The Autobiography of a Species in Twenty-three Chapters.* New York: HarperCollins, 1999. Ridley explores knowledge gained through the Human Genome Project, from cancer to sex, and takes on the ethics of this world-altering knowledge.

Tagliaferro, Linda, and Mark V. Bloom. *The Complete Idiot's Guide to Decoding Your Genes.* New York: Macmillan, 1998. This book, written for the lay person, gives clear and succinct information on genes, genetic technologies, and the Human Genome Project.

Wade, Nicholas, ed. *The Science Times Book of Genetics.* New York: Lyons Press, 1998. This series of science essays from *The New York Times* provides an excellent background on the genetic processes and the ethical issues associated with the Human Genome Project.

HUMAN IMMUNODEFICIENCY VIRUS (HIV)

DISEASE/DISORDER

ANATOMY OR SYSTEM AFFECTED: Immune system

SPECIALTIES AND RELATED FIELDS: Immunology, internal medicine, public health, virology

DEFINITION: HIV is the virus responsible for acquired immunodeficiency syndrome (AIDS) and AIDS-related complex (ARC). Although the virus has been found in various body fluids—such as saliva, tears, and breast milk—only blood and semen have been associated with its transmission. Therefore, any activities involving blood or semen can spread HIV, including sexual intercourse, the sharing of needles, blood transfusions, kidney transplantations, and artificial insemination; the risk of transmission from the last three activities has been virtually eliminated through testing procedures. There is an unpredictable lag between exposure to HIV and a positive test result for HIV antibodies (although it is usually within one year), and another lag until the HIV-positive individual develops AIDS (which may range from eighteen months to many years). Infection with HIV increases the chances of developing dermatitis, thrush, shingles, herpes simplex infection, and tuberculosis.

—Jason Georges and Tracy Irons-Georges

See also Acquired immunodeficiency syndrome (AIDS); Autoimmune disorders; Immune system;

Immunodeficiency disorders; Immunology; Immuno-pathology; Sexually transmitted diseases; Viral infections.

FOR FURTHER INFORMATION:

Levy, Jay A. "Pathogenesis of Human Immunodeficiency Virus Infection." *Microbiological Reviews* 57 (March, 1993): 183-289.

Miller, Roger, and Nava Sarver. "HIV Accessory Proteins as Therapeutic Targets." *Nature Medicine* 3, no. 4 (April, 1997): 389-394.

Petrow, Steven, ed. *HIV Drug Book*. New York: Pocket Books, 1995.

HUNTINGTON'S DISEASE. *See* BRAIN DISORDERS.

HYDROCELECTOMY

PROCEDURE

ANATOMY OR SYSTEM AFFECTED: Genitals, reproductive system

SPECIALTIES AND RELATED FIELDS: General surgery, urology

DEFINITION: The removal of a hydrocele, a collection of fluid between the lining membranes protecting the testicle in the scrotum.

INDICATIONS AND PROCEDURES

Hydrocelectomy is primarily indicated for hydroceles in adults which produce discomfort, objectionable scrotal enlargement, or an uncertainty regarding underlying testicular abnormalities upon scrotal ultrasound or physical examination. The presence of a hydrocele does not necessarily require surgical intervention, drainage, or other intervention; it must be accompanied by some significant abnormality to require surgery.

Hydroceles occur in 1 percent of adult males. In patients between the ages of eighteen and thirty-five, the presence of an underlying testicular tumor must be ruled out. Accurate diagnosis can be carried out through physical examination. A hydrocele is a smooth, cystlike mass completely surrounding the testicle such that only the mass can be palpated; the testis, inside, cannot be felt. Hydroceles do not involve the spermatic cord. When a light is shined through the cyst, the light is readily transmitted. If the hydrocele is large or tense and the testis cannot be examined, ultrasound examination can eliminate the diagnosis of a testicular abnormality.

Surgical excision is the most effective method for treatment and can be done on an outpatient basis. A 5.0- to 7.6-centimeter (2.0- to 3.0-inch) incision is made in the scrotum, and the wall of the hydrocele is identified and dissected free. The hydrocele sac is removed and its edges sewn or cauterized to eliminate bleeding. The testis is then returned to the scrotum, and the incision is closed. For large hydroceles, a small drainage tube is introduced into the scrotum to limit swelling.

USES AND COMPLICATIONS

The most frequent complication of hydrocele surgery is scrotal swelling, which may continue for eight weeks. Most patients return to full activity within seven to ten days of surgery, however, and recurrences are rare.

In addition to surgical removal, other treatment options include needle aspiration and aspiration with the injection of sclerosing agents. Needle aspiration is rarely effective and increases infection risk. Fluid usually reaccumulates within three months of aspiration. Aspiration with the injection of sclerosing agents such as tetracycline is successful in fewer than 50 percent of patients and usually requires multiple treatments.

—*Culley C. Carson III, M.D.*

See also Abscess drainage; Cyst removal; Reproductive system; Testicular surgery.

FOR FURTHER INFORMATION:

Glenn, James F., ed. *Glenn's Urologic Surgery*. 5th ed. Philadelphia: J. B. Lippincott, 1998.

Kay, K. W., R. V. Clayman, and P. H. Lange. "Outpatient Hydrocele and Spermatocele Repair Under Local Anesthesia." *Journal of Urology* 130, no. 2 (August, 1983): 269-271.

HYDROCEPHALUS

DISEASE/DISORDER

ANATOMY OR SYSTEM AFFECTED: Brain, head, nervous system, psychic-emotional system

SPECIALTIES AND RELATED FIELDS: Critical care, general surgery, neonatology, neurology, perinatology

DEFINITION: A collection of excessive amounts of cerebrospinal fluid (CSF) within the cranial cavity, which can cause increased pressure within the brain and skull, leading to brain tissue damage and, in infants, enlargement of the skull.

cerebrospinal fluid (CSF): the fluid that bathes and nourishes the inner and outer surfaces of the brain and spinal cord

shunt: a tube that is surgically inserted to drain excess fluid away from an area such as the brain

"water on the brain": a common term for hydrocephalus

CAUSES AND SYMPTOMS

Frequently referred to as "water on the brain," hydrocephalus is a disorder most commonly seen in newborns and infants but sometimes occurring in older children and adults. The water is actually a relatively small amount (about 10 cubic centimeters for every kilogram of body weight) of cerebrospinal fluid (CSF), which surrounds and cushions the brain and spinal cord on both the inside and the outside. Within the brain are four CSF-filled spaces called ventricles. The CSF is continuously formed here and then moves down through the central canal, a tube that runs the length of the spinal cord. From the base of the spine, the fluid moves upward on the outside of the spinal cord, returning to the skull, where it covers the outer surfaces of the brain. Here it is absorbed by the brain's outer lining. If interference occurs in any part of this process, CSF continues to accumulate in the brain. This usually causes increased pressure to develop within the skull. Abnormally high pressure can lead to permanent brain damage and even death. In the infant, this accumulation also causes the skull to enlarge, since the growth regions of the skull have not yet become firm.

Excessive CSF may develop due to overproduction of fluid in the brain, a blockage of the fluid's circulation, or a blockage of fluid reabsorption on the brain's surface. Hydrocephalus can be congenital or may develop as a result of a head injury, infection, brain hemorrhage, or tumor. Congenital hydrocephalus and most hydrocephalus that begins in infancy are characterized by an enlarged head, which continues to grow at an abnormally rapid pace.

Symptoms and signs that accompany congenital hydrocephalus include lethargy, vomiting, irritability, epilepsy, rigidity of the legs, and the loss of normal reflexes. If left untreated, the condition causes drowsiness, seizures, and severe brain damage, leading to death possibly within days or weeks. Hydrocephalus is also often associated with other anomalies of the brain and nervous system, such as spina bifida.

When hydrocephalus develops in older children and adults, the head size will not increase since the growth lines in the bones of the skull have hardened. If the CSF pressure increases, resulting symptoms include headaches, vomiting, vision problems, problems with muscle coordination, and a progressive decrease in mental activity.

Hydrocephalus

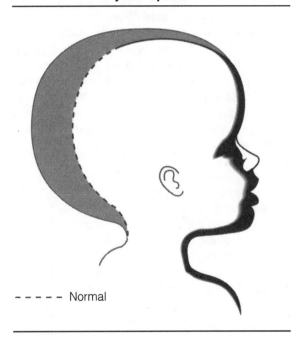

----- Normal

Normal head size vs. size of head with hydrocephalus.

TREATMENT AND THERAPY

Diagnosis of hydrocephalus and related nervous system defects sometimes can be made before birth, either by fetal ultrasound or by testing for the presence of an abnormal amount of a brain-associated protein, alpha-fetoprotein, in the pregnant woman's blood. However, even with early diagnosis and surgical intervention promptly after birth, the prognosis is guarded.

Older children and adults suspected of having hydrocephalus should be examined by a neurologist. A computed tomography (CT) scan or magnetic resonance imaging (MRI) of the brain can visualize the structure of the brain and the extent of the hydrocephalus.

Surgical correction is the primary treatment for hydrocephalus. The excess pressure must be drained from within the brain, or a balance between the production and elimination of CSF must be established. In some cases, a combination of surgery and medication is successful. For example, the drugs furosemide (Lasix) and acetazolamide (Diamox), when used for increased CSF pressure from brain hemorrhage, may reduce the amount of CSF fluid produced and thereby decrease the amount of swelling.

Relieving the CSF pressure within the brain is generally achieved by the surgical insertion of a tube, called a shunt, through brain tissue into one of the cerebral ventricles. A one-way valve is attached to the tube; this allows CSF to escape from the skull cavity when the pressure exceeds a certain level. The tubing is then passed beneath the skin into either the right side of the heart or the abdominal cavity, where the excessive CSF can be absorbed safely. Complications of this procedure are fairly common and include repeated infections, septicemia, peritonitis, or meningitis.

PERSPECTIVE AND PROSPECTS

The outcome of treated patients with hydrocephalus has improved over the years, but the condition is still associated with long-term problems. A modest percentage of newborns with congenital hydrocephalus will survive and achieve normal intelligence.

—*Cynthia Beres*

See also Birth defects; Brain; Brain disorders; Childbirth complications; Critical care, pediatric; Meningitis; Mental retardation; Neonatology; Nervous system; Neurology, pediatric; Pediatrics; Shunts; Spina bifida; Spinal cord disorders; Surgery, pediatric.

FOR FURTHER INFORMATION:

Clayman, Charles B., ed. *The American Medical Association Encyclopedia of Medicine.* New York: Random House, 1994. A concise presentation of numerous medical terms and illnesses. A good general reference.

Professional Guide to Diseases. 7th ed. Springhouse, Pa.: Springhouse, 2001. A comprehensive yet concise medical reference covering more than six hundred disorders.

Toporek, Chuck, and Kellie Robinson. *Hydrocephalus: A Guide for Patients, Families, and Friends.* Sebastopol, Calif.: O'Reilly & Associates, 1999. Provides clear advice on living with hydrocephalus.

HYDROTHERAPY

PROCEDURE

ANATOMY OR SYSTEM AFFECTED: All

SPECIALTIES AND RELATED FIELDS: Alternative medicine, physical therapy, rheumatology, sports medicine

DEFINITION: The application of water in any form in the treatment of disease is known as hydrotherapy. Immersion in water can take many forms, including hot tubs, whirlpools, saunas, foot baths, and spas. In all cases, the healing properties of water stem from its buoyancy and its temperature. Buoyancy makes movement easier and allows patients who are recuperating from injury or surgery to prevent muscle atrophy by beginning an early pro-

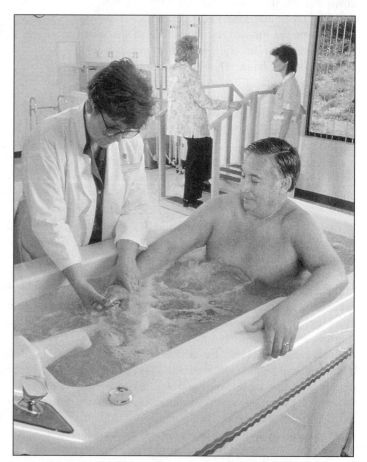

A patient receives a therapeutic bath. (Digital Stock)

gram of stretching and strengthening the muscles without the full stress of gravity. The warm temperature of water immersion promotes relaxation and circulation and decreases pain. The resistance provided by water presents an added challenge to an individual's movements, thereby giving an intensive aerobic workout which is cushioned by the water's buoyancy. In many cases, the use of hydrotherapy following trauma has reduced recovery time by up to 50 percent. Immersion hydrotherapy is effective in the relief of pain from back injuries and has been used to alleviate pain and encourage the healing process in burn patients and those with asthma, hypertension, headaches, and arthritis, among many other illnesses.

—*Karen E. Kalumuck, Ph.D.*

See also Alternative medicine; Exercise physiology; Healing; Pain management; Physical rehabilitation; Sports medicine.

FOR FURTHER INFORMATION:

Goldberg, Burton, comp. *Alternative Medicine: The Definitive Guide.* Puyallup, Wash.: Future Medicine, 1993.

Jacobs, Jennifer, ed. *The Encyclopedia of Alternative Medicine: A Complete Family Guide to Complementary Therapies.* Rev. ed. Boston: Journey Edition, 1997.

Kastner, Mark, and Hugh Burroughs. *Alternative Healing: The Complete A-Z Guide to Over 160 Different Alternative Therapies.* New York: Henry Holt, 1996.

Mills, Simon, and Steven J. Finando. *Alternatives in Healing.* London: Grange Books, 1995.

HYPERADIPOSIS

DISEASE/DISORDER

ALSO KNOWN AS: Severe obesity, extreme obesity

ANATOMY OR SYSTEM AFFECTED: All

SPECIALTIES AND RELATED FIELDS: Biochemistry, endocrinology, family practice, genetics, nutrition

DEFINITION: Having excess body fat; exceeding 200 percent of standard body weight as defined on a height-weight table.

CAUSES AND SYMPTOMS

Obesity results from consuming more calories than the body uses. Severe obesity accounts for less than 1 percent of all obesity in the United States but is linked to a large number of deaths each year, many of them due to heart disease or diabetes. Genetics, socioeconomic status, and emotional disturbances may all contribute to severe obesity.

One leading theory proposes that body weight is regulated by a set point in the hypothalamus (a section of the brain), similar to a thermostat setting. A higher-than-normal set point would explain why some people are obese and why losing weight and maintaining weight loss are difficult for them. It is also well established that an increase in the size and/or number of fat cells adds to the amount of fat stored by the body. Those who become obese during early childhood may have up to five times as many fat cells as people of normal weight. Because the number of cells cannot be reduced, weight loss can come about only by decreasing the amount of fat stored in each cell.

Accumulation of excess fat below the diaphragm and in the chest wall places pressure on the lungs, leading to shortness of breath and difficulty in breathing, even with minimal exertion. This may also seriously interfere with sleep. Low back pain and osteoarthritis, especially in the hips, knees, and ankles, may be seen, and skin disorders are common, owing to moisture retention in the folds of the fatty skin. Because of a low ratio of surface area to body weight in severe obesity, the body has a hard time getting rid of excess body heat, leading to excessive sweating and fluid accumulation in the ankles and feet.

Fat tends to accumulate in the abdomen in males, and in the thighs and buttocks in females. Abdominal obesity in particular is linked with a high incidence of coronary artery disease, high blood pressure, adult onset diabetes, hyperlipidemia, and gallbladder disease. In addition, an increase in menstrual disorders and in breast, uterine, and ovarian cancer is seen in women. Men have higher rates of colorectal and prostate cancer.

TREATMENT AND THERAPY

Self-help and nonclinical weight loss programs rarely work in individuals with severe obesity. Clinical programs that combine supervised weight loss, behavior modification, and exercise have shown good results. Drugs such as amphetamines (ephedrine) have questionable value in cases of severe obesity. Total fasting produces a risk of ketonemia and electrolyte imbalances, leading to cardiac arrhythmias.

Surgery has become an increasingly popular form of treatment. Vertical banded gastroplasty (stomach stapling) and gastric bypass are the most common procedures. Both produce satiety with small food intake and, if coupled with exercise, can result in weight losses approximating one-half of the excess weight (80 to 160 pounds). Jejunoileal bypass is also effective but produces a permanent malabsorption syndrome that may lead to other metabolic problems. Liposuction, where a small incision is made and fatty deposits are suctioned out, produces only moderate results in the severely obese. Because of potential risks to blood vessels and nerves, only a small amount of fat can be removed from each location.

Leptin, the protein hormone product of the ob gene, has been suggested as a useful new treatment for severe obesity. However, only about 5 percent of obese individuals fail to produce leptin on their own, and in those individuals either daily injections of leptin or gene therapy to correct the chromosomal defect would be required. Neither is currently considered a practical solution.

PERSPECTIVE AND PROSPECTS

Since 1900, the incidence of severe obesity in the United States has more than doubled, despite the fact that the average number of calories consumed per day has decreased by 10 percent. The most likely explanation is a decrease in physical activity among the population at large. While everyone needs to be conscious of dietary intake and exercise needs, parents of young children in particular need to be careful not to use food as either reward or punishment, as the early years of development appear to be most crucial in setting the stage for later obesity.

—*Kerry L. Cheesman, Ph.D.*

See also Eating disorders; Glands; Leptin; Malnutrition; Nutrition; Obesity; Weight loss and gain; Weight loss medications.

FOR FURTHER INFORMATION:

Bennett, J. Claude, et al., eds. *Cecil Textbook of Medicine*. 21st ed. Philadelphia: W. B. Saunders, 2000. This textbook offers a brief review of all aspects of the problem of obesity by a recognized authority in the field.

Bjorntorp, Per, and Bernard N. Brodoff, eds. *Obesity*. Philadelphia: J. B. Lippincott, 1992. A very comprehensive, multiauthored book on all aspects of obesity, from basic considerations of metabolism, body composition, and etiology, to practical questions of the psychological and medical consequences and the various methods of treatment.

Consensus Development Conference Panel. "Gastrointestinal Surgery for Severe Obesity: Consensus Development Conference Statement." *Annals of Internal Medicine* 115, no. 12 (1991): 956-961. Describes a consensus reached by leading surgeons, gastroenterologists, endocrinologists, psychiatrists, and nutritionists on the status of surgical procedures for the treatment of severe and intractable obesity.

HYPERCHOLESTEROLEMIA

DISEASE/DISORDER

ANATOMY OR SYSTEM AFFECTED: Blood vessels, circulatory system

SPECIALTIES AND RELATED FIELDS: Cardiology, family practice, hematology, internal medicine, nutrition, preventive medicine, serology, vascular medicine

DEFINITION: Found in animal oils and fats, tissues, bile, blood, and egg yolk, cholesterol is used by the body in the production of steroids, including sex hormones and hormones of the adrenal glands. Excessive amounts of cholesterol in the blood, called hypercholesterolemia, have been shown to increase the risk of atherosclerosis, which is the deposit of fatty plaques on the inside of blood vessels. The replacement of animal fat in the diet with vegetable oil containing polyunsaturated fats will cause blood cholesterol levels to fall. Hypercholesterolemia is also responsible for the majority of gallstone cases.

—*Jason Georges and Tracy Irons-Georges*

See also Arteriosclerosis; Blood and blood disorders; Cholesterol; Gallbladder diseases; Heart disease; Hyperlipidemia; Steroids

FOR FURTHER INFORMATION:

Brook, Robert H. *Hypercholesterolemia*. Santa Monica, Calif.: Rand, 1981.

Gotto, Antonio M., Jr. *Hypercholesterolemia: New Findings and Clinical Applications*. Newton, Mass.: Cahners, 1991.

Grundy, Scott M. *Cholesterol-Lowering Therapy: Evaluation of Clinical Trial Evidence*. New York: Marcel Dekker, 2000.

Hunninghake, Donald B. *Hypercholesterolemia: Reducing the Risk*. Secaucus, N.J.: Network for Continuing Medical Education, 1989.

Rifkind, Basil M., ed. *Lowering Cholesterol in High-Risk Individuals and Populations*. New York: Marcel Dekker, 1995.

HYPERLIPIDEMIA

DISEASE/DISORDER

ANATOMY OR SYSTEM AFFECTED: Blood

SPECIALTIES AND RELATED FIELDS: Family practice, hematology, internal medicine, serology, vascular medicine

DEFINITION: The presence of abnormally large amounts of lipids (fats) in the blood.

CAUSES AND SYMPTOMS

Although elevated triglyceride levels have been implicated in clinical ischemic diseases, most investigators believe that cholesterol-rich lipids are a more significant risk factor. Although measurements of both cholesterol and triglyceride levels have been used to predict coronary disease, studies suggest that the determination of the alpha-lipoprotein/beta-lipoprotein ratio is a more reliable predictor. Because the alpha-lipoprotein has a higher density than the beta-lipoprotein, they are more often designated as high-density lipoprotein (HDL) and low-density lipoprotein (LDL), respectively. HDL is often referred to as "good cholesterol," and LDL is referred to as "bad cholesterol." The latter is implicated in the development of atherosclerosis.

Atherosclerosis is a disease that begins in the innermost lining of the arterial wall. Its lesions occur predominantly at arterial forks and branch openings, but they can also occur at sites where there is injury to the arterial lining. The initial lesion usually appears as fatty streaks or spots, which have been detected even at birth. With passing years, more of these lesions appear, and they may develop into elevated plaques that obstruct the flow of blood in the artery. The lesions are rich in cholesterol derived from beta-lipoproteins in the plasma. In addition to elevated blood lipids, other risk factors associated with atherosclerosis include hypertension, faulty arterial structure, obesity, smoking, and stress.

TREATMENT AND THERAPY

The treatment of hyperlipidemia involves both dietary and drug therapies. Although studies in nonhuman primates indicate that the reduction of hyperlipidemia results in decreased morbidity and mortality rates from arterial vascular disease, studies in humans are less conclusive. Initial treatment involves restricting the dietary intake of cholesterol and saturated fat. Drug therapy is instituted when further lowering of the serum lipids is desired. Among the drugs that have been used as antihyperlipidemic agents are lovastatin and its analogs, clofibrate and its analogs (particularly gemfibrozil), nicotinic acid, D-thyroxine, cholestyramine, probucol, and heparin. A simplified diagram of the endogenous biosynthesis and biotransformation of cholesterol is given below.

acetate ⟶ acetyl SCoA ⟶ HMGCoA ⟶ MVA ⟶
squalene ⟶ desmosterol ⟶ cholesterol ⟶ bile acids

Lovastatin blocks the synthesis of cholesterol by inhibiting the enzyme (HMGCoA reductase) that catalyzes the conversion of beta-hydroxy-beta-methyl glutaryl coenzyme A (HMGCoA) to mevalonic acid (MVA), the regulatory step in the biosynthesis of cholesterol. Both lovastatin and MVA are beta, delta-dihydroxy acids, but lovastatin has a much more lipophilic (fat-soluble) group attached to it. Clofibrate and gemfibrozil block the synthesis of cholesterol prior to the HMGCoA stage. For this reason, they are likely to inhibit triglyceride formation as well. Nicotinic acid inhibits the synthesis of acetyl coenzyme A (acetyl SCoA) and thus would be expected to block the synthesis of both cholesterol and the triglycerides. To be effective in lowering the serum level of lipids, nicotinic acid must be taken in large amounts, which often produces an unpleasant flushing sensation in the patient. A way to inhibit the synthesis of cholesterol at the post-MVA stages has also been sought. Agents such as triparanol, which inhibit biosynthesis near the end of the synthetic sequence, have been developed. Although they are effective in lowering serum cholesterol, they had to be withdrawn from clinical use because of their adverse side effects on the muscles and eyes. Moreover, the penultimate product in the biosynthesis of cholesterol proved to be atherogenic. Investigations are being conducted on the inhibition of cholesterol synthesis at both the immediate presqualene and immediate postsqualene stages. The effects of such inhibitors on the production of steroid hormones and ubiquinones, as well as on cholesterol and triglycerides, are expected to be of considerable interest.

D-thyroxine promotes the metabolism of cholesterol in the liver, transforming it into the more hydrophilic (water-soluble) bile acids, thereby facilitating its elimination from the body. An approach to reducing the serum level of cholesterol by a process involving the sequestering of the bile acids utilizes the resin cholestyramine as the sequestrant. The sequestered bile acids cannot be reabsorbed into the entero-hepatic system and are eliminated in the feces. Consequently, more cholesterol is oxidized to the bile acids, resulting in the reduction of the serum level of cholesterol. Unfortunately, a large quantity of cholestyramine is required. Sequestration of cholesterol with beta-sitosterol prevents both the absorption of dietary cholesterol and the reabsorption of endogenous cholesterol in the intestines. Here, too, a large quantity of the sequestrant needs to be administered.

Probucol is an antioxidant. Because, structurally, it is a sulfur analog of a hindered hydroquinone, it acts as a free radical scavenger. Evidence suggests that the antihyperlipidemic effect of probucol is attributable to its ability to inhibit the oxygenation of LDL. The oxygenated LDL is believed to be the atherogenic form of LDL. Heparin promotes the hydrolysis of triglycerides as it activates lipoprotein lipase, thereby reducing lipidemia. Because of its potent anticoagulant properties, however, its use in therapy must be closely monitored. Cholesterol that is present in atherosclerotic plaques is acylated, generally by the more saturated fatty acids. The enzyme catalyzing the acylation process is acyl-CoA cholesterol acyl transferase (ACAT). The development of regulators of ACAT and the desirability of reducing the dietary intake of saturated fatty acids are based on this rationale.

Cholesterol within the cell is able to inhibit further synthesis of cholesterol by a feedback mechanism. Cholesterol that is associated with LDL is transported into the hepatic cell by means of the LDL receptor on the surface of the cell. In individuals who are afflicted with familial hypercholesterolemia, an inherited disorder that causes death at an early age, the gene that is responsible for the production of the LDL receptor is either absent or defective. Studies in gene therapy have shown that transplant of the normal LDL receptor gene to such an individual results in a dramatic decrease in the level of the "bad cholesterol" in the serum. Cholesterol derivatives that are oxygenated at various positions have also been found to regulate the serum level of cholesterol by either inhibiting its synthesis or promoting its catabolism. More studies need to be done, however, in order to demonstrate their effectiveness in humans and to establish that they themselves do not induce atherosclerosis.

—Leland J. Chinn, Ph.D.

See also Arteriosclerosis; Blood and blood disorders; Cholesterol; Heart disease; Hypercholesterolemia; Hypertension; Metabolism; Obesity.

FOR FURTHER INFORMATION:

Ball, Madeleine, and Jim Mann. *Lipids and Heart Disease: A Guide for the Primary Care Team.* 2d ed. Oxford, England: Oxford University Press, 1994. Topics include the function of lipids, plasma lipids and coronary heart disease, atherosclerosis, and hyperlipidemia.

Farnier, Michel, and Jean Davignon. "Current and Future Treatment of Hyperlipidemia: The Role of Statins." *The American Journal of Cardiology* 82, no. 4B (August 27, 1998): 3J-10J. Hyperlipidemia is recognized as one of the major risk factors for the development of coronary artery disease and progression of the atherosclerotic lesions. Dietary therapy together with hypolipidemic drugs is central to the management of hyperlipidemia.

Haffner, Steven M. "Diabetes, Hyperlipidemia, and Coronary Artery Disease." *The American Journal of Cardiology* 83, no. 9B (May 13, 1999): 17F-21F. Type 2 diabetes is associated with a marked increase in the risk of coronary artery disease. Dyslipidemia is believed to be a major source of this increased risk.

Larsen, Scott D., and Charles H. Spilman. "New Potential Therapies for the Treatment of Atherosclerosis." *Annual Reports in Medicinal Chemistry* 28 (1993): 217.

Rifkind, Basil M., ed. *Drug Treatment of Hyperlipidemia.* New York: Marcel Dekker, 1991. Discusses such topics as hyperlipoproteinemia and antilipemic agents. Includes bibliographical references and an index.

Safeer, Richard S., and Cynthia L. Lacivita. "Choosing Drug Therapy for Patients with Hyperlipidemia." *American Family Physician* 61, no. 11 (June 1, 2000): 3371-3382. Almost thirteen million American adults require drug therapy to meet the low-density lipoprotein goals set by the National Cholesterol Education Program.

Witiak, D. T., H. A. I. Newman, and D. R. Feller, eds. *Antilipidemic Drugs: Medicinal, Chemical, and Biochemical Aspects.* Amsterdam: Elsevier, 1991. Discusses such topics as antilipemic agents, lipids, and lipoproteins. Includes bibliographical references.

HYPERPARATHYROIDISM AND HYPOPARATHYROIDISM

DISEASE/DISORDER

ANATOMY OR SYSTEM AFFECTED: Endocrine system, glands, musculoskeletal system, neck

Hyperparathyroidism

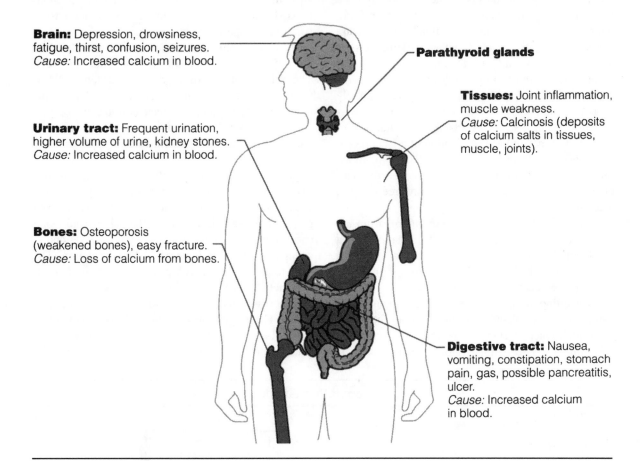

Brain: Depression, drowsiness, fatigue, thirst, confusion, seizures. *Cause:* Increased calcium in blood.

Parathyroid glands

Tissues: Joint inflammation, muscle weakness. *Cause:* Calcinosis (deposits of calcium salts in tissues, muscle, joints).

Urinary tract: Frequent urination, higher volume of urine, kidney stones. *Cause:* Increased calcium in blood.

Bones: Osteoporosis (weakened bones), easy fracture. *Cause:* Loss of calcium from bones.

Digestive tract: Nausea, vomiting, constipation, stomach pain, gas, possible pancreatitis, ulcer. *Cause:* Increased calcium in blood.

SPECIALTIES AND RELATED FIELDS: Endocrinology

DEFINITION: Excessive, uncontrolled secretion (hyperparathyroidism) or reduced secretion (hypoparathyroidism) of parathyroid hormone.

CAUSES AND SYMPTOMS

The precise regulation of calcium is vital to the survival and well-being of all animals. Approximately 99 percent of the calcium in the body is found in bones and teeth. Of the remaining 1 percent, about 0.9 percent is packaged within specialized organelles inside the cell. This leaves only 0.1 percent of the total body calcium in blood. Approximately half of this calcium is either bound to proteins or complexed with phosphate. The other half of blood calcium is free to be utilized by cells. For this reason, it is critical that calcium inside the cell be rigorously maintained at extremely low concentrations. Even a slight change in calcium outside the cell can have dramatic consequences.

The function and regulation of calcium. Calcium plays a vital role in many different areas of the body. For example, the entry of calcium into secretory cells, such as nerve cells, triggers the release of neurotransmitters into the synapse. A fall in blood calcium results in the overexcitability of nerves, which can be felt as a tingling sensation and numbness in the extremities. Similarly, calcium entry into cells is essential for muscle contraction in both heart and skeletal muscle.

Free calcium is thus one of the most tightly regulated substances in the body. The key player in the moment-to-moment regulation of calcium is parathyroid hormone (PTH). PTH is synthesized in the parathyroid glands, a paired gland located in the neck, and released in response to a fall in blood calcium.

PTH serves several functions: to increase blood calcium, to decrease blood phosphate, and to stimulate the conversion of vitamin D into its active form, which can then stimulate the uptake of calcium across the digestive tract. Together these actions result in an increase in free calcium, which returns calcium concentrations in the blood to normal.

PTH binds to specific receptors located primarily in bone and kidney tissue. Since most calcium is stored in bone, it serves as a bank for withdrawal of calcium in times of need. Activation of a PTH receptor on osteoclasts, or bone-cutting cells, results in the production of concentrated acids that dissolve calcium from bone, thereby making more free calcium available to the blood supply. PTH also acts on the kidney, where it stimulates calcium uptake from the urine while promoting phosphate elimination. As a result, more calcium is made available to the blood and less phosphate is available to form complexes with the free calcium.

By exerting these effects on its target organs, PTH can restore low calcium concentrations in the blood to normal. Once calcium has returned to a particular set point, PTH secretion is slowed dramatically. If PTH release is not controlled, however, the imbalance in calcium can lead to life-threatening situations. These conditions are termed hyperparathyroidism and hypoparathyroidism.

Hyperparathyroidism. This disorder is defined as the excessive and uncontrolled secretion of PTH. The release of a closely related substance, PTH-related protein, from cancer cells can also cause this condition. Hyperparathyroidism is found in 0.1 percent of the population and is more common in the elderly, who have an incident rate of approximately 2 percent.

There are two types of hyperparathyroidism, primary and secondary. Primary hyperparathyroidism is caused by disease or damage to the parathyroid glands. For example, cancer of the parathyroid gland can result in the uncontrolled release of PTH and is characterized by an increase in blood calcium. The symptoms associated with primary hyperparathyroidism include osteoporosis, muscle weakness, nausea, and increased incidence of kidney stones and peptic ulcers. These symptoms can all be linked to the presence of excess calcium, which is a result of the oversecretion of PTH.

Hypoparathyroidism

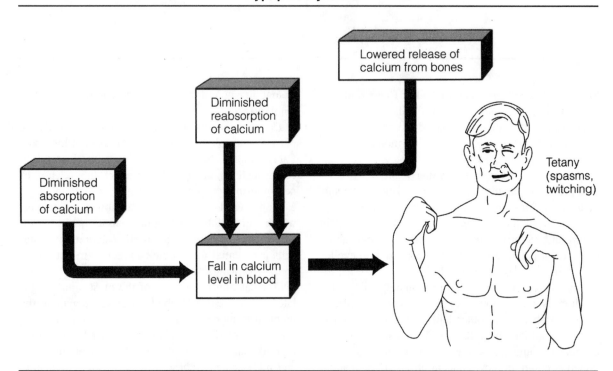

Secondary hyperparathyroidism often results when PTH cannot function normally, such as in kidney failure or insensitivity of target tissues to PTH. Secondary hyperparathyroidism is usually characterized by an overall decrease in blood calcium levels, even though there is a marked increase in the amount of PTH being released. Its symptoms may include muscle cramps, seizures, paranoia, depression, and, in severe cases, tetany (the tonic spasm of muscles). These symptoms are a direct result of the decline in available calcium.

Hypoparathyroidism. Less common than hyperparathyroidism, hypoparathyroidism is defined by a reduction in the secretion of PTH. This condition is normally characterized by low calcium levels and elevated phosphate levels in response to the lack of PTH. Not only are calcium levels unusually low, but phosphate levels are unusually high as well, which complicates this condition because phosphate ties up some of the free calcium.

Hypoparathyroidism can also have primary and secondary causes. Primary hypoparathyroidism is known to have two separate origins. The most common is a decrease in PTH release caused by accidental removal of the parathyroid gland. The other is damage of the blood supply around the parathyroid glands. Both occur after there has been some type of surgery or other medical procedure in the neck area. Consequently, the decline in PTH results in low calcium and elevated phosphate concentrations.

Secondary hypoparathyroidism is a frequent complication of cirrhosis and is characterized by a decrease in both calcium and magnesium concentration. Because magnesium is essential for the release of PTH, this condition can be corrected with magnesium replacement.

Complications associated with all types of hypoparathyroidism include hyperventilation, convulsions, and in some cases tetany of the muscle cells.

TREATMENT AND THERAPY

The treatments for primary hyperparathyroidism vary and are dependent on the severity of the condition. Specific drugs can be prescribed that lower elevated blood calcium. Hormone therapy, which includes the administration of estrogen, also acts to restore calcium to normal. Other treatments include dietary calcium restriction and/or surgery to remove the abnormal parathyroid tissue.

Treatment of secondary hyperparathyroidism often involves correcting the problems associated with kidney failure. This can be done by administration of a dietary calcium supplement to restore plasma calcium levels or, in more severe cases, by kidney transplantation. Vitamin D therapy has also been attempted for those patients diagnosed in the early stages of renal failure.

Hypoparathyroidism is usually treated with dietary calcium and vitamin D supplementation. Both of these treatments promote calcium absorption and decrease calcium loss. The duration of the treatment depends on the severity of the condition and may last a lifetime.

—*Jeffrey A. McGowan and Hillar Klandorf, Ph.D.*

See also Endocrine disorders; Endocrinology; Endocrinology, pediatric; Glands; Hormones; Osteoporosis; Stones; Vitamins and minerals.

FOR FURTHER INFORMATION:

Al Zarani, Ali, and Michael A. Levine. "Primary Hyperparathyroidism." *The Lancet* 349, no. 9060 (April 26, 1997): 1233-1238. The authors discuss primary hyperparathyroidism (PHP), a common endocrine disorder characterized by excessive secretion of parathyroid hormone and consequent hypercalcaemia.

Burch, Warner M. *Endocrinology.* 3d ed. Baltimore: Williams & Wilkins, 1994. A handbook of endocrine diseases designed for the house officer. Includes bibliographical references and an index.

Gardner, David, and Francis Greenspan. *Basic and Clinical Endocrinology.* East Norwalk, Conn.: Appleton & Lange, 2000. This resource superbly reviews contributions of molecular biology to endocrinology and the practical implications of these advances. Each chapter includes advances in molecular biology and the diagnosis and management of the various syndromes.

Neal, J. Matthew. *Basic Endocrinology: An Interactive Approach.* Oxford, England: Blackwell Science, 1999. Meant to supplement existing textbooks, this guide to the basic clinical principles and physiology of clinical endocrinology is for medical students, residents, and others needing a review of clinical endocrinology.

HYPERTENSION

DISEASE/DISORDER

ANATOMY OR SYSTEM AFFECTED: Blood vessels, brain, circulatory system, heart, kidneys, urinary system

SPECIALTIES AND RELATED FIELDS: Cardiology, family practice, internal medicine

DEFINITION: An abnormally high blood pressure, an often silent cardiovascular condition that may lead to heart attack, stroke, and major organ failures.

KEY TERMS:

cardiovascular: of, relating to, or involving the heart and blood vessels

cerebrovascular: of, or involving, the cerebrum (brain) and the blood vessels supplying it

diastolic blood pressure: the pressure of the blood within the artery while the heart is at rest

hypertension: abnormally high blood pressure, especially high arterial blood pressure; also the systemic condition accompanying high blood pressure

peripheral vascular: of, relating to, involving, or forming the vasculature in the periphery (the external boundary or surface of a body); usually referring to circulation not involving cardiovascular, cerebrovascular, or major organ systems

side effect: a secondary and usually adverse effect (as of a drug); also known as an adverse effect or reaction

sphygmomanometer: a device that uses a column of mercury to measure blood pressure force; pressure is measured in millimeters of mercury

systolic blood pressure: the pressure of the blood within the artery while the heart is contracting

CAUSES AND SYMPTOMS

Hypertension is a higher-than-normal blood pressure (either systolic or diastolic). Blood pressure is usually measured using a sphygmomanometer and a stethoscope. The stethoscope is used to hear when the air pressure within the cuff of the sphygmomanometer is equal to that in the artery. When taking a blood pressure, the cuff is pumped to inflate an air bladder secured around the arm; the pressure produced will collapse the blood vessels within. As cuff pressure decreases, a slight thump is heard as the artery snaps open to allow blood to flow. At this point, the cuff pressure equals the systolic blood pressure. As the cuff pressure continues to fall, the sound of blood being pumped will continue but become progressively softer. At the point where the last sound is heard, the cuff pressure equals the diastolic blood pressure.

In hypertension, both systolic and diastolic blood pressures are usually elevated. Blood pressures are reported as the systolic pressure over the diastolic

pressure, such as 130/80 millimeters of mercury. It is important to recognize there are degrees of seriousness for hypertension. The higher the blood pressure, the more rigorous the treatment may be. When systolic pressures are in the high normal range, the individual should be closely monitored with annual blood pressure checks. Persistently high blood pressures (greater than 140-159/90-99 millimeters of mercury) require closer monitoring and may result in a decision to treat the condition with medication or other types of intervention.

The blood pressure in an artery is determined by the relationship among three important controlling factors: the blood volume, the amount of blood pumped by the heart (cardiac output), and the contraction of smooth muscle within blood vessels (arterial tone). To illustrate the first point, if blood volume decreases, the result will be a fall in blood pressure. Conversely, the body cannot itself increase blood pressure by rapidly adding blood volume; fluid must be injected into the circulation to do so.

A second controlling factor of blood pressure is cardiac output (the volume of blood pumped by the heart in a given unit of time, usually reported as liters per minute). This output is determined by two factors: stroke volume (the volume of blood pumped with each heartbeat) and the heart rate (beats per

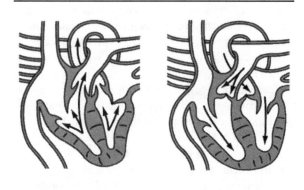

Blood Pressure

Systolic   Diastolic

Blood pressure is measured in two numbers: systolic pressure (the pressure of the blood as it flows out when the heart contracts) over diastolic pressure (the pressure of the blood within the artery as it flows in when the heart is at rest). Readings greater than 140 systolic over 90 diastolic indicate the presence of hypertension.

Blood Pressure and Hypertension	
Status	*Systolic/Diastolic*
Normal (maximum)	130/85
High normal	131-139/86-89
Stage I hypertension (mild)	140-159/90-99
Stage II (moderate)	160-179/100-109
Stage III (severe)	180-209/110-119
Stage IV (very severe)	210/120+

minute). As heart rate increases, output generally increases and blood pressure may rise as well. If blood volume is low, such as with excessive bleeding, the blood returning to the heart per beat is lower and could lead to decreased output. To compensate, the heart rate increases to prevent a drop in blood pressure. Therefore, as cardiac output changes, blood pressure does not necessarily change.

Last, a major controlling factor of blood pressure is arterial tone. Arteries are largely tubular, smooth muscles that can change their diameter based on the extent of contraction (tone). This contraction is largely under the control of a specialized branch of the nervous system called the sympathetic nervous system. An artery with high arterial tone (contracted) will squeeze the blood within and increase the pressure inside. There is also a relaxation phase that will allow expansion and a decrease in blood pressure. Along with relaxation, arteries are elastic to allow some stretching, which may further help reduce pressure or, more important, help prevent blood pressure from rising.

There are two general types of hypertension: essential and secondary. Secondary hypertension is attributable to some underlying identifiable cause, such as a tumor or kidney disease, while essential hypertension has no identifiable cause. Therefore, essential hypertension is a defect that results in excessive arterial pressure secondary to poor regulation by any one of the three controlling factors discussed above. Each factor can serve as a focal point for treatment with medications.

The negative consequences of hypertension are mainly manifested in the deteriorating effect that this condition has on coronary heart disease (CHD). Cardiovascular risk factors for CHD are described as two types, unmodifiable and modifiable. Unmodifiable risk factors cannot be changed. This group includes gender, race, advanced age, and a family history of heart disease (hypertensive traits can be inherited). The modifiable risk factors are cigarette smoking (or other forms of tobacco abuse), high blood cholesterol levels, control over diabetes, and perhaps other factors not yet discovered. For example, additional factors are now recognized for their adverse effects on hypertension, including obesity, a lack of physical activity, and psychological factors.

There is no definitive blood pressure level at which a person is no longer at risk for CHD. While any elevation above the normal range places the person at increased risk for CHD, what are considered high normal blood pressures were previously defined as normal. (Looking back at older data, researchers noted that persons able to maintain pressures at or below 139/89 millimeters of mercury had less severe CHD.) The definition of "normal" blood pressure may change again in the future as new information is discovered. There is a practical limit as to how low pressure can be while maintaining day-to-day function.

In coronary heart disease, the blood supply to the heart is reduced and the heart cannot function well. The common term for arteriosclerosis, "hardening of the arteries," indicates the symptom of reduced blood flow, which is a major component of CHD. When the heart cannot supply itself with the necessary amount of blood (a condition known as ischemia), a characteristic chest pain called angina may be produced. The hardening aspect of this disease is the result of cholesterol deposits in the vessel, which decrease elasticity and make the vessel wall stiff. This stiffness will force pressures in the vessel to increase if cardiac output rises. As pressures advance, the vessel may develop weak spots. These areas may rupture or lead to the development of small blood clots that may clog the vessel; either problem will disrupt blood flow, making the underlying CHD worse. Eventually, if the blood supply is significantly reduced, a myocardial infarction (heart attack) may occur. Where the blood supply to the heart muscle itself is functionally blocked, that part of the heart will die.

Besides contributing to an increased risk of heart attack and coronary heart disease, hypertension is a major risk for other vascular problems, such as stroke, kidney failure, heart failure, and visual disturbances secondary to the effects on the blood vessels within the eye. Hypertension is a major source of premature death in the United States and by all estimates affects more than sixty million Americans. Forty percent of all African Americans and more than half of those over the age of sixty are affected. Public awareness of hypertension is increasing, yet less than half of all patients diagnosed are treated. More important, only one in five identified hypertensives have the condition under control. This lack of control is particularly important when one considers the organs influenced by hypertension, most notably the brain, eyes, kidneys, and heart.

Although causative factors of hypertension cannot be identified, many physiological factors contribute to hypertension. They include increased sympathetic nervous activity (part of the autonomic nervous system), which promotes arterial contraction; overproduction of an unidentified sodium-retaining hormone or chronic high sodium intake; inadequate dietary intake of potassium or calcium; an increased or inappropriate secretion of renin, a chemical made by the kidney; deficiencies of arterial dilators, such as prostaglandins; congenital abnormalities (birth defects) of resistance vessels; diabetes mellitus or resistance to the effects of insulin; obesity; increased activity of vascular growth factors; and altered cellular ion transport of electrolytes, such as potassium, sodium, chloride, and bicarbonate.

The kidneys are greatly responsible for blood pressure control. They have a key role in maintaining both blood volume and blood pressure. When kidney function declines, secondary to problems such as a decrease in renal blood flow, the kidney will release renin. High renin levels result in activation of the renin-angiotensin-aldosterone system. The resulting chemical cascade produces angiotensin II, a potent arterial constrictor. Another chemical released is aldosterone, an adrenal hormone which causes the kidney to retain water and sodium. These two actions add to blood volume and increase arterial tone, resulting in higher blood pressure. Normally, the renin-angiotensin-aldosterone system protects kidney function by raising blood pressure when it is low. In hypertensives, the controlling forces seem to be out of balance, so that the system does not respond appropriately. The renin-angiotensin-aldosterone system has a negative effect on bradykinin, a chemical which protects renal function by producing vasodilating prostaglandins that help maintain adequate

renal blood flow. This protection is especially important in elderly individuals, who may depend on this system to maintain renal function. The system can be inhibited by medications such as aspirin or ibuprofen, resulting in a recurrence of hypertension or less control over the existing disease.

Arteries are largely smooth muscles under the control of the autonomic nervous system, which is responsible for organ function. Yet there is often no conscious control of organs; for example, one can "tell" the lungs to take a breath, but one cannot "tell" the heart to beat. The autonomic nervous system has two branches, sympathetic and parasympathetic, that essentially work against each other. The sympathetic system exerts much control over blood pressure. Many chemicals and medicines, such as caffeine, decongestants, and amphetamines, affect blood pressure by mimicking the effects of increased sympathetic stimulation of arteries.

Numerous factors associated with blood pressure elevations will affect one or more of the key determinants of blood pressure; they affect one another as well. An example will show the extent of their relationship. Sodium and water retention will increase blood volume returning to the heart. As this return increases, the heart will increase output (to a point) to prevent heart failure. This higher cardiac output may also raise blood pressure. If arterial vessels are constricted, pressures may be even higher. This elevated pressure (resistance) will force the heart to try to increase output to maintain blood flow to vital organs. Thus, a vicious cycle is started; hypertension can be perceived as a merry-go-round ride with no exit.

TREATMENT AND THERAPY

Blood pressure reduction has a protective effect against cardiovascular disease. Generally, as blood pressure decreases, arteries are less contracted and are able to deliver more blood to the tissues, maintaining their function. Further, this decreased blood pressure will help reduce the risk of heart attack in the patient with heart disease. With lower pressures, the heart does not need to work as hard supplying blood to itself or the rest of the body. Therefore, the demand for cardiac output to supply blood flow is less. This reduced workload lowers the incidence of angina.

Treatment of hypertensive patients may involve using one to four different medications to achieve the goal of blood pressure reduction. There are many types of medications from which to choose: diuretics, sympatholytic agents (also known as antiadrenergic drugs), beta-blockers (along with one combined-action alpha-beta blocker), calcium-channel blockers, peripheral vasodilators, angiotensin-converting enzyme inhibitors, and the newest class, angiotension receptor inhibitors. The list of available drugs is extensive; for example, there are fourteen different thiazide-type diuretics and another six diuretics with different mechanisms of action. So many choices may present the physician with a confusing set of alternatives.

Patients prone to sodium and water retention are treated with diuretics, agents that prevent the kidney from reabsorbing sodium and water from the urine. Diuretics are usually added to other medications to enhance those medications' activity. Research into thiazide-type diuretics has shown that these agents possess mild calcium-channel blocking activity, aiding their ability to reduce hypertension.

Beta-blocking agents are used less often than when they were first developed. They work by decreasing cardiac output through reducing the heart rate. Although they are highly effective, the heart rate reduction tends to produce side effects. Most commonly, patients complain of fatigue, sleepiness, and reduced exercise tolerance (the heart rate cannot increase to adapt to the increasing demand for blood in tissues and the heart itself). These agents are still a good choice for hypertensive patients who have suffered a heart attack. Their benefit is that they reduce the risk of a second heart attack by preventing the heart from overworking.

Calcium-channel blockers were originally intended to treat angina. These agents act primarily by decreasing arterial smooth muscle contraction. Relaxed coronary blood vessels can carry more blood, helping prevent the pain of angina. When calcium ions enter the smooth muscle, a more sustained contraction is produced; therefore, blocking this effect will produce relaxation. Physicians noted that this relaxation also produced lower blood pressures. The distinct advantage to these agents is that they are well tolerated; however, some patients may require increasing their fiber intake to prevent some constipating effects.

Peripheral vasodilators have been a disappointment. Theoretically, they should be ideal since they work directly to cause arterial dilation. Unfortunately, blood pressure has many determinants and patients seem to become "immune" to direct vasodilator effects. Peripheral vasodilators are useful, however, when added to other treatments such as beta-blockers or sympatholytic medications.

The sympatholytic agents are divided into two broad categories. The first group works within the brain to decrease the effects of nerves that would send signals to blood vessels to constrict (so-called constrict messages). They do this by increasing the relax signals coming out of the brain to offset the constrict messages. The net effect is that blood vessels dilate, reducing blood pressure. Many of these agents have fallen into disfavor because of adverse effects similar to those of beta-blockers. The second group of sympatholytics works directly at the nerve-muscle connection. These agents block the constrict messages of the nerve that would increase arterial smooth muscle tone. Overall, these agents are well tolerated. Some patients, especially the elderly, may be very susceptible to their effect and have problems with low blood pressure; this issue usually resolves itself shortly after the first dose.

The renin-angiotensin-aldosterone system is a key determinant of blood pressure. Angiotensin-converting enzyme inhibitors (ACE inhibitors) work by blocking angiotensin II and aldosterone and by preserving bradykinin. They have been found quite effective for reducing blood pressure and are usually well tolerated. Some patients will experience a first-dose effect, while others may develop a dry cough that can be corrected by dose reductions or discontinuation of the medication. The angiotension receptor inhibitors work, instead, by blocking the effects of this substance on the target cells of the arteries themselves. They are proving to be excellent substitutes for people who cannot tolerate the related class of ACE inhibitors.

Unfortunately, and contrary to popular belief, no one can reliably tell when his or her own blood pressure is elevated. Consequently, hypertension is called a "silent killer." It is extremely important to have regular blood pressure evaluations and, if diagnosed with hypertension, to receive treatment.

From 1950 through 1987, as advances in understanding and treating hypertension were made, the United States population enjoyed a 40 percent reduction in coronary heart disease and a more than 65 percent reduction in stroke deaths. (By comparison, noncardiovascular deaths during the same period were reduced little more than 20 percent.)

It is evident that blood pressure can be reduced without medications. Research in the 1980's led to a nonpharmacologic approach in the initial management of hypertension. This strategy includes weight reduction, alcohol restriction, regular exercise, dietary sodium restriction, dietary potassium and calcium supplementation, stopping of tobacco use (in any form), and caffeine restriction. Often, these methods can produce benefits without medication being prescribed. Using this approach, medication is added to the therapy if blood pressure remains elevated despite good efforts at nonpharmacologic control.

Other aspects of hypertension and hypertensive patients have been identified to help guide the clinician to the proper choice of medication. With this approach, the clinician can focus therapy at the most likely cause of the hypertension: sodium and water retention, high cardiac output, or high vascular resistance. This pathophysiological approach led to the abandonment of the rigid step-care approach described in many texts covering hypertension. The pathophysiological approach to hypertension management is based on a series of steps that are taken if inadequate responses are seen (see figure).

Hypertension Management

Nonpharmacologic therapy
↓
(inadequate response)
↓
Continue nonpharmacologic therapy
with medication
↓
(inadequate response)
↓
Increase dose
or   change medication
or add second medication
↓
(inadequate response)
↓
Add second or third medication
↓
(inadequate response)
↓
Add a diuretic
if not already prescribed

By far, the best strategy for controlling hypertension is to be informed. Each person needs to be aware of his or her personal risk for developing hypertension. One should have regular blood pressure evaluations, avoid eating excessive salt and sodium, increase exercise, and reduce fats in the diet. Maintaining ideal body weight may be a key control factor. Studies have shown that patients who have been successful at losing weight will require less stringent treatment. The benefits could be a need for fewer medications, reduced doses of medications, or both.

—*Charles C. Marsh, Pharm.D.;*
updated by Connie Rizzo, M.D.

See also Angina; Arteriosclerosis; Cardiology; Cholesterol; Circulation; Claudication; Embolism; Heart; Heart attack; Heart disease; Hyperadiposis; Hypercholesterolemia; Hyperlipidemia; Kidney disorders; Kidneys; Phlebitis; Physical examination; Strokes; Thrombolytic therapy and TPA; Thrombosis and thrombus; Vascular medicine; Vascular system.

FOR FURTHER INFORMATION:

Dorland, W. A. Newman. *Dorland's Illustrated Medical Dictionary.* 28th ed. Philadelphia: W. B. Saunders, 1994. A standard work for the explanation of medical terms. It is well illustrated and should help any reader gain more understanding of complex medical terms. Reviewing this reference is an educational experience in itself.

Messerli, Franz H., ed. *Cardiovascular Disease in the Elderly.* 3d ed. Boston: Kluwer Academic, 1993. An excellent book for detailed discussions regarding cardiovascular disease in older persons. Issues such as aging, multiple illnesses, and the social challenges seen in the elderly are discussed.

_____. *The Heart and Hypertension.* New York: Yorke Medical Books, 1987. An excellent reference work edited by one of the most distinguished clinicians and researchers in hypertension. This text's strength is its discussion of the pathophysiology of hypertension.

Seeley, Rod R., Trent D. Stephens, and Philip Tate. *Anatomy and Physiology.* St. Louis: Mosby Year Book, 2000. A well-illustrated, easy-to-read basic reference text for the general reader. The text's obvious strengths are its discussions of the heart, arteries, and veins and their roles in cardiovascular function.

Tierney, Lawrence M., Jr., et al., eds. *Current Medical Diagnosis and Treatment: 2001.* 39th ed. New

York: McGraw-Hill, 2000. This text, updated yearly, is the point of reference for physicians and other health care practitioners. It incorporates each year's biomedical research discoveries that have immediate, relevant, and applicable use for the patient.

HYPERTHERMIA AND HYPOTHERMIA
DISEASE/DISORDER

ANATOMY OR SYSTEM AFFECTED: All

SPECIALTIES AND RELATED FIELDS: Anesthesiology, critical care, emergency medicine, environmental health, internal medicine

DEFINITION: Hyperthermia is the elevation of the body core temperature of an organism, while hypothermia is a decrease in that temperature; both conditions are medical emergencies when not intentionally induced, and both can be useful when applied to surgical and treatment techniques.

KEY TERMS:

ambient temperature: the temperature of the surrounding environment

body temperature: the temperature that reflects the level of heat energy in an animal's body; a consequence of the balance between the heat produced by metabolism and the body's exchange of heat with the surrounding environment

frostbite: injury that results from exposure of skin to extreme cold, most commonly affecting the ears, nose, hands, and feet

hibernation: a condition of dormancy and torpor that occurs in poikilotherm vertebrates and invertebrates; as the environmental temperatures drop, the inner core temperature of such animals also drops to decrease the metabolic rate and physiological functions

homeotherms: animals, such as birds and mammals, that have the ability to maintain a high body core temperature despite large variations in environmental temperatures

hyperthermia: an abnormally elevated body temperature that leads to fever and muscle rigidity

hypothermia: an abnormally low body temperature that leads to drastic metabolic changes and eventual death

CAUSES AND SYMPTOMS

Body temperature reflects the level of heat energy in the body of an animal or human being. It is the consequence of the balance between the heat generated by metabolism and the body's heat exchange with the surrounding environment (ambient temperature). Generally, animal life can be sustained in the temperature range of 0 degrees Celsius (32 degrees Fahrenheit) to 45 degrees Celsius (113 degrees Fahrenheit), but appropriate processes can store animal tissues at much lower temperature. Homeotherms, such as birds and most mammals, have the ability to maintain their high body core temperature despite large variations in environmental temperatures. Poikilotherms have slow metabolic rates at rest and, as a result, difficulty in maintaining their inner core temperatures. Such a form of thermal regulation is called ectothermic ("outer heated") and is directly affected by the uptake of heat from the environment; such organisms are often termed cold-blooded. On the other hand, homeotherms are endothermic ("inner heated") and depend largely on their fast and controlled rates of heat production; such organisms are termed warm-blooded. Thus, the lizard, an example of ectotherm, maintains its body temperature by staying in or out of shade and by assuming a posture toward the sun that would maximize the adjustment for its body heat. At night, the lizard burrows, but its body temperature still drops considerably until the next morning, when it increases with the rising sun.

Body core temperatures vary considerably among mammals and birds. For example, the sparrow's inner core temperature is about 43.5 degrees Celsius (110.3 degrees Fahrenheit), the turkey's 41.2 degrees Celsius (106.2 degrees Fahrenheit), the cat's 36.4 degrees Celsius (97.5 degrees Fahrenheit), and the opossum's 34.7 degrees Celsius (94.5 degrees Fahrenheit). In humans, although the temperature of the inner organs varies by only 1 to 2 degrees Celsius (1.8 to 3.6 degrees Fahrenheit), the skin temperature may vary 10 to 20 degrees Celsius (18 to 36 degrees Fahrenheit) below the core temperature of 37 degrees Celsius (98.6 degrees Fahrenheit), depending on the ambient temperature. This is possible because the cells of the skin, muscles, and blood vessels are not as sensitive as are those of the vital organs.

An elevation in core temperature of homeotherms above the normal range is called hyperthermia, while a corresponding decrease is called hypothermia. Both can be brought about by extremes in the environment. Although the human body can withstand a lack of food for a number of weeks and that of water for several days, it cannot survive a lack of thermoregulation, which is the maintaining of the inner core temperature. The core temperature has to be kept within strict limits; otherwise, the brain and heart will be compromised and death will result. Clinically, the inner core temperature can be monitored by recording the temperature of the rectum, the eardrum, the mouth, and the esophagus. In elderly people, the body's ability to cope with extreme temperatures may be impaired. Exposure to even mildly cold temperatures may lead to accidental hypothermia that can be fatal if not detected and treated properly.

All animals produce heat by oxidation of substrates to carbon dioxide. On the average, about 75 percent of food energy is converted to heat during adenosine triphosphate (ATP) formation and its transfer to the functional systems of the cells. In defense against heat, sweating is the primary physiological mechanism in mammals. Dogs, cats, and other furred carnivores increase evaporative heat loss by panting, while small rodents spread saliva. Human beings have two to three million glands that can produce up to 23 liters of sweat per hour for a short period of time.

Fever may occur for at least four main reasons. Infection by microorganisms is the most familiar because of its large variety of causes. Such an infection may be bacterial (as with septicemia and abscesses), viral (in measles, mumps, and influenza), protozoal (in malaria), or spichaetal (in syphilis). Fever can also take place because of immunological conditions, such as drug allergies and incompatible blood transfusions. The last two reasons are malignancy, which can lead to Hodgkin's disease and leukemia, and noninfective inflammation, which results in gout and thrombophlebitis.

Antipyretics are medicines whose consumption results in the lowering of fever. The bark of trees provides antipyretics such as spiraeic acid and its derivatives (aspirin). The mechanism of action of the nonnarcotic antipyretics remains a subject of research. Two hypotheses are considered to justify the suppression of fever. One involves inhibition of the formation of arachidonic acid metabolites, which leads to the formation of pain-reducing substances. The other postulates that a modification of the physiological membrane properties takes place, with subsequent incorporation of drug molecules into the tertiary structure of proteins.

Temperature regulation involves the brain and spinal cord, which monitor the difference between the internal and peripheral (skin and muscle) temperature, with physiological and psychological adjustments to maintain a constant internal temperature. The brain records the various body temperatures via specialized nerve endings called thermal receptors. Heat transfer occurs between the skin surface and the environment via conduction (which takes place by means of physical contact) or convection (which occurs through the movement of air).

During cold weather, hikers and climbers are particularly at risk for hypothermia; in extreme cases, body functions are depressed to the extent that victims may be mistaken for dead. Injuries that result from skin exposure to extreme cold are described as frostbite. Frostbite most commonly affects outer organs such as the nose, ears, hands (especially the fingertips), and feet, which first turn unusually red and then unnaturally white. Early symptoms include feelings of coldness, tingling, pain, and numbness. Frostbite takes place when ice crystals form in the skin and (in the most serious cases) in the tissue beneath the skin. If not treated, frostbite may lead to gangrene, the medical term for tissue death. The freezing-thawing process causes mechanical disruption (from ice), intracellular and extracellular biochemical changes, and the disruption of the blood corpuscles. Frostbite treatment involves the use of warm water to restore blood circulation and heat to the affected body part.

There are several types of hypothermia. Immersion hypothermia occurs when a person falls into cold water. Any movement of the body leads to loss of heat, and the drastic temperature change may trigger a heart attack. Generally, a person can withstand immersion in water that is 10 degrees Celsius (50 degrees Fahrenheit) for about ten minutes before succumbing to death. Divers are equipped with wet suits to minimize heat loss, but they cool themselves rapidly when they move in cold water and, at the same time, breathe dry air mixtures. Submersion hypothermia is actual drowning in cold water. Although a person cannot last more than a few minutes without oxygen, drowning in cold water is more survivable than in water of other temperatures. As the cold water enters the lungs and bathes the skin, the body's metabolic rate decreases, which allows the individual (especially a child) up to forty-five minutes of oxygen debt before death occurs.

Clinical reports also indicate hypothermia in alcohol-intoxicated individuals. Shivering, which is common to people suffering from hypothermia, is a sequence of skeletal muscle contractions which lead to coordinated movements and produce a maximum amount of heat. Other conditions of heat loss that deteriorate the already hypothermic person include tight and wet clothing, injury causing hemorrhage, fatigue, and even psychosis.

TREATMENT AND THERAPY

Nature protects poikilotherm vertebrates and invertebrates in winter by means of hibernation. Hibernation, which is a condition of dormancy and torpor, occurs when the body temperatures of such animals drop in repsonse to a decrease in environmental temperatures. Animals such as bears, raccoons, badgers, and some birds become drowsy in winter because ambient temperature drops of a few degrees considerably decrease their metabolic rates and physiological functions. For example, the body temperature of a bear is 35.5 degrees Celsius (96 degrees Fahrenheit) at an air temperature of 4.4 degrees Celsius (40 degrees Fahrenheit) and only 31.2 degrees Celsius (88 degrees Fahrenheit) at an air temperature of 31.2 degrees Celsius (25 degrees Fahrenheit).

In humans, however, a significant decrease in body temperature is always a medical emergency requiring immediate attention. The treatment for mild cases of hypothermia may consist only of covering the head and offering the victim a warm drink. More serious cases may involve immersing the victim in a warm bath. Severe hypothermia requires hospitalization in an intensive care unit, where the body temperature is returned to normal by placing the patient under special heat-reflecting blankets, by injecting warm fluid into the abdominal cavity, or by bypassing the circulating blood through a machine to heat it.

Hyperthermia is often termed heat stroke, while mild elevations in temperature can produce heat exhaustion. Heat stroke is a serious condition treated with emergency procedures. The victim is wrapped naked in a cold, wet sheet or blanket or sponged with cold water and fanned constantly. Salt tablets or a weak salt solution is given to conscious patients.

Both hyperthermia and hypothermia can be used medically. Although cancer treatment consists primarily of radiation therapy, surgery, and chemotherapy, experimental approaches include immunotherapy and hyperthermia. In the latter case, heat is used to destroy cancer cells. In all cases, except surgery, the tumor cells have to be killed in situ, meaning that their reproductive ability has to be inhibited without affecting irreversibly the normal tissues.

First Aid for Hypothermia

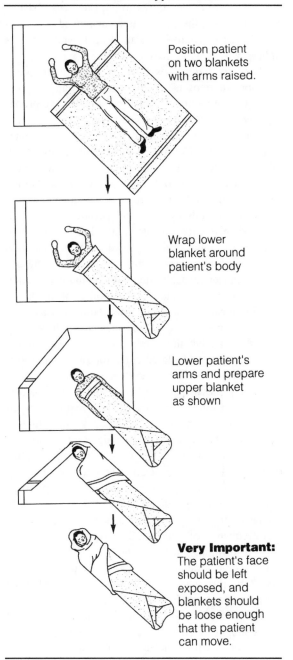

Position patient on two blankets with arms raised.

Wrap lower blanket around patient's body

Lower patient's arms and prepare upper blanket as shown

Very Important: The patient's face should be left exposed, and blankets should be loose enough that the patient can move.

A study of cell exposure to high temperatures has demonstrated that the circulation of blood decreased as temperature treatment at 42.5 degrees Celsius continued. The electron microscope showed that after about three hours, a vascular collapse (seen as cloudiness) took place in most of the located vessels. At

1172 • Hyperthermia and hypothermia

that point, the high-temperature treatment ended and the cells were cooled down to 33.5 degrees Celsius. Two days later, the central areas displayed an extensive degree of necrosis (tissue death), while the periphery was largely unaffected.

There are indications that malignant tumor cells are more thermosensitive than the surrounding normal cells from which the malignant cells have probably developed. Although some scientists believe that brain neurons are damaged by temperature greater then 42 degrees Celsius, in most cases neurons can tolerate temperatures in the range of 42.5 to 43 degrees Celsius for up to thirty minutes. Chemotherapy has been found to be much more potent upon exposure of the tumor cells to higher temperatures. Although the mechanisms responsible are not fully understood, there are several possible explanations. Some scientists believe that hyperthermia may increase the drug uptake by cancer cells, alter the intracellular distribution of the drug, or even alter the metabolism of the drug.

In brain cancer patients, it was common practice to induce brain hyperthermia by means of whole body hyperthermia, but this method has been substituted by several others. Isolated perfusion of the appropriate artery and vein has produced excellent results. Radiofrequency capacitive heating (in which paddle-shaped transmitters are placed next to the exposed brain) and interstitial radiofrequency (in which a gold-plated brass electrode provides tumor temperatures of 44 degrees Celsius while holding the surroundings at 42 degrees Celsius) are also extensively used. Microwave hyperthermia, magnetic loop induction, and ferromagnetic seeds (which are surgically implanted into the tumor and later heated by external radiofrequency of 300 to 3,000 megahertz) are also applied to brain cancer patients.

Ultrasonic irradiation, which uses a thin, stainless steel tube to induce hyperthermia, is believed to be the promising technique of the future. The heat generated by the energy produced improves the local blood supply by dilating the blood vessels. This dilation, together with an acceleration of enzyme activity, helps cells to obtain fresh nutrients and, at the same time, rid themselves of waste products. The other advantage of ultrasonic irradiation is the vibrations that it creates. In a hardened and calcified brain tumor, for example, these vibrations can crush the tumor, which can then be removed via vacuum.

Hypothermia began to be used extensively in modern surgery in the 1970's and 1980's. In certain operations, the patient's body temperature is lowered by wrapping the already anesthetized patient in a rubber blanket that contains coils through which cold water is circulated. When the temperature is sufficiently low, as determined by an electrical rectal thermometer, general anesthesia is discontinued. As a result, much less bleeding occurs in both brain and heart surgery. Under conditions of hypothermia, breathing is slower and shallower, and the brain requirements for blood and oxygen are drastically reduced. This situation allows an intentional stoppage of the heart for prolonged periods of time in order to complete the surgical repairs of that organ.

There is a point, however, below which the human body temperature cannot be lowered. In cold-blooded animals, the loading and unloading of oxygen can be carried out adequately only within a certain temperature range; thus an octopus's blood becomes fully saturated with oxygen at 0 degrees Celsius but little oxygen is unloaded by hemoglobin, which results in the animal's oxygen starvation. In humans, little oxygen is delivered to the tissues at 20 degrees Celsius, which sets a natural limit to the possibility of lowering body temperature during surgical procedures. The lack of dissociation of oxyhemoglobin at low temperature accounts for the red color of ears and noses on cold days.

PERSPECTIVE AND PROSPECTS

Both hypothermia and hyperthermia have had a commanding role in medicine. An Egyptian papyrus roll which can be dated back to 3000 B.C.E. describes the treatment of a breast tumor with hyperthermia. Heat has been used as a therapeutic agent since the days of Hippocrates (c. 460-c. 370 B.C.E.), who stated that a patient who could not be cured by heat was actually incurable. In the seventeenth century, the Japanese performed hyperthermia to treat syphilis, arthritis, and gout, using hot water to increase the body temperature to about 39 degrees Celsius.

The medical use of hyperthermia owes much of its modern-era development to Georges Lakhovsky (1880-1942), a Russian Jew who had a brilliant physics background and did most of his work in Paris, France. Although he is not generally given the credit for it, he was the first person to design and build a "short wave diathermy" machine, which created artificial fever for the first time in 1923. His work was done primarily on patients with malignant tumors at the Hospital de la Salpetriere and the Hospital Saint-

Louis. The first machine that he developed used frequencies from 0.75 megahertz to 3,000 megahertz, a range very much in use in today's clinical hyperthermia. In 1931, he started using a new machine that emitted radio waves of multiple wavelengths. He had partial success with his treatment, as reported to the Pasteur Institute and the French Academy of Sciences. Other scientists in this field include the German physicians W. Busch and P. Bruns, who applied it to erysipelas infection in 1886, and the Swedish gynecologist N. Westermark, who applied it with partial success to nonoperable carcinomas of the cervix uteri in 1898. The combination of hyperthermia and immunotherapy was applied by William B. Coley, a New York surgeon who managed to cause complete regression of malignant melanoma in patients by inducing artificial fever created by inoculation of infected erysipelas cells.

The application of hyperthermia to serious cases of cancer will take a gigantic leap once it is firmly established that the cancer cells have a greater thermosensitivity than normal cells. At this time, it is generally used in combination with surgery and radiation. Hyperthermia is applied to the cancer cells left behind following surgery, and it can kill those cells that tend to be radioresistant. Unlike radiation, hyperthermia has no known cumulative toxicity, and it can be safely reapplied to recurrent lesions. Ultrasound-induced hyperthermia has produced encouraging results, and it is hoped to be as useful as ultrasound is to the removal of kidney stones.

The application of hyperthermia in cases of acquired immunodeficiency syndrome (AIDS) has not yet provided decisively positive results. The process has involved circulating the patient's blood through a chamber heated to approximately 10 degrees Fahrenheit higher than the body temperature. Although the AIDS virus is killed, many of the patients' other enzymes are found to lose their activity. Consequently, United States health officials have opposed and criticized blood-heating therapy for this disease until more convincing results are produced.

The role of hyperthermia in treating metastatic cancer, in combination with radiation and drugs that are heat and radiation cell sensitizers, is increasing. This technique has been made feasible by the technological advancements in deep-heating machines, such as the Magnetrode and the BSO annular array, which allow the sequential regional hyperthermia of large body regions such as the thorax and the abdomen.

Hypothermic brain operations have the great advantage of reduced swelling. As a result, during the surgery the brain rarely bulges out of the opening in the skull, which is not the case when the operation is performed at room temperature. This advantage has led to reduced hospital stays and faster recovery times. The requirements of the tissues for oxygen and the rate at which they produce waste products fall as temperature drops.

—*Soraya Ghayourmanesh, Ph.D.*

See also Anesthesia; Anesthesiology; Critical care; Critical care, pediatric; Emergency medicine; Fever; Frostbite; Gangrene; Heat exhaustion and heat stroke; Surgery, general.

FOR FURTHER INFORMATION:

Ballester, J. Michael, and Fred P. Harchelroad. "Hyperthermia: How to Recognize and Prevent Heat-Related Illness." *Geriatrics* 54, no. 7 (July, 1999): 20-24. Older patients are predisposed to heat illness secondary to factors such as impaired thermoregulation, reduced sweating response to thermal stress, cardiovascular disease, diabetes, medications, and impaired mobility.

Bicher, Haim I., J. R. McLaren, and G. M. Pigliucci, eds. *Consensus on Hyperthermia for the 1990s*. New York: Plenum Press, 1989. A series of research papers presented at the Twelfth International Symposium on Clinical Hyperthermia in Rome in 1989. Topics include the clinical use and instrumentation for hyperthermia types (including ultrasound) and applications in liver, brain, and ovarian cancer.

Bloomfield, Molly M. *Chemistry and the Living Organism*. 6th ed. New York: John Wiley & Sons, 1996. An excellent allied health text. Perspective 9-2 discusses hypothermia and death.

Gautherie, Michel, ed. *Biological Basis of Oncologic Thermotherapy*. Berlin: Springer-Verlag, 1990. An advanced treatise on cancer thermotherapy that discusses heat transfer to tissues, types of hyperthermia treatment, mechanisms of heat and radiosensitization action in the killing of cells, and temperature distribution in tumors.

Gierach, John. "The Life Threatening Cold: Hypothermia." *Sports Afield* 223, no. 4 (April, 2000): 84. Gierach discusses the perils of hypothermia, a condition in which one's core body temperature drops below the body's ability to bring itself back up to normal. Provides tips for raising core temperature.

Hickey, Robert W., et al. "Hypothermia and Hyperthermia in Children After Resuscitation from Cardiac Arrest." *Pediatrics* 106, no. 1 (July, 2000): 118-122. In experimental models of ischemic-anoxic brain injury, changes in body temperature after the insult have a profound influence on neurologic outcome.

HYPERTROPHY

BIOLOGY

ANATOMY OR SYSTEM AFFECTED: All

SPECIALTIES AND RELATED FIELDS: Endocrinology, family practice, internal medicine

DEFINITION: The growth of a tissue or organ as the result of an increase in the size of the existing cells within that tissue or organ; this process is responsible for the growth of the body as well as for increases in organ size caused by increased workloads on particular organs.

KEY TERMS:

atrophy: the wasting of tissue, an organ, or an entire body as the result of a decrease in the size and/or number of the cells within that tissue, organ, or body

compensatory hypertrophy: an increase in the size of a tissue or an organ in response to an increased workload placed upon it

growth: the increase in size of an organism or any of its parts during the developmental process; caused by increases in both cell numbers and cell size

hyperplasia: the increase in size or growth of a tissue or an organ as a result of an increase in cell numbers, with the size of the cells remaining constant

PROCESS AND EFFECTS

The growth and development of the human body and all its parts requires not only an increase in the number of body cells as the body grows, a process known as hyperplasia, but also an increase in the size of the existing cells, a process known as hypertrophy. It is true that as humans grow, they increase the number of cells in their bodies, resulting in an increase in the size of tissues, organs, systems, and the body. For some tissues, organs, and systems, however, the number of cells is genetically set; therefore, the number of cells will increase minimally if at all after birth. Thus, if growth is to occur in those tissues, organs, and systems, it must take place by means of an increase in the size of the existing cells.

The process of hypertrophy occurs in nearly all tissues in the body but is most common in those tissues in which the number of cells is set at the time of birth. Among such tissues are adipose tissue, which is composed of fat cells, and nervous tissue, which is found in the brain, in the spinal cord, and in skeletal muscle tissue. Other tissues, such as cardiac tissue and smooth muscle tissue, also show the ability to undergo hypertrophy.

It is generally true that the number of fat cells within the human body is set at birth. Therefore, an increase in body fat is thought to result primarily from an increase in the amount of fat stored within the fat cells. An increase in the amount of fat consumed in the diet increases the amount of fat that is placed inside a fat cell, resulting in an increase in the fat cell's size.

The number of nerve cells within the brain and spinal cord also is set at birth. The cerebellum of the human brain, however, increases in size about twentyfold from birth to adulthood. This increase is brought about by an increase in the size of the existing nerve cells, and particularly by an increase in the number of extensions protruding from each nerve cell and the length to which the extensions grow. Furthermore, there is an increase in the number of the components within the cell. Specifically, there is an increase in the number of mitochondria within the cell, which provide a usable form of energy so that the cell can grow.

The number of skeletal muscle cells is also, in general, preset at the time of birth. The skeletal muscle mass of the human body increases dramatically from birth to adulthood. This increase is accomplished primarily by means of individual skeletal muscle cell hypertrophy. This increase in the diameter of the individual muscle cells is brought about by increases in the amounts of the contractile proteins, myosin and actin, as well as increases in the amount of glycogen and the number of mitochondria within individual cells. As each muscle cell increases in size, it causes an increase in the size of the entire muscle of which it is a part.

Each of the above-mentioned examples occurs naturally as part of the growth process of the human body. Some tissues, however, are capable of increasing in size as the result of an increased load or demand being placed upon them. This increased load or demand is usually brought about by an increased use of the muscle. This increase in the size of cells in response to an increased demand or use is called compensatory hypertrophy. The most common tissues that show the phenomenon of compensatory hypertrophy are the skeletal, cardiac, and smooth muscles.

Skeletal muscle is particularly responsive to being utilized. This response, however, is dependent upon the way in which the skeletal muscle is used. It is well known that an increase in the size of skeletal muscle can be brought about by such exercises as weight lifting. Lifting heavy weights or objects requires strong contractions of the skeletal muscle that is doing the lifting. If this lifting continues over a long period of time, it eventually results in an increase in the size of the existing muscle fibers, leading to an increase in the size of the exercised muscle. Because the strength of a muscle is dependent upon its size, the increase in the muscle's size results in an increase in its strength. The extent to which the size of the muscle increases is dependent upon the amount of time spent lifting the objects and the weight of the objects. The size that a muscle can reach is, however, limited.

Unlike exercises such as weight lifting, endurance types of exercise, such as walking, jogging, and aerobics, do not result in larger skeletal muscles. These types of exercise do not force the skeletal muscles to contract forcibly enough to produce muscle hypertrophy.

In the same way that an increased load or use will cause compensatory hypertrophy in skeletal muscle, a decreased use of skeletal muscle will result in its shrinking or wasting away. This process is referred to as muscle atrophy. This type of atrophy commonly occurs when limbs are broken or injured and must be immobilized. After six weeks of the limb being immobilized, there is a marked decrease in muscle size. A similar type of atrophy occurs in the limb muscles of astronauts, since there is no gravity present in space to provide resistance against which the muscles must work. If the muscles remain unused for more than a few months, there can be a loss of about one-half of the muscle mass of the unused muscle.

Cardiac muscle, like skeletal muscle, can also be caused to hypertrophy by increasing the resistance against which it works. Although endurance exercise does not cause hypertrophy in skeletal muscle, it does result in an increased size of the heart because of the hypertrophy of the existing cardiac muscle cells in this organ. In fact, the heart mass of marathon runners enlarges by about 40 percent as a result of the

Hypertrophy

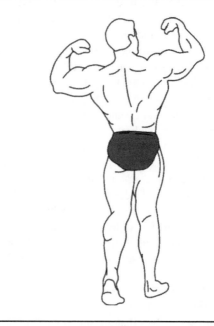

Weight lifters and body builders take advantage of the process of hypertrophy to increase the size of their muscles.

increase in endurance training. This increase occurs because the heart must work harder to pump more blood to the rest of the body when the body is endurance exercising. Only endurance forms of exercise result in the hypertrophy of the cardiac muscle. Weight lifting, which causes hypertrophy of skeletal muscle, has no effect on the cardiac muscle.

Smooth muscle also is capable of compensatory hypertrophy. Increased pressure or loads on the smooth muscle within arteries can result in the hypertrophy of the muscle cells. This in turn causes a thickening of the arterial wall. Smooth muscle, however, unlike skeletal and cardiac muscle, is capable of hyperplasia as well as hypertrophy.

COMPLICATIONS AND DISORDERS

Hypertrophy also occurs as a result of some pathological and abnormal conditions. The most common pathological hypertrophy is enlargement of the heart as a result of cardiovascular disease. Most cardiovascular diseases put an increased workload on the heart, making it work harder to pump the blood throughout the body. In response to the increased workload, the heart increases its size, a form of compensatory hypertrophy.

The left ventricle of the heart is capable of hypertrophying to such an extent that its muscle mass may increase four- or fivefold. This increase is the result of improper functioning of the valves of the left heart. The valves of the heart work to prevent the backflow of blood from one chamber to another or from the arteries back to the heart. If the valves in the left heart are not working properly, the left ventricle contracts and blood that should leave the ventricle to go out to the body instead returns to the left ventricle. The enlargement of the left ventricle increases the force with which it can pump the blood out to the body, thus reducing the amount of blood that comes back to the left ventricle despite the damaged heart valves. There is, however, a point at which the enlargement of the left ventricle can no longer help in keeping the needed amount of blood flowing through the body. At that point, the left ventricle finally tires out and left heart failure occurs.

The same type of hypertrophy can and does occur in the right side of the heart as well. Again, this is the result of damaged valves that are supposed to prevent the backflow of blood into the heart. Should the valves of both sides of the heart be damaged, hypertrophy can occur on both sides of the heart.

High blood pressure, also known as hypertension, may also lead to hypertrophy of the ventricles of the heart. With high blood pressure, the heart must work harder to deliver blood throughout the body because it must pump blood against an increased pressure. As a result of the increased demand upon the heart, the heart muscle hypertrophies in order to pump more blood.

The hypertrophy of the heart muscle is beneficial in the pumping of blood to the body in individuals who have valvular disease and hypertension; however, an extreme hypertrophy sometimes leads to heart failure. One of the reasons this may occur is the inability of the blood supply of the heart to keep up with the growth of the cardiac muscle. As a result, the cardiac cells outgrow their blood supply, resulting in the loss of blood and thus a loss of oxygen and nutrients needed for the cardiac cells to survive.

Smooth muscle, like cardiac muscle, may also hypertrophy under the condition of high blood pressure. Smooth muscle makes up the bulk of many of the arteries and smaller arterioles found in the body. The increased pressure on the arterial walls as a result of high blood pressure may cause the hypertrophy of the smooth muscles within the walls of the arteries and arterioles. This increases the thickness of the walls of the arteries and arterioles but also decreases the size of the hollow spaces within those vessels, which are known as the lumina. In the kidneys, the narrowing of the lumina of the arterioles may result in a decreased blood supply to these organs. The reduced blood flow to the kidneys may eventually cause the kidneys to shut down, leading to renal failure.

Smooth muscle may also hypertrophy under some unique conditions. During pregnancy, the uterus will undergo a dramatic hypertrophy. The uterus is a smooth muscle organ that is involved in the housing and nurturing of the developing fetus during pregnancy. Immediately prior to the birth of the fetus, there is marked hypertrophy of the smooth muscle within this organ. This increase in the size of the uterus is beneficial in providing the strong contractions of this organ that are needed for childbirth.

Skeletal muscle also may be caused to hypertrophy in some diseases in which there is an increase in the secretion of male sex hormones, particularly testosterone. Men's higher levels of testosterone, a potent stimulator of muscle growth, are responsible for the fact that males have a larger muscle mass than do females. Furthermore, synthetic testosterone-like hormones have been used by some athletes to increase muscle size. These synthetic hormones are called anabolic steroids. The use of these steroids does result in the hypertrophy of skeletal muscle, but these steroids have been shown to have harmful side effects.

Obesity is another condition that results largely from the hypertrophy of existing fat cells. In children, however, obesity is thought to result not only from an increase in the size of fat cells but also from an increase in their number. In adults, when weight is lost, it is the result of a decrease in the size of the existing fat cells; the number of fat cells remains constant. Thus, it is important to prevent further weight increases in overweight children to prevent the creation of fat cells that will never be lost.

In the onset of diseases that result in muscle degeneration, such as muscular dystrophy, there is a hypertrophy of the affected muscles. This hypertrophy differs from other forms of muscle hypertrophy in that the muscle cells do not increase in size because of an increase in the contractile protein, mitochondria, or glycogen, but because the muscle cells are being filled with fat. As a result of the contractile protein being replaced with fat, the affected muscles are no longer useful.

PERSPECTIVE AND PROSPECTS

The exact mechanisms that bring about and control the hypertrophy of cells and tissues are not well understood. During the growth and developmental periods, however, the hypertrophy of many tissues is thought to be under the control of blood-borne chemicals known as hormones. Among these hormones is one that promotes growth and is thus called growth hormone. Growth hormone brings about an increase in the number and size of cells. Growth hormone causes the hypertrophy of existing cells by increasing the protein-making capability of these cells. Thus, there is an increase in the number of organelles, such as mitochondria, within the cell, which leads to an increase in cell size.

Growth hormone also causes the release of chemicals known as growth factors. There are several different growth factors, but one of particular importance is nerve growth factor. Nerve growth factor is involved with the increase in number of cell processes of single nerve cells. Such chemicals have been shown to enhance the growth of damaged nerve cells in the brains of animals. As a result, it is possible that nerve growth factor could be used in the treatment of nerve damage in humans by causing the nerves to grow new cell processes and form new connections to replace those that were damaged. This may be of great importance for the treatment of those suffering from brain or spinal cord damage.

Other hormones may have similar effects on tissues other than nervous tissue. For example, the hypertrophy of the smooth muscle in the uterus is thought to be brought about hormonally. Immediately prior to birth, when the hypertrophy of the uterus is occurring, there is an increased amount of estrogen, the primary female hormone, in the blood. It is this increase in estrogen that is thought to lead to the great enlargement of the uterus during this time. Some hormones have the effect of preventing or inhibiting the hypertrophy of body tissues. The enlargement of the uterus prior to birth is brought about not only by an increase in estrogen but also as a result of a decrease in another hormone known as progesterone. Progesterone levels are high in the blood throughout pregnancy. Immediately prior to birth, however, there is a dramatic decrease in the level of progesterone in the blood. Thus, it is believed that the high level of progesterone prevents or inhibits the hypertrophy of the smooth muscle cells in the uterus, since the hypertrophy of this organ will not occur until estrogen levels are high and progesterone levels are low.

It has been suggested that compensatory hypertrophy, such as that which occurs in skeletal, smooth, and cardiac muscle, occurs as a result of the stretching of muscle. Some studies have shown that the stretching of skeletal, cardiac, and smooth muscle does lead to hypertrophy. American astronauts and Russian cosmonauts, however, showed a loss in muscle mass even though they exercised and stretched their muscles as much as three hours per day, seven days per week. This suggests that mechanisms other than the stretching of muscles may be involved in compensatory muscle hypertrophy.

Through an understanding of the mechanisms involved in muscle hypertrophy, it may one day be possible to prevent the atrophy that occurs during space flights, prolonged bed rest, and immobilization necessitated by the injury of limbs. Furthermore, the understanding of the mechanisms that control hypertrophy may help to alleviate the effects of disabling diseases such as muscular dystrophy by reversing the effects of muscle atrophy.

—David K. Saunders, Ph.D.

See also Endocrinology; Endocrinology, pediatric; Exercise physiology; Growth; Hormones; Muscles; Muscular dystrophy; Obesity; Pregnancy and gestation; Steroid abuse; Steroids.

FOR FURTHER INFORMATION:

Guyton, Arthur C., and John E. Hall. *Textbook of Medical Physiology.* 10th ed. Philadelphia: W. B. Saunders, 2000. An easily read textbook that provides much information on compensatory hypertrophy and other forms of hypertrophy. Provides an in-depth look at hypertrophy and the mechanisms that bring it about, particularly the effects of exercise on the hypertrophy of skeletal and cardiac muscle.

Hole, John W., Jr. *Essentials of Human Anatomy and Physiology.* 6th ed. Dubuque, Iowa: Wm. C. Brown, 1993. An introductory college anatomy and physiology text that is easily read and understood. Provides a good general overview of the processes of hypertrophy and atrophy.

Marieb, Elaine N. *Human Anatomy and Physiology.* 5th ed. Redwood City, Calif.: Benjamin/Cummings, 2000. Provides an in-depth look at how obesity occurs as a result of both hypertrophy and hyperplasia. Also provides an overview of the hormones that can cause hypertrophy and the mechanisms by which they bring about changes in size.

Shostak, Stanley. *Embryology: An Introduction to Developmental Biology.* New York: HarperCollins, 1991. Provides an introduction to the growth and development of the human body. It provides a good discussion of the role that hypertrophy plays in the development of the human body. It also points out those tissues that grow primarily by hypertrophy rather than by hyperplasia.

Tortora, Gerard J., and Sandra R. Grabowski. *Principles of Anatomy and Physiology.* 9th ed. New York: John Wiley & Sons, 2000. This textbook does a good job of explaining hypertrophy in skeletal, cardiac, and smooth muscle. It provides several examples of pathological conditions in which hypertrophy occurs and may be harmful.

HYPNOSIS

PROCEDURE

ANATOMY OR SYSTEM AFFECTED: Brain, nervous system, psychic-emotional system

SPECIALTIES AND RELATED FIELDS: Alternative medicine, anesthesiology, immunology, psychiatry, psychology

DEFINITION: The induction of an altered state of consciousness.

KEY TERMS:

hypnotherapy: a therapeutic method in which hypnosis works in conjunction with the psychotherapeutic process

hypnotic depth: a state frequently measured by the degree of suggestibility possessed by a presumably hypnotized individual

hypnotic induction: the production of hypnosis by means of precise rules and patterns (formal) or rules and patterns that permit limited flexibility (informal)

operator: the person who induces a hypnotic state; synonymous with "hypnotist" and "suggestor"

suggestion: a communication that evokes a nonvoluntary response reflecting the ideational content of the communication

INDICATIONS AND PROCEDURES

The term "hypnosis" comes from the Greek word *hypnos,* meaning sleep. While scientists and researchers do not understand the exact nature of hypnosis, theorists agree that it is an altered state of consciousness occurring on a continuum of awareness. Hypno-

sis may occur naturally and spontaneously, as in the case of a daydream. The daydreamer is alert and awake but focuses attention inward rather than outward.

The trance state, often synonymous with the hypnotic state, is characterized by an altered psychological state and minimal motor functioning. A trance can be recognized by the individual's glassy-eyed stare, lack of mobility, and unresponsiveness to external stimuli. A person in a trance state has a heightened receptivity to suggestion. Hypnosis, then, is a natural state that can be induced by another or by oneself (self-hypnosis) for a specific purpose. As a method of treatment, hypnosis, which is often used in conjunction with other approaches to alter psychophysiological states, promotes an understanding that allows for creative problem solving.

In the hypnotic state, the subject is not necessarily docile or submissive and may, because of unconscious processes, reject a suggestion given by even the most expert hypnotist. Four basic types of suggestion have been described: verbal, which includes words and any kind of sound; nonverbal, which applies to body language and gestures; intraverbal, which relates to the intonation of words; and extraverbal, which utilizes the implications of words and gestures that facilitate the acceptance of ideas. Suggestions are also described as being direct or indirect. Suggestibility is a behavior that is not hindered by the individual's logical processes but is enhanced by the subject's motivation, expectation, and trust in the operator as well as by the frequency and manner in which a suggestion is given.

Typically, prior to hypnosis, a subject is seated comfortably opposite or alongside the operator. The operator and subject generally have already discussed what will occur during the hypnotic process. The subject is encouraged to talk about his or her attitudes regarding hypnosis and the operator, as well as any previous experience with hypnosis. If the situation is a clinical one, a full psychiatric history and evaluation will already have been completed. For a positive hypnotic experience to emerge, a comfortable and trusting relationship between subject and operator must exist. There must be a willingness to undergo the experience on the part of the subject and a sensitive, observant, and supportive attitude on the part of the operator. Not all subjects are hypnotizable, but it is believed that most individuals, under appropriate circumstances, can respond to simple suggestions.

The induction process can be one of many types, ranging from directing the subject to close his or her eyes and think of a peaceful scene to having the subject gaze at a particular spot, shiny object, or swinging pendulum until the subject's eyes become heavy and close. Focusing on an object or scene leads the subject to redistribute his or her attention so as to withdraw it from the general surroundings and focus it on a circumscribed area. In the meantime, the subject is encouraged to relax and to allow events to unfold naturally. This induction procedure is sometimes followed, or even replaced, by what are described as deepening techniques. The direction is given to imagine gradually descending a staircase or elevator, or drifting on a boat past a slowly disappearing landscape. Counting forward or backward is another deepening or induction technique. Throughout this procedure, the operator offers comments or suggestions in a slow, repetitive, monotonous voice, exhorting the subject to feel relaxed and calm or to float and drift.

After a period generally lasting from one to several minutes, the operator gives the subject motor and sensory suggestions. For example, the operator may ask the subject to concentrate on the feelings in his or her fingers and hand, to feel the small muscles in the fingers begin to twitch and the arm and forearm begin to feel light. The operator states that these muscles will eventually feel so light that they will lift up off the armrest of the chair and, continually floating upward, ultimately reach the side of the subject's face. The operator might add that the higher the hand floats, the deeper the hypnosis will become, and the deeper the hypnosis becomes, the higher the hand will float. The operator then adds that when the hand reaches the side of the face, the subject will be deeply hypnotized.

When this point is reached, and the hand and arm have "levitated," the operator assumes that the subject is well hypnotized and then adds suggestions that are appropriate to the situation. Not all subjects, however, respond to hypnosis to the same extent or at the same rate.

There is no evidence to support the view that the operator in hypnosis is able to control the experience and behavior of the subject against the latter's wishes. It is the subject's motivation to behave in accordance with the wishes and directions of the operator that creates that erroneous impression. Moreover, there is no evidence to support the idea that a hypno-

tized subject can transcend his or her normal volitional capacity because of the hypnosis; despite persuasive clinical reports of altered somatic structures in hypnosis, no physiological changes uniquely associated with hypnosis have been demonstrated. Hypnosis is not so much a way of manipulating behavior as of creating increased perception and memory.

USES AND COMPLICATIONS

Because the mind, body, and emotions are interdependent, factors that influence one influence the others as well. The roles of the mind and emotions in functional or psychophysiological (psychosomatic) illness are widely recognized, but in cases of organic illness, their importance is often underestimated.

Regardless of etiology (causes), there are physical and psychological components to all illness. Emotional states that continue over extended periods can produce physiological changes. The fear, resentment, or depression that often accompanies illness may prolong or exacerbate it and interfere with a patient's willingness or ability to participate in treatment. Addressing such issues through hypnosis can greatly improve the overall medical management of a patient, from the initial diagnosis through all forms of treatment, including the treatment of unconscious and critically ill patients.

One advantage of modern clinical hypnosis is that it requires the practitioner to approach the patient as a whole person rather than as a collection of parts, one or more of which may be diseased. For the physician using hypnosis, a medical history goes beyond a list of past illnesses, allergies, and hospitalizations. A more comprehensive picture is developed that includes an understanding of a patient's personality, present state of mind, and life history and the positive aspects as well as the stresses and strains of the patient's present environment.

The use of hypnosis in most, if not all, medical specialties has been well documented. Hypnosis can be used alone or in combination with other approaches to overcome a variety of habit disorders. While some problems, such as thumb-sucking, can be resolved relatively quickly, others, such as overeating, sometimes require extended treatment or a multidimensional approach. Smoking and bed-wetting are examples of habit disorders that can be managed through hypnosis.

There is much evidence that children as a group are more responsive to hypnosis than adults, and that infants and young children frequently experience hypnosis as a natural part of their lives. Children can often be helped in a remarkably short period of time. Hypnosis has been used with children in the treatment of such diverse ailments as bed-wetting, soiling, asthma, epilepsy, learning difficulties, some behavioral and delinquency problems, stuttering, and nailbiting.

Hypnosis has been used effectively as an adjunct to the treatment of numerous problems with autonomic (internal) nervous system components. For example, there have been many controlled studies and successful case reports on the use of hypnosis in the treatment of asthma, which is the most common of the psychophysiological respiratory disorders. Through hypnosis, a patient can be helped to break the vicious cycle in which anxiety and emotional upsets can trigger an acute asthma attack, which in turn can produce anxiety and fear of other attacks.

Hypnosis has also been used effectively in the control and relief of pain. Because pain is experienced psychologically as well as physiologically, hypnosis can help people alter the perception of pain. A patient can learn to block pain to specific areas of the body, lessen the sensation of pain, or move pain from one area of the body to another. This ability is useful in the management of many types of pain, including chronic back pain, postoperative pain, and the pain associated with illness, migraine headache, burns, childbirth, and medical procedures.

In addition to being used to treat chronic conditions such as hypertension, hypnosis has been used to provide symptomatic relief of other chronic conditions, such as musculoskeletal disorders (for example, rheumatoid arthritis, osteoarthritis, fractures, and bursitis) and hemophilia.

Hypnosis has been used in dentistry for the relief of anxiety as well as pain and has been found to be helpful in teeth grinding (bruxism) and gagging. Modern hypnodontics is not primarily concerned with producing a surgical hypoanalgesia except in rare instances in which chemical anesthesia cannot be tolerated. The dentist is concerned with making visits to his or her office more tolerable and less threatening.

In obstetrics and surgery, hypnosis has been used to induce relaxation and relieve anxiety and to reduce the amount of anesthetic necessary. Occasionally, no anesthetic is required. This is sometimes desirable in childbirth, when the mother prefers to be aware of the birth process, or in other surgical procedures in which a minimum of anesthetic is desirable.

Hypnosis has also been utilized by the police in what has been termed "investigative hypnosis." Witnesses to crimes are interrogated in an effort to improve their memory retrieval.

Hypnosis has also been helpful in increasing athletic effectiveness. It has been utilized by both team and individual athletes to increase self-confidence and other factors such as self-image and the ability to assess the competition. Hypnosis thus applied to maximize performance in sports has been very effective, but the principles involved are essentially no different from those applied to other areas of living, such as increasing the efficiency of performance in the home, school, or workplace.

Since the mid-1970's, there has been much research into immune system functioning. Studies of the effects of stress on immune system functioning are lending scientific support to anecdotal reports that indicate that hypnosis may be effective in altering the disease process in cancer and AIDS patients. Researchers have found that unless treatments for these illnesses are based on the premise that the mind, body, and emotions are all striving to achieve health, physical intervention alone (radiation or chemotherapy, for example) will not be effective.

PERSPECTIVE AND PROSPECTS

Although medical hypnosis is considered to have had its beginnings with the Viennese physician Franz Anton Mesmer (1733-1815) in the latter half of the eighteenth century, hypnosis, or something very similar to it, has been practiced by religious and other healers in various ways for centuries in most cultures. The earliest evidence of its existence was found among shamans, who were also referred to as "witch doctors," "medicine men," or "healers."

In preparation for healing, a shaman adhered to certain practices that allowed his or her powers of concentration to be heightened. Placing himself or herself in isolation, the shaman began a descent into the "lower world." This often meant visualizing an opening in the earth and a journey downward into that opening. The journey was frequently accompanied by rhythmic drumming, chanting, singing, or dancing. The monotonous rhythm and constancy allowed the shaman's subconscious mind to become strongly focused, seek out the sick spirit of the patient, make it whole, and bring it back to the patient. The shaman actually engaged in a powerful process of visualization and suggestion during which the shaman willed the sick person to be healed.

In the eighteenth century, Mesmer recognized this ancient healing phenomenon and incorporated it into a theory of animal magnetism. Mesmer believed that a "cosmic fluid" could be stored in inanimate objects, such as magnets, and transferred to patients to cure them of illness.

Mesmer dressed flamboyantly. His consulting rooms were dimly lit and hung with mirrors, and he kept soft music playing in the background. The doctor's patients sat in a circle around a vat that contained such elements as powdered glass or iron filings. Then the patients grasped iron rods that were immersed in the vat and were believed to transmit a curing force.

Mesmer's first success was with a twenty-nine-year-old woman who suffered from a convulsive malady, a condition commonly called a "nervous disorder." Her symptoms consisted of blood rushing to her head and a tremendous pain in her ears and head. This state was followed by delirium, rage, vomiting, and fainting. During one of the woman's attacks, Mesmer applied three magnets to the patient's stomach and legs while she concentrated on the positive effects of the "cosmic fluid." In a short time, her symptoms subsided. When her symptoms resurfaced the next day, Mesmer gave her another treatment and achieved similar results. Mesmer believed that the "cosmic fluid," stimulated by the magnets, was directed through his patient's body. Her energy flow was restored, and as a result she regained her health.

Eventually Mesmer discarded the magnets. He began to regard himself as a magnet through which a fluid life force could be conducted and then transmitted to others as a healing force. This is what Mesmer described as "animal magnetism."

Despite the fact that no scientific evidence supported the existence of Mesmer's "cosmic fluids" or the concept of "animal magnetism," he had a tremendous rate of success. Thousands flocked to him for treatment. The only explanation for his success is that his patients were literally "mesmerized" into the belief and expectation that they would be cured. "Mesmerism" was a forerunner of the concept of hypnotic suggestion.

During this same period, a new slant on Mesmer's theories was introduced by one of his disciples, the Marquis de Puységur. He believed that the "cosmic fluid" was not magnetic but electric. This electric fluid was generated in all living things—in plants as well as animals. Puységur used the natural environ-

ment to fill his patients with the healing electric fluid that was expected to end their suffering. His clinic was held outdoors, where the sick were received under an elm tree in the center of the village green. Puységur believed that the tree had an innate healing power and that the force would travel through the trunk and branches to cords that he hung from the tree. At the foot of the tree, patients sat in a circle on stone benches with the cords wrapped around the diseased parts of their bodies. They were "connected" to one another when they touched their thumbs together, which made it possible for the "fluid" to circulate from person to person and to heal.

During this activity, Puységur noticed a strange phenomenon. Some of the patients entered a state of deep sleep as a result of being mesmerized. In this state, the patient could still communicate and be lucid and responsive to the suggestions of the mesmerist. The marquis had discovered the hypnotic trance but had not identified it as such.

In the mid-1800's, the hypnotic trance was used to relieve pain. An eminent London physician, John Elliotson (1791-1868), reported 1,834 surgical operations performed painlessly. In India, a Scottish surgeon named James Esdaile (1808-1859) performed many major operations, such as amputation of limbs, using mesmerism (or, as he called it, "magnetic sleep") as the sole anesthetic. One procedure involved conditioning the patient weeks prior to surgery. This was accomplished by inducing a trance state in the patient and offering posthypnotic suggestions to numb the part of the body on which the surgery was to be performed. In a second method, the hypnotist attended to the patient in the operating room, inducing a trance state and suggesting disassociation from any pain. It was possible for the patient to be completely lucid during this state and also to be oblivious to pain, as though completely anesthetized.

Mesmerism continued to provoke new theories and uses. During the late nineteenth century, an English physician, James Braid (1795-1860), gave mesmerism a scientific explanation. He believed mesmerism to be a "nervous sleep" and coined the word "hypnosis," which was derived from the Greek word *hypnos*, meaning sleep. Braid showed that hypnotized subjects are often abnormally susceptible to impressions on the senses and that much of the subjects' behavior was caused by suggestions made verbally.

Soon, other theories began to emerge. Jean Martin Charcot (1825-1893), a neurologist who taught in

Paris, explained hypnosis as a state of hysteria and categorized it as an abnormal neurological activity.

In France, Auguste Ambroise Leibeault (1823-1904) and Hippolyte Bernheim (1837-1919) were the first to regard hypnosis as a normal phenomenon. They asserted that expectation is a most important factor in the induction of hypnosis, that increased suggestibility is its essential symptom, and that the hypnotist works on the patient by means of mental influences.

As hypnosis began to receive serious study and could be explained rationally, it began to gain acceptance in the scientific community. It was no longer relegated to the realm of the bizarre.

Sigmund Freud became interested in hypnosis at this same time and visited Leibeault and Bernheim's clinic to learn their induction techniques. As Freud observed patients enter a hypnotic state, he began to recognize the existence of the unconscious. Although he was not the first to make this observation, he was the first to recognize the unconscious as a major source of psychopathology. Early in his research, however, Freud rejected hypnosis as the tool to unlock repressed memories, favoring instead his technique of free association and dream interpretation. With the rise of psychoanalysis in the first half of the twentieth century, hypnosis declined in popularity.

Then, however, a reversal occurred. During World War II, interest in hypnosis was regenerated by the need for short-term therapy (it was often applied in cases of "battle fatigue") and by the combination of hypnosis and more traditional analytic approaches. Mind control and "brainwashing" techniques that surfaced during the Korean War again sparked interest in the power of suggestion, especially when the subject was under duress. In the late 1960's and early 1970's, with the rise of public interest in alternative forms of mental health (Transcendental Meditation, biofeedback, yoga) and ways of coping with the stress of the modern world, hypnosis experienced a rebirth. Researchers found new and potent uses for it in therapy, and the trance state began to be recognized as a highly effective tool for modifying behavior and for healing.

—*Genevieve Slomski, Ph.D.*

See also Alternative medicine; Anesthesia; Anesthesiology; Anxiety; Asthma; Bed-wetting; Brain; Meditation; Pain management; Psychiatry; Psychosomatic disorders; Stress; Stress reduction.

FOR FURTHER INFORMATION:

Brown, Peter. *The Hypnotic Brain*. New Haven, Conn.: Yale University Press, 1991. This scholarly work examines how communication in human beings arose, the importance of nonverbal communication, the rise in oral cultures, and evidence for the common "everyday" trance.

Forrest, Derek, and Anthony Storr. *The Evolution of Hypnotism*. Forfar, England: Black Ace Books, 1999. This book offers a history of hypnotism and its predecessor, mesmerism. Traces the major figures of mesmerism, leading up through Sigmund Freud and hypnotism's influence in the twentieth century.

Hadley, Josie, and Carol Staudacher. *Hypnosis for Change*. 3d ed. New York: Ballantine Books, 1996. This popular account provides step-by-step details on the practice of self-hypnosis. It also offers a brief historical sketch of hypnosis, explores all facets of induction, and examines various aspects of hypnotic communication. Includes a bibliography.

Zahourek, Rothlyn P., ed. *Clinical Hypnosis and Therapeutic Suggestion in Patient Care*. New York: Brunner/Mazel, 1990. Representing a variety of disciplines, the contributors to this book argue that hypnosis is a natural, noninvasive tool that can be of use in patient care.

HYPOCHONDRIASIS
DISEASE/DISORDER

ANATOMY OR SYSTEM AFFECTED: Psychic-emotional system, all bodily systems

SPECIALTIES AND RELATED FIELDS: Psychiatry, psychology

DEFINITION: Unwarranted belief about or anxiety over having a serious disease which is based on one's subjective interpretation of physical symptoms or sensations; the belief or anxiety is maintained in spite of appropriate medical assurances that there is no serious disease.

KEY TERMS:

defense mechanisms: automatic, unconscious mental processes that become activated in the presence of emotional distress and anxiety; these processes work to maintain inner harmony by preventing mental awareness of that which would be otherwise too emotionally painful to endure

hypochondria: an earlier term for hypochondriasis; from classical Greek, it means the abdominal region of the body below the rib cage, from which black bile was believed to cause melancholy and yellow bile was believed to cause ill-temper

hypochondriacal neurosis: an earlier, but still-used, term for hypochondriasis; because experts have disagreed about what "neurosis" means precisely, the term is considered less descriptive than "hypochondriasis"

hypochondriacal reaction: another earlier term for hypochondriasis; experts who still prefer this term view hypochondriasis as a transient reaction to life stress and tend not to see it as a mental-emotional disorder in its own right

primary hypochondriasis: hypochondriasis as a disorder in its own right, and not accompanied by another psychiatric disorder such as generalized anxiety or panic

secondary hypochondriasis: the experience of hypochondriacal symptoms as part of an underlying, causal condition such as panic disorder, generalized anxiety disorder, schizophrenia, or major depression with psychotic features

somatization disorder: the somatoform disorder most similar to hypochondriasis; in somatization, the preoccupation is primarily with symptoms that one experiences and not with a disease that one is fearful of getting, an important distinction when these conditions are treated

somatoform disorders: the grouping of disorders that includes hypochondriasis; these disorders feature symptoms that suggest physical disease but that are actually caused by psychological upset

CAUSES AND SYMPTOMS

With hypochondriasis, the real problem is the patient's excessive worry and mental preoccupation with having or developing a disease, not the disease about which the patient is so worried. While concern about contracting a serious disease is common and normal, and may even make one more prudent, excessive worry, endless rumination, and obsessive interpretation of every symptom and sensation can disable and prevent effective functioning. A diagnosis of hypochondriasis is made when the patient's dread about the disease or diseases impairs normal activity and persists despite appropriate medical reassurances and evidence to the contrary. Even though hypochondriacs can acknowledge intellectually the possibility that their fears might be without rational foundation, the acknowledgment itself fails to bring any relief.

Researchers estimate that a low of 3 percent to a high of 14 percent of all medical (versus psychiatric) patients have hypochondriasis. Just how prevalent it is in the population as a whole is unknown. What is known is that the disorder shows up slightly more in men than in women, starts at any age but most often between twenty and thirty, shows up most often in physicians' offices with patients who are in their forties and fifties, and tends to run in families.

Most clinicians believe that hypochondriasis has a primary psychological cause or causes but that, in general, hypochondriacs have only a vague awareness that they are doing something that perpetuates and worsens their hypochondriacal symptoms. Hypochondriacs do not feign illness; they genuinely believe themselves to be sick, or about to become so.

Clinicians usually favor one of four hypotheses about how hypochondriasis starts. The hypotheses are based on anecdotal, clinical experience with patients who have gotten better when treated specifically for hypochondriasis. Researchers have rarely studied hypochondriasis using strict experimental methods. Nevertheless, the anecdotal evidence is important, because it gives clinicians a way to think about how to treat the condition.

The most popular view among mental health professionals sees hypochondriacs as essentially angry, but deep down inside. Because their life experience is of hurt, disappointment, rejection, and loss, they engage in a two-stage process to make up for their sad state of affairs. Though they believe themselves unlovable and unacceptable as they are, they solicit attention and caring by presenting themselves either as ill or as dangerously close to becoming ill. Their fundamental anger fosters their development of an interpersonal pattern in which they bite the emotional hands which seek to feed them. Endless worry and rumination soon render ineffective others' concern. No amount of reassurance allays their preoccupation and anxiety. In this way, those moved to show concern tire, grow impatient, and finally give up their efforts to help, proving to the worried hypochondriacs that no one really does care about them after all. Meanwhile, the hypochondriacs remain sad and angry.

This view often assumes that hypochondriasis is actually a form of defense mechanism which transfers angry, hostile, and critical feelings felt toward others into physical symptoms and signs of disease. Because hypochondriacs find it too difficult to admit that they feel angry, isolated, and unloved, they hide from the emotional energy associated with these powerful feelings and transfer them into bodily symptoms. This process seems to occur most often when hypochondriacal people harbor feelings of reproach because they are bereaved and lonely. In effect, they are angry at being left alone and left uncared for, and they redirect the emotion inwardly as self-reproach manifested in physical complaints.

Others hypothesize that hypochondriasis enables those who either believe themselves to be basically bad and unworthy of happiness or feel guilty for being alive ("existential guilt") to atone for their wrongdoings and, thereby, undo the guilt that they are always fighting not to feel. The mental anguish, emotional sadness, and physical pain so prevalent in hypochondriasis make reparation for the patients' real, exaggerated, or imagined badness.

A third view is sociological in orientation. Health providers who endorse it see hypochondriasis as society's way of letting people who feel frightened and overwhelmed by life's challenges escape from having to face those challenges, even if temporarily. Hypochondriacs take on a "sick role" which removes societal expectations that they will face responsibilities. In presenting themselves to the world as too sick to function, they also present themselves as excused from doing so. A schoolchild's stomachache on the day of a big test provides a relatively common and potentially harmless example of this role at work. Non-physically disabled adults who seek refuge from life stress by staying in bed, and who find themselves with true physical paralysis years later, provide a more serious and regrettable example.

A fourth view utilizes some experimental data which suggest that hypochondriacal people may have lower thresholds for (and lower tolerances of) emotional and physical pain. The data suggest that hypochondriacs experience physical and/or emotional sensations that are a magnification of what is normal experience. Thus, sensation that what would be sinus pressure for most people would be experienced as severe sinus headache in the hypochondriac. Hypersensitivity (lower threshold) to bodily sensations keeps hypochondriacs ever on watch for these upsetting, intense sensations because of how amplified the physical and emotional experiences are. What seems to most people an exaggerated concern with symptoms is simply prudent, self-protective vigilance to hypochondriacs.

Regardless of why the disorder develops, the majority of hypochondriacs go to their physicians with concerns about stomach and intestinal problems or heart and blood circulation problems. These complaints are usually only part of broader concerns about other organ systems and other anatomical locations. The key clinical feature of the disorder of hypochondriasis, however, is not where and how many bodily complaints there are but the patients' belief that they are seriously sick, or are just about to become so, and that the disease has yet to be detected. Laboratory tests that reveal healthy organs, physician reassurances that they are well, and long periods in which the dreaded disease fails to manifest itself are not reassuring at all. In fact, before the hypochondriasis itself is treated psychologically, it seems that nothing can stop the frantic rumination and accompanying nervousness, even the patients' acknowledgment that they may be exaggerating their reaction to their heartbeat, headache, diarrhea, morning cough, or perspiration. Hypochondriacs seem genuinely unable not to worry.

Hypochondriacs typically present their medical history in great detail and at great length. Often, they have an elaborate, exotic, and complex pathophysiological theory to explain how they acquired the disease and what it is doing, or will soon do, to them. At times, they cite recent research and give great importance to other causes, tests, or treatments that they and their health providers have not yet tried. Because their actual problem is not, strictly speaking, medical (or not only medical) and because they usually frustrate professional caretakers such as physicians, as well as nonprofessional caretakers such as family and friends, breakdown in the helping process is common. Worried patients tax physicians' time and resources, while busy physicians feel increasingly drained for what they believe is no good reason. The hypochondriacal patients sense that their concerns are not respected or taken seriously; they start to sense resentment. Phone calls to physicians' offices go unreturned for longer and longer periods. The perceived lack of access to their health providers makes the hypochondriac worry even more frenetically. The physicians increasingly believe that these patients are unappreciative—that they are, in fact, healthy and that they are not cooperating with treatment goals. Instead, these hypochondriacal patients are seen as excessively demanding. Anger builds on both sides, relationships deteriorate, and the hypochondriacs begin to "doctor-shop," while the physicians lose them as patients.

Although hypochondriasis is usually chronic, with periods in which it is more and less severe, temporary hypochondriacal reactions are also commonly seen. Such reactions most often occur when patients have experienced a death or serious illness of someone close to them or some other major life stressor, including their own recovery from a life-threatening illness.

When these reactions persist for less than six months, the technical diagnosis is a condition called "somatoform disorder not otherwise specified," and not hypochondriasis. When external stressors cause the reaction, the hypochondriacal symptoms usually remit when the stressors dissipate or are resolved. The important exception to this rule occurs when family, friends, or health professionals inadvertently reinforce the worry and preoccupation through inappropriate amounts of attention. In effect, they reward hypochondriacal behavior and increase the likelihood that it will persist: A mother may never have received more support and help at home than following breast cancer surgery; a father may never have felt his children's affection as much as when he recuperated from having a heart attack; an employee may have never obtained special allowances on the job or received so many calls from coworkers as when recovering from herniated disk surgery; or a student may never have gotten as special treatment or as many gifts from teammates as when treated for rheumatic fever. What began as a transient hypochondriacal reaction can become chronic, primary hypochondriasis.

The life of hypochondriacs is unhappy and unrewarding. Nervous tension, depression, hopelessness, and a general lack of interest in life mark the fabric of the hypochondriacs' daily routines. Actual clinical, depressive disorders can easily coexist with hypochondriasis, to the point that even antidepression medications will simultaneously alleviate hypochondriacal symptoms.

Hypochondriasis often accompanies physical illness in the elderly. As a group, the elderly have declining health, experience diminished physical capacities, and are at increased risk for contracting and developing disease. Sometimes, earlier tendencies toward hypochondriasis simply intensify with age. Sometimes, old age is simply when it first appears. Hypochondriasis is not, however, a typical or expected aspect of normal aging; most elderly people are not hypochondriacal. In those who are, however, hypochondriasis is most likely a symptom of depression, abandonment, or loneliness, and these are the conditions that should first be treated.

TREATMENT AND THERAPY

The most important aspect of treating hypochondriasis is assessing whether true organic disease exists. Many diseases in their early stages are diffuse and affect multiple organ systems. Neurologic diseases (such as multiple sclerosis), hormonal abnormalities (such as Graves' disease), and autoimmune/connective tissue diseases (such as systemic lupus) can all manifest themselves early in ways that are difficult to diagnose accurately. The frantic and obsessive reporting of hypochondriacal patients can just as easily be the worried and detailed reporting of patients with early parathyroid disease; both report symptoms that are multiple, vague, and diffuse. The danger of hypochondriasis lies in its being diagnosed in place of true organic disease, which is exactly the kind of event hypochondriacs fear will happen.

Of course, there is nothing to prevent someone with true hypochondriasis from getting or having true physical illness. Worrying about illness neither protects from nor prevents illness. Moreover, barring a sudden, lethal accident or event, every hypochondriac is bound to develop organic illness sooner or later. Physical illness can coexist with hypochondriasis— and does so when attitudes, symptoms, and mental and emotional states are extreme and disproportionate to the medical problem at hand.

The goal in treating hypochondriasis is care, not cure. These patients have ongoing mental illness or chronic maladaptation and seem to need physical symptoms to justify how they feel. Neither surgical nor medical interventions will ameliorate a psychological need for symptoms. The best treatments (when hypochondriasis cannot itself be the target of treatment, which is most of the time) are long term in orientation and seek to help patients tolerate and accommodate their symptoms while health providers learn to understand and adapt to these difficult-to-treat patients.

Medications have proved useful in treating hypochondriasis only when accompanied by pharmacotherapy-sensitive conditions such as major depression or generalized anxiety. When hypochondriasis coexists with either mental or physical disease, the latter must be treated in its own right. Secondary hypochondriasis means that the primary disorder warrants primary treatment.

The course of hypochondriasis is unclear. Clinicians' anecdotal experience tends to endorse the perception that these people are impossible as patients. Outcome studies, however, belie the pessimism. The research suggests that many who are treated get better, and the more the following conditions are present, the better the outcome is likely to be: coexisting anxiety or depressive disorder, rapid onset, onset at a younger age, higher socioeconomic status, absence of organic disease, and absence of a personality disorder.

A fifty-six-year-old married male, for example, recounted his history as never having been in really good health at any time in his life. He made many physician office visits and had, over the years, seen many physicians, though without ever feeling emotionally connected to them. Over the past several months, he felt increasingly concerned that he was having headaches "all over" his head and that they were caused by an undetected tumor in the middle of his brain, "where no X ray could detect it." He had read about magnetic resonance imaging (MRI) in a health letter to which he subscribed and said that he wanted this procedure performed "to catch the tumor early." Various prescribed medications for his headache usually brought no relief.

While productive at work and promoted several times, he had been passed over for his last promotion because, he believed, his superiors did not like him. He also stated that he believed that many on the job saw him as cynical and pessimistic but that no one appreciated the "pain and mental anxiety" he endured "day in and day out."

His spouse of thirty-two years had advanced significantly at a job she had begun ten years earlier, and she seemed to him to be closer to their three children than he was. She was increasingly involved with outside voluntary activities, which kept her quite busy. She reported that she often asked him to join her in at least some of her activities but he always said no. She said that when she arrived home late, he was often in a state of physical upset, but for which she could never seem to do the "right thing to help him." In their joint interview, each admitted often feeling angry at and frustrated with the other. She could never determine why he was sick so often and why her efforts to help only seemed to make his situation worse.

He could not understand how she could leave him all alone feeling as physically bad as he did. He believed that she never seemed to worry that something might happen to him while she was out being "a community do-gooder." The husband was suffering from a classic case of hypochondriasis.

Perspective and Prospects

Both the concept and term "hypochondriasis" have ancient origins and reflect a view that all persons are subject to their own humoral ebb and flow. Humors were once thought to be bodily fluids that maintained health, regulated physical functioning, and caused certain personality traits. In classical Greek, *hypochondria*, the plural of *hypochondrion*, referred to both a part of the anatomy and the condition known today as hypochondriasis. *Hypo* means "under," "below," or "beneath," and *chondrion* means literally "cartilage" but in this case refers specifically to the bottom tip of cartilage at the breastbone (the xiphoid or, more formally, xiphisternum). Here, below the breastbone but above the navel, two humors were thought to flow in excess in the hypochondriacal person. The liver, producing black bile, made people melancholic, depressed, and depressing; the spleen, producing yellow bile, made people bilious, cross, and cynical. This view, or a variant of it, persisted until the middle to late eighteenth century.

Sigmund Freud and other psychiatrists treated hypochondriacal symptoms with some success while approaching the disorder as a defense mechanism rather than as an excess of bodily fluids. Their treatment for the first time cast a psychological role for what had been seen as a physical problem. Mental health professionals whose theoretical orientation is psychoanalytic or psychodynamic continue to deal with hypochondriasis as they deal with other defense mechanisms.

In the 1970's, some researchers began to suggest that hypochondriasis was being incorrectly applied to describe a discrete disorder, when it was really only an adjective that described a cluster of nonspecific behaviors. They argued that hypochondriasis is not a real diagnosis. Other researchers disagreed and argued for differentiating between primary and secondary hypochondriasis. Their view has proved to have significant pragmatic utility in treating the wide range of patients who exhibit symptoms of hypochondriasis, and it remains the prevailing view.

Given the general unwillingness of patients with

hypochondriasis to admit that they have a psychological problem and not some yet-to-be-found organic condition, the interpersonal difficulties that often arise between health providers and these patients, and the serious potential of concurrent organic disease, it is not surprising why hypochondriasis continues to challenge both persons afflicted with this disorder and those who treat them.

—*Paul Moglia, Ph.D.*

See also Anxiety; Bipolar disorder; Depression; Factitious disorders; Midlife crisis; Neurosis; Obsessive-compulsive disorder; Panic attacks; Phobias; Psychiatric disorders; Psychiatry; Psychiatry, child and adolescent; Psychiatry, geriatric; Psychosomatic disorders; Stress; Stress reduction.

FOR FURTHER INFORMATION:

Barsky, Arthur J. "Somatoform Disorders." In *Comprehensive Textbook of Psychiatry VI*. Vol. 1, edited by Harold I. Kaplan and Benjamin J. Sadock. 6th ed. Baltimore: Williams & Wilkins, 1995. While Kaplan and Sadock's book remains the standard psychiatric reference for psychiatrists and nonpsychiatric physicians alike, Barsky's chapter includes an excellent discussion of hypochondriasis that is readily intelligible to laypeople.

Ben-Tovim, David I., and Adrian Esterman. "Zero Progress with Hypochondriasis." *The Lancet* 352, no. 9143 (December 5, 1998): 1798-1799. Despite behavioral research on patients suffering from hypochondriasis, no acceptable treatment for this condition has been discovered. It is important for doctors to adequately examine these patients, however, because even hypochondriacal patients can fall ill.

De Jong, Peter J., Marie-Anne Haenen, Anton Schmidt, and Birgit Mayer. "Hypochondriasis: The Role of Fear-Confirming Reasoning." *Behaviour Research and Therapy* 36, no. 1 (January, 1998): 65-74. This article investigates whether hypochondriacal patients are prone to selectively search for danger-confirming information when asked to judge the validity of conditional rules in the context of general and health threats.

Hill, John. *Hypochondriasis: A Practical Treatise.* New York: AMS Press, 1992. Originally published in 1766, this well-regarded and readable work presents the world of the hypochondriac in ways that challenge stereotypical and biased views of them.

HYPOGLYCEMIA

DISEASE/DISORDER

ANATOMY OR SYSTEM AFFECTED: Blood, endocrine system, glands

SPECIALTIES AND RELATED FIELDS: Endocrinology, family practice, hematology, internal medicine, serology

DEFINITION: The condition in which concentration of glucose in the blood is too low to meet the needs of key organs, especially the brain; this condition limits treatments for diabetes mellitus.

KEY TERMS:

fasting hypoglycemia: hypoglycemia that occurs when no food is available from the intestinal tract; usually caused by failure of the neural, hormonal, and/or enzymatic mechanisms that convert stored fuels (primarily glycogen) into glucose

glucagon: a pancreatic hormone which signals an elevated concentration of glucose in the circulation

gluconeogenesis: the synthesis of molecules of glucose from smaller carbohydrates and amino acids

glucose: a simple sugar, readily converted to metabolic energy by most cells of the body and essential for the welfare of brain cells

glycogen: a storage form of carbohydrate, composed of many molecules of glucose linked together; found in many tissues of the body and serves as a major source of circulating glucose

glycogenolysis: the cleavage of glycogen into its constituent molecules of glucose

hypoglycemic unawareness: the occurrence of hypoglycemia without the warning symptoms of trembling, palpitations, hunger, or anxiety

hypoglycemic unresponsiveness: inadequate recovery of the circulating glucose concentration after an episode of hypoglycemia

insulin: a pancreatic hormone which signals a reduced concentration of glucose in the circulation

neuroglycopenia: abnormal function of the brain, caused by an inadequate supply of glucose from the circulation

reactive hypoglycemia: hypoglycemia that occurs within a few hours after ingestion of a meal

CAUSES AND SYMPTOMS

The condition known as hypoglycemia exists when the concentration of glucose in the bloodstream is too low to meet bodily needs for fuel, particularly those of the brain. Ordinarily, physiological compensatory mechanisms are called into play when the circulating concentration of glucose falls below about 3.5 millimoles. Activation of the sympathetic nervous system and the secretion of glucagon are especially important in promoting glycogenolysis and gluconeogenesis. Symptoms of sympathetic nervous activation normally become apparent with glucose concentrations that are less than about 3 millimoles. Brain function is usually demonstrably abnormal at glucose concentrations below about 2 millimoles; sustained hypoglycemia in this range can lead to permanent brain damage.

Some of the symptoms of hypoglycemia occur as by-products of activation of the sympathetic nervous system. These symptoms include trembling, pallor, palpitations and rapid heartbeat, sweating, abdominal discomfort, and feelings of anxiety and/or hunger. These symptoms are not dangerous in themselves; in fact, they may be considered to be beneficial, as they alert the individual to obtain food. Meanwhile, the sympathetic nervous system signals compensatory mechanisms. The manifestations of abnormal brain function during hypoglycemia include blunting of higher cognitive functions, disturbed mentation, confusion, loss of normal control of behavior, headache, lethargy, impaired vision, abnormal speech, paralysis, neurologic deficits, coma, and epileptic seizures. The individual is usually unaware of the appearance of these symptoms, which can present real danger. For example, episodes of hypoglycemia have occurred while individuals were driving motor vehicles, leading to serious injury and death. After recovery from hypoglycemia, the patient may have no memory of the episode.

There are two major categories of hypoglycemia: fasting and reactive. The most serious, fasting hypoglycemia, represents impairment of the mechanisms responsible for the production of glucose when food is not available. These mechanisms include the functions of cells in the liver and brain that monitor the availability of circulating glucose. Additionally, there is a coordinated hormonal response involving the secretion of glucagon, growth hormone, and other hormones and the inhibition of the secretion of insulin. The normal consequences of these processes include the addition of glucose to the circulation, primarily from glycogenolysis, as well as a slowing of the rate of utilization of circulating glucose by many tissues of the body, especially the liver, skeletal and cardiac muscle, and fat. Even after days without food, the body normally avoids hypoglycemia through breakdown of stored proteins and activation of gluco-neogenesis. There is considerable redundancy in the systems that maintain glucose concentration, so that the occurrence of hypoglycemia often reflects the presence of defects in more than one of these mechanisms.

The other category of hypoglycemia, reactive hypoglycemia, includes disorders in which there is disproportionately prolonged and/or great activity of the physiologic systems that normally cause storage of the glucose derived from ingested foods. When a normal person eats a meal, the passage of food through the stomach and intestines elicits a complex and well-orchestrated neural and hormonal response, culminating in the secretion of insulin from the beta cells of the islets of Langerhans in the pancreas. The insulin signals the cells in muscle, adipose tissue, and the liver to stop producing glucose and to derive energy from glucose obtained from the circulation. Glucose in excess of the body's immediate needs for fuel is taken up and stored as glycogen is or utilized for the manufacture of proteins. Normally, the signals for the uptake and storage of glucose reach their peak of activity simultaneously with the entry into the circulation of glucose from the food undergoing digestion. As a result, the concentration of glucose in the circulation fluctuates only slightly. In individuals with reactive hypoglycemia, however, the entry of glucose from the digestive tract and the signals for its uptake and storage are not well synchronized. When signals for the cellular uptake of glucose persist after the intestinally derived glucose has dissipated, hypoglycemia can result. Although the degree of hypoglycemia may be severe and potentially dangerous, recovery can take place without assistance if the individual's general nutritional state is adequate and the systems for activation of glycogenolysis and gluconeogenesis are intact.

DIAGNOSIS AND TREATMENT

The diagnostic evaluation of an individual who is suspected of having hypoglycemia begins with verification of the condition. Evaluation of a patient's symptoms can be confusing. On one hand, the symptoms arising from the sympathetic nervous system and those of neuroglycopenia may occur in a variety of nonhypoglycemic conditions. On the other hand, persons with recurrent hypoglycemia may have few or no obvious symptoms. Therefore, it is most important to document the concentration of glucose in the blood.

To establish the diagnosis of fasting hypoglycemia, the patient is kept without food for periods of time up to seventy-two hours, with frequent monitoring of the blood glucose. Should hypoglycemia occur, blood is taken for measurements of the key regulatory neurosecretions and hormones, including insulin, glucagon, growth hormone, cortisol, and epinephrine, as well as general indices of the function of the liver and kidneys. If there is suspicion of an abnormality in an enzyme involved in glucose production, the diagnosis can be confirmed by measurement of the relevant enzymatic activity in circulating blood cells or, if necessary, in a biopsy specimen of the liver.

Fasting hypoglycemia may be caused by any condition that inhibits the production of glucose or that causes an inappropriately great utilization of circulating glucose when food is not available. Insulin produces hypoglycemia through both of these mechanisms. Excessive circulating insulin ranks as one of the most important causes of fasting hypoglycemia, most cases of which result from the treatment of diabetes mellitus with insulin or with an oral drug of the sulfonylurea class. If the patient is known to be taking insulin or a sulfonylurea drug for diabetes, the cause of hypoglycemia is obvious; appropriate modification of the treatment should be made. Hypoglycemia caused by oral sulfonylureas is particularly troublesome because of the prolonged retention of these drugs in the body. The passage of several days may be required for recovery, during which time the patient needs continuous intravenous infusion of glucose.

Excessive insulin secretion may also result from increased numbers of pancreatic beta cells; the abnormal beta cells may be so numerous that they form benign or malignant tumors, called insulinomas. The preferred treatment of an insulinoma is surgery, if feasible. When the tumor can be removed surgically, the operation is often curative. Unfortunately, insulinomas are sometimes difficult for the surgeon to find. Magnetic resonance imaging (MRI), computed tomography (CT) scanning, ultrasonography, or angiography may help localize the tumor. Some insulinomas are multiple and/or malignant, rendering total removal impossible. In these circumstances, hypoglycemia can be relieved by drugs that inhibit the secretion of insulin.

Malignant tumors arising from various tissues of the body may produce hormones that act like insulin with respect to their effects on glucose metabolism.

In some cases, these hormones are members of the family of insulin-like growth factors, which resemble insulin structurally. Malnutrition probably has an important role in predisposing patients with malignancy to hypoglycemia, which tends to occur when the cancer is far advanced.

Fasting hypoglycemia can be caused by disorders affecting various parts of the endocrine system. One such disorder is adrenal insufficiency; continued secretion of cortisol by the adrenal cortex is required for maintenance of normal glycogen stores and of the enzymes of glycogenolysis and gluconeogenesis. Severe hypothyroidism also may lead to hypoglycemia. Impairment in the function of the anterior pituitary gland predisposes a patient to hypoglycemia through several mechanisms, including reduced function of the thyroid gland and adrenal cortices (which depend on pituitary secretions for normal activity) and reduced secretion of growth hormone. Growth hormone plays an important physiologic role in the prevention of fasting hypoglycemia by signaling metabolic changes that allow heart and skeletal muscles to derive energy from stored fats, thereby sparing glucose for the brain. Specific replacement therapies are available for deficiencies of thyroxine, cortisol, and growth hormone.

Hypoglycemia has occasionally been reported as a side effect of treatment with medications other than those intended for treatment of diabetes. Drugs which have been implicated include sulfonamides, used for treatment of bacterial infections; quinine, used for treatment of falciparum malaria; pentamidine isethionate, given by injection for treatment of pneumocystosis; ritodrine, used for inhibition of premature labor; and propranolol or disopyramide, both of which are used for treatment of cardiac arrhythmias. Malnourished patients seem to be especially susceptible to the hypoglycemic effects of these medications, and management should consist of nutritional repletion in addition to discontinuation of the drug responsible. In children, aspirin or other medicines containing salicylates may produce hypoglycemia.

Alcohol hypoglycemia occurs in persons with low bodily stores of glycogen when there is no food in the intestine. In this circumstance, the only potential source of glucose for the brain is gluconeogenesis. When such an individual drinks alcohol, its metabolism within the liver prevents the precursors of glucose from entering the pathways of gluconeogenesis. This variety of fasting hypoglycemia can occur in persons who are not chronic alcoholics: It requires the ingestion of only a moderate amount of alcohol, on the order of three mixed drinks. Treatment involves the nutritional repletion of glycogen stores and the limitation of alcohol intake.

Severe infections, including overwhelming bacterial infection and malaria, can produce hypoglycemia by mechanisms that are not well understood. Patients with very severe liver damage can develop fasting hypoglycemia, because the pathways of glycogenolysis and gluconeogenesis in the liver are by far the major sources of circulating glucose in the fasted state. In such cases, the occurrence of hypoglycemia usually marks a near-terminal stage of liver disease. Uremia, the syndrome produced by kidney failure, can also lead to fasting hypoglycemia.

Some types of fasting hypoglycemia occur predominantly in infants and children. Babies in the first year of life may have an inappropriately high secretion of insulin. This problem occurs especially in newborn infants whose mothers had increased circulating glucose during pregnancy. Children from two to ten years of age may develop ketotic hypoglycemia, which is probably related to insufficient gluconeogenesis. These disorders tend to improve with time. Fasting hypoglycemia is also an important manifestation of a variety of inherited disorders of metabolism characterized by the abnormality or absence of one of the necessary enzymes or cofactors of glycogenolysis and gluconeogenesis or of fat metabolism (which supplies the energy for gluconeogenesis). Most of these disorders become evident in infancy or childhood. If there is a hereditary or acquired deficiency of an enzyme of glucose production, the problem can be circumvented by provision of a continuous supply of glucose to the affected individual.

There are several other rare causes of fasting hypoglycemia. A few individuals have had circulating antibodies that caused hypoglycemia by interacting with the patient's own insulin, or with receptors for insulin on the patient's cells. Although the autonomic (involuntary) nervous system has an important role in signaling recovery from hypoglycemia, diseases affecting this branch of the nervous system do not usually produce hypoglycemia; presumably, hormonal mechanisms can substitute for the missing neural signals.

Reactive hypoglycemia can occur when there is unusually rapid passage of foodstuffs through the upper intestinal tract, such as may occur after partial or total removal of the stomach. Persons predisposed to maturity-onset diabetes may also have reactive hypoglycemia, probably because of the delay in the secretion of insulin in response to a meal. Finally, reactive hypoglycemia need not indicate the presence of any identifiable disease and may occur in otherwise normal individuals.

Diagnosis of reactive hypoglycemia is made difficult by the variability of symptoms and of glucose concentrations from day to day. Adding to the diagnostic uncertainty, circulating glucose normally rises and falls after meals, especially those rich in carbohydrates. Consequently, entirely normal and asymptomatic individuals may sometimes have glucose concentrations at or below the levels found in persons with reactive hypoglycemia. Therefore, the glucose tolerance test, in which blood samples are taken at intervals for several hours after the patient drinks a solution containing 50 to 100 grams of glucose, is quite unreliable and should not be employed for the diagnosis of reactive hypoglycemia. Proper diagnosis of reactive hypoglycemia depends on careful correlation of the patient's symptoms with the circulating glucose level, preferably measured on several occasions after ingestion of ordinary meals. Some persons develop symptoms such as weakness, nausea, sweating, and tremulousness after meals, but without a significant reduction of circulating glucose. This symptom complex should not be confused with hypoglycemia.

When rapid passage of food through the stomach and upper intestine causes reactive hypoglycemia, the administration of drugs that slow intestinal transit may be helpful. When reactive hypoglycemia has no evident pathological cause, the patient is usually advised to take multiple small meals throughout the day instead of the usual three meals and to avoid concentrated sweets. These dietary modifications can help avoid hypoglycemia by reducing the stimulus to secretion of insulin.

Two rare inherited disorders of metabolism can produce reactive hypoglycemia after the ingestion of certain foods. In hereditary fructose intolerance, the offending nutrient is fructose, a sugar found in fruits as well as ordinary table sugar. In galactosemia, the sugar responsible for hypoglycemia is galactose, a major component of milk products. Management of these conditions, which usually become apparent in infancy or childhood, consists of avoidance of the foods responsible.

Perspective and Prospects

Fasting hypoglycemia is uncommon, except in the context of treatment of diabetes mellitus. The most serious public health problem associated with hypoglycemia is that it limits the therapeutic effectiveness of insulin and sulfonylurea drugs. Evidence suggests that elevation of the circulating glucose concentration (hyperglycemia) is responsible for much of the disability and premature death among patients with diabetes. In many of these patients, therapeutic regimens consisting of multiple daily injections of insulin or continuous infusion of insulin through a small needle placed under the skin can reduce the average circulating glucose to normal. Frequent serious hypoglycemia is the most important adverse consequence of such regimens. Persons with diabetes seem to be at especially high risk for dangerous hypoglycemia for two reasons. First, there is often a failure of the warning systems that ordinarily cause uncomfortable symptoms when the circulating glucose concentration declines, a situation termed hypoglycemic unawareness. As a consequence, when a patient with diabetes attempts to control his or her blood sugar with more frequent injections of insulin, there may occur unheralded episodes of hypoglycemia that can lead to serious alterations in mental activity or even loss of consciousness. Many patients with diabetes also have hypoglycemic unresponsiveness, an impaired ability to recover from episodes of hypoglycemia. Also, diabetes can interfere with the normal physiologic responses that cause the secretion of glucagon in response to a reduction of circulating glucose, thus eliminating one of the most important defenses against hypoglycemia. If both hypoglycemic unawareness and hypoglycemic unresponsiveness could be reversed, intensive treatment of diabetes would become safer and more widely applicable.

Reactive hypoglycemia, although seldom a clue to serious disease, has attracted public attention because of its peculiarly annoying symptoms. These symptoms, which reflect activation of the sympathetic nervous system, resemble those of fear and anxiety. The symptoms are not specific, and many patients with these complaints do not have hypoglycemia.

In summary, hypoglycemia indicates defective regulation of the supply of energy to the body. When severe or persistent, hypoglycemia can lead to serious behavioral disorder, obtunded consciousness, and even brain damage. Fasting hypoglycemia may be a clue to significant endocrine disease. Reactive hypoglycemia, while annoying, usually responds to simple dietary measures. The study of hypoglycemia has led to many important insights into the regulation of energy metabolism.

—*Victor R. Lavis, M.D.*

See also Blood and blood disorders; Diabetes mellitus; Endocrine disorders; Endocrinology; Endocrinology, pediatric; Hormones; Metabolism; Obesity; Pancreas; Pancreatitis; Vitamins and minerals.

For Further Information:

Cryer, Philip E. "Glucose Homeostasis and Hypoglycemia." In *Williams Textbook of Endocrinology*, edited by Jean D. Wilson and Daniel W. Foster. 9th ed. Philadelphia: W. B. Saunders, 1998. A complete and definitive chapter. Delineates especially well the coordination of the nervous and hormonal systems in physiologic defense against hypoglycemia, as well as the special problems of hypoglycemia in patients with diabetes mellitus.

Davidson, Mayer B. "Hypoglycemia." In *Diabetes Mellitus: Diagnosis and Treatment*. 8th ed. New York: John Wiley & Sons, 1986. The author has made an important contribution to the study of diabetes and metabolism. The chapter offers clear explanations of the physiological abnormalities in hypoglycemia and emphasizes the importance of fasting hypoglycemia as an index of serious illness.

Kahn, Ronald C., and Gordon C. Weir, eds. *Joslin's Diabetes Mellitus*. 13th ed. Philadelphia: Lea & Febiger, 1994. The definitive American textbook of diabetes. Covers all causes of hypoglycemia, not simply those related to diabetes.

Hypoparathyroidism. *See* Hyperparathyroidism and Hypoparathyroidism.

Hypospadias repair and urethroplasty

Procedure

Anatomy or system affected: Genitals, reproductive system

Specialties and related fields: General surgery, urology

Definition: Urethroplasty is any plastic surgery performed on the urethra; one of these procedures is the repair of hypospadias, the presence of an abnormal opening in the male urethra.

INDICATIONS AND PROCEDURES

Urethroplasty is performed to correct defects of the urethra, the tube leading from the bladder to the outside of the body through which urine exits the body. Hypospadias is a congenital defect of the distal end of the urethra in which it opens on the underside of the penis instead of at the tip. Less commonly, the opening can occur lower down on the underside of the penis or in the scrotum. Hypospadias is also associated with abnormalities in the kidneys.

The correction of hypospadias involves a technique known as a "flip-flap" repair: Two incisions on the undersurface of the glans and shaft of the penis are made, and skin from the glans is fashioned into an opening that is anatomically normal. The operation is usually done under general anesthesia.

The lines for both incisions are drawn and incisions carefully made to avoid damaging adjacent structures and erectile tissue. The prepuce is released from the body of the penis. A V-shaped flap is cut from the skin immediately below the hypospadias. The flap is rotated, and one side is sutured into one of the incisions made in the glans. The other side is similarly inserted into the other incision and sutured in place, forming a tube that extends the urethra. Excess skin from the prepuce is removed; the prepuce is sutured back into position on the shaft of the penis. The skin from the underside of the penis is brought together over the repaired urethra and sutured together. A catheter is frequently (but not universally) placed in the urethra and kept in place for up to three weeks. Some surgeons believe that the presence of a catheter helps to establish the new urethra. Others think that it only contributes to postoperative holes (fistulas) and do not use it, allowing the patient to urinate immediately through the newly constructed tube. The patient returns to the surgeon's office in a week for a postoperative check and the removal of sutures.

Another type of urethroplasty is the surgical repair of a discontinuity in the male urethra. Most commonly, this defect occurs on the underside of the penis and is attributable to the incomplete closure of the skin portions that normally fuse over the urethra during embryonic development. The technique is similar to that described above. Under general anesthesia, skin is removed from the prepuce of the penis and is sutured in place over the defect, closing the opening. A catheter may or may not be inserted. The patient returns to the surgeon's office in a week for a postoperative check and the removal of sutures.

USES AND COMPLICATIONS

The techniques associated with urethroplasty are used to repair congenital defects. Complications from these procedures are unusual, but they may include infection and stricture. Such problems can be avoided with careful attention to the finer details of the surgery.

The need for urethroplasty and hypospadias repair is unlikely to disappear. From a psychological standpoint, it benefits the patient to repair a hypospadias as early in life as possible, preferably before the age of three.

—*L. Fleming Fallon, Jr., M.D., Ph.D., M.P.H.*

See also Fistula repair; Genital disorders, male; Neonatology; Pediatrics; Reproductive system; Surgery, pediatric; Urinary system; Urology; Urology, pediatric.

FOR FURTHER INFORMATION:

Berkow, Robert, and Andrew J. Fletcher, eds. *The Merck Manual of Diagnosis and Therapy*. 17th ed. Rahway, N.J.: Merck Sharp & Dohme Research Laboratories, 1999.

Montague, Drogo K. *Disorders of Male Sexual Function*. Chicago: Year Book Medical, 1988.

Swanson, Janice M., and Katherine A. Forrest. *Men's Reproductive Health*. New York, N.Y.: Springer, 1984.

HYPOTHERMIA. *See* HYPERTHERMIA AND HYPOTHERMIA.

HYSTERECTOMY

PROCEDURE

ANATOMY OR SYSTEM AFFECTED: Reproductive system, uterus

SPECIALTIES AND RELATED FIELDS: Endocrinology, general surgery, gynecology, oncology

DEFINITION: The removal of the uterus and sometimes the ovaries and surrounding tissues, which is usually performed as a treatment for invasive cancer.

KEY TERMS:

adhesion: the "gluing" together by scar tissue of internal organs and tissues, often caused by endometriosis or infections; a common cause of pelvic pain

adrenal gland: a small organ located near the kidney that is responsible for the production of certain sex hormones, including testosterone and small amounts of estrogen

estrogen: the female sex hormone produced by the ovaries and the adrenal gland that is responsible for the development of female secondary sex characteristics; the three types naturally produced by the body are estradiol, estrone, and estriol

Fallopian tubes: the structures located between the uterus and ovaries that are responsible for the transport of the egg; also called the oviducts

laparoscopy: a surgical procedure in which an optical instrument called a laparoscope is inserted through a small incision in the abdomen

progesterone/progestin: a hormone produced in the ovaries, adrenal gland, and placenta (of pregnant women) that prepares for and sustains pregnancy

INDICATIONS AND PROCEDURES

The term "hysterectomy" comes from the Greek *hystera,* meaning "uterus," and *ektome,* meaning "to cut out." While hysterectomy refers to the removal of the uterus and, most commonly, the attached Fallopian tubes, there are several types of hysterectomies. Total hysterectomy, contrary to popular belief, does not mean that the ovaries are removed with the uterus. Rather, the term indicates the removal of the uterus and cervix. Subtotal, or partial, hysterectomy is the excision of the uterus above the cervix; the cervix is left in place. Either one or both ovaries may be removed with the uterus (oophorectomy or bilateral oophorectomy). Salpingo oophorectomy refers to the removal of one of the Fallopian tubes along with the accompanying ovary, while bilateral salpingo oophorectomy refers to the removal of both Fallopian tubes and ovaries.

Most frequently, the surgery is accomplished through a 6- to 8-inch midline incision running either down from the navel or across the lower abdomen near or below the hairline (known as a "bikini incision"). This procedure is referred to as an abdominal hysterectomy. Vaginal hysterectomy is the removal of the uterus through the vaginal canal, rather than through a surgical opening of the abdomen. This procedure is most often performed to resolve prolapse (because the uterus has already descended into the vaginal canal) or when the uterus is not enlarged and can be pulled down and out through the vagina. If the hysterectomy is performed because of fibroid tumors, the abdominal approach is usually advised. Tumors so large that they require the removal of the uterus are generally too large to pass safely through the vagina.

Hysterectomy

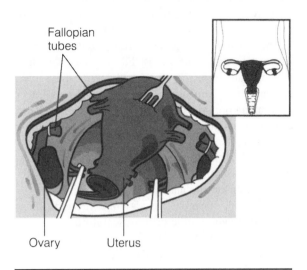

Fallopian tubes

Ovary   Uterus

The uterus, and sometimes such accompanying organs as the ovaries and Fallopian tubes, may be removed to treat disease conditions or as a contraceptive measure; the inset shows the location of the uterus.

Fibroids are responsible for approximately two hundred thousand hysterectomies per year and are the most common and troublesome gynecologic complaint of women. The most common benign disease entities of the female reproductive tract, they are present in anywhere from 30 to 50 percent of all women between forty and fifty years of age, afflicting twice as many African American women as white women. Women who have never had children and nonsmokers also seem to be at greater risk of developing fibroids, although the reason for this is uncertain. It has been noted that estrogen may play a role in their growth and development, since fibroids are never seen before puberty and seem to shrink after the menopause. In addition, fibroids tend to worsen during pregnancy, when estrogen levels are high. In the early days of higher-dose birth control pills, users seemed to be more predisposed to fibroids, although more recent studies indicate that this may no longer be the case.

The term "fibroid" refers to the fact that the composing tissue is fibrouslike, but fibroids are actually smooth muscle in origin. Therefore, the more precise but less commonly used medical term, leiomyoma, is actually more appropriate (*leio* meaning "smooth," *my* meaning "muscle," and *oma* meaning "tumor" or "growth").

Why or how fibroids develop is uncertain, but they are believed to start out as a smooth muscle cell that goes awry in the myometrium (the middle layer of the uterus). From there, a myoma may remain within the myometrium or intrude into the outermost or innermost layers of the uterus. Fibroids can occasionally migrate from the uterus and invade the cervix, surrounding ligaments, or, on rare occasions, other abdominal organs containing smooth muscle. They can occur singularly, but multiple fibroids are more common. They can be so tiny that they are visible only under a microscope or so large as to weigh thirty pounds. Furthermore, the symptoms may have no direct bearing on the number or size of the tumors; a woman could have one the size of a full-term pregnancy that causes little or no discomfort.

Generally speaking, when a woman does have symptoms from her fibroids, those symptoms are heavier flow and perhaps more painful menstrual periods. Fibroids can also cause an abnormal pattern of bleeding, however, such as spotting between periods or bleeding after the menopause. Depending on its location, a fibroid may cause inflammation and pain. In addition, many women with fibroids suffer from a sensation of pressure in the back, legs, or lower abdominal region. Yet only 0.5 percent of fibroids become malignant. A cancerous fibroid, called a leiomyosarcoma, is suspected when a fibroid is observed to enlarge at an unusually rapid rate.

Myomectomy is a surgical procedure whereby the fibroid tumors are removed and the remainder of the uterus is preserved and reconstructed. Because this surgery is complex and time-consuming, traditional physicians most often recommend hysterectomy, sometimes with oophorectomy, to women in their forties as a more appealing and permanent solution to their fibroids. Traditional physicians claim that myomectomy may cause greater blood loss, thus increasing the chance of a transfusion. Yet a woman, regardless of her childbearing plans, often has emotional reasons for wanting to preserve her uterus.

Hysterectomy is often recommended as a definitive treatment for endometriosis and adenomyosis (in which the endometrial tissue invades the deeper muscle layers of the uterus). From 1964 to 1984, the number of hysterectomies performed for endometriosis increased by 176 percent, more than for any other diagnosis, despite the fact that successful surgical techniques and drugs which can conserve organs were developed during this twenty-year period.

Endometriosis refers to the growth of small portions of the normal tissue that line the uterus (the endometrium) outside their normal location. These bits of misplaced tissue, called endometrial implants, survive within the pelvic cavity—on the Fallopian tubes, ovaries, or bowels—and in rare cases, as far away as the lungs, thighs, chest, arms, or any other part of the body.

Endometrial growths are not malignant. Each month, these foreign colonies of uterine tissue build up and then break down and bleed, as if they were still within the uterus. The result is internal bleeding, degeneration of the blood and tissue, inflammation of the surrounding areas, and the formation of scar tissue and adhesions. In rare cases, intestinal bleeding and obstruction, bladder difficulties, and kidney obstruction can occur. Endometriosis is a frequent cause of infertility.

Traditionally, hysterectomy and oophorectomy were considered the definitive answer to this problem if childbearing was not an issue. Increasingly, however, female reconstructive surgery—microsurgery (surgery using needles, sutures, and other surgical materials that cause a minimum of tissue damage and using fingers rather than instruments), laser surgery (in which a light beam is used to excise or burn away the tissue), or electrocautery (which employs a high-heat electrical current)—coupled with medication has been used successfully in the treatment of endometriosis.

Hysterectomy has been the treatment of choice for a variety of life-threatening cancers: endometrial hyperplasia (overgrowth of uterine lining, in which the thickened cells may cause spotting or abnormal bleeding), endometrial cancer, cervical cancer, and ovarian cancer.

While hysterectomy has been the standard treatment for uterine prolapse (the descent of the uterus), prolapsed uteri can be repositioned and repaired. It is thought that in the majority of cases prolapse results from pregnancy and childbirth. When the uterus and surrounding support tissues expand to accommodate pregnancy and delivery, they may lose their ability to contract back to their normal position and elasticity. Prolapse also occurs, however, in women who have never been pregnant, perhaps because of the passage of time, hormone deprivation, the long-term effects of gravity, or a genetic predisposition to having less collagen and elastin in the tissue.

Various other medical conditions, including excessive bleeding, cramps, problems after tubal ligation (in which the Fallopian tubes are cut and tied for the purpose of sterilization), and other menstrual or pelvic problems, have also been treated by hysterectomy.

USES AND COMPLICATIONS

The short-term operative complications of hysterectomy vary. Blood transfusion is common during hysterectomy. Some gynecologists routinely perform a transfusion before surgery if a woman is anemic. Other patients require transfusion during surgery. The average blood loss during a hysterectomy is estimated at between 400 and 500 cubic centimeters (about a pint). Massive bleeding, however, can occur and may cause varying degrees of shock. Abdominal bleeding may occur as late as ten to fourteen days following a hysterectomy. In addition, blood clots may form one week after the hysterectomy.

Urinary tract complications are most frequently caused by gynecological surgery; the rate varies from 1 to 10 percent of all cases. Retention of urine is a common complication of hysterectomy, particularly after a vaginal approach with anterior repair. Because the urine is not adequately expelled, bacteria can multiply within the bladder and cause cystitis, or bladder infection.

Other complications include peritonitis (an infection of the membrane lining the abdominal cavity), ovarian infections, lung infections, bowel complications, severe adhesions, and general prolapse of other pelvic organs (including the intestines, bowels, bladder, and vagina).

Among the long-term physical effects of hysterectomy is loss of ovarian function. With the loss of the ovaries following a hysterectomy-oophorectomy, the female hormones that stimulate the menstrual cycle, including estrogen and progesterone, stop circulating abruptly. The body is forced into a state of "surgical menopause." Even ovaries left intact may fail in 30 to 50 percent of hysterectomy cases.

Osteoporosis, the gradual thinning and weakening of the skeletal system, is one major consequence of the loss of ovarian function. It is one of the most common bone diseases in the United States, affecting ten million women and 26 percent of all women over the age of sixty. Women suffer from osteoporosis more frequently than men because, in women, the absorption of calcium into the bones is dependent on estrogen. Bone calcium content declines with the menopause because of the gradual loss of this hormone, and women become more prone to fractures, often of the spine and hip.

Many studies have confirmed a link between premenopausal hysterectomy and cardiovascular disease (including heart attacks and high cholesterol). While the reasons for this link are uncertain, the loss of the ovaries appears to be a factor because estrogen may protect the circulatory system. In addition, the chemical prostacyclin may be created in the uterus and may provide some protection against coronary artery disease.

Hot flashes are the most common reason that postmenopausal women seek medical attention. Changes in skin temperature, skin resistance, core temperature, and pulse rate have been measured during these episodes. At night, hot flashes contribute to insomnia, which can create great emotional distress. Most clinicians have observed that hot flashes and heavy sweating in women who have undergone hysterectomy-oophorectomy are more severe and more sudden in onset than those seen in the natural menopause. For some women, hot flashes and night sweats increase significantly after hysterectomy, even when the ovaries are preserved.

In addition to physiological complications, hysterectomy also has emotional complications. Much research has been conducted linking hysterectomy with psychiatric problems. The likelihood of hysterectomy causing severe psychological problems, including depression, depends on the reason for the surgery (women who undergo surgery because of cancer are less likely to be depressed); the woman's psychological state prior to surgery; the woman's relationship to her husband/partner and her general sense of well-being; and her desire to bear children. In addition, the absence of the uterus and menstruation may represent a loss of youth, strength, vitality, and self-esteem to some women; there is often grief over this loss.

Depression results not only from the surgical procedure but also from the loss of hormones following oophorectomy or ovarian failure. Some studies suggest that an imbalance in certain neurohormones is associated with such mood changes as crying spells, irritability, nervousness, and changes in sexual desire (libido). The metabolism of these hormones within the brain is believed to depend on estrogen levels. Scientists have found that depression and anxiety, as well as bone loss and decreased cardiovascular functioning, are alleviated in some women by hormone replacement therapy.

As early as the Renaissance, physicians recognized the loss of sexual satisfaction that can be brought on by a hysterectomy. Modern research shows deterioration in sexual activities after the operation. Frequent complaints include a decreased libido, decrease in coital activity, loss of orgasms, loss of lubrication (atrophic vaginitis), and painful intercourse (dyspareunia).

Perspective and Prospects

In ancient times, the complaints of women and the illnesses of the female organs were viewed as coming from an "unhappy uterus." It was believed that the uterus had the primary purpose of childbearing and that, when the uterus was not occupied with this function, it might show its wrath by abnormal bleeding and pain. These beliefs prevailed for centuries; early medical history indicates that women's gynecologic complaints were largely ignored. Moreover, no safe surgical procedures had been developed.

A noteworthy event in early American medical history was the operation attempted and documented by a frontier physician and surgeon, Ephraim McDowell. In 1809 in Danville, Kentucky, this daring young doctor carried out experimental surgery on a middle-aged woman to remove a huge ovarian tumor. Without the benefit of anesthesia and a sterile technique, he successfully performed abdominal surgery on four out of five other patients.

Myomectomy, or removal of a fibroid tumor of the uterus, was the next procedure to be performed—first in France and later (about 1850) in Massachusetts by Washington Atlee. The first hysterectomy was successfully performed by Walter Burnham in the same decade, but he lost twelve of his next fifteen hysterectomy patients.

In the text *Operative Gynecology* (1898), Howard A. Kelly of Baltimore voices concern over hysterectomy. He describes one hundred hysterectomies that he performed in the late nineteenth century, all done because of pelvic infection. He lost only four patients, though convalescence for some survivors was prolonged.

Remarkable medical progress occurred in the twentieth century in abdominal and vaginal surgical techniques. In the 1850's, Marion Sims of South Carolina was the first to perform vaginal surgery in the United States. He successfully repaired a vesicovaginal fistula, an opening between the bladder and the vagina through which urine escapes into the vagina. In the late nineteenth century, the "Manchester" operation

for uterine prolapse was performed by A. Donald in Manchester, England. Prior to this procedure, uterine prolapse was treated with a pessary, a device inserted into the vagina to hold the uterus in place.

In the early part of the twentieth century, hysterectomy was considered a relatively dangerous procedure; many of the medical advances necessary for its success (such as anesthesia, asepsis, and blood banks) were not yet available or perfected. Later, hysterectomy became one of the safer surgical procedures; mortality figures have dropped to between 0.2 and 0.5 percent, usually resulting from a pulmonary embolism (a blood clot in the lungs).

In the 1930's, N. Sproat Heany of Chicago devised the present-day technique of vaginal hysterectomy. Vaginal (as opposed to abdominal) hysterectomy, it was believed, resulted in a less complicated procedure with shorter convalescence and more cosmetically pleasing results for most patients.

For some time, vaginal hysterectomy was viewed as superior to abdominal hysterectomy. In the 1970's, between 25 and 40 percent of all hysterectomies were accomplished vaginally, depending on the age of the woman at the time of surgery. In 1981, however, a landmark study published by the U.S. Congress, weighing the costs, risks, and benefits of hysterectomy, stated that women undergoing vaginal hysterectomy are more likely to have postoperative fever and to receive antibiotic treatment. Other studies have shown a significantly greater risk of bleeding and infection of the ovary. Moreover, vaginal hysterectomy patients may undergo further surgery at a rate as high as 5 to 10 percent.

The vaginal hysterectomy is performed by grabbing the cervix and literally pulling the uterus out through the vagina. As the physician pulls, the ligaments and supporting structures alongside the uterus are cut until all the supporting structures are free. These ligaments are drawn down and eventually sewn into the vaginal closure. The original pelvic configuration and angle is never reapproximated. With the internal support structures gone, other pelvic organs can collapse inward, often causing vaginal vault prolapse.

By the late 1980's and early 1990's, the trend among many gynecologists had shifted away from hysterectomy to more conservative treatments. Physicians, many of them women, began to question whether hysterectomies were, in some or even in most cases, medically necessary. This trend became apparent even in the treatment of cancers of the uterus and ovaries. While most conservative gynecologists who did not normally treat cancer considered this condition to be the one instance in which they could unequivocally recommend hysterectomy, gynecological cancer specialists began to revolutionize the field by giving women the option of keeping at least some of their reproductive organs.

As more information became available to women regarding alternatives to hysterectomy (a major revenue-producing surgical procedure in the United States), many women asserted their right to challenge their physicians when told that hysterectomy was the only possible solution to their gynecological problems.

—*Genevieve Slomski, Ph.D.*

See also Cancer; Cervical, ovarian, and uterine cancers; Contraception; Dysmenorrhea; Ectopic pregnancy; Endometriosis; Ethics; Genital disorders, female; Gynecology; Hormone replacement therapy; Hormones; Menorrhagia; Oncology; Sex change surgery; Sterilization; Tubal ligation.

FOR FURTHER INFORMATION:

Clark, Jan. *Hysterectomy and the Alternatives: How to Ask the Right Questions and Explore Other Options*. London: Vermilion, 2000. Discusses the treatment of uterine fibroids and menstrual disorders and offers alternatives to radical hysterectomy.

Cutler, Winnifred B. *Hysterectomy: Before and After.* Rev. ed. New York: Harper & Row, 1990. Written by a reproductive biologist, this book discusses the extensive medical evidence showing the vital role of the uterus and ovaries in a woman's well-being. Explains why, in most cases, hysterectomy should be avoided, how to obtain an accurate diagnosis, and when surgery is necessary.

Dennerstein, Lorraine, Carl Wood, and Ann Westmore. *Hysterectomy: New Options and Advances.* 2d ed. New York: Oxford University Press, 1995. This popular work on hysterectomy addresses all aspects of the procedure. Includes a bibliography and an index.

IATROGENIC DISORDERS

DISEASE/DISORDER

ANATOMY OR SYSTEM AFFECTED: All

SPECIALTIES AND RELATED FIELDS: All

DEFINITION: Health problems caused by medical treatments.

CAUSES AND SYMPTOMS

Iatrogenic disorders may be attributable to inefficient or uncaring physicians or to the risks inherent in medical procedures that are necessary to prevent death or crippling disease. Such disorders are usually divided into those caused by medications, surgery, and medical misdiagnosis.

The average patient of any age expects physicians and the medical infrastructure to deliver perfect cures for all diseases. This is not possible because some diseases have no cure and because medical treatment always involves some potential risk to the persons being treated. In fact, a percentage—usually a small one—of the patients treated for any disease develop unexpected health problems (adverse reactions) which can be diseases themselves.

The term "iatrogenic disorder" is a catchall used to encompass the many different adverse reactions that accompany the practice of modern medicine. The number of such problems has grown as medical science has become more sophisticated. They are often blamed entirely on physicians and other medical staff involved in cases producing iatrogenic disorders.

This blame is correctly directed in instances where a physician and other staff involved are uncaring, inattentive, careless, or incompletely educated. However, iatrogenic disorders often result from the nature of modern medicine. Doctors frequently attempt therapeutic methods (such as surgery) that are innovative efforts which cure serious diseases but have some inherent risk of failure. They may also use therapeutic drugs that are powerful agents for cure of specific disease processes but that have side effects causing other health problems in some people who take them. In addition, doctors will very often utilize complicated overall therapy having adverse consequences that patients may not acknowledge despite physicians' attempts to explain them orally and with consent forms.

TREATMENT AND THERAPY

Despite careful efforts of most physicians—who are informed, caring, and efficient—iatrogenic disorders accompany many medical procedures. Public attention is, however, focused most on the effects of therapeutic agents, drugs and vaccines, because patients are often unaware that no therapeutic agent in use is ever perfectly safe. Even a clear physician description of the dos and don'ts associated with such therapy may be flawed by biological variation among patients, causing problems in one individual but not others. Furthermore, the explosion of new diseases and new versions of old diseases since the late 1980's has led to much more complex treatment regimens Consequently, iatrogenic disorders occur much more often.

This has become particularly germane in treatment of the aged, acquired immunodeficiency syndrome (AIDS) victims, and the very young. Hence, several rules must be followed concerning therapeutic agents. First, wherever possible, these medications should be used only after other means fail and the benefits to be gained clearly outweigh the risks entailed. Second, therapy should begin with the lowest possible effective dose, and all dose increases should be accompanied by frequent symptom relief and toxicity monitoring. Third, patients and responsible family members must be made aware of all possible adverse symptoms, how to best counter them, and the foods or other medications to be avoided to diminish iatrogenic potential. Such problems, in the aged, are due to biochemical changes which alter their tolerance for many medications.

Many iatrogenic disorders are caused by the presence of bacterial contamination in wounds and the fact that surgical maintenance of sterility is not absolutely perfect. For example, iatrogenesis occurs after 30 percent of surgical procedures carried out at heavily contaminated surgical sites (such as emergency surgery of abdominal wounds). In addition, the use of antibiotics can be problematic. In many cases, the large doses of these therapeutic agents required to fight primary bacterial infection will cause superinfection by other microbes, such as fungi. Furthermore, wide antibiotic use in hospitals has led to the creation of antibiotic-resistant bacteria.

For these reasons, treatment of surgical sites requires individualized attention. Clean wounds can be closed up immediately without high risk of infection, but deep wounds known to be contaminated prior to surgery are often best handled by closing up interior tissues and leaving skin and subcutaneous tissues open until it is clear that infection is under control. Many patients are frightened by such procedures and the pain involved, not understanding that it is in their best interest. Hence, they may resist treatment and accuse conscientious physicians of causing iatrogenic disorders. Such treatment is most crucial in the aged and in young children. In elderly patients the cause is diminution of body defenses against infection (for example, the immune system). It has been reported that the elderly experience a doubled or tripled chance of experiencing postoperative complications that may be seen as iatrogenic by their families. Young children are also more at risk than postpubertal individuals and "younger" adults, for reasons related to their incompletely developed immune systems.

Iatrogenesis resulting from misdiagnosis is too complicated an issue to be considered in depth here. In some cases, it is caused by physician inadequacy, but more often such problems are attributable to the great difficulty in diagnosing any disease absolutely.

It is essential for patients and physicians to communicate effectively. Such interaction lowers the occurrence of iatrogenic disorders because patients can decide to forgo treatment or to learn how to comply exactly with complex treatment protocols. Patients who do not receive adequate answers to questions posed to physicians should seek treatment elsewhere. Physicians should completely explain potential problems associated with therapeutic procedures by oral communication, informative consent forms, and well-educated counselors.

Because of the many iatrogenic disorders associated with medical therapy, physicians often believe that the best course of treatment—where a symptom is unclear and severe danger to patients is not imminent—is to allow nature to take its course so as to do no harm. This approach is often misunderstood by patients. To clarify the issue and to satisfy them, it should be explained—by the physician—that treatment can often be more dangerous than a perceived health problem.

It is hoped that the continued development of medical science, careful and complete therapy explanations by medical staffs, and better medical understanding and better treatment compliance by patients will decrease the incidence of iatrogenic disorders.

—Sanford S. Singer, Ph.D.

See also Antibiotics; Bacterial infections; Ethics; Hospitals; Law and medicine; Malpractice; Nausea and vomiting; Surgery, general; Surgical procedures; Wounds.

FOR FURTHER INFORMATION:

Apfel, Roberta J., and Susan M. Fisher. *To Do No Harm: DES and the Dilemmas of Modern Medicine.* New Haven, Conn.: Yale University Press, 1984. The book is well written and has a glossary of medical terms, twenty pages of footnotes, a bibliography of four hundred references, and an index, all of which enhance its usefulness.

Carroll, Paula. *Life Wish: One Woman's Struggle Against Medical Incompetence.* Alameda, Calif.: Medical Consumers, 1986. This personal narrative of a woman struggling to overcome breast cancer offers warnings of malpractice and surgical errors.

Preger, Leslie, ed. *Iatrogenic Diseases.* 2 vols. Boca Raton, Fla.: CRC Press, 1986. Offers helpful advice on diagnosing iatrogenic diseases. Includes bibliographical references and an index.

Sharpe, Virginia F., and Alan I. Faden. *Medical Harm: Historical, Conceptual, and Ethical Dimensions of Iatrogenic Illness.* New York: Cambridge University Press, 1998. Of the many seekers after a healthier life or of relief from suffering who rightfully expect benefit from the health care system, some are more harmed than helped. This book deals mostly with harmful medical events which happen in hospitals.

Vincent, Charles, Maeve Ennis, and Robert J. Audley, eds. *Medical Accidents.* Oxford, England: Oxford University Press, 1993. Covers such topics as diagnostic errors, iatrogenic disease, and medical malpractice. Also discusses liability insurance.

ILEOSTOMY AND COLOSTOMY

PROCEDURES

ANATOMY OR SYSTEM AFFECTED: Abdomen, gastrointestinal system, intestines

SPECIALTIES AND RELATED FIELDS: Gastroenterology

DEFINITION: Surgical procedures that reroute the intestines to a hole, or stoma, in the abdomen after the removal of all or part of the colon.

KEY TERMS:

anastomosis: the surgical connection of one tubular organ to another

appliance: any device for collecting or removing stool from a stoma

colon: the last section of the intestines, where most fluids are absorbed, located between the ileum and the rectum; also called the large bowel or intestine

ileum: the lower third of the small intestine, which joins with the colon

ostomy: a popular term for any operation that results in a stoma

rectum: the intestinal storage area for feces between the colon and anus

stoma: a surgically created passage between the intestines and the outer skin

stool: the waste matter of digestion excreted from the body through the anus or stoma

INDICATIONS AND PROCEDURES

Despite great advances in drugs and nonsurgical procedures, doctors can cure some disabling or life-threatening diseases of the intestines only on the operating table. Common procedures of this type are the colostomy and ileostomy, both of which replace the anus with a stoma on the abdominal wall. Such surgery stresses patients considerably, and, in the aftermath, when they must entirely relearn the once-simple act of defecation, some drift into depression, despair, and withdrawal as their bowel functions consume their attention and disturb their social lives. Even for the large majority who adjust, and for whom the procedures are a life-lengthening boon, their postsurgical body, in most cases, requires a permanent, profound change in habits and a complete reliance on technology.

Colostomy and ileostomy are medical terms compounding *stoma* (from Greek, "mouth") and a prefix identifying the section of gut that ends in the newly created "mouth." If a portion of the colon is retained and ends in a stoma, the operation constructing it is called a colostomy. If the entire colon is removed and the lower section of the small bowel, or ileum, ends in a stoma, the operation constructing it is called an ileostomy. Nonmedical support groups for patients commonly use the back-formation "ostomy" to refer to any operation that creates a stoma (including a urostomy, in which a stoma is created for the excretion of urine) and to such patients as "ostomates," although neither term belongs to medical technical vocabulary.

Physicians determine that an ileostomy or a colostomy is necessary after inspecting the damaged intestinal segments by endoscopy, by imaging, or during surgery. In consultation with a surgeon, the patient agrees to undergo the procedure. The patient fasts before the surgery and receives laxatives and enemas (except in the case of obstructions or severe ulcerative colitis) to clean as much feces from the intestines as possible and thus reduce the chance of infec-

tion during surgery. The surgeon, often with the advice of an enterostomal therapist (ET), examines the patient's abdomen carefully, checking where the skin naturally folds and stretches when the patient assumes various common body positions, and a spot for the stoma is selected that is convenient for the patient and free of stress from muscles and skin tension. That place is marked. An area to the right and below the navel is the usual location for an ileostomy. The left side is commonly chosen for a colostomy.

In ileostomy, the surgeon makes the opening incision to the left of the navel, starting a few centimeters above it and continuing to the pelvic area. After the abdominal cavity is exposed, the tissues connecting the colon to surrounding structures are severed, starting at the cecum; the blood supply is cut and tied off; and clamps are placed over the ileum and rectum. Then the colon is cut free of the small intestine and rectum and is removed. If the operation is a "subtotal" procedure, the rectum is sutured shut and left in place or the open end is pulled through the abdominal wall as a "mucous stoma." (Such a second stoma is sometimes fashioned because the surgeon plans to connect the ileum and rectum in a later operation.) If the surgeon performs a proctocolectomy, the rectum is removed after the stoma is made and the anus is sutured shut.

The stoma is built by cutting a small round opening first in the skin and then in the abdominal wall and pulling the end of the ileum through the hole. The end sticks above the skin, is folded back over itself, and is sutured to the edges of the hole, leaving the stoma protruding two to three centimeters. This basic ileostomy is called a Brooke ileostomy, after the English surgeon Bryan Brooke.

Variations on this basic procedure are employed depending on the wishes and health of the patient. A Kock pouch, named after its inventor, Nils Kock of Sweden, can be fashioned just behind the stoma in the abdominal cavity to act as an artificial rectum, collecting liquid waste until the ostomate wishes to void it; because this arrangement gives the patient control over defecation, it is called a continent ileostomy. The surgeon uses about 45 centimeters of ileum to form the pouch and adjusts the stoma so that it acts as a valve until a tube is inserted for drainage. In other procedures, the surgeon operates twice more on the ostomate, first detaching the ileum and closing the stoma and then reconnecting the bowel either to the rectum or to the anus.

If the ileum and rectum are joined, the procedure is called an ileorectal anastomosis. The rectum resumes its old job as a feces reservoir, and the patient defecates normally through the anus. This arrangement is seldom employed for ulcerative colitis patients, however, since the disease usually persists in the rectum. If the ileum is sutured directly to the anus, the procedure is called an ileoanal anastomosis. Because there is no rectum to collect feces, the surgeon must construct one. The pouch is made from loops of ileum that are slit along their length and stitched together. If not enough ileum remains from which to make a pouch, the surgeon pulls the end through the rectum and ties it directly to the anus, a procedure called an

endorectal ileal pull-through. The anastomosis procedures require two operations—one for the temporary stoma and construction of the pouch, one to connect the pouch and the rectum, or anus— to give the artificial rectum a chance to heal properly and so prevent leaking.

Colostomies feature somewhat more variety of stoma placement than ileostomies, but since removal of the rectum, sigmoid colon, or both are the most common reasons for the creation of the stoma, it is usually placed on the lower left of the abdomen, near the hipbone. If more of the colon is removed, the stoma may be higher up toward the rib cage. The operation begins much as for an ileostomy, except that

The Results of Colostomy

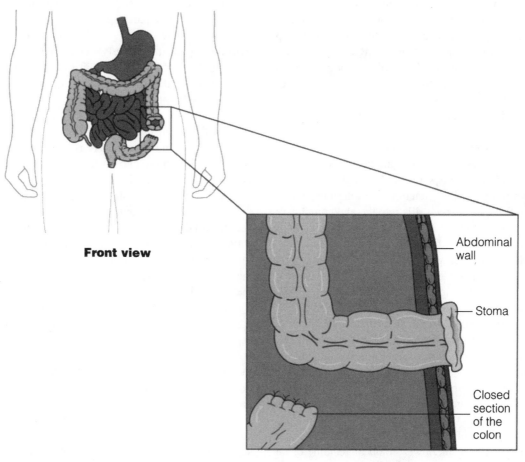

Front view

Abdominal wall

Stoma

Closed section of the colon

Side view

In colostomy, the colon is severed, the uppermost end of the intestine is extended through the abdominal wall to create a stoma through which fecal matter will be expelled, and the remaining section of the colon is closed off with sutures.

only the portion of the colon from the damaged or diseased area to the anus is removed; and the initial incision begins near that damaged section. The remaining, healthy colon is pulled through holes in the abdomen and skin, and its end is rolled back and fastened. The stoma protrudes out about two to three centimeters, so that an appliance for storing waste, if needed, can be attached.

There are three varieties of colostomy. The first, a single-barreled end colostomy, is the classical configuration. The rectum and anus are removed, and a single circular stoma, about 25 millimeters in diameter, is the permanent exit for stool. If, however, the surgeon believes that the colon and rectum can be rejoined, the rectum is left intact and closed. Either of two procedures can be used to give the colon a rest period between the removal of the diseased section and reconnection to the rectum. A double-barreled colostomy involves slicing through the colon and making side-by-side stomas from the ends. In a loop colostomy, the colon is not cut through; instead, a slit is made in one side, which is pulled through the skin and made into an oval stoma, usually larger than other stomas. In both cases, the upper colon discharges stool, and the lower length passes mucus.

USES AND COMPLICATIONS

Both colostomy and ileostomy are last-resort or emergency treatments. When a wound, such as one caused by a knife or gunshot, punctures the intestines, waste matter, full of bacteria, spills into the abdominal cavity. The severe infection that is sure to follow can kill a patient in days; thus, an emergency operation is required. The surgeon pulls healthy bowel through the abdominal wall and forms a temporary stoma (so that no more waste can leak out of the intestines), cleans out the spillage, and repairs the damaged bowel. In many cases, it is possible to reconnect the healthy bowel to the damaged portion after the wound has healed; at the same time, the stoma is closed, and the patient resumes defecation through the anus.

Emergency operations, however, account for only a small percentage of colostomies and ileostomies. About two-thirds of surgeries to form stomas are colostomies, most of which follow operations removing cancer (usually in the lower colon or rectum) or an obstruction. Diverticulitis, the inflammation of little pouches in the colon wall, may also require a colostomy; the diversion of wastes allow the inflammation to subside and the colon wall to heal, after which the stoma may be removed and the colon reconnected. Additionally, repair of some rare birth defects may entail a colostomy.

Ileostomies account for about one-quarter of stoma-creating procedures. Most are performed to eradicate ulcerative colitis, a chronic inflammation of the colon that begins in the rectum and may spread upward until the whole colon is involved. No drug or dietary treatment cures ulcerative colitis; when the condition becomes too unbearable for a patient to endure, an ileostomy removes the source of trouble: the colon itself. Long-standing ulcerative colitis is particularly likely to become cancerous, and the colon may be removed for that reason alone. Likewise, familial polyposis, a hereditary disease which dots the colon with toadstool-shaped lumps that are likely to become cancerous, may require removal of the colon and ileostomy.

Wounds, diverticulitis, familial polyposis, and birth defects, while not particularly rare, are the reasons for relatively few stomas. Together, colorectal cancer (particularly in the elderly) and ulcerative colitis (commonly disabling patients in their twenties) lead to hundreds of thousands of stoma operations yearly in the United States. As the average age of the population increases, so does the incidence of colon cancer and the need for ostomies.

Recovery from stoma surgery is prolonged. Surgery shocks the intestines, and several days pass before the gut resumes the wavelike contractions (called peristalsis) that enable digestion and push wastes toward the stoma. In the meantime, patients live on intravenous fluid nourishment. When bowel motion restarts and wastes begin coming through the stoma, the ileostomate must develop new habits to cope with the flow of wastes (which are always fluid because the ileum does not remove sufficient water to solidify the waste matter) by learning to attach and empty appliances and to keep the stoma clean. Colostomates, especially those who have lost only their sigmoid colon, can look forward to passing firm stools and may eventually be able to live without an appliance, but months of diarrhea occur before the bowel regains full operation.

Many complications can plague the new anatomy, some of which require surgical correction. The most serious include intestinal obstruction, scar adhesions that distort the shape of the bowel, retraction of the stoma, abscesses, prolapse (more of the bowel pushing out of the body), and kidney stones (which form because persistent diarrhea can dehydrate ostomates).

Less threatening, but demanding attention, are offensive odors, diarrhea, skin irritation, and bowel inflammation. Steady advances in surgical technique have lowered the complication rates, and few patients die because of the surgery.

Ostomates often must live with the stoma for the rest of their lives. Feces exit through the stoma, rather than the anus, forcing patients to "toilet train" themselves all over again. Some stomas are continent; that is, they hold back wastes until the patient is ready to defecate by draining them with a tube. Many, however, are not, and stool and gas steadily seep through the opening, where the waste matter is collected in an appliance, usually a plastic bag that seals over the stoma.

Having a plastic bag of stool on the abdomen and needing to empty it periodically to prevent it from leaking, instead of defecating by sitting down on a toilet, proves a difficult adjustment for some patients, both physically and psychologically. Several aid resources help new ostomates adjust. Specially trained registered nurses called enterostomal therapists teach patients how to manage their new stomas and how to attach appliances or insert catheters to drain continent stomas; they also help care for the stomas after the operation and periodically review their patients' progress. Gastroenterologists, physicians who specialize in the intestinal tract, can provide medical guidance and directly inspect the bowel wall behind the stoma through an endoscope, a flexible fiber-optic tube, should trouble develop. For those ostomates who feel isolated and depressed because of the stoma, the United Ostomy Association, a support group with branches throughout the United States, organizes social events and provides information and encouragement, often sending representatives to meet patients soon after surgery.

It is unfortunate that the widely felt repugnance for surgery involving the intestines and the social taboo against discussing defecation and excrement in polite conversation have obscured the triumph of stoma procedures. Much riskier and less rehabilitating surgeries, such as cardiac bypasses and organ transplantations, occupy the limelight, while ileostomies and colostomies, which prolong or improve more lives, receive scant popular attention. Medical journalists report that many patients, when told that they need a colostomy, know little or nothing of the procedure. After the doctor explains, they typically are dismayed and horrified. Nevertheless, few refuse the operation.

On the other hand, potential ileostomates who suffer from ulcerative colitis are almost always better informed and look forward to the operation as the end to years of intense abdominal distress and fears about cancer.

Out of the hospital, ostomates literally face a new and different life. As well as learning to handle appliances or irrigate artificial rectums, they must face the fact that a major organ of their bodies is changed. The need for the stoma may anger or depress them, and this fixation on the change, if unalleviated, can evolve into loss of self-esteem and attendant social withdrawal. Many ostomates experience guilt in the belief that the disease and stoma, as well as the effects of the stoma on their families, are somehow their own fault.

These reactions require social and psychological therapy, extending care well beyond that afforded by the surgeon and the hospital. Support groups and the enterostomal supply therapist supply the majority of this care, but occasionally professional psychological help is required. The repulsion that patients feel for stomas and the consequent chance of morbid psychological reactions have encouraged surgeons to prefer anastomoses to stomas when possible, even though anastomoses are more difficult, have higher failure rates, and require a longer recovery period.

Moreover, the impression lingers, encouraged by popular accounts of research linking diet to disease, that most serious intestinal maladies (cancer in particular) result solely from poor eating habits. This type of reasoning sometimes leads to the insinuation that a stoma amounts to a kind of punishment for those habits, which is a hasty and erroneous conclusion that can worsen the guilt some ostomates feel. More often, factors over which people may have no control, such as genetic susceptibility and environmental toxins, contribute to the diseases that make stomas necessary.

Fortunately, the great majority of ostomates do adjust to their new lives; they seldom have any other alternative. Providing that the original need for surgery has been eliminated—the cancer has been removed, for example—they can look forward to an undiminished life span and few if any restrictions upon appetite, sexual function, or exercise. About 95 percent of ostomates recover completely, returning to their previous occupations after recovery, and of these the majority believe themselves to be in good or excellent health. Without the operations, all of them would have led drastically impaired lives, and many would have died. The high success rate places the ileostomy and colostomy procedures among the ranks of surgical interventions that rescue the seriously ill from otherwise incurable organic diseases.

PERSPECTIVE AND PROSPECTS

Although drastic techniques requiring much skill from surgeons and stamina from patients, ostomies did not originate with modern medicine and its sophisticated technology for sustaining patients during operations. Some colostomies date from the last quarter of the eighteenth century. In the nineteenth century, the number of operations creating a stoma—then called "artificial" or "preternatural" anus—increased, although without antiseptic conditions or anesthesia a patient's chances for survival were not good. Surgeons sometimes placed the stomas on the back instead of the abdomen. In 1908, William Ernest Miles conducted the first operation to remove a cancerous rectum; since the patient's intestines were still moving waste matter, which needed an exit, Miles created a stoma, thereby establishing one of the most common surgeries of the twentieth century.

Still, colostomies and ileostomies did not proliferate until after World War II. Since then, refinements in surgical techniques and postoperative care have steadily reduced the chance of complications and the length of the recovery period. At the same time, several variations of permanent and temporary stomas have been developed.

Like many other extreme surgical interventions, the ileostomy and colostomy testify to the limits of biomedical knowledge: Most of these surgeries are performed because other remedies fail. Until researchers discover the mechanisms causing cancer, ulcerative colitis, and other deadly lower bowel diseases and develop nonsurgical cures, ileostomies and colostomies will remain common, especially among the elderly.

—*Roger Smith, Ph.D.*

See also Bypass surgery; Cancer; Colitis; Colon and rectal surgery; Colon cancer; Crohn's disease; Digestion; Diverticulitis and diverticulosis; Gastrectomy; Gastroenterology; Gastroenterology, pediatric; Gastrointestinal disorders; Gastrointestinal system; Intestinal disorders; Intestines.

FOR FURTHER INFORMATION:

Brandt, Lawrence J., and Penny Steiner-Grossman, eds. *Treating IBD: A Patient's Guide to the Medical and Surgical Management of Inflammatory Bowel Disease*. Reprint. New York: Raven Press, 1996. Although devoted to inflammatory bowel disease (IBD) in general, this book contains a section on surgical cures for ulcerative colitis and Crohn's disease. Types of ileostomy and anastomosis are described thoroughly in lay terms, and drawings and photographs depict the bowel reconstructions.

Fries, Colleen Farley. "Managing an Ostomy." *Nursing* 29, no. 8 (August, 1999): 26. Ostomies are used to assist patients with conditions like ulcerative colitis and bowel obstruction. The selection of an ostomy should be based on the patient's needs and is available in one- or two-piece devices and a number of sizes.

Kelly, Michael P. *Colitis*. New York: Routledge, 1992. Kelly, a sociologist, presents the experiences of colitis patients in England. Although his book passes quickly over types of surgical cures, he has included an excellent chapter on the psychological effects of the surgery on patients' lives.

Mullen, Barbara Dorr, and Kerry Anne McGinn. *The Ostomy Book: Living Comfortably with Colostomies, Ileostomies, and Urostomies*. Rev. ed. Palo Alto, Calif.: Bull, 1992. An amusingly written, inspirational account of the most typical of ostomy cases: a colostomy necessitated by rectal cancer. It is Mullen's own story, and she relates her emotional turmoil with candor, making her account invaluable reading for anyone who must undergo a colostomy.

Way, Lawrence W., ed. *Current Surgical Diagnosis and Treatment*. 11th ed. Norwalk, Conn.: Appleton and Lange, 1998. A reference work on general surgery for physicians, this tome is nevertheless comprehensible to laypersons familiar with medical terminology. Presents succinct overviews of the stoma procedures and their potential complications and contains finely detailed illustrations.

IMAGING AND RADIOLOGY

PROCEDURE

ANATOMY OR SYSTEM AFFECTED: All

SPECIALTIES AND RELATED FIELDS: Nuclear medicine, radiology

DEFINITION: Radiology is a branch of medicine that uses ionizing radiation (such as X rays) and non-ionizing radiation (such as ultrasound, microwaves, and magnetic fields) to create visual images that allow physicians to see the anatomy and morphology of organs, viscera, bones, blood vessels, and soft tissues.

KEY TERMS:

angiography: an imaging procedure in which a substance (contrast material) that is opaque to X rays is injected into blood vessels, allowing images of the opacified vessels to be made

computed tomography (CT) scanning: an imaging technique that uses X rays, sensitive radiation detectors, and computers to produce images of the entire body for diagnosis

detector: a device or substance that can sense the presence of ionizing radiation and produce an indication of its presence for visual display; examples are photographic film, certain phosphors such as calcium tungstate, and crystals such as sodium iodide

ionizing radiation (X rays): a form of electromagnetic radiation that occurs in a wide range of wavelengths, from about 0.04 Å to more than 1,000 Å; the useful range for radiographic imaging is between 0.1 Å and 0.5 Å (the symbol Å stands for a scientific unit of measure called the angstrom; one angstrom is one one-hundred-millionth of a centimeter in length)

magnetic resonance imaging (MRI): an imaging technique that uses microwave energy, powerful magnetic fields, and computers to produce images of the entire body for diagnosis; MRI is particularly useful in examining soft tissue structures such as the brain, the spinal cord, the liver, the pancreas, and the spleen

ultrasonography: an imaging technique that uses ultrasonic waves to produce diagnostic images of certain soft tissue structures in the body; it is also used to study dynamic processes such as blood flow

X-ray tube: a high-voltage electronic device used to produce X rays; X-ray tubes are used in X-ray machines, fluoroscopes, and CT scanners

INDICATIONS AND PROCEDURES

Diagnostic radiology uses X rays and other forms of radiation, such as ultrasound, microwaves, and powerful magnetic fields, to produce images of structures and processes in the human body. X rays are a form of ionizing electromagnetic radiation. The term "ionizing" means being able to add or remove electrons from atoms, thus producing ions. An ion is an atom that has had one or more electrons added or removed. Other forms of electromagnetic radiation that are not ionizing are visible light, infrared light, ultraviolet light, and radio waves. Some other forms of ionizing radiation are cosmic rays and gamma rays. The factors that distinguish one type of electromagnetic radiation from another are frequency and wavelength.

X rays can penetrate solid matter. When an object or individual is exposed to X rays, that exposure produces ions in the atoms of the object or person exposed. This is one of the principal reasons that X-ray exposure is harmful to living beings. When X-ray diagnostic radiology procedures are used judiciously and applied by professionals, however, the benefit of their use far outweighs the risk factors associated with exposure.

The diagnostic radiology procedures with which people are most familiar are chest X rays and dental X rays. Most radiographic examinations are performed by registered radiologic technologists. The examinations are then interpreted by a physician specializing in diagnostic radiology. These physicians are called radiologists.

When a technologist takes an X ray, he or she places a cassette containing radiographic film beneath the area of interest of the patient being examined. The technologist then positions the X-ray tube directly over the same area. After adjusting technical factors and the size of the X-ray field, the technologist produces an X-ray exposure. X rays emanating from the X-ray tube pass through the patient's body and are selectively absorbed by the tissues of varying density through which they pass. When they exit the patient's body, they form an "image in space" composed of differential absorption patterns. When the X rays encounter dense tissue such as bone, they are mostly absorbed. When they encounter soft tissue such as muscle or fat, they pass through easily with little or no absorption. It is this process that produces the differential absorption pattern. As the X rays pass through the cassette, the absorption pattern is captured by the film in the cassette. When the film is processed, a permanent image of that differential absorption pattern is produced, resulting in what is commonly called an "X ray" but is more properly called a radiograph. The information contained in the radiographs that radiologic technologists produce is interpreted by radiologists when they "read" them. Their "readings" are dictated, recorded, and transcribed. The transcription process results in a final written report that is sent to the physician who referred the patient to radiology for the examination.

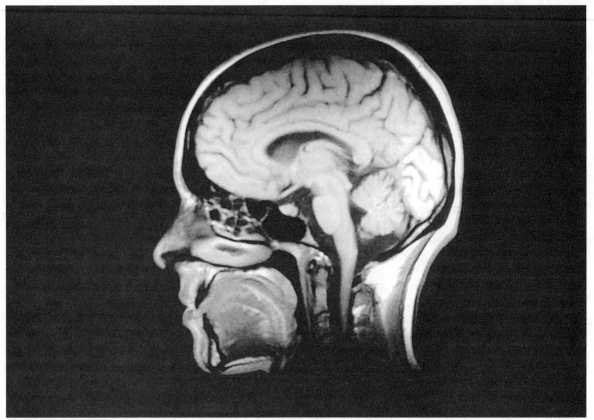

An MRI allows physicians to visualize soft tissues inside the body, such as the brain and nasopharyngeal tissues. (Digital Stock)

Newer radiographic techniques employ electronic detectors and photostimulable phosphors instead of film to capture radiographic images. A photostimulable phosphor is a substance whose atomic structure becomes semipermanently altered when exposed to ionizing radiation. Once altered, the phosphor can be scanned electronically. This scanning process records the information contained in the altered atoms of the phosphor and makes it possible to produce images that can be displayed and viewed on television monitors and manipulated with computers. If desired, these same images can be recorded on film.

Fluoroscopy is a procedure that uses X rays to view and record dynamic processes such as swallowing, the movement of food through the gastrointestinal tract, defecation, and urination. A fluoroscope is an X-ray machine configured with an X-ray tube and an image intensifier that are mechanically aligned one behind the other. The arrangement allows the user (usually a radiologist) to vary the distance between the X-ray tube and the image intensifier while ensuring that they re-

main constantly aligned. It also allows the user to move the fluoroscope up and down, positioning it at any point between the patient's head and feet. An image intensifier is a large electronic tube that contains phosphors that produce electrons and light when bombarded by X rays. When X rays pass through the input phosphor, electrons are produced. Those electrons are then accelerated through the tube and focused on the output phosphor, resulting in substantial amplification. When a patient is placed between the X-ray tube and image intensifier and the X-ray beam is turned on, an "image in space" is once again produced. This image is captured by the image intensifier and recorded on the output phosphor. A television camera is focused on the output phosphor, allowing the fluoroscopic image to be displayed and viewed on a television monitor. When the radiologist turns on the X-ray beam, he or she is able to see inside the patient. The fluoroscope is connected to an X-ray table, and fluoroscopic examinations can be conducted with the patient in a standing position, a recumbent position, and positions between standing and recumbent. All these procedures represent "traditional" radiograph imaging.

More sophisticated imaging techniques involve the use of powerful computers and different means of signal detection. Computed tomography (CT) scanning is one such technique. A CT scanner employs an array of multiple detectors that sense discrete levels of radiation passing through a patient's body. The X-ray beam is moving, producing a pattern of signals that represent the absorption levels of a single point from different perspectives. This entire process produces millions of signals. The computer uses the information contained in those signals in ways that ultimately allow the system to draw a picture of what the patient's anatomy looks like. This process is very different from traditional radiographic imaging because, while traditional imaging techniques produce images that are direct representations of the anatomy examined, CT yields pictures that are drawn by the computer. This is a subtle but important distinction. When one looks at a traditional radiograph, such as a chest X ray, one sees a one-to-one analogue representation of the anatomy. In that sense, it is very much like a photograph. When one looks at a CT scan, however, it is very much like looking at an artist's rendition of the anatomy. The artist, in this case, is the computer that is part of the CT scanner.

This is also true for imaging modalities such as magnetic resonance imaging (MRI) and positron emission tomography (PET) scanning.

Magnetic resonance imaging (MRI) is one of radiology's newest modalities. It does not use ionizing radiation. Instead, it relies on powerful magnetic fields in the range of 0.3 to 2.0 kilogauss. (A gauss is a unit of magnetic strength. The earth's magnetic field exerts a force of approximately 1 gauss.)

The key components of an MRI scanner are a cylindrical magnet large enough to accommodate a patient's body, a powerful and highly controllable radio-frequency generator, and a computer. For an MRI scan, the patient is positioned inside the magnet. Because the magnetic field is so strong, all the hydrogen atoms in the patient's body align themselves with the magnetic field. In order to visualize what this means, imagine that each hydrogen atom is a tiny arrow. When not in a powerful magnetic field, all those little arrows are in disarray, pointing in every possible direction. Since the human body is mostly water, and that water is composed of one part oxygen and two parts hydrogen, innumerable arrows are involved.

When the patient is placed in the magnet, those arrows point in the same direction. Next, the radio-frequency generator is turned on and tuned to a highly specific frequency that will cause all the arrows to vibrate or resonate. When that happens, their orientation is changed—for example, from pointing up to pointing down. Then the radio-frequency pulse is turned off and the arrows (hydrogen atoms) once again align themselves with the magnetic field. As they do, they emit tiny pulses of extremely faint energy. Because the magnetic field is so powerful, the magnet in essence listens for and is able to hear, or detect, those pulses. The information contained in those hundreds of millions of tiny pulses is sent to the computer, which then processes it. Much as with the CT scanner, the computer performs hundreds of millions of calculations. Then, using powerful mathematical algorithms, it draws a representation of what the tissue should look like based on the information gleaned from all those pulses. The information is displayed on television monitors and can be manipulated in innumerable ways.

USES AND COMPLICATIONS

A common examination that employs both fluoroscopy and radiography is the upper gastrointestinal tract examination, or upper GI, which is used to examine the esophagus, stomach, and small bowel.

During an examination of the upper gastrointestinal tract, the X-ray table is put in an upright position. The patient is positioned on a foot rest at the bottom of the table, which places the patient between the X-ray tube and the image intensifier. A technologist then hands the patient a cup of barium sulfate liquid, which is opaque to X rays and which the radiologist can see with the fluoroscope. The radiologist asks the patient to drink the barium sulfate. As the patient drinks, the radiologist turns on the X-ray beam and watches the barium as it moves from the patient's mouth, through the esophagus, and into the stomach. The radiologist can move the fluoroscope and follow the path of the barium. While watching the barium move, the radiologist can also capture hard-copy images, either electronically or on film. During an upper GI, the radiologist also watches the stomach empty into the small bowel and records hard-copy images of the process. The radiologist can record the dynamic aspects of the examination on videotape.

During a fluoroscopic examination of the colon, or lower intestinal tract, the patient is asked to lie down on the X-ray table. The technologist and radiologist then administer an enema, using barium sulfate. The procedure is that used in the upper gastrointestinal examination. As the barium fills the patient's colon, the radiologist uses the fluoroscope to watch the process and record hard-copy images. After the procedure has been completed, the radiologist interprets the hard-copy images.

Fluoroscopy is also used to guide radiologists when they are attempting to perform biopsy procedures. A biopsy is the acquisition of a small piece of tissue that can be examined by a pathologist for the presence of disease or abnormality. Radiologists usually use specially designed needles that can be inserted into the tissue or organ of interest. A fluoroscope is extremely helpful in achieving the proper placement of biopsy needles.

Fluoroscopy is commonly used during surgical procedures to provide "X-ray control." This means that it is used to guide the placement of such items as the pins used to fix fractures and artificial hip and knee replacements.

Angiography, or examination of the blood vessels, is the most complex procedure performed using conventional radiographic and fluoroscopic imaging techniques. When doing an angiogram, a radiologist injects contrast material into the vessels of interest. Using a fluoroscope, the radiologist positions a small tube called a catheter in the patient's femoral artery through a small puncture in the groin. Once the end of the tube is in the area of interest, the radiologist injects a contrast material that opacifies the vessels being examined.

Since blood is constantly coursing through a patient's blood vessels, it is necessary to inject quickly an adequate amount of contrast material (a bolus) to opacify the vessels being studied for several seconds. Of critical importance to the angiographic process is the ability to capture and record images of those vessels as they fill with and subsequently empty of contrast material.

This is accomplished using serial film changers that can move film rapidly. The film changer is placed under the area of interest and an X-ray tube is placed above. The X-ray machine and film changer are synchronized with a power injector that is used to deliver the bolus of contrast material. When everything has been positioned properly and all the technical radiographic exposure factors have been set, the angiographic series is triggered. Once triggered, the injector

injects the contrast material, the X-ray machine produces a series of exposures, and the serial film changer moves film in and out of the area being examined. The result is a series of radiographs that show the vessels filling with contrast material and subsequently emptying.

Digital subtraction angiography (DSA) is a type of angiography that uses a fluoroscope instead of a film changer. The television camera attached to the fluoroscope is specially designed to capture images and send them to a computer. The computer then digitizes the images, essentially turning them into pictures made up of hundreds of thousands of tiny rectangular picture elements called pixels. This digitizing process makes possible powerful image manipulation, because each pixel can be analyzed and controlled by the computer. Before injecting the contrast material, using the DSA machine, the technologist captures a series of images with no contrast material. Contrast material is then injected, and the angiographic series is captured. Since the computer associated with the DSA device provides such exquisite control of each image, it is possible to electronically subtract information that is extraneous or that blocks what the radiologist wishes to see. Bony structures such as the skull and the spine often get in the way of vessels radiologists want to see on angiographic series. Using the DSA computer, the technologist simply subtracts those bony structures electronically. The result is quite spectacular. Only the vessels are displayed on the subtracted images.

During angiography, radiologists are also able to perform therapeutic procedures. Sometimes, patients' vessels become narrowed, or occluded, from the buildup on those vessel walls of fatty deposits known as plaque. Using a special catheter with a small, sausage-shaped balloon on the end, a radiologist is able to position the balloon in the area of occlusion. When the balloon is gently inflated, the plaque is compressed, thus opening the previously occluded vessel and allowing blood to flow freely once again. The procedure is known as angioplasty. Before angioplasty became available, patients with occluded vessels had no choice but to have surgery to correct the occlusion.

The contrast sensitivity of the CT scanning process is orders of magnitude greater than that available with conventional film radiography. To gain an understanding of how and why that is important, consider that a conventional X ray of the skull will yield only information about the skull, whereas a CT scan of the skull will also provide much information about the brain. The introduction of CT scanning to radiology's array of imaging modalities was a watershed event for medicine and humanity. CT scanning has become so integral to the practice of medicine that it is considered blatant malpractice not to order a CT scan on a patient who arrives in a hospital emergency room with severe head trauma.

PERSPECTIVE AND PROSPECTS

X rays were discovered by Wilhelm Conrad Röntgen in 1895. With that discovery, the art and science of radiology and radiography were born, changing forever the way in which medicine is practiced. It also expanded the horizons of medicine and health care far beyond what anyone, at the time, imagined possible. Since 1895, radiology has become highly technology intensive and capital intensive. It advances when its practitioners push the edge of the technological envelope, which is defined by the branches of science that form the foundation of radiology.

Radiology has become so integral to medicine and health care that, without it, contemporary medical efforts would be, at best, primitive. Early developments allowed physicians to see inside their patients' bodies for the first time without surgery. While late nineteenth century imaging techniques were crude by today's standards, they nevertheless permanently changed the way in which physicians practiced medicine. As the capability of medical imaging expanded, physicians came to rely even more heavily on the information that it made available. Each new modality yields more and better information that physicians can use to make more accurate diagnoses.

Imaging techniques are beginning to take the place of traditional surgical procedures. New developments will continue to rely heavily on computers. As the speed and power of computers increase, radiology's horizons will expand further. The general practice of medicine is so intertwined with the kinds of images that radiology provides that, without it, physicians could not practice acceptable medicine.

—Stephen J. Hage

See also Angiography; Angioplasty; Computed tomography (CT) scanning; Magnetic resonance imaging (MRI); Mammography; Noninvasive tests; Nuclear medicine; Nuclear radiology; Positron emission tomography (PET) scanning; Radiation therapy; Radiopharmaceuticals; Ultrasonography.

FOR FURTHER INFORMATION:

Cullinan, John Edward. *Illustrated Guide to X-Ray Technics*. 2d ed. Philadelphia: J. B. Lippincott, 1980. An excellent and extremely well written text that thoroughly covers the information required by any working radiologic technologist. It is written in easy-to-understand prose, and its approach to the subject is ultimately practical.

Ravin, Carl E., ed. *Imaging and Invasive Radiology in the Intensive Care Unit*. New York: Churchill Livingstone, 1993. This text addresses critical care management using diagnostic imaging techniques and interventional radiology. Includes a bibliography and an index.

Snopek, Albert Michael. *Fundamentals of Special Radiographic Procedures*. 4th ed. Philadelphia: W. B. Saunders, 1999. The focus of this text is "special procedures," which are defined as procedures that are much more complex than normal radiographic procedures. Examples are angiography, myelography, cardiac angiography, bronchography, arthrography, and hysterosalpingography.

IMMUNE SYSTEM

BIOLOGY

ANATOMY OR SYSTEM AFFECTED: Blood, cells, circulatory system, glands, liver, lymphatic system, spleen

SPECIALTIES AND RELATED FIELDS: Cytology, hematology, immunology, microbiology, preventive medicine, serology

DEFINITION: A system—including the thymus, spleen, lymphatic system, and specialized cells—that protects the body from foreign substances.

KEY TERMS:

antibody: any of the proteins produced in the body during an immune response; recognizes and attacks foreign antigen substances

antigen: a substance within the human body recognized as foreign either by antibodies or by special immune cells; the cause behind the stimulation of the immune response

autoimmunity: an abnormal immune reaction against antigens

immunosuppression: a decrease in the effectiveness of the immune system

pathogen: any disease-causing organism, including a virus, bacterium, protozoan, mold or yeast, or other parasite

STRUCTURE AND FUNCTIONS

The immune system is capable of recognizing and identifying many different substances foreign to the human body. To function properly, this system must receive, interpret, and transmit large amounts of information about invaders from outside or within the body. These constant and ever-changing threats to the body must be met and destroyed by one complex system—namely, the human immune system. Many organs and parts of the body play a major role in maintaining resistance; some have more important roles than others, but all parts must work in unison. The circulatory and lymphatic systems, along with specific organs, are of primary importance in the overall workings of the immune system.

Blood. Besides the outer protective layer of the skin and mucous membranes, the first line of defense in the immune system includes the blood in the circulatory system. About 50 percent of human blood is made up of a fluid called plasma, which contains water, proteins, carbohydrates, vitamins, hormones, and cellular waste. The other half of blood is composed of white cells, red cells, and platelets. The red blood cells, called erythrocytes, are responsible for moving oxygen from the lungs to the other parts of the body. The special platelet cells, called thrombocytes, enable the blood to form clots, thus preventing severe bleeding. An unborn child produces red and white blood cells in the spleen and liver, while a newborn makes blood in the center of bones, called the marrow. After maturity, all red and most white blood cells are produced in the bone marrow. Although the red cells and platelets are vital, it is the white cells that play a major role in the immune system.

In a broad sense, white blood cells surround and engulf foreign matter and adjacent dying cells in a process called phagocytosis. The function is possible since the white blood cells can move, unlike red corpuscles, by pushing their bodies out and pulling forward. Red corpuscles move because of the flow of the blood within the circulatory system. White blood cells move in the lymph vessels, where they work to defend the body against disease, but are also transported through the blood. Bacteria and other foreign material can remain alive within a white corpuscle, but sometimes the corpuscle dies from the toxins produced by the bacteria. The resulting formation of pus is actually an accumulation of dead white blood cells. At other times, the white corpuscles win and the foreign matter is destroyed.

Three major types of white blood cells, known collectively as leukocytes, are involved in immune responses. All three—granulocytes, monocytes, and lymphocytes—arise from areas in either bone marrow, the spleen, or the liver.

The granulocytes, each of which is about twice the size of a red blood cell, originate from red bone marrow and live only about twelve hours. Under the classification of granulocytes, distinct cells have different structures, sizes, and shapes. These specialized granulocytes include the neutrophils, eosinophils, and basophils. None of these cells has a specific memory for future immune responses. The neutrophil granulocyte eats and digests small foreign matter with the help of special enzymes. Between 40 and 75 percent of the white blood cells in the human body are neutrophils. When these highly mobile neutrophil cells arrive at an injury site, they burst, releasing their enzymes and melting away the surrounding tissues. Eosinophils are similar to neutrophils but seem to be specialized in fighting infection caused by parasites, because of the seven toxic proteins that they use to fight. They are also effective against fungal, bacterial, viral, or protozoan infections. Basophils, which are smaller in size, move from the bone marrow through the body and act as a control by preventing overreactions during an immune response. Basophils prevent coagulation, but they cannot destroy foreign matter. These cells account for less than 1 percent of the white blood cells found in the blood.

The second group of leukocytes includes the monocytes, the largest cells found in the blood. Monocytes are two to three times as large as red cells, yet they are not very numerous, making up to 3 to 9 percent of all the leukocytes in the blood. After only a few days in the blood, they move to areas between tissues. Over the course of months or years, the monocytes enlarge ten times in size in order to specialize in phagocytosis. After this growth, they are called macrophages. They are also referred to as terminal cells since they cannot divide, and thus do not reproduce.

The third type of leukocyte, and the most sophisticated of the white blood cells, are called lymphocytes because they come from the lymph system as well as bone marrow. The T lymphocytes, which are primarily responsible for immunity, can change into helper, killer, and suppressor cells. Besides being able to recognize foreign matter precisely, they can live freely in the blood, grow larger and divide, and then change back to their original form after working against the invader. Lymphocytes circulate throughout the body, moving from the bloodstream through the lymph fluid and back into the blood. The two major types of lymphocytes are T lymphocytes (also called T cells) and B lymphocytes (also called B cells). Both T and B cells can recognize foreign matter and hook onto it. Some of these special "memory" cells remain in the body for life, preventing a specific invader from causing illness when it is encountered again in the future. These specialized cells must have a way to travel through the body; one of these transport systems is the lymphatic system.

The lymphatic system. This system is a closed network of vessels that help in circulating fluids from the body and returning them to the bloodstream. The lymphatic system also defends against disease-causing foreign materials, known as antigens. The smallest components of the lymph system are the lymphatic capillaries that run parallel to the blood capillaries. The fluid inside these capillaries, which has come across the thin wall membrane from tissues all across the body, is called lymph. These capillaries merge into larger lymphatic vessels, which then merge into a type of collecting area called a lymph node. The lymph fluid is drained into trunks that join one of two collecting ducts. The larger left thoracic duct collects lymph from the upper arm, head, and neck of the left side of the body before emptying into a vein near the neck and shoulder. The right lymphatic duct does the same for the right side of the body. After leaving the collecting ducts, the lymph fluid becomes part of the blood plasma in the veins and returns to the right atrium of the heart. Lymph does not flow like blood in veins and arteries; instead, it is controlled by muscular activity.

The spleen. This largest lymphatic organ is located in the upper left part of the abdominal cavity, behind the stomach and under the diaphragm. The hollow spaces within the spleen are filled with blood, making it soft and elastic. The white blood cells in the lining of these hollow cavities engulf and destroy foreign materials, as well as damaged red blood cells that pass through the spleen.

The thymus. This gland is located between the lungs and above the heart, just behind the upper part of the breastbone. It contains large numbers of white cells; some are inactive, but others develop and leave the thymus to become functional in the immune system.

The liver. Located in the upper right part of the abdominal cavity below the diaphragm, the liver is well protected by the ribs. Since it is the largest gland in the body, it plays a major role in metabolism while also aiding the body's ability to clot blood. In addition, various liver cells, called macrophages, help in destroying damaged red blood cells. The liver's connection to the immune system is its ability to also destroy foreign substances through phagocytosis.

Bone marrow. Marrow is located in the center of bones. It can be divided into two types, red or yellow marrow. It is the red marrow that aids in the formation of white and red blood cells. The yellow marrow stores fat and is not involved in producing blood cells. Some white blood cells come from bone marrow cells. They are released into the blood and are carried to the thymus gland, where they undergo special processing that changes them into T lymphocytes (the letter *T* shows that they came from the thymus gland). The other lymphocytes that do not reach the thymus after leaving the bone marrow are named B lymphocytes (*B* because they came from bone marrow). These B lymphocytes are abundant in lymph nodes, the spleen, bone marrow, secretory glands, intestinal lining, and in the reticuloendothelial tissue.

THE RESPONSES OF THE IMMUNE SYSTEM

Failures of the immune system can lead to devastating diseases, either because the immune system attacks itself or because it fails to defend against outside foreign antigen matter. An antigen can be any substance that stimulates the body to fight, ranging from a bacterial infection to the virus that causes acquired immunodeficiency syndrome (AIDS).

When the body fights against an antigen, the immune system can produce two types of response, either a cellular immune response or a humoral immune response. The cellular response involves specific types of cells that recognize, attack, and destroy the invading antigen. The humoral immune response is actually the body's main defense against a bacterium, virus, or fungus in the blood or body fluids. This response involves various chemicals in the bloodstream that fight against the invaders.

Another way of looking at how the body fights to keep itself healthy is to separate the immune responses into either primary or secondary responses. The second time that a given antigen enters the body, the immune system attacks with what is called the secondary immune response stored in special immune memories, making it faster and more extensive than the primary response that occurred when the antigen was first encountered. This immune memory must be built for each antigen before the body becomes immune to the wide variety of diseases and conditions to which one is exposed on a daily basis.

The body begins to build this memory prior to birth by making an inventory of all the molecules within the body. Foreign substances not in this memory are considered to be antigens, which will activate an immune response. When an antigen is first encountered, the primary response occurs, producing lymphocytes that are sensitized to the invader. Many types of lymphocytes can respond in order to create the appropriate antibody molecules, which are then released into the lymph and transported to the blood. This process may last several weeks. During this primary immune response, the B cells and T cells serve as memory cells. Because a memory for the antigen has been stored, if this antigen is encountered in the future the memory cells can react more quickly and effectively. In this secondary immune response, the antibodies are ready to react by attaching themselves to the surfaces of the antigens. There must be a specific type of antibody produced for every type of antigen. These new antibodies may survive only a few months, but the memory cells live much longer.

There are four main ways that an antibody can bind to an antigen. The antibody can pull together clusters of invading organisms to prevent the antigens from spreading. Another possibility is for this special component of the blood to punch a hole in the invader and destroy it. The antibody can also combine with the antigen, which makes it easier to destroy. In the case of a virus or a toxin, the antibody can neutralize the harmful activity by covering the outside of the antigen. With so many ways for an antibody to attach to an antigen, it is equally important for the antibody memory to be established. It is this special memory that leads to future immunity.

These memory cells are responsible for the four different types of immunity, two of which are acquired actively and two of which are acquired passively. The first type is naturally acquired active immunity, which results after the body is exposed to a live pathogen and develops the disease. The second type is artificially acquired active immunity, such as that gained after a vaccination. The immune response is triggered after an injection of weakened or dead pathogens is received, but the body does not suffer the severe symptoms of the disease. An example would be a smallpox vaccination. The third type of immunity is artificially acquired passive immunity, gained through an injection of prepared antibodies. This method is considered passive since the antibodies, called gamma globulin, were made by another person. This type of immunity usually does not last more than a few weeks, and the person will be susceptible to that pathogen in the future. Naturally ac-

In the News: MHCPs, Immune Responses, and Genes

The cellular immune system operates due to complex interactions between several kinds of leukocytes. Its first step is engulfment of an antigen molecule by an amoeba-like macrophage. Engulfment leads the macrophage partially to digest the antigen and causes attachment of antigen fragments to its surface. Fragment attachment is due to Class I major histocompatibility proteins (I-MHCPs). All the I-MHCPs holding an antigen fragment can attach to certain immature T cells. Once such a T cell and I-MHCP-antigen complex hook up, the T cell reproduces many times.

Its offspring, killer T cells, recognize the antigen whenever it is associated with invader cells, bind to such cells, and destroy them. Destruction is caused by adding a substance called perforin to the cell membrane of a cell to be killed. Perforin

produces abnormal cell membrane pores that cause cells to burst. The huge importance of the cellular immune system and I-MHCPs has been shown in recent times by the epidemic of fatal human acquired immunodeficiency syndrome (AIDS), which kills T cells.

Class II MHCPs (II-MHCPs) interact similarly in antibody production by the humoral immune system. Understanding of the genes used in production of the I-MHCPs and the II-MHCPs has led to great hope for methods to control their production, possibilities for eventual cure of acquired immunodeficiency syndrome (AIDS), emerging cancer treatments, and better understanding of the production of antibodies.

—*Sanford S. Singer, Ph.D.*

quired passive immunity occurs when the antibodies pass to the fetus from the mother, but it includes only those antibodies available in the blood of the mother. This process gives an infant certain short-term immunities for the first year of life.

These types of immunity are usually desirable, but there are occasions when an immune response is not wanted, such as after an organ transplant. When tissue or organs are transplanted from one person to another, the body may reject the foreign tissue, triggering an immune response and possibly destroying the new organ. Consequently, attempts are made to match the tissue between recipient and donor. In an effort to halt the immune response, immunosuppressive drugs are given to interfere with the recipient's ability to form antibodies, and drugs can be administered to destroy the lymphocytes that produce these antibodies. Unfortunately, the recipient is often left unprotected against infections, since the immune system is not functioning normally.

Perspective and Prospects

In the same way that the discovery of penicillin shocked the world, immunology has created endless possibilities in medicine. When surgeons found that they could transplant an organ from one person to another, the interest in immunology exploded.

This field of medicine has discovered that the immune system's power and effectiveness can be lessened because of several factors. Improper diet, stress, disease, and excessive physical activity levels can depress the immune system. Other factors that can modify immunity include age, genetics, and metabolic and environmental factors. The anatomical, physiological, and microbial factors are shown in the susceptibility of the young and the very old to infections. For the young, the system is immature, while the aged have suffered a lifetime of assaults from pathogens. The impact of psychological stress is difficult to measure, yet it holds the potential for negatively affecting the immune system.

Before immunology can be fully understood, more knowledge must be gained about how antibodies are made and how they develop memories. Lymphocytes must be examined to discover what role they play in the immune response. Studies must look at not only the whole picture of the immune system but also its smaller parts—the organs and how each participates. Such studies could lead to better success in transplanting these organs. Unanswered questions remain about how the immune system relates to other body systems. The relationships among the brain and nervous system, hormones, and the respiratory system leave many areas ripe for further study.

Additional information is needed on defects in the system, as are explanations for its dysfunctions. With greater knowledge of immunology, it may be possible to conquer AIDS, allergies, and asthma and to develop birth control methods based on the immune response. Doctors may be able to cure cancer, diabetes, herpes, infertility, multiple sclerosis, and rheumatoid arthritis. The possibilities are endless and could also include perfecting transplants of organs and skin grafts and preventing birth defects and even obesity. Through human gene therapy, those at risk for genetic disorders could be diagnosed and those with existing genetic conditions could be treated. Genetically engineered drugs and gene replacement therapy could relieve the stress on the human immune system. Until these methods become feasible, however, individuals must protect the natural immunity supplied by their bodies.

—*Maxine M. Urton, Ph.D.*

See also Acquired immunodeficiency syndrome (AIDS); Allergies; Antioxidants; Autoimmune disorders; Blood and blood disorders; Bone marrow transplantation; Cells; Chemotherapy; Circulation; Cytology; Cytopathology; Dialysis; Endocrinology; Endocrinology, pediatric; Glands; Healing; Hematology; Hematology, pediatric; Homeopathy; Hormones; Host-defense mechanisms; Human immunodeficiency virus (HIV); Immunization and vaccination; Immunodeficiency disorders; Immunology; Immunopathology; Infection; Liver; Lymphatic system; Multiple chemical sensitivity syndrome; Oncology; Preventive medicine; Serology; Skin; Stress reduction; Systems and organs; Transfusion; Transplantation.

For Further Information:

Berger, Stuart. *Dr. Berger's Immune Power Diet.* New York: New American Library, 1985. Although most of the text covers special diets, information about the workings of the immune system is spread throughout. The author explains how to build an effective immune system through a special diet.

Hole, John W. *Essentials of Human Anatomy and Physiology.* 6th ed. Dubuque, Iowa: Wm. C. Brown, 1993. One entire chapter is devoted to the lymphatic system, and another covers the blood. A bit technical, but a comprehensive source for those interested in this topic.

Life, Death, and the Immune System. New York: W. H. Freeman, 1994. This comprehensive collection of articles from *Scientific American* provides basic information and research directions on AIDS, autoimmune disorders, and allergies, as well as an excellent discussion of the immune system in general.

Marieb, Elaine N. *Essentials of Human Anatomy and Physiology.* 6th ed. Redwood City, Calif.: Benjamin/Cummings, 2000. This introductory anatomy and physiology textbook, easily accessible to those with little science background, is richly illustrated with diagrams and photographs, which help to illuminate body systems and processes.

Mizel, Steven, and Peter Jaret. *In Self-Defense.* San Diego, Calif.: Harcourt Brace Jovanovich, 1985. The layperson's guide for understanding the components of the immune system. A helpful glossary of terms is included.

IMMUNIZATION AND VACCINATION
PROCEDURE

ANATOMY OR SYSTEM AFFECTED: Blood, cells, immune system

SPECIALTIES AND RELATED FIELDS: Immunology, microbiology, preventive medicine, public health

DEFINITION: Immunization is the process by which exposure to an infectious agent or chemical confers an organism with resistance to that agent; vaccination involves the injection of a killed or attenuated microorganism, with the intention of inducing immunity.

KEY TERMS:

active immunity: immunity resulting from antibody production following exposure to an antigen

antibody: a protein secreted by lymphocytes in response to antigen stimuli, such as bacteria or viruses; also referred to as immunoglobulin

antigen: any chemical substance that stimulates the production of antibodies

attenuation: the weakening or elimination of the pathogenic properties of a microorganism; ideally, the organism is rendered harmless

passive immunity: immunity resulting from the introduction of preformed antibodies

serotype: a subgroup member within a larger species that is similar, but not identical, to other members of the species

toxoid: a toxin that has been chemically treated to eliminate its toxic properties but that retains the same antigens as the original

vaccinia: a virus which causes a poxlike illness in cattle (cowpox) and serves as smallpox vaccine in humans because of its similarity to the smallpox virus

THE FUNDAMENTALS OF IMMUNIZATION

The major day-to-day function of the immune response is to protect the body from infection. Exposure to foreign antigens such as infectious agents results in the stimulation of either of two components of the immune system: the humoral (or antibody) immune response or the cellular immune response. Although no clear division exists between these two facets of the immune system, the antibody response deals primarily with organisms such as bacteria that live outside the cell. The cellular response deals primarily with microbes that live within a cell, such as intracellular bacteria or viral-infected cells.

A specialized class of white cells called B lymphocytes carries out the production of antibodies. Stimulation of these cells results from a complicated interaction between a variety of cells, including antigen-presenting cells (macrophage and dendritic cells) and both T and B lymphocytes. The response is specific in that each type of T or B cell can interact with only a single antigen. The B cell that produces antibodies against a particular characteristic or shape on the surface of a bacterium reacts only with that particular determinant. In turn, the antibodies secreted by that B cell can interact only with specific determinants.

Antibodies secreted by B cells are themselves inert proteins. A variety of effects can result, however, when an antibody binds an antigen. The specific results depend on the nature of the antigen. For example, binding of an antibody to a toxin results in the neutralization of that substance. If the antigen is on the surface of a bacterial cell, the antibody can act as a flag that attracts other chemicals circulating in the blood. The technical term for an antibody bound to a bacterium is an opsonin. The antibody-bacterium complex becomes much more likely to be ingested and destroyed by a specialized cell called a phagocyte than if the antibody were not present. Likewise, if the antigen is an extracellular virus particle, binding of the antibody may inhibit the ability of the virus to infect a cell.

The cellular immune system also reacts in a specific manner. A subclass of T lymphocytes called cytotoxic T cells reacts with specific antigenic deter-

Immunization and the Action of Vaccines

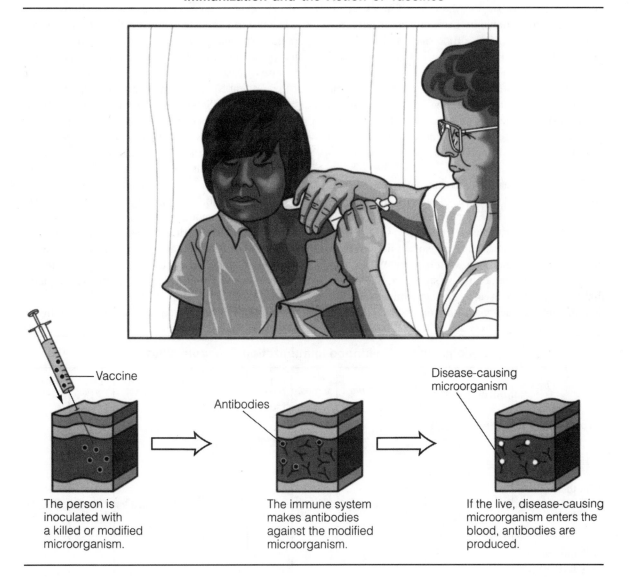

Vaccine

The person is
inoculated with
a killed or modified
microorganism.

Antibodies

The immune system
makes antibodies
against the modified
microorganism.

Disease-causing
microorganism

If the live, disease-causing
microorganism enters the
blood, antibodies are
produced.

minants on the surface of infected cells. When the T cells bind to a target, the result is the local release of toxic chemicals that ultimately kill the target.

The development of vaccines against specific infectious microbial agents resulted in the control or elimination of many diseases caused by these agents. The first formal vaccine developed for the prevention of disease was that used by Edward Jenner against smallpox during the 1790's. Another century would pass before the molecular basis for vaccine function would begin to be understood.

Immunity to an antigen or disease may be induced using either of two methods. If preformed antibodies produced in another human or animal are inoculated into an individual, the result is passive immunity. Passive immunity can be advantageous in that the recipient achieves immunity in a short period of time. For example, if a person has been exposed to a toxin or has come into contact with an infectious agent, passive immunity can provide a rapid, short-term protection. Yet, since the individual does not generate the capacity to produce that antibody and the preformed antibodies are gradually removed from the body, no long-range protection is achieved.

The stimulation of antibody production through exposure to antigens, such as those found in a vaccine, results in active immunity. Development of effective active immunity requires a time span of several days to several weeks. The immunity is long-term, however, often lasting for the life span of the individual. Furthermore, each additional exposure to that same antigen, either through a vaccine booster or through natural exposure, results in a more rapid, greater response than those achieved previously. This increased rate of reaction is referred to as an anamnestic response.

The actual material utilized in a vaccine is variable, depending on the form of antigen. The earliest vaccine, that utilized by Jenner against smallpox, consisted of a virus that caused a disease in cattle called cowpox. The word "vaccination" is itself derived from this use; *vacca* is the Latin word for cow. While cowpox is distinct from the disease smallpox, the viruses that cause the two diseases contain similar antigenic determinants. Jenner made this observation. He ex-

ploited the fact that exposure to the cowpox virus results in active immunization against smallpox.

The use of attenuated strains of bacteria or viruses applies the same principle of cross-reaction. Attenuated organisms are mutants that have lost the ability to cause disease but that retain the antigenic character of the virulent strain. The most notable application of attenuation is the Sabin oral poliovirus vaccine (OPV). By testing hundreds of virus isolates for the ability to cause polio in monkeys, Albert Sabin was able to isolate certain strains that did not cause disease. These strains formed the basis for his vaccine. Similar testing resulted in the development of attenuated virus vaccines against a wide variety of agents, including those against measles, mumps, and rubella. Likewise, the Bacillus Calmette-Guerin (BCG) strain of *Mycobacterium tuberculosis* serves as a vaccine against the agent that causes tuberculosis. Unfortunately, the vaccine does not always result in immunity for the recipient. It is not used in the United States.

In some cases, the isolation of attenuated strains of

Recommended Childhood Immunization Schedule (2001)

	Birth	1 mo.	2 mos.	4 mos.	6 mos.	12 mos.	15 mos.	18 mos.	4-6 yrs.	11-12 yrs.	14-16 yrs.
Hepatitis B	Dose 1	Dose 1	Dose 2		Dose 3	Dose 3	Dose 3	Dose 3		Catch-up	
Diphtheria, pertussis, tetanus (DPT)			Doses 1, 2, 3	Doses 1, 2, 3	Doses 1, 2, 3		Dose 4	Dose 4	Dose 5	Tetanus and Diphtheria Booster	Tetanus and Diphtheria Booster
***H. influenzae* type B (HiB)**			Doses 1, 2, 3	Doses 1, 2, 3	Doses 1, 2, 3	Dose 4	Dose 4				
Polio			Doses 1, 2	Doses 1, 2	Dose 3	Dose 3	Dose 3	Dose 3	Dose 4		
Measles, mumps, rubella (MMR)						Dose 1	Dose 1		Dose 2	Dose 2	
Chickenpox						Dose 1	Dose 1	Dose 1		Catch-up	
Pneumococcal vaccine (PCV)			Doses 1, 2, 3	Doses 1, 2, 3	Doses 1, 2, 3	Dose 4	Dose 4				

Approved by the Advisory Committee on Immunization Practices, the American Academy of Pediatrics, and the American Academy of Family Physicians.

microorganisms has proved difficult. For this reason, inactivated or killed microorganisms often serve as the basis for vaccine production. The Salk inactivated poliovirus vaccine represents the best-known example. By treating poliovirus with a solution of the chemical formalin, Jonas Salk was able to inactivate the organism. The virus retained its antigenic potential and served as an effective vaccine. A similar process has resulted in vaccines to protect against other bacterial diseases, such as bubonic plague, cholera, and pertussis (whooping cough), and against viral influenza.

In some cases, the vaccine is not directed against the etiological agent itself but against toxic materials produced by the agent. This is the case with diphtheria and tetanus. The vaccines are produced by treating the diphtheria and tetanus toxins secreted by these bacteria with formalin. The toxoids that result are antigenically similar to the actual toxins and so are able to induce immunity. They are incapable, however, of causing the deleterious effects of the respective diseases.

Only those determinants of a virus or bacterium that stimulate neutralizing antibodies are necessary in most vaccines. For this reason, the use of genetically engineered vaccines was begun in the 1980's. The first example put into use was the production of a vaccine against the hepatitis B virus (HBV). The gene that encodes the surface antigen of HBV was isolated and inserted into a piece of genetic material within the yeast *Saccharomyces*. The HBV antigen produced by the yeast was purified and subsequently found to be as effective in a vaccine as the whole virus. Since no live virus is involved, there is no danger of an attenuated strain reverting to its virulent parent. Recently, similar technology has been applied to produce vaccines that protect against chickenpox and hepatitis A virus.

THE HISTORY OF VACCINATION AND ITS MAJOR SUCCESSES

Since the first use of vaccination by Edward Jenner in the 1790's for the prevention of smallpox, immunization techniques have been developed for protection against most major infectious illnesses. The term "vaccination" was originally applied to immunization against smallpox, but its definition has long been expanded to include most immunization techniques. "Vaccination" and "immunization" are used interchangeably, although there are technical differences in the definitions of the words.

The nineteenth century improvements in public health measures, combined with the passage of laws for compulsory vaccination, resulted in a steady decrease in the number of smallpox cases in the United States and most countries of Europe. Even as late as 1930, however, approximately 49,000 cases were reported in the United States. In the 1950's, large numbers of cases were still being reported in areas of Africa and Asia. At that time, the World Health Organization (WHO) of the United Nations decided on a plan for the elimination of smallpox based on the fact that humans served as the sole reservoir for the smallpox virus; animals are not naturally infected with smallpox. Through the use of mass immunization techniques, the plan was to isolate areas of infection into smaller and smaller pockets.

Ironically, the origins of the vaccine in use during the 1960's are unknown. The original strain of cowpox used by Jenner was lost sometime during the nineteenth century. The strain used in the vaccine during the twentieth century, called vaccinia virus, may have originated from an isolate obtained during the Franco-Prussian War in the 1870's.

The plan for the elimination of smallpox developed by WHO ultimately proved completely successful. There are actually two different forms of smallpox. The last known natural case of variola major was reported in Bangladesh in 1974. The last known case of variola minor was reported in Somalia in 1976. Although an outbreak of smallpox resulting from a laboratory accident was reported in Great Britain, there were no additional naturally caused cases of smallpox. In 1978, WHO declared the world to be free of smallpox.

Although vaccination was effective in immunizing most persons against smallpox, use of the vaccine itself was associated with some risk. Serious complications were rare but did occasionally occur. With the disappearance of the disease, the need for routine immunization lessened, and, in 1971, compulsory vaccination of children in the United States was discontinued. In 1976, the routine vaccination of hospital employees was also discontinued. By the 1990's, the only known sites of existence of smallpox virus were freezers in four laboratories.

The use of vaccines for the elimination of poliomyelitis represents another success story. Although sporadic outbreaks of polio occurred in earlier centuries and probably as long ago as the time of ancient Egypt, the first epidemics appeared in the late nineteenth century. Ironically, this increase in the incidence of polio was caused by improvements in public health. Poliovirus is easily transmitted through a fecal-oral route, but the majority of cases, particularly in young children, are without symptoms, or asymptomatic. With improvements in sanitation, the first exposure to polio was often delayed until later childhood or, as in the case of President Franklin Delano Roosevelt, in the adult years. Under these circumstances, the disease is often more severe.

In 1955, the inactivated poliovirus vaccine developed by Jonas Salk was introduced for general use; in 1961, Albert Sabin's oral poliovirus vaccine was licensed for use. By the 1990's, polio had been eliminated from the Western Hemisphere and from developed countries elsewhere. Nevertheless, WHO estimated that 250,000 cases of polio occurred yearly throughout developing countries of the world. For this reason, the American Academy of Pediatrics (AAP) recommends that children receive immunizations by their first birthday and boosters at eighteen months of age and again prior to starting school. Adults who plan to travel to areas of the world in which polio is found should also be immunized.

The WHO campaign to eliminate polio has been largely successful in the Western Hemisphere. New cases are still being reported in parts of Asia and Africa. Money to fund the program has been a problem. Civil strife has prevented medical teams from entering some areas and providing immunizations. Experts have remained optimistic that polio can be eliminated by the year 2003.

The most significant advancement in twentieth century health care in the United States has been the elimination of most major childhood diseases. In addition to poliovirus immunization, children routinely receive a variety of early immunizations. Measles, mumps, and rubella (MMR) vaccines are administered in a single preparation at fifteen months of age. All three contain live attenuated viruses. The measles vaccine was first introduced in 1966 and resulted in a decline in reported measles cases of nearly 99 percent by the 1980's. Beginning about 1986, however, increasing numbers of cases of measles were reported among young adults who had been previously immunized. For this reason, the AAP recommends that children receive boosters of measles vaccine prior to entering high school, at approximately eleven to twelve years of age. A series of the diphtheria, pertussis, and tetanus (DPT) vaccine is administered at two, four, six, and eighteen months, with tetanus and diphtheria boosters recommended at ten-year intervals throughout the remainder of life.

With the elimination of most other major childhood illnesses, *Hemophilus influenzae* type B infections moved into the dubious position of being among the most significant causes of illness and death among young children. In 1985, a vaccine developed from the outer coat of the bacterium was licensed for use. The vaccine worked poorly in children under the age of two, the major population at risk. Consequently, an improved vaccine was developed and licensed by 1987. The second vaccine consisted of a portion of the influenza coat joined to diphtheria toxoid. It was found to immunize children effectively at eighteen months of age; immunization with the vaccine is recommended by the age of fifteen months.

By 1991, a total of nineteen vaccines had been licensed in the United States by the Food and Drug Administration (FDA) for uses in either children or adults. Aside from the eight previously described vaccines for children, eleven vaccines (five viral and six bacterial) are recommended for special circumstances. For example, in 1986, a genetically engineered hepatitis B virus vaccine was developed and licensed. The gene that encodes the virus surface antigen was placed in a small piece of deoxyribonucleic acid (DNA), a plasmid, and inserted into the common baker's yeast *Saccharomyces cerevisiae*. The antigen that is produced is used in a three-dose series to immunize individuals at risk for the disease: health care workers, institutional staff persons, and anyone else who is likely to come into contact with the virus.

Although routine vaccination of children has worked virtually to eliminate most health-threatening infectious disease from that population, immunization of adults against preventable diseases has not been as successful. It was estimated that, in the early 1990's, 50,000 to 70,000 adults died yearly from diseases that were preventable through immunization, such as pneumococcal pneumonia, influenza, and hepatitis B.

Historically, pneumococcal pneumonia, caused by the bacterium *Streptococcus pneumonia*, has been a killer of adults. In the 1990's, an estimated 40,000 persons, primarily the elderly, died from this disease. The available vaccine is a polysaccharide vaccine, representing serotypes for twenty-three of the major strains of the bacterium. When administered by the age of fifty, the vaccine provides a significant degree of protection against the organism.

Between 1957 and 1993, nineteen influenza epidemics each resulted in more than 10,000 deaths from the disease in the United States alone. Two of the epidemics each resulted in more than 40,000 deaths. Most of these deaths were in elderly adults. Although the usefulness of vaccination among the elderly is limited, immunization against influenza will often lessen the severity of the disease, even if it fails to prevent infection.

Some specialized vaccines are recommended only for international travelers. Both killed and live attenuated oral vaccines against typhoid are licensed. The ease of administration of an oral vaccine has made this form the preferred choice. In addition, vaccines against cholera, dengue fever, plague, and yellow fever may be used in appropriate circumstances.

Although active immunization in most circumstances remains the preferred method of protection through vaccination, situations occur in which passive immunization may provide therapeutic treatment. Individuals may be immunosuppressed or lack a functional immune system. This condition may result from infection (acquired immunodeficiency syndrome, or AIDS), medical intervention (chemotherapy), or congenital reasons (severe combined immunodeficiency disease, or SCID). Whatever the cause, active immunization does not develop. In addition, there are circumstances in which the necessary time for the development of immunity through active immunization is not available, such as with exposure to tetanus toxin, the hepatitis virus, or rabies. For passive immunization or replacement therapy in immunodeficiency disorders, immunoglobulin is usually prepared from pools of plasma obtained from large numbers of blood donors. Specific immunoglobulins, directed against specific targets such as rabies or tetanus, are prepared from plasma containing high concentrations of these antibodies.

PERSPECTIVE AND PROSPECTS

The elimination of smallpox represents the classic example in which the efficacy of a vaccine resulted in the eradication of disease. Smallpox was an ancient disease, with origins as early as the twelfth century B.C.E. It appeared in the Middle East in the sixth century C.E., with subsequent dissemination into northern Africa and southern Europe as a result of the Arab invasions from the sixth to the eighth centuries. The disease spread throughout Europe with the return of the Crusaders during the eleventh and twelfth centuries and reached the Americas as a result of the African slave trade in the sixteenth century. It has been estimated that, at its peak during the eighteenth century, smallpox killed 400,000 persons each year and caused more than one-third of all cases of blindness. It has also been estimated that smallpox or other diseases killed approximately 85 percent of the American Indians who died during colonial periods, certainly far more than the number who died from bullet wounds.

In the News: Vaccine for Childhood Pneumococcal Meningitis and Septicemia

In February, 2000, the Food and Drug Administration (FDA) approved conjugate pneumococcal vaccine (Prevnar) for use in children under the age of two years for the prevention of pneumococcal infections. The American Academy of Pediatrics (AAP) recommended Prevnar for use in all children twenty-three months of age and younger. The AAP also recommended Prevnar for all immunocompromised children twenty-four to fifty-nine months of age who are at high risk for invasive pneumococcal infection. Prevnar may be administered in a series of four inoculations given at two, four, six, and twelve to fifteen months of age. Pneumococcal infections are a major cause of meningitis and septicemia in infants and children.

In clinical trials in which nineteen thousand children received the vaccine, Prevnar was 100 percent effective in preventing invasive pneumococcal disease. The reported side effects have been generally mild injection site reactions, irritability, drowsiness, decreased appetite, and fever higher than 100.3 degrees Fahrenheit. According to Dr. Jane Henney, Commissioner of Food and Drugs, in a U.S. Department of Health and Human Services newsletter published in 2000, "When we prevent these infections, we are also preventing brain damage and mortality from pneumococcal diseases."

—Sharon W. Stark, R.N.

The principle of immunization in prevention did not originate with Edward Jenner, the English physician credited with development of the smallpox vaccine in the 1790's. A practice called variolation was well known in China and parts of the Middle East for centuries prior to Jenner. Variolation consisted of the inhalation of dried crust prepared from the pocks obtained from individuals suffering from mild cases of smallpox. A variation involved removing small amounts of fluid from an active smallpox pustule and scratching the liquid into the skin of children. Lady Mary Wortley Montagu, wife of the British ambassador to the Ottoman Empire, introduced the practice of variolation into Great Britain during the early eighteenth century. Use of variolation was empirical: The practice was often successful. The possibility remained, however, that immunization might actually introduce the disease.

Born in 1749, Jenner first became aware of the protective effects of cowpox from the story of a local dairymaid who had been exposed to the disease. After years of study and observation, he became convinced of the story's validity. In 1796, he immunized an eight-year-old boy with material from a cowpox lesion. No ill effects were seen. Further immunizations supported the theory that cowpox protected against smallpox. Jenner called this material variolae vaccinae. Richard Dunning, a Plymouth physician, in an 1800 analysis of the procedure, was the first to use the term "vaccination."

Wider application of the principle of vaccination followed from Louis Pasteur's studies during the 1870's and 1880's. With his attenuation of the bacterium that caused chicken cholera, Pasteur demonstrated that one could manipulate the virulence of a microorganism. This practice soon led to his development of vaccines against both anthrax and rabies. It is ironic that no clinical trials have ever been conducted to test rabies vaccine.

The twentieth century saw the development of effective vaccines against most major childhood diseases. Use of the DPT toxoid became routine in the United States about 1945. Development of the oral Sabin vaccine and inactivated Salk vaccines during the 1950's resulted in the complete elimination of poliomyelitis from the Western Hemisphere by the 1990's. The use of genetic engineering, in which only the genes necessary to synthesize specific antigens are utilized, was first applied to the hepatitis B vaccine. It has recently been applied successfully to create vaccines against chickenpox and hepatitis A virus. A vaccine against hepatitis C virus is under development. This technology provides the potential for manufacturing vaccine "cocktails," or combinations of such genes from a variety of infectious agents in a single vaccine.

Many experts are trying to develop a vaccine to protect against AIDS. This is difficult because the very mechanism that has been exploited by other vaccines, namely the stimulation of T cells to produce antibodies that protect a recipient, is nonfunctional in AIDS. The successful development of a vaccine against AIDS will require scientific ingenuity.

—Richard Adler, Ph.D.;
updated by L. Fleming Fallon, Jr.,
M.D., Ph.D., M.P.H.

See also Acquired immunodeficiency syndrome (AIDS); Anthrax; Antibiotics; Bacterial infections; Bacteriology; Chickenpox; Childhood infectious diseases; Cholera; Diphtheria; Disease; Environmental health; Hepatitis; Host-defense mechanisms; Immune system; Immunology; Influenza; Measles; Microbiology; Mumps; Pathology; Plague; Poliomyelitis; Preventive medicine; Rubella; Smallpox; Tuberculosis; Viral infections; Whooping cough; World Health Organization.

FOR FURTHER INFORMATION:

Behbehani, Abbas. *The Smallpox Story in Words and Pictures.* Kansas City: University of Kansas Medical Center, 1988. The book includes the history of Edward Jenner and his use of cowpox in the first smallpox vaccine. The drawings and photographs are of particular interest.

Bittle, J. L., and F. A. Murphy, eds. *Vaccine Biotechnology.* San Diego, Calif.: Academic Press, 1989. A discussion of the use of techniques in molecular biology and genetic engineering in vaccine development. The style and depth of coverage is appropriate to anyone with basic knowledge of biology.

Brock, Thomas D., ed. *Microorganisms: From Smallpox to Lyme Disease.* New York: W. H. Freeman, 1990. A collection of readings from *Scientific American* magazine. Included is a section on the role of vaccines in the prevention of disease, including their role in the elimination of smallpox. Also found are articles on synthetic vaccines and vaccination in Third World countries.

Plotkin, Stanley A., and Edward Mortimer, Jr., eds. *Vaccines.* 3d ed. Philadelphia: W. B. Saunders,

1999. An excellent description of the role of vaccines in the prevention of disease. The book begins with a history of immunization practices. Each subsequent chapter deals with a specific disease and the role and history of vaccine production in its prevention. While enough detail is provided to interest someone in the field, the text is appropriate for nonscientists.

Roitt, Ivan. *Roitt's Essential Immunology.* 9th ed. Boston: Blackwell Scientific, 1997. An excellent textbook on the subject of immunology. Much of the book is detailed and requires some background in biology. Nevertheless, the chapters which deal with infection and immunization are clear and contain much that will interest nonscientists. Numerous graphs illustrate material from the text.

IMMUNODEFICIENCY DISORDERS
DISEASE/DISORDER

ANATOMY OR SYSTEM AFFECTED: Immune system

SPECIALTIES AND RELATED FIELDS: Genetics, immunology

DEFINITION: Genetic or acquired disorders that result from disturbances in the normal functioning of the immune system.

KEY TERMS:

antibody: protein immunoglobulin secreted by B lymphocytes; the production of antibodies is induced by specific foreign invaders, and they combine with and destroy only those invaders

B lymphocytes: also referred to as B cells; white cells of the immune system that produce antibodies; produced within the bone marrow

phagocytes: white cells of the immune system that destroy invading foreign bodies by engulfing and digesting them in a nonspecific immune response; includes macrophages and neutrophils

stem cells: multipotential precursor cells within the bone marrow that develop into white cell populations, including lymphocytes and phagocytic cells

T lymphocyte: a type of immune cell that kills host cells infected by bacteria or viruses and secretes chemicals (interleukins) that regulate the immune response

CAUSES AND SYMPTOMS

The defense of the body against foreign invaders is provided by the immune system. In nonspecific immunity, phagocytic cells engulf and destroy invading particles. Specific immunity consists of very specialized cell types that are synthesized in response to a particular type of foreign invader. Self-replicating stem cells within the bone marrow give rise to lymphocytes, which mediate specific immunity. Lymphocytes establish self-replacing colonies within the thymus, spleen, and lymph nodes. The various categories of T lymphocytes are derived from the thymus colonies, while B lymphocytes develop and mature within the bone marrow. B lymphocytes secrete highly specific antibodies that attack bacteria and some viruses. T lymphocytes do not secrete antibodies but instead either attack the body cells that have been infected with a bacterium or virus or produce chemical compounds that aid other types of T cells in destroying the infected cells. In immunodeficiency disorders, some or all of these defenses are compromised, which can have life-threatening consequences. Less commonly, immunodeficiency diseases are the result of genetic abnormalities and are present from birth; others are acquired through infection or exposure to damaging drug or radiation treatments.

The most severe immunodeficiency disorder is attributable to the absence of stem cells, which results in a total lack of both B and T lymphocytes. This rare genetic condition is referred to as severe combined immunodeficiency syndrome (SCID). Affected infants show a failure to thrive from birth and can easily die from common bacterial or viral infections. The most common cause of SCID is a deficiency in the enzyme adenosine deaminase. This deficiency disrupts the normal deoxyribonucleic acid (DNA) synthesis in the stem cells. A variant of SCID is Swiss-type agammaglobulinemia, in which the thymus is absent and few lymph nodes exist.

Major syndromes that involve defects specific to the T lymphocyte population are characterized by recurrent viral and fungal infections. Di George syndrome results from improper development of the thymus, which in turn results in insufficient production of T lymphocytes, often accompanied by other structural abnormalities in the infant. Death usually results prior to age two from overwhelming viral infections.

The most common disorders affecting B lymphocytes are forms of hypogammaglobulinemia. This condition is characterized by insufficient levels of antibody. The cause is generally associated with increased rates of antibody breakdown or loss in the urine secondary to kidney malfunction. Bruton's agammaglobulinemia is a rare, sex-linked form of the condition, in which B cells fail to mature properly. Severe bacterial infections are the most common symptom. When the disorder is left untreated, infants generally die of severe pneumonia prior to six months of age.

Several immunodeficiency disorders may be the result of partial defects in the production and/or function of B and T lymphocytes. Wiskott-Aldrich syndrome is a genetically inherited disease manifested by recurrent infections and an itchy, scaly inflammation of the skin. Certain classes of antibodies are absent or scarce. Chronic mucocutaneous candidiasis is characterized by chronic fungal infection of the skin and mucous membranes; reduced levels of T cells are responsible for this disfiguring disorder.

Immunodeficiency disorders may also be the result of defects in phagocytic cells; the underlying cause of most of these disorders is ill-defined but often involves deficiencies in hydrolytic enzymes. In chronic granulomatosis, an inherited enzyme deficiency prevents the immune system from destroying bacteria that have been phagocytized. Infants affected by this disorder develop severe infections and chronic inflammations of internal organs and bones. The bacteria responsible for these infections are generally common flora that are not considered pathogens in healthy individuals.

Most of the disorders that affect the immune system are not inherited but develop sometime during the person's life. They are either the result of an infection or a consequence of another disease or its treatment. The use of corticosteroids to treat inflammations, or the illicit use of them in muscle-building, can interfere with the proper production and function of T lymphocytes. Other immunosuppressive drugs used to diminish the possibilities of graft or transplant rejection, or in the treatment of autoimmune diseases, can severely depress antibody production. Chemotherapeutic agents used in the treatment of cancer can affect DNA replication and severely compromise the entire immune system. Whole-body radiation can damage or destroy bone marrow stem cells.

Major trauma, surgery, and burns all lead to an increased risk of infection. These experiences result in depressed function of both the nonspecific and specific immune responses. The effect is temporary, however, and immune responses generally return to normal during the recuperative process. Advanced malignancies (cancer) are frequently associated with a depressed immune response, perhaps because of tumor proliferation and interference with the development and maturation of B and T lymphocytes.

Acquired immunodeficiency syndrome (AIDS) is caused by the human immunodeficiency virus (HIV). HIV specifically infects one type of regulatory T lymphocyte, resulting in severe immune depression. The virus may be harbored in an individual for years without symptoms. Initial symptoms may be quite mild but generally progress so that the affected individual becomes susceptible to a host of unusual bacterial and fungal infections, including a rare form of cancer called Kaposi's sarcoma. AIDS produces neurological damage in about one-third of infected individuals. HIV is transmitted primarily through unprotected sexual contact, sharing of needles for intravenous drug use, transfusion with contaminated blood products, or other contact with contaminated body fluids.

TREATMENT AND THERAPY

Treatment of immunodeficiency disorders is targeted at the source of the deficiency. For example, in Di George syndrome, characterized by the congenital absence of the thymus, fetal thymus transplants may correct the problem, with improvement in lymphocyte levels seen within hours after the transplants. The use of thymus extracts has also been beneficial. Syndromes such as hypogammaglobulinemia can be managed by injection with mixtures of antibodies. Drug therapy to substitute for some absent immune components of Wiskott-Aldrich syndrome has been shown to have variable effects. The most effective treatment for chronic mucocutaneous candidiasis is aggressive antifungal medication to eradicate the causative organism; treatment must continue for several months because fungal infections are slow to respond to therapy and frequently recur. Chronic granulomatosis is notoriously difficult to treat, and the most effective therapy has been antibiotic and antifungal agents used aggressively during an overt infection.

Because of the magnitude of the defects, many inherited immunodeficiency disorders are difficult to treat successfully and are commonly fatal early in life. Chronic granulomatosis is usually fatal within the first few years of life, and only about 20 percent of patients reach the age of twenty. SCID is a serious disorder in which affected infants can die before a proper diagnosis is made. For individuals with these and other serious immunodeficiency disorders, maintenance in an environment free of bacteria, viruses, and fungi, such as a sterile "bubble," has been the best means to prevent life-threatening infections. Such an approach, however, precludes the possibility of a normal life. The most effective treatment for individuals with severely compromised immune systems is bone marrow transplantation. In this procedure, bone marrow from a compatible individual is introduced into the bone marrow of the patient. If the procedure works—and the success rate is high—in approximately one to six months the transplant recipient's immune system will be reconstituted and functional. Bone marrow transplantation is a permanent cure for these disorders, since the transplanted marrow will contain stem cells that produce all the cell types of the immune system. The difficulties in transplantation include finding a compatible donor and preventing infections during the period after the transplant. Individuals are particularly susceptible to infection prior to the activation of the transplanted bone marrow. Such patients are frequently kept in sterile bubbles to limit the possibility of infection.

Drug therapy for AIDS utilizes treatments that interfere with replication of the virus. The first drug to be approved for use was zidovudine (formerly AZT), a DNA analogue, but its success was somewhat limited, as it was associated with severe side effects and the creation of resistant virus. More recent treatments utilize drug "cocktails," combinations of drugs that act at different stages of viral replication. Vaccines and antibiotic therapy are used to prevent or treat the opportunistic illnesses that accompany AIDS. Various drugs may also help to ease symptoms of AIDS such as appetite disturbances, nausea, pain, insomnia, anxiety, depression, fever, and diarrhea. A combination of therapies has been shown to increase life expectancy in AIDS patients. Many patients choose to participate in clinical trials of experimental drugs not approved for general use in the hope that the new drug will be more effective at alleviating the disease. Others seek out alternative or nontraditional medical treatments that have a long history of use in non-Western cultures. These treatments include acupuncture, herbology, meditation, and homeopathy. An important aspect of therapy for AIDS patients is maintaining mental health through support groups and supportive caregivers.

Illicit use of corticosteroids can seriously compromise the immune system and may lead to permanent damage. The best therapy for this type of acquired immunodeficiency is prevention—that is, to not misuse the drugs. In their supervised use to control inflammation or other disease symptoms, normal immune function will return after treatment has been completed. A huge risk to cancer patients who are being treated with chemotherapy and/or radiation therapy is the depression of the immune system, which can lead to a host of infections being contracted and not easily fought off by the body's compromised immune system. These individuals should avoid exposure to infectious agents when possible and be attentive to lifestyle modifications that can strengthen the immune

---

In the News: New Treatment for Di George Syndrome

Di George syndrome is a rare genetic disorder which results in improper development of the thymus gland. Approximately two thousand children each year are diagnosed with the disorder in the United States, with between five and ten of these children completely lacking a thymus. In order to survive, these children must receive T cells from a closely matched sibling; most do not have such a match.

In a seven-year study, a team of physicians from Duke University was able to "cure" Di George syndrome in several children by transplanting thymus tissue from unrelated donors. These donors were children who had undergone pediatric heart surgery. At this stage of neonatal development, the thymus gland is so large relative to the size of the heart that small portions of the gland must be removed to carry out such surgery. Previously, the thymic tissue was discarded. Instead, the physicians placed pieces of the tissue, likened to "slabs of bacon," in culture dishes in the laboratory for two weeks, enabling the mature T cells which might react against a new host to die. The remaining cells from the thymic tissue, mainly epithelial cells which function to "educate" immature T cells migrating from the bone marrow, were transplanted into the thigh muscles of children with Di George syndrome. Several of these children subsequently produced normal T cells, reversing the immune defects associated with the syndrome.

—Richard Adler, Ph.D.

system and encourage its speedy recovery, including a nutritious diet, plenty of rest, and avoidance of stress. Close monitoring for any signs of infection facilitates rapid antibiotic therapy, which can prevent serious complications.

PERSPECTIVE AND PROSPECTS

Prior to the gains in scientific knowledge about the mechanics of the immune system, individuals with genetic immunodeficiency disorders would die of serious infections during their first few years of life. Even when it was finally realized that these individuals suffered from defects of the immune system, little could be done for most of the disorders, except to treat infections as they developed and to avoid contact with potential disease-causing organisms—a near impossibility if one is to lead a normal life. Housing persons with SCID in sterile bubbles was uncommon because of the expense and impracticality. During the 1970's, bone marrow transplants were first developed; by the 1990's they had progressed to a greater than 80 percent success rate. As a result of improved transplant-rejection drugs, transplants from donors with less-than-perfect tissue matches are now possible. Bone marrow transplantation has been a source of cure for many individuals with immune disorders.

Bone marrow transplantation is not suitable or possible in every case of immunodeficiency disorder, and scientists have long sought a means to cure the genetic defects themselves. In 1992, French Anderson of the National Institutes of Health conducted the first gene therapy trial on a young girl suffering from SCID. Some of the girl's bone marrow cells were removed from her body and exposed to an inactivated virus containing a normal gene for ADA, the defective enzyme. Some of the stem cells in the marrow incorporated the healthy gene, and the engineered cells were returned to her body. The cells lodged in her bone marrow, where they produced healthy immune cells. The procedure was repeated successfully in three other children shortly afterward.

Gene therapy is being considered for a variety of immunodeficiency conditions. In the future, bone marrow cells may be engineered to be resistant to chemotherapy and radiation therapy; therefore, patients could be given more frequent dosages of cancer-fighting therapies without destroying their ability to fight infections. Bone marrow cells may also be engineered for resistance to infection by the AIDS virus; in this way, individuals with AIDS may be given a population of cells that will reverse the immunodeficiency associated with AIDS. Aging individuals develop depressed immune systems, and medical research is searching for ways to prevent this decline. These efforts toward curing immunodeficiency diseases with the tools of contemporary molecular biology are promising.

—*Karen E. Kalumuck, Ph.D.;*
updated by Richard Adler, Ph.D.

See also Acquired immunodeficiency syndrome (AIDS); Allergies; Arthritis; Asthma; Autoimmune disorders; Blood and blood disorders; Bone marrow transplantation; Cells; Cytology; Cytopathology; Gene therapy; Hematology; Hematology, pediatric; Host-defense mechanisms; Human immunodeficiency virus (HIV); Immune system; Immunology; Immunopathology; Serology.

FOR FURTHER INFORMATION:

Bartlett, John G., and Ann K. Finkbeiner. *The Guide to Living with HIV Infection.* Baltimore: The Johns Hopkins University Press, 1991. This informative book developed at The Johns Hopkins University AIDS Clinic is a great resource for information about the disease and a guide for patients and caregivers in living with the disease.

Dwyer, John M. *The Body at War: The Story of Our Immune System.* 2d ed. New York: Penguin Books, 1993. This easy-to-read text is an excellent introduction to the functions of the immune system and such related topics as immune disorders, allergies, and immunology research.

Fox, Stuart I. *Perspectives on Human Biology.* Dubuque, Iowa: Wm. C. Brown, 1991. An understandably written and beautifully illustrated text. Includes an extensive chapter on the immune system and diseases.

Life, Death, and the Immune System. New York: W. H. Freeman, 1994. This comprehensive collection of articles from *Scientific American* provides basic information and research directions on AIDS, autoimmune disorders, and allergies, as well as an excellent discussion of the immune system in general.

Petrow, Steven, ed. *HIV Drug Book.* New York: Pocket Books, 1995. This book was produced by Project Information, the leading community-based AIDS treatment information and advocacy organization in the United States. Its user-friendly guide provides information on the most-used HIV/AIDS treatments.

Roitt, Ivan. *Roitt's Essential Immunology*. 9th ed. Boston: Blackwell Scientific, 1997. A thorough introduction to the science of immunology. Well illustrated. Includes an extensive section on immunodeficiency disorders.

Stine, Gerald J. *AIDS Update: 2000*. Upper Saddle River, N.J.: Prentice Hall, 2000. An overview of AIDS, its cause, and methods of treating it. Included are sections outlining the immunodeficiency disorders that are sequelae to HIV infection.

IMMUNOLOGY

SPECIALTY

ANATOMY OR SYSTEM AFFECTED: Blood, cells, immune system

SPECIALTIES AND RELATED FIELDS: Cytology, hematology, microbiology, preventive medicine, serology

DEFINITION: The study of the immune system, its protection of the body from foreign agents, and its malfunction in autoimmune diseases, in which the body's defenses react against the body's own cells or tissues.

KEY TERMS:

antibody: a protein produced by lymphocytes in response to an antigen; binds only to a specific antigen

antigen: any substance perceived by immunological defenses to be foreign and against which antibody is produced; generally a protein

autoantibody: an antibody produced against tissue antigens within a host—that is, self-antigens

complement: a series of about twenty serum proteins that, when sequentially activated by immune complexes, may trigger cell damage

determinant: a region on the surface of an antigen capable of creating an immune response or of combining with an antibody produced by an immune response

Hashimoto's disease: thyroiditis; among the earliest characterized autoimmune diseases

lupus: systemic lupus erythematosus; a chronic inflammatory disease characterized by an arthritic condition and a rash

lymphocyte: a small white blood cell constituting about 25 percent of all blood cells; two basic types are B cells (antibody production) and T cells (cellular immunity)

tolerance: the state in which an organism does not normally react against its own tissue

SCIENCE AND PROFESSION

The field of immunology deals with the ability of the immune system to react against an enormous repertoire of stimulation by antigens. In most instances, these antigens are foreign infectious agents such as viruses or bacteria. Inherent in this process is the ability to react against nearly any known determinant, whether natural or artificially produced. The most reactive antigenic determinants are proteins, though to a lesser degree, other substances such as carbohydrates (sugars), lipids (fats), and nucleic acids may also stimulate a response.

In general, the body exhibits tolerance during the constant exposure to its own tissue. The precise reasons behind tolerance are vague, but the basis for the lack of response lies in two major mechanisms: the elimination during development of immunological cells capable of responding to the body's own tissue and the active prevention of existing reactive cells from responding to self-antigens. When this regulation fails, autoimmune disease may result.

There are two major types of immunological defense: humoral immunity and cell-mediated immunity. Humoral immunity refers to the soluble substances in blood serum, primarily antibody and complement, while cellular immunity refers to the portion of the immune response that is directly mediated by cells. Though these processes are sometimes categorized separately, they do in fact interact with and regulate each other.

Antibodies are produced by cells called B lymphocytes in response to foreign antigens. These proteins bind to the antigen in a specific manner, resulting in a complex that can be removed readily by phagocytic white blood cells. More important in the context of autoimmunity, antibody-antigen complexes also activate the complement pathway, a series of some twenty enzymes and serum proteins. The end result of activation is the lysis of the antigenic targets. In general, the targets are bacteria; in autoimmune disease, the target may be any cell in the body.

The cellular response utilizes any of several types of cytotoxic cells. These can include a specialized lymphocyte called the T cell (so named because of its development in the thymus) or another unusual type of large granular lymphocyte called the natural killer (NK) cell. NK and cytotoxic T cells function in a similar manner—by binding to the target and releasing toxic granules in apposition to its cell membrane.

Though autoimmune diseases differ in scope, they do tend to exhibit certain common factors. The pathologies associated with most of these illnesses result in part from the production of autoantibodies, which are antibodies produced against the body's own cells or tissues. If the antibody binds to tissue in a particular organ, complement is activated in the tissue, causing the destruction of those regions of the organ. For example, Goodpasture's syndrome is characterized by the deposition of autoantibodies directed against the membrane of the glomerulus in the kidneys. Complement activation can result in severe organ pathology and subsequent kidney failure.

If the autoantibody binds to soluble material in blood serum, the resultant antibody-antigen complexes are carried along in the circulation, and there is the possibility that they will lodge in various areas of the body. For example, systemic lupus erythematosus (SLE, or lupus) results from the production of autoantibodies against soluble nucleoprotein, which is released from cells as they undergo normal death and lysis. The immune complexes frequently lodge in the kidney, where they can cause renal failure.

This is not to say that all autoimmune diseases result solely from autoantibody production. Though a precise role for either cytotoxic T cells or NK cells in human autoimmune disease has not been fully confirmed, several observations make such an association likely. First, large numbers of T cells are found in certain organ-specific diseases, including thyroiditis and pernicious anemia. Second, animal models of similar diseases show a specific role for such cells in the pathology of these diseases. Thus, it is likely that these cells do participate in the organ destruction.

Autoimmune disorders can be categorized in the form of a disease spectrum. At one end of the spectrum one can place organ-specific diseases. For example, Hashimoto's disease is an autoimmune thyroid disorder characterized by the production of autoantibodies against thyroid antigens. The extensive infiltration and proliferation of lymphocytes is observed (although, as described above, their roles are unproved), along with the subsequent destruction of follicular tissue.

Likewise, diabetes mellitus, Type I (formerly called juvenile-onset diabetes) may be an organ-specific autoimmune disease. In this case, however, autoantibodies are directed against the beta cells of the pancreas, which produce insulin. In pernicious (or megaloblastic) anemia, antibodies are produced against intrinsic

factor, a molecule necessary for uptake of vitamin B_{12}. Subsequent pathology results from lack of absorption of the vitamin. Addison's disease, from which U.S. president John F. Kennedy suffered, is a potentially life-threatening condition resulting from antibody production against the adrenal cortex. Myasthenia gravis is characterized by severe heart or skeletal muscle weakness caused by antibodies directed against neurotransmitter receptors on the muscle. In fact, cells from any organ may be potential targets for production of an autoantibody.

Certain organ-specific autoimmune diseases in the spectrum are characterized not by antibodies directed against any specific organ, but by cellular infiltration triggered in some manner by less specific autoantibodies. For example, biliary cirrhosis, an inflammatory condition of the liver, is characterized by the obstruction of bile flow through the liver ductules. Though extensive cellular infiltration is observed, serum antibodies are directed against mitochondrial antigens, which are found within all cells. Certain types of chronic hepatitis also exhibit an analogous situation.

In some cases, antibodies may be directed against circulatory cells. Antibodies directed against red blood cells may cause subsequent lysis of the cells, leading to hemolytic anemia. Often, these are temporary conditions that have resulted from the binding of a pharmacologic chemical such as an antibiotic to the surface of the cell, which triggers an immune response. A more serious condition is hemolytic disease of the newborn (HDN), one example being erythroblastosis fetalis, or Rh disease. In this case, a mother lacking the Rh protein on her blood cells may produce an immune response against that protein, which is present in the blood of the fetus she is carrying during pregnancy. Prior to 1967, when an effective preventive measure became available, HDN was a serious problem for many pregnancies. Antibodies directed against blood platelets can cause a reduction in the number of those cells, resulting in thrombocytopenia purpura. An analogous situation can be seen with other cell types.

At the other end of the autoimmune spectrum are those diseases that are not cell- or organ-specific but result in widespread lesions in various parts of the body. Lupus received its name from the butterfly rash often seen on the faces of patients, which resembles a wolfbite (*lupus* is Latin for "wolf"). Pathologic changes can be found at various sites in the body, however, including the kidneys, joints, and blood vessels. Likewise, rheumatoid arthritis is characterized by the production of rheumatoid factor, an antibody molecule directed against other antibodies in blood serum. The resultant immune complexes lodge in joints, causing the joint pain and destruction associated with severe arthritis.

In most cases, the specific reason for the production of autoantibodies is unknown. Genetic factors are certainly involved, since some autoimmune diseases run in families. Some may be triggered by bacterial or viral infections. Viral antigens may be expressed on the surfaces of certain cells or the virus itself may be attached to the cell. Heart muscle appears to express antigenic determinants in common with certain streptococcal bacteria. A mild "strep throat" may be followed several weeks later by severe rheumatic fever.

The binding of drugs to cell surfaces may trigger an immune response. For example, penicillin may bind to the surfaces of red blood cells, triggering a hemolytic anemia. Likewise, sedormid may bind to the membrane of platelets.

Most cases of autoimmune disease, however, are triggered by no apparent cause. They may "simply" involve a breakdown of the normal regulatory mechanisms associated with the immune response.

DIAGNOSTIC AND TREATMENT TECHNIQUES

The regulation of self-reactive lymphocytes is necessary for the maintenance of tolerance by the immune system. When regulation breaks down or is otherwise defective, either humoral or cellular immunity is generated against the cells or tissues. The resultant pathology may be simply a painful nuisance or may have potentially fatal consequences. The difference relates to the extent of damage to particular organs, in the case of organ-specific autoimmune reactions, or to the level of tissue damage in systemic disease.

Despite differences in pathology, the mechanisms of tissue damage are similar in most autoimmune diseases. Most involve the formation of immune complexes. Either antibodies bind to cell surfaces or immune complexes form in the circulation. In either case, the result is complement activation. Components of the complement pathway, in turn, can either directly damage cell membranes or trigger the infiltration of a variety of cytotoxic cells.

Because the damage associated with most autoimmune diseases results from parallel processes, methods of treatment vary little in theory from one illness to another. Most involve the treatment of resultant symptoms; for example, the use of aspirin to reduce minor inflammation and, when necessary, the use of steroids to reduce the level of the immune response.

The treatment of autoimmune diseases does not eliminate the problem. The disease remains, but under ideal conditions, it is held under control. At the same time, there exists the danger of side effects of treatment. For example, most methods that reduce the level of the immune response are nonspecific; reducing the severity of the autoimmune disease may cause the patient to become more susceptible to infections by bacteria or viruses.

Certain approaches have been successful in the palliative treatment of some forms of autoimmune disease. For example, patients with myasthenia gravis (MG) exhibit significant muscle weakness. A myasthenia gravis patient may have difficulty breathing and may experience extreme fatigue, in severe cases being unable to open his or her mouth or eyelids. Associated with the disease are autoantibodies produced against the receptor for the neurotransmitter acetylcholine (ACh), the chemical utilized by nerves in regulating movement by the muscle. By blocking the ACh receptor, these antibodies inhibit the ability of nerves to control muscle movement. In effect, the patient loses control of the muscles.

Patients with myasthenia gravis often exhibit abnormalities of the thymus, the gland associated with T-cell production. In addition, there is evidence that the thymus contains ACh receptors that are particularly antigenic (perhaps exacerbating the illness). Removal of the thymus, even in adults, often aids in reducing the symptoms of the disease. The thymus, though not superfluous in adults, carries out its main functions during the early years of life, through adolescence. Thus, its removal generally has few major implications.

Often, MG will respond to more conventional forms of treatment. Steroid treatment will often reduce symptoms. Metabolic controls may also aid in reducing symptoms. For example, during normal nerve transmission of ACh, the enzyme cholinesterase is present to break down ACh, thereby regulating muscle movement. The use of anticholinesterase drugs to prolong the presence of ACh at the site of the receptor on the muscle has also been of benefit to some patients.

Systemic lupus erythematosus is among the most common of systemic autoimmune diseases. The disease usually strikes women in the prime of life, between the ages of twenty and forty. It is characterized by a butterfly rash over the facial region, weakness, fatigue, and often a fever. In many respects, the symptoms are those of severe arthritis. As the disease progresses, tissue or organ degradation may occur in the kidney or heart.

The specific cause of the symptomology is the formation of immune complexes, which consist of antibodies against cell components such as DNA or nucleoprotein. Complexes in the kidney have been large enough to observe with the electron microscope, particularly when the complexes contain cell nuclei. Similar complexes have been observed in regions of the skin characterized by inflammation and a rash. The immune complexes are sometimes ingested (phagocytized) by scavenger neutrophils, which make up the largest proportion (65 percent) of white blood cells. The presence of these so-called LE cells, white cells with ingested antibody-bound nuclei, was at one time used for the diagnosis of lupus.

As is true for many autoimmune diseases, the control of lupus often involves the use of steroids as immunosuppressive drugs. These have included drugs such as cyclosporin, which blocks T-cell function, and antimitotic drugs such as azathioprine or methotrexate, which block the proliferation of immune cells. Generalized immunosuppression as a side effect is a concern. Often, using combinations of steroids and immunosuppressives makes it possible to use lower concentrations of each, increasing the drugs' effectiveness and reducing the danger of toxicity.

Other palliative treatments of symptomology can increase patient comfort. For example, aspirin may be used to reduce inflammation or joint pain. Topical steroids can reduce the rash. Since lupus may significantly increase the photosensitivity of the skin, staying out of direct sunlight, or at least covering the surface of the skin, may reduce skin lesions. It should be emphasized again that these treatments deal only with symptoms; none will cure the disease.

Since some systemic diseases result from immune complex disorders, a reduction of the levels of such complexes has been found to be beneficial to some patients. Treatment involves a process called plasmapheresis. Plasma, the liquid portion of the blood, is removed from the patient (a small proportion at a time), after which the immune complexes are separated from the plasma. Though a temporary measure, since additional complexes continue to form, the process does prove useful.

Rheumatoid arthritis is another common autoimmune disorder. As is true of most autoimmune diseases, rheumatoid arthritis is primarily a disease of women. Symptomology results from the lodging of immune complexes in joints, resulting in the inflammation of those joints. Many cases result from the formation of antibodies directed against other antibody molecules—a case of the immune system turning against itself. Pathology results both from complement activation and from the infiltration of a variety of cells into the joint; the result is damage to both cartilage and bone.

Medical treatment usually begins with the anti-inflammatory drug of choice: aspirin. Other common treatments are those that increase patient comfort: rest, proper exercise, and weight loss, if necessary. In severe cases, steroids may be prescribed.

In general, autoimmune diseases are characterized by alternating periods of symptomology and remission. Treatments are generally similar in their approach of reducing inflammation as the first line of intervention, with the use of immunosuppression being the last resort. Since the precise origin of most of these disorders is unknown, prevention remains difficult.

PERSPECTIVE AND PROSPECTS

During the 1950's, F. Macfarlane Burnet published his theory of clonal selection. Burnet believed that antibody specificity was predetermined in the B cell as it underwent development and maturation. Selection of the cell by the appropriate antigen resulted in proliferation of that specific cell, a process of clonal selection.

Burnet also had to account for tolerance, however, the inability of immune cells to respond against their own antigens. Burnet theorized that during prenatal development, exposure to self-antigens, or determinants, resulted in the abortion of any self-reactive cells. Only those self-reactive immune cells that were directed against sequestered antigens survived.

Though Burnet's theories have reached the level of dogma in the field of immunology, they fail to account for certain autoimmune disorders. In the "correct" circumstances, the body does react against itself. Though they were not recognized at the time as such, autoimmune disorders were recognized as early as 1866. In that year, W. W. Gull demonstrated the link between chilling and a syndrome called paroxysmal hemoglobinuria. When external tissue such as skin is exposed to cold, large amounts of hemoglobin are discharged into the urine. In 1904, Karl

Landsteiner established the autoimmune basis for the disease by demonstrating the role of complement in the lysis of red blood cells, causing the release of hemoglobin and the symptomology of the disorder. Further, he demonstrated that one could cause the lysis of normal cells by mixing them with sera from hemoglobinurics.

Hashimoto's disease was among the first organ-specific autoimmune diseases to be described. The disease was first described in 1912 by Hakaru Hashimoto, a Japanese surgeon, and the immune basis for the disease was established independently by Ernest Witebsky and Noel Rose in the United States, and by Deborah Doniach and Ivan Roitt in Great Britain, in 1957.

Since the 1950's, dozens of autoimmune disorders have been described. Treatment of these disorders remains, for the most part, nonspecific. Research in the area, in addition to attempts to define the precise trigger for autoimmune disease, has attempted to develop ways to suppress specifically those immune reactions responsible for the symptomology. Successes have been associated with vaccines directed against components involved with the reactions under investigation. For example, since the production of autoantibodies is the basis for some forms of disease, the generation of additional antibody molecules directed against determinants on the autoantibodies at fault could serve to neutralize the effects of those components. This procedure could be likened to a police department that arrests its own dishonest officers. There is a precedent for such an operation. Newborn children of mothers suffering from myasthenia gravis synthesize just such antibodies against the inappropriate MG antibodies that have crossed the placenta. Synthesis does seem to ameliorate the symptoms of the disease.

There is no question that autoimmune disorders represent an aberrant form of immune response. Nevertheless, an understanding of the underlying mechanism will shed light on exactly how the immune system is regulated. For example, it remains unclear how antibody production is controlled following a normal immune response. In the presence of an antigen, antibody levels increase for a period of days to weeks, reach a plateau, and then slowly decrease as additional production comes to a halt. The means by which the shutdown takes place remains nebulous.

Tolerance does not result solely from an absence of T or B cells that respond to antigens; it involves an active suppression of the process. A more detailed understanding of the process will lead to a more thorough understanding of the immune system in general.

—Richard Adler, Ph.D.

See also Acquired immunodeficiency syndrome (AIDS); Allergies; Autoimmune disorders; Blood and blood disorders; Bone marrow transplantation; Cells; Chemotherapy; Circulation; Cytology; Cytopathology; Dialysis; Endocrinology; Endocrinology, pediatric; Glands; Healing; Hematology; Hematology, pediatric; Homeopathy; Hormones; Host-defense mechanisms; Human immunodeficiency virus (HIV); Immune system; Immunization and vaccination; Immunodeficiency disorders; Immunopathology; Infection; Liver; Lymphatic system; Multiple chemical sensitivity syndrome; Oncology; Serology; Skin; Transfusion; Transplantation.

FOR FURTHER INFORMATION:

Dwyer, John M. *The Body at War: The Story of Our Immune System.* 2d ed. London: J. M. Dent, 1993. Dwyer provides a basic discussion of the immune system for the layperson. Though their coverage is not particularly detailed, topics include the basis for immune tolerance and autoimmunity. Clearly written and accessible to the nonscientific public.

Fettner, Ann G. *Viruses: Agents of Change.* New York: McGraw-Hill, 1990. Though argumentative in her approach, Fettner provides a simple discussion of the role of viruses in disease. Included are sections on autoimmunity and the possible roles played by viruses.

Roitt, Ivan. *Roitt's Essential Immunology.* 9th ed. Boston: Blackwell Scientific, 1997. A textbook written by a leading authority in the field. Several chapters deal specifically with immune disorders. Concise, with a large number of illustrations, but does require a basic knowledge of biology.

Roitt, Ivan, J. Brostoff, and D. K. Male. *Immunology.* 3d ed. London: Mosby, 1996. A concise, thorough, well-written textbook on immunology. Chapters are exceptionally descriptive, with easily understood diagrams and photographs. The section on autoimmune disease requires only a basic scientific background.

Rose, Noel R., and I. R. Mackay, eds. *The Autoimmune Diseases.* 3d ed. San Diego, Calif.: Academic Press, 1998. A well-written textbook containing thorough discussions of autoimmune disorders. Primarily for those with a background in immunology, but does provide much basic information.

IMMUNOPATHOLOGY

SPECIALTY

ANATOMY OR SYSTEM AFFECTED: All

SPECIALTIES AND RELATED FIELDS: Forensic medicine, immunology, pathology

DEFINITION: The medical field that studies hypersensitivity reactions or tissue damage resulting from an immune response against one's own tissues.

SCIENCE AND PROFESSION

Immunopathology is the subdiscipline of immunology that deals with diseases resulting from the body reacting against itself. In its mildest form, immunopathology may deal with allergies that, while a nuisance, are rarely life-threatening. In more severe forms, hypersensitivity to tissue antigens may result in damage to one's own cells or organs. The process may result in a wide variety of autoimmune diseases, including arthritis, lupus erythematosus, or rheumatic fever. Physicians who deal with such disorders are trained in immunology and/or pathology. In general, the tendency toward developing an autoimmune disease has a genetic basis; in turn, exposure to a particular environmental antigen may trigger the phenomenon in the susceptible individual.

DIAGNOSTIC AND TREATMENT TECHNIQUES

Autoimmune disease falls into four major categories: immediate hypersensitivities (allergies), antibody-dependent autoimmune reactions (transfusion reactions), immune complex disease (lupus), and delayed hypersensitivities (poison ivy). Treatment is determined by the specific form of the disease. In its simplest form, treatment consists of avoidance or removal of the allergen. In some cases, the injection of small quantities of the material into the patient may result in desensitization. In more severe situations, involving autoimmune or immune complex disease, treatment may consist of steroid derivatives that decrease the activity of immune cells. Since such inhibition is of a general nature, there exists the danger that the person may become increasingly susceptible to infection by common environmental microbes. Treatment may also be directed against the inflammatory process that leads to pathology, such as the use of aspirin in limiting the pain or inflammation of arthritis.

PERSPECTIVE AND PROSPECTS

Immunopathology studies immunologically mediated reactions against one's own tissue. A better under-standing of the reasons behind such a loss of tolerance to "self" antigens is necessary for prevention of the phenomenon. Such understanding will allow the development of treatments aimed either at reestablishing self-tolerance or at controlling the immune response in a manner that does not leave the individual as vulnerable to other forms of infection.

—*Richard Adler, Ph.D.*

See also Allergies; Autoimmune disorders; Arthritis; Blood and blood disorders; Bone marrow transplantation; Cells; Chemotherapy; Cytology; Cytopathology; Endocrinology; Endocrinology, pediatric; Glands; Healing; Hematology; Hematology, pediatric; Homeopathy; Hormones; Host-defense mechanisms; Immune system; Immunization and vaccination; Immunology; Lupus erythematosus; Lymphatic system; Oncology; Rheumatic fever; Serology; Skin; Transfusion; Transplantation.

FOR FURTHER INFORMATION:

Dwyer, John M. *The Body at War: The Story of Our Immune System.* 2d ed. London: J. M. Dent, 1993.

Feiden, Karyn. *Hope and Help for Chronic Fatigue Syndrome.* New York: Prentice Hall, 1990.

Life, Death, and the Immune System. New York: W. H. Freeman, 1994.

Nilsson, Lennart. *The Body Victorious.* New York: Delacorte Press, 1987.

IMPETIGO

DISEASE/DISORDER

ANATOMY OR SYSTEM AFFECTED: Skin

SPECIALTIES AND RELATED FIELDS: Bacteriology, dermatology, immunology, microbiology

DEFINITION: One of several severe skin infections caused by bacteria.

CAUSES AND SYMPTOMS

The most common form of impetigo begins as a small inflamed region on the skin, which becomes a small blister as much as 0.5 inch in diameter. The blister eventually becomes pustular and ruptures. A thick, yellow, encrusted scab develops. The lesions are superficial and painless, but they itch. Most cases of impetigo are caused by *Streptococcus pyogenes*, but a few cases are caused by *Streptococcus agalactiae*. Approximately 20 percent of women carrying *S. agalactiae* transmit it to their newborn babies. A few babies develop impetigo from the bacteria; others develop neonatal meningitis.

Bullous impetigo of the skin is characterized by large pustules about 1 inch in diameter surrounded by reddish, inflamed zones. The pustules contain a clear, yellowish fluid. The dried lesions develop a crust. This form of impetigo is caused by certain strains of *Staphylococcus aureus* that produce an exfoliative toxin. *S. aureus* accounts for approximately 10 percent of all impetigo cases. Bullous impetigo is an extremely contagious disease that is spread by direct contact or contact with contaminated objects. *S. aureus* is carried by up to 40 percent of all humans in the nose. Hospital outbreaks of *S. aureus* are common in infant nurseries, in burn units, and among patients recovering from surgery.

TREATMENT AND THERAPY

Impetigo caused by streptococci is treated most effectively with injected penicillin or erythromycin. Oral antibiotics are not as effective against streptococci as injected drugs. An ointment called mupirocin has been found to be as effective as oral penicillin or erythromycin. Bullous impetigo can be treated effectively with oral penicillin, cephalosporin, or erythromycin.

PERSPECTIVE AND PROSPECTS

Impetigo is generally associated with young children between two and five years of age. Untreated impetigo caused by streptococci may lead to a serious kidney disease called acute glomerulonephritis. In about 1 percent of children with impetigo, many different antibodies develop against the bacteria. Some of the antibodies may cross-react with kidney tissue or simply accumulate in the kidney. These antibodies activate complement, a group of proteins that normally kill bacteria. Activated complement in the kidneys damages these organs, leading to renal failure and death. Prompt treatment of impetigo with injected penicillin or erythromycin and topical mupirocin has been very effective in preventing acute glomerulonephritis in infants and children.

—*Jaime S. Colomé, Ph.D.*

See also Antibiotics; Bacterial infections; Dermatology; Dermatology, pediatric; Glomerulonephritis; Kidney disorders; Kidneys; Rashes; Renal failure; Skin; Skin disorders; Streptococcal infections.

FOR FURTHER INFORMATION:

Biddle, Wayne. *Field Guide to Germs*. New York: Henry Holt, 1995.

Finegold, Sydney M., and William J. Martin. *Bailey and Scott's Diagnostic Microbiology*. 6th ed. St. Louis: C. V. Mosby, 1998.

Pelczar, Michael J., Jr., E. C. S. Chan, and Noel R. Krieg. *Microbiology*. 5th ed. New York: McGraw-Hill, 1986.

Schlegel, Hans G. *General Microbiology*. 6th ed. Cambridge, England: Cambridge University Press, 1986.

IMPOTENCE. *See* SEXUAL DYSFUNCTION.

IN VITRO FERTILIZATION
PROCEDURE

ANATOMY OR SYSTEM AFFECTED: Cells, reproductive system, uterus

SPECIALTIES AND RELATED FIELDS: Embryology, genetics, gynecology

DEFINITION: The collection of eggs and sperm and their mixture in a dish in order to achieve fertilization, followed by the introduction of the resulting embryos into the uterus.

KEY TERMS:

capacitation: a change that the sperm goes through when in the female reproductive tract which causes it to swim more vigorously and enables it to fertilize the egg

chromosome: one of a pair of delicate filaments in the nucleus or a cell; each chromosome carries a specific portion of the total genetic information in the nucleus

diploid: containing a paired set of chromosomes, bearing two complete copies of nuclear genetic information for a cell

flagellum: a long, whiplike structure at the base of the sperm that propels it forward

gamete: a germ cell; an egg (ovum or oocyte) or sperm (spermatozoan)

haploid: containing only a single set of chromosomes; mature gametes are haploid

in vitro: a Latin term used in modern biology to indicate a process that has been taken from an organism and placed in a laboratory container (such as a test tube or dish) for observation

in vivo: a Latin term used in modern biology to indicate a process as it occurs naturally in a living organism

polyspermy: entry of more than one sperm into an egg, resulting in too many sets of chromosomes

zygote: the single cell formed after fertilization that has the capacity to develop into a new individual

Fertilization as a Natural Process

The goal of fertilization is to create a new individual that has the same number of chromosomes as the parent individuals, but who has a unique mixing of genetic traits from both the mother and father. A simple fusion of any two cells, one from each parent, would not achieve fertilization, since this would double the number of chromosomes in the new individual. Instead, specialized cells must be used that are haploid; that is, they have halved their number of chromosomes through a series of special cell divisions called meiosis. These haploid cells are the gametes (eggs and sperm) that reside in the gonads (the ovaries and testes). When two of these mature gametes fuse, they restore the normal, or diploid, number of chromosomes to the zygote that is formed.

Gametes are further specialized to carry out their specific tasks. The sperm is compact and motile in order to deliver its genetic material to the egg, or ovum. Its head, a somewhat flattened oval, contains its tightly packed haploid nucleus, topped off by an acrosomal cap. This cap is a bag of enzymes which will be used by the sperm when it reaches the egg. The narrow midpiece of the sperm contains its powerhouse, the mitochondria, which are surrounded by a carbohydrate energy source that will fuel the sperm's long journey. This is followed by a long tail, or flagellum, whose whiplike motion will propel the sperm toward its goal.

The egg is specialized to support and direct early development, for it is the egg that, after receiving the sperm, must divide to form the many cells that will finally mold themselves into the new organism. The egg, therefore, must be large. The human egg, only a tenth of a millimeter in diameter, is one of the largest cells in the body and is hundreds of times larger than a sperm. In its outer cytoplasm are huge numbers of cortical granules, which will be used at the time of fertilization. Surrounding the egg is a translucent layer, secreted by the follicular cells, called the zona pellucida.

In vivo fertilization, the normal process by which an egg and sperm meet and fuse to produce a zygote, is certainly a successful method of uniting two haploid set of chromosomes, a maternal set and a paternal set. In human in vivo fertilization, sperm start their long trip toward the egg in the female reproductive tract from the vagina. Substances contained in the secretions of the female reproductive tract alter the sperm, making them vigorous, straight swimmers. This process, called capacitation, although not thoroughly understood, is required for fertilization. From the vagina, the sperm move up through the uterus and into the 3-millimeter channel of the two Fallopian tubes that lead out to the ovaries. The sperm must travel to the far reaches of the Fallopian tubes, to a region called the ampulla, before meeting an egg. Three hundred million sperm will start the journey, and only several hundred will arrive. The entire trip takes about seventy minutes, and the sperm will remain alive in the female reproductive tract for approximately one to two days.

If fertilization is to take place, an egg must be available in the ampulla of one of the Fallopian tubes, where it will wait for about one day after being released. Ovulation of the egg is induced by two pituitary gland hormones, follicle-stimulating hormone (FSH) and luteinizing hormone (LH), which reach a peak of production around the fourteenth day of a woman's twenty-eight-day reproductive cycle. At ovulation, the egg bursts from its ovarian follicle, the fluid-filled compartment where it has been growing, and is picked up by the gently sweeping fingers of the Fallopian tube, the fimbria, which ensure safe passage of the egg from the ovary into the mouth of the Fallopian tube. The released egg is surrounded by several layers of follicle cells.

When a sperm encounters an egg in the ampulla, it must traverse several barriers before reaching the egg's surface. The first barrier is the layer of follicle cells around the egg called the corona radiata; this layer is loose and easily penetrated. The sperm then encounters the zona pellucida, which plays a critical role. One of the sugar-containing proteins in the zona pellucida, ZP3, captures the sperm by binding to its head and causes the acrosome, a cap on the head of the sperm that contains enzymes, to burst. This action releases acrosomal enzymes, which then coat the head of the sperm and digest a trail for the sperm through the rest of the zona pellucida. This acrosomal reaction must occur for fertilization to follow. When a sperm reaches the membrane of the egg, it settles on the surface broadside. The membranes of the sperm and egg fuse, and the chromosomes of the sperm enter the egg; fertilization has taken place.

Once the egg has permitted the entrance of one sperm, it is crucial that it then quickly bar any further sperm from entering. If polyspermy, or multiple-sperm entrance, occurs, havoc is wreaked by the extra sets of chromosomes, and usually death of the embryo ensues. The egg's mechanisms against polyspermy are swift and are mobilized as soon as the first sperm binds to the egg membrane. These changes are permanent and protect the egg from the entry of any further sperm.

The egg is now activated, and development begins by the division of the egg into many cells. As this proceeds, the egg slowly moves down the Fallopian tube to the uterus, where it will implant itself. It arrives in the uterus about four days after fertilization and implants on the sixth or seventh day. Only about one third of the eggs that are fertilized will actually survive the entire nine months of pregnancy. The other two thirds are spontaneously aborted, often without the woman ever having known that she was pregnant. This is nature's kind intervention, since most of these embryos are genetically or developmentally abnormal.

In Vitro Fertilization Techniques

An alternative to in vivo fertilization is in vitro fertilization, which allows sperm and eggs to meet in a culture dish; it has become a successful method of overcoming infertility. Since the procedure must mimic in vivo events, its development was dependent upon detailed knowledge of in vivo fertilization. The first task is to collect a number of eggs by inducing multiple ovulations using the hormones that normally regulate the process of ovulation. Usually a mixture of FSH and LH is used, followed by a large dose of human chorionic gonadotropin, which stimulates a surge of LH and causes the maturation of multiple eggs within their follicles.

Eggs are collected just prior to ovulation from their ripe follicles, using a small suction needle inserted through the vagina into the pelvic cavity. The needle is guided by ultrasonography (the use of ultrasonic waves to create a two-dimensional image). Eggs that are recovered are put into a culture medium and incubated at body temperature (37 degrees Celsius) for six to twenty-four hours, until they mature. They are then combined with sperm. The sperm have been freshly collected or previously collected and held in frozen storage. It is critical that the sperm are artificially capacitated before they are used. Though it is not clear what specifically causes capacitation, it is fortunate that the culture medium used to wash the sperm serves this function. After several washes, the sperm that swim up through the culture medium are collected, ensuring that only vigorous swimmers are used and providing a concentrated sample of about two hundred thousand sperm.

The Process of In Vitro Fertilization

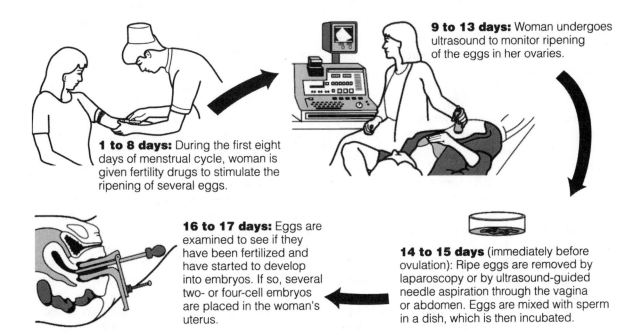

1 to 8 days: During the first eight days of menstrual cycle, woman is given fertility drugs to stimulate the ripening of several eggs.

9 to 13 days: Woman undergoes ultrasound to monitor ripening of the eggs in her ovaries.

14 to 15 days (immediately before ovulation): Ripe eggs are removed by laparoscopy or by ultrasound-guided needle aspiration through the vagina or abdomen. Eggs are mixed with sperm in a dish, which is then incubated.

16 to 17 days: Eggs are examined to see if they have been fertilized and have started to develop into embryos. If so, several two- or four-cell embryos are placed in the woman's uterus.

Once fertilization takes place, the embryos are observed in vitro through the course of several cell divisions to ensure that development is taking place and that it appears to be normal. One of the problems that has been observed is polyspermy. Eggs that are immature or too old apparently are less able to mobilize their defenses against polyspermy. When healthy embryos reach the eight- to sixteen-cell stage, several embryos are introduced into the woman's uterus. Though this method poses a risk of multiple births, it also provides a better chance for success.

For many couples who are infertile, the disappointment of being unable to conceive children is too great to bear. For these people, in vitro fertilization has provided a welcome alternative route to conception. It has been estimated that one out of every eight couples of childbearing age is infertile. The causes are many. Often, the delicate Fallopian tubes are blocked or even missing. These tubes are easily damaged by inflammation, with about 40 percent of blocked Fallopian tubes resulting from the two most common sexually transmitted diseases, gonorrhea and chlamydia. Endometriosis, a condition in which cells from the lining of the uterus spread to other regions of the body, can also cause infertility, as can the presence of antibodies against sperm in the female reproductive tract or alterations in the cervical mucus. Up to 40 percent of infertility is attributable to low sperm counts or sperm deficiencies in the male. Though in vitro fertilization was originally designed to overcome infertility caused by blocked Fallopian tubes, it has been found to be effective in overcoming infertility in each of the causes listed above.

Couples normally face an average of six to nine years of infertility before turning to an in vitro fertilization clinic. The demand for this technique is certainly great, and the success rate of live births is 21 percent, about that achieved naturally; some clinics have a much higher success rate. In 1994 alone, there were 294 such clinics registered in the United States; 39,390 procedures were performed, and 9,573 births occurred.

Clinics concentrate on improving success rates and consequently have developed a number of variations in the technique. Improvements have been made in the method of transferring the embryo into the patient. Often, two to four embryos, which have been developing in culture for less than two days, are transferred into the uterus using a narrow gauge plastic catheter passed through the cervix and into the uterus. This is a safe, nonsurgical procedure. The disadvantage is that the embryos are being placed in the uterus at least two days prior to the time that they would arrive with in vivo fertilization. To overcome the problems that this early arrival might pose, new techniques have been developed, such as zygote intrafallopian transfer (ZIFT) and gamete intrafallopian transfer (GIFT), in which the embryos or gametes are transferred to the Fallopian tubes rather than to the uterus. This procedure only works, however, if the patient's Fallopian tubes are functional. Moreover, it has the disadvantage of requiring two surgical procedures: one for obtaining the eggs and the second for inserting the embryos into the Fallopian tubes.

In situations in which the male partner has abnormal sperm that cannot penetrate an egg, laboratory scientists may use a microneedle to inject a single sperm directly into the egg. This fertilization method, called intracytoplasmic sperm injection or ICSI (pronounced "ick-see"), is highly successful even with sperm surgically removed from the male reproductive tract.

In situations that require specific knowledge of the embryo's genetics, one or two cells called blastomeres can be removed from the eight- or sixteen-cell-stage embryo. Genetic material in the removed blastomeres can be chemically evaluated by a procedure called polymerase chain reaction (PCR). This evaluation can be very useful when there is a high probability that the embryo may have a life-threatening genetic disease. Embryos determined to be free of such disease can be selected for uterine transfer, none the worse for the lost blastomere.

With microsurgery, it is even possible to remove the nucleus from an egg and replace it with the diploid nucleus from another cell of the organism providing the egg. This procedure enables duplicate copies called clones to be made of the animal providing the transplanted nucleus. This procedure offers great commercial promise for animal breeders, but its use in human medicine has been ethically renounced.

The development of cryopreservation, or freezing, techniques have dramatically improved the process of in vitro fertilization. Embryos can be safely preserved at extremely low temperatures (approximately minus 200 degrees Celsius) and then thawed for implantation. Generally, many more embryos are produced in an in vitro fertilization procedure than can be used. With cryopreservation, the unused embryos can be preserved and used in a second attempt at implantation, if the first fails. Success is often better in a second attempt, since the uterus has recovered from the hormonal barrage required for the collection of eggs and has been prepared for implantation by the woman's own natural cycle. Ethical complications can occur, for example, when frozen embryos remain after the death of the intended parents.

In vitro fertilization methods are extraordinarily safe. There is no increase in birth defects or mortality for the babies that are conceived using this technique. There is a marked increase in multiple births, however, which occur in 1 percent of in vivo fertilization cases and in 15 to 20 percent of in vitro fertilization cases. This increase can be avoided as techniques improve, making it less necessary to place multiple embryos in the patient.

In vitro fertilization has opened the door to many combinations of solutions to the problems of infertility. For example, if a woman can produce normal eggs but is unable to carry a fetus as a result of a malfunctioning uterus, then this technique allows her eggs to be combined with her partner's sperm and the embryos implanted into a surrogate mother. If she is unable to produce eggs but has a healthy uterus, a donor can be used to supply eggs, and the recipient can then carry the embryos to term. Women in their fifties or sixties who have gone through the menopause have received fertilized eggs donated by younger women and have given birth. Such variations in parenthood, however, lead to complex legal and ethical questions.

PERSPECTIVE AND PROSPECTS

It was on July 25, 1978, that the first baby conceived through in vitro fertilization was born. Louise Brown was born to a couple in England who had tried in vain for more than nine years to have a child before they turned to a clinic started by Patrick Steptoe, a surgeon from Oldham Hospital, and Robert Edwards, a reproductive physiologist from the University of Cambridge. Their clinic was the first in the world to adapt in vitro fertilization techniques to humans.

Steptoe and Edwards had started their work in the late 1960's, building on a string of successes and failures with in vitro fertilization. Attempts at using this technique in mammals date back to the nineteenth century. No successes could occur, however, until the discovery of capacitation in 1951; once it was known that mammalian sperm had to be capacitated artificially before they could be used in vitro, progress

could be made. The first successful in vitro fertilization of mammalian eggs followed in 1959, using rabbit gametes. The 1960's saw a rapid increase in the use of in vitro fertilization techniques applied to animal breeding. Work on human in vitro fertilization did not start until 1965, when Edwards reported that he had successfully induced maturation of a human egg in vitro. Edwards teamed up with Steptoe, and they, along with coworker Jean Purdy, reported in 1970 that they had achieved in vitro fertilization and cleavage in human eggs. A year later, they reported success in growing a human embryo in vitro up to the stage of implantation. Cryopreservation of a mammalian embryo came in 1972, when two independent studies reported that mouse embryos had been frozen and thawed without damage. All the pieces were then in place.

In vitro fertilization clinics are now found in many countries all over the world. The first one in the United States was started by Georgeanna Jones, a reproductive endocrinologist, and her husband Howard Jones, a gynecological surgeon. Facing retirement, they instead found themselves caught up in the possibilities of in vitro fertilization solutions for infertile couples and established their own clinic in Norfolk, Virginia, in 1979. Their first success came in 1981 in the form of a baby named Elizabeth Carr. The first successful use of a previously frozen human embryo occurred in Australia in 1984; two years later, a similar procedure was employed successfully in the United States.

In vitro fertilization and its many permutations have opened many doors of opportunity and led to many heated controversies. What is to be done with unused frozen embryos? What are the rights of gamete donors to the child that is born? What are the rights of a surrogate mother or the rights of a child to knowledge of his or her parentage? Some countries, such as Australia, Norway, Spain, and the United Kingdom, have already responded by passing extensive legislation regulating IVF. Other countries have been slower to respond. This vacuum of social consensus leaves decisions involving in vitro fertilization to physicians, scientists, and the courts.

—Mary S. Tyler, Ph.D.;
updated by Armand M. Karow, Ph.D.

See also Bionics and biotechnology; Conception; Embryology; Ethics; Genetic engineering; Gynecology; Infertility in females; Infertility in males; Multiple births; Obstetrics; Pregnancy and gestation; Reproductive system.

FOR FURTHER INFORMATION:

Bonnicksen, Andrea L. *In Vitro Fertilization: Building Policy from Laboratories to Legislature.* New York: Columbia University Press, 1989. An excellent discussion of the history of in vitro fertilization and the ethical questions raised. An appendix includes a detailed but concise description of the technique.

Harkess, Carla. *The Infertility Book: A Comprehensive Medical and Emotional Guide.* Berkeley, Calif.: Celestial Arts, 1992. Harkness, a professional writer, describes IVF from a patient's viewpoint. The book also includes a bibliography, four line drawings, a glossary, a resource directory, and an index.

Seibel, Machelle M., and Susan L. Crockin, eds. *Family Building Through Egg and Sperm Donation.* Sudbury, Mass.: Jones and Bartlett, 1996. A physician and an attorney have assembled a collection of essays written by and for their peers on IVF procedures and their social, ethical, religious, and legal issues. The authors gaze into the future of genetic implications. This book will be heavy reading for the nonprofessional but provides great rewards for the effort.

Sher, Geoffrey, Virginia Marriage Davis, and Jean Stoess. *In Vitro Fertilization.* Rev. ed. New York: Facts on File, 1998. Dr. Sher and his clinical associates describe for patients in words and line drawings the process of evaluating patients and the procedures involved in IVF. The book also includes a glossary and an index.

Stephenson, Patricia, and Marsden G. Wagner, eds. *Tough Choices: In Vitro Fertilization and the Reproductive Technologies.* Philadelphia: Temple University Press, 1993. The editors assembled an international group of academic authorities to present an analysis of the effects of IVF on social structure.

Weschler, Toni. *Taking Charge of Your Infertility.* New York: HarperPerennial, 1995. This book encourages women to become responsible consumers of their own reproductive health. Includes excellent discussions of infertility, natural birth control, and achieving pregnancy.

Wisot, Arthur, and David Meldrum. *Conceptions and Misconceptions.* Vancouver: Harley and Marks, 1997. Written by two leading fertility experts, this book is an excellent guide through the maze of in vitro fertilization and other assisted reproductive techniques. Includes an excellent discussion of the basic physiology of conception and reproduction.

INCONTINENCE
DISEASE/DISORDER

ANATOMY OR SYSTEM AFFECTED: Abdomen, bladder, gastrointestinal system, urinary system

SPECIALTIES AND RELATED FIELDS: Family practice, geriatrics and gerontology, gynecology, internal medicine, obstetrics, pediatrics, psychiatry, urology

DEFINITION: Involuntary loss of urine or feces, primarily a social and hygienic problem that particularly affects the older population.

KEY TERMS:

atonic bladder: a bladder characterized by weak muscles

enuresis: bed-wetting

frequency: urination at short intervals; a common problem accompanying incontinence

micturition: the act of urinating

nocturia: nighttime urination

sphincter: a ring-shaped muscle that surrounds a natural opening in the body and can open or close it by expanding or contracting

urge incontinence: a strong desire to urinate followed by leakage of urine

urgency: a strong desire to void urine immediately

CAUSES AND SYMPTOMS

Continence is skill acquired in humans by the interaction of two processes: socialization of the infant and maturation of the central nervous system. Without society's expectation of continence, and without broadly accepted definitions of appropriate behavior, the concept of "incontinence" would be meaningless. There are many causes for urinary incontinence. Three broad (interrelated and often overlapping) categories are physiologic voiding dysfunction, factors directly influencing voiding function, and factors affecting the individual's capacity to manage voiding.

The causes of physiologic voiding dysfunction involve an abnormality in bladder or sphincter function, or both. The bladder and sphincter have only two functions: to store urine until the appropriate time for urination and then to empty it completely. Voiding dysfunction involves the failure of one or both of these mechanisms. Four basic types of voiding dysfunction can be distinguished: detrusor instability, genuine stress incontinence, outflow obstruction, and atonic bladder.

Detrusor instability is a condition characterized by involuntary bladder (detrusor muscle) contraction during filling. While all the causes of bladder instability are not fully understood, it can be associated with the following: neurologic disease (brain and spinal cord abnormalities), inflammation of the bladder wall, bladder outlet obstruction, stress urinary incontinence, and idiopathic (spontaneous or primary) dysfunction. Detrusor instability usually causes symptoms of frequency, urgency, and possibly nocturia or enuresis.

Genuine stress incontinence is caused by a failure to hold urine during bladder filling as a result of an incompetent urethral sphincter mechanism. If the closure mechanism of the bladder outlet fails to hold urine, incontinence will occur. This is usually manifested during physical exertion or abdominal stress (such as coughing or sneezing). It can occur in either sex, but it is more common in women because of their shorter urethra and the physical trauma of childbirth. Men can experience stress incontinence following traumatic or surgical damage to the sphincter.

Obstruction of the outflow of urine during voiding can produce various symptoms, including frequency, straining to void, poor urinary stream, preurination and posturination dribbling, and a feeling of urgency with resulting leakage (urge incontinence). In severe cases, the bladder is never completely emptied and a volume of residual urine persists. Overflow incontinence can result. Common causes of bladder outlet obstruction are prostatic enlargement, bladder neck narrowing, or urethral obstruction. Functional obstruction occurs when a neurologic lesion prevents the coordinated relaxation of the sphincter during voiding. This phenomenon is termed detrusor-sphincter dyssynergia.

An atonic bladder—one with weak muscle walls—does not produce a sufficient contraction to empty completely. Emptying can be enhanced by abdominal straining or manual expression, but a large residual volume persists. The sensation of retaining urine might or might not be present. If sensation is present, frequency of urination is common because only a small portion of the bladder volume is emptied each time. Sensation is often diminished, and the residual urine volume can be considerable (100 to 1,000 milliliters). Overflow incontinence often occurs.

An acute urinary tract infection can cause transient incontinence, even in a fit, healthy young person who normally has no voiding dysfunction. Acute frequency and urgency with disturbed sensation and pain can result in the inability to reach a toilet in time or to detect when incontinence is occurring. If an underlying voiding dysfunction is also present, an acute urinary tract infection is likely to cause incontinence.

Many drugs can also disturb the delicate balance of normal functioning. The most obvious category consists of diuretics, those drugs which increase urinary discharge; a large, swift production of urine will give most people frequency and urgency. If the bladder is unstable, it might not be able to handle a sudden influx of urine, and urge incontinence can result. Sedation can affect voiding function directly (for example, diazepam can lower urethral resistance) or can make the individual less responsive to signals from the bladder and thus unable to maintain continence. Other commonly prescribed drugs have secondary actions on voiding function. Not all patients, however, will experience urinary side effects from these drugs.

Various endocrine disorders can upset normal voiding function. Diabetes can cause polydypsia (extreme thirst), requiring the storage of a large volume of urine. Glycosuria (sugar in the urine) might encourage urinary tract infection. Thyroid imbalances can aggravate an overactive or underactive bladder. Pituitary gland disorders can result in the production of excessive urine volumes because of an antidiuretic hormone deficiency. Estrogen deficiency in postmenopausal women causes atrophic changes in the vaginal and urethral tissues and will worsen stress incontinence and an unstable bladder.

Several bladder pathologies can also cause incontinence by disrupting normal functioning. A patient with a neoplasm (abnormal tissue growth), whether benign or malignant, or a stone in the bladder occasionally experiences incontinence as a symptom. These are infrequent causes of incontinence.

Often it takes something else in addition to the underlying problem to tip the balance and produce incontinence. This is especially true for elderly and disabled persons who are delicately balanced between continence and incontinence. For example, immobility—anything that impedes access—is likely to induce incontinence. Immobility can be the result of the gradual worsening of a chronic condition, such as arthritis, multiple sclerosis, or Parkinson's disease, until eventually the individual simply cannot reach a toilet in time. The condition may be acute—an accident or illness that suddenly renders a person immobile might be the start of failure to control the bladder.

In the case of children, most daytime wetting persists until the child reaches school age. It is less common than bed-wetting (enuresis), and the two often go together. One in ten five-year-old children, however, still wets the bed regularly. With no treatment, this figure gradually falls to 5 percent of ten-year-olds and to 2 percent of adults. It is twice as common in boys as in girls, has strong familial tendencies, and is associated with stressful events in the third or fourth year of life. A urinary tract infection is sometimes the cause.

Fecal, as opposed to urinary, incontinence is generally caused by underlying disorders of the colon, rectum, or anus; neurogenic disorders; or fecal impaction. Severe diarrhea increases the likelihood of having fecal incontinence. Some of the more common disorders that can cause diarrhea are ulcerative colitis, carcinoma, infection, radiation therapy, and the effect of drugs (for example, broad-spectrum antibiotics, laxative abuse, or iron supplements). Fecal incontinence tends to be a common, if seldom reported, accompaniment.

The pelvic floor muscles support the anal sphincter, and any weakness will cause a tendency to fecal stress incontinence. The vital flap valve formed by the anorectal angle can be lost if these muscles are weak. An increase in abdominal pressure would therefore tend to force the rectal contents down and out of the anal canal. This might be the result of congenital abnormalities or of later trauma (for example, childbirth, anal surgery, or direct trauma). A lifelong habit of straining at stool might also cause muscle weakness.

The medulla and higher cortical centers of the brain have a role in coordinating and controlling the defecation reflex. Therefore, any neurologic disorder that impairs the ability to detect or inhibit impending defecation will probably result in a tendency to incontinence, similar in causation to the uninhibited or unstable bladder. For example, the paraplegic can lose all direct sensation of and voluntary control over bowel activity. Neurologic disorders such as multiple sclerosis, cerebrovascular accident, and diffuse dementia can affect sensation or inhibition, or a combination of both. Incontinence occurs with some demented people because of a physical inability to inhibit defecation. With others, it occurs because the awareness that such behavior is inappropriate has been lost.

Severe constipation with impaction of feces is probably the most common cause of fecal incontinence, and it predominates as a cause among the elderly and those living in extended care facilities. Chronic constipation leads to impaction when the fluid content of the feces is progressively absorbed by the colon, leaving hard, rounded rocks in the bowel. This hard matter promotes mucus production and bacterial activity, which causes a foul-smelling brown fluid to accumulate. If the rectum is overdistended for any length of time, the internal and external sphincters become relaxed, allowing passage of this mucus as spurious diarrhea. The patient's symptoms usually include fairly continuous leakage of fluid stool without any awareness of control.

Most children are continent of feces by the age of four years, but 1 percent still have problems at seven years of age. More boys than girls are incontinent, suggesting that developmental factors can be relevant because boys mature more slowly. Fecal incontinence or conscious soiling in childhood (sometimes referred to as encopresis) has, like nocturnal enuresis, long been regarded as evidence of a psychiatric or psychologic disorder in the child. The evidence, however, does not support the claim that most fecally incontinent children are disturbed.

Such children usually have fastidious, overanxious parents who are intent on toilet training. The child is punished for soiling, so defecation tends to be inhibited, both in the underwear and in the toilet. When toilet training is attempted, the child may be repeatedly seated on the toilet in the absence of a full rectum and be unable to perform. The situation becomes fraught with anxiety, and bowel movements become associated with unpleasantness in the child's mind. The child therefore retains feces and becomes constipated. Defecation then becomes difficult and painful as well.

TREATMENT AND THERAPY

The two primary methods of treating urinary incontinence involve medical and surgical intervention (drug therapy and surgery) and bladder training.

Many drugs can be prescribed to help those with urinary incontinence. Often the results are disappointing, although some drugs can be useful for carefully selected and accurately diagnosed patients. Drugs are often used to control detrusor instability and urge incontinence by relaxing the detrusor muscle and inhibiting reflex contractions. This therapy is helpful in some patients. Sometimes when the drug is given in large enough doses to be effective, however, the side effects are so troublesome that the therapy must be abandoned. Drugs that reduce bladder contractions must be used cautiously in patients who have voiding difficulty, since urinary retention can be precipitated. Careful assessment must be made of residual urine.

Drug therapy is also used with caution in patients with a residual volume greater than 100 milliliters. Some drugs are used in an attempt to prevent stress incontinence by increasing urethral tone. Phenylpropanolamine and ephedrine, those most often used, are thought to act on the alpha receptors in the urethra.

Drug therapy can also be used to relieve outflow obstruction. Phenoxybenzamine is most commonly used, but this drug can have dangerous side effects, such as tachycardia (an abnormally fast heartbeat) or postural hypotension. If the bladder does not contract sufficiently to ensure complete emptying, drug therapy can be attempted to increase the force of the voiding contractions. Carbachol, bethanechol, and distigmine bromide have all been used with some success. Other drugs might be useful in treating factors affecting incontinence—for example, antibiotics to treat a urinary tract infection or laxatives to treat or prevent constipation.

Many drugs can exacerbate a tendency to incontinence. For those who are prone to incontinence, medications and dosage schedules are chosen that will have a minimal effect on bladder control. For example, a slow-acting diuretic, in a divided dose, can help someone with urgency and weak sphincter tone to avoid incontinence. An analgesic might be preferable to night sedation for those who need pain relief but who wet the bed at night if they are sedated.

Turning to surgical intervention, none of the several surgical approaches that have been used in an attempt to treat an unstable bladder has gained widespread use. Cystodistention (stretching the bladder under general anesthesia) and bladder transection, for example, are presumed to act by disturbing the neurologic pathways that control uninhibited contractions. Many vaginal and suprapubic procedures are available to help correct genuine stress incontinence in women. Surgery can also be used to relieve outflow obstruction—for example, to remove an enlarged prostate gland, divide a stricture, or widen a narrow urethra.

In cases of severe intractable incontinence, major surgery is an option. For those with a damaged urethra, a neourethra can be constructed. For those with a nonfunctioning sphincter, an artificial sphincter can be implanted. In some patients, a urinary diversion with a stoma (outlet) is the only and best alternative for continence. Although a drastic solution, a urostomy might be easier to cope with than an incontinent urethra, because an effective appliance will contain the urine.

Urinary incontinence is occasionally the result of surgery, usually urologic or gynecologic but sometimes a major pelvic or spinal procedure. Such iatrogenic incontinence can be caused by neurologic or sphincter damage, leading to various dysfunctional voiding patterns.

Several different types of bladder training or retraining are distinguishable and can be used in different circumstances. The most important element for success is that the correct regimen be selected for each patient and situation. A thorough assessment identifies those patients who will benefit from bladder training and determines the most appropriate method. Other factors that contribute to the incontinence should also be treated (for example, a urinary tract infection or constipation), because ignoring them will impair the success of a program.

Bladder training is most suitable for people with the symptoms of frequency, urgency, and urge incontinence (with or without an underlying unstable bladder) and for those with nonspecific incontinence. The elderly often have these symptoms. Patients with voiding dysfunction, other than an unstable bladder, are unlikely to benefit from bladder training.

The aim of bladder training is to restore the patient with frequency, urgency, and urge incontinence to a more normal and convenient voiding pattern. Ultimately, voiding should occur at intervals of three to four hours (or even longer) without any urgency or incontinence. Drug therapy is sometimes combined with bladder training for those with detrusor instability.

Bladder training aims to restore an individual's confidence in the bladder's ability to hold urine and to reestablish a more normal pattern. Initially, a patient keeps a baseline chart for three to seven days, recording how often urine is passed and when incontinence occurs. This chart is reviewed with the program supervisor, and an individual regimen is developed. The purpose is to extend the time between voiding gradually, encouraging the patient to practice delaying the need to void, rather than giving in to the feeling of urgency. Initially, the times chosen can be at set intervals throughout the day (for example, every one or two hours) or can be variable, according to the individual's pattern as indicated by the baseline chart. When the baseline chart reveals a definite pattern to the incontinence, it might be possible to set voiding times in accordance with and in anticipation of this pattern.

A pattern of voiding is set for patients throughout the day (timed voiding). Usually no pattern is set at night, even if nocturia or nocturnal enuresis is a problem. Patients are instructed to pass urine as necessary during the night. Sometimes the provision of a suitable pad or appliance helps to increase confidence and means that, if incontinence does occur, the results will not be disastrous. If urgency is experienced, patients are taught to sit or stand still and try to suppress the sensation rather than to rush immediately to the toilet. A normal fluid intake is encouraged because the goal is to have the patient continent and able to drink fluids adequately.

As patients achieve the target intervals without having to urinate prematurely or leaking, the intervals can gradually be lengthened. The speed of progress depends on the individual and on other variables, such as the initial severity of symptoms, motivation, and the amount of professional support. Patients usually remain at one time interval for one to two weeks before it is increased by fifteen to thirty minutes for another two weeks. Once the target of three- to four-hour voiding without urgency has been achieved, it is useful to maintain the chart and set times for at least another month to prevent relapse.

Some people find that practicing pelvic muscle exercises helps to suppress urgency. Any weakness in the pelvic floor muscles will cause a tendency not only to urinary incontinence but also to fecal stress incontinence. Mild weakness can respond to pelvic muscle exercises similar to those used in alleviating the symptoms of stress incontinence, but with a concentration on the posterior rather than the anterior portion of the pelvic muscles. Rectal tone is assessed by digital examination, during which the patient is instructed to squeeze. Regular contractions on the posterior portion of the pelvic muscles are then practiced often for at least two months (usually in sets of twenty-five, three times a day).

In cases of fecal impaction, a course of disposable phosphate enemas—one or two daily for seven to ten days, or until no further return is obtained—is the treatment of choice. A single enema is seldom efficient, even if an apparently good result is obtained, because impaction is often extensive: The first enema merely clears the lowest portion of the bowel. If fecal incontinence persists once the bowel has been totally cleared (a plain abdominal X ray can be helpful in confirming this), the condition is assumed to be neurogenic in origin rather than caused by the impaction.

PERSPECTIVE AND PROSPECTS

Historically, most health professionals have been profoundly ignorant of the causes and management of incontinence. Incontinence was often regarded as a condition over which there was no control, rather than as a symptom of an underlying physiologic disorder or as a symptom of a patient with a unique combination of problems, needs, and potentials. The unfortunate result of such limited understanding was passive acceptance of the symptom of incontinence. Incontinence, often viewed as repulsive, is often a condition that is merely tolerated. As public recognition of the implications of incontinence has increased, however, the stigma associated with it has slowly decreased. It has become common knowledge that millions of Americans suffer from incontinence, and most pharmacies and supermarkets have a section for incontinence products.

At one time, incontinence was primarily regarded as a "nursing" problem, with nurses providing custodial care—keeping the patient as clean and comfortable as possible and preventing pressure ulcers from developing. Gradually, nurses were not alone in acknowledging that incontinence was a symptom requiring investigation and intervention; those in other health professions also began to realize this need. In the 1980's, research dollars began to be allocated for the study of incontinence. In 1988, U.S. Surgeon General C. Everett Koop estimated that 8 billion dollars was being spent by the federal government on incontinence in the United States annually.

As incontinence began to be recognized by the public as a health problem rather than as an inevitable part of aging, more people admitted having the symptoms of incontinence and sought medical attention. It has been estimated that, of all cases of incontinence, more than one-third can be cured, another one-third can be dramatically improved, and most of the remainder can be significantly improved.

—*Genevieve Slomski, Ph.D.*

See also Bed-wetting; Constipation; Diarrhea and dysentery; Digestion; Sphincterectomy; Stone removal; Stones; Urinary disorders; Urinary system; Urology; Urology, pediatric.

FOR FURTHER INFORMATION:

Dierich, Mary, and Felecia Froe. *Overcoming Incontinence: A Straightforward Guide to Your Options.* New York: John Wiley & Sons, 2000. The authors present no-nonsense, practical advice on incontinence. Readers will learn how the urinary system works and how and when to seek professional help.

Gartley, Cheryle, ed. *Managing Incontinence*. Ottawa, Ill.: Jameson Books, 1985. An overview of the basic treatment options for urinary incontinence, including surgical and nonsurgical methods. Although somewhat technical, this work is accessible to the general reader. Includes a bibliography.

Jeter, Katherine, et al., eds. *Nursing for Continence*. Philadelphia: W. B. Saunders, 1990. This work, written by a group of nurses, addresses the diagnosis, treatment, and management of incontinence in all age groups and in special populations and circumstances in a practical, thorough, and sensitive manner.

Lucas, Malcolm, Simon Emery, and John Beynon, eds. *Incontinence*. Malden, Mass.: Blackwell Science, 1999. This book's editors are consultant surgeons at Swansea NHS Trust, and they have combined their expertise in this volume, in which they describe the various operations they perform to counteract urinary and fecal incontinence.

Raz, Sholomo, ed. *Female Urology*. 2d ed. Philadelphia: W. B. Saunders, 1996. The book begins with fundamentals of the female genitourinary tract, then analyzes the dynamics of continence mechanisms. Female urinary incontinence is treated as a multifaceted subject.

INDIGESTION
DISEASE/DISORDER
ANATOMY OR SYSTEM AFFECTED: Abdomen, gastrointestinal system, intestines, stomach

SPECIALTIES AND RELATED FIELDS: Family practice, gastroenterology, internal medicine

DEFINITION: Indigestion, which is also known as dyspepsia, is a digestive disorder that is often mistaken for heartburn. This burning sensation in the chest and throat is one of the symptoms of indigestion, but the patient may have other complaints as well, such as abdominal pain, belching, a bloated feeling, nausea, vomiting, and sometimes diarrhea. There is usually no organic cause for this disorder; it may be attributable to stress, the consumption of certain foods and beverages, and the excessive swallowing of air while eating. Sometimes, however, an underlying disease may be present, such as inflammation of the esophagus, a peptic ulcer, disease of the gallbladder or liver, and bacterial or viral infections. A psychological factor may also exist.

—*Jason Georges and Tracy Irons-Georges*

See also Abdomen; Abdominal disorders; Appendicitis; Cholecystitis; Cirrhosis; Colitis; Constipation; Crohn's disease; Diarrhea and dysentery; Digestion; Diverticulitis and diverticulosis; Gallbladder diseases; Gastroenterology; Gastroenterology, pediatric; Gastrointestinal disorders; Gastrointestinal system; Heartburn; Intestinal disorders; Liver; Liver disorders; Nausea and vomiting; Nutrition; Stress; Ulcer surgery; Ulcers.

FOR FURTHER INFORMATION:
Hunter, J. O., and V. Alun Jones, eds. *Food and the Gut*. Philadelphia: Bailliere Tindall, 1985.

Janowitz, Henry D. *Indigestion: Living Better with Upper Intestinal Problems*. New York: Oxford University Press, 1992.

_____. *Your Gut Feelings: A Complete Guide to Living Better with Intestinal Problems*. Rev. ed. New York: Oxford University Press, 1994.

Wolfe, M. Michael, and Sidney Cohen. *Therapy of Digestive Disorders: A Companion to Sleisenger and Fordtran's Gastrointestinal and Liver Disease*. Philadelphia: W. B. Saunders, 2000.

INFARCTION. *See* HEART ATTACK.

INFECTION
DISEASE/DISORDER
ANATOMY OR SYSTEM AFFECTED: All

SPECIALTIES AND RELATED FIELDS: Bacteriology, family practice, hematology, internal medicine, virology

DEFINITION: Invasion of the body by disease-causing organisms such as bacteria, viruses, fungi, and parasites; symptoms of infection may include pain, swelling, fever, and loss of normal function.

KEY TERMS:
antibiotic: a substance that destroys or inhibits the growth of microorganisms, such as bacteria

antibody: a small protein secreted from specialized white blood cells which binds to and aids in the destruction of pathogens

antigen: a substance found on pathogens to which the antibodies bind; also, any substance considered foreign by the body

bacteria: small microorganisms; some bacteria found normally in and on the body have helpful functions, while others that invade the body or disrupt the normal bacteria are harmful and often infectious

edema: an abnormal accumulation of fluid in the body tissues; tissue with edema is swollen in appearance

infectious: referring to a microorganism which is capable of causing disease, often with the ability to spread from one person to another

inflammation: a tissue reaction to injury which may or may not involve infection; pain, heat, redness, and edema are the usual signs of inflammation

pathogen: a microorganism or substance capable of producing a disease, such as a bacterium causing an infection

phagocytosis: the ingestion and destruction of a pathogen or abnormal tissue by specialized white blood cells known as phagocytes

virus: a very small organism which is dependent upon a host cell to meet its metabolic needs and to reproduce

PROCESS AND EFFECTS

Healthy people live with potential pathogens; that is, people have on and in their bodies non-disease-causing bacteria. They live in harmony with these organisms and in fact benefit from their presence. For example, some of the bacteria found in the intestinal tract supply vitamin K, which is important in blood-clotting reactions.

The human body has several features which prevent disease-causing organisms from inducing an infection. These features include anatomical barriers, such as unbroken skin, and the mucus in the nose, mouth, and lungs, which can trap pathogens. Another defense is the acid within the stomach, and even bacteria that are normally present in certain areas of the body can force out more harmful bacteria. The immune system is specially developed to ward off intruders.

Immune cells and factors secreted from these cells provide the next line of defense against invading organisms. Antibodies are secreted from specialized white blood cells known as plasma cells. These antibodies are very specific for the recognition of pathogens. For example, one antibody will recognize a particular strain of bacteria but not another. Antibodies attach themselves to the part of the bacterium called the antigen. Once bound to the antigen, they aid in the destruction of the pathogen. In addition to plasma cells, other white blood cells help in combating infections. These include the phagocytes called macrophages and neutrophils. Both of these immune cells have the ability to eat and digest pathogens such as bacteria in a process known as phagocytosis.

Microorganisms that cause disease must, in some way, overwhelm the body's natural defenses and immune system. Bacteria capable of causing infections may even be naturally occurring organisms that have left their normal environment and overcome the elements that normally hold them at bay. For example, some normal bacteria that reside in the mouth may cause pneumonia (inflammation of the lungs) if they gain access to the lungs.

Other infections can be caused by pathogens that do not normally reside in the body. One can "catch" a cold or the flu, or even a sexually transmitted disease. These kinds of infections are called communicable or transmissible infections. Similarly, a physician treating someone who has been bitten by a bat, skunk, or dog will want to know whether the animal has rabies. Rabies is a viral infection which is transmitted via a bite which breaks the skin and contaminates the wound with infectious saliva.

No matter what the route of infection, the body must mount a response to the intruding microorganism. Often the signs and symptoms one observes are not caused by the direct action of the infecting pathogen, but rather reflect the immune system's response to the infection. The most frequent signs and symptoms include inflammation and pain at the site of infection, as well as fever.

The inflammatory response is a nonspecific defense that is triggered whenever body tissues are injured, as in the case of infection. The goal of the inflammatory response is to prevent the spread of the infectious agent to nearby tissues, destroy the pathogens, remove the damaged tissues, and begin the healing process.

The signs of inflammation include redness, edema (tissue swelling), heat, pain, and loss of normal function. At first glance, these reactions do not appear to be beneficial to the body, but they do help fight the infection and aid in the healing process. The redness is attributable to an increase in blood flow to the area of infection. This increase in blood to the site of infection helps provide nutrients to the tissue, as well as removing some of the waste products that develop as the immune system fights the infection. With this increase in blood flow comes an increase in the temperature and the amount of blood that leaks out of blood vessels into the tissue spaces, causing edema at the site of infection. Some of the blood that leaks into the site of infection contains clotting proteins that help form a clot around the infected area, thereby reducing the chances that the pathogen could escape

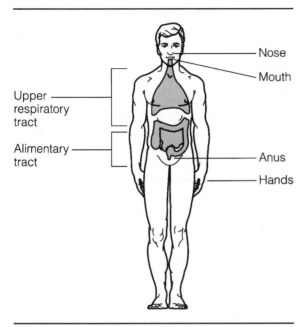

Common sites for entry of infection into the body; in addition, a break in the skin anywhere on the body is an invitation to infection.

into the bloodstream or uninfected tissue nearby. Pain is present when the damaged tissue releases waste products and the pathogen releases toxins. The swelling of the injured area and the pain associated with infections keep the patient from using that area of the body and thus aid in healing. It is interesting to note that while some painkillers such as aspirin reduce the inflammatory reaction by stopping the production of some of the chemicals released during inflammation, the aspirin-like drugs do nothing to harm the pathogen, only the body's response to the microorganism.

Some of the same chemicals that are found in inflamed tissues also cause fever. This abnormally high body temperature represents the body's response to an invading microorganism. The body's thermostat, located in a region of the brain known as the hypothalamus, is set at 37 degrees Celsius (98.6 degrees Fahrenheit). During an infection, the thermostat is reset to a higher level. Chemicals called pyrogens are released from white blood cells called macrophages. Once again, aspirin-like drugs can be used to reduce the fever by inhibiting the action of some of these chemicals in the hypothalamus.

The body responds to viral infections in a similar way. Virally infected cells, however, secrete interferon,

exerting an antiviral action which may provide protection to uninfected neighboring cells. It appears that interferon acts to inhibit the virus from replicating. Therefore, cells that are already infected must be destroyed to rid the body of the remaining virus.

In addition to being part of the inflammatory response, certain white blood cells play an important role in attempting to remove the pathogen. Soon after inflammation begins, macrophages already present at the site of infection start to destroy the microorganism. At the same time, chemicals are being released from both the damaged tissue and the macrophages, which recruit other white blood cells such as neutrophils. The neutrophils, like the macrophages, are effective at attacking and destroying bacteria but, unlike the macrophages, they often die in the battle against infection. Dead neutrophils are seen as a white exudate called pus.

Other manifestations of infection include systemic (whole-body) effects in addition to changes at the site of infection. As noted, fever is a systemic effect mediated by chemicals from the site of infection. Some of these same factors have the ability to act on the bone marrow to increase the production of white blood cells. Physicians look for fever and an increase in white blood cell number as a sign of infection. If the infection is severe, the bone marrow may not be able to keep up with the demand and an overall decrease in white blood cell number is found.

COMPLICATIONS AND DISORDERS

Physicians and other health care workers must use patient history, signs and symptoms, and laboratory tests to determine the type of infection and the most appropriate treatment. Patient history can often tell the examiner how and when the infection started. For example, the patient may have cut himself or herself, been exposed to someone with an infectious disease, or had intimate contact with someone carrying a sexually transmitted disease. Signs of infection—edema, pain, fever—are usually rather easy to detect, but some symptoms may be rather vague, such as feeling tired and weak. These general signs and symptoms may indicate to a physician that the patient has an infection, but they will not provide information about the type of microorganism causing the infection. Nevertheless, some microorganisms do cause specific symptoms. For example, the herpes zoster virus that causes chickenpox or the paramyxovirus that causes measles leave characteristic rashes.

When the microorganism does not have a characteristic sign, physicians must use laboratory tests to determine the pathogen involved. Diagnosis of the disease relies on identifying the causative pathogen by microscopic examination of a specimen of infected tissue or body fluid, by growing the microorganism using culture techniques, or by detecting antibodies in the blood that have developed against the pathogen.

Once the physician determines what type of microorganism has caused the infection, he or she will have to determine the best treatment to eradicate the disease. Drug therapy usually consists of antibiotics and other antimicrobial agents. The selection of the appropriate drug is important, as certain pathogens are susceptible only to certain antibiotics. Unfortunately, few effective antiviral drugs are available for many infectious viruses. In these cases, drugs can be used to treat symptoms such as fever, pain, diarrhea, and vomiting rather than to destroy the virus.

Anti-infective drugs are commonly used by physicians to treat infections. Agents that kill or inhibit the growth of bacteria are known as antibiotics and can be applied directly to the site of infection (topical), given by mouth (oral), or injected. The latter two modes of administration allow the drug to be carried throughout the body by way of the blood. Some antibiotic drugs are effective against only certain strains of infectious bacteria. Antibiotics that act against several types of bacteria are referred to as broad-spectrum antibiotics. Some bacteria develop resistance to a particular antibiotic and require that the physician switch agents or use a combination of antibiotics. Antibiotic therapy for the treatment of infections should be used when the body has been invaded by harmful bacteria, when the bacteria are reproducing at a more rapid rate than the immune system can handle, or to prevent infections in individuals with an impaired immune system.

Some serious common bacterial infections include gonorrhea, which is sexually transmitted and treatable with penicillin; bacterial meningitis, which causes inflammation of the coverings around the brain and is treatable with a variety of antibiotics; pertussis (or whooping cough), which is transmitted by water droplets in air and treatable with erythromycin; pneumonia, which causes shortness of breath, is transmitted via the air, and can be treated with antibiotics; tuberculosis, which infects the lungs and is treatable with various antibiotics; and salmonella (or typhoid fever), which is transmitted in food or water contaminated with fecal material, causes fever, headaches, and digestive problems, and is treated with antibiotics. It should be noted that antibiotics are not effective in viral infections; only bacterial infections are treated with antibiotics.

Antiviral drugs such as acyclovir, amantadine, and zidovudine (formerly known as azidothymide, or AZT) are used in the treatment of infection by a virus. These drugs have been difficult to develop. Most viruses live within the cells of the patient, and the drug must in some way kill the virus without harming the host cells. In fact, antiviral agents cannot completely cure an illness, and infected patients often experience recurrent disease. Nevertheless, they do reduce the severity of these infections.

There are several common viral infections. Human immunodeficiency virus (HIV) infection, which causes acquired immunodeficiency syndrome (AIDS), is transmitted by sexual contact or contaminated needles or blood products; it is often treated with zidovudine but remains lethal. Chickenpox (herpes zoster virus), which is transmitted by airborne droplets or direct contact, is treated with acyclovir. The common cold is caused by numerous viruses that are transmitted by direct contact or air droplets and has no effective treatment other than drugs that reduce the symptoms. Hepatitis is transmitted by contaminated food, sexual contact, and blood; it causes flulike symptoms and jaundice (a yellow tinge to the skin caused by liver problems) and may be helped with the drug interferon. Influenza viruses ("the flu") are transmitted by airborne droplets; the only treatment for the flu is of its symptoms. Measles is transmitted by virus-containing water droplets and causes fever and a rash; treatment consists of alleviating the symptoms. Mononucleosis is transmitted via saliva and causes swollen lymph nodes, fever, a sore throat, and generalized tiredness; a patient with mononucleosis can only receive treatment for the symptoms, as no cure is available. Poliomyelitis (polio) is transmitted by fecally contaminated material or airborne droplets and can eventually cause paralysis; no treatment is available. Rabies is caused by a bite from an infected animal, as the virus is present in the saliva; the major symptoms include fever, tiredness, and spasms of the throat, and there is no effective treatment for rabies after these symptoms have appeared. Rubella is transmitted by virus-containing air droplets and is associated with a fever and rash; there is no treatment other than for the symptoms.

A major problem with infectious diseases is that there is almost always lag time between when the microorganism has entered the body and the onset of signs and symptoms. This gap may last from a few hours or days to several years. A patient without noticeable symptoms is likely to spread the pathogen. Thus a cycle is set up in which individuals unknowingly infect others who, in turn, pass on the disease-causing agent. Large numbers of people can quickly become infected.

One way to prevent the spread of infectious agents is to vaccinate patients. Diseases such as diphtheria, measles, mumps, rubella, poliomyelitis, and pertussis are rare in the United States because of an aggressive immunization program. When a patient is vaccinated, the vaccine usually contains a dead or inactive pathogen. After the vaccine is administered (usually by injection), the immune system responds by making antibodies against the antigens on the microorganism. Since the pathogen in the vaccine is unable to cause disease, the patient has no symptoms after immunization. The next time that the person is exposed to the infectious agent, his or her immune system is prepared to fight it before symptoms become evident.

In addition to immunization to prevent infection, individuals can largely avoid serious infectious diseases through good hygiene with respect to food and drink, frequent washing, the avoidance of contact with fecal material and urine, and the avoidance of contact with individuals who are infected and capable of transmitting the disease. When such avoidance is impractical, other protective measures can be taken.

Sexually transmitted diseases are usually preventable by using barrier contraceptives and practicing "safe sex." The most common of these diseases include chlamydial infections, trichomoniasis, genital herpes, and HIV infections. Prevention is particularly important in the viral infections of herpes and HIV, as there are no known cures.

Some infections can be acquired at birth, including gonorrhea, genital herpes, chlamydial infections, and salmonella. These microorganisms exist in the birth canal, and some infectious agents can even pass from the mother to the fetus via the placenta. The more serious infections transmitted in this manner are rubella, syphilis, toxoplasmosis, HIV virus, and the cytomegalovirus. The risk of transmitting these infections can be reduced by treating the mother before delivery or performing a cesarean section (surgical delivery from the uterus), thereby avoiding the birth canal.

Perspective and Prospects

The ancient Egyptians were probably the first to recognize infection and the body's response to the introduction of a disease-causing microorganism: Some hieroglyphics appear to represent the inflammatory process. Sometime in the fifth century B.C.E., the Greeks noted that patients who had acquired an infectious disease and survived did not usually contract the same illness a second time.

More solid scientific evidence about infections was provided in the nineteenth century by Edward Jenner, an English physician and scientist. Jenner was able to document that milkmaids seemed to be protected against smallpox because of their exposure to cowpox. With this knowledge, he vaccinated a boy with material from a smallpox pustule. The boy had a typical inflammatory response, but he showed no symptoms of the disease after being injected with smallpox a second time. His immune system protected him from the virus. Since that time, scientists have reached a much better understanding of how the body deals with infection.

Many scientists are focusing their attention on how pathogens are transmitted from the source of infection to susceptible individuals. Epidemiology is the study of the distribution and causes of diseases that are prevalent in humans. Since some infectious diseases are communicable (transmittable), epidemiologists gather data when an outbreak occurs in a population. These data include the source of infectious agents (the tissues involved), the microorganisms causing the disease, and the method by which the pathogens are transmitted from one person to another. Physicians and other health care workers help in the battle against infections by identifying susceptible individuals; developing and evaluating sources, methods, and ways to control the spread of the pathogens; and improving preventive measures, which usually includes extensive educational efforts for the general population. With this knowledge, scientists and physicians attempt to eradicate the disease.

While scientists and physicians have made great advances in the understanding of infection, many problems remain. The spread of certain diseases, such as sexually transmitted diseases, is difficult to control except by modifying human behavior. The most difficult to treat are viral illnesses in which the drugs that are used are ineffective in completely eradicating the virus, and bacterial diseases in which the bacteria have developed drug resistance. Because these microorganisms evolve rapidly, new strains continually emerge. When a new infectious agent develops, it is often years before scientists can devise an effective drug or vaccine to treat the disease. In the meantime, large numbers of patients may become ill and even die. Perhaps the most effective way to combat infection is to use preventive measures whenever practical.

—Matthew Berria, Ph.D.

See also Arthropod-borne diseases; Bacterial infections; Bites and stings; Childhood infectious diseases; Disease; Ear infections and disorders; Fever; Fungal infections; Iatrogenic disorders; Inflammation; Lice, mites, and ticks; Parasitic diseases; Prion diseases; Staphylococcal infections; Streptococcal infections; Viral infections; Zoonoses; *specific diseases.*

FOR FURTHER INFORMATION:

Clayman, Charles B., ed. *The American Medical Association Encyclopedia of Medicine.* New York: Random House, 1994. Covers, in alphabetical order, medical terms, diseases, and medical procedures. Lists all major infectious illnesses, with their causes and treatments. Does an excellent job of explaining rather complex medical subjects for a nonprofessional audience.

Diseases. 3d ed. Springhouse, Pa.: Springhouse, 2000. This text provides excellent descriptions of disease states. Chapter 2 specifically deals with infections; their causes, signs and symptoms, complications, and prevention; and the types of therapies that can eliminate the disease-causing agent.

The Incredible Machine. Washington, D.C.: National Geographic Society, 1994. A colorful book which describes, in layperson's terms, how the body works and how humans alter their own health. The chapter on how the immune system combats infectious agents is very well written and contains exciting pictures and drawings of inflammatory processes.

Shaw, Michael, ed. *Everything You Need to Know About Diseases.* Springhouse, Pa.: Springhouse Press, 1996. This well-illustrated consumer reference, compiled by more than one hundred doctors and medical experts, describes five hundred illnesses and conditions, their causes, symptoms, diagnosis, treatment, and prevention. A valuable reference book for everyone interested in health and disease. Of particular interest is chapter 19, "Infection."

INFERTILITY IN FEMALES
DISEASE/DISORDER

ANATOMY OR SYSTEM AFFECTED: Genitals, reproductive system, uterus

SPECIALTIES AND RELATED FIELDS: Endocrinology, gynecology

DEFINITION: The inability to achieve a desired pregnancy as a result of dysfunction of female reproductive organs.

KEY TERMS:

cervix: the bottom portion of the uterus, protruding into the vagina; the cervical canal, an opening in the cervix, allows sperm to pass from the vagina into the uterus

endometriosis: a disease in which patches of the uterine lining, the endometrium, implant on or in other organs

follicles: spherical structures in the ovary that contain the maturing ova (eggs)

hormone: a chemical signal that serves to coordinate the functions of different body parts; the hormones important in female reproduction are produced by the brain, the pituitary, and the ovaries

implantation: the process in which the early embryo attaches to the uterine lining; a critical event in pregnancy

ovaries: the pair of structures in the female that produce ova (eggs) and hormones

oviducts: the pair of tubes leading from the top of the uterus upward toward the ovaries; also called the Fallopian tubes

ovulation: the process in which an ovum is released from its follicle in the ovary; ovulation must occur for conception to be possible

pelvic inflammatory disease: a general term that refers to a state of inflammation and infection in the pelvic organs; may be caused by a sexually transmitted disease

uterus: the organ in which the embryo implants and grows

vagina: the tube-shaped organ that serves as the site for sperm deposition during intercourse

CAUSES AND SYMPTOMS

Infertility is defined as the failure of a couple to conceive a child despite regular sexual activity over a period of at least one year. Studies have estimated that in the United States 10 percent to 15 percent of couples are infertile. In about half of these couples, it is the woman who is affected.

The causes of female infertility are centered in the reproductive organs: the ovaries, oviducts, uterus, cervix, and vagina. The frequency of specific problems among infertile women is as follows: ovarian problems, 20 percent to 30 percent; damage to the oviducts, 30 percent to 50 percent; uterine problems, 5 percent to 10 percent; and cervical or vaginal abnormalities, 5 percent to 10 percent. Another 10 percent of women have unexplained infertility.

The ovaries have two important roles in conception: the production of ova, culminating in ovulation, and the production of hormones. Ovulation usually occurs halfway through a woman's four-week menstrual cycle. In the two weeks preceding ovulation, follicle-stimulating hormone (FSH) from the pituitary gland causes follicles in the ovaries to grow and the ova within them to mature. As the follicles grow, they produce increasing amounts of estrogen. Near the middle of the cycle, the estrogen causes the pituitary gland to release a surge of luteinizing hormone (LH), which causes ovulation of the largest follicle in the ovary.

Anovulation (lack of ovulation) can result either directly—from an inability to produce LH, FSH, or estrogen—or indirectly—because of the presence of other hormones that interfere with the signaling systems between the pituitary and ovaries. For example, the woman may have an excess production of androgen (testosterone-like) hormones, either in her ovaries or in her adrenal glands, or her pituitary may produce too much prolactin, a hormone that is normally secreted in large amounts only after the birth of a child.

Besides ovulation, the ovaries have another critical role in conception since they produce hormones that act on the uterus to allow it to support an embryo. In the first two weeks of the menstrual cycle, the uterine lining is prepared for a possible pregnancy by estrogen from the ovaries. Following ovulation, the uterus is maintained in a state that can support an embryo by progesterone, which is produced in the ovary by the follicle that just ovulated, now called a corpus luteum. Because of the effects of hormones from the corpus luteum on the uterus, the corpus luteum is essential to

Common Causes of Female Infertility

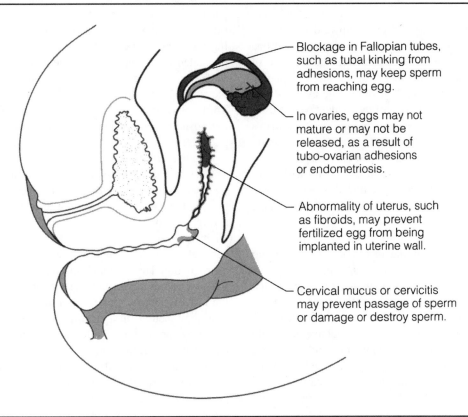

Blockage in Fallopian tubes, such as tubal kinking from adhesions, may keep sperm from reaching egg.

In ovaries, eggs may not mature or may not be released, as a result of tubo-ovarian adhesions or endometriosis.

Abnormality of uterus, such as fibroids, may prevent fertilized egg from being implanted in uterine wall.

Cervical mucus or cervicitis may prevent passage of sperm or damage or destroy sperm.

the survival of the embryo. If conception does not occur, the corpus luteum disintegrates and stops producing progesterone. As progesterone levels decline, the uterine lining can no longer be maintained and is shed as the menstrual flow.

Failure of the pregnancy can result from improper function of the corpus luteum, such as an inability to produce enough progesterone to sustain the uterine lining. The corpus luteum may also produce progesterone initially but then disintegrate too early. These problems in corpus luteum function, referred to as luteal phase insufficiency, may be caused by the same types of hormonal abnormalities that cause lack of ovulation.

Some cases of infertility may be associated with an abnormally shaped uterus or vagina. Such malformations of the reproductive organs are common in women whose mothers took diethylstilbestrol (DES) during pregnancy. DES was prescribed to many pregnant women from 1941 to about 1970 as a protection against miscarriage; infertility and other problems occurred in the offspring of these women.

Conception depends on normal function of the oviducts (or Fallopian tubes), thin tubes with an inner diameter of only a few millimeters; they are attached to the top of the uterus and curve upward toward the ovaries. The inner end of each tube, located near one of the ovaries, waves back and forth at the time of ovulation, drawing the mature ovum into the opening of the oviduct. Once in the oviduct, the ovum is propelled along by movements of the oviduct wall. Meanwhile, if intercourse has occurred recently, the man's sperm will be moving upward in the female system, swimming through the uterus and the oviducts. Fertilization, the union of the sperm and ovum, will occur in the oviduct, and then the fertilized ovum will pass down the oviduct and reach the uterus about three days after ovulation.

Infertility can result from scar tissue formation inside the oviduct, resulting in physical blockage and inability to transport the ovum, sperm, or both. The most common cause of scar tissue formation in the reproductive organs is pelvic inflammatory disease (PID), a condition characterized by inflammation that spreads throughout the female reproductive tract. PID may be initiated by a sexually transmitted disease such as gonorrhea and chlamydia. Physicians in the United States have documented an increase in infertility attributable to tubal damage caused by sexually transmitted diseases.

Damage to the outside of the oviduct can also cause infertility, because such damage can interfere with the mobility of the oviduct, which is necessary to the capture of the ovum at the time of ovulation. External damage to the oviduct may occur as an aftermath of abdominal surgery, when adhesions induced by surgical cutting are likely to form. An adhesion is an abnormal scar tissue connection between adjacent structures.

Another possible cause of damage to the oviduct, resulting in infertility, is the presence of endometriosis. Endometriosis refers to a condition in which patches of the uterine lining implant in or on the surface of other organs. These patches are thought to arise during menstruation, when the uterine lining (endometrium) is normally shed from the body through the cervix and vagina; in a woman with endometriosis, for unknown reasons, the endometrium is carried to the interior of the pelvic cavity by passing up the oviducts. The endometrial patches can lodge in the oviduct itself, causing blockage, or can adhere to the outer surface of the oviducts, interfering with mobility.

Endometriosis can cause infertility by interfering with organs other than the oviducts. Endometrial patches on the outside of the uterus can cause distortions in the shape or placement of the uterus, interfering with embryonic implantation. Ovulation may be prevented by the presence of the endometrial tissues on the surface of the ovary. Yet the presence of endometriosis is not always associated with infertility. Thirty percent to forty percent of women with endometriosis cannot conceive, but the remainder appear to be fertile.

Another critical site in conception is the cervix. The cervix, the entryway to the uterus from the vagina, represents the first barrier through which sperm must pass on their way to the ovum. The cervix consists of a ring of strong, elastic tissue with a narrow canal. Glands in the cervix produce the mucus that fills the cervical canal and through which sperm swim en route to the ovum. The amount and quality of the cervical mucus changes throughout the menstrual cycle, under the influence of hormones from the ovary. At ovulation, the mucus is in a state that is most easily penetrated by sperm; after ovulation, the mucus becomes almost impenetrable.

Cervical problems that can lead to infertility include production of a mucus that does not allow sperm passage at the time of ovulation (hostile mucus syndrome) and interference with sperm transport caused by narrowing of the cervical canal. Such narrowing may be the result of a developmental abnormality or the presence of an infection, possibly a sexually transmitted disease.

TREATMENT AND THERAPY

The diagnosis of the exact cause of a woman's infertility is crucial to successful treatment. A complete medical history should reveal any obvious problems of previous infection or menstrual cycle irregularity. Adequacy of ovulation and luteal phase function can be determined from records of menstrual cycle length and changes in body temperature (body temperature is higher after ovulation). Hormone levels can be measured with tests of blood or urine samples. If damage to the oviducts or uterus is suspected, hysterosalpingography will be performed. In this procedure, the injection of a special fluid into the uterus is followed by X-ray analysis of the fluid movement; the shape of the uterine cavity and the oviducts will be revealed. Cervical functioning can be assessed with the postcoital test, in which the physician attempts to recover sperm from the woman's uterus some hours after she has had intercourse with her partner. If a uterine problem is suspected, the woman may have an endometrial biopsy, in which a small sample of the uterine lining is removed and examined for abnormalities. Sometimes, exploratory surgery is performed to pinpoint the location of scar tissue or the location of endometriosis patches.

Surgery may be used for treatment as well as diagnosis. Damage to the oviducts can sometimes be repaired surgically, and surgical removal of endometrial patches is a standard treatment for endometriosis. Often, however, surgery is a last resort, because of the likelihood of the development of postsurgical adhesions, which can further complicate the infertility. Newer forms of surgery using lasers and freezing offer better success because of a reduced risk of adhesions.

Some women with hormonal difficulties can be treated successfully with so-called fertility drugs. There are actually several different drugs and hormones that fall under this heading: Clomiphene citrate (Clomid), human menopausal gonadotropin (HMG), gonadotropin-releasing hormone (GnRH), bromocriptine mesylate (Parlodel), and menotropins (Pergonal) are commonly used, with the exact choice depending on the woman's particular problem. The pregnancy rate with fertility drug treatment varies from 20 per-

cent to 70 percent. One problem with some of the drugs is the risk of multiple pregnancy (more than one fetus in the uterus). Hyperstimulation of the ovaries, a condition characterized by enlarged ovaries, can be fatal as a result of severe hormone imbalances. Other possible problems include nausea, dizziness, headache, and general malaise.

Artificial insemination is an old technique that is still useful in various types of infertility. A previously collected sperm sample is placed in the woman's vagina or uterus using a special tube. Artificial insemination is always performed at the time of ovulation, in order to maximize the chance of pregnancy. The ovulation date can be determined with body temperature records or by hormone measurements. In some cases, this procedure is combined with fertility drug treatment. Since the sperm can be placed directly in the uterus, it is useful in treating hostile mucus syndrome and certain types of male infertility. The sperm sample can be provided either by the woman's partner or by a donor. The pregnancy rate after artificial insemination is highly variable (14 percent to 68 percent), depending on the particular infertility problem in the couple. There is a slight risk of infection, and, if donated semen is used, there may be no guarantee that the semen is free from sexually transmitted diseases or that the donor does not carry some genetic defect.

Another infertility treatment is gamete intrafallopian transfer (GIFT), the surgical placement of ova and sperm directly into the woman's oviducts. In order to be a candidate for this procedure, the woman must have at least one partially undamaged oviduct and a functional uterus. Ova are collected surgically from the ovaries after stimulation with a fertility drug, and a semen sample is collected from the male. The ova and the sperm are introduced into the oviducts through the same abdominal incision used to collect the ova. This procedure is useful in certain types of male infertility, if the woman produces an impenetrable cervical mucus, or if the ovarian ends of the oviducts are damaged. The range of infertility problems that may be resolved with GIFT can be extended by using donated ova or sperm. The success rate is about 33 percent overall, but the rate varies with the type of infertility present.

In vitro fertilization is known colloquially as the "test-tube baby" technique. In this procedure, ova are collected surgically after stimulation with fertility drugs and then placed in a laboratory dish and combined with sperm from the man. The actual fertilization, when a sperm penetrates the ovum, will occur in the dish. The resulting embryo is allowed to remain in the dish for two days, during which time it will have acquired two to four cells. Then, the embryo is placed in the woman's uterine cavity using a flexible tube. In vitro fertilization can be used in women who are infertile because of endometriosis, damaged oviducts, impenetrable cervical mucus, or ovarian failure. As with GIFT, in vitro fertilization may utilize either donated ova or donated sperm, or extra embryos that have been produced by one couple may be implanted in a second woman. The pregnancy rate with this procedure varies from 15 percent to 25 percent.

Embryo freezing is a secondary procedure that can increase the chances of pregnancy for an infertile couple. When ova are collected for the in vitro fertilization procedure, doctors try to collect as many as possible. All these ova are then combined with sperm for fertilization. No more than three or four embryos are ever placed in the woman's uterus, however, because a pregnancy with a large number of fetuses carries significant health risks. The extra embryos can be frozen for later use, if the first ones implanted in the uterus do not survive. This spares the woman additional surgery to collect more ova if they are needed. The freezing technique does not appear to cause any defects in the embryo.

Some women may benefit from nonsurgical embryo transfer. In this procedure, a fertile woman is artificially inseminated at the time of her ovulation; five days later, her uterus is flushed with a sterile solution, washing out the resulting embryo before it implants in the uterus. The retrieved embryo is then transferred to the uterus of another woman, who will carry it to term. Typically, the sperm provider and the woman who receives the embryo are the infertile couple who wish to rear the child, but the technique can be used in other circumstances as well. Embryo transfer can be used if the woman has damaged oviducts or is unable to ovulate, or if she has a genetic disease that could be passed to her offspring, because in this case the baby is not genetically related to the woman who carries it.

Some infertile women who are unable to achieve a pregnancy themselves turn to the use of a surrogate, a woman who will agree to bear a child and then turn it over to the infertile woman to rear as her own. In the typical situation, the surrogate is artificially inseminated with the sperm of the infertile woman's husband. The surrogate then proceeds with pregnancy and delivery as normal, but relinquishes the child to the infertile couple after its birth.

PERSPECTIVE AND PROSPECTS

One of the biggest problems that infertile couples face is the emotional upheaval that comes with the diagnosis of the infertility. Bearing and rearing children is an experience that most women treasure. When a woman is told that she is infertile, she may feel that her femininity and self-worth are diminished. In addition to the emotional difficulty that may come with the recognition of infertility, more stress may be in store as the couple proceeds through treatment. The various treatments can cause embarrassment and sometimes physical pain, and fertility drugs themselves are known to cause emotional swings. For these reasons, a couple with an infertility problem is often advised to seek help from a private counselor or a support group.

Along with the emotional and physical trauma of infertility treatment, there is a considerable financial burden as well. Infertility treatments, in general, are very expensive, especially the more sophisticated procedures such as in vitro fertilization and GIFT. Since the chances of a single procedure resulting in a pregnancy are often low, the couple may be faced with submitting to multiple procedures repeated many times. The cost over several years of treatment—a realistic possibility—can be staggering. Many health insurance companies in the United States refuse to cover the costs of such treatment and are required to do so in only a few states.

Some of the treatments are accompanied by unresolved legal questions. In the case of nonsurgical embryo transfer, is the legal mother of the child the ovum donor or the woman who gives birth to the child? The same question of legal parentage arises in cases of surrogacy. Does a child born using donated ovum or sperm have a legal right to any information about the donor, such as medical history? How extensive should governmental regulation of infertility clinics be? For example, should there be standards for ensuring that donated sperm or ova are free from genetic defects? In the United States, some states have begun to address these issues, but no uniform policies have been set at the federal level.

The legal questions are largely unresolved because American society is still involved in religious and philosophical debates over the proprieties of various infertility treatments. Some religions hold that any interference in conception is unacceptable. To these denominations, even artificial insemination is wrong. Other groups approve of treatments confined to a husband and wife, but disapprove of a third party being involved as a donor or surrogate. Many people disapprove of any infertility treatment to help an individual who is not married. The basic problem underlying all these issues is that these technologies challenge the traditional definitions of parenthood.

—*Marcia Watson-Whitmyre, Ph.D.*

See also Conception; Contraception; Ectopic pregnancy; Endocrinology; Endometriosis; Gynecology; Hormones; Hysterectomy; In vitro fertilization; Infertility in males; Menopause; Menstruation; Miscarriage; Obstetrics; Ovarian cysts; Pelvic inflammatory disease (PID); Pregnancy and gestation; Sexual dysfunction; Sperm banks; Sterilization; Stress; Tubal ligation.

FOR FURTHER INFORMATION:

Fathalla, Mahmoud F., et al., eds. *Reproductive Health: Global Issues.* Vol. 3 in *The FIGO Manual of Human Reproduction.* 2d ed. Park Ridge, N.J.: Parthenon, 1990. Chapter 4 in this text deals with infertility—its causes, diagnosis, and treatment—in a concise and understandable manner.

Harkness, Carla. *The Infertility Book: A Comprehensive Medical and Emotional Guide.* Berkeley, Calif.: Celestial Arts, 1992. Written as a guide for the infertile couple, this book offers emotional support as well as medical information. The text is augmented by firsthand accounts of individuals' reactions to their infertility and the treatments.

Quilligan, Edward J., and Frederick P. Zuspan, eds. *Current Therapy in Obstetrics and Gynecology.* 5th ed. Philadelphia: W. B. Saunders, 1999. This excellent handbook provides detailed information on procedures for various infertility causes and treatments, arranged alphabetically amid other gynecological subjects.

Speroff, Leon, Robert H. Glass, and Nathan G. Kase, eds. *Clinical Gynecologic Endocrinology and Infertility.* 6th ed. Baltimore: Williams & Wilkins, 1999. A good basic textbook that can help the reader understand the normal functioning of the female reproductive system and the events associated with infertility.

Weschler, Toni. *Taking Charge of Your Infertility.* New York: HarperPerennial, 1995. This book encourages women to become responsible consumers of their own reproductive health. Includes excellent discussions of infertility, natural birth control, and achieving pregnancy.

Wisot, Arthur, and David Meldrum. *Conceptions and Misconceptions.* Vancouver: Harley and Marks, 1997. Written by two leading fertility experts, this book is an excellent guide through the maze of in vitro fertilization and other assisted reproductive techniques. Includes an excellent discussion of the basic physiology of conception and reproduction.

Yeh, John, and Molly Uline Yeh. *Legal Aspects of Infertility.* Boston: Blackwell Scientific, 1991. The authors, a practicing physician and a lawyer, wrote this text as a guide for doctors, but it makes fascinating reading for anyone interested in the governmental regulation of infertility treatments.

INFERTILITY IN MALES
DISEASE/DISORDER

ANATOMY OR SYSTEM AFFECTED: Genitals, reproductive system

SPECIALTIES AND RELATED FIELDS: Endocrinology, urology

DEFINITION: The inability to achieve a desired pregnancy as a result of dysfunction of male reproductive organs.

KEY TERMS:

antibody: a chemical produced by lymphocytes (blood cells) that enables these cells to destroy foreign materials, such as bacteria

cryopreservation: a special process utilizing cryoprotectants that enables living cells to survive in a frozen state

cryoprotectant: one of several chemicals that enables living cells to survive in a frozen state; some cryoprotectants are made by animals that survive freezing

epididymis: an organ attached to the testis in which newly formed sperm reach maturity (that is, become capable of fertilizing an egg)

infertility: the inability to produce a normal pregnancy after one year of intercourse in the absence of any contraception; it may be caused by male and/or female factors

insemination: the placement of semen in the female reproductive tract, which may occur naturally as a result of sexual intercourse or artificially as a result of a medical procedure

testis: either of two male gonads that are suspended in the scrotum and produce sperm
varicocele: a swollen testicular vein in the scrotum occurring as a result of improper valvular function

CAUSES AND SYMPTOMS

To create a baby requires three things: normal sperm from a man, a normal egg from a woman, and a normal, mature uterus. Anything that blocks the availability of the sperm, egg, or uterus can cause infertility. Infertility can be thought of as an abnormal, unwanted form of contraception.

Many different factors may be responsible for infertility. In general, these factors may be infectious, chemical (from inside or outside of the body, such as illegal drugs, pharmaceuticals, or toxins), or anatomical. Genetic factors may be responsible as well, since genes control the formation of body chemicals (such as hormones and antibodies) and body structures (one's anatomy). The way that these factors work is illustrated by male infertility.

The process by which sperm are made begins in a man's testis (or testicle). Because the transformation of testis cells into sperm is controlled by genes and hormones, abnormalities can cause infertility. Sperm released from the testis become mature in the epididymis. Sperm travel from the testis to the epididymis through ducts (tubes) in the male reproductive tract. A blockage of these ducts or premature release of sperm from the epididymis can cause infertility.

A blockage of reproductive ducts can occur as a result of a bodily enlargement, such as swollen tissue, a tumor, or cancer. An infection usually causes tissue swelling and can leave ducts permanently scarred, narrowed, or blocked. Infection can have a direct detrimental effect on the production of normal sperm. Cancer and the drugs or chemicals used to treat cancer can also damage a man's reproductive tract.

Another factor that may be important to male fertility is scrotal temperature. The temperature in the scrotum, the sac that holds the testis, is somewhat cooler than body temperature. The normal production of sperm seems to be dependent upon a cool testicular environment.

The leading cause of male infertility may be varicoceles, which occur when one-way valves fail in the veins that take blood away from the testicles. When these venous valves become leaky, blood flow becomes sluggish and causes the veins to swell. Many men with varicoceles are infertile, but the exact reason

for this association is unknown. The reasons sometimes given are increased scrotal temperature and improper removal of materials (hormones) from the testis.

Mature sperm capable of fertilizing an egg are normally placed in the female reproductive tract by the ejaculation phase of sexual intercourse. The sperm are accompanied by fluid called seminal plasma; together, they form semen. A blockage of the ducts that transport the semen into the woman or toxic chemicals, including antibodies, in the semen can cause infertility.

For conception to take place—that is, for an egg to be fertilized after sperm enters the female tract—a normal egg must be present in the portion of the tract called the Fallopian tube, and sperm must move through the female tract to that egg. If the egg is absent or is abnormal, or if normal sperm cannot reach the egg, female infertility will result. The female factors that determine whether sperm fertilize an egg are the same as the male factors: anatomy, chemicals, infection, and genes.

There are many ways to treat infertility. Female infertility may be treated, depending upon the cause, by surgery, hormone therapy, or in vitro fertilization. Treatment of male infertility may be by surgery, hormone therapy, or therapeutic (artificial) insemination. Therapeutic insemination is often performed when the couple is composed of a fertile woman and an infertile man.

The first step for therapeutic insemination is for a physician to determine when an egg is ovulated or released into the Fallopian tube of the fertile woman. At the time of ovulation, semen is placed with medical instruments in the woman's reproductive tract, either on her cervix or in her uterus.

The semen used by the physician is obtained through masturbation by either the infertile man (the patient) or a fertile man (a donor), depending on the cause of the man's infertility. The freshly produced semen from either source usually undergoes laboratory testing and processing. Tests are used to evaluate the sperm quality. An effort may be made to enhance the sperm from an infertile patient and then to use these sperm for therapeutic insemination or in vitro fertilization. Other tests evaluate semen for transmissible diseases. During testing, which may require many days, the sperm can be kept alive by cryopreservation. Freshly ejaculated sperm remains fertile for only a few hours in the laboratory if it is not cryopreserved.

There are several processes that might enhance sperm from an infertile man. If the semen is infertile because it possesses too few normal sperm, an effort can be made to eliminate the abnormal sperm and to increase the concentration of normal sperm. Sperm may be abnormal in four basic ways: They may have abnormal structure, they may have abnormal movement, they may be incapable of fusing with an egg, or they may contain abnormal genes or chromosomes. Laboratory processes can often eliminate from semen those sperm with abnormal structure or abnormal movement. These processes usually involve replacing the seminal plasma with a culture medium. Removing the seminal plasma gets rid of substances that may be harmful to the sperm. After the plasma is removed, the normal sperm can be collected and concentrated. Pharmacologic agents can be added to the culture medium to increase sperm movement.

Testing for transmissible diseases is especially important if donor semen is used; these diseases may be genetic or infectious. There are many thousand genetic disorders. Most of these disorders are very rare and can be transmitted to offspring only if the sperm and the egg both have the same gene for the disorder. It is impossible, therefore, to test a donor for every possible genetic disorder; he is routinely tested only for a small group of troublesome disorders that are especially likely to occur in offspring. Tests for other disorders that the donor might transmit can be performed at the woman's request, usually based upon knowledge of genetic problems in her own family.

Much of the genetic information about a person is based on family history. Special laboratory procedures allow the genetic code inside individual cells to be interpreted. For this reason, it is important to store a sample of donor cells, not necessarily sperm, for many years after the procedure. These cells provide additional genetic information that might be important to the donor's offspring but not known at the time of insemination.

Semen can also be the source of infectious disease. Syphilis, gonorrhea, and acquired immunodeficiency syndrome (AIDS) are examples of venereal or sexually transmitted diseases (STDs). Tests for STDs can be done on blood and semen from a donor. These tests must be conducted in an approved manner, and the results must be negative before donor semen can be used therapeutically. In some cases, a test must be repeated in order to verify that the semen is not infectious.

Common Causes of Male Infertility

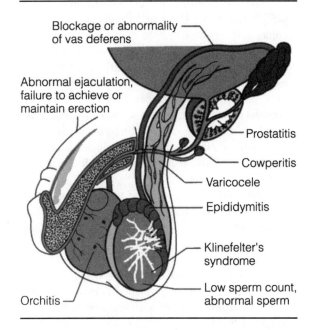

Blockage or abnormality of vas deferens

Abnormal ejaculation; failure to achieve or maintain erection

Prostatitis

Cowperitis

Varicocele

Epididymitis

Klinefelter's syndrome

Low sperm count, abnormal sperm

Orchitis

Cryopreservation of sperm is important to therapeutic insemination for two major reasons. First, it gives time to complete all necessary testing. Second, it allows an inventory of sperm from many different donors to be kept constantly available for selection and use by patients. Sperm properly cryopreserved for twenty years, when thawed and inseminated, can produce normal babies.

Cryopreservation involves treating freshly ejaculated sperm with a cryoprotectant pharmaceutical that enables the sperm to survive when frozen; the cryoprotectant for sperm is usually glycerol. Survival of frozen sperm is also dependent upon the rate of cooling, the storage temperature, and the rate of warming at the time of thawing. Sperm treated with a cryoprotectant have the best chance of survival if they are cooled about 1 degree Celsius per minute and stored at a temperature of –150 degrees Celsius or colder. An environment of liquid nitrogen is often used to attain these storage temperatures. The storage temperature must be kept constant to avoid the damaging effects of recrystallization. When sperm are to be thawed, survival is enhanced if they are warmed at 10 to 100 degrees Celsius per minute.

The cryopreservation procedure involves the actual formation of ice, although the ice is confined to the extracellular medium. Intracellular ice is lethal. Ice formation during cryopreservation causes the cells to lose water and to shrink. The cryoprotectant seems to replace intracellular water and thereby maintain cell volume.

An alternative process for low-temperature preservation of sperm is called vitrification. Vitrification uses temperatures as cold as cryopreservation, but it avoids ice formation altogether. Instead of using one cryoprotectant, vitrification uses a mixture of several. It employs a much slower cooling rate and a much faster warming rate. Technically, vitrification is more difficult to perform; therefore, it is seldom used by clinical sperm banks.

Human sperm can be shipped to almost any location for therapeutic insemination. Sperm is usually cryopreserved before shipment and thawed at the time of insemination.

TREATMENT AND THERAPY

The use of therapeutic insemination to treat two kinds of male infertility will be considered here. The first example is male infertility that cannot be treated by other means. The second example is a fertile man at high risk for becoming infertile because of his lifestyle or because he is receiving treatment for a life-threatening disease.

The first example might occur when a heterosexual couple, having used no contraception for a year or longer, has been unsuccessful in conceiving a baby. In 40 percent of infertility cases, the woman has the major, but not necessarily the only, problem preventing the pregnancy. In 40 percent of the cases, the man is the major factor. In 20 percent, each person makes a substantial contribution to the problem. Therefore, both partners must deal with the infertility and be involved in the treatment.

The solution to a couple's infertility involves evaluation and therapy. The couple will be evaluated in regard to their present sexual activity and history, such as whether either one has ever contributed to a pregnancy. The medical evaluation of both partners will include a physical examination, laboratory tests, and even imaging techniques such as X rays, ultrasonography, or magnetic resonance imaging (MRI). For the man, the physical examination will include a search for the presence of varicoceles, and the laboratory tests will include a semen analysis. About 15 to 30 percent of couples entering an infertility program achieve pregnancy during the evaluation phase of the program, before any therapy is begun.

Varicoceles are probably the most readily detected problem that may cause male infertility. They are three times more common in infertile men than in men with proved fertility. This association does not prove that varicoceles cause infertility, however, because surgery that corrects a varicocele does not always correct infertility.

If the medical evaluation determines that the female partner has a normal reproductive tract and is ovulating on a regular basis, and if it determines that the male partner has too few normal sperm to make a pregnancy likely, the couple may be asked to consider adopting a baby or undergoing therapeutic insemination. With therapeutic insemination, the woman actually becomes pregnant, and half of the baby's genes come from the mother. The other half of the genes come from the sperm donor, usually a person unknown to the couple. The physician performing therapeutic insemination may provide the couple with extensive information on several possible donors. Such information might include race, ethnic origin, blood type, physical characteristics, results of medical and genetic tests, and personal information, but the donor usually remains anonymous. The semen from each donor has undergone laboratory testing and cryopreservation. The frozen semen is thawed at the time of insemination.

Although the idea of therapeutic insemination is simple, it usually involves some very complicated emotions. Although a couple may be very happy about all other aspects of their lives together, they are usually deeply disturbed to learn of the man's infertility. It may be extremely difficult for them to discuss his infertility with anyone else. Some people ridicule infertile men as being less virile or even being impotent. (This is not the case: The majority of infertile or sterile men have normal sex lives.) These feelings will influence the couple's selection of a sperm donor. Later, they must decide whether to tell the child about the circumstances of his or her birth. Sometimes, a child who originated through therapeutic insemination will try to learn the identity of the donor.

The donor must be considered as well. In a typical sperm bank, persons are subjected to a variety of tests before they are accepted as donors. Sperm donors are typically in their second decade of life, but some are older. These men are primarily, but not solely, motivated to be sperm donors by financial compensation. Payment effectively maintains donor cooperation for a period of several years. In addition to payment, the donor usually wants an assurance that he will not be held responsible, financially or legally, for the offspring produced by his semen. As a donor grows older, however, his attitude about his donation may change: He may wonder about the children he has helped to create.

Although male-factor infertility is the situation that benefits most from insemination and semen cryopreservation procedures, these procedures might be requested by a fertile couple that is at risk for male-factor infertility. Such couples may fear that the man's lifestyle, such as working with hazardous materials (solvents, toxins, radioisotopes, or explosives), may endanger his ability to produce sperm or may harm his genetic information. The man could be facing medical therapy that will cure a malignancy, such as Hodgkin's disease or a testicular tumor, but may render him sterile. A man facing such a situation may benefit from having some of his semen cryopreserved for his own future use, in the event that he actually becomes infertile.

Therapeutic insemination with a husband's semen is usually not as effective as with donor semen, especially when cryopreservation is involved. Although cryopreservation keeps cells alive in the frozen state, not all the cells survive. Men selected to be semen donors have sperm that survive freezing much better than the sperm of most men (although the reason for this ability is unknown). If a man undergoing medical treatment is already sick at the time that the decision is made to store his sperm, his concentration of functioning sperm may be less than normal.

There are ways to compensate for decreased semen quality. The semen may be processed in ways to increase the concentration of normal sperm. The processed semen may be placed directly into the woman's uterus (intrauterine insemination) rather than on her cervix, or in vitro fertilization may be used. In this procedure, the sperm and eggs are mixed in a laboratory and the resulting embryo is implanted in the woman. All these techniques have proved helpful to infertile couples wanting children.

PERSPECTIVE AND PROSPECTS

It has been estimated that infertility affects 8 to 15 percent of American marriages, which means that three to nine million American couples would like to, but cannot, have children without medical assistance. By the early 1990's, therapeutic insemination produced more than thirty thousand American babies yearly.

This procedure advanced in the United States during the latter half of the twentieth century in large measure because of changes in attitudes, not because of new medical knowledge.

The medical knowledge to treat male infertility has been available for several centuries, even when the biological basis for pregnancy was not understood. The importance of sexual intercourse in reproduction was probably recognized by prehistoric humans. The Bible records stories of patriarchal families that knew the problem of infertility (Abraham and Sarah, Jacob and Rachel) and even indicates, in the story of Onan and Tamar (Genesis 38:9), that semen was understood to be important to reproduction. The possibility of therapeutic insemination was mentioned in the fifth century Talmud. Arabs used insemination in horse breeding as early as the fourteenth century, and Spaniards used it in human medicine during the fifteenth century.

The presence of sperm in semen was first observed by Antoni van Leeuwenhoek in the seventeenth century, but their importance and function in the fertilization process was not recognized until the nineteenth century. In 1824, Jean Louis Prévost and J. A. Dumas correctly guessed the role of sperm in fertilization, and in 1876, Oskar Hertwig and Hermann Fol proved that the union of sperm and egg was necessary to create an embryo.

Therapeutic insemination became an established but clandestine procedure in the late nineteenth century in the United States and England. Compassionate physicians pioneering therapeutic insemination encouraged secrecy to protect the self-esteem of the infertile man, his spouse, the offspring, and the donor. In an uncertain legal climate, the offspring might have been viewed as the illegitimate product of an adulterous act. Even by the beginning of the twenty-first century, many Americans continued to stigmatize masturbation and therapeutic insemination. Social attitudes, especially machismo, have limited the acceptability of therapeutic insemination to many infertile couples worldwide.

Cryopreservation of sperm became practical with the discovery of chemical cryoprotectants, reported in 1949 by Christopher Polge, Audrey Smith, and Alan Parkes of England. In 1953, American doctors R. G. Bunge and Jerome Sherman were the first to use this procedure to produce a human baby. Cryopreservation made possible the establishment of sperm banks; prior to this development, sperm donors had to provide the physician with semen immediately before insemination was to take place.

Recent research has shown a few promising new techniques: intracytoplasmic injection, which involves the placement of sperm into the ovum itself, and electroejaculation, which involves electrical stimulation of the penis to promote ejaculation. Intracytoplasmic injections are useful when the sperm are immotile or the woman's own immune system aggressively rejects the man's sperm. It is not always successful, however, and is affected by age and cycle. Electroejaculation has been successfully used in men with vascular compromise, as might be caused by diabetes mellitus, or with spinal cord injuries. It is also helpful in cases where men are unable to ejaculate for psychological reasons.

Therapeutic insemination and other alternative means of reproduction give rise to thorny issues of personal rights of various "parents" (social, birth, and genetic) and their offspring. In the United States, a few states have addressed these issues by enacting laws, usually to grant legitimacy to offspring of donor insemination. In the United Kingdom, Parliament established a central registry of sperm and egg donors. Offspring in the United Kingdom have access to nonidentifying donor information; these children are even able to learn whether they are genetically related to a prospective marriage partner.

—Armand M. Karow, Ph.D.;
updated by Paul Moglia, Ph.D.

See also Conception; Genital disorders, male; In vitro fertilization; Infertility in females; Pregnancy and gestation; Reproductive system; Sexual dysfunction; Sperm banks; Sterilization; Stress; Testicular surgery; Vasectomy.

FOR FURTHER INFORMATION:

Baran, Annette, and Reuben Pannor. *Lethal Secrets.* New York: Warner Books, 1993. The authors, medical social workers, discuss the possible consequences of secrecy in donor insemination using a series of case histories.

Glover, Timothy D., and C. L. R. Barratt, eds. *Male Fertility and Infertility.* New York: Cambridge University Press, 1999. The editors have assembled a collection of essays by experts in the field. Includes bibliographical references and an index.

Schover, Leslie R., and Anthony J. Thomas. *Overcoming Male Infertility: Understanding Its Causes and Treatments.* New York: John Wiley & Sons, 2000. Clinical psychologist Schover has long worked with infertile couples, as urologist Thomas has with male infertility. Their combined skills and knowledge make this a valuable book. Patient-oriented, it conveys a vast amount of information understandably and maintains an underlying sense of humor.

Warnock, Mary. *A Question of Life.* New York: Basil Blackwell, 1993. This report, commissioned by the British Parliament, discusses medical procedures for alleviating infertility and social issues of family formation and inheritance.

INFLAMMATION

DISEASE/DISORDER

ANATOMY OR SYSTEM AFFECTED: All
SPECIALTIES AND RELATED FIELDS: Family practice, internal medicine, pathology, rheumatology
DEFINITION: The reaction of blood-filled living tissue to injury.

In inflammation, the following changes are seen locally: redness, swelling, heat, pain, and loss of function. These changes are chemically mediated. Inflammation may be caused by microbial infection; physical agents such as trauma, radiation, and burns; chemical toxins; caustic substances such as strong acids or bases; decomposing or necrotic tissue; and reactions of the immune system. Acute inflammation is of relatively short duration (from a few minutes to a day or so), while chronic inflammation lasts longer. The local changes associated with inflammation include the outflow of fluid into the spaces between cells and the inflow or migration of white blood cells (leukocytes) to the area of injury. Chronic inflammation is characterized by the presence of leukocytes and macrophages, as well as by the proliferation of new blood vessels and connective tissue.

Inflammation is a protective mechanism for the body. Redness is attributable to increased blood flow to the injured area. Swelling is caused by the flow of fluid into the spaces between cells. Heat is produced by a combination of increased blood flow and chemical reactions in the local area. Pain results from the presence of two main chemicals found in the bloodstream: prostaglandins and bradykinin. Loss of function is a result of pain (the body limits movement to reduce discomfort) and swelling (interstitial fluid limits movement).

Acute inflammation. Many chemicals are involved in acute inflammation. Mediators of inflammation originate from blood plasma and from both damaged and normal cells. Vasoactive amines are a class of chemicals that increase the permeability of blood vessel and cell walls. The most well studied of these are histamine and serotonin. Histamine is stored in granules in mast cells that are found in both tissue and basophils, the latter being a type of cell found in the blood. Serotonin is found in mast cells and platelets; it is another type of cell found in the bloodstream. These substances cause vasodilation (expansion of the walls of blood vessels) and increased vascular permeability (leakage through the walls of small vessels, especially veins). Histamine and serotonin can be released by trauma or exposure to cold. Other chemicals that circulate in the blood can release histamine. Two of these are part of the complement system; another is called interleukin-1. The effects of histamine diminish after approximately one hour.

Plasma proteases comprise three interrelated systems that explain much that is known about inflammation: the complement, kinin, and clotting systems. The complement system is composed of twenty different proteins involved in reactions against microbial agents that invade the body. The various chemicals act in a cascade, similar to falling dominoes: Each one sets off another in sequence. The result of these chemical actions is to increase vascular permeability, promote chemotaxis (the attraction of living cells to specific chemicals), engulf invading microorganisms, and destroy pathogens through a process called lysis.

The kinin system is responsible for releasing bradykinin, a chemical substance that causes contraction of smooth muscle tissue, dilation of blood vessels, and pain. The duration of action for bradykinin is brief because it is inactivated by the enzyme kininase. Bradykinin does not promote chemotaxis.

The clotting system is made up of a series of chemicals that result in the formation of a solid mass. The most commonly encountered example is the scab that forms at the site of a cut in the skin. Like the complement system, the clotting system is a cascade of thirteen different chemicals. In addition to producing a solid mass, the clotting system also increases vascular permeability and promotes chemotaxis for white blood cells.

Other substances are involved in acute inflammation. Among the most important of these is a class called prostaglandins. Several different prostaglandin molecules have been isolated; they are derived from the membranes of most cells. Prostaglandins cause pain, vasodilation, and fever. Aspirin counteracts the effects of prostaglandins, which explains the antipyretic (fever-reducing) and analgesic (pain-reducing) properties of the drug.

Another group of substances involved in acute inflammation are leukotrienes. The primary sources for these molecules are leukocytes, and some leukotrienes are found in mast cells. This group promotes vascular leakage but not chemotaxis. They also cause vasoconstriction (a decrease in the diameter of blood vessels) and bronchoconstriction (a decrease in the diameter of air passageways in the lungs). The effect of these leukotrienes is to slow blood flow and restrict air intake and outflow. A different type of leukotriene is found only in leukocytes. This type enhances chemotaxis but does not contribute to vascular leakage. In addition, leukotrienes cause white blood cells to stick to damaged tissues, speeding the removal of bacteria and promoting healing.

Other chemical substances are known to be involved with inflammation: platelet-activating factor, tumor necrosis factor, interleukin-1, cationic (positively charged) proteins, neutral proteases (enzymes that break down proteins), and oxygen metabolites (molecules resulting from reactions with oxygen). The sources of these are generally leukocytes, although some are derived from macrophages. They reinforce the effects of prostaglandins and leukotrienes.

There are four different outcomes for acute inflammation. There may be complete resolution in which the injured site is restored to normal; this outcome usually follows a mild injury or limited trauma where there has been only minor tissue destruction. Healing with scarring may occur, in which injured tissue is replaced with scar tissue that is rich in collagen, giving it strength but at the cost of normal function; this outcome follows more severe injury or extensive destruction of tissue. There may be the formation of an abscess, which is characterized by pus and which follows injuries that become infected with pyogenic (pus-forming) organisms. The fourth outcome is chronic inflammation.

Chronic inflammation. Acute inflammation may be followed by chronic inflammation. This reaction occurs when the organism, factor, or agent responsible for the acute inflammation is not removed or when the normal processes of healing fail to occur. Repeated episodes of acute inflammation may also lead to chronic inflammation, in which the stages of acute inflammation seem to remain for long periods of time. In addition, chronic inflammation may begin insidiously, such as with a low-grade infection that does not display the usual signs of acute inflammation; tuberculosis, rheumatoid arthritis, and chronic lung disease are examples of this third alternative.

Chronic inflammation typically occurs in one of the following conditions: prolonged exposure to potentially toxic substances such as asbestos, coal dust, and silica that are nondegradable; immune reactions against one's own tissue (autoimmune diseases such as lupus and rheumatoid arthritis); and persistent infection by an organism that is either resistant to drug therapy or insufficiently toxic to cause an immune reaction (such as viruses, tuberculosis, and leprosy). The characteristics of chronic inflammation are similar to those of acute inflammation but are less dramatic and more protracted.

—*L. Fleming Fallon, Jr., M.D., Ph.D., M.P.H.*

See also Abscess drainage; Abscesses; Arthritis; Burns and scalds; Bursitis; Disease; Healing; Infection; Wounds; *specific diseases.*

FOR FURTHER INFORMATION:

Gallin, John I., Ira M. Goldstein, and Ralph Snyderman, eds. *Inflammation: Basic Principles and Clinical Correlates.* 3d ed. New York: Raven Press, 1999. This well-written book is for the reader who wants to know about inflammation in great detail.

Majno, Guido, Ramzi Cotran, and Nathan Kaufman, eds. *Current Topics in Inflammation and Infection.* Baltimore: Williams & Wilkins, 1982. This specialized monograph provides extensive details on the subject. It assumes that the reader is familiar with the basics of inflammation.

Robbins, Stanley L., Ramzi S. Cotran, and Vinay Kumar, eds. *Robbins' Pathologic Basis of Disease.* 6th ed. Philadelphia: W. B. Saunders, 1999. A widely used pathology text which contains a good discussion of inflammation. Written for health professionals, but the serious nonspecialist will find a wealth of material.

INFLUENZA

DISEASE/DISORDER

ANATOMY OR SYSTEM AFFECTED: Lungs, respiratory system

SPECIALTIES AND RELATED FIELDS: Epidemiology, family practice, internal medicine, public health, virology

DEFINITION: Any one of a group of commonly experienced respiratory diseases caused by viruses, responsible for many major, worldwide epidemics.

KEY TERMS:

antibody: a protein substance produced by white blood cells (lymphocytes) in response to an antigen; combats bacterial, viral, chemical, or other invasive agents in the body

antigen: a chemical substance, often on a bacterial or viral surface, containing substances that activate the body's immune response

pneumonia: a respiratory tract infection that can be caused by bacteria or viruses; it is the major complication of influenza and the major cause of influenza deaths

ribonucleic acid (RNA): the material contained in the core of many viruses that is responsible for directing the replication of the virus inside the host cell

CAUSES AND SYMPTOMS

Epidemics of what scientists believe was influenza have been reported in Europe and Asia for at least a thousand years. Epidemics of what could have been influenza were reported by ancient Greek and Roman historians. Influenza epidemics still occur, striking isolated societies, entire nations, or, as with pandemics, the entire world. Among the great plagues that have afflicted the world over the centuries, influenza is the one that remains active today. Smallpox has been conquered, and bubonic plague (the Black Death), yellow fever, and typhus no longer erupt every few years as they once did. Cholera still breaks out, but rarely as a major epidemic. Before acquired immunodeficiency syndrome (AIDS), influenza was called "the last of the great plagues."

The term "influenza" is from the Italian and refers to the fact that some early scientists thought that the disease was caused by the malevolent influence of the planets, stars, and other heavenly bodies. To others, this "influence" was a miasma or poisonous effluvium carried in the air—a theory which is closer to the truth.

In the eighteenth and nineteenth centuries, there were about twenty major epidemics of influenza in Europe and America. They were of varying severity—some mild, some harsh. In 1918, a pandemic of influenza became one of the worst afflictions ever endured by humankind. It came in three waves, the first in the spring of 1918. This wave was relatively mild and mortality rates were low, and it spread evenly through

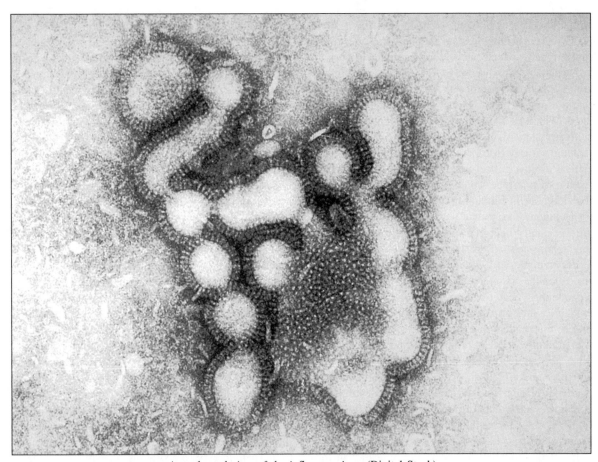

An enlarged view of the influenza virus. (Digital Stock)

all age groups of the population. The second wave came in the fall, and it was the most devastating outbreak of disease seen since the great plagues of the Middle Ages. Up to 20 percent of its victims died, and about half the deaths were of people in the prime of life, twenty to forty years of age. The last wave came in the winter and was not as severe. By the time that the pandemic was over, more than 20 million people worldwide had died from it, with more than 500,000 deaths in the United States alone.

In 1918, scientists understood enough about microbiology to realize that a microorganism caused influenza, but they originally thought that it was a bacterium, *Haemophilus influenzae*, because this organism was isolated from some of the victims. *H. influenzae* causes many diseases, but influenza is not among them, as researchers found when infection from it failed to produce influenza symptoms in test subjects. It soon became apparent that the organism responsible for influenza was unlike any bacterium that sci-

ence had yet encountered. Bacteria were easily seen in the microscope and could be collected in filters. Whatever it was that caused influenza was invisible to the microscope, and it could not be trapped in filters. So, scientists postulated that the influenza pathogen was far smaller than bacteria. They used the term "filtrable virus" to describe it—an interesting locution, because what they meant was that the organism could *not* be filtered by the devices that they were using. "Filter-passing virus," another term used at the time, is more accurate.

It was not until 1931, thirteen years after the great pandemic, that the first influenza virus was isolated. It was found in swine, and the methods used to discover it formed the basis for the techniques used to isolate the human influenza virus, a major event in microbiology that occurred in 1933.

It was later found that there were not one but three kinds of human influenza virus: type A, which is the major cause of severe influenza outbreaks; type B, which also causes influenza epidemics but less often and which is usually less severe than type A; and the rarest, type C, which causes a mild, coldlike illness.

Further, it was discovered that there are different strains of virus within type A and type B, subtypes that are not identical to one another but that are related. Within each subtype there are variants. As these subtypes and variants began to appear, it became clear that the virus was capable of mutation. This was a critical discovery because it meant that influenza infection of one type would not necessarily immunize the victim against influenza of another type. This ability to mutate means that new influenza virus strains are constantly being developed—and are constantly threatening new waves of disease.

For example, in 1957, a new strain of influenza virus called the Asian flu came out of China and started a pandemic. Asian flu, or variants of it, caused the flu epidemics in the years from 1957 to 1968, but immunity to it spread so that the severity of the epidemics was gradually reduced. Then the Hong Kong flu, another new strain from the Far East, appeared. People had no immunity to it, so it caused another major pandemic. Hong Kong flu and its variants caused the epidemics that occurred in the next nine years. Then, in 1977, still another pandemic arose from a newer strain, also from Eastern Asia.

In 1976, another type, swine flu, appeared in the United States. This virus infects pigs and humans and is apparently a distant descendant of the virus that caused the 1918 pandemic. It was evidently not as hardy as the 1977 virus, because that one replaced it and swine flu disappeared, although some experts predict its return.

The reason that the influenza virus can mutate readily is related to its physiological structure. The virus is usually spherical, but the shape can vary. It is extremely small, about 0.0001 millimeter in diameter. Its surface is covered with spikes of protein, hemagglutinin and neuraminidase. They are the two major antigens that trigger the body's immune system to repel the virus and provide immunity against future infection. Hemagglutinin (H) causes red blood cells to agglutinate, or clump together. Neuraminidase (N) is an enzyme.

Inside the core of the virus are two additional antigens that trigger the production of antibodies, but these antibodies do not protect against future infection. Also in the core is a feature unique to influenza virus: Instead of a single strand of ribonucleic acid (RNA), there are eight individual strands, each one a single gene. Genes are said to be "encoded" to produce specific characteristics within an organism. When the virus invades a host cell, the RNA directs a process of replication in which components of the cell are used to make new viruses. The new viruses are then released to enter other cells and continue replicating.

The H and N antigens mutate gradually over the years because of changes in the RNA genes that encode for them. This process is called antigenic drift, and it refers to slight variations that appear in the influenza virus and account for minor and localized epidemics of the disease. When a particular strain of virus has been prevalent for some time, a "herd immunity" develops in the populations exposed to it, and incidence of disease from it declines. When the H or N antigen changes radically, the process is called antigenic shift. It creates a new subtype of the virus, one that can cause a major pandemic because there is no immunity to it. There are at least thirteen variants of H (labeled H1 to H13) and at least nine variants of N (labeled N1 to N9).

Before 1968, most influenza A viruses in circulation had H2N2 antigens on its surface. This virus was the Asian flu; it had been around for some years, so the world population had become relatively immune to it. Then, in 1968, a new virus appeared in Southeast Asia, with a combination of H3N2. The H antigen had changed completely, while the N antigen remained the same, but the combination was essentially a new virus; it gave rise to the worldwide epidemic of the Hong Kong flu.

It is known that influenza viruses from animals influence the structure of the human viruses and contribute the variations that become new strains capable of causing pandemics. There is an interesting theory of how the 1957, 1968, and 1977 pandemics that came out of China developed. The Chinese people not only eat an enormous amount of duck but also keep large flocks to eat insects that attack rice crops. Ducks carry a wide variety of influenza viruses in their intestines, and they live in close proximity to humans. This theory suggests that the influenza viruses from duck droppings modified the human influenza virus and created the new strains that caused the pandemics that emanated from China. Other animals, such as pigs, which gave the world swine flu, also harbor influenza viruses that can interact with the human influenza virus.

To cause disease, the virus must be inhaled, which is why the "influence" of poisonous effluvium carried in the air is a more correct attribution of the actual cause of the disease than the influence of heavenly bodies. Inside the upper respiratory tract, there is a layer of cilia-bearing cells (cells with small, hairlike filaments) that acts as a barrier against infection. Ordinarily, the tiny cilia spread a layer of mucus over respiratory tissues. The mucus collects infectious organisms and carries them to the stomach, where they are destroyed by stomach acids. The influenza virus causes the cilia-bearing cells to disintegrate, exposing a layer of cells beneath. The virus invades these and other host cells in the respiratory tract and begins replicating. Invasion and replication by the virus destroy the host cells. Destruction of the cells starts the inflammatory process that causes the symptoms of disease.

Influenza infection grows rapidly, and symptoms can appear in only a few hours, although the incubation period in most people is two days or so. Fever, malaise, headache, muscular pain (particularly in the back and legs), coughing, nasal congestion, shivering, and a sore throat are common symptoms. The disease can spread quickly among populations because the virus is airborne. There is good reason to believe that the virus can remain infective in the air for long periods of time. It has been reported that the crew members on a ship sailing past Cuba during an epidemic there were infected with the disease, presumably from virus-laden particles carried from shore by the wind.

The major complication of influenza is pneumonia, which can be caused by the influenza virus itself (primary influenza viral pneumonia), by infection from bacteria (secondary bacterial pneumonia), or by mixed viral and bacterial infection. Pneumonia is the major cause of death from influenza. In the severe pandemic of 1918, up to 20 percent of patients developed pneumonia and, of these, about half died.

Primary influenza viral pneumonia can come on suddenly, and it often progresses relentlessly with high fever, rapidly accumulating congestion in the lungs, and difficulty in breathing. Pneumonia caused by secondary bacterial infection can be caused by a large number of pathogens. In nonhospitalized patients, both children and adults, the common causes are pneumococci, streptococci, and *Haemophilus influenzae*. In older, infirm, or hospitalized patients, the common causes are pneumococci, staphylococci, and *Klebsiella pneumoniae*.

When influenza B is the pathogen, Reye's syndrome can develop, most often in children under eighteen. This disease, which causes brain and liver damage, is fatal in about 21 percent of cases.

TREATMENT AND THERAPY

There are two main goals of therapy for the patient with influenza: treatment and preventing the spread of the disease. The first aim of therapy is to keep the patient comfortable, address the symptoms of the disease that can be treated, and deal with any complications that may arise. Bed rest is recommended, particularly during the most severe stages of the disease. Exertion is to be avoided, in order to prevent excessive weakness that could encourage further infection. Aspirin, acetaminophen, and other drugs are given for fever, and painkillers are given to relieve aches and pains. Cough suppressants and expectorants can relieve the hacking coughs that develop. Drinking large amounts of liquids is advised to replace the fluids lost as a result of high fever and sweating.

Amantadine hydrochloride is sometimes given to patients with influenza A infection. It reduces fever and relieves respiratory symptoms. An analogue of amantadine, rimantadine, works similarly. In severe cases of influenza caused by either A or B virus, an antiviral drug called ribavirin can be administered as a mist to be breathed in by the patient. Ribavirin shortens the duration of fever and may alleviate primary influenza viral pneumonia.

Primary influenza viral pneumonia is usually treated in the intensive care unit of a hospital, where the patient is given oxygen and other procedures are used to give respiratory and hemodynamic support. Secondary bacterial pneumonia must be treated with appropriate antibiotics. Identifying the precise bacterium will help the physician decide which antibiotic to prescribe. This identification is not always feasible, however, in which case broad-spectrum antibiotics will be used. They are effective against the most common bacteria that cause these secondary infections: *Streptococcus pneumoniae*, *Staphylococcus aureus*, and *Haemophilus influenzae*.

In preventing the spread of influenza, the first line of defense is to isolate the patient from susceptible persons and to initiate a program of vaccination. Because the influenza virus is constantly mutating, vaccines are regularly reformulated to confer immunity to the current pathogens. For the most part, the differences are not great between one year's virus and the one causing the next year's disease. Current vaccines may confer immunity or may require adjustment. If a major antigenic mutation has occurred, however, immunity cannot be conferred unless a new vaccine is developed against the new strain. Because it can take months to develop a new vaccine, there is the danger that the epidemic will have run its course and infected entire populations by the time that the vaccine is ready. Fortunately, major pandemics of influenza usually start slowly, so researchers have the time to identify the new strain, create a vaccine, and disseminate it.

The usual recommendation is to vaccinate people who are at highest risk of complications from the disease. These people include those over sixty-five years of age; residents of nursing homes or other patients with chronic medical conditions; adults and children with chronic pulmonary or cardiovascular diseases, including children with asthma; adults and children who have been hospitalized during the previous year for metabolic disorders, such as diabetes mellitus, or for renal diseases, blood disorders, or immunosuppression; teenagers and children who are receiving long-term aspirin therapy (who may be at risk of developing Reye's syndrome as a result of influenza infection); and pregnant women whose third trimester occurs in winter.

When a family member brings influenza into the household, other members should be vaccinated. After vaccination, it usually takes about two weeks for immunity to develop. Amantadine may protect against influenza A in the meantime; it can be discontinued after immunity has been achieved. If, for any reason, a person cannot be vaccinated, amantadine should be given throughout the entire length of the epidemic, which may last six to eight weeks.

A history of influenza vaccine development beginning with the identification of the virus in 1933 illustrates how constant vigilance is required to combat the disease. Various influenza vaccines were developed from 1935 to 1942, but they were all unsatisfactory. Building on the work that had gone before them, Thomas Francis and Jonas Salk (who later developed the first polio vaccine) produced a vaccine in 1942 that conferred immunity against the current strains of both influenza A and influenza B. Intensive animal testing and human trials showed that the vaccine was effective for about a year.

In 1947, however, many people who had been vaccinated came down with the disease: A new strain of influenza A virus had surfaced. The old vaccine had no effect on it, and a new vaccine had to be developed. This pattern has been repeated constantly: The original vaccine of 1942 was effective until a new

In the News: New Influenza Medications

In 1999, the Food and Drug Administration (FDA) approved for general use two new anti-influenza medications: Relenza (zanamivir) and Tamiflu. Both drugs act in a similar manner, by inhibiting the activity of the viral neuraminidase, an enzyme on the surface of the virus which is necessary for spread from an infected cell. Tamiflu, manufactured by Roche Laboratories, can be taken as a capsule; Relenza, produced by GlaxoSmithKline, is used as an inhalant.

Though each of the drugs has been found effective in shortening the duration and severity of influenza in some patients, their usefulness is limited. Relenza must be taken within forty-eight hours of the onset of symptoms, and treatment must continue for about five days. Patients with asthma or other forms of bronchoconstriction should use caution if choosing the drug. Further-

more, the symptoms associated with influenza are often similar to those found in other types of respiratory infections, including colds. Therefore the window of time necessary for antiviral treatment may be too short for even a proper diagnosis.

Tamiflu has been on the market for a shorter period than Relenza. Though there is no evidence for significant side effects following use of the drug, in the absence of long-term studies, similar precautions should be followed.

A new nasal mist has also become available for protection against influenza and the accompanying ear infections often seen as a complication. FluMist has proven to be more than 90 percent effective in protecting children against flu variants not found in current vaccines.

—Richard Adler, Ph.D.

strain appeared and a new vaccine had to be developed. That one was satisfactory until the next new strain, the Asian flu, appeared in 1957, and the process had to be repeated to find a vaccine that would protect against it. Similarly, in 1968 and in 1977, new vaccines had to be developed, and these have had to be modified to match the changes in the virus.

The World Health Organization (WHO) maintains reference laboratories around the world to keep up with the mutations of the influenza viruses. Their vigilance discovers new varieties as they appear. The new variants are studied, and vaccines are prepared to immunize against those strains that seem likely to cause extensive epidemics. This activity blunts the force of new pandemics and saves millions of lives.

PERSPECTIVE AND PROSPECTS

Researchers are constantly working to prevent the recurrent epidemics and pandemics of influenza, or at least to make them less severe. The fact that vaccines have to be modified periodically, and new ones developed from time to time, will probably not change.

It is theoretically possible for a pandemic of the severity of 1918 to occur. If a new subtype of the influenza virus were to arise and its initial spread were rapid, it could rage around the globe before an effective vaccine could be developed and made available. Mass devastation and death could result.

Another major concern is the enormous number of influenza virus strains that are living in animals. Hundreds of different types of influenza virus have been isolated from birds alone. These strains have the potential of causing mutations in the human influenza virus, as the Chinese ducks did in causing the Asian flu, the Hong Kong flu viruses, and the virus that caused the pandemic of 1977.

So far, medical science has been able to produce vaccines capable of protecting against the new mutant viruses as they arise. Even when a significant portion of any society is vaccinated, however, some people still become infected and there are no agents available that can kill the influenza virus. Furthermore, there are few therapeutic measures that can do any more than alleviate individual symptoms. Basically, the body's own immune system is the best therapy currently available.

Chemoprophylaxis (prevention of a disease by the use of a drug) with amantadine is effective in limiting the spread of disease caused by influenza A, but amantadine has some undesirable side effects, and the drug seems to have no effect on the virus itself. Rimantadine, a closely related compound, is equally effective as a chemoprophylactic agent and seems to be better tolerated. It is still considered an experimental drug, however, and it has not been licensed.

No chemotherapeutic agent (a drug capable of curing a disease) has yet been developed that will kill an influenza virus in the same way that an antibiotic destroys bacteria and other microorganisms. The search for antiviral agents is among the most urgent activities in medical science, and the problems are enormous. Yet the science is young. As researchers learn more about the structure, physiology, and activities of viruses, they will also develop means of controlling them.

When an agent is discovered that is safe and effective against influenza virus, it could be subject to the same limitations as the vaccines; that is, it may have to be modified periodically to remain effective against the new strains of influenza virus that are continually developing, and it may be necessary to develop new agents to deal with radically new mutants.

—C. Richard Falcon

See also Antibiotics; Bacterial infections; Centers for Disease Control and Prevention (CDC); Epidemiology; Fever; Lungs; Microbiology; Nausea and vomiting; Pneumonia; Pulmonary diseases; Pulmonary medicine; Pulmonary medicine, pediatric; Respiration; Reye's syndrome; Viral infections; World Health Organization; Zoonoses.

FOR FURTHER INFORMATION:

Biddle, Wayne. *Field Guide to Germs*. New York: Henry Holt, 1995. This comprehensive book is easily accessible to the nonspecialist and includes a discussion of nearly every virus, bacterium, and fungus known to cause human and nonhuman animal disease. The history of the microbe and the treatment of diseases are included.

Kiple, Kenneth F., ed. *The Cambridge World History of Human Disease*. New York: Cambridge University Press, 1993. The section on influenza gives a useful account of the epidemics and pandemics of influenza throughout the years.

Kolata, Gina. *Flu: The Story of the Great Influenza Pandemic of 1918 and the Search for the Virus That Caused It*. New York: Farrar, Straus and Giroux, 1999. Kolata's book vividly describes how the 1918 influenza outbreak, the most deadly pandemic the United States has ever faced, affected society. It not only offers an apocalyptic vision of the course of the disease but also details the ongoing efforts to track down its source.

Larson, David E., ed. *Mayo Clinic Family Health Book*. 2d ed. New York: William Morrow, 1996. A good general medical text for the layperson. The section on influenza is short but thorough.

Sahelian, Ray, and Victoria Dolby Toews. New York: Avery, 1999. *The Common Cold Cure: Natural Remedies for Colds and Flu*. The miseries of the common cold are many, and while a definitive medical cure remains elusive, its most annoying symptoms can certainly be addressed and, as Sahelian and Toews maintain, its duration shortened without the use of over-the-counter pharmaceuticals.

INSECT BITES. *See* BITES AND STINGS.

INSOMNIA. *See* SLEEP DISORDERS.

INSULIN RESISTANCE SYNDROME
DISEASE/DISORDER

ANATOMY OR SYSTEM AFFECTED: All
SPECIALTIES AND RELATED FIELDS: All
DEFINITION: A reduced sensitivity to the action of insulin, which brings glucose into body tissues to be used as a source of energy.

KEY TERMS:

glucose: blood sugar

insulin: a peptide hormone secreted by the pancreas; it helps the body by promoting glucose utilization, protein synthesis, and the formation and storage of neutral lipids by regulating the sugar metabolism

syndrome: a cluster of symptoms

CAUSES AND SYMPTOMS

Normally, after a meal, the body digests food, nutrients are absorbed into the blood, and the level of glucose (sugar) in the blood rises. Glucose is then quickly transported into cells for use, as glucose is the principal energy source in the human body. Most tissues, particularly skeletal muscle tissue, require insulin action to transport glucose into cells. Insulin, a hormone secreted by the pancreas, helps transport glucose into cells by binding with receptors on cells as a key would fit into a lock. Once the key—insulin— has fitted into the lock and unlocked the door, the cell allows the entry of glucose, and the glucose can pass from the bloodstream into the cell. Inside cells, glucose is either used for energy, or stored for future use in the form of glycogen in liver or muscle cells.

Insulin resistance occurs when the normal amount of insulin secreted by the pancreas is not able to unlock the door for glucose entering into cells. In some cases, the pancreas secretes additional insulin to maintain a normal blood glucose level. In other cases, when the body cells do not respond to even higher levels of insulin, glucose builds up in the blood resulting in a high blood glucose (sugar) level, or Type II diabetes (non-insulin-dependent diabetes). Thus, the consequences of insulin resistance include decreased insulin function throughout the body, and hyperinsulinemia (a high insulin level in the blood).

However, insulin resistance does not occur alone. People with insulin resistance often have some other abnormalities, including an increased level of triglycerides (blood fat), a decreased level of HDL cholesterol (good cholesterol), hypertension (high blood pressure), and obesity (overweight). This cluster of abnormalities, together with hyperinsulinemia and hyperglycemia (high blood glucose), is called insulin resistance syndrome, which is also known as Syndrome X or Deadly Quartet. The syndrome is a cluster of risk factors for heart disease, and insulin resistance may be the common factor linking other risk factors.

The cause of insulin resistance is still not clear as of today. Some scientists believe that a defect in specific genes may result in insulin resistance and Type II diabetes. What is currently known is that insulin resistance is aggravated by obesity and physical inactivity.

As a consequence of hyperinsulinemia, additional fat is stored in the body, because the body is trying to protect itself by turning excess insulin into triglyceride. High insulin levels in the blood also contribute to high levels of low-density lipoprotein (LDL) cholesterol (so-called bad cholesterol), low levels of high-density lipoprotein (HDL) cholesterol, and hypertension. Obesity, associated with insulin resistance, often shows as upper body obesity.

Because insulin resistance syndrome does not have any outward physical signs, 20 to 25 percent of the "healthy" population may be insulin resistant but are not aware of it. Almost all individuals with Type II diabetes and many with hypertension, cardiovascular disease, and obesity are insulin resistant.

TREATMENT AND THERAPY

Insulin resistance often goes unrecognized until later in life when metabolic abnormalities develop. Thus, the first step of the treatment for this disorder is to identify those who may be at risk, including those who are overweight, have a parent or sibling with Type II diabetes, and have high blood pressure. Women who had diabetes during pregnancy also have a higher risk for this disorder. To diagnose this disorder, the oral glucose tolerance test can be used.

It is possible to reduce insulin resistance by caloric restriction, weight loss, exercise, and drug therapy. The multiple risk factor intervention treatment is usually recommended, aiming aggressively at reducing all cardiac risk factors that may exist. The key of this multiple risk factor intervention treatment is the modification of lifestyle. Lowering calorie intake can reduce insulin resistance within a few days. A diet low in saturated fat (less than 10 percent of total calories) and more moderate in total fat content (less than 40 percent of total calories) is beneficial. Concentrated sweets should be cut down. Weight loss, maintenance of ideal body weight, and regular exercise are essential. This kind of behavioral intervention is recommended for all those who have hypertension, high cholesterol, simple obesity, heart disease, diabetes, or insulin resistance syndrome.

If medical treatment is necessary, a variety of drugs are available, such as metformin and troglitazone. Metformin is a drug which enhances insulin sensitivity without affecting insulin secretion (not effective in the absence of insulin). It lowers glucose by decreasing glucose production in the liver. In addition, metformin decreases blood pressure, induces weight loss, and has a beneficial effect on lowering LDL cholesterol and triglyceride levels. Metformin has several gastrointestinal side effects, including diarrhea, nausea, and anorexia. These symptoms often improve with dosage reduction. Metformin also impairs absorption of vitamin B_{12} and folic acid but rarely causes clinical symptoms. In patients with kidney or heart disease, the use of metformin can increase the risk of lactic acidosis.

Troglitazone increases glucose transport. The treatment effect from troglitazone may not occur until two to three weeks after initiation of the drug. Troglitazone decreases the concentration of blood glucose and triglycerides, but increases HDL cholesterol. Some clinical trials have also shown that troglitazone decreases blood pressure. One important side effect of troglitazone is liver dysfunction. Thus, the liver function should be checked each month for the first six months of therapy, every two months for the next

six months, and periodically thereafter. Often a combined therapy (using two or more drugs) plus behavioral intervention are used together for the treatment of insulin resistance.

PERSPECTIVE AND PROSPECTS

No data are currently available to determine if long-term drug therapy aimed at reducing insulin resistance can prevent the development of diabetes and, consequently, heart disease. To investigate this issue, the Diabetes Prevention Program was recently initiated. This large randomized trial will compare four treatment groups—intensive lifestyle intervention, metformin, or troglitazone with standard diet and exercise, and a control group—to determine the effectiveness of these interventions on the prevention of Type II diabetes among high-risk people with insulin resistance. The United Kingdom Prospective Diabetes Study is a multicenter, prospective, randomized intervention trial, in which the combination effect of diet and drug therapy is being evaluated.

Insulin resistance syndrome is more common in well-developed countries, such as the United States, where the population is becoming more sedentary and more obese. As both physical inactivity and obesity aggravate insulin resistance, more effective prevention and treatment of obesity should have a major impact on reducing the development of this "deadly quartet."

—*Kimberly Y.-Z. Forrest, Ph.D., M.P.H.*

See also Diabetes mellitus; Endocrine disorders; Endocrinology; Endocrinology, pediatric; Hormones; Obesity.

FOR FURTHER INFORMATION:

Granberry, Mark C., and Vivian A. Fonseca. "Insulin Resistance Syndrome: Options for Treatment." *Southern Medical Journal* 92 (January, 1999): 2-15.

Opara, James U., and John H. Levine. "The Deadly Quartet—The Insulin Resistance Syndrome." *Southern Medical Journal* 90 (December, 1997): 1162-1169.

Reaven, Gerald M., Terry Kristen Strom, and Barry Fox. *Syndrome X: Overcoming the Silent Killer That Can Give You a Heart Attack.* New York: Simon & Schuster, 2000.

INTENSIVE CARE. *See* CRITICAL CARE; CRITICAL CARE, PEDIATRIC.

INTERNAL MEDICINE

SPECIALTY

ANATOMY OR SYSTEM AFFECTED: Abdomen, bladder, gallbladder, gastrointestinal system, glands, heart, intestines, kidneys, liver, lungs, pancreas, reproductive system, respiratory system, spleen, stomach, urinary system, uterus

SPECIALTIES AND RELATED FIELDS: Cardiology, endocrinology, gastroenterology, gynecology, nephrology, proctology, pulmonary medicine

DEFINITION: The field of medicine concerned with the diagnosis and treatment of disease of the body's inner organs and structures, usually including surgery on these organs.

KEY TERMS:

acute: referring to a short-term disease process

cellular biology: the study of the processes that take place within a cell

chronic: referring to a long-term disease process

inflammation: redness, pain, and heat resulting from trauma or infection; often the first step in the body's self-healing process

molecular biology: study of the interactions that occur among the molecules that make up living organisms

pathogen: any microorganism that can cause disease, including bacteria, viruses, fungi, yeasts, and parasites

trauma: physical injury to bodily tissue

SCIENCE AND PROFESSION

Internists, or practitioners of internal medicine, are skilled in the diagnosis and treatment of disease conditions that can occur virtually anywhere within the human body. They must be expert in human biology and anatomy and in pathophysiology (that is, the study of the processes that lead to disease conditions). By its nature, internal medicine embraces many other medical specialties, such as cardiology or gastroenterology. In fact, many internists become certified in related specialties.

The original model for the modern internist was Sir William Osler (1849-1919), a Canadian physician who practiced in the United States for much of his life. Osler was deeply beloved and respected for his compassion and humanity as well as his extraordinary skills in anatomy and diagnosis and in effecting cures for his patients. In his long career as physician and teacher of medicine, Osler formulated many of the guiding principles in the practice of internal medicine.

Knowledge of many scientific disciplines is required of internists. They must understand the physical and biological basis of disease. This involves knowledge of genetics, cellular biology, immunology, and the activities and nature of the various microorganisms that cause disease, such as bacteria, viruses, fungi, yeasts, and parasites.

Internists must understand the components and role of each type of cell in the human body and know how the cell functions. Human cells are not simple entities, but complex miniature organisms with many activities going on simultaneously, particularly metabolic processes. Just as important, internists must understand what happens within and outside of the cell in the disease process. For example, they must know how individual bacteria cause infection and how viruses invade cells, use them for their replication, and then destroy them. Internal medicine involves all the body's organ systems and structures, such as the heart and circulatory system, the gastrointestinal system, the genitourinary system, the respiratory system, the skin, the brain, and the skeletal system.

Internists must also be able to examine patients and diagnose the presence or absence of disease. This process involves a wide variety of techniques and procedures. It usually begins with an introductory interview, followed by physical examination of the patient. Pain is the most common symptom of disease, and manifestation of it is investigated thoroughly.

DIAGNOSTIC AND TREATMENT TECHNIQUES

Internists understand the intricate pathways of pain throughout the body and know that proper explanation of a pain will often lead directly or indirectly to a correct diagnosis of the underlying disorder. Much of the diagnostic skill of the internist, however, is in the understanding that pain may be ambiguous. Headache can point to the possibility of many disorders, ranging from sinusitis to severe pathologies within the brain. Pain in the chest can be caused by upper-respiratory tract infection or heart disease. Pain in the limbs and/or joints may indicate physical trauma as a result of accidents or overexercising, or it may be attributable to arthritic or rheumatic disease or other causes. Abdominal pain can be present in literally dozens of different conditions. Similarly, back and neck pain can be caused simply by physical exertion or may point to a serious underlying disease.

Blood pressure and pulse are checked in the physical examination, and the doctor listens to heart and chest sounds through a stethoscope. The ears, mouth, and nose are examined. Body temperature is an important diagnostic consideration. Excess body heat or fever often accompanies infection and may also be present in other disease conditions. The doctor also checks for enlargement of lymph nodes and other signs that might suggest infection or other disorders.

Blood or urine samples are often taken for laboratory analysis. The internist will specify the tests he or she wants in the laboratory workup. These will include standard assays to give the internist a general picture of the patient's health and may include special tests for individual functions that the doctor may suspect are impaired.

Changes in the function of different body systems can lead the physician through the process of diagnosis. For example, such symptoms as dizziness; fainting; numbness; vision, speech, or hearing disturbances; or coma may be caused by dysfunction of the nervous system or may point to heart disease or other disorder. Abnormalities in respiratory function have specific meaning to the internist and may lead to a diagnosis ranging from a common cold to a more serious respiratory disease or a disease of other organs, such as the heart. Alterations in the skin may indicate a dermatological disorder or may suggest some internal condition.

Sometimes, a diagnosis is easy to make: The presenting symptoms are obvious signs of a specific disease. Sometimes, a group of symptoms, called a syndrome, may be ambiguous and could be related to any of a number of conditions. If the exact nature of a disease or its cause is uncertain, the internist will conduct a differential diagnosis in which possible causes of the disease are investigated in order to eliminate those that are not candidates and to pinpoint the actual cause.

Internists treat a wide variety of disorders. Among the most significant are the infectious diseases. They must study the pathogenesis (from *pathos*, meaning "disease" and *genesis*, meaning "origin" or "source") of infectious diseases in order to know how to diagnose and treat them. Harmful bacteria cause disease in different ways, but one way or another, they damage and destroy body cells and tissue. Some cause infection at the point where they enter the body, such as at the site of a wound, or in the respiratory tract when they are breathed into the body. Sometimes, bacteria are carried from their site of entry to other parts of the body, where they colonize and cause infection.

The range of bacterial infections is enormous, but one thing that they often have in common is inflammation. Inflammation is the beginning of the immune process by which the body defends itself against invading pathogens. It starts when the body recognizes that the invading organism is a foreign entity by detecting foreign antigens (substances on the surfaces of invading organisms such as bacteria and viruses). The body then releases certain white blood cells, called leukocytes, that are specific for producing antibodies that can destroy the organism. Once the body has identified a foreign organism and created antibodies for it, the immune system will retain a memory of the organism and destroy it whenever it enters the body again.

When confronted with bacterial infection, internists may recognize the organism that causes it from the patient's symptoms, or they may have to take specimens from the site of inflammation and test them in order to identify the organism involved. Sometimes, the organism is identified by microscopic examination, often using a dye that stains certain bacteria. Sometimes, it is necessary to grow the organism in a culture medium in order to identify it. The organism may also be identified by its antigen or by the type of antibody that the immune system produces to fight it.

The signs of viral infection are often exactly the same as those of bacterial infection. The main difference is that the causative organism cannot be isolated and identified as easily. Unlike bacteria, viruses cannot be seen through a microscope or otherwise identified by many of the methods used for bacteria. They can be cultured, however, or antigens or antibodies may be detectable.

In addition to infectious diseases, internists are called on to treat dysfunction in all parts of the body. They treat many patients suffering from heart disease, the major killer of Americans. The heart is actually subject to a wide range of disorders, the most common and the most deadly of which is coronary artery disease. Internists have many means of both diagnosing heart diseases and, often, predicting them. The patient's presenting symptoms and an analysis of the patient's lifestyle will often suggest the possibility of heart disease. Various in-office and laboratory procedures will inform the internist of the precise status of the patient's heart function and help direct the course of therapy.

Cancer, the second most common cause of mortality in the United States, is often seen by internists.

Lung cancer is the leading cause of cancer death, followed by cancer of the colon or rectum, breast, prostate gland, urinary tract, and uterus. The lymph system, blood, mouth, pancreas, skin, stomach, and ovary are also common sites. The term "cancer" describes a large number of disorders. What all cancers have in common is that the cells of an organ multiply uncontrollably. As the cancer cells proliferate, they crowd out other cells and interfere with organ function. Sometimes cancer cells from one organ spread to neighboring organs or are carried to other parts of the body. This process is called metastasis, and it can indicate that the cancer has spread or is spreading throughout the body. Internists may be responsible for treating cancer patients throughout the disease process or may refer them to oncologists, or cancer specialists.

Diseases of the respiratory system are major concerns of the internist. In addition to bacterial and viral infections, there are many acute and chronic respiratory conditions. One major example is asthma. Its cause is unknown, but it is believed to be at least partially attributable to allergy. When an asthma attack occurs, airways in the lungs swell and constrict. Mucus builds up and airflow is restricted, causing the patient to wheeze and gasp for air. Many internists have become skilled in helping asthmatic patients, alleviating symptoms, and preventing attacks.

All parts of the body harbor the potential for disease, infectious and otherwise. They are all, to some degree, the province of internists. The kidneys and the urinary system, the gastrointestinal system, the immune system, the endocrine glands, the brain and the nervous system, and the skeletal system are all within the internist's broad purview. Often disorders in these various organs and systems can be treated fully by internists. When they believe that a patient needs a physician with greater knowledge in a particular area of medicine, however, internists will refer the patient to an appropriate specialist.

In addition to their diagnostic skills, internists must possess a wide knowledge of modern treatment modalities. Surgery is rarely among the procedures mastered by the internist, so surgical procedures are routinely referred to surgeons specializing in the particular techniques involved.

Primary among the internist's tools for fighting infectious diseases are the antibiotics. These are the mainstays of therapy for infections caused by bacteria and other nonviral microorganisms. Since the first antibiotics were developed in the 1930's and 1940's, literally hundreds more have been developed. Scores of these are in use, and new agents are constantly being introduced.

It is vital for internists to keep abreast of new antibiotics because disease-causing organisms are often able to develop resistance against antibiotic agents that have been in use for a long time. For example, many strains of bacteria that were susceptible to penicillin have developed the ability to counteract its antibiotic effect. Other agents had to be found to destroy these resistant strains. This phenomenon occurs across virtually the entire range of the available antibiotics: Prolonged use of a given agent often allows the target organism to develop resistance to it. Internists must also be skilled in the proper use of antibiotics. Knowing which agent or combination of agents to prescribe, in what amounts, and for how long are important considerations in developing the patient's treatment plan. Antibiotics are not useful for treating viral infections, but there are a limited number of antiviral agents available for treating certain diseases.

Immunization against infectious diseases can be an important concern of the internist. The most extensive immunization programs in the United States are directed toward the vaccination of children and thus are generally carried out by pediatricians and family practitioners. Internists are often responsible, however, for the immunization of adult patients. Immunization against influenza is recommended for the elderly, particularly when a new strain of influenza virus arises. It is also recommended that elderly hospitalized patients be vaccinated against pneumococcal pneumonia. Internists are a primary avenue of immunization against hepatitis B, particularly among high-risk target populations, such as medical personnel, intravenous drug abusers, and adult male homosexuals. Internists are also involved in immunizing patients who require special vaccinations because of exposure to disease or for travel to foreign countries.

Patients who require long-term or lifelong therapy for noninfectious diseases include individuals with heart diseases, high blood pressure, diabetes, cancer, respiratory disorders, and a host of other conditions. The challenge to the internist is to develop a regimen that is both efficacious and safe. Drug therapy is prominent in the internist's treatment armamentarium. In either short-term or long-term drug therapy, problems may arise. The patient may develop significant side effects or adverse reactions. The drug may lose its effectiveness after months or years of therapy. The condition may change and require dosage adjustments, additional medications, or a complete change of regimen.

Consistent monitoring of the patient's condition is an important part of therapy. The internist wants to ensure that the prescribed regimen is working and that the therapy is comfortable for the patient. For example, the earliest agents for high blood pressure, or hypertension, often had such disagreeable side effects that patients would stop taking them. Hypertension has virtually no symptoms. After the patient started taking medication, however, he or she could experience loss of energy, listlessness, impotence, dream disturbances, and many other unwelcome effects. Similarly, diabetes patients who are dependent on regular insulin injections sometimes neglect their therapy. They may balk against sticking themselves with needles three or four times a day, and they may not monitor their blood sugar adequately. Preventing the devastating and potentially fatal consequences of diabetes depends on rigorous compliance with all aspects of the diabetes regimen, including diet, insulin, and monitoring.

Thus, patient compliance with therapy becomes one of the major tasks of the internist and virtually any other physician: If the patient does not cooperate with the regimen that the doctor prescribes, the therapy is not likely to be effective. For this reason, many internists now make patient counseling part of their practice. The modern internist recognizes that patients must understand their therapeutic goals, why they are being given certain medicines, and what these drugs can be expected to accomplish. Further, many internists find that it is wise to alert their patients to possible adverse reactions, although they understand the necessity of not frightening the patient. Some internists find the time to discuss their therapeutic regimens thoroughly with their patients. Others use nursing staff or other health care workers to educate patients.

Treatment modalities change constantly, and internists are required to be aware of the latest advances in order to modify their therapy programs to take advantage of improvements in drugs or procedures. Not only are new drugs constantly being approved for use, but modern medical science is continually learning new facts about old diseases as well, and these new insights often radically alter the way a given disease is treated. A good example is a stomach ulcer. For years,

it was thought that certain ulcers in the stomach were caused by erosion of the stomach wall by gastric juices. A group of investigators found, however, that a significant number of ulcer patients were also infected with the bacterium *Campylobacter pylori*. It has been suggested that infection may play a role in the development of these ulcers and that, therefore, therapy should be amended to include an antibacterial agent that is effective against *C. pylori*.

Furthermore, the internist's patient load is changing. Most internal medicine practices are treating increasing numbers of elderly patients, who have special needs. Internists must be aware of the constant advances in geriatric medicine in order to modify therapy for older patients.

PERSPECTIVE AND PROSPECTS

In the last decades of the twentieth century, internal medicine became somewhat fragmented as more and more physicians elected to practice in narrower specialties, such as cardiology, gastroenterology, hematology, or oncology, among many others. Specialties are still very much needed, but the practice of medicine seems to be headed back to the broader range of the internist.

As in the past, internists are at the forefront of progress in treatment. Recent generations have seen a far-reaching revolution in an understanding of the basic chemistry of life. As scientists elucidate the activities that occur at the molecular level of physical processes, insights are gained into exactly how the body works, as well as how antagonistic pathogens function. From this knowledge, new treatments have been devised for managing disease states.

A good example is the treatment of hypertension, one of the most common conditions seen by internists. Years ago, the only medications for high blood pressure were essentially sedatives and diuretics. It was not fully understood exactly what occurred at the cellular and molecular level that caused vasoconstriction, which is the main physical characteristic of hypertension. Researchers discovered complex biochemical activities that contributed to vasoconstriction and other aspects of high blood pressure. They were then able to develop agents that could treat the condition more effectively than anything available before. Internists now have a wealth of antihypertensive agents with which to work. Some reduce blood pressure by reducing heart activity, some dilate blood vessels by direct action, and some interfere with the biochemical processes that cause vasoconstriction. In addition, most of the agents that internists and other physicians use for hypertension cause many fewer side effects and adverse reactions than their predecessors.

In the fight against infectious diseases, new research is combining genetics with molecular biology to elucidate the exact biochemical processes by which pathogenic organisms invade and damage body cells and tissues. This research is having an enormous impact on the understanding of bacteria and viruses: how they work, how they mutate, and, perhaps most important, in what ways they are vulnerable. With increased knowledge comes increased capability to design more efficient antibiotics and to find agents that will inhibit the pathogen's ability to develop resistant strains. Internists are among the leaders in the application of these technologies. Because they see such a wide range of disease conditions, internists often function as the main channel by which new medications and treatments reach the patient.

—*C. Richard Falcon*

See also Abdomen; Abdominal disorders; Angina; Arrhythmias; Arteriosclerosis; Bacterial infections; Beriberi; Bleeding; Bronchitis; Candidiasis; Cardiology; Cardiology, pediatric; Cholecystitis; Cirrhosis; Colitis; Colonoscopy; Constipation; Coughing; Crohn's disease; Diabetes mellitus; Dialysis; Diarrhea and dysentery; Digestion; Diverticulitis and diverticulosis; *E. coli* infection; Emphysema; Endocarditis; Endoscopy; Gallbladder diseases; Gangrene; Gastroenterology; Gastroenterology, pediatric; Gastrointestinal disorders; Gastrointestinal system; Glands; Glomerulonephritis; Guillain-Barré syndrome; Gynecology; Heart; Heart attack; Heart disease; Heart failure; Heartburn; Hepatitis; Hernia; Incontinence; Indigestion; Influenza; Intestinal disorders; Intestines; Ischemia; Kidney disorders; Kidneys; Legionnaires' disease; Leprosy; Liver; Liver disorders; Lungs; Mitral insufficiency; Multiple sclerosis; Nephritis; Nephrology; Nephrology, pediatric; Palpitations; Pancreas; Pancreatitis; Parasitic diseases; Peristalsis; Peritonitis; Pneumonia; Proctology; Pulmonary medicine; Pulmonary medicine, pediatric; Renal failure; Reproductive system; Reye's syndrome; Rheumatic fever; Rheumatoid arthritis; Roundworm; Scarlet fever; Schistosomiasis; Staphylococcal infections; Stone removal; Stones; Streptococcal infections; Tapeworm; Tumor removal; Tumors; Ulcer surgery; Ulcers; Urinary system; Urology; Urology, pediatric; Viral infections; Whooping cough; Worms.

FOR FURTHER INFORMATION:

Braunwald, Eugene. *Harrison's Principles of Internal Medicine*. New York: McGraw-Hill, 2000. A standard text on internal medicine. Includes bibliographical references and an index.

Kiple, Kenneth, ed. *The Cambridge World History of Human Disease*. New York: Cambridge University Press, 1993. This text is useful for tracing the progress in medical practice through the years.

Larson, David E., ed. *Mayo Clinic Family Health Book*. 2d ed. New York: William Morrow, 1996. This text from the world-renowned medical facility was written for the layperson. Its coverage of medical practice in general and the diseases treated by the internist are clear and thorough.

Wagman, Richard J., ed. *The New Complete Medical and Health Encyclopedia*. 4 vols. Chicago: J. G. Ferguson, 1993. A good general medical reference work for the layperson. Its coverage of internal medicine is useful for clarifying the nature of the internist's practice and contrasting it with the subspecialties often practiced by internists.

INTERNET MEDICINE

SPECIALTY

ALSO KNOWN AS: Telehealth, telemedicine, e-medicine

ANATOMY OR SYSTEM AFFECTED: All

SPECIALTIES AND RELATED FIELDS: All

DEFINITION: The use of World Wide Web-based and other electronic long-distance communication technologies for health information, assessment, service delivery, training, and public health administration.

KEY TERMS:

anonymous: of unknown authorship, unidentified by a singular identity

assessment: a thorough physical and/or psychiatric examination; a process of systematically collecting comprehensive information about health care behavior, physical and psychiatric conditions, and general well-being for the purpose of diagnosis or treatment planning

clinical trials: scientifically based research examinations of new treatment procedures, techniques, devices, or pharmaceuticals that are considered state of the art in the treatment of diseases and other medical disorders

confidential: a situation distinguished by the willing disclosure of intimate information because of assurances that the information will be protected from general distribution or unauthorized disclosure; information which, if disclosed, has the potential to be damaging or dangerous to the person providing the information, their reputation, status, or their associates

diagnosis: a process of distinguishing knowledge about symptoms and problems that leads to the rendering of conclusions about physical and psychiatric illness; a label used to communicate specific health information among professionals, researchers, health systems, and insurance providers; a label which informs the process of treatment

Internet: a worldwide electronic system connecting individual computer users, computer networks, Web sites, and computer facilities for business, government, and organizational purposes

privacy: the state of being free from unwanted or unauthorized observation, company, or other intrusion

professional licensing: state-granted privileges to health care and other professionals allowing them to deliver services or to participate in certain activities; a privilege that is revokable and subject to censure; a privilege usually only granted after thorough examination of the skill and practice of a person seeking licensure

profiling: the collection of data to summarily categorize and track the behavior of individual users or types of users, through electronic or other tracking systems, to learn more about their behavior, usually for the purpose of prediction, done either with or without the knowledge or consent of the user

screening: a triage process; a process of asking a few questions of an individual, as opposed to an assessment, in order to determine whether there is sufficient risk of a problematic condition being present to justify completing a detailed evaluation or, instead, to justify assigning that individual to a category of lesser or no risk

Web site: a location on the Internet that has an individual address and that presents information, usually in the form of individual pages, or webpages, that the owner of the Web site wishes to make available to Internet users

SCIENCE AND PROFESSION

The Internet is a computer-based tool that is facilitating communication among vast numbers of individuals, groups, businesses, and governments. In addition to purely social and business-related ventures, the Internet is proving to be a valuable tool for improving the state of public health. This is because a new type of medical care and medical services has developed. These services, typically called telehealth, telemedicine, and e-medicine, use the Internet as a key tool in their dispensation, organization, and evaluation of health care services. Such services have taken the form of a variety of health care-related Web sites that provide services once only available through a face-to-face visit with a doctor or other health or social services professional. The Web sites are valuable in that they provide almost instantaneous information and other communications assistance to patients, their families, treatment professionals, trainers, trainees in the health care and social service professions, and also medical researchers.

In terms of assisting patients, Internet-based medical approaches provide a variety of services to individual Internet users. First, they provide a wealth of information on different symptoms and medical conditions. They also allow for screening of such conditions to see if they warrant further attention from medical professional and advice on how to handle minor health ailments and medical emergencies. They also help consumers to find medical advice, health care providers, self-help or support groups, and therapy over the Internet, all of which may or may not be supervised by medical professionals. Finally, they can give patients and their families information on different treatment options, including common procedures, the latest in alternative medicine, and even current clinical trials information.

Internet medicine can also be very helpful for family members of individuals having medical problems. Often, family members do not know how best to help their signficant others in times of medical need. To meet this need, Web sites may post a wide variety of information that can help people understand the conditions, the requirements of treatment, the limits of treatment, and things they can do to be helpful to the ill family member. Additionally, Web sites sometimes offer online support for family members through mechanisms such as e-mail and e-mail lists, also known as listservs, or other ongoing support groups in settings such as Internet chat rooms.

Health care and social service providers also find the Internet beneficial for their work. For some, it might be as simple as using the Internet to schedule appointments, or to communicate test results, reminder information about treatment procedures, or appointment reminders via e-mail with clients. For others, it might involve using special Web sites to conduct assessments of clients for the purpose of tracking their treatment success or progress. Professionals may also use telemedicine in order to learn about new treatments and procedures, or to learn about new drugs and other pharmaceutical products. In addition, health care and social service providers may benefit their general practice by using the Internet to keep abreast of new clinical trials to test state-of-the-art treatments, changes in licensing laws affecting their practice, and the development of new health care databases for tracking, triage, and communication with insurance companies. Finally, some providers are actually using the Internet for health services delivery.

Health care providers in training and their trainers also benefit greatly from telemedicine. To trainees living in remote areas or those who might be highly mobile, such as those in the armed forces, the Internet provides immediate access to large online libraries, knowledgeable online teachers, and databases full of important medical information. Both long-established

and new institutions interested in telemedicine increasingly are translating typical face-to-face training approaches into distance-based training programs utilizing the Internet. Encyclopedias, descriptions of techniques, pictures of what different conditions might look like both inside and outside the body, and even video of actual procedures are available online. Similarly, instruction in the use of such material is available online through training programs that lead to certificates of training and actual accredited degrees, ranging from bachelors to doctoral degrees and post-doctoral training. In addition to helping individuals who are at remote locations, such material also can be used to reach a larger number of trainees than might typically be able to observe or attend such training. The increased ability to teach, show procedures, or give supervision at a distance using pictoral, written, oral, and video information greatly facilitates continuing education and improvement of general health care practice. It also helps to facilitate the evaluation of those practices and training sessions. Since all of the work takes place over the Internet, different aspects of the work can be monitored and evaluated electronically.

Much of the evaluation of this kind of information is done by researchers who are studying client, trainer, provider, or even health care system behavior and organization. This is done by evaluating information, also known as data, in individual sessions or visits to Web sites, as well as by examining data that is collected over time, across multiple visits. For instance, a person might first go to a Web site for information on a specific medical condition and then, at a later time or times, come back and look up different treatment approaches, or visit online discussion groups. What they do from time to time would be evaluated by researchers to see how individuals use the site, how long they stay on it, or what things they try searching for which may not yet be on the site. The process of watching behavior over time is called tracking. Tracking allows researchers to profile the users of Web sites to learn more about their behavior, usually for the purpose of predicting their behavior

One of the disadvantages of the Internet is the ease with which illegal or dangerous substances, such as this home manufacturing kit for the "date rape" drug gamma hydroxybutyrate (GHB), can be distributed. (AP/Wide World Photos)

and response to treatment. By creating tracking databases of what happens with Web site users, the information gathered can be used to improve services and to decrease long-term health care service, training, and administration costs on a continuing basis.

Because of all the data being collected on how individuals are using different Web sites or other Internet-based services, there has been some concern over the individual's right to privacy and the protection of the information collected. For instance, some people have been concerned that if they are searching for information related to the human immunodeficiency virus (HIV) or substance use, they might be identified as being at risk for having that condition whether they do or not. Further, many individuals do not want that information linked to their identities or medical records. On one hand, they may be wishing to avoid solitication of business from sellers of medical services or products because of their association with the condition; they do not want their personal information sold for that purpose to the providers of such products or services. On the other hand, they may also wish to maintain privacy and keep their information confidential so as to avoid having any threat to their future insurability or their ability to get health care coverage. As an example, if a health care provider such as a health maintenance organization (HMO) tracked users' information on a Web site and discovered, through the database, that someone who was now applying for coverage had certain medical conditions, that person might have a greater risk of being refused coverage if their time on the Web site was not completely anonymous. In sum, given these concerns, users of Internet medicine need to understand that there are differences between the terms privacy, confidentiality, and anonymity, as well as in the legal issues and protections one can exercise when using this type of medicine. Each Web site may be operating under different constraints, and so it is always important for users of these services to be sure they understand how the Web sites handle privacy. Finding out how a Web site protects or does not protect the privacy of its users is the only way a user can determine how safe it is to reveal confidential information when they use a specific Web site.

DIAGNOSTIC AND TREATMENT TECHNIQUES
One of the biggest opportunities offered by Internet medicine is that of increasing the ability of individuals to do self-screening for medical conditions to see if they need medical assistance. Likewise, the ability of service providers to do screening and assessment for a larger number of people is increased relative to what can be done in person. This is because the assessments can be administered via the computer, saving valuable provider time. Additionally, assessments can be completed online and sent to providers in advance for immediate evaluation. While it may be some time before conclusive diagnoses can be offered via online technology, such advances are not far off; the differences between online and in-person assessments are being studied.

Intervention via the Internet is also much improved because large quantities of information can be dispensed electronically, printed out by clients or their families, or distributed to large numbers of individuals. Such informational interventions can be important for facilitating proper compliance with medical prescription regimens, helping clients to avoid bad drug interactions, or providing reminders about other things needed to facilitate wellness. Informational interventions can also be used for primary prevention, or preventing problems from happening in the first place. By providing suggestions for problem prevention, much suffering could be spared and many health care dollars can be saved. This is especially true for teenagers and college-age populations, who are often savvy Internet users.

Treatment also takes place on the Internet via simultaneous online interactions such as in chat rooms, communicating via videoconferencing as in a normal conversation but using video cameras, and simple asynchronous e-mail between the client and the provider. Generally this type of treatment is a complement to face-to-face treatment. For instance, some HMOs use online support groups as additional treatment for persons already receiving therapy. Others are using programs such as self-guided online courses that clients can work through to benefit their health. In general, practitioners are permitted to do this so long as they are properly licensed. This usually requires being licensed by the state in which they are practicing and/or where the client is receiving the services.

PERSPECTIVE AND PROSPECTS
The Internet continues to grow on a daily basis, with an increasing number of computer owners and Web sites taking advantage of its capabilities. Communications technologies are also improving on a near daily

basis, allowing for almost instant individual communication of written, oral, print, and video information at distances and speeds that were inconceivable in the past. As a result of these developments, as well as increases in health care costs, and the potential economic and health benefits provided by Internet medicine, this specialty area is here to stay. Commitment by governments to examine such developments in health care underscore this likelihood. In 1998, for example, the Health Resources and Service Administration of the United States Department of Health and Human Services established the Office for the Advancement of Telehealth. This office is devoted to advancing the use of telehealth and Internet-based medicine to facilitate improvement in the state of public health and research on public health. The ability of such approaches to provide more services with streamlined administrative procedures and decreased costs holds much promise for improving the state of public health.

—*Nancy A. Piotrowski, Ph.D.*

See also Allied health; Alternative medicine; Clinical trials; Education, medical; Family practice; Health maintenance organizations (HMOs); Herbal medicine; Noninvasive tests; Nursing; Pharmacology; Pharmacy; Physical examination; Screening; Self-medication.

FOR FURTHER INFORMATION:

Armstrong, Myrna L. *Telecommunications for Health Professionals: Providing Successful Distance Education and Telehealth*. New York: Springer, 1998. Provides strategies for using distance education and resources. Legal and ethical issues are discussed to inform patients, providers, students, and legislators.

Bauer, Jeffrey C., and Marc A. Ringel. *Telemedicine and the Reinvention of Healthcare*. New York: McGraw-Hill, 1999. History, technical, social, and policy-oriented issues are reviewed in this book that discusses telemedicine as a revolution in a series of scientific advances affecting health care.

Coiera, Enrico. *Guide to Medical Informatics, the Internet, and Telemedicine*. New York: Oxford University Press, 1997. The boundaries of appropriate communication of medical information via the Internet are outlined in this book tailored to the general reader, student, or trainer of health care provision.

Darkins, Adam William, and Margaret Ann Cary. *Telemedicine and Telehealth: Principles, Policies, Performance, and Pitfalls*. New York: Springer, 2000. Defines and examines telemedicine, discussing how it is organized, provided, and managed, along with its medical, social, economic, and cultural significance.

Davis, James B., Maureen Lynch, and Kathryn Swanson. *Health and Medicine on the Internet 2000*. Los Angeles: Health Information Press, 2000. Provides an annual guide for individuals interested in Internet-based health care.

Goldstein, Douglas E. *E-Healthcare: Harness the Power of the Internet, e-Commerce, and e-Care*. Gaithersburg, Md.: Aspen, 2000. An easy to understand resource, for patients, service providers, and entrepreneurs interested in online health care, describing the types of services provided and important legal issues (helpful CD-ROM included).

Kinsella, Audrey. *Home Telehealth in the Twenty-first Century: A Resource Book About Improved Services That Work*. Kensington, Md.: Information for Tomorrow, 2000. Provides an in-depth discussion of how telemedicine can help with chronic medical concerns.

Price, Joan. *Complete Idiot's Guide to Online Medical Resources*. Indianapolis, Ind.: Que, 2000. Provides information on traditional and alternative medicine approaches, helping readers evaluate Internet-based information so as to avoid bad or unreliable advice or recommendations.

INTERSTITIAL PULMONARY FIBROSIS (IPF)

DISEASE/DISORDER

ANATOMY OR SYSTEM AFFECTED: Chest, lungs, respiratory system

SPECIALTIES AND RELATED FIELDS: Environmental health, occupational health, pulmonary medicine

DEFINITION: In IPF, scarring and thickening (fibrosis) of the lung tissue occurs, causing difficulties in breathing. Its symptoms include chest pain, coughing, and shortness of breath (dyspnea). The disease is sometimes termed idiopathic or diffuse, which indicates that the cause is not known. The disease may be an autoimmune disorder, and it may be attributable to radiation therapy, lung cancer, and drug reactions. IPF has also been linked to occupational hazards, such as the repeated inhalation of organic dust (as from minerals) and chemical fumes. Such exposure may result in extrinsic allergic alveolitis (or hypersensitivity pneumonitis), which may in turn develop into IPF after several years. In IPF, the lungs may become increasingly stiff until heart failure or bronchopneumonia develops.

—Jason Georges and Tracy Irons-Georges

See also Lungs; Occupational health; Pneumonia; Pulmonary diseases; Pulmonary medicine; Pulmonary medicine, pediatric; Respiration.

FOR FURTHER INFORMATION:

Fishman, Alfred, ed. *Update: Pulmonary Diseases and Disorders.* 2d ed. New York: McGraw-Hill, 1992.

Fraser, Robert G., and J. A. Peter Pare. *Diagnosis of Diseases of the Chest.* 3d ed. Philadelphia: W. B. Saunders, 1990.

James, D. Geraint, and Peter R. Studdy. *A Color Atlas of Respiratory Disease.* 2d ed. St. Louis: Mosby Year Book, 1992.

Victor, Lyle, ed. *Clinical Pulmonary Medicine.* Boston: Little, Brown, 1992.

West, John B. *Pulmonary Pathophysiology: The Essentials.* 4th ed. Baltimore: Williams & Wilkins, 1992.

INTESTINAL CANCER. *See* STOMACH, INTESTINAL, AND PANCREATIC CANCERS.

INTESTINAL DISORDERS
DISEASE/DISORDER

ANATOMY OR SYSTEM AFFECTED: Abdomen, anus, gastrointestinal system, intestines

SPECIALTIES AND RELATED FIELDS: Family practice, gastroenterology, internal medicine

DEFINITION: Diseases or disorders of the small intestine, large intestine (or colon), liver, pancreas, and gallbladder.

KEY TERMS:

acute: the stage of a disease or presence of a symptom that begins abruptly, with marked intensity, and subsides after a short time

chronic: the stage of a disease or presence of a symptom that develops slowly and usually lasts for the lifetime of the individual

diarrhea: the passage of approximately six loose stools within a twenty-four-hour period caused by a variety of circumstances, such as infection, malabsorption, or irritable bowel

diverticulitis: inflammation or swelling of one or more diverticula, caused by the penetration of fecal material through thin-walled diverticula and the collection of bacteria or other irritating agents there

diverticulosis: the presence of diverticula in the colon, which may lead to diverticulitis

diverticulum: an outpouching through the muscular wall of a tubular organ, such as the stomach, small intestine, or colon

electrolytes: elements or compounds found in blood, interstitial fluid, and cell fluid that are critical for normal metabolism and function

peristalsis: the involuntary, coordinated, rhythmic contraction of the muscles of the gastrointestinal tract that forces partially digested food along its length

stricture: an abnormal narrowing of an organ because of pressure or inflammation

villi: folds within the small intestine that are important for the absorption of nutrients into the blood

PROCESS AND EFFECTS

Intestinal diseases and disorders are sometimes included with those of the digestive system. For the sake of clarity, this article makes the distinction between the structures of the digestive and intestinal tracts. The entire digestive tract, which includes the intestinal tract and is approximately 7.6 to 9.1 meters in length in adults, begins in the mouth and ends with the anus. It includes organs specific to digestion, such as the esophagus and stomach and their substructures. The intestinal tract, which constitutes the major part of the digestive tract, includes the small intestine, the large intestine (also known as the colon), and the organs that branch off these structures (the liver, pancreas, and gallbladder). The function of the small and large intestines is to break down food, absorb its nutrients into the bloodstream, and carry off waste products of digestion as feces.

The small intestine is approximately 6.1 meters long and 3.8 centimeters in diameter and is made up of the duodenum, the jejunum, and the ileum. It is where the process of digestion begins in full. The smaller products broken down by the stomach are received by the small intestine, where they are absorbed into the bloodstream through its lining by villi combined with bile (from the liver) and pancreatic juices.

Almost all food nutrients are absorbed in the small intestine. What passes into the large intestine is a mix of unabsorbed nutrients, water, fiber, and electrolytes. Most of the moisture from this process is removed as the mix passes through the large intestine, leaving solid waste products. Before excretion as feces, approximately 90 percent of the liquid that entered the large intestine has been reabsorbed. This reabsorption

Intestinal Disorders

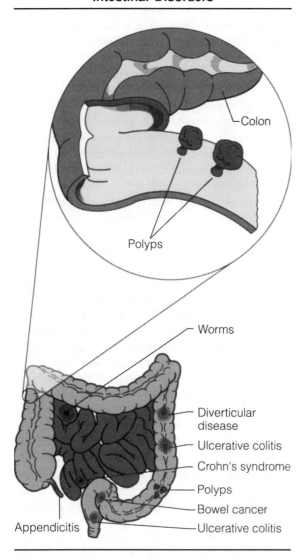

is necessary for health because it contains sodium and water.

The large intestine is approximately 1.5 meters long and connected to the small intestine at the ileocecal valve. Waste products from the digestive process pass through this valve into a large holding area of the large intestine called the cecum. The appendix is attached to this structure. The large intestine consists of the ascending colon (which begins on the right side of the abdomen and moves up toward the liver), the transverse colon (which crosses the abdomen), and the descending colon (which moves down the left side of the abdomen). The sigmoid colon is an S-shaped

structure which connects to the descending colon and joins the rectum, a tube 12 to 20 centimeters long that leads to the anus. Small microorganisms in the large intestine break down waste products not broken down by the stomach and small intestines, resulting in gas (also known as flatus).

COMPLICATIONS AND DISORDERS

Diseases and disorders of the intestinal tract constitute a major health problem affecting many individuals at one point or another in their lives. The common diseases and disorders that affect the intestinal tract are those of acute inflammatory disorders (appendicitis), diverticular disorders (diverticulosis and diverticulitis), chronic inflammatory bowel disease (Crohn's disease and ulcerative colitis), intestinal infections (intestinal parasites and bacterial infections with *Salmonella*, *Shigella dysenteriae*, and *Escherichia coli*), intestinal obstructions, cancers or tumors of the rectum and colon, and polyps.

The most common acute inflammatory disorder is appendicitis. Its symptoms usually affect individuals between the ages of ten and thirty and include abdominal pain and tenderness, nausea and vomiting, loss of appetite, rapid heart rate, fever, and an elevated white blood cell count. Normally, the appendix, whose function is not clearly understood, fills and empties with food as regularly as does the cecum, of which it is a part. It sometimes becomes inflamed because of either kinking or obstruction, producing pressure and initiating symptoms. The most common major complication associated with appendicitis is perforation, which causes severe pain and an elevation of temperature. In these cases, a physician must be notified immediately. Treatment consists of surgical removal of the appendix.

Diverticular disorders include diverticulosis and diverticulitis. Diverticulosis is the presence of diverticula without any inflammation or symptoms. Diverticulitis is the result of an inflammation or infection of the intestine produced when food or bacteria are retained in a diverticulum. Some signs of diverticulosis include cramplike pain in the left lower part of the abdomen, bowel irregularity, diarrhea, constipation, or thin stools. There may be some intermittent rectal bleeding with diverticulitis.

Inflammatory bowel disease (IBD) of unknown cause is most common in whites (usually female) between the ages of fifteen and thirty-five, occurring most frequently in the American Jewish population.

The two types of IBD are Crohn's disease, which is also known as regional enteritis, and ulcerative colitis. Both disorders are considered to be separate diseases with similar characteristics.

Crohn's disease may affect any part of the intestinal tract but often affects the small intestine. The inflammation usually involves the entire thickness of the intestinal wall. Treatment for Crohn's disease depends on the presence or absence of symptoms. If there are no symptoms, treatment is not necessary. If there is evidence of inflammation, however, anti-inflammatory medication may be prescribed. Vitamin and mineral replacement may be given because of the problems of absorption associated with this disease. Surgery may be required at some point in the disease process because of its associated complications, such as obstruction.

Ulcerative colitis is characterized by tiny ulcers and abscesses in the inner lining of the colon, where it is usually confined. There is a tendency for these ulcerations to bleed, causing bloody diarrhea. The chronic nature of inflammatory bowel disease may cause a stricture, which can result in an obstruction requiring surgical intervention. As with Crohn's disease, the treatment for ulcerative colitis depends on the type of symptoms and may consist of medication, nutrition, or surgery. Anti-inflammatory drugs are used for flare-ups of the disease. Liquid food supplements may be given to compensate for nutrients lost in diarrhea. Intravenous therapy may be prescribed if the colon is considered too diseased to tolerate food.

There are many types of infections that affect the intestinal tract. The most common bacterial infections are caused by microorganisms such as *Salmonella* and *Shigella*. *Salmonella* bacteria are commonly found in meats, fruits (through contaminated fertilizer), poultry, eggs, dairy products, and contaminated marijuana. Pet turtles are also a source of this bacteria. The source of infections for *Shigella* bacteria is feces from an infected person, with the route of transmission being oral-fecal—for example, changing the soiled diaper of an infant, or having a bowel movement, and then eating or preparing food without properly washing the hands.

Intestinal parasites may also cause infection. The most common of these parasites, *Giardia lamblia*, is present where water supplies are contaminated by raw sewage. The primary treatment for these conditions consists of replacement of lost fluids and essential electrolytes. Although not normally used because they

may interfere with the elimination of the causative agent, antidiarrheal medications may be prescribed.

Intestinal obstruction occurs when the normal flow of the intestine is partially or totally impeded because of an accumulation of contents, gas, or fluid. It may also be caused by the intestine's inability to propel contents along the intestinal tract in the process called peristalsis. Peristalsis may be obstructed by scars that bind together two normally separate anatomic surfaces (adhesions), hernias, or tumors. Another cause may be a paralytic ileus, a paralysis of the peristaltic movement of the intestinal tract caused by the effect of trauma or toxins on the nerve endings that regulate intestinal movement. Conservative treatment consists of decompression of the bowel using a nasogastric tube. Surgical treatment may be indicated if the bowel is completely obstructed.

While tumors of the small intestine are rare, tumors of the colon are common. Cancer of the colon and rectum is the second most common type of cancer in the United States (with lung cancer being the most common). The majority of intestinal tumors are benign (noncancerous) and discovered between the ages of forty and sixty. There are several types of benign tumors, which do not spread. They include lipomas, leiomyomas, angiomas, and adenomas. A small percentage of tumors of the small intestine is malignant (cancerous). The most common are adenocarcinomas, leiomyosarcomas, carcinoid tumors, and lymphomas. The symptoms of these tumors include weight loss, abdominal pain, nausea and vomiting, and bleeding. Treatment is dependent upon the stage and location of the tumor. Surgical removal of the tumor may be coupled with chemotherapy and/or radiation therapy.

Polyps are benign tumors of the large intestine and are common to individuals over the age of sixty. They arise from the lining of the colon and are usually found during tests to diagnose other conditions. Polyps include several different varieties, the most common of which is a hyperplastic polyp. Hyperplastic polyps are less than one-half of a centimeter in diameter and do not pose a health risk. Juvenile polyps can occur in childhood, and inflammatory polyps are believed to result from injury or inflammation, such as after an episode of ulcerative colitis. Neither of these conditions poses a health risk. There is a major category of polyps known as adenomas, however, which have the potential for malignancy. These types of polyps are generally removed to prevent the development of cancer.

Rectal cancer and colon cancer are two types of cancer common among both men and women. Factors that predispose an individual to these types of cancer include family history or a prior history of adenomatous colon polyps, colon cancer, or ulcerative colitis. The precise cause of these cancers is unknown, but diet is believed to play a significant role, specifically diets low in fiber and high in animal fat. One of the key symptoms of these conditions requiring immediate attention (especially for individuals over the age of forty) is rectal bleeding. Treatment consists of surgery to remove the affected part of the colon. The physician may prescribe additional treatment in the form of chemotherapy and/or radiation therapy.

PERSPECTIVE AND PROSPECTS

Problems associated with the intestinal tract are characterized by a variety of symptoms and treatments. These problems may be temporary in nature or may be manifestations of more serious underlying conditions interfering with the normal functions of absorption, fluid and electrolyte balance, and elimination. Symptoms are signs of malfunction and should not be ignored or go untreated.

Preventing problems associated with the intestinal tract may not always be possible because the causes of some intestinal diseases and disorders are unknown. Nevertheless, there has been substantial research related to intestinal diseases and disorders to support a strong correlation between nutrition and intestinal tract health. For example, there is evidence to support the relationship between the consumption of sugars, high amounts of animal protein and fat, and cholesterol and cancer-causing agents in the intestinal tract. Stress and its resulting influence on stomach acidity also contribute to intestinal ill health. Smoking and lack of regular exercise may also negatively influence normal peristalsis.

The prevention of these and other problems related to intestinal health are important not only to general health but also to work productivity. In the United States, for example, intestinal problems account for a large percentage of lost work time. Education about intestinal health and health issues beginning early in one's life will lower the incidence of some of the more common intestinal diseases and disorders.

—*John A. Bavaro, Ed.D., R.N.*

See also Abdomen; Abdominal disorders; Appendectomy; Appendicitis; Bacterial infections; Bypass surgery; Celiac sprue; Cholecystitis; Cirrhosis; Colic; Colitis; Colon and rectal polyp removal; Colon and rectal surgery; Colon cancer; Colon therapy; Colonoscopy; Constipation; Crohn's disease; Diarrhea and dysentery; Digestion; Diverticulitis and diverticulosis; Enemas; Enterocolitis; Fistula repair; Food poisoning; Gallbladder diseases; Gastroenterology; Gastroenterology, pediatric; Gastrointestinal disorders; Gastrointestinal system; Hemorrhoid banding and removal; Hemorrhoids; Hernia; Hernia repair; Hirschsprung's disease; Ileostomy and colostomy; Indigestion; Internal medicine; Intestines; Irritable bowel syndrome (IBS); Jaundice; Lactose intolerance; Liver cancer; Liver disorders; Malabsorption; Malnutrition; Nutrition; Obesity; Obstruction; Pancreatitis; Parasitic diseases; Peristalsis; Pinworm; Proctology; Renal failure; Roundworm; Soiling; Stomach, intestinal, and pancreatic cancers; Tapeworm; Tumor removal; Tumors; Worms.

FOR FURTHER INFORMATION:

Clayman, Charles B., ed. *The American Medical Association Encyclopedia of Medicine*. New York: Random House, 1994. Written in an encyclopedic format, this book is an authoritative guide to all aspects of medical and health topics. Contains many illustrations of various body systems and organs that are clearly presented and simple to understand.

Larson, David E., ed. *Mayo Clinic Family Health Book*. 2d ed. New York: William Morrow, 1996. This comprehensive medical guide was written for the general public by experts in the field of medicine. It can be used as an excellent basic source of authoritative health and medical information.

Mullen, Kathleen D., et al. *Connections for Health*. 3d ed. Madison, Wis.: Wm. C. Brown/Benchmark, 1993. A basic personal health textbook used in introductory college-level health courses. It is easily read and incorporates the concepts of wellness and disease prevention. Excellent references and recommended readings can be found at the end of each chapter.

Payne, Wayne A., and Dale B. Hahn. *Understanding Your Health*. 6th ed. St. Louis: Mosby Year Book, 2000. An introductory textbook that is easy to read. Focuses on overall health and disease prevention. Each chapter offers a list of references and recommended readings related specifically to its content.

Tapley, Donald F., et al., eds. *The Columbia University College of Physicians and Surgeons Complete Home Medical Guide*. Rev. 3d ed. New York: Crown,

1995. An outstanding reference guide organized by each organ system and its function. Written in easily understandable terms and avoids the use of medical jargon. Part 3 provides in-depth information on how the body works and includes a full-color atlas showing major organ systems.

INTESTINES
ANATOMY

ANATOMY OR SYSTEM INVOLVED: Abdomen, anus, gastrointestinal system

SPECIALTIES AND RELATED FIELDS: Gastroenterology, internal medicine

DEFINITION: The portion of the gastrointestinal tract from the lower end of the stomach to the anus, which consists of the small intestine and the colon (large intestine).

KEY TERMS:

amylase: the enzyme responsible for breaking down carbohydrates in the small intestine; amylase enters the intestinal tract from the salivary glands and the pancreas

colon: the large intestine, divided from the small intestine by the cecum (a controlled passageway) and ending at the sigmoid, which leads food waste into the rectum

fiber: food material derived from plant substances that retain the full structure of their cell walls despite the chemical effects of the digestive process

lipases: enzymes secreted by the pancreas into the small intestine; these serve to break down fatty materials (triglycerides) in the first intestinal stage of digestion

peristalsis: the muscular contraction in the walls of the intestines that propels food material forward through the bowels

STRUCTURE AND FUNCTIONS

After the initial process of digestion takes place in the stomach, food passes into the intestines, where the chemical action of several gastric juices separates out the nutritive content of fats, carbohydrates, and proteins. This nutritive material is then absorbed into the bloodstream through the walls of the intestines, while waste material is collected for excretion.

In adult humans, the small intestine and large intestine together represent a total length of nearly 9 meters (30 feet). Both small and large intestines are hoselike muscular organs; the former is much longer, but substantially narrower, than the latter. The two in-

testines are joined at the cecum, which is located in the right-lower abdominal cavity. The appendix, which is sometimes called a "blind pouch" because it is unessential to the main processes performed in the gastrointestinal tract, projects from the cecum.

The physical disposition and function of the large intestine, or colon, are distinct from those of the small intestine. As the large intestinal tube leaves the cecum, it assumes a specific shape, following horizontal and vertical lines within the abdominal cavity. This is not the case with the small intestine, whose extensive length (some 7 meters, or 23 feet) takes an intertwined "nesting" shape in the limited abdominal space available. By contrast, the colon, which is about 1.5 meters (5 feet) in length, has three easily identifiable sections: the ascending colon on the right side of the abdominal cavity, the transverse colon, and the descending colon on the left side of the abdomen. A final leftward bend in the colon at the sigmoid provides for its attachment to the rectum.

The two parts of the intestines carry out distinct functions in the overall digestive process. As food material passes from the lower end, or pylorus, of the stomach, only a part of the digestive process has occurred. Once partially digested food enters the small intestine, it is propelled through the intestine by means of a process of muscular contraction in the intestinal wall, which is called peristalsis.

As the food moves forward, different substances, some secreted from the lining of the intestine itself, and others—principally, bile and pancreatic fluid, which enter the upper intestine (duodenum) from the liver and pancreas—contribute to a further breaking down of food material.

Very small projections called villi are found along the interior surface of the small intestine. The villi absorb those portions of the food material that have been altered by the digestive process. From the villi, nutritive material is passed into the blood and lymphatic system for distribution to cells throughout the body. This process continues in the middle and end portions (jejunum and ileum, respectively) of the small intestine until, passing through the cecum, the remaining residue enters the large intestine.

The mixture of material contained in the large intestine, or colon, consists of indigestible food, bacteria, and substantial amounts of water. Most of the water is absorbed into the body through the walls of the colon, while the remaining waste material, or feces, is excreted through the rectum.

In order to understand how food materials are actually absorbed by the villi inside the small intestine and passed into the bloodstream, one must consider several chemical processes, according to the nature of the material in question.

For example, the triglyceride components of fat, chains of fatty acids attached to glycerol, are chemical compounds that do not dissolve in water (a major part of the main bloodstream). The pancreatic enzymes called lipases split the triglycerides into separate units of fatty acid. Once separated, these fatty acids become coated with bile salts secreted by the liver, a process that allows them to pass into the mucous cells lining the intestine. As this passage occurs, the coated fatty acids (micelles) resume their chainlike form as triglycerides. At this point, however, the triglycerides have assumed an altered chemical state. In this altered form, fats can be absorbed into the blood and carried throughout the body to be used as body "fuel" or, if unused, stored in fatty tissues.

Carbohydrates must be broken down into simple sugars (glucose, galactose, and fructose) before they can be absorbed by the cell linings of the small intestine. This process occurs when the more complex carbohydrates (both starches and sugars) are split by the chemical effects of the enzyme amylase, which enters the small intestine from the salivary glands and the pancreas.

Finally, proteins, which contain the amino acids so essential for the process of tissue formation in the body, must be split in several stages, the first of which occurs in the stomach itself. Here, proteins are partially broken down by the action of the gastric juices, mainly pepsin. Once protein material passes into the upper part of the small intestine, or duodenum, the process is accelerated by the influence of two main pancreatic enzymes: trypsin and chymotrypsin. These secretions cause the proteins to release amino acids in three forms: simple, dual, or triplicate bodies. It is not until these three forms are actually inside the cell walls of the small intestine that other enzymes split the dual and triplicate amino acids into their simplest single form, which can be absorbed into the veins that carry nourishment to the various organs of the body.

In the overall chemical process leading to the absorption of various body nutrients by the small and large intestines, there is a certain "absorptive specialization" in different zones of the gastrointestinal tract. Iron and calcium, for example, are absorbed in the duodenum, while proteins, fats, sugars, and all vitamins except vitamin B_{12} are absorbed in the jejunum. Finally, in the ileum, salt, vitamin B_{12}, and bile salts are processed.

DISORDERS AND DISEASES

Doctors have always known that the digestive processes of the intestines can be affected in either positive or negative ways by the nature of the food that is consumed. In the simplest terms, negative reactions are manifested by the obvious effects of indigestion and diarrhea. The control of such symptoms of improper or incomplete digestion may appear to the layperson to be a simple matter of using "over-the-counter" tablets such as laxatives or "antigas" pills. Treatment of the symptoms of indigestion, however, may provide only a superficial solution to a problem that is much more serious.

An area of important medical concern that goes beyond the general discomfort caused by imbalanced digestive functioning of the intestines involves peptic ulcers. A peptic ulcer is an open sore on the mucous membrane lining the gastrointestinal tract. The general label "peptic ulcer" was applied to this condition since the discovery, in the mid-1830's, of pepsin, the first clearly identified enzyme known to contribute to the chemical breakdown of ingested foods. Although later stages of research into the digestive process yielded much more extensive knowledge of the component elements of gastric juices, the specific name has remained attached to the general phenomenon of intestinal ulceration. The term "gastric ulcer" refers specifically to ulceration in the stomach lining.

Generally speaking, peptic ulcers occur when there is an imbalance between the task of digestion to be accomplished by the intestines and the amounts and levels of concentration of the gastric juices secreted into the gastrointestinal tract. When the amounts or concentrated strengths of gastric juices in the intestines exceed the level required for digestion (or flow into the intestine when no food has been ingested), these agents actually begin to digest the membranes of the intestine itself.

Various forms of treatment for intestinal ulcers have been developed, including both therapeutic drugs that have the capacity to counteract the corrosive effects of excessive gastric juices and, in the preventive vein, diets that contain natural combatants against intestinal disorders, especially high-fiber, unprocessed, or lightly processed foods.

In recent years, research into the causes of ulcers has extended into the field of gastrointestinal hormonal secretions originating not in the pancreas itself but in the intestine or stomach. These secretions reach the pancreas later through the bloodstream and stimulate its production of digestive juices. Such secretive processes may, if they fail to communicate properly balanced "codes" concerning the task of digestion that needs to take place in the intestines, cause an excessive supply (in volume or strength) of gastric juices, which can cause ulcerations to develop.

The most serious pathological condition that can affect the intestines is cancer of the colon. Thought to develop from a degenerative process originating in benign polyps (stem-based tumors that may develop in areas of the organism lined with mucous membrane, such as the nose, colon, and, in females, the uterus), cancer of the colon has registered a survival rate that is statistically higher than those of cancers in other vital organs of the abdominal cavity (the liver and stomach, in particular). This is partly because—if the cancer is discovered in time—substantial areas of the colon that have been attacked by cancer can be removed surgically without endangering the continued essential functioning of the intestines.

Almost all questions relating to the pathology of the intestinal tract are somehow connected with the type of food that is eaten. Thus, medical science has turned increasingly to publicizing preventive dietary practices that can have a bearing on all functions of the intestines, from the simplest level of discomfort to the most serious level of chronic diseases.

As stated above, a relatively recent and valuable contribution to the knowledge of natural ways to aid in the absorptive work of both the small intestine and the colon—and to reduce the dangers of ulceration and/or intestinal cancer—involves the role of the fiber content of foods. Fiber is generally described as consisting of polysaccharides and lignin, two plant substances that, more than any other nutritive material, retain their natural forms as plant cell walls and are not broken down by human digestive enzymes. The plant food that is richest in these materials is wheat bran, which contains about 40 percent fiber. As fiber-rich foodstuffs such as bran pass through the gastrointestinal tract, the fiber material they contain is subject to fermentation by anaerobic bacteria in the colon. Two chemical results of this complex process seem to be the removal of deoxycholic acid from the

bile and the reduction of the cholesterol saturation level of the bile. Both effects are deemed beneficial, since the reduction of deoxycholic acid and cholesterol in intestinal bile tends, at the very least, to reduce the likelihood of developing gallstones. Fiber-rich diets in combination with the reduction of excess weight became standard symbols of preventive health care by the 1990's.

By the mid-twentieth century, typical personal diets in the Western world contained commercially refined foodstuffs that were rich in sugars and syrups, which are mainly fiber depleted. In addition to the specific disease-related factors mentioned above, medical cience has noted that high consumption of fiber-depleted foods results in higher levels of energy intake (absorption of Calories) during the digestive process that occurs in the intestines. In simple terms, when Calorie intake exceeds the level required by the normally exercised body, the result is weight gain that may continue to the point of obesity.

PERSPECTIVE AND PROSPECTS

Medical science began to become aware of the various digestive functions of hormonal secretions only in the first decades of the twentieth century. Although the early nineteenth century American army surgeon William Beaumont was the first doctor to discover the presence of gastric juices in the intestines, his analysis of digestive fluids remained quite elementary. Beaumont could easily identify hydrochloric acid in stomach secretions. He also took samples of bile from the intestinal tract and performed laboratory experiments that proved the role of bile in breaking down fatty materials. What remained unsolved were the identity and origins of other components of gastric juice and an explanation for their controlled secretion from surrounding organs in the abdominal cavity into the intestines. Beaumont's view that mental concentration (including "negative mental concentration," or anxiety) induced the flow of gastric juices proved eventually to be only partially correct.

It was only in 1902 that the British doctors Ernest Henry Starling and Sir William Maddock Bayliss were able to show that, in addition to nerve "signals," certain chemical factors induced the flow of gastric juices, specifically from the pancreas into the intestinal tract. These doctors found that, in fact, the small intestine released into the bloodstream a "chemical transmitter" that, as it circulated to the other vital organs, stimulated the production and flow of the pancreatic juices necessary for digestion. They called this "chemical transmitter" secretin. To this initial agent would be added a whole category of secretions that are called "hormones," a term taken from the Greek word for "urging on."

A discovery was made in 1928 that helped to clarify the complex relationship of hormones, gastric juice secretion, and the carrying out of the digestive process by the small and large intestines. This was the discovery of pancreozymin, the second main "chemical transmitter" affecting the pancreas, by the American researcher Andrew Ivy. Pancreozymin was found to cause the release by the pancreas of an enzyme-rich fluid made up of three agents: trypsin, lipase, and amylase. Each agent proved to be an activator in the process of breaking down different nutrients (protein, fats, and carbohydrates, respectively).

Although the intestines are the ultimate destination of and seat of activity for the pancreatic juices released by command of this hormone (as well as of the last major digestion-linked hormone, gastrin, which was discovered in 1955), secretin alone has its origin in the intestines themselves. Both pancreozymin and gastrin are secreted from the stomach.

In time, researchers found that most gastrointestinal hormones are secreted by specialized cells that line the interior of the stomach. Such cells react at various levels according to the composition of the food that has been ingested, sending chemical signals, via the hormones they secrete, that determine the relative amounts and strengths of the several gastric juices that enter the intestines from the pancreas. A similar question of varied amounts and strengths of gastric juices was linked to the so-called vagus nerve function, which also activates pancreatic flow to the intestinal tract.

The functional relationship between these two activator agents—the one nervous and the other chemical—has become one of the primary interests of researchers who deal with the most common ailment attacking the intestinal organs: peptic ulceration.

—*Byron D. Cannon, Ph.D.*

See also Abdomen; Abdominal disorders; Bypass surgery; Colitis; Colon and rectal surgery; Colonoscopy; Digestion; Endoscopy; Enemas; Gastroenterology; Gastroenterology, pediatric; Gastrointestinal disorders; Gastrointestinal system; Hemorrhoids; Hernia; Internal medicine; Intestinal disorders; Laparoscopy; Malnutrition; Nutrition; Obstruction; Peristalsis; Proctology.

FOR FURTHER INFORMATION:
Janowitz, Henry D. *Good Food for Bad Stomachs.* New York: Oxford University Press, 1997. A popular work on indigestion and diseases of the gastrointestinal system that suggests diet therapy. Includes an index.

_____. *Indigestion: Living Better with Upper Intestinal Problems from Heartburn to Ulcers and Gallstones.* New York: Oxford University Press, 1994. An extension of the combination of scientific and "commonsense" approach of *Your Gut Feelings* (see next listing) to several other areas and organs involved in the process of digestion.

_____. *Your Gut Feelings: A Complete Guide to Living Better with Intestinal Problems.* Rev. ed. New York: Oxford University Press, 1994. This book uses scientific precision to develop a semi-popular approach to the most common health problems associated with the gastrointestinal tract. Such problems are either externally simple ones (stomach gas, diarrhea, and so forth) or more complex questions of the effects of aging and chronic conditions (such as peptic ulcers and cancer of the colon).

Wolfe, M. Michael, and Sidney Cohen. *Therapy of Digestive Disorders: A Companion to Sleisenger and Fordtran's Gastrointestinal and Liver Disease.* Philadelphia: W. B. Saunders, 2000. This resource is divided into sections that discuss such topics as esophageal, gastroduodenal, pancreaticobiliary, hepatic, intestinal, and miscellaneous disorders.

INTOXICATION
DISEASE/DISORDER
ANATOMY OR SYSTEM AFFECTED: All
SPECIALTIES AND RELATED FIELDS: Emergency medicine, psychiatry, toxicology
DEFINITION: Intoxication is the general term for poisoning of the body by toxins, such as drugs, including alcohol. It commonly refers to alcohol intoxication, or drunkenness. Of the amount of alcohol ingested, 95 percent will be absorbed directly into the wall of the stomach or small intestine and pass quickly into the bloodstream. If too much alcohol is consumed in a short period of time, the extreme slowdown of breathing and circulation can cause death; however, vomiting or coma generally precedes such an event. Intoxication decreases motor ability, reaction time, depth perception, and night vision; causes poor judgment; impairs sexual function; and may result in mood swings. If a comatose

state is not reached, the intoxication will eventually resolve itself; no other method, such as coffee or cold showers, can counteract the effects of alcohol.

—Jason Georges and Tracy Irons-Georges
See also Addiction; Alcoholism; Club drugs; Coma; Poisoning; Toxicology.

FOR FURTHER INFORMATION:

Julien, Robert M. *A Primer of Drug Action*. 9th ed. New York: W. H. Freeman, 2000.

Miller, William R., and Nick Heather, eds. *Treating Addictive Behaviors: Processes of Change*. 2d ed. New York: Plenum Press, 1998.

Schlaadt, Richard G., and Peter T. Shannon. *Drugs of Choice: Current Perspectives on Drug Use*. 2d ed. Englewood Cliffs, N.J.: Prentice Hall, 1986.

Weil, Andrew, and Winifred Rosen. *From Chocolate to Morphine: Everything You Need to Know About Mind-Altering Drugs*. Rev. ed. Boston: Houghton Mifflin, 1998.

INVASIVE TESTS

PROCEDURES

ANATOMY OR SYSTEM AFFECTED: All

SPECIALTIES AND RELATED FIELDS: All

DEFINITION: Tests that require the passage of an instrument through the body's protective barriers.

INDICATIONS AND PROCEDURES

Skin, sphincters, and gag and cough reflex systems are some of the defenses that can be penetrated to gather important diagnostic information. Invasive tests provide medical insights that are unattainable by noninvasive or laboratory tests. Invasive tests are typically performed last in a diagnostic protocol, however, because penetration of the body defenses is not without risk. An anesthetic agent is commonly used to minimize any discomfort or pain that may arise during the tests. Although invasive, these tests often circumvent the trauma of exploratory surgery.

In general, invasive tests may be classified as those that allow the physician to obtain samples of fluid, tissue, or tumors directly from their site of origin (through aspiration, lumbar puncture, and biopsy) or those that allow direct viewing of specific areas of the body through endoscopy. Some test procedures allow both direct viewing and sample collection; bronchoscopy is one such example.

One of the more familiar aspiration tests is amniocentesis. Amniocentesis involves removing 20 to 30 milliliters of fluid from the amniotic sac for analysis. This test is used in prenatal care at weeks fifteen to eighteen in order to assess the genetic makeup of the fetus or to detect developmental abnormalities.

Fluid from effusions can also be aspirated for analysis. Effusions are collections of an abnormally large quantity of fluid within a serous or synovial cavity. While a small amount of fluid is normal in these cavities, a large amount indicates a pathology that should be identified and treated. Once an effusion is tapped, the fluid is grossly examined for color and for clarity or turbidity. Microscopic investigations of the fluids are performed to assess the types of cells present (such as immune cells or malignant cells) and to identify microorganisms that may be present. Paracentesis is the removal of fluid from effusions within the abdominal, or peritoneal, cavity. If the effusion in this region is large, it is called ascites. Removal of fluid from the lung cavity, called thoracentesis, requires penetration of the chest wall between the ribs (intercostal spaces). Common causes of effusions include infections, congestive heart failure, kidney disease, and malignancy.

Synovial fluid is most commonly aspirated from the knee, but other joints can be investigated in this manner. Red blood cells, inflammatory cells, or crystals may be identified by microscopic evaluation of the aspirated fluid. Osteoarthritis, rheumatoid arthritis, and gout are some diseases that can be diagnosed through synovial fluid aspiration.

Cerebrospinal fluid (CSF) is housed within the bony cranium and spinal column. Fluid from this space is collected by lumbar puncture (spinal tap) and is drawn when a viral, bacterial, or fungal meningitis is suspected. Lumbar puncture may also be performed when a tumor or leukemia of the central nervous system is suspected, or to determine whether a subarachnoid hemorrhage is present.

Fine needle aspiration (FNA) is a specific kind of percutaneous (through-the-skin) needle biopsy. FNA can be used to collect a sample of cells from any palpable mass. By directly inserting a needle into the mass and then washing, or flushing, the region, some cells can be eroded from the tissue surface. These cells are set adrift in the fluid, which is sucked back into the flushing syringe. Microscopic evaluation of the cells can then be performed. Breast, neck, abdominal, and lymph nodes are some of the places where FNA is utilized.

Alternative biopsy techniques include gently scraping off a small surface, as in the Papanicolaou (Pap) smear of the cervix, or removing a deeper tissue sample, as in the punch biopsy of the cervix. Biopsy can sometimes require small surgical incisions to reach a certain organ, such as muscle, skin, breast, bone, or renal (kidney) biopsy.

Tissue biopsies may be taken directly from an organ without surgical incisions; one way to do this is with endoscopy. Typically, endoscopes are flexible probing instruments fitted with fiber-optic viewing devices. Often, a tool attachment allows the use of tiny cutting and sampling devices. Small pieces of tissue can be removed from some otherwise inaccessible areas of the body. Different kinds of endoscopes are used to accommodate the unique structural features of body regions, such as the bronchi, stomach, or colon. Sterile techniques are implemented in all cases.

Bronchoscopy is utilized in diagnosing pulmonary infections and lung cancers or in locating and removing foreign objects found in the airways. Esophagealgastroscopy is used to determine the source of upper gastrointestinal problems such as gastric or peptic ulcers, esophageal varices, esophageal reflux, or malignancy. Colonoscopy is similarly used to evaluate the origins of lower gastrointestinal problems. Colon polyps can be identified, and the mucosal lining of the colon can be evaluated for ulcerative colitis, diverticula, or adenocarcinomas.

Finally, arteriography (including angiography) and cardiac catheterization are important and frequently used invasive tests. These tests are used to evaluate the cardiovascular system. Angiography combines radiographic techniques with the injection of dyes into arteries. This combination allows the physician to determine whether an artery is blocked (occluded). Angiography is particularly useful in patients who have heart conditions, such as angina, and can be used to evaluate renal (kidney) arteries, aortic dissection, or cerebral aneurysms. The result of arteriography is a critical component in determining whether surgery or drug intervention is best for a given patient.

As a diagnostic tool, cardiac catheterization provides insight into the health of a heart. Pictures of the heart can be taken as the catheter is advanced into the right and then the left sides of the heart. A dye is injected into the heart so that the flow can be traced as the heart pumps. The heart chambers, valves, and blood vessels can be evaluated. Additionally, pressures within the heart chambers can be recorded.

USES AND COMPLICATIONS

The greatest health risk with any invasive test is infection. For this reason, sterile methods are used to keep infections and mortality caused by infections to a minimum. With proper care, the risks of invasive testing are surpassed by the benefits of the early and proper diagnosis that such tests provide.

—*Mary C. Fields, M.D.*

See also Amniocentesis; Angiography; Arthroscopy; Biopsy; Blood testing; Breast biopsy; Catheterization; Chorionic villus sampling; Colonoscopy; Cystoscopy; Endometrial biopsy; Endoscopy; Laparoscopy; Magnetic resonance imaging (MRI); Positron emission tomography (PET) scanning; Radiopharmaceuticals.

FOR FURTHER INFORMATION:

Cavanaugh, Bonita Morrow. *Nurse's Manual of Laboratory and Diagnostic Tests*. 2d ed. Philadelphia: F. A. Davis, 1995. Provides information on hundreds of laboratory and diagnostic tests, with each test presented in two distinct, cross-referenced sections: "Background Information" sections provide a complete description of each test and its purposes; "Clinical Application Data" sections focus on the information nurses most commonly need while caring for clients.

Dublin, Arthur B., ed. *Outpatient Invasive Radiologic Procedures: Diagnostic and Therapeutic*. Philadelphia: W. B. Saunders, 1989. Discusses such topics as radiography, radiotherapy, and diagnostic imaging. Also covers interventional radiography. Includes bibliographical references and an index.

Ravin, Carl E., ed. *Imaging and Invasive Radiology in the Intensive Care Unit*. New York: Churchill Livingstone, 1993. Discusses such topics as critical care medicine, diagnostic imaging, and interventional radiology. Includes bibliographical references and an index.

Zaret, Barry L., ed. *Yale University School of Medicine Patient's Guide to Medical Tests: Detailed Descriptions of the Most Common Diagnostic Procedures*. Boston: Houghton Mifflin, 1998. Written and edited by Yale University School of Medicine faculty, this resource provides detailed information on types of diagnostic tests, how doctors use them, and what patients can do for themselves.

IPF. *See* INTERSTITIAL PULMONARY FIBROSIS (IPF).

Irritable bowel syndrome (IBS)
Disease/disorder

Also known as: Colitis, spastic colon

Anatomy or system affected: Abdomen, intestines, gastrointestinal system, anus, nervous system

Specialties and related fields: Alternative medicine, gastroenterology, nutrition

Definition: A common intestinal disorder characterized by abdominal pain and cramps, altered bowel habits, bloating, and nausea.

Key terms:

biofeedback: the technique of making unconscious or involuntary bodily processes perceptible to the senses in order to manipulate them by conscious mental control

Crohn's disease: a disease characterized by inflammation of the intestines, whose early symptoms may resemble those of irritable bowel syndrome

defecation: passage of feces through the anus

endoscopy: the use of a small-diameter, flexible tube of optical fibers with an external light source to examine visually the interior of the body

feces: undigested food and other waste that is eliminated through the anus

gastroenterology: diagnosis and treatment of diseases and disorders of the digestive tract

lactose: a sugar found in milk and milk products; some people cannot digest lactose, causing lactose intolerance, which can produce symptoms that resemble those of irritable bowel syndrome

peristalsis: a series of muscular contractions that move food through the intestines during the process of digestion

ulcerative colitis: an inflammatory disease that causes ulcers in the large intestine

Causes and Symptoms

Although the causes of irritable bowel syndrome (IBS) are not understood, it is believed to result from changes in activity of the major part of the large intestine, or colon. Following food digestion by the stomach and the small intestine, the undigested material is pushed toward the rectum by peristalsis. When peristalsis becomes disrupted by IBS, the flow becomes too slow, causing constipation, or too fast, causing diarrhea.

Some foods and drinks appear more likely to trigger IBS attacks by disrupting peristalsis. Fatty foods, fried foods, milk products, chocolate, drinks with caffeine, and alcohol can exacerbate the symptoms of IBS, as well as some fruits or vegetables, such as cabbage, broccoli, cauliflower, asparagus, or brussels sprouts. In some cases, however, no specific foods cause specific symptoms, as any food intake seems to worsen symptoms. Often, IBS-aggravating foods vary from person to person.

The nervous system's links between the brain and the intestines suggest that stress may be culprit in IBS. Many IBS sufferers report symptoms following a meal when they experience stress. Female reproductive hormones are thought to trigger IBS attacks, because IBS is sometimes accentuated during menstruation.

IBS is more commonly seen in women than in men, with up to 20 percent of the American population affected. Although it can occur at any time, it generally appears in teens and twenties, and is frequently found in members of the same family.

Although symptoms vary in intensity, they do not grow steadily worse over time. Abdominal pain is always present, or discomfort associated with constipation, diarrhea, or alternating constipation with diarrhea. Other symptoms include bloating, passage of mucus, nausea, gas, an increased urge to defecate, and a feeling of incomplete rectal evacuation.

Diagnosis of IBS is an involved process that is accomplished through a standard evaluation called the Rome criteria. Symptoms present for three months of the year are considered, along with the results of physical examination, laboratory tests, stool sample, and endoscopy—all of which rule out serious diseases such as colon cancer.

Treatment and Therapy

Generally, a low-fat, high-fiber diet lessens symptoms, although the tolerance of fiber as well as of all foods varies from person to person. Dietary changes vary according to the severity of the patient's symptoms. In mild cases of IBS, known aggravating foods should be identified and avoided. Symptoms may be eased by eating smaller meals or eating smaller portions. Since no diet has been found that controls all symptoms, a diary of symptoms and food intake is valuable in determining which foods are offensive. Constipation and diarrhea can be alleviated by taking one tablespoon of Metamucil or Fiberall daily. Establishment of fixed times for meals and bathroom visits help regulate bowel habits.

For more severe symptoms, dietary changes should be supplemented with antispasmodic drugs for abdominal pain. Psychological counseling, behavioral

In the News: The Debate over a New IBS Drug

In February, 2000, following a seven-month "fast track" review process, the FDA approved a new type of medication to treat irritable bowel syndrome (IBS). Alosetron hydrochloride, sold by GlaxoWellcome under the brand name Lotronex, was designed for women with diarrhea-predominant IBS and associated abdominal pain and discomfort. It was the first medication shown in well-controlled, large clinical trials to address multiple symptoms of this disease. Lotronex was reported to be generally well tolerated, the most common side effect being constipation.

Although many patients taking the drug experienced substantial or complete relief of their IBS symptoms, others suffered severe side effects. Out of about 450,000 prescriptions, 70 cases were reported of intestinal damage from ischemic colitis or of severely obstructed or ruptured bowels, a complication of severe constipation. Some patients required hospitalization or surgical intervention, and a few died. GlaxoWellcome suggested label modifications, restricted distribution, ongoing patient education, new clinical and epidemiological research, and review by an independent board. The FDA found these proposals inadequate; in November, 2000, GlaxoWellcome withdrew Lotronex from the market.

Controversy surrounding the drug continued. Some criticized the speed of the FDA's initial approval process or claimed improprieties by the manufacturer. A group of patients who had been helped by Lotronex, however, lobbied the FDA for access to the medication under stricter guidelines.

—*Tracy Irons-Georges*

therapy, including hypnosis and biofeedback, and relaxation techniques are recommended to reduce anxiety and encourage learning to cope with the pain of IBS. Severe pain from IBS can be blocked with antidepressants. Moderate exercise has also been shown to be beneficial.

In addition to dietary changes prescribed by doctors, alternative practitioners advise herbal remedies such as ginger and peppermint oil or the antispasmodic ingredients in chamomile, valerian, or rosemary. Aromatherapy, hydrotherapy, acupuncture, chiropractic, and osteopathy may also be useful.

PERSPECTIVE AND PROSPECTS

IBS was once believed to be a psychological disorder, but more contemporary researchers believe it is a physical disorder that has specific characteristics and causes real pain. Although there is no cure for IBS, it is not a life-threatening condition. It has not been shown to cause intestinal bleeding or inflammation, as in Crohn's disease, ulcerative colitis, or cancer. Long-term management, though frustrating, involves commitment to therapy for six months or more to find the best combinations of medicine, diet, counseling, and support for control of IBS symptoms. Recent research has discovered a genetic link to panic and anxiety that may be a link to IBS. Other studies stress a mind-body connection to assist in minimizing the symptoms of IBS.

—*Mary Hurd*

See also Abdominal disorders; Colitis; Constipation; Crohn's disease; Diarrhea and dysentery; Gastroenterology; Gastrointestinal disorders; Gastrointestinal system; Intestinal disorders; Intestines; Lactose intolerance; Peristalsis.

FOR FURTHER INFORMATION:

Clayman, Charles B., ed. *American Medical Association Family Medical Guide.* 3d rev. ed. New York: Random House, 1994.

"Irritable Bowel Syndrome." In *Gale Encyclopedia of Medicine.* Detroit: Gale Research, 1999.

Salt, William B., II. *Irritable Bowel Syndrome and the Mind-Body/Brain-Gut Connection: Eight Steps for Living a Healthy Life with a Functional Bowel Disorder or Colitis.* Columbus, Ohio: Parkview, 1999.

ISCHEMIA

DISEASE/DISORDER

ANATOMY OR SYSTEM AFFECTED: Blood, blood vessels, circulatory system, all other systems

SPECIALTIES AND RELATED FIELDS: Cardiology, hematology, internal medicine, vascular medicine

DEFINITION: Ischemia occurs when the blood supply to an organ or tissue is interrupted, usually by a narrowing of the arteries from deposits of plaque. Other causes may include blood vessel injury, an inefficient heartbeat, and spasms in the vessel wall that result in constriction. The major sites of ischemia are the eyes, kidneys, heart, brain, and legs. Insufficient blood supply to the legs or heart causes pain; ischemia in the kidneys, eyes, and brain can result in renal failure, blindness, and stroke, respectively. The circulation can be restored with vasodilator drugs or surgery, such as angioplasty or a bypass. The temporary induction of ischemia in the legs can be used to reduce bleeding in operations on the extremities.

—*Jason Georges and Tracy Irons-Georges*

See also Angioplasty; Arteriosclerosis; Bypass surgery; Cardiology; Claudication; Heart; Heart attack; Heart disease; Heart failure; Hyperlipidemia; Hypertension; Renal failure; Strokes; Thrombosis and thrombus; Vascular medicine; Vascular system.

FOR FURTHER INFORMATION:

Ernst, Calvin B., and James C. Stanley, eds. *Current Therapy in Vascular Surgery.* 4th ed. St. Louis: Mosby, 2000.

Hershey, Falls B., Robert W. Barnes, and David S. Sumner, eds. *Noninvasive Diagnosis of Vascular Disease.* Pasadena, Calif.: Appleton Davies, 1984.

Rutherford, Robert B., ed. *Vascular Surgery.* 5th ed. Philadelphia: W. B. Saunders, 2000.

ITCHING

DISEASE/DISORDER

ALSO KNOWN AS: Pruritus

ANATOMY OR SYSTEM AFFECTED: Skin

SPECIALTIES AND RELATED FIELDS: Dermatology, otorhinolaryngology, pharmacology, psychiatry

DEFINITION: An unpleasant sensation on or in the skin that causes a desire to scratch or rub the affected area.

CAUSES AND SYMPTOMS

Itching is elicited by the physical or chemical stimulation of nerve receptors in the skin. It can be caused by a wide variety of problems in a variety of different organ systems.

Nearly any skin lesion may itch; skin-related causes include such varied problems as eczema, psoriasis, contact dermatitis, insect bites, bacterial infections, fungal infections, sunburn, and exposure to wool. Viral infections such as chickenpox can cause intense itching. Itching of the eyes and nose are commonly associated with allergies. Itching with4out a skin rash may be caused by a number of internal problems. Various endocrine problems in children associated

with itching include liver disease, kidney failure, thyroid disease, and diabetes. Some malignancies, particularly lymphomas, may cause itching. Hookworms and pinworms are both internal causes of itching, as are certain drugs. Finally, some women experience generalized itching during pregnancy.

Certain psychiatric problems are associated with itching. Patients may scratch hard enough to create deep ulcers. The intensity of the itching seems to be related to the degree of nervous tension. In addition, patients who suffer from certain psychotic states or those who abuse drugs such as cocaine may experience a deep itching sensation that they describe as bugs crawling beneath the skin.

Itching may rarely be associated with neurologic disease in which changes in sensation are interpreted by the patient as itching. Occasionally, circulatory problems will cause itching, primarily on the legs. Both of these conditions are more common in the older adults than in children or young adults.

TREATMENT AND THERAPY

Treatment should be directed toward the cause of the itching. Hydration (bathing followed by moisturizing lotion) may be helpful in providing relief. When itching is the result of an allergen such as poison ivy, however, a drying agent should be used. Various medications (primarily antihistamines) may relieve itching, but most also cause significant sleepiness.

—*Rebecca Lovell Scott, Ph.D.*

See also Allergies; Athlete's foot; Bacterial infections; Bites and stings; Candidiasis; Chickenpox; Dermatitis; Dermatology; Dermatology, pediatric; Diabetes mellitus; Eczema; Endocrine system; Endocrinology; Endocrinology, pediatric; Fungal infections; Hemorrhoids; Hepatitis; Hives; Impetigo; Lice, mites, and ticks; Liver; Liver disorders; Parasitic diseases; Pinworm; Pityriasis rosea; Poisonous plants; Psoriasis; Rashes; Renal failure; Ringworm; Scabies; Sexually transmitted diseases; Skin; Skin disorders; Sunburn; Thyroid disorders; Viral infections; Worms.

FOR FURTHER INFORMATION:

Bernhard, Jeffrey D., ed. *Itch: Mechanisms and Management of Pruritus.* New York: McGraw-Hill, 1994.

Fleischer, Alan B., Jr. *The Clinical Management of Itching.* New York: Parthenon, 2000.

Rodale, J. I. *The Itch and What to Do Besides Scratching.* Emmaus, Pa.: Rodale Books, 1971.

JAUNDICE

DISEASE/DISORDER

ANATOMY OR SYSTEM AFFECTED: Blood, eyes, liver, skin

SPECIALTIES AND RELATED FIELDS: Hematology, internal medicine, neonatology

DEFINITION: Jaundice is a liver disorder characterized by a yellowish discoloration of the skin, the whites of the eyes, and other tissues; the urine may also darken in hue. The condition is caused by excessive amounts of bile pigments, called bilirubin, in the bloodstream. The liver excretes bilirubin in the process of breaking down red blood cells. Excess bile pigments are produced if too many red blood cells are destroyed (hemolytic jaundice), the bile ducts are blocked by a tumor or gallstones (obstructive jaundice), or the liver becomes inflamed in the condition known as hepatitis (hepatocellular jaundice). Treatment is for the underlying cause.

—Jason Georges and Tracy Irons-Georges
See also Cirrhosis; Hepatitis; Jaundice, neonatal; Liver; Liver disorders.

FOR FURTHER INFORMATION:

Avery, Gordon B., Mary A. Fletcher, and Mhairi G. MacDonald. *Neonatology: Pathophysiology and Management of the Newborn.* 5th ed. Philadelphia: J. B. Lippincott, 1999.

Fanaroff, Avroy A., and Richard J. Martin. *Neonatal-Perinatal Medicine: Diseases of the Fetus and Infant.* 6th ed. St. Louis: C. V. Mosby, 1997.

Levy, Joseph. "Newborn Jaundice." *Parents Magazine* 69, no. 7 (July, 1994): 59-60.

Maisels, Jeffrey M. "Neonatal Jaundice." *Clinics in Perinatology* 17, no. 2 (June, 1990).

JAUNDICE, NEONATAL

DISEASE/DISORDER

ANATOMY OR SYSTEM AFFECTED: Blood, bones, brain, liver, spleen

SPECIALTIES AND RELATED FIELDS: Hematology, neonatology, neurology

DEFINITION: A yellowish coloration visible on the skin that is the most frequent physical finding in newborn infants.

KEY TERMS:

bilirubin encephalopathy: disease resulting from damage to the brain cells by bilirubin; also called kernicterus

exchange transfusion: the removal of an individual's blood and its replacement with a donor's blood

hyperbilirubinemia: a condition in which the bilirubin concentration in the blood reaches a level that is higher than that generally found in umbilical cord blood (1.5 milligrams per 100 milliliters)

hypertonia: an increase in muscle tone

hypotonia: a decrease in muscle tone

phototherapy: a treatment consisting of exposure to light from a bank of fluorescent or other types of lamps

CAUSES AND SYMPTOMS

Most jaundice found in children is neonatal nonhemolytic jaundice, a yellowish pigmentation of the skin of some infants. The term "nonhemolytic" is used to differentiate this condition from jaundice caused by blood group incompatibilities (such as Rh or ABO groups) or other enzyme abnormalities of the red blood cells.

Neonatal nonhemolytic jaundice is the result of an excess of the pigment bilirubin. Bilirubin is derived from two major sources. One source is the normal destruction of circulating red blood cells (erythrocytes). The normal life span of the erythrocytes varies from eighty to one hundred twenty days. Old erythrocytes are removed and destroyed in specific tissues in the spleen and liver, where the hemoglobin of the red blood cells is broken down and converted to bilirubin. This accounts for 75 percent of the daily production of bilirubin, and 1 gram of hemoglobin yields 35 milligrams of bilirubin. The remaining 25 percent of bilirubin is derived from ineffective erythropoiesis (red blood cell formation) in the bone marrow and other tissue heme or heme proteins from the liver.

The bilirubin formed is transported in the plasma of the blood and bound reversibly to albumin, a protein in the blood and tissues. This bilirubin-albumin complex is then transported to the liver, where it is converted into a water-soluble compound (or conjugated) by the enzyme glucuronyl transferase in the interior of the liver cells. The conjugated bilirubin is excreted into the bile capillaries and then into the intestine. Once in the small intestine, the conjugated bilirubin is converted by bacteria in the colon into a colorless compound known as urobilinogen. In the newborn infant, because of the lack of bacteria in the colon and the presence of the enzyme B-glucuronidase in the gut wall, a significant amount of the conjugated bilirubin is deconjugated and reabsorbed back into the plasma pool, a process known as the entero-hepatic shunt.

Chemical hyperbilirubinemia can be defined as a serum concentration of bilirubin that exceeds 1.5 milligrams per 100 milliliters. Visible yellowing (icterus) of the skin is caused by the combination of skin color, bilirubin-albumin complexes located outside the blood vessels, and precipitated bilirubin acid in the membranes of the cell walls. It first becomes visible when serum bilirubin reaches from 3 to 6 milligrams per deciliter, depending on the infant's skin texture and pigmentation and on the observer. In the neonate, jaundice is detected by blanching the skin over a bony structure with digital pressure, thus revealing the underlying color of the skin and subcutaneous tissue. Jaundice is first seen in the face and then progresses toward the trunk and extremities.

In general, infants whose jaundice is restricted to the face and trunk and does not extend below the umbilicus have serum bilirubin levels of about 12 milligrams per deciliter or less, while those whose hands and feet are jaundiced have serum bilirubin levels in excess of 15 milligrams per deciliter. A more objective way to estimate the depth of jaundice in neonates is with the use of an icterometer, a strip of transparent plastic with five transverse yellow strips in different shades. The baby's skin is blanched using pressure, and the resulting shade of yellow is matched against a color scale. In recent years, a transcutaneous bilirubinometer has been developed, which provides an electronic readout of an index that corresponds with a serum bilirubin concentration. A more precise way to judge jaundice is to draw a small amount of blood (usually less than a tablespoon) from the baby and to measure its serum concentration in a laboratory.

A transient rise in serum bilirubin concentration is almost universally seen in healthy newborns. This type of jaundice, called physiologic jaundice, may be attributable to several factors. First, this condition may result from increased bilirubin load on liver cells caused by increased red blood cell volume, decreased red blood cell survival time, increased heme from muscles, or increased enterohepatic circulation of bilirubin. Second, the condition may result from decreased liver uptake of bilirubin from plasma caused by a decrease in specific proteins in liver cells (termed Y and Z proteins) for the transport of bilirubin. Third, it may result from defective bilirubin conjugation caused by decreased enzyme activity. Fourth, physiologic jaundice can result from defective bilirubin excretion.

The serum bilirubin level in newborns reaches its peak between forty-eight and seventy-two hours after birth and then decreases, so that the yellowish pigmentation may not be visible by the fifth to seventh day. The peak level of serum bilirubin in physiologic jaundice varies from a mean of 5 to 15 milligrams per 100 milliliters. A number of factors will confound the level of serum bilirubin present with this condition. They include maternal pregnancy history, complications, drugs, gestational age, early initiation of feeding, type of feeding (breast milk or formula), and ethnicity. The heterogeneity of the human population makes it difficult to apply a particular serum bilirubin level to the definition of physiologic jaundice. No jaundice should be dismissed as physiologic, however, without at least a review of maternal and neonatal history, an examination of the infant for signs of illness, and further laboratory investigation when indicated.

In some cases, excess bilirubin can cause neurotoxicity leading to brain damage known as bilirubin encephalopathy or kernicterus. This damage can result in either neonatal death or the development of long-term abnormal neurologic findings, such as cerebral palsy, a low intelligence quotient (IQ), lower school achievement, hyperactivity, and deafness. The identification of jaundiced newborn infants at risk for kernicterus is difficult. The data suggest that healthy infants with serum bilirubin levels as high as 25 to 30 milligrams per 100 milliliters may not have adverse neurologic effects, since the bilirubin is bound to adequate albumin and the blood-brain barrier formed by cerebral blood vessels is intact in these infants. Early hospital discharge policies practiced in many maternity centers, however, make it difficult to assess the evolution of physiologic as well as pathologic jaundice, or confounding factors such as infection. Clinicians, practitioners, and home health visitors need to pay special attention to the degree of jaundice and when it is associated with danger signs such as sleepiness, lethargy, irritability, poor feeding, vomiting, fever, high-pitched or shrill cry, hypertonia or hypotonia (depending on whether the infant is asleep or awake), neck and trunk arching, dark urine, or light stools.

TREATMENT AND THERAPY

The treatment of jaundice depends on the underlying pathology. For clinical purposes, the two major types need to be separated: jaundice resulting from hemolytic disease (Rh, ABO, and other blood group incompatibilities) and nonhemolytic jaundice. Nonhemolytic jaundice may be physiologic or an accentuation of physiologic jaundice, such as jaundice caused by polycythemia (an increased number of red blood cells), cephalhematoma (the collection of blood in the scalp between the bone and bone lining), bruising, cerebral or other hemorrhages, swallowed blood, increased enterohepatic shunting (because of breast-feeding, delayed passage of stools, or gastrointestinal tract obstruction), and infection or sepsis.

Although no general consensus exists concerning the management of nonhemolytic jaundice, infants with this condition are generally treated with phototherapy when the serum bilirubin level reaches between 15 and 18 milligrams per 100 milliliters, using the upper value for uncomplicated physiologic jaundice and the lower value when the jaundice has accentuating factors. Phototherapy consists of exposure of the baby's skin to light energy from a bank of fluorescent or other special lamps. The light converts the fat-soluble bilirubin, which cannot be excreted, into a water-soluble bilirubin, which can be easily excreted in the bile, thus lowering the serum concentration of bilirubin.

When the serum bilirubin level reaches between 20 and 25 milligrams per 100 milliliter—some clinicians advocate between 25 and 30 milligrams per 100 milliliters—exchange transfusion is generally recommended. In this method, all of the baby's bilirubin-containing blood is removed and exchanged with compatible blood, without bilirubin, from a donor. Both forms of treatment, phototherapy and exchange transfusion, aim to reduce or remove bilirubin from the baby's system, thereby preventing brain injury.

PERSPECTIVE AND PROSPECTS

Jaundice was identified as a major problem in newborn infants in the nineteenth century. Its association with brain injury was first described by German pathologist Johannes J. Orth in 1875. Fifty years later, brain damage was further identified with increased destruction of red blood cells because of hemolysis caused by Rh and ABO blood group incompatibilities.

It was also realized, however, that jaundice is encountered in normal newborn infants. The major problem has been to identify which infant is at risk for brain damage when bilirubin is at a particular level. Since there are multiple confounding factors, better means are being developed for identifying risks, such as laboratory methods to identify free (unbound) bili-

rubin and noninvasive clinical methods such as auditory evoked potential to measure brain waves in response to sound, the use of computers to analyze the shrillness of the baby's cry, and nuclear magnetic resonance (a form of X ray) to measure the energy metabolism of brain cells. In addition, methods to prevent the formation of bilirubin or to reduce its levels by decreasing the activity of the enzyme heme oxygenase are being studied.

—*Paul Y. K. Wu, M.D.*

See also Anemia; Blood and blood disorders; Cerebral palsy; Hematology, pediatric; Hemolytic disease of the newborn; Hepatitis; Jaundice; Light therapy; Liver; Liver disorders; Neonatalogy.

FOR FURTHER INFORMATION:

Appleby, Julie. "Jaundice-Caused Brain Damage Is on the Rise." *USA Today*, October 26, 2000, p. D10. Because babies are being sent home from the hospital earlier, many cases of jaundice are missed. There have been eighty-eight cases of jaundice-caused brain damage in the United States since 1984, the majority since 1990.

Avery, Gordon B., Mary A. Fletcher, and Mhairi G. MacDonald, eds. *Neonatology: Pathophysiology and Management of the Newborn*. 5th ed. Philadelphia: J. B. Lippincott, 1999. A standard textbook on the pathophysiology and management of the major disease processes affecting the neonate, first published in 1975. Two coeditors have joined Avery in bringing out this edition, now with sixty-one chapters.

Fanaroff, Avroy A., and Richard J. Martin. *Neonatal-Perinatal Medicine: Diseases of the Fetus and Infant*. 6th ed. St. Louis: C. V. Mosby, 1997. This classic reference work is one of the most comprehensive to date and features discussions on the diverse practice of neonatal-perinatal medicine, pregnancy disorders and their impact on the fetus, delivery room care, provisions for neonatal care, and the development and disorder of organ systems.

Kirchner, Jeffrey T. "Clinical Assessment of Neonatal Jaundice." *American Family Physician* 62, no. 8 (October 15, 2000): 1880. Neonatal jaundice is a common condition, most often caused by normal physiologic mechanisms and not usually of significant concern. The decision to obtain a serum bilirubin level in a newborn usually is based on the child's appearance and the clinical judgment of the physician.

Jaw wiring

Procedure

Anatomy or system affected: Bones, gums, mouth, musculoskeletal system, teeth

Specialties and related fields: Dentistry, emergency medicine, nutrition, orthodontics, plastic surgery, speech pathology

Definition: A surgical procedure in which the upper and lower teeth are brought closely together and secured with wire in order to immobilize the jaw.

Key terms:

arch bar: a pliable piece of metal with small hooked attachments; one is fitted along the upper teeth, another is fitted along the lower teeth, the two pieces are connected to the teeth with wires, and other wires are looped around the hooks and brought together to prevent jaw movement

facial edema: swelling of the facial tissue

intermaxillary fixation: the medical term for jaw wiring

mandible: the lower jawbone

maxilla: the upper jawbone

oral hygiene: care of the teeth and mouth

orthognathic surgery: jaw reconstruction

reduction: the restoration of a fractured bone to its normal position

zygoma: the cheekbone

Indications and Procedures

Jaw wiring is often necessary to repair fractures in the jaw. The principles of treatment for facial fractures, in which bones need to be lined up and held in position until healing takes place, are the same as for a fractured arm or leg. Whereas an arm or leg fracture is reduced and casted to hold the bones in proper alignment, however, this method cannot be used for fractures of the face. Instead, once the fractures have been reduced (the bones have been restored to their proper positions), the jaws are wired shut to prevent the displacement of bone or bone fragments until they have healed.

Fractures of the face can involve any of the facial bones. The lower jawbone (mandible) is the most commonly fractured facial bone. Nevertheless, the upper jawbone (maxilla), the cheekbone (zygoma), the nasal bones, or the orbits (formed from bones of the cranium and face around the eyes) may also suffer fractures. A fracture may involve an individual bone or a combination of bones. One of the most common causes of facial fractures is blunt trauma. A blow to the face, the impact from an automobile or motorcycle accident, and a gunshot wound to the face are some examples of such trauma.

When considering fractures of the face, more than simply the bony structures must be evaluated. The skeletal structure encapsulates and protects organs that are vital to the functions of seeing, breathing, eating, talking, and swallowing. Early identification and treatment of fractures of the face are necessary to maintain maximum function of these delicate organs. Therefore, even though facial fractures and related injuries to soft tissue are seldom fatal, they must be treated immediately, since improper care could result in disfigurement, permanent sensory impairment, and lifelong disabilities.

In addition to facial fractures, jaw wiring is sometimes performed to correct malformations of the facial bones, certain birth defects, and acquired disfigurements as a result of trauma or growth-related imperfections. At times, jaw wiring is performed to correct malformations that have caused headaches, chewing disorders, and breathing and speech impairments. This type of surgery is referred to as orthognathic or jaw reconstruction surgery, part of which may involve jaw wiring. This procedure may also be performed as a weight-loss treatment for obese persons.

When a patient is hospitalized for elective facial surgery involving jaw wiring, or intermaxillary fixation, ample time can be given to preparing the patient for the surgical procedure and both preoperative and postoperative care. For the patient who sustains facial trauma, however, the same opportunity for surgical preparation may not be possible.

Facial fractures can often be reduced and immobilized by jaw wiring on the day of the injury. When there is marked facial edema (swelling), when other serious injuries are present, or when the person has eaten within a certain period of time prior to the trauma, however, the surgery will need to be delayed until a general anesthetic can be administered safely and the patient's condition has stabilized to the point that the surgical procedure can be tolerated.

The purpose of jaw wiring is to reduce and stabilize the fracture in such a manner that proper alignment of the bone will be maintained until it has healed. If the surgery is for jaw reconstruction, then the bone is fractured and positioned by the surgeon. These surgical fractures also require stabilization so that they will heal in the intended position. Interosseous wiring (the wiring of one portion of bone to another) using stainless steel wire may be necessary to maintain proper bone alignment. Sometimes, compression plates are used to secure the bones together. At other times, a bite block splint is inserted between the teeth to provide stabilization. This splint resembles a denture plate. An appliance called an external fixation device may be needed to keep the bones in proper alignment until they are healed.

If the patient wears dentures, then the denture plates are wired to the bone, the lower plate to the mandible, and the upper plate to the maxilla, prior to the jaw-wiring procedure. If the patient has no teeth at all, a bite block splint must be wired to the mandible and the maxilla, similar to the way in which dentures would be wired into place.

Jaw wiring is accomplished by first attaching arch bars to the base of the teeth. Arch bars are pliable pieces of metal with small hooked attachments on one side. They come in pre-cut lengths and can also be cut to fit the individual's mouth. One fits along the base of the lower dental arch, and the other fits along the base of the upper dental arch. Thin pieces of stainless steel wire are passed around the base of each tooth and brought out, then hooked around the arch bar and twisted firmly into place to secure the arch bar itself. The wires are cut, and their edges are tucked down between the teeth to prevent them from poking into gum or cheek tissue. If the patient wears dentures, the arch bar is either wired or glued to the denture plate with a special glue before the plate is wired to the bone structure.

Once the arch bars are positioned and secured, then special rubber bands are drawn around the hooked attachments from the upper to the lower bar. These bands are what actually hold the jaw tightly together. They are usually replaced with thin wires a few days after surgery, when the danger of nausea and vomiting have passed. Wire cutters need to be kept within easy reach at all times, in the event of vomiting. Should this happen, only the wires that hold the teeth together are clipped, and they will need to be reapplied by the physician.

USES AND COMPLICATIONS

Until the 1970's, orthognathic surgery carried a purely cosmetic connotation among the general public. Gradually, with surgical practice, documentation, research, and reports of the results of orthognathic surgery, people have come to understand the importance of such surgery in terms of proper physical functioning, as well as psychological and social functioning. Surgical reconstruction of the face can produce amazing results, but it also comes with a price. The process sometimes takes several years and teamwork by dentists, orthodontists, oral and/or plastic surgeons, and sometimes even psychiatrists to achieve these results. It can also be very costly because some insurance companies still consider orthodontia and corrective surgery cosmetic rather than functional and do not accept claims for these services.

Whatever the reason for jaw wiring, this process involves much more than a simple surgical procedure. Patients are usually hospitalized. Many of them are young, and others have had little hospital experience and may be anxious about the outcome. Lack of family support or financial concerns may increase this anxiety. Other injuries may be present in addition to the facial ones, some of which could be life-threatening and need to be attended to first.

Since jaw wiring usually means that the jaws are tightly wired shut, careful immediate postoperative monitoring by a nurse is needed to ensure that respiratory functioning is adequate, nausea and vomiting are controlled, mouth care is performed, nutritional intake of an all-liquid diet is satisfactory, and facial swelling and pain are reported to the surgeon, if necessary.

Before being discharged from the hospital, patients need to be shown proper mouth care techniques. Primary among them is the use of an electrical appliance that delivers pulsating jets of water, saline, or a mouth care solution to areas between the teeth and under the gumline. It rinses out food debris and harmful bacteria from the mouth. Mouth care is very important during the period of time when the jaws are wired, so that healing is promoted and dental caries (cavities) are prevented.

Good nutritional habits are also important during this time. Since the patient's diet must be liquid in form, concerns about weight loss, adequate food variations, appropriate nutrients for healing, management of food preparation, and possible nutritional supplementation need to be addressed and resolved before a patient is discharged. Patients should have a written diet plan to use at home. Medications needed for pain, nausea, vitamins, and sometimes antibiotics will also need to be obtained in liquid form. Instructions regarding how to administer emergency care, when to call the doctor, and how to cut wires if vomiting occurs must be given.

Followup care with the physician will be needed to evaluate progress and to arrange for the clipping of wires and the removal of the arch bars. These procedures are usually done in the physician's office.

PERSPECTIVE AND PROSPECTS

It is likely that attempts were made to treat fractures of the face from the time of the cave dwellers, but no records of such attempts were kept. The earliest known records relating to the treatment of jaw fractures are found in the Smith Papyrus, which is thought to have been written about 25 to 30 centuries B.C.E. The author advises against the treatment of compound (open) fractures but recommends that the dislocation of the mandible be treated. Definite proof of the art of dentistry was found among the Etruscans, an ancient people living in what is now Tuscany and part of Umbria, in about 600 to 500 B.C.E.: Skeletal remains with the teeth bound with gold wire have been discovered.

In the time of Hippocrates (c. 460-c. 370 B.C.E.), the Greek physician known as the Father of Medicine, writings bear evidence that facial injuries or fractures were treated with some method of wiring. A section of the Corpus Hippocraticum reads:

> If the jaw is broken right across, which rarely happens, one should adjust it in the manner described [one thumb inside the mouth and the fingers outside, for reduction]. After adjustment one should fasten the teeth together as was described above [with gold wire or, lacking that, with linen thread], for this will contribute greatly to immobility, especially if one joins them properly and fastens the ends as they should be.

The use of bandages to treat facial maladies was also practiced by some ancient cultures. Galen of Pergamum (129-c. 199 C.E.) and Soranus of Ephesus (98-138 C.E.) describe such methods. An ancient manuscript by Soranus of Ephesus illustrates the types of bandages used by the ancients to treat head and facial injuries.

Greek writings even suggested dietary practices in cases of jaw injury. When the mandible was fractured, liquid nourishment was recommended, and solid foods were withheld until bone healing was definite. Patients were also advised not to talk for a certain period of time.

In the thirteenth century, Italian surgeon Guglielmo da Saliceto (c. 1210-c. 1277), also known as William of Saliceto, performed one of the first documented cases of jaw wiring, attaching the teeth of the lower jaw to the corresponding teeth of the upper jaw. He used linen and silk thread, twisting them together and then waxing the twist to keep it in place. In the next several centuries, however, the medieval literature lacks any references to the management of facial bone fractures. Whether the work of earlier surgeons was unknown or whether such surgical practices remained standard during these years, without notable progress, remains a mystery.

It was toward the end of the nineteenth century that the development of intermaxillary fixation by wiring was developed by an American physician and dentist, Thomas Lewis Gilmer (1849-1931). Gilmer carried out the jaw wiring procedure "by twisting wires around the necks of the teeth of the upper and lower jaws, by adjusting the lower teeth to the occlusion of the upper jaw, and by twisting together the connecting upper and lower wires for stabilization."

Many great names are associated with the twentieth century contributions to improved and refined methods of jaw wiring techniques and patient care during this process. Much was learned about the nature of facial fractures themselves from the work of French physician Rene LeFort. LeFort conducted a series of experiments in the early twentieth century to study facial fracture combinations. He subjected cadaver skulls to violent blows under many conditions and at various angles and then described the outcomes.

A survey of the progress made in jaw wiring would be incomplete without recognition of the impact that antibiotic therapy, advanced anesthetic techniques, and blood replacement therapy have had on this procedure and on medical science as a whole. These achievements paved the way for open surgical procedures and internal fixation, which have led to dramatic results and remarkable changes for individuals undergoing jaw wiring.

—*Karen A. Mattern*

See also Bones and the skeleton; Dentistry; Emergency medicine; Fracture and dislocation; Fracture repair; Hyperadiposis; Nutrition; Obesity; Orthodontics; Orthopedic surgery; Orthopedics; Orthopedics, pediatric; Plastic surgery.

FOR FURTHER INFORMATION:

Fonseca, Raymond J., and Robert V. Walker, eds. *Oral and Maxillofacial Trauma*. 2d ed. Philadelphia: W. B. Saunders, 1997. This text discusses wounds and injuries to the face, mouth, and jaw, as well as therapies to treat them. Includes a bibliography and an index.

Niamtu, Joseph, III. "Cosmetic Oral and Maxillofacial Surgery Options." *The Journal of the American Dental Association* 131, no. 6 (June, 2000): 756-764. A global diagnosis and treatment plan which includes facial esthetics can enhance cosmetic dentistry and serve to frame the work of the restorative dentist.

Watts, V., S. Madick, J. Pepperney, and C. Petras. "When Your Patient Has Jaw Surgery." *RN* 48 (October, 1985): 44-47. This article written for health care professionals focuses on jaw surgery as a result of facial deformities rather than fractures, describing some deformities. Also includes postoperative care of the patient.

JOINT DISEASES. *See* **ARTHRITIS.**

JOINT REPLACEMENT. *See* **ARTHROPLASTY; HIP REPLACEMENT.**

KAPOSI'S SARCOMA

DISEASE/DISORDER

ANATOMY OR SYSTEM AFFECTED: Intestines, liver, lungs, skin

SPECIALTIES AND RELATED FIELDS: Internal medicine, oncology

DEFINITION: A disease in which cancer cells are found in tissues, causing lesions on the skin and/or mucous membranes and spreading to other organs in the body.

CAUSES AND SYMPTOMS

It is uncertain whether Kaposi's sarcoma is actually cancer because, unlike cancer, it arises from several cell types. Although there is no accepted staging system for Kaposi's sarcoma, patients are grouped by the type that they have. The three types are classic, epidemic, and recurrent.

Classic Kaposi's sarcoma usually occurs in older men of Mediterranean heritage. It progresses slowly (over ten to fifteen years), with progression bringing lower limb swelling, impeded blood flow, possible spread to other organs, and other types of cancer in later life. Epidemic Kaposi's sarcoma, found in people with acquired immunodeficiency syndrome (AIDS), is a more virulent, fast-spreading, and fatal form, with symptoms of painless, either flat or raised, pink or purple plaques on the skin and mucosal surfaces. This type usually spreads to the lungs, liver, spleen, lymph nodes, digestive tract, and other internal organs. Recurrent Kaposi's sarcoma comes back after it has been treated in the original area where it started. Sometimes, it appears in another part of the body.

TREATMENT AND THERAPY

Four kinds of treatment are usually used: surgery (taking out the cancer), chemotherapy (using drugs to kill cancer cells), external beam radiation therapy (using high-dose X rays to kill cancer cells), and biological therapy (using the body's immune system to fight the cancer).

Classic Kaposi's sarcoma may be treated by radiation therapy, local excision (cutting out the lesion and some of the tissue around it), systemic chemotherapy

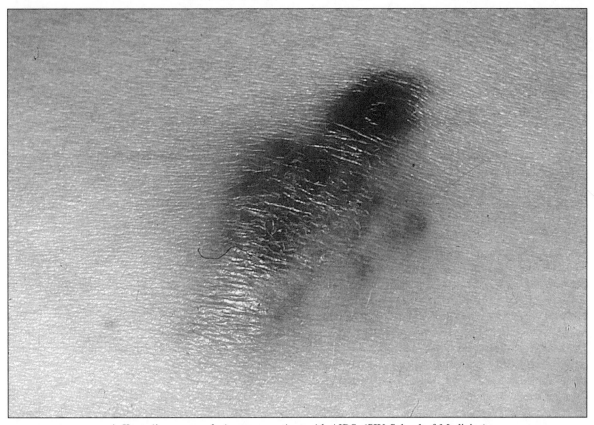

A Kaposi's sarcoma lesion on a patient with AIDS. (SIU School of Medicine)

(in which the drug enters the bloodstream, travels through the body, and kills cancer cells outside the original site), intralesional chemotherapy (in which the drug is injected into the lesion), or a combination of these treatments.

Epidemic Kaposi's sarcoma is treated by surgery, including electrodesiccation and curettage (burning the lesion and removing it with a sharp instrument) and cryotherapy (killing the tumor by freezing it). It can also be treated with chemotherapy or biological therapy.

PERSPECTIVE AND PROSPECTS
Until the early 1980's, Kaposi's sarcoma was found mainly in older male patients who had received organ transplants. The AIDS epidemic gave rise to cases that spread quickly among homosexual men and African men. Recovery depends on the type of Kaposi's sarcoma, age, general health, and whether the condition is accompanied by AIDS.

—*Patricia A. Ainsa, M.P.H., Ph.D.*

See also Acquired immunodeficiency syndrome (AIDS); Biopsy; Cancer; Chemotherapy; Cryotherapy and cryosurgery; Malignancy and metastasis; Oncology; Radiation therapy; Sarcoma.

FOR FURTHER INFORMATION:
Corey, Lawrence, ed. *AIDS: Problems and Prospects.* New York: W. W. Norton, 1993.

Feigal, Ellen G., Alexandra M. Levine, and Robert J. Biggar. *AIDS-related Cancers and Their Treatment.* New York: Marcel Dekker, 2000.

Gottlieb, Geoffrey J., and A. Bernard Ackerman. *Kaposi's Sarcoma: A Text and Atlas.* Philadelphia: Lea & Febiger, 1988.

Shepherd, Frances A. *Management of Kaposi's Sarcoma Associated with Human Immunodeficiency Virus Infection.* Ottawa: Health and Welfare Canada, 1991.

Ziegler, John L., and Ronald F. Dorfman, eds. *c: Pathophysiology and Clinical Management.* New York: Marcel Dekker, 1988.

KERATOSES
DISEASE/DISORDER
ANATOMY OR SYSTEM AFFECTED: Skin

SPECIALTIES AND RELATED FIELDS: Dermatology

DEFINITION: Keratoses, wartlike growths, are caused by the excessive production of the skin protein keratin; they usually occur in elderly people. Solar keratoses result from repeated exposure to the sun-

light and thus appear on the face, arms, and hands. They are small and may be red or uncolored. Seborrheic keratoses, which are of unknown origin, may be small, dark brown, flat, or rough; they are generally greasy and crusted over. Seborrheic keratoses are benign, but solar keratoses may, on rare occasions, develop into a squamous cell carcinoma or other skin cancer. Both types can be removed if the patient desires, usually with cryosurgery.

—*Jason Georges and Tracy Irons-Georges*

See also Carcinoma; Dermatology; Skin; Skin cancer; Skin disorders; Warts.

FOR FURTHER INFORMATION:
Lamberg, Lynne. *Skin Disorders.* Philadelphia: Chelsea House, 2001.

Mackie, Rona M. *Clinical Dermatology.* 4th ed. New York: Oxford University Press, 1997.

Siegel, Mary-Ellen. *Safe in the Sun.* Rev. ed. New York: Walker, 1995.

KIDNEY DISORDERS
DISEASE/DISORDER
ANATOMY OR SYSTEM AFFECTED: Kidneys, urinary system

SPECIALTIES AND RELATED FIELDS: Internal medicine, nephrology, urology

DEFINITION: Disorders, from structural abnormalities to bacterial infections, that can affect the kidneys and may lead to renal failure.

KEY TERMS:

creatinine: the breakdown product of creatine, a nitrogenous compound found in muscle, blood, and urine

cystinosis: a congenital disease characterized by glucose and protein in the urine, as well as by cystine deposits in the liver and other organs, rickets, and growth retardation

hematuria: the abnormal presence of blood in the urine

hydronephrosis: the cessation of urine flow because of an obstruction of a ureter, allowing urine to build up in the pelvis of the kidney; can cause renal failure

oliguria: the diminished capacity to form and pass urine, so that metabolic products cannot be excreted efficiently

reflux: the abnormal backward flow of urine

toxemia: blood poisoning

uremia: the presence of excessive amounts of urea and other nitrogenous waste products in the blood

CAUSES AND SYMPTOMS

Disorders of the kidney can occur for a variety of reasons. The cause may be congenital (present from birth) or may develop very quickly and at any age. Many of these problems and disorders can be easily treated. The main areas of kidney disorders are classified as malformations in development of the kidney, part of the kidney, or the ureter; glomerular disease; tubular and interstitial disease or disruption; vascular (other than glomerular) disease; and kidney dysfunction that occurs secondary to another disease.

The kidney frequently exhibits congenital anomalies, some of which occur during specific developmental stages. Agenesis occurs when the ureteric bud fails to develop normally. When the tissue does not develop, the ureter itself fails to form. If there is an obstruction where the ureter joins the pelvis of the kidney, there may be massive hydronephrosis (dilation). One or both kidneys may be unusually small, containing too few tubules. The kidneys may be displaced, too high or offset to one side or the other. They may even be fused. All these conditions could seriously affect the manufacture of urine, its excretion, or both.

Glomerulonephritis refers to a diverse group of conditions that share a common feature—primary involvement of the glomerulus. The significance of glomerulonephritis is that it is the most common cause of end-stage renal failure. Its features include urinary casts, high protein levels (proteinuria), hematuria, hypertension, edema (swelling), and uremia. The two forms of glomerulonephritis are primary and secondary. In the primary form, only the kidneys are affected, but in the secondary form, the lesion (affected area) is only one of a series of problems.

Nephrotic syndrome is usually defined as an abnormal condition of the kidney characterized by the presence of proteinuria together with edema and high fat and cholesterol levels. It occurs in glomerular disease, in thrombosis of a renal vein, and as a complication of many systemic diseases. Nephrotic syndrome occurs in a severe, primary form characterized by anorexia, weakness, proteinuria, and edema.

Interstitial nephritis is inflammation of the interstitial tissue of the kidney, including the kidneys. Acute interstitial nephritis is an immunologic, adverse reaction to certain drugs; drugs especially associated with it are nonsteroidal anti-inflammatory drugs (NSAIDs) and some antibiotics. Acute renal failure, fever, rash, and proteinuria are indicative signs of this condition. If the medication is stopped, normal kidney function returns. Chronic interstitial nephritis is defined as inflammation and structural changes associated with such conditions as ureteral obstruction, pyelonephritis, exposure of the kidney to a toxin, transplant rejection, or certain systemic diseases.

Kidney stones (calculi) are commonly manufactured from calcium oxalate and/or phosphate, triple phosphate, uric acid (urate), or a mixture of these. Calcium stones are not necessarily the result of high serum calcium, although they can be. Struvite calculi of magnesium ammonium (triple) phosphate mixed with calcium are bigger but softer than other types; they grow irregularly, filling much of the kidney pelvis. They arise from infection with urea-splitting organisms that cause alkaline urine. Urate stones are a complication of gout.

Those who have a tendency to develop stones may experience concomitant infection known as pyonephrosis. Pyonephrosis is a result of not only blockage at the junction of the ureter and kidney pelvis but also any constricture at this location. Bacteria from the bloodstream collect and cause an abscess to form. If the tube is completely blocked, the inflammation produces enough pus to rupture a portion of the kidney, and more of the abdominal cavity becomes involved.

Pyelonephritis is inflammation of the upper urinary tract. Acute pyelonephritis may be preceded by lower tract infection. The patient complains of lethargy, fever, and back pain. The major symptoms are fever, renal pain, and body aches accompanied by nausea and toxemia. Chronic pyelonephritis often affects the renal tubules and the small spaces within the kidney. Fibrous tissue may take over these areas and cause gradual shrinking of the functional kidney. The chronic form may also result from previous bacterial infection, reflux, obstruction, overuse of analgesics, X rays, and lead poisoning.

Obstruction may be caused by inadequate development of the renal tissue itself, closing off one or both ureters. Other malformations and certain calculi can also obstruct urine flow. Reflux may occur when the contraction of the bladder forces urine backward, up toward and into the kidney. Lesser degrees of reflux do not damage the kidney, but the greater the reflux, the more likely damage will occur. Bacterial infection is often attributable to *Escherichia coli*, but other bowel bacteria may also infect the area. They generally move upward from outside the body through the urinary organs, but they may move inward from the bloodstream.

Acute renal failure is defined as a sudden decline in normal renal function that leads to an increase in blood urea and creatinine. The onset may be fast (over days) or slow (over weeks) and is often reversible. It is characterized by oliguria and rapid accumulation of nitrogenous wastes in the blood, resulting in acidosis. Acute renal failure is caused by hemorrhage, trauma, burns, toxic injury to the kidney, acute pyelonephritis or glomerulonephritis, or lower urinary tract obstruction. Occasionally, it will progress into chronic renal failure.

Chronic renal failure may result from many other diseases. Its signs are sluggishness, fatigue, and mental dullness. Patients also display other systemic problems as a result of chronic renal failure. Almost all such patients are anemic; three-fourths of them develop hypertension. The skin becomes discolored; the muddy coloration is caused by anemia and the presence of excess melanin.

Renal symptoms suggestive of renal dysfunction include increases in frequency of urination, color changes in urine, areas of edema, and hypertension. The patient may experience only one symptom but is more likely to have a series of complaints. To determine the cause of renal disease, several diagnostic tools can be used to distinguish the type of pathogenic process affecting the kidney. The degree to which other body systems are involved determines whether the disease process is systemic or confined to the kidneys. Other valuable clues may be gathered from medical history, family history, and physical examination. The key factors, however, are renal size and renal histopathology.

Examination of the urine can reveal important data relative to renal health. Stick tests may show the abnormal presence of blood, glucose, and/or protein. Assaying the kind and amount of protein may pinpoint the cause of the disease. Urine contaminated with bacteria has always been used as an indication of some form of urinary tract infection. Microscopic examination of urine sediment may help diagnose acute renal failure. Blood tests may also indicate the source of a renal disorder. A series of blood tests might reveal rising urea and creatinine levels. The urea-to-creatinine ratio may aid in determining if and which type of acute renal failure may be present. A high red cell count might suggest kidney stones, a tumor, or glomerular disease; a high white cell count would hint at inflammation and/or infection. Cells cast from the kidney tubules may indicate acute interstitial nephritis, while red cell breakdown products may mean glomerulonephritis. The diagnostician should also be diligent in tracking down possible septic causes. Repeated cultures of blood and urine should help ascertain if there is an abscess anywhere near the kidney.

X rays can provide useful information. An abdominal X ray may show urinary stones and abnormalities in the renal outline. Ultrasound will measure renal size, show scarring, and reveal dilation of the tract, perhaps as a result of an obstructive lesion. Abdominal ultrasound has become the investigation of choice because it can be performed at the patient's bedside.

Renal biopsy can give an accurate diagnosis of acute renal failure but may be more dangerous to the patient than the condition itself. The main indications for biopsy would be suspected acute glomerulonephritis and renal failure that has lasted six weeks.

TREATMENT AND THERAPY

If glomerulonephritis is suspected or diagnosed, its treatment seeks to avoid complications of the illness. The patient is monitored daily for fluid overload; as long as the patient is retaining fluid, blood tests that measure urea, creatinine, and salt balance are also run daily. The patient should stay in bed and restrict fluid as well as potassium intake. Medications may be prescribed: diuretics, vasodilators for hypertension, and calcium antagonists. If the cause is bacterial, a course of oral antibiotics may be given. If these measures are unsuccessful, short-term dialysis may be needed. Some urinary abnormalities may last for as long as a year.

The first measure undertaken to treat acute renal failure is to rebuild depressed fluid volumes: blood if the patient has hemorrhaged, plasma for burn patients, and electrolytes for a patient who is vomiting and has diarrhea. If infection is suspected as the underlying cause, an appropriate antibiotic should be administered when blood cultures confirm the presence of bacteria. After fluid volumes have been replenished, a diuretic may be necessary to reduce swelling of tissues within the kidney.

In chronic renal failure, the major undertaking is to relieve the obstruction of the urinary tract. If the blockage is within the bladder, simple catheterization may relieve it. If a stone or some similar obstacle is blocking a ureter, however, surgery to remove it may be necessary. A tube may be inserted to allow urine drainage, and the stone will pass or be removed.

In sufferers of recurrent stones, maintaining a high urine output is important, which requires the patient to drink fluids throughout the day and even at bedtime. Those enduring intense pain may need to be hospitalized. Analgesics for pain are administered, as well as forced fluid intake to increase urine output so that the stone might be passed. If these measures do not work, surgical intervention may be necessary.

Patients suffering from progressive, incurable renal failure need medical aid managing conservation of, substitution for, and eventual replacement of nephron function. Conservation attempts to prolong kidney function for as long as possible; renal function is aided by drug treatment. Substitution means the maintenance of kidney function by dialysis, especially hemodialysis. Replacement is the restoration of renal function by a kidney transplant. By this third stage of treatment, urine formation is independent of further drug treatment, and kidney function must be achieved by other means. Patients suffering from end-stage renal failure have two options: dialysis and transplantation. A patient may go from dialysis to transplantation. In fact, if a compatible donor (preferably a sibling) is available, a transplant is advisable. For those without a suitable donor, long-term hemodialysis is the first option.

Dialysis is defined as the diffusion of dissolved molecules through a semipermeable membrane. Several types of dialysis are available. Hemodialysis filters and cleans the blood as it passes through the semipermeable membranous tube in contact with a balanced salt solution (dialysate). Hemodialysis can be performed in a dialysis unit of a hospital or at home. It must usually be done two or three times a week, with each session lasting from three to six hours, depending on the type of membranes used and the size of the patient. Hemodialysis can lead to acute neurological changes. Lethargy, irritability, restlessness, headache, nausea, vomiting, and twitching may all occur. In some patients, neurological complications occur after dialysis is terminated. Convulsions are the most common of these consequences. In continuous abdominal peritoneal dialysis, a fresh amount of dialysate is introduced from a bag attached to a permanently implanted plastic tube. Wastes and water pass into the dialysate from the surrounding organs; then the fluid is collected four to eight hours later.

Peritoneal dialysis is performed by the patient. It is continuous, so the clearance rate of wastes is higher. The most important neurological complications of peritoneal dialysis are worsening of urea-induced brain abnormalities accompanied by twitching and, rarely, psychosis and convulsions.

Transplantation of a kidney is considered for patients with primary renal diseases as well as end-stage renal failure resulting from any number of systemic and metabolic diseases. Success rates are highest for those suffering from lupus nephritis, gout, and cystinosis. If a kidney is received from a close relative, there is a 97 percent one-year survival rate. Even if the organ transplant comes from a nonrelative, the survival rate is still 90 percent.

—*Iona C. Baldridge*

See also Dialysis; Edema; Genital disorders, male; Glomerulonephritis; Incontinence; Kidney transplantation; Kidneys; Lithotripsy; Nephrectomy; Nephritis; Nephrology; Nephrology, pediatric; Renal failure; Stone removal; Stones; Urethritis; Urinary disorders; Urinary system; Urology; Urology, pediatric.

FOR FURTHER INFORMATION:

Catto, Graeme R. D., and David A. Power. *Nephrology in Clinical Practice*. London: Edward Arnold, 1988. This book addresses health care professionals in particular. Its goal is to educate practitioners in methods of recognition and diagnosis and of treatment.

Dalton, John R., and Erick J. Bergquist. *Urinary Tract Infections*. London: Croom Helm, 1987. One of a series written to update clinicians' and health care workers' knowledge of urinary dysfunction. That infection anywhere in the tract can ultimately affect renal health is noted, but most attention is paid to lower tract infection.

Dische, Frederick E. *Concise Renal Pathology*. 2d ed. Oxford, England: Oxford University Press, 1995. For those in training for medical fields, this book describes renal anatomy and pathology. The terminology is somewhat simplified so that the descriptions are more understandable.

Tierney, Lawrence M., Jr., et al., eds. *Current Medical Diagnosis and Treatment: 2001*. 39th ed. New York: McGraw-Hill, 2000. This reference volume covers all aspects of internal medicine. It is readable and concisely describes more than one thousand diseases and disorders, as well as their medical management.

KIDNEY REMOVAL. *See* **NEPHRECTOMY.**

KIDNEY STONES. *See* **KIDNEY DISORDERS; STONE REMOVAL; STONES.**

KIDNEY TRANSPLANTATION
PROCEDURE
ANATOMY OR SYSTEM AFFECTED: Abdomen, kidneys, urinary system

SPECIALTIES AND RELATED FIELDS: General surgery, nephrology

DEFINITION: A surgical procedure that replaces the recipient's diseased, nonfunctioning kidney with a donated one.

KEY TERMS:

end-stage renal disease: the final phase of long-standing kidney disease, characterized by a nearly complete loss of function

hemodialysis: the use of an external apparatus to filter the blood of patients with end-stage renal disease

immunosuppression: the use of a variety of drugs to depress the immune system's response to foreign tissue; lowers the probability of rejection of transplanted organs

rejection: a cellular and chemical attack by the immune system on a transplanted organ, which is recognized as foreign to the body

renal: referring to the kidneys

INDICATIONS AND PROCEDURES

Transplantation of a human kidney from a donor to a recipient has been used since the middle of the twentieth century to improve the quality and length of life for people with renal failure. While hemodialysis—or the use of an artificial kidney machine, as it is commonly known—can be used satisfactorily for years, transplantation is often the ultimate goal because it can return the patient to a near-normal life.

The kidneys play a pivotal role in maintaining a stable internal environment by controlling fluid levels, excreting waste products, and regulating the blood concentration of acids and bases and of ions such as sodium and potassium. The kidneys are also responsible for regulating blood pressure by secreting substances that constrict the blood vessels. Clearly, the derangement of such complex functions, as occurs in renal disease, is life-threatening.

There are many reasons for renal failure, but the most frequent are inherited disorders, severe infections, toxic substances, allergic reactions, diabetes mellitus, and hypertension. The latter two, which are common illnesses in the United States, result in renal damage because of long-term injury to the blood vessels. The symptoms of minimally or nonfunctioning kidneys reflect an accumulation of toxic waste products and dramatic changes in the chemical composition of the blood. Every system is affected until coma and death ensue. The process of hemodialysis is used intermittently to cleanse the blood and maintain life. Transplantation in the otherwise healthy person, however, is preferred.

An extraordinary amount of cooperation and preparation is necessary for successful kidney transplantation. The donor organ may come from a living blood relative or from a cadaver within minutes of death. The organ is removed and maintained at low temperature in a special preservative solution for up to forty-eight hours. A suitable recipient is located through a national registry that can rapidly pair a cadaver organ to a waiting patient. The chosen candidate is immediately prepared for surgery, and through an abdominal incision, the kidney is placed in the abdomen and connected to the blood supply by its artery and vein. The ureter, the urine-collecting duct, is attached to the bladder. The recipient's own diseased kidneys may or may not be removed; their presence does not interfere with the transplanted organ. Within hours, the newly transplanted organ begins to form urine.

Kidney Transplantation

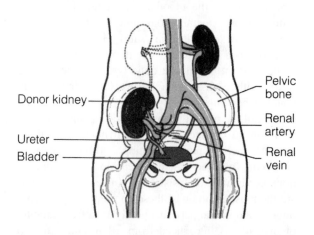

Donor kidney

Ureter

Bladder

Pelvic bone

Renal artery

Renal vein

The donor kidney is usually attached in front of the pelvic bone, rather than in the location of the nonfunctioning kidney, which is not removed in some cases.

USES AND COMPLICATIONS

All transplanted organs and tissues face both immediate and long-term rejection by the recipient's immune system. Recognizing the donated kidney as foreign, or "nonself," the immune system attacks it both physically and chemically. The injury can be so severe as to result in the organ's death and the need for its surgical removal. In an attempt to prevent this reaction, certain steps are taken both before and after transplantation surgery.

Matching a donor and recipient involves careful selection that must minimize the physiological differences that exist between people. The blood types (the ABO and Rh systems) should be the same. Advanced testing of the gene sequences on the sixth chromosome that code for immune system components are also matched as closely as possible in a process known as human leukocyte antigen (HLA) compatibility. Living, first-degree relatives, such as parents or siblings, often provide the best survival rates because of the genetic similarities between donor and recipient. The loss of one kidney in a healthy individual does not appear to affect the body.

The excellent success rates that have been achieved—nearly 80 percent—are attributable both to preoperative matching and to immunosuppression, which is begun shortly before surgery and continued for many months afterward. Potent drugs are used to inhibit the recipient's immune system, thereby protecting the new kidney from attack and significantly reducing rejection. Eventually, the drugs are tapered off and stopped, having allowed the body time to adjust to the foreign tissue and the kidney time to heal.

As can be expected in a procedure as difficult as kidney transplantation, the risks and complications are many. In the immediate postoperative period, hemorrhaging from the attached renal artery or vein, leakage from the ureter, organ malfunction, and immediate rejection can occur. Often, difficulties begin weeks or even months later, because of both rejection damage to the kidney and side effects related to severe immunosuppression. Immunosuppression leaves the body prey to bacterial, viral, and fungal infections, as well as cancer. Sometimes, a vicious cycle begins, in which life-threatening infections require the discontinuation of the immunosuppressive drugs, and the probability of organ rejection and irreparable kidney damage is heightened. Continual patient monitoring is absolutely essential to maintain the delicate balance between the risks and benefits involved in this procedure.

PERSPECTIVE AND PROSPECTS

Prior to 1962, when immunosuppressive drugs were unavailable and matching could only be based on blood type, kidney transplantation was an experimental procedure usually involving the organ of a living, first-degree relative. In the following decades, an extraordinary surge in information about the immune system and the genes that control the rejection response, as well the discovery of powerful drugs, made transplantation a successful alternative for patients supported by hemodialysis. It also significantly increased the donor pool of organs by allowing unrelated cadaver kidneys to be used. It is in both areas, more precise matching and the development of less toxic postoperative drugs, that research continues. Contributions made in this field are readily used for research in all other organ transplantation as well.

—*Connie Rizzo, M.D.*

See also Circulation; Cysts; Dialysis; Internal medicine; Kidney disorders; Kidneys; Nephrectomy; Nephritis; Nephrology; Nephrology, pediatric; Renal failure; Transplantation; Urinalysis; Urinary disorders; Urinary system; Urology; Urology, pediatric.

FOR FURTHER INFORMATION:

Brezis, M., et al. "Renal Transplantation." In *Brenner and Rector's The Kidney*, edited by Barry M. Brenner and Floyd C. Rector, Jr. 6th ed. Philadelphia: W. B. Saunders, 1999. A chapter in a treatise which, at more than two thousand pages, is the most comprehensive and authoritative source on the normal and diseased human kidney.

Carpenter, C., and M. Lazarus. "Dialysis and Transplantation in Renal Failure." In *Harrison's Principles of Internal Medicine*, edited by Kurt Isselbacher et al. 14th ed. New York: McGraw-Hill, 1998. A chapter in a standard text on internal medicine. Includes bibliographical references and an index.

Schrier, Robert W., and Carl W. Gottschalk, eds. *Diseases of the Kidney*. 6th ed. Boston: Little, Brown, 1997. Addresses the spectrum of systemic diseases and the kidney, covering malignancies, paraproteinemias, HIV, hepatitis, cryoglobulimea, sickle cell disease, sarcoidosis, and tropical diseases, in an atlas format.

KIDNEYS

ANATOMY

ANATOMY OR SYSTEM AFFECTED: Abdomen, circulatory system, urinary system

SPECIALTIES AND RELATED FIELDS: Hematology, nephrology, urology

DEFINITION: The organs that control the amount and composition of body water by separating the blood into waste products (which leave the body as urine) and nutrients (which are returned to the blood).

KEY TERMS:

Bowman's capsule: the group of renal cells that forms the cup of a nephron; fluids that seep from glomerular capillaries into the hollow wall of the capsule will be transformed into urine during their passage through the renal tubule leading from the capsule

glomerulus: a tuft or ball of capillaries contained within a Bowman's capsule

nephron: the almost-microscopic functional unit of the kidney, composed of special capillary blood vessels and of a Bowman's capsule connected to a renal tubule; each kidney has approximately 1.2 million nephrons

renal: of or relating to the kidneys

renal pelvis: the central pocket or sac of each kidney, which collects urine from all nephrons and channels it into the ureter

renal tubule: the tubular portion of a nephron that allows renal fluid to flow from the Bowman's capsule to the renal pelvis; these tubules, shaped like hairpins, are crucially important in the production of urine

ureter: the tube that transports urine from the renal pelvis to the urinary bladder

STRUCTURE AND FUNCTIONS

The normal human body has two kidneys, fist-sized organs located behind the abdomen and under the diaphragm. Each kidney, shaped like a bean, has a notch called the hilum, and the backbone separates the two kidneys. The kidneys make urine from blood. The renal artery transports blood into the kidney, while the renal vein transports blood out of the kidney. The blood vessels and the ureter connect with the kidney at its hilum.

The two kidneys are essentially identical in structure and function; consequently, kidney function can be discussed in the singular. The kidneys are a major functional unit of the circulatory system—unlike organs such as the brain, skin, or uterus, which are merely supported by that circulation. The kidney controls the environment of all cells of the body, an activity which is essential to life. That environment is salt water, and to understand the structure and function of

Anatomy of a Kidney

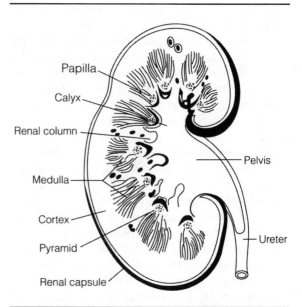

the kidney, it is necessary to understand the nature of salt water in the body.

The human body is about 56 percent water, and the composition of this fluid is very important. One-third of this water is outside the cells; some of this extracellular fluid is between cells, and some of it is the liquid in blood vessels (blood is composed of liquid and cells). Two-thirds of the body's water is inside cells. The cell membrane surrounding each cell retains the intracellular fluid, but the water molecules move freely across the cell membrane. The size of each cell is determined by its water content. Cells swell or shrink based on the accumulation or loss of water molecules. The concentration of substances dissolved in the water determines whether water will accumulate inside or outside cells. Some of these dissolved substances are gases such as oxygen and carbon dioxide; some are minerals such as hydrogen, sodium, and calcium; some are sugars or proteins; and others are nutrients and waste products.

The amount and the composition of body water is controlled by the kidneys. Two other organs that aid in controlling the composition of body water are the lungs and the digestive tract; they can add or remove materials from the body water. The kidneys control the composition of body water primarily by removing materials from body water. Unlike the lungs and the digestive tract, however, the kidneys also regulate the amount of body water. The kidneys carry out both of these functions by acting on the blood. The kidney has three other important functions: It helps to control blood pressure, helps to control the manufacture of red blood cells, and participates in the manufacture of vitamin D. This article focuses on function of the normal kidney and what can make the kidney function abnormally.

Each kidney contains more than a million nephrons, its functional units, arranged in cones. A nephron is composed of blood vessels and a Bowman's capsule, a cup of renal cells containing the capillary tuft called a glomerulus and attached to a renal tubule.

A kidney has between eight and eighteen cones of nephrons. The base of each cone is near the surface of the kidney, and the peak of each cone is pointed at the renal pelvis, the central sac that collects and channels urine. Each nephron acts like a very sophisticated filtration system for the blood. Approximately 20 to 25 percent of all the blood in the body flows through the blood vessels of the kidneys every minute.

The action of the nephron actually begins with a porous filter, the glomerulus, that separates particles from a liquid. In this case, the liquid is blood plasma and the particles are blood cells and those protein molecules that are too large to pass through the glomerular pores. About 20 percent of the liquid in the blood seeps through the wall of glomeruli and into the inner space of Bowman's capsules. This liquid that crosses into a Bowman's capsule contains water, minerals, sugars, amino acids, and products of cell metabolism. The body needs to retain many of these substances, including water, so they must be recaptured by nephrons and returned to the blood.

The recapturing process occurs in the renal tubules. This is the process in which the nephron differs from an ordinary filter. The tubules have special cells that are capable of selectively reabsorbing those materials that must be retained by the body. These materials are passed from the liquid inside the tubules, through the tubule cells, and into blood capillaries that are laced or braided around the outside wall of the tubules. About 99 percent of the water molecules that seep into the renal tubules from the glomeruli are returned to the blood. The substances that do not need to be retained by the body continue to flow through the tubules and eventually leave the kidney as urine.

The mechanism in the renal tubular cells that selectively reabsorbs substances from the tubular liquid is quite special. The membrane of each cell contains proteins that act as chemical pumps. These pump proteins pick up substances to be reabsorbed from the tubular liquid and pass those substances into and through the tubular cells, where they enter renal capillaries. The reabsorbed substances may be salts or electrolytes, such as sodium or bicarbonate, or they may be sugars or even amino acids. As these substances are reabsorbed, much of the tubular water is also reabsorbed.

The pump proteins can work in the opposite direction as well. They can move substances from the renal capillaries surrounding the tubules, through the wall of the tubules, and into the tubular liquid. This process is called tubular secretion. Substances that commonly undergo tubular secretion are potassium, ammonium, and acid.

The remarkable action of the pump proteins requires fuel—in this case, adenosine triphosphate (ATP). ATP is made by living cells from oxygen, sugar, fatty acids, and nucleic acids in the blood. Pump proteins stop working when cells are unable to make ATP.

The pressure of the blood flow through the glomeruli and the reabsorption process of the renal tubules are closely controlled. This control takes place directly in the kidney, which contains sensing mechanisms that respond to changes in fluid composition. The kidney makes a hormone, called renin, that increases blood pressure. Other sensors that respond to changes in fluid composition are located in the brain. When these sensors detect changes that require action, the brain, acting through the pituitary gland, releases hormones, such as antidiuretic hormone (ADH), that act on the kidney. Another important hormone that controls kidney function, aldosterone, comes from the adrenal gland. The actual means by which these hormones control kidney function, however, is only partially understood.

By other mechanisms, the kidney detects whether the blood contains sufficient red blood cells (erythrocytes). Red blood cells are responsible for carrying oxygen to all the other cells in the body. When more red blood cells are needed, the kidney makes a hormone called erythropoietin, which stimulates the bone marrow and causes it to make more red blood cells.

DISORDERS AND DISEASES
The advantage of having a pair of kidneys becomes obvious if renal function becomes impaired. A person

does quite well with one kidney; in fact, half of one kidney is sufficient to keep an individual alive.

A kidney problem may be suspected if an individual experiences changes in urination, such as pain on urination, changes in frequency of urination (more often or less often than usual), or changes in the urine that is formed (such as in its amount, appearance, or odor). Puffiness of the skin all over the body, but especially of the hands, feet, ankles, and face, may indicate abnormal renal function. This puffiness signifies water retention. Kidney disease can also be manifested by severe pain in the lower back, side, abdomen, or sex organs. The pain may be long-lasting or may occur with startling suddenness.

A person can be born with abnormal kidneys; this is a form of kidney disease. Normal kidneys, however, can malfunction because of a problem in the kidney itself, a problem in the blood circulation, or a problem in the flow of urine from the kidneys. Examples of abnormal kidneys at birth, abnormal urinary flow (kidney stones), and kidney infection will be discussed.

The formation of the kidneys by a fetus is quite complex and is controlled by genes. The development of the kidneys, other parts of the urinary tract (the ureters, bladder, and urethra), and the sex organs are all closely related. There are many opportunities for the developmental process to go wrong. Sometimes no kidneys are formed; sometimes the two kidneys are fused together; and sometimes more than one pair of kidneys is formed.

One of the most common malformations of the kidney is polycystic kidney disease, a hereditary (genetic) disorder affecting about 2 in 1,000 people. In the United States, it is ten times more common than sickle-cell disease and fifteen times more common than cystic fibrosis. In polycystic kidney disease, each kidney contains numerous fluid-filled sacs, or cysts, scattered throughout the organ. The cysts are of different sizes, some very small and some the size of a grape. Polycystic kidneys are noticeably enlarged.

The cysts are caused by a malformation of the renal tubules. A cyst is formed when a renal tubule develops a branch from the main tubule. Tubules are not supposed to form branches; if this occurs, however, then the branch may become sealed off from the original tubule so that it has no entrance or exit. These sealed-off tubules are the cysts. They are capable of secretory activity because their cells contain pump proteins. The cysts enlarge as they accumulate fluid,

putting pressure on the blood vessels, their capillaries, and the nephrons. The flow of blood and of urine is hindered. Patients with polycystic kidney disease often develop high blood pressure, kidney stones, and kidney infections. The disease can begin before birth, but symptoms may not occur until childhood or early adulthood. The intensity or severity of the disease varies greatly, from symptomless to life-threatening. Treatment of mild polycystic kidney disease may consist of relieving the pain, curing the infection, and controlling the blood pressure. Treatment of severe or life-threatening polycystic renal disease requires dialysis or kidney transplantation.

Stones in the urinary tract are very common. About 1 in 100 Americans have stones, and 1 in 1,000 adults experience such severe symptoms that they require hospitalization. Kidney stones are caused by a prolonged high concentration of certain minerals in the urine, usually calcium, oxalate, or urate. The stones usually consist of crystals bound together by proteins.

The size and shape of kidney stones vary greatly. They may be microscopic or the size of a pea or even larger; they may be smooth or jagged. The stones may be passed from the urinary tract during urination, but some require removal by a urologist. Microscopic stones may not cause any symptoms, while larger stones can be very painful and may produce blood in the urine. Because stones hinder the flow of urine, their presence can allow bacteria to grow in the urinary tract, producing an infection.

Kidney stones that produce symptoms and are not passed by the patient must be removed. Some stones may be removed with a ureteroscope while the patient is under general anesthesia. A ureteroscope is a urological instrument like a hollow tube. It is inserted into the urinary tract through the external opening of the urethra and passed through the bladder and into the ureter. The tube can actually be inserted into the renal pelvis. The optical system of the ureteroscope allows the physician to see inside the urinary tract. Through the ureteroscope, kidney stones may be broken up by applying ultrasonic, laser, or electrohydraulic (acoustic shock-wave) energy.

An alternative means of removing large kidney stones is extracorporeal shock-wave lithotripsy, or ESWL. ESWL is desirable because it uses shock waves to break up the stones, thus eliminating the need to insert medical instruments into the patient. In one method of ESWL, the anesthetized patient is placed in a tub of water. X-ray imaging locates and monitors the stones as shock waves crush them. The patient's tissues are not damaged, and the sandy remains of the stones are then passed with urine. The development of ESWL has offered a useful means of treating kidney stones, but it has not eliminated the need for surgical or ureteroscopic removal of these stones from some patients. Each patient and each stone is different; they require the professional evaluation of a urologist.

Urinary tract infections are common, affecting 10 to 20 percent of women at some point in their lives; they are less common in men. Pathogens usually infect the kidneys by ascending the urinary tract via the urethra, bladder, and ureters. The normal bladder is an effective barrier to these infections, but any obstruction to the flow of urine, such as enlarged prostate, renal cysts, pregnancy, or a urinary stone, will weaken this barrier. Sometimes, pathogens infect the kidneys through the blood. Most urinary tract infections can be effectively treated with antibiotics. It is important for the physician to choose an antibiotic that is effective against the causative pathogen. Each antibiotic is effective against only a few types of bacteria, and many different bacteria can cause urinary tract infections.

Infections involving the kidney are especially serious. Because the kidneys are essential to life, these infections must be treated promptly and completely. Some infections affect the kidney even after the infection is cured. The body reacts to pathogens by producing proteins called antibodies, which circulate in the bloodstream. Antibodies in the blood can coat and damage the glomerular filters in Bowman's capsules. This reduces the effectiveness of the filters, allowing blood and protein to enter the urine and causing the body to become puffy. The medical term for this serious kidney disease is glomerulonephritis. Treatment is available, but it is better to prevent the disease from occurring. If left untreated, the kidney damage may be so extensive that dialysis or transplantation is required to prevent death.

PERSPECTIVE AND PROSPECTS

The ancient Greeks seem to be the earliest people whose writings about the kidney have survived. They had no regard for the importance of this organ, mainly because their frame of reference consisted of four "humors." Even before 500 B.C.E., the Greeks were developing the doctrine of the four elements of the inanimate universe: air, fire, water, and earth. From

this idea, Polybus, the son-in-law of Hippocrates, created the corollary of the four "humors" responsible for life: yellow bile (choler), blood, phlegm (pituita), and black bile (melancholia). The concept of humors dominated the thinking of Aristotle (384-322 B.C.E.) when he wrote about his study of the anatomy of kidneys in several animals, including humans. This approach delayed an understanding of even the basic concept that kidneys and urine are related, an idea finally proposed about 290 B.C.E. by Erasistratus of Ceos.

Knowledge of Erasistratus comes mainly from Galen (129-c. 199 C.E.). Galen, rather than applauding the advances of his forebears, ridiculed unfounded assertions. He conducted physiological experiments on living animals, such as observing the effect of cutting and tying one ureter while leaving the opposite one intact. His experiments yielded much information about renal physiology. The writings of Galen formed the foundation of medical knowledge for the next four hundred years. Students and teachers, rather than building upon the experimental process, accepted the proclamations of Galen as dogma.

The next great advance in renal knowledge came from the Italian anatomist Bartolommeo Eustachio (1520-1574), who, without the benefit of a microscope, discovered the renal tubules and their relationship to the renal vascular system. His descriptions and drawings of 1564 were lost in the Vatican library until 1714. In the meantime, another Italian, Lorenzo Bellini (1643-1704), independently discovered the renal tubules and discerned their function. A contemporary, Marcello Malpighi (1628-1694), discovered glomeruli and their relationship to tubules.

Subsequent advances had to wait until the nineteenth century, when knowledge of all aspects of human biology and medicine began a rapid advance. Many independent advances in the nineteenth and twentieth centuries—in surgery, pharmacology, and immunology—made the transplantation of kidneys and other major organs possible. General anesthesia was developed independently by two Americans: by Crawford Long in 1842 and by William T. G. Morton in 1846. Antiseptic procedures were originated in 1867 by the Englishman Joseph Lister, and vascular surgical techniques were developed in 1902 by French surgeon Alexis Carrel and Hungarian surgeon Emerich Ullman. Anticoagulants were developed in 1914 and 1915, and systemic antibiotics were developed in the 1930's and 1940's. Blood typing was begun in Europe by Karl Landsteiner (1868-1943). Tissue immunology was first explained in 1953, and tissue typing was introduced in France and the United States in the 1960's. Immunosuppressive drugs were developed during this same period. Kidney transplantation is also possible because of extracorporeal support devices such as the dialysis machine, the heart-lung machine, and the organ perfusion machine.

The first transplant of a human kidney between identical twins was performed on December 23, 1954, by Joseph E. Murray. He later performed the first human kidney transplant between unrelated persons on April 5, 1962. By the 1990's, tens of thousands of kidney transplants were being performed in the United States every year. There are many more persons waiting for a transplant than there are kidneys available for transplantation. The solution to this problem is unclear. Transplants between living persons in the same family may be encouraged, and transplants from animals to humans may be perfected. It is even possible that a transplantable artificial kidney can be developed, but this task will be enormously difficult, considering all the functions of a natural kidney.

—*Armand M. Karow, Ph.D.*

See also Adrenalectomy; Blood and blood disorders; Circulation; Cysts; Dialysis; Glomerulonephritis; Internal medicine; Kidney disorders; Kidney transplantation; Laparoscopy; Lithotripsy; Nephrectomy; Nephritis; Nephrology; Nephrology, pediatric; Renal failure; Stone removal; Stones; Systems and organs; Transplantation; Urinalysis; Urinary disorders; Urinary system; Urology; Urology, pediatric.

FOR FURTHER INFORMATION:

Andreoli, Thomas E., et al., eds. *Cecil Essentials of Medicine*. 5th ed. Philadelphia: W. B. Saunders, 2001. This paperback book, written for physicians, describes diseases and their treatment in humans. Contains a good section on the kidneys.

Brenner, Barry M., and Floyd C. Rector, Jr., eds. *Brenner and Rector's Kidney*. 2 vols. 6th ed. Philadelphia: W. B. Saunders, 1999. This treatise, at more than two thousand pages, is the most comprehensive and authoritative source on the normal and diseased human kidney.

Davidson, Bill. *Gary Coleman: Medical Miracle*. New York: Coward, McCann & Geoghegan, 1981. Davidson, a professional writer, provides a biography of a thirteen-year-old television comedian and kidney transplant recipient. Coleman's story, told from the perspective of family members, presents heartaches and triumphs.

Gottschalk, Carl W., Robert W. Berliner, and Gerhard H. Giebisch, eds. *Renal Physiology: People and Ideas*. Bethesda, Md.: American Physiological Society, 1987. This collection of scholarly essays traces the historical development of renal physiology. While the work is exhaustive and comprehensive, emphasis is placed on the nineteenth and twentieth centuries.

Vander, Arthur J. *Renal Physiology*. 5th ed. New York: McGraw-Hill, 1995. This paperback book, written for medical students, describes the anatomy and physiology of the normal human kidney. Provides extensive, exhaustive information in a comprehensible format. The text may be somewhat challenging for those who have not taken introductory college-level courses in chemistry and biology.

KINESIOLOGY

SPECIALTY

ANATOMY OR SYSTEM AFFECTED: Brain, cells, circulatory system, heart, lungs, muscles, musculoskeletal system, nervous system, psychic-emotional system, respiratory system, spine

SPECIALTIES AND RELATED FIELDS: Cardiology, exercise physiology, orthopedics, physical therapy, psychology, sports medicine

DEFINITION: The applied science of human movement, which combines the general areas of anatomy (the study of structure) and physiology (the study of function).

SCIENCE AND PROFESSION

In 1989, the American Academy of Physical Education endorsed the term "kinesiology" to describe the entire field traditionally known as physical education, which includes the following subdisciplines: exercise physiology, biomechanics, motor control and learning, sports nutrition, sports psychology, sports sociology, athletic training programs, pedagogy, adapted physical education, cardiac rehabilitation, and physical therapy.

Exercise physiology describes the body's muscular, cardiovascular, and respiratory functioning during both short-term and long-term exercise. Research has focused on muscle fiber typing, oxygen uptake assessment, lactic acid metabolism, thermoregulation, body composition, and muscle hypertrophy. Biomechanics applies Isaac Newton's laws of physics to improve the mechanical efficiency of muscle movement patterns; using high-speed video and computer analysis, flaws in joint and limb dynamics can be assessed and changed to optimize performance. Motor control and learning pinpoint the areas of the brain and spinal cord that are responsible for the acquisition and retention of motor skills. Understanding the neurological basis of reflex and voluntary muscle movements helps to refine teaching strategies and describe the mechanisms of fatigue.

Sports nutrition describes how the body stores, circulates, and converts nutrients for aerobic and anaerobic energy production through carbohydrate loading and other strategies. Sports psychology explores the workings of the mind before, during, and after exercise and competition. Sports sociology examines aspects such as cultural, ethnic, and gender differences, dynamics in small and large groups, and the role of sports in ethical and moral development. Athletic trainers work with sports physicians and surgeons to prevent and rehabilitate injuries caused by overuse, trauma, or disease. Physical therapists use clinical exercise therapy and other modalities in a variety of rehabilitation settings.

Allied health areas under the kinesiology umbrella include pedagogy (teaching progressions for movement skills), adapted physical education (activities for the physically and mentally challenged), and cardiac rehabilitation (recovery stages for those disabled by heart disease). Professional organizations in the field of kinesiology include the American College of Sports Medicine, the American Physical Therapy Association, the National Athletic Trainers Association, the National Strength and Conditioning Association, and the American Alliance for Health, Physical Education, Recreation, and Dance.

—*Daniel G. Graetzer, Ph.D.*

See also Allied health; Anatomy; Cardiac rehabilitation; Exercise physiology; Muscles; Nervous system; Neurology; Physical rehabilitation; Physiology; Respiration; Sports medicine.

For Further Information:

Brooks, George A., and Thomas D. Fahey. *Fundamentals of Human Performance.* New York: Macmillan, 1987.

Costill, David L. *Inside Running: Basics of Sports Physiology.* Indianapolis: Benchmark, 1986.

Sharkey, Brian J. *Physiology of Fitness.* 3d ed. Champaign, Ill.: Human Kinetics Books, 1990.

KLINEFELTER SYNDROME
DISEASE/DISORDER

ANATOMY OR SYSTEM AFFECTED: Breasts, endocrine system, genitals, hair, psychic-emotional system, reproductive system

SPECIALTIES AND RELATED FIELDS: Embryology, endocrinology, genetics, psychology

DEFINITION: A male chromosomal disorder causing infertility and significant femaleness.

CAUSES AND SYMPTOMS

Klinefelter syndrome is caused by a variation in the number of sex chromosomes. Normal males possess one X and one Y chromosome, while females have two X chromosomes. When an embryo has two X chromosomes and one Y chromosome (XXY), normal development and reproductive function are hampered and the boy shows the symptoms of Klinefelter syndrome. These symptoms include breast development, incomplete maleness, and school or social difficulties. The major symptom is sterility or very reduced fertility. The testes remain small after puberty and produce few, if any, sperm.

In adolescence, breast tissue develops significantly in about 50 percent of all cases. In addition, normal facial and pubic hair may not develop in these boys. Although their average height is six feet, young men with Klinefelter syndrome are often unathletic and less physically strong or coordinated than their peers. Some affected individuals exhibit some degree of subnormal intelligence. Others appear passive and without self-confidence or experience difficulties learning language and speech.

TREATMENT AND THERAPY

Klinefelter syndrome is diagnosed using a karyotype, an analysis of the chromosomes from blood or cheek cells. It can determine the presence of forty-seven chromosomes, including one Y and two X. Although Klinefelter syndrome is genetic and cannot be cured, treatment in the form of a monthly injection of testosterone can be administered to supplement the usually insufficient amount produced by the boy's own testes. This therapy should enhance male physical development by increasing the size of the penis and causing pubic and facial hair growth and greater muscle bulk.

Hormone therapy cannot increase the size of the testes, however, nor can it cure sterility. It cannot reverse breast tissue development, which can only be treated by surgical removal. It may, however, increase self-esteem and a sense of maleness, thereby easing social interactions.

PERSPECTIVE AND PROSPECTS

Found in one or two in every thousand males born, Klinefelter syndrome is the most common human chromosomal variation. Described by Harry Klinefelter in 1942, its cause was discovered by Patricia Jacobs and John Strong in 1959. Affected males have normal erections and may suffer no major effects other than those mentioned above.

—*Grace D. Matzen*

See also Genetic diseases; Genetics and inheritance; Gynecomastia; Hermaphroditism and pseudohermaphroditism; Puberty and adolescence; Reproductive system; Sexual diffentiation.

FOR FURTHER INFORMATION:

Bandmann, H.-J., and R. Breit., eds. *Klinefelter's Syndrome.* New York: Springer-Verlag, 1984.

Theilgaard, Alice, et al. *A Psychological-Psychiatric Study of Patients with Klinefelter's Syndrome.* Aarhus, Denmark: Universitetsforlaget i Aarhus, 1971.

Zuppinger, Klaus. *Klinefelter's Syndrome: A Clinical and Cytogenetic Study in Twenty-Four Cases.* Copenhagen: Periodica, 1967.

KNEECAP REMOVAL

PROCEDURE

ANATOMY OR SYSTEM AFFECTED: Bones, joints, knees, legs, muscloskeletal system, tendons

SPECIALTIES AND RELATED FIELDS: General surgery, orthopedics

DEFINITION: The surgical removal of the kneecap.

INDICATIONS AND PROCEDURES

The kneecap, or patella, is the triangular bone at the front of the knee. It is held in position by the lower end of the quadriceps muscle, which surrounds the patella and is attached to the upper part of the tibia by the patellar tendon. The role of the kneecap is to protect the knee.

Kneecap removal surgery, or patellectomy, is performed as a result of fracture, frequent dislocation, or painful arthritis in the kneecap. Fracture is usually caused by a direct or sharp blow to the knee. Dislocation of the patella is often linked to a congenital abnormality, such as the underdevelopment of the lower end of the femur or excessive laxity of the lig-

aments that support the knee. Painful degenerative arthritic conditions, such as retropatellar arthritis and chondromalacia patelae, inflame and roughen the undersurface of the kneecap. Arthritic pain often worsens with the climbing of stairs or bending of the knee.

Before surgery begins, a clinical examination is conducted including blood and urine studies, and X rays of both knees. The knee is thoroughly cleansed with antiseptic soap. Anesthesia is administered either by local injection or spinal injection or by inhalation and injection (general anesthesia).

Surgery begins with an incision made around the kneecap. The skin is pulled back, exposing the muscle-covered kneecap. Surrounding muscle and connecting tendons attached to the kneecap are cut, and the kneecap is carefully removed. The remaining muscle is then sewn back together with strong suture material. Surgery is completed with the closing of the skin with sutures or clips. Full recovery takes about six weeks.

USES AND COMPLICATIONS

Following surgery, a scar will form along the incision. As the incision heals, the scar will recede gradually. Pain from the incision can be alleviated with heating pads. The affected leg should be elevated with pillows. Frequent movement of legs while resting in bed will decrease the likelihood of deep vein blood clots. General activity and returning to work is encouraged as soon as possible. Standing for prolonged periods of time, however, is not recommended during recovery. Following the approximate six-week recovery time, physical therapy is often used to restore strength to the knee.

Possible complications associated with kneecap removal include excessive bleeding and surgical wound infection. Additional complications can occur during recovery if general postoperative guidelines are not followed. Some loss of function can be expected.

—*Jason Georges*

See also Arthritis; Bones and the skeleton; Fracture and dislocation; Lower extremities; Orthopedic surgery; Orthopedics; Orthopedics, pediatric; Physical rehabilitation.

FOR FURTHER INFORMATION:

Bentley, George, and Robert B. Greer, eds. *Orthopaedics.* 4th ed. Oxford, England: Linacre House, 1993.

Tapley, Donald F., et al., eds. *The Columbia University College of Physicians and Surgeons Complete*

Home Medical Guide. Rev. 3d. ed. New York: Crown, 1995.

Tierney, Lawrence M., Jr., Stephen J. McPhee, and Maxine A. Papadakis, eds. *Current Medical Diagnosis and Treatment: 2001*. 39th ed. New York: McGraw-Hill, 2000.

Way, Lawrence W., ed. *Current Surgical Diagnosis and Treatment*. 11th ed. Norwalk, Conn.: Appleton & Lange, 1998.

KNOCK-KNEES
DISEASE/DISORDER

ALSO KNOWN AS: Genu valgum

ANATOMY OR SYSTEM AFFECTED: Bones, knees, legs

SPECIALTIES AND RELATED FIELDS: Orthopedics, physical therapy

DEFINITION: Knock-knees refers specifically to the bending out of the lower legs so that the knees touch but the ankles do not. It generally does not occur in children before puberty unless the child is obese. Knock-knees may develop throughout puberty, usually manifesting itself in girls rather than in boys. This bending occurs as a result of the widening of a young woman's hips through puberty. In some cases, patellar (kneecap) tracking problems may occur; therapeutic exercises or surgery may be needed to alleviate the problem.

—Alan J. Coelho, Ed.D.

See also Bones and the skeleton; Growth; Lower extremities; Obesity; Orthopedics; Orthopedics, pediatric; Puberty and adolescence.

FOR FURTHER INFORMATION:

Crouch, James E. *Functional Human Anatomy*. 4th ed. Philadelphia: Lea & Febiger, 1985.

Thompson, George H., "Common Orthopedic Problems of Children." In *Nelson Essentials of Pediatrics*, edited by Richard E. Behrman and Robert M. Kliegman. 3d ed. Philadelphia: W. B. Saunders, 1998.

Wenger, Dennis R., and Mercer Rang. *The Art and Practice of Children's Orthopaedics*. New York: Raven Press, 1993.

KWASHIORKOR
DISEASE/DISORDER

ANATOMY OR SYSTEM AFFECTED: Gastrointestinal system, intestines, stomach

SPECIALTIES AND RELATED FIELDS: Nutrition, pediatrics, public health

DEFINITION: Its name derived from a Ghanaian word, kwashiorkor is a protein-deficiency disease that usually affects young children in developing countries. When children in these countries are weaned, they may suddenly be placed on protein-poor diets that cannot provide adequate nutrients. The results of this severe malnutrition are stunted growth, weakness, and apathy. With kwashiorkor, the child suffers from edema, a swelling of the tissues, even though dehydration may be present. Serious complications of this disease include an enlarged liver, jaundice, and an ineffective immune system; a severe infection may prove fatal. Kwashiorkor can be treated with supplements to control the edema, followed by a high-protein diet; most children recover.

—Jason Georges and Tracy Irons-Georges

See also Bleeding; Edema; Jaundice; Malnutrition; Nutrition.

FOR FURTHER INFORMATION:

Garrow, J. S., and W. P. T. James, eds. *Human Nutrition and Dietetics*. 10th ed. New York: Churchill Livingstone, 2000.

Kreutler, Patricia A., and Dorice M. Czajka-Narins. *Nutrition in Perspective*. 2d ed. Englewood Cliffs, N.J.: Prentice Hall, 1987.

Wardlaw, Gordon M., Paul M. Insel, and Marcia F. Seyler. *Contemporary Nutrition*. St. Louis: Mosby Year Book, 1991.

Winick, Myron, Brian L. G. Morgan, Jaime Rozovski, and Robin Marks-Kaufman, eds. *The Columbia Encyclopedia of Nutrition*. New York: G. P. Putnam's Sons, 1988.

KYPHOSIS
DISEASE/DISORDER

ANATOMY OR SYSTEM AFFECTED: Back, bones

SPECIALTIES AND RELATED FIELDS: Orthopedics

DEFINITION: A marked increase of the normal curvature of the thoracic vertebrae or upper back, sometimes referred to as dowager's hump because of its prevalence in elderly women.

CAUSES AND SYMPTOMS

Patients with kyphosis appear to be looking down with their shoulders markedly bent forward. They are unable to straighten their backs, their body height is reduced, and their arms therefore appear to be disproportionately long. The increased curvature of the thoracic vertebrae tilts the head forward, and the patient has to raise her head and hyperextend her neck in order to look forward. This posture increases the strain on the neck muscles and leads to discomfort in the neck, shoulders, and upper back. It limits the field of vision and increases the patient's chances of tripping over an object not directly in the line of vision. It also shifts forward the body's center of gravity and increases the chances of falling.

In severe cases, kyphosis limits chest expansion during breathing. As a result, less air gets into the lungs, which become underventilated and prone to infections. Pneumonia is a common cause of death in these patients. In very severe cases, the curvature of the thoracic vertebrae is so pronounced that the lower ribs lie over the pelvic cavity. Patients with severe kyphosis are not able to lie flat on their backs, and many spend most of their time sitting up in a chair or in bed, propped by a number of pillows. Unless the patient changes positions frequently, the pressure exerted by the vertebrae on the skin and subcutaneous tissue may precipitate pressure sores (bed sores) on the upper back. Pressure sores may also develop on the buttocks. The sores often become infected, and the infection may spread to the blood, leading to septicemia and death.

The most common cause of kyphosis is osteoporosis, a disease in which the bone mass is reduced. As a result, the bones become mechanically weak and are unable to sustain the pressure of the body weight. The vertebrae gradually become wedged and partially collapsed, more so in the front (anteriorly) than in the back (posteriorly), thus increasing the forward curvature of the thoracic vertebrae. Sometimes, the compression of a vertebra is associated with sudden, very severe, and incapacitating pain that is usually relieved spontaneously after about four weeks. In most cases, however, the compression is a gradual process associated with slowly worsening back discomfort. The discomfort is caused by the strain imposed on the muscles on either side of the vertebrae. In rare instances, the nerves exiting the spinal cord become trapped by the wedged or collapsed vertebrae, and the patient experiences severe pain that tends to radiate to the area supplied by the entrapped nerve.

Less common causes of kyphosis include the compression of a vertebra as a result of tumors or infections. In these cases, the angulation of the thoracic curvature is very prominent.

TREATMENT AND THERAPY

The availability of medications to treat and prevent osteoporosis should reduce significantly the prevalence of both that disease and kyphosis.

—*Ronald C. Hamdy, M.D.*

See also Bone disorders; Bones and the skeleton; Osteoporosis; Pneumonia; Safety issues for the elderly; Spinal cord disorders; Spine, vertebrae, and disks.

FOR FURTHER INFORMATION:

Byyny, Richard, and Leonard Speroff. *A Clinical Guide for the Care of Older Women*. Baltimore: Williams & Wilkins, 1990.

Crystal, Stephen. *America's Old-Age Crisis*. New York: Basic Books, 1982.

Heaney, Robert P. "Osteoporosis." In *Nutrition in Women's Health*, edited by Debra A. Krummel and Penny M. Kris-Etherton. Gaithersburg, Md.: Aspen, 1996.

Meredith, C. M. "Exercise in the Prevention of Osteoporosis." In *Nutrition of the Elderly*, edited by Hamish Munro and Gunter Schlierf. Nestle's Nutrition Workshop Series 29. New York: Raven Press, 1992.

LABORATORY TESTS

PROCEDURES

ANATOMY OR SYSTEM AFFECTED: Blood, cells

SPECIALTIES AND RELATED FIELDS: Bacteriology, cytology, endocrinology, epidemiology, forensic medicine, genetics, hematology, histology, immunology, microbiology, oncology, pathology, pharmacology, serology, toxicology, virology

DEFINITION: The collection and analysis of body fluids such as blood and urine in order to establish a diagnosis or to monitor a treatment regimen.

KEY TERMS:

antibody: a protein produced in the body by the immune system that recognizes and binds selectively to foreign material (antigens) to facilitate their elimination; antibodies can be cultivated in animals or by artificial means in the laboratory and chemically altered for use as reagents in immunoassays

clinical chemistry: a chemistry specialty which deals with an analysis of the chemical components of body fluids

clinical laboratory: a general term for those areas of a medical facility where analyses of body fluids are performed

clinical microbiology: the scientific discipline involving the study of microscopic organisms (such as bacteria, fungi, and viruses) that cause disease

coagulation: the process of blood clotting, a very complicated process that can be affected by many disease states; the clotting process is inhibited for specimen collection purposes using substances called anticoagulants

hematology: the medical specialty dealing with the detection and diagnosis of blood-related diseases

immunoassay: the use of antibody-antigen recognition as the basis of a medically useful method of detecting and measuring a substance in body fluids

pathology: the medical specialty that deals with the structural and biochemical changes that are produced by disease

INDICATIONS AND PROCEDURES

Clinical laboratory testing is a vital element in diagnosis. After physical examination and the taking of the patient's medical history, the physician will often request that specific tests be performed on blood, urine, or other body fluids. Appropriate specimens are collected and forwarded to the laboratory for specimen processing.

Blood is the most common specimen submitted for testing in the clinical laboratory. In a hospital or large referral laboratory, there may be special personnel, called phlebotomists, employed to collect blood. In a small office laboratory, blood may be collected by the attending physician or nurse. Blood is collected in a syringe or in special tubes which may contain anticoagulants.

Urine is the next most common laboratory specimen and is collected as a result of a single void (random urine specimen) or for a time period of twenty-four hours or more. In the latter case, the collection container may also contain substances that act as a preservative. If a long-term urine specimen is necessary, it is very important for the patient to follow the directions regarding collection. Failure to follow these directions can lead to erroneous laboratory results.

Less commonly collected specimens include cerebrospinal fluid, gastric (stomach) fluid, and amniotic fluid. Cerebrospinal fluid is usually collected by a physician by direct sampling with a needle (lumbar puncture, or spinal tap). Gastric fluid is obtained by the insertion of a gastric collection tube. Amniotic fluid is collected by an obstetrician in the process called amniocentesis, in which a sample of the fluid surrounding the fetus is removed by the insertion of a needle through the mother's abdomen. Frequently, laboratory tests are also ordered on infectious material associated with a wound or surgical incision.

A major aspect of specimen collection is ensuring that the sample is correctly labeled and that no mixup of specimens has occurred. Part of this process may involve checking identification armbands or asking patients or nursing staff to confirm identification. While this procedure may be exasperating to the patient or nursing personnel, it is a necessary part of detecting errors.

Immediately after the specimen is received in the laboratory, documentation of time of receipt and the tests requested is made, which is referred to as logging in the specimen. Each sample receives a special code called an accession number. The test performance and results are tracked with this number, since multiple specimens can be received on a single patient in a given day. This process is usually computerized and may utilize bar code labeling in a process very similar to that used for automatic cash-register pricing of grocery items.

In large hospital or referral laboratories, the processing center is responsible for distributing the sample to the laboratory sections, where various tests are performed. Since each test requires a specific amount of sample, specimen processing also involves determining that the correct amount of fluid has been collected and reserved for proper performance of the test.

For blood specimens, many laboratory determinations are made regarding plasma, or serum, which is the liquid component of blood that contains no cells. The whole blood specimen is separated into cellular and liquid components by centrifugation. The sample is spun rapidly so that the force of the spin sediments the cells, with the serum or plasma layer on top.

Once the specimen is distributed to the pertinent laboratory sections, testing is done using a variety of analytical techniques. The testing methodology is almost as varied as the types of analyses requested. A few general statements, however, are applicable. Automation is the guiding force behind laboratory test methodology development. Routinely ordered tests are done with instruments specifically designed to perform a group or panel of tests, rather than each test

being performed individually by a technologist using manual chemistry methods. Automation coupled with computerization has greatly increased laboratory efficiency, decreased turnaround time (the time required for a test to be performed and results to be reported to the physician), eliminated human errors, and allowed more tests to be performed on smaller test sample material. The latter advantage is particularly important for pediatric specimens, in which sample size is usually an important consideration. Automation also eliminates much of the technologist's contact with the specimen, considerably reducing the risk of spreading infectious diseases.

Each section of the laboratory is responsible for a specific set of tests. The chemistry section performs chemical analyses of body fluids. Panels of tests related to kidney, heart, and liver function are also done. In addition, tests to measure amounts of therapeutic drugs, hormones, blood proteins, and cancer-related proteins are accomplished with immunoassay techniques. The development of antibody-related techniques has revolutionized testing in all areas of the clinical laboratory. The ability to customize antibody

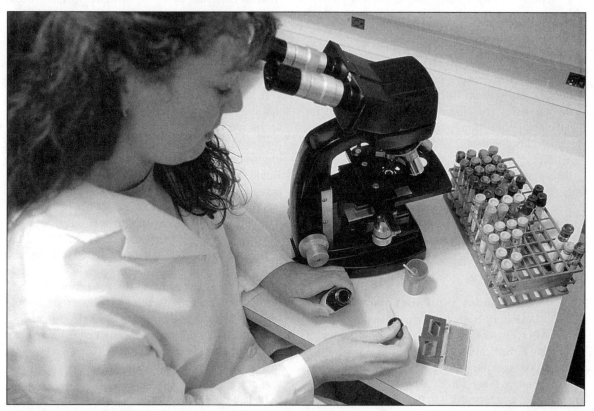

Laboratory tests are vital in the diagnosis of disease. A scientist examines samples with a microscope. (PhotoDisc)

production and adapt it to specific analytical requirements has allowed the continual development of new tests and methodologies.

The hematology section is responsible for monitoring the level of blood cells and clotting factors. Other specialized tests to diagnose cancer of the blood cells may also be done. Blood typing and donor testing are technically hematology-related tests, but they are usually reserved for a separate section designated as blood bank or transfusion services. Transfusion service is a specialty in its own right and is almost always reserved for hospital-associated laboratories.

Microbiology is the section where body fluids are checked for infectious microorganisms. Once an organism is identified, the section can also determine which antibiotics may be useful for treatment by performing antibiotic susceptibility tests.

As the laboratory tests are performed, the results are recorded and reported to the physician. Computerization has permitted the transfer of patient results directly from the instrument performing the test to the patient's file, eliminating many tedious and error-prone clerical functions.

For hospital and reference laboratories, a laboratory director—either a physician (usually a pathologist) who specialized in laboratory medicine or a scientist with doctoral level training in a laboratory specialty—monitors the performance of the laboratory, helps physicians with the interpretation of ambiguous or complex laboratory results, and provides guidance on the introduction of new tests or instrumentation. Most laboratories also have a section supervisor or administrator who is an experienced medical technologist to oversee the daily laboratory routine.

In the United States, hospital and reference laboratories are inspected periodically by federal and state government agencies as well as professional medical societies to check the quality of the work performed. The most commonly used proficiency testing program is that administered by the College of American Pathology (CAP), which also sponsors a program of peer inspection of laboratories. Many state and federal agencies will accept CAP approval of a laboratory as a substitute for a detailed inspection by its own agency.

USES AND COMPLICATIONS
Because of the variety of laboratory testing, it is impractical to cover its applications in depth in a brief review. Instead, a few illustrative tests which are per-

formed often or which are associated with familiar disorders will be presented. The most frequently ordered laboratory tests are serum glucose tests, serum electrolyte (salt) level measurements, and complete blood count (CBC) tests.

The maintenance of blood glucose (sugar) levels is essential for body activity and brain function. The laboratory measurement of blood glucose is one of the oldest known procedures performed in the clinical laboratory. It is part of the diagnostic procedures used to monitor and test for diabetes mellitus. Glucose and electrolyte testing are performed in the chemistry section of the laboratory, while a CBC takes place in hematology. Certain levels of electrolytes—sodium, chloride, potassium, and calcium—are needed for proper cardiac function. An abnormal level of these salts could also indicate possible hormonal or kidney malfunction. The CBC is a measure of the cell populations that carry oxygen (red blood cells), fight infection or invasion by foreign substances (white blood cells), and activate the blood-clotting mechanism (platelets). The white cell population is elevated in infections but also in cases of leukemia (malignant growth of a white cell population). More specialized testing is needed when leukemia is suspected. An instrument called a flow cytometer can be used to count and detect subtypes of white cells. These data, along with a pathologist's microscopic examination of a blood smear and the results of clinical examination, are used to arrive at a diagnosis of the specific type of leukemia present. The identification of the cell population causing the cancer is important for determining treatment and prognosis.

A deficiency of red cells or their oxygen-carrying hemoglobin molecule is called anemia. It can be caused by iron deficiency and other impairments of red cell production, chronic bleeding, or accelerated red cell destruction (hemolysis). Each of the causes must be either confirmed or ruled out through additional testing or by clinical examination.

Platelet deficiency is a major cause of clotting disorders, although many other causes of bleeding disorders are possible. The specific defect can be determined by measuring the clotting time and by using special immunoassays to measure clotting substances in the blood.

Many hormonal (endocrine) disorders can be diagnosed through laboratory testing. For example, the thyroid, the regulator gland for body metabolism, can produce a variety of symptoms when it is not functioning properly. Thyroid testing is the most common endocrine-related laboratory procedure requested by physicians. The blood levels of thyroid hormone and of the pituitary factor that stimulates the thyroid gland are measured in the laboratory using immunoassay methods. These types of assays can also be used to monitor other hormones involved in fertility, growth, and the function of the adrenal gland (the gland that helps maintain sugar metabolism and electrolyte balance).

Immunoassay methodology has also permitted the routine laboratory testing of therapeutic drugs as well as of drugs of abuse. In the past, the technology for analyzing drugs in biological fluids involved expensive, labor-intensive techniques that were impractical for routine laboratory use. With the introduction of immunologically based testing for drugs, however, it became possible to monitor patients on antibiotics, immunosuppressive agents, cardiac drugs, and anti-seizure medication. Testing has been automated so that these drug levels can be performed as routine laboratory procedures. Assay results can be used to establish an individual dosage schedule so that dosage is maintained in the therapeutic range and does not exceed the concentration threshold leading to toxic effects or decline to values too low to achieve adequate treatment (subtherapeutic levels).

A continuing research effort is directed toward developing specific diagnostic cancer tests. These tests could be used to screen patients for tumors in order to detect them early, when therapy would be most effective. Substances that appear in body fluids coincident with the growth of tumors are referred to as tumor markers. The ideal tumor marker would appear only in patients afflicted with a specific type of cancer. Its concentration would reflect the size of the tumor as well as the presence of metastasis, in which tumor cells migrate from the initial cancer site to other sites in the body.

The ideal tumor marker has not yet been discovered. Most have not been specific or sensitive enough to use as a screening tool for detecting tumors, although they have been useful for monitoring the effects of therapy. One example of a useful marker is prostate-specific antigen (PSA). The level of this protein in serum is very low when the prostate gland is normal. When prostate cancer is present, however, the serum level, as measured by immunoassay, is elevated. The test can also be used for screening, provided that any positive result is confirmed by clinical examination. It is also used following prostate surgery or radiation therapy in order to determine the completeness of tumor removal. Continually high or rising levels of PSA in the serum following treatment indicate that residual tumor is still present.

In the microbiology department, the culturing of body fluids and antibiotic susceptibility studies allow the selection of the most appropriate antibiotic for treatment. The course and duration of treatment can then be followed in the chemistry laboratory using the therapeutic drug monitoring techniques discussed above. When an infection is suspected, body fluids are cultured or incubated with media selected to grow only specific microorganisms. Antibiotic susceptibility studies are performed by culturing the organism with various antibiotics until growth is arrested. Many strains of bacteria and other microorganisms will become resistant to an antibiotic which had proven effective previously, and patients who are allergic to some antibiotics may need to be treated with an alternative regimen.

The detection and identification of viruses has become a subspecialty in microbiology with distinctly different culturing techniques. Newer immunoassay methods and other biotechnologically based methods have made virus diagnosis easier. Acquired immunodeficiency syndrome (AIDS) testing is a prime example of the application of immunoassay techniques to virology testing. A detection technique which required growth of the human immunodeficiency virus (HIV) in the laboratory would be extraordinarily difficult and tedious. It would also be prohibitively expensive and time-consuming to screen large populations such as blood donors and high-risk groups. Instead, laboratory screening for HIV utilizes an automated immunoassay technique based on the detection of patient antibodies to virus-specific antigens. Although this test is very specific, the possibility of false positives is greatly minimized by confirming all positive screening results with another antibody test called a Western blot. In this test, a serum sample from a suspected HIV-positive patient is applied to a membrane impregnated with virus proteins. The virus proteins are localized at a characteristic position determined by their migration rate when the membrane coated with virus proteins is subjected to an electric field in a process called protein electrophoresis. After the membrane has been treated with patient serum and color development reagents, the presence in the patient sample of an antibody to one or more of these proteins is revealed as a colored stripe on the membrane. A combination of the two tests is a cost-efficient and extremely accurate procedure to confirm a suspected diagnosis of HIV infection.

PERSPECTIVE AND PROSPECTS

According to a study of the history of the clinical laboratory by J. Büttner, the concept of the modern hospital laboratory was first documented in 1791 when French physician and chemist Antoine-François de Fourcroy, wrote that in hospitals "a chemical laboratory should be set up not far away from a ward having twenty or thirty beds." Büttner asserts that the two suppositions necessary for the creation of these laboratories were the idea that the results of laboratory examinations can be used as "chemical signs" in medical diagnosis and a new concept of disease which was the result of the "birth of the clinic" at the end of the eighteenth century.

During this phase of laboratory development, investigations were performed at patients' bedsides by physicians themselves. In the period from 1840 to 1855, clinical laboratories were established as operations distinct from hospitals and clinics. Most of these laboratories were developed in German-speaking countries and staffed by scientists who performed tests for the hospitals and taught medical students physiological chemistry. From 1855 onward, the concept of the clinical laboratory spread rapidly, with clinicians assuming directorship roles. The laboratory ultimately serving as a model for clinical laboratories in the United States was established by the renowned pathologist Rudolf Virchow at Berlin University. As the chair for pathological anatomy, he set up a "chemical department" within the institute for pathology in 1856. This laboratory represented a center of clinical chemistry research and established the clinical laboratory as integral to pathology.

Laboratories have evolved as essential but distinctly separate specialties of medical services. Although there is little or no participation in the analytical process by the physicians ordering the tests, a major part of a physician's diagnostic skill is knowing which tests to order as a supplement to examination and medical history. Laboratory tests cost money and time and may be useless in the diagnostic process if not ordered in a judicious fashion. The old medical admonishment to "treat the patient, not the laboratory result" is still an appropriate consideration. Moreover, responsibility for the correct interpretation of the results lies with the attending physician, who has access to all the pertinent patient data.

Laboratory results are usually interpreted with the help of a reference range. Reference ranges ideally represent laboratory values characteristic of a sample population which is free of known disease. If the results lie within this range, however, the laboratory result cannot always be assumed to rule out a specific diagnosis. Since considerable biological variation exists for most laboratory values, diseased individuals can sometimes yield test values in the normal range and, conversely, healthy individuals can occasionally have low or elevated values.

In order to verify a diagnosis, all laboratory results and clinical impressions should complement one another. The detection of blood-clotting deficiencies by the hematology department could be related to a poorly functioning liver, which will also be reflected in changes in enzymes and blood proteins measured in the chemistry laboratory. Cardiac disorders are diagnosed not only by examining an electrocardiograph (EKG or ECG) but also by measuring the levels of specific cardiac-related enzymes which rise to abnormally high levels when cardiac blood supply is diminished (such as with myocardial infarction, or heart attack). In summary, the clinical laboratory provides a valuable tool for physicians, but it should never displace clinical examination and medical history as methods of determining the final diagnosis.

—*David J. Wells, Jr., Ph.D.*

See also Amniocentesis; Bacteriology; Biopsy; Blood and blood disorders; Blood testing; Breast biopsy; Cells; Cytology; Cytopathology; DNA and RNA; Endometrial biopsy; Forensic pathology; Genetic engineering; Genetics and inheritance; Gram staining; Hematology; Hematology, pediatric; Histology; Hormones; Microbiology; Microscopy; Pathology; Screening; Serology; Toxicology; Urinalysis.

FOR FURTHER INFORMATION:

Bennington, James L., ed. *Saunders Dictionary and Encyclopedia of Laboratory Medicine and Technology.* Philadelphia: W. B. Saunders, 1984. An excellent reference to laboratory vocabulary and terminology. Gives detailed information about complicated procedures and topics, rather than a simple dictionary definition.

Henry, John B., ed. *Clinical Diagnosis and Management by Laboratory Methods.* 20th ed. Philadelphia: W. B. Saunders, 2001. The classic text on the clinical laboratory. Multiple authors cover all aspects of laboratory operations, including management and administration. The most recent edition should be consulted.

Price, Christopher P., and David J. Newman, eds. *Principles and Practice of Immunoassay.* 2d ed. New York: Stockton Press, 1997. This work covers all aspects of immunoassays, including assay development, laboratory quality assurance, and test methodology.

Tietz, Norbert W. *Clinical Guide to Laboratory Tests.* 3d ed. Philadelphia: W. B. Saunders, 1995. A paperback condensation of the vital information needed for the interpretation of clinical laboratory tests. Tests are arranged alphabetically in tabular form for easy reference.

LACERATION REPAIR

PROCEDURE

ANATOMY OR SYSTEM AFFECTED: Skin

SPECIALTIES AND RELATED FIELDS: Emergency medicine, general surgery, plastic surgery

DEFINITION: The closure of an irregular skin wound.

INDICATIONS AND PROCEDURES

A laceration is a jagged, torn, mangled, or ragged wound. This type of wound is most commonly encountered in the skin, although any tissue may be lacerated. Lacerations are caused by sharp objects such as a piece of metal, glass, or a stick, or they may occur in accidents involving machinery or animals.

The first priority in laceration repair is to stop bleeding, thereby minimizing blood loss. This is usually accomplished by pressure either directly on the wound or on the injured blood vessel nearest the injury site.

The second priority with a laceration is to clean the wound, which involves the removal of any foreign material or debris. With penetrating injuries, this cleaning must be done carefully lest the removal of the object initiate bleeding. Tissue that has been destroyed beyond the body's ability to repair it must also be removed; this process is called debridement. Devitalized tissue is removed to prevent infection. The wound site is then cleaned through irrigation with saline and a disinfectant, usually a mild soap or a chemical.

Lacerations may then be treated for bacterial or other pathogenic contamination. Aqueous solutions

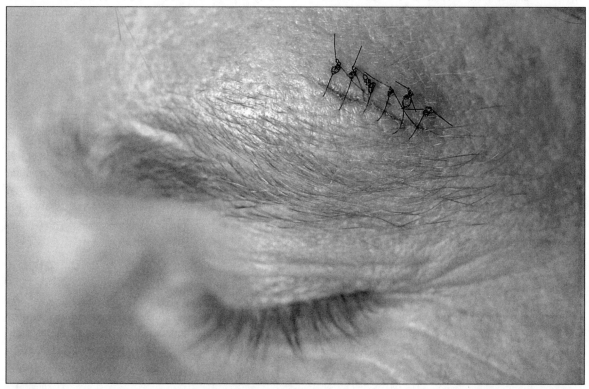

Stitches or sutures may be required to hold together the edges of lacerations that are large, deep, or ragged. (PhotoDisc)

containing an antibiotic are used with most wounds. If contamination with other pathogens is suspected, appropriate agents are used to rinse the wound. Antibiotic powders may be employed in field conditions, although this form of treatment is unusual in a hospital setting. Other than soap and water, there is no special treatment for viral contamination.

Closure of the wound is then completed. The edges are brought together and may be held in place with forceps. Sutures, or stitches, are inserted to hold the edges together while the tissue heals. On skin surfaces, these sutures are usually nonabsorbable and are later removed. The amount of time that sutures are kept in place varies with the location of the wound and the age of the patient: Mucous membranes heal more quickly than the palm, for example, and children's skin heals more rapidly than that of adults. Removable sutures are made of nylon or a similar material. Sutures that are used beneath the skin cannot be removed and are made of material that will break down within the body. Wound closure may also be accomplished with wire, staples, or adhesive tape. These materials have some advantages—durability (wire), ease of placement (staples), and minimal pain (tape)—and disadvantages—potential contamination (wire) and premature, accidental removal (tape). Lacerations should be rechecked by a physician when sutures or other means of wound closure are removed.

USES AND COMPLICATIONS

The techniques of laceration repair are used on all parts of the body where such wounds occur. Plastic surgery may be required to improve the appearance of the repaired tissue and to reduce scars when the patient believes that cosmetic results are an issue. In addition to scarring, other complications that may be associated with the repair of lacerations include infection and tetanus. All these problems can be minimized through good surgical techniques, the use of antibiotics, and careful postoperative care. The repair of lacerations on the face of all exposed areas of skin are especially important. Careful technique minimizes scarring, as do some new methods of wound closure.

—*L. Fleming Fallon, Jr., M.D., Ph.D., M.P.H.*

See also Bleeding; Emergency medicine; Grafts and grafting; Healing; Plastic surgery; Skin; Wounds.

FOR FURTHER INFORMATION:

Crosby, Lynn A., and David G. Lewallen, eds. *Emergency Care and Transportation of the Sick and In-jured.* 6th ed. Rosemont, Ill.: American Academy of Orthopaedic Surgeons, 1997.

Handal, Kathleen A. *The American Red Cross First Aid and Safety Handbook.* Boston: Little, Brown, 1992.

Thygerson, Alton L. *First Aid and Emergency Care Workbook.* Boston: Jones and Bartlett, 1987.

LACTOSE INTOLERANCE
DISEASE/DISORDER

ANATOMY OR SYSTEM AFFECTED: Gastrointestinal system, intestines, stomach

SPECIALTIES AND RELATED FIELDS: Gastroenterology, nutrition

DEFINITION: Lactose intolerance is an inability to break down and absorb milk sugar, known as lactose, resulting in stomach pain, gas, and diarrhea if lactose is consumed.

CAUSES AND SYMPTOMS

Lactose is a complex sugar commonly found in dairy products. It is composed of two simple sugars, glucose and galactose. In babies and young children, a gene produces an enzyme called lactase that breaks down lactose into its two component sugars, which are then absorbed into the bloodstream through the intestinal wall. In many people, sometime after early childhood, the lactase gene is "turned off." It no longer synthesizes lactase, which prevents the digestion and absorption of lactose.

Normal bacterial inhabitants of the intestines synthesize lactase and break down the lactose molecules, producing large quantities of gas as a by-product. This can lead to cramping for the lactose-intolerant individual. The presence of lactose in the large intestine causes excessive amounts of water to move into the intestine, which can lead to diarrhea. Symptoms subside one to two days after the last lactose-containing food has been consumed.

TREATMENT AND THERAPY

Lactose intolerance can often be misdiagnosed as a host of gastrointestinal disorders, largely as a result of the commonness of its major symptoms, cramps and diarrhea. Typically, a dietary history must be kept. Patients with lactose intolerance will note an association between their symptoms and the consumption of milk products containing lactose. After elimination of these products from the diets, symptoms should not recur.

There is no treatment for lactose intolerance; prevention of symptoms is the general course of action. Avoidance of foods that contain lactose—including milk, ice cream, and cheese—is usually the best recourse. For those who wish to indulge in these products, over-the-counter lactase pills are available; their use usually prevents symptoms of the disorder.

PERSPECTIVE AND PROSPECTS

The vast majority of the world's population is lactose intolerant, yet this disorder was not recognized in the United States until the latter third of the twentieth century. Today, lactase supplements are available to help prevent symptoms for lactose-intolerant people who choose to consume dairy products. Alternatively, more and more dairy products are being manufactured as lactose-free; they can be consumed safely by the lactose-intolerant population.

—*Karen E. Kalumuck, Ph.D.*

See also Diarrhea and dysentery; Digestion; Enzymes; Gastroenterology; Gastroenterology, pediatric; Gastrointestinal disorders; Gastrointestinal system; Irritable bowel syndrome (IBS); Nutrition.

FOR FURTHER INFORMATION:

Gracey, Michael, ed. *Diarrhea.* Boca Raton, Fla.: CRC Press, 1991.

Greenberger, Norton J. *Gastrointestinal Disorders: A Pathophysiologic Approach.* 4th ed. Chicago: Year Book Medical, 1989.

Janowitz, Henry D. *Your Gut Feelings: A Complete Guide to Living Better with Intestinal Problems.* Rev. ed. New York: Oxford University Press, 1994.

LAMINECTOMY AND SPINAL FUSION

PROCEDURES

ANATOMY OR SYSTEM AFFECTED: Back, bones, spine
SPECIALTIES AND RELATED FIELDS: General surgery, orthopedics
DEFINITION: Surgical procedures that join two or more vertebrae, the arching bones that make up the spine.

INDICATIONS AND PROCEDURES

Laminectomies, which are designed to relieve pressure on the spinal cord, are often performed as the initial surgery in cases of extreme back pain caused by the compression of the spinal canal. An incision is made in the patient's back to expose the laminae, the flattened portions of the vertebral arch, and one or more adjacent laminae are chipped away. On occasion, several laminae are excised.

In such cases, spinal fusion, which involves the immobilization of the spine with steel rods or bone grafts, is indicated. Spinal fusion, like laminectomy a major surgery done under general anesthesia, is performed if X rays reveal unusual motion between adjacent vertebrae.

The causes of the severe back pain that usually precedes laminectomy or spinal fusion may be related to three conditions: osteoarthritis, which causes deterioration of the spinal joints; scoliosis caused by an injury or tumor that is destroying vertebrae; or spondylolisthesis, the dislocation of facet joints. In spinal fusion, when the damaged vertebrae are exposed, joint fusion is sometimes performed by using bone chips from the patient's pelvis. Following surgery, the vertebrae are held in place with plates or screws.

USES AND COMPLICATIONS

Both laminectomy and spinal fusion usually relieve the persistent back pain that has caused patients to seek treatment. Such surgery involves distinct risks, inasmuch as the spinal cord is exposed and there is often considerable blood loss. In the hands of a seasoned orthopedic surgeon, however, the risk is minimized.

Recovery from the surgery can be slow and often involves up to six weeks of confinement in bed. After this confinement, patients are usually required to wear a plaster cast until final vertebral fusion has occurred. This process can take half a year.

Fusion sometimes places an additional burden on the rest of the spinal column. In some cases, this pressure results in renewed back pain in other areas of the spine. Additional surgery may be indicated to control this pain.

—*R. Baird Shuman, Ph.D.*

See also Bone grafting; Bones and the skeleton; Disk removal; Fracture and dislocation; Grafts and grafting; Orthopedic surgery; Orthopedics; Orthopedics, pediatric; Osteoarthritis; Scoliosis; Spinal cord disorders; Spine, vertebrae, and disks.

FOR FURTHER INFORMATION:

Cotler, J. M., and H. B. Cotler, eds. *Spinal Fusion: Science and Technique.* New York: Springer-Verlag, 1990.

Hitchon, Patrick W., Setti Rengachary, and Vincent

C. Traynelis. *Techniques in Spinal Fusion and Stabilization*. New York: Thieme Medical, 1994.

Szpalski, Marek, et al., eds. *Instrumental Fusion of the Degenerative Lumbar Spine: State of the Art, Questions, and Controversies*. Philadelphia: Lippincott-Raven, 1996.

Watkins, Robert G., and John S. Collis, Jr. *Lumbar Discectomy and Laminectomy*. Rockville, Md.: Aspen, 1987.

Yonenobu, K., K. Ono, and Y. Takemitsu, eds. *Lumbar Fusion and Stabilization*. New York: Springer, 1993.

LAPAROSCOPY

PROCEDURE

ANATOMY OR SYSTEM AFFECTED: Abdomen, gallbladder, gastrointestinal system, intestines, kidneys, reproductive system, urinary system, uterus

SPECIALTIES AND RELATED FIELDS: Endocrinology, gastroenterology, general surgery, gynecology

DEFINITION: The examination of the abdominal organs with a laparoscope, a fiber-optic tube which can also be used to perform surgery to correct several disease conditions.

KEY TERMS:

abdomen: the area of the body between the diaphragm and the pelvis; it contains the visceral organs

cholecystectomy: the surgical removal of the gallbladder

ectopic pregnancy: the development of a fertilized egg in a Fallopian tube instead of the uterus; can be fatal to the mother unless it is corrected surgically

endometriosis: a female reproductive disease in which cells from the uterine lining (the endometrium) grow outside the uterus, causing severe pain and infertility and sometimes the need for hysterectomy

Fallopian tubes: the two tubes through which eggs pass on the way from the ovaries to the uterus

general anesthesia: anesthesia that induces unconsciousness

implant: a section of endometrial tissue found outside the uterus

local anesthesia: anesthesia that numbs the feeling in a body part, administered by injection or direct application to the skin

INDICATIONS AND PROCEDURES

Laparoscopy is a surgical technique for examining the abdominal organs and for treating surgically many diseases of these organs. The instrument used is called a laparoscope. It is a flexible tube that contains fiber optics for visualization purposes and a channel through which physicians can pass special surgical instruments into the abdominal cavity.

Upon insertion of a laparoscope into the abdomen through a small surgical incision (usually near the navel), physicians can observe the liver, kidneys, gallbladder, pancreas, spleen, and exterior aspects of the intestines in both sexes. Hence the technique is useful for detecting cirrhosis of the liver, the presence of stones and tumors, and many other diseases of the abdominal organs. The female reproductive organs can also be examined in this manner.

Before laparoscopy can be carried out, the patient must fast for at least twelve hours. The patient is given a local or general anesthetic, depending on the purpose of the procedure. In exploratory abdominal examinations, the instrument is inserted into the abdomen through a small incision in the abdominal wall after local anesthesia has numbed it. Often, especially when extensive surgery is anticipated, the procedure begins after general anesthesia produces unconsciousness. Upon the completion of exploration or surgery, the laparoscope is withdrawn and the incision is closed.

Laparoscopic abdominal examination is often used to detect endometriosis, the presence of endometrial cells outside the uterus. This procedure begins with the administration of local anesthesia when only exploration or biopsy is planned. General anesthesia is used when the removal of implants (endometrial tissue) is anticipated. The entry incision is made near the navel, and the laparoscope is inserted. The fiber-optics system is used to search the abdominal organs for implants. Visibility of the abdominal organs is usually enhanced by pumping in a harmless gas, such as carbon dioxide, to distend the abdomen. After the confirmation of endometriosis, surgical implant removal is carried out immediately, unless the decision is made to institute drug therapy instead. Full recovery from this surgery requires only a day of postoperative bed rest and a week of curtailing activities.

Laparoscopy can also be employed for female sterilization. The patient is given a general anesthetic. After laparoscopic visualization of the Fallopian tubes in the gas-distended abdomen is achieved, surgical instruments for tube cauterization or cutting are introduced and the sterilization is carried out. The entire procedure often requires only thirty minutes, which is

Laparoscopy

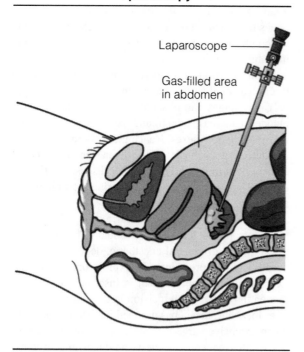

Laparoscope

Gas-filled area
in abdomen

Many surgical procedures involving the abdomen, such as appendectomy or the removal of eggs from the ovaries for in vitro fertilization, can be performed using laparoscopy. Gas is pumped into the abdominal cavity, and a fiber-optic scope and instruments are inserted through a small hole in the skin.

one reason for its popularity. In addition, patients can go home in a few hours and have fully recovered after a day or two of bed rest and seven to ten days of curtailing activities.

USES AND COMPLICATIONS

Common laparoscopic surgeries are cholecystectomy (the removal of the gallbladder), the removal of gallstones and kidney stones, tumor resection, female sterilization by cutting or blocking the Fallopian tubes, the treatment of endometriosis through the removal of implants from abdominal organs, and the removal of biopsy samples from abdominal organs. Traditional uses of laparoscopy in female reproductive surgery are to identify and correct pelvic pain resulting from endometriosis, ectopic pregnancy, and pelvic tumors.

Laparoscopy has several advantages. There is rarely a need for patients on chronic drug therapy to discontinue medication before laparoscopy. In addition, the use of laparoscopy dramatically lowers surgical inci-

sion size, surgical trauma, length of hospital stay, and recovery time. Laparoscopy should be avoided, however, in cases of advanced abdominal wall cancer, severe respiratory or cardiovascular disease, or tuberculosis. Extreme obesity does not disqualify a patient from undergoing laparoscopy but makes the procedure much more difficult to perform.

As laparoscopic surgery has increased in scope, more procedures yield surgical tissues that are larger in size than the laparoscope channel (for example, the removal of gallbladders, gallstones, and ovaries). In many cases these organs and structures are cut into small pieces for removal. If potentially dangerous items are involved—such as malignancies that can spread on dissection—larger, more conventional incisions are often combined with laparoscopy.

PERSPECTIVE AND PROSPECTS

Since the 1970's, the uses of laparoscopy have constantly expanded. Once confined to the exploratory examination of the abdomen, the methodology has been applied to a large number of different types of surgery in addition to those already mentioned. Such versatility is attributable to the development of better laparoscopes, advanced instrumentation for diverse surgeries, and improved fiber-optic and video technologies.

As a consequence of these advances, many surgeons predict that most future abdominal surgery will be laparoscopic. The driving force for such innovation includes the public demand for quicker recovery times. In the United States, this desire is intensified by the requirements of insurance companies, employers, and the federal government for shorter hospital stays. Both changes are made possible by decreased severity of surgical trauma in laparoscopy when compared to traditional surgery, a result of the smaller incisions. The dramatic trend toward laparoscopy can be seen with cholecystectomies: Of those done in 1992, 70 percent were laparoscopic, compared to less than 1 percent in 1989.

—Sanford S. Singer, Ph.D.

See also Abdomen; Abdominal disorders; Appendectomy; Appendicitis; Biopsy; Cholecystectomy; Ectopic pregnancy; Endometriosis; Endoscopy; Gynecology; Internal medicine; Sterilization; Stone removal; Stones; Tubal ligation; Tumor removal; Tumors.

FOR FURTHER INFORMATION:

Graber, John N., et al., eds. *Laparoscopic Abdominal Surgery.* New York: McGraw-Hill, 1993. A text for surgery residents and practicing surgeons wishing to gain an understanding of the theory and technique of laparoscopic surgery, written by experts in each area who were instrumental in the development of laparoscopic approaches. Abundantly illustrated with clear, detailed line drawings and color photographs.

Lauersen, Niels H., and Constance DeSwaan. *The Endometriosis Answer Book: New Hope, New Help.* New York: Rawson Associates, 1988. Endometriosis is one of the most insidious diseases of our time—and the leading cause of infertility in America today. Often misdiagnosed and undetected in its early stages, it is painful and debilitating and dramatically disrupts a woman's career and family life.

Reddick, Eddie Joe, ed. *An Atlas of Laparoscopic Surgery.* New York: Raven Press, 1993. Discusses such topics as cholecystectomy and peritoneoscopy. Includes an index.

Zucker, Karl A. *Surgical Laparoscopy.* Philadelphia: Lippincott, Williams & Wilkins, 2000. Discusses the gastrointestinal system, peritoneoscopy, and the methods of biliary tract surgery and endoscopic surgery.

LARYNGECTOMY
PROCEDURE

ANATOMY OR SYSTEM AFFECTED: Respiratory system, throat

SPECIALTIES AND RELATED FIELDS: General surgery, oncology, otorhinolaryngology

DEFINITION: The removal of all or part of the voice box, or larynx.

INDICATIONS AND PROCEDURES

Continued hoarseness and coughing can indicate laryngeal disorders. Polyps, which may be caused by excessive smoking or drinking, can form on the larynx. Children sometimes develop warts on it. Although these polyps and warts are generally benign, they should be removed and subjected to biopsy to preclude the presence of cancer.

Polyps, warts, and tumors are all detected quite easily with a laryngoscopic examination carried out by an otorhinolaryngologist with a mirror, an endoscope (a flexible fiber-optic tube), or a combination of the two. Such an examination, in addition to determining whether a growth is benign or cancerous, can detect signs of cancer in the lining of the larynx.

If cancer is detected early enough, radiation can usually control it. If the disease has advanced significantly, however, a laryngectomy may be necessary. In this surgical procedure, performed under general anesthesia, an incision is made in the neck and the larynx is removed. The windpipe directly below the larynx is then sewn to the skin around the surgical opening to form a permanent opening, or stoma, through which the patient breathes.

USES AND COMPLICATIONS

This surgery is used when cancer is sufficiently advanced that radiation therapy cannot destroy it. The major complication is that the patient's air supply is now taken through the stoma, meaning that swimming is precluded and that bathing must be undertaken with considerable caution.

A more apparent complication is that, with the loss of the larynx, one cannot speak. Through an extensive and painstaking course of speech therapy, however, esophageal speech can be achieved. This involves swallowing air and expelling it in such a way that it can be shaped by the palate, lips, and tongue into understandable words and sentences. An electronic larynx is also available. It makes a buzzing sound which, when pressed against the top of the throat, permits the patient to convert the sound into words.

—*R. Baird Shuman, Ph.D.*

See also Cancer; Endoscopy; Otorhinolaryngology; Speech disorders; Tumors; Warts.

FOR FURTHER INFORMATION:
Blom, Eric D., Mark I. Singer, and Ronald C. Hamaker. *Tracheoesophageal Voice Restoration Following Total Laryngectomy.* San Diego, Calif.: Singular, 1998.

Edels, Yvonne, ed. *Laryngectomy: Diagnosis to Rehabilitation.* Rockville, Md.: Aspen Systems, 1983.

Sataloff, Robert T. *Reflux Laryngitis and Related Disorders.* San Diego, Calif.: Singular, 1999.

Serafini, I. *Restoration of Laryngeal Function After Laryngectomy.* New York: Karger, 1969.

LARYNGITIS
DISEASE/DISORDER

ANATOMY OR SYSTEM AFFECTED: Respiratory system, throat

SPECIALTIES AND RELATED FIELDS: Family practice, otorhinolaryngology

DEFINITION: An inflammation of the larynx, or voice box, laryngitis may be chronic or acute. Its most distinguishing characteristic is a hoarseness in the voice; eventually, the ability to speak may be lost. Coughing, pain, and discomfort on swallowing may also occur. Acute laryngitis is caused by an infection, either viral or bacterial. Resting the voice, drinking warm liquids, and taking antibiotics if bacteria are to blame should restore the voice. Chronic laryngitis is caused by irritation, such as that produced by alcohol, tobacco, and chemical fumes; by overuse of the voice, as sometimes found with singers; by chronic coughing; or (rarely) by a malignant tumor.

—*Jason Georges and Tracy Irons-Georges*
See also Common cold; Laryngectomy; Multiple chemical sensitivity syndrome; Nasopharyngeal disorders; Otorhinolaryngology; Pharyngitis; Sore throat; Strep throat; Tonsillectomy and adenoid removal; Tonsillitis; Voice and vocal cord disorders.

FOR FURTHER INFORMATION:

Colton, Raymond H., and Janina K. Casper. *Understanding Voice Problems: A Physiological Perspective for Diagnosis and Treatment.* 2d ed. Baltimore: Williams & Wilkins, 1996.

Greene, Margaret C. L. *The Voice and Its Disorders.* 5th ed. London: Whurr, 1989.

Tucker, Harvey M. *The Larynx.* 2d ed. New York: Thieme Medical, 1993.

LASER USE IN SURGERY

PROCEDURE

ANATOMY OR SYSTEM AFFECTED: Eyes, skin

SPECIALTIES AND RELATED FIELDS: Dermatology, oncology, ophthalmology, urology

DEFINITION: The application of laser technology to surgical procedures, such as the vaporization of blood clots or arterial plaque, the breaking up of kidney stones into small fragments, the removal of birthmarks, and the stoppage of hemorrhaging in the retina of the eye.

KEY TERMS:

ionization: a process in which a neutral atom loses one or more of its orbital electrons because of light, heat, or electrical collisions

laser: an acronym for light amplification by stimulated emission of radiation; a laser produces a very-high-intensity light beam at a single wavelength

optical fiber: a very thin thread made of high-purity glass, plastic, or quartz; used to transmit light from a laser into the body

photon: a particle of light whose energy depends on its wavelength (that is, its color); many billions of individual photons make up a light beam

pulsed laser: a laser technique used to deliver a light beam of high power for a very short time in order to localize the heating effect without damaging surrounding tissue

shock wave: a miniature explosion caused by intense local heating with a laser beam; used to fragment stones in the kidney or gallbladder

stimulated emission of radiation: the process in a laser whereby an avalanche of photons is created, all of which are synchronized in wavelength and direction of travel

wavelength: a property used to measure colors in the spectrum of light from infrared to ultraviolet; usually expressed in units of microns (one micron is equal to one-millionth of a meter)

THE FUNDAMENTALS OF LASER TECHNOLOGY

The first successful laser was built in 1960 by Theodore H. Maiman at the Hughes Aircraft Research Laboratory in Palo Alto, California. Since then, many applications have been developed for lasers. These include the compact disc player, telephone systems with fiber optics, guidance systems for military weapons, supermarket checkout scanners, quality control in industry, entertainment with laser light shows, and numerous medical applications.

Ordinary light sources such as flashlights, flames, and the sun do not emit laser light. The individual atoms emit their light waves in a random, uncoordinated manner, in the same way that water waves spread out at random when a handful of pebbles is thrown into a pool. In contrast, a laser beam consists of light waves that are all synchronized; they all have the same wavelength and remain in step as they travel in the same direction. Synchronizing the light emission from billions of atoms in a light source is the chief difficulty in building a laser.

The key idea for solving this problem had been proposed in an article on the general theory of light absorption and emission by atoms written by the famous physicist Albert Einstein in the 1920's. When an atom absorbs a burst of light energy (a photon), an electron in the atom is raised from a lower energy level to a higher one. A short time later, the electron spontaneously falls back down to the lower energy level, emitting a photon of light in the process. Einstein's contribution was to suggest a third mechanism

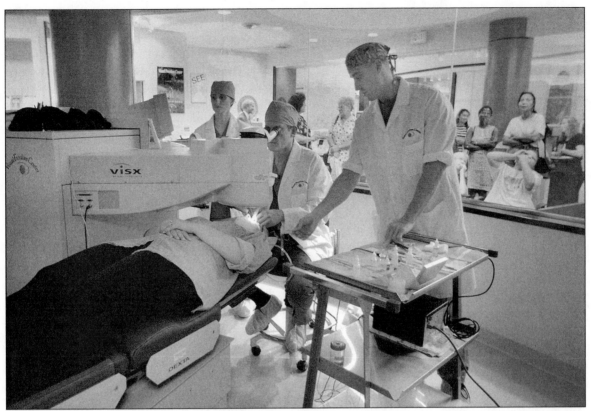

Lasers are taking a more prominent role in many procedures, especially eye surgery. Some worry that the popularity of laser vision correction—here a patient is treated at a shopping mall as spectators look on—has compromised safety. (AP/Wide World Photos)

in addition to ordinary absorption and emission. Based on theoretical arguments of symmetry and the conservation of energy, he proposed a new process called "stimulated emission of radiation." (The word "laser" is an acronym for light amplification by stimulated emission of radiation.)

To understand stimulated emission, consider an atom whose electron has been raised to a higher energy level, called an "excited state." This state is unstable, and the electron ordinarily will fall back down to the lower energy level in a short time. Suppose, however, that a photon of precisely the right energy strikes the atom while the electron is still in its temporary excited state. This photon cannot be absorbed because the electron is already in its excited state. Einstein reasoned that the incoming photon would cause the excited electron to fall to the lower energy level. A photon would then be emitted from the atom and would join the incoming photon. The two photons would be exactly synchronized in wavelength and direction.

If there were many atoms whose electrons had previously been raised to excited states, the process of stimulated emission would continue. The two photons could strike two other excited atoms and stimulate them to emit light energy, making a total of four photons. These four would trigger four more atoms, making eight photons, and so forth. Eventually, a so-called photon avalanche consisting of a huge number of synchronized light waves would be generated, which is the desired laser beam.

To make a successful laser, some additional requirements must be met. For one thing, a source of energy must be provided to raise most of the electrons to their excited states. For a gas laser, this energy is normally supplied by a high voltage. Examples of gas lasers are those using carbon dioxide, argon, or a mixture of helium and neon. A solid crystal, such as a clear ruby rod, would be excited by a bright burst of light from a device similar to a camera flash attachment. A solid-state diode laser is energized by a flow of electric current across a diode junction. In each case, it is necessary to "pump" the laser so that many atoms are in their excited state, ready and waiting to be triggered by an incoming photon to release their energy.

Another requirement for a successful laser is that the electrons must remain in their excited state for a longer-than-normal time. The problem with most materials is that electrons fall spontaneously to their lower energy level almost instantaneously, in less than one-millionth of a second. The photon avalanche effect requires that a substantial majority of the atoms be in their excited state. For very short-lived excited states, it is not possible to maintain this condition. Experimenters have no way to control the lifetime of excited states, so they must search for those atoms and molecules that already have the appropriate longer lifetime supplied by nature. It has not been possible to build a laser using hydrogen gas, for example, because hydrogen does not have any long-lived excited states. The spontaneous emission of light takes place so quickly that there is no time for a photon avalanche to develop.

Another condition for laser action is to have two parallel mirrors at the ends of the laser material. The laser beam bounces back and forth many times between the mirrors at the speed of light, gaining or maintaining its energy from the excited atoms of the laser material. One of the mirrors is made slightly less than 100 percent reflecting, so that a small portion of the laser energy is allowed to exit in a narrow beam. For most medical applications, a thin optical fiber is joined directly to the end of the laser in order to transmit the beam to the desired location in the body.

Much research has been done to develop good optical fibers. The fiber should transmit a laser beam with very little loss of energy along the way. The technology of drawing thin glass fibers with few impurities or imperfections has become quite sophisticated. A fiber must be thin and uniform so that the laser beam will be forced to travel down its center, thus avoiding the loss of light energy through the walls.

For an ultraviolet laser, glass fibers cannot be used because of absorption. (The sun's ultraviolet radiation is absorbed by ordinary eyeglasses.) Special quartz fibers with low absorption have been developed for lasers in the ultraviolet region of the spectrum. In the infrared region of the spectrum, new optical materials are still under continuing investigation.

The wavelength (color) of a laser is determined entirely by the energy levels of the atoms or molecules being used. For example, a carbon dioxide laser always has a wavelength of 10.6 microns, which is infrared. The helium-neon gas laser always produces visible red light at a wavelength of 0.63 microns. A wide range of laser wavelengths has become available as a result of extensive research efforts by physicists and optical engineers. Since 1960, lasers have become much more rugged and dependable in construction. Some lasers operate with a continuous beam, while others produce very short pulses, depending on the desired application. Also, lasers can be designed to operate at a low power level for diagnostic purposes or a high power level for surgery.

Safety precautions must be followed when working with a laser. Not only the patient but also the surgical team must be protected from possible harmful radiation. The eyes must be protected from laser beam reflections from a shiny surface. Ultraviolet light is a special hazard because its high-energy photons can cause cell damage and genetic mutations. The great benefits of laser surgery can be negated by an inexperienced or careless surgeon.

USES AND COMPLICATIONS

The first medical use of a laser beam was for surgery on the retina of the eye, in 1963. Diabetic patients in particular frequently develop excessive blood vessels in the retina that give their eyes a typically reddish color. In advanced cases, the blood vessels can hemorrhage and eventually cause blindness. The green light of an argon laser will pass through the clear cornea and lens of the eye, but when it hits the dark brown melanin pigment of the retina, it will be absorbed and cause a tiny hot spot. The physician uses a series of laser pulses, carefully focused on affected areas of the retina, to burn away the extra blood vessels. The remarkable property of the laser beam in this procedure is that its energy penetrates to the rear of the eye, leaving the clear fluid unaffected.

In a greenhouse, light from the sun comes in through the glass but infrared radiation cannot get back out. This example illustrates that some materials, such as glass, are transparent for visible light but opaque for infrared light. Similarly, the front of the eye is transparent for visible light but absorbs infrared light. Therefore, an infrared laser such as the YAG (yttrium-aluminum-garnet) laser can be used for surgery near the front of the eye because its light energy is selectively absorbed there.

A particular problem following cataract surgery is that a secondary cataract may develop on the membrane behind the implanted artificial lens. About one-third of patients with such a lens implant require a second surgery to remove the secondary cataract. A YAG laser beam will pass through the cornea and artificial lens but can be focused to produce a hot spot at the site of the secondary cataract to destroy it. More than 200,000 such procedures are performed each year in the United States, and the result is a dramatic, almost instantaneous improvement of vision.

A third form of laser eye surgery, LASIK (laser in-situ keratomileusis), became quite popular at the end of the twentieth century; it has, in fact, become the most commonly performed surgery in the country. In LASIK surgery, the cornea of the eyeball is reshaped to help patients overcome myopia (nearsightedness), hyperopia (farsightedness) or astigmatism. The procedure is done with a cool beam laser that can be used to remove thin layers of tissue from selected sites on the cornea to change its curvature. Success rates for the surgery are high: 90 to 95 percent of the patients get 20/40 vision, and 65 to 75 percent of the patients get 20/20 vision or better. The surgery is not without its problems, however. Because of its popularity and the large fee charged for a quick and fairly simple procedure, unqualified or less experienced physicians are oftentimes performing the delicate procedure; approximately 5 percent of patients receiving LASIK surgery receive less-than-satisfactory results. Two other corrective procedures for eyesight involving lasers are Kera-Vision Intacs (intrastomal corneal rings), which involves placing a lens in the cornea, and PRK (photorefractive keratectomy), where the cornea is scraped without LASIK's actual incision into the cornea.

Another dramatic medical application of the laser is the breaking up of stones in the kidney, ureter, or gallbladder. Such calcified, hard deposits previously could only be removed by surgery. It is now possible, for example, to insert an optical fiber of less than half a millimeter in diameter through the urethra and then transmit the laser beam to the site of the stone. High-power light pulses of very short duration (less than one-billionth of a second) create a shock wave that breaks the stone into small fragments that the body can eliminate.

Another promising application of laser surgery that has received much publicity is laser angioplasty, which is used to open up a blood vessel near the heart that is partially or wholly blocked by a deposit of plaque. The hope is that the laser procedure may be able to replace heart bypass surgery, but the results are still preliminary.

Laser angioplasty involves inserting a catheter that contains a fiberscope, an inflation cuff, and an optical fiber into the artery of the arm and advancing it into the coronary artery. The fiberscope enables the physician to see the blockage, the cuff is used to stop the blood flow temporarily, and the optical fiber transmits the laser energy that vaporizes the plaque. Sometimes, the laser method is used only to open up a small channel, after which balloon angioplasty is used to stretch the walls of the blood vessel.

The main risk in using the laser beam is that the alignment of the optical fiber inside the artery may be deflected and cause a puncture of the blood vessel wall. Improvements in the imaging system are needed. Also, further work must be done to see which light wavelengths are most effective in removing plaque and preventing recurrence of the obstruction.

The heating effect of a laser beam has been used by surgeons to control bleeding. For example, bleeding ulcers in the stomach, intestine, and colon have been successfully cauterized with laser light transmitted through an optical fiber. A similar procedure has been used to treat emphysema patients. An optical fiber is inserted through the wall of the chest, and the laser's heat is used to shrink the small blisters that are present on the surface of the lungs. Also, the heat from a laser has been used during internal surgery to seal the surrounding capillaries that contribute to bleeding.

For the preceding procedures, a carbon dioxide gas laser that emits infrared light is normally used. The reason is that water molecules in the tissue absorb the infrared wavelengths most efficiently. The optical fibers used to transmit infrared light are not as efficient and reliable as those used for visible or ultraviolet light, however, so further research on fiber materials is in progress.

One notable success of laser surgery has been the removal of birthmarks. Because of their typically reddish-purple coloration, birthmarks are commonly called port-wine stains. They can be quite unsightly, especially when located on the face of a person with an otherwise light complexion. To remove such a birthmark, the laser beam has to burn out the network of extra blood vessels under the skin. A similar procedure can be used to remove unwanted tattoos.

The color of the laser must be chosen so that its wavelength will be absorbed efficiently by the dark purple stain. What would happen if a purple laser beam were used? Its light would be reflected rather than absorbed by a purple object, and it would not produce the desired heating. Yellow or orange is most effectively absorbed by a purple object. The surgeon must be careful that the laser light is absorbed primarily by the purple birthmark without harming the normal, healthy tissue around it.

Experimental work is being done to determine whether laser surgery can be applied to cancer. Small malignant tumors in the lungs, bladder, and trachea have been treated with a technique called photodynamic therapy. The patient is injected with a colored dye that is preferentially absorbed in the tumor. Porphyrin, the reddish-brown pigment in blood, is one substance that has been known for many years to become concentrated in malignant tissue. The suspected site is irradiated with ultraviolet light from a krypton laser, causing it to glow like fluorescent paint, which allows the surgeon to determine the outline of the tumor. To perform the surgery, an intense red laser is focused on the tumor to kill the malignant tissue. Two separate optical fibers must be used for this procedure, one for the ultraviolet diagnosis and one for the red laser therapy.

The three traditional cancer treatments of surgery, chemotherapy, and radiation therapy all seek to limit damage to healthy tissue surrounding a tumor. Photodynamic surgery by laser must develop its methodology further to accomplish the same goal.

Much has already been accomplished in applying laser surgery to various body organs. Future developments are likely to emphasize microsurgery on smaller structures, such as individual cells or even genetic material in DNA molecules.

PERSPECTIVE AND PROSPECTS

Some inventions, such as the printing press, the steam engine, and the electric light bulb, were made by innovators who were trying to solve a particular practical problem of their time. Other inventions, such as the microscope, radio waves, and low-temperature superconductivity, initially were scientific curiosities arising from basic research, and their later applications were not at all anticipated. The laser belongs to this second category.

The first successful laser, built by Theodore Maiman, consisted of a small cylindrical ruby rod with shiny

mirrored ends and a bright flash lamp to excite the atoms in the rod. His goal was to determine whether the separately excited atoms could be made to release their absorbed energy almost simultaneously in one coordinated burst of monochromatic (single wavelength) light.

No one could have foreseen the wide range of technological applications that resulted from Maiman's experiment. It is important to appreciate that he did not set out to improve telephone communication or eye surgery; those developments came about after the laser became available.

It is worthwhile here to summarize some of the general uses for lasers in modern technology. The tremendous advances in medical applications could not have happened without the concurrent development of new types of lasers, with a variety of wavelengths and power levels, needed for other industrial products.

Among laser applications are the following: the compact disc (CD) player, in which the laser beam replaces the LP record needle; optical fibers that can carry several thousand simultaneous telephone calls; supermarket check-out scanners, in which a laser beam reads the universal product code on each item; three-dimensional pictures, called holograms, that are displayed at many art museums; military applications, such as guided weapons and Star Wars technology; surveying, bridge building, and tunneling projects in which exact alignment is critical; and nuclear fusion research, in which high-power lasers can produce nuclear reactions that may become a future source of energy as coal and oil resources are depleted. Sophisticated advances in using lasers to control specific chemical reactions and to predict earthquakes are under development.

The future of laser technology in medicine will continue to advance as biologists, electrical and optical engineers, physicians, biophysicists, and people from related disciplines share this common interest.

—*Hans G. Graetzer, Ph.D.;*
updated by Cassandra Kircher, Ph.D.

See also Angioplasty; Astigmatism; Bionics and biotechnology; Bleeding; Blurred vision; Cataract surgery; Cataracts; Cervical procedures; Dermatology; Electrocauterization; Eye surgery; Eyes; Malignant melanoma removal; Myopia; Neurosurgery; Ophthalmology; Skin; Skin disorders; Skin lesion removal; Stone removal; Stones; Tattoo removal; Ulcer surgery; Ulcers.

FOR FURTHER INFORMATION:

Berns, Michael W. "Laser Surgery." *Scientific American* 264, no. 6 (June, 1991): 84-90. Contains photographs showing blood vessels in the retina before and after surgery, a urinary tract stone being fragmented by a laser, colored dye being made to fluoresce with laser light to diagnose malignant cancer, and other applications.

Cameron, John R., James G. Skofronick, and Roderick M. Grant. *Medical Physics: Physics of the Body.* Madison, Wis.: Medical Physics, 1992. A well-written textbook for college students planning a career in the health professions. The section on lasers in medicine gives an excellent discussion of eye surgery, relating the laser beam spot size, power level, wavelength, exposure time, and resulting tissue damage.

Ehrlich, Matthew. *How to See Like a Hawk When You're Blind as a Bat.* Venice, Fla.: Doctor's Advice Press, 1999. Ehrlich, an opthalmologist, provides a thorough description of various eye problems and whether Lasik eye surgery can be used to correct them. He draws on statistics from a group of Lasik patients to show final outcomes and the proportion of people who experience various complications.

Fitzpatrick, Richard E., and Mitchel P. Goldman. *Cosmetic Laser Surgery.* St. Louis: Mosby, 2000. Discusses methods of cosmetic surgery using lasers. Includes bibliographical references and an index.

IEEE Journal of Quantum Electronics 26, no. 12 (December, 1990). A special issue on lasers in biology and medicine. This journal is the professional publication of the Institute of Electrical and Electronic Engineers. The articles require some technical background on the part of the reader.

LAW AND MEDICINE

ETHICS

DEFINITION: The use of medicine in legal contexts—to determine whether a person has been injured by the act of another, the extent of such an injury and its treatment, and whether a defendant was physically or emotionally capable of committing a crime or tort—and in related ethical and philosophical contexts—to determine when life begins (in the abortion debate) or how one evaluates "quality of life" (the euthanasia debate).

KEY TERMS:

compensable injury: an injury for which damages may be awarded

competency: the capacity to understand and act reasonably under given circumstances

diminished capacity: partial insanity; a legal determination that a defendant does not have the ability to achieve the state of mind required to commit a crime

DNA testing: a technique for identifying a person based on matching unique gene-bearing proteins (deoxyribonucleic acid, or DNA) from an organic sample taken from that person (such as hair, blood, or tissue) with another organic sample retrieved from the scene of a crime

emotional distress: damage to a plaintiff's emotional state caused by fear, anger, anxiety, stress, depression, or other negative emotions; such damage may be judged "compensable," or deserving of material compensation

euthanasia: the act of putting a person or other living being to death in order to end incurable pain or disease; popularly called "mercy killing"

forensic: having to do with a court of justice; forensic medicine and its various subspecialties apply medical science to the purposes of the law

insanity: a mental disease or defect that renders a person incapable of appreciating the wrongfulness of certain acts or of conforming to the requirements of the law

tort: a wrongful act for which civil courts, rather than criminal courts, are empowered to render justice

THE ROLE OF MEDICINE IN LEGAL AND ETHICAL DEBATES

Medicine as it relates to law is referred to as forensic medicine. Forensic medicine plays a part in three basic areas of the law. The first two involve the practical application of medicine in civil law and in criminal law. The third area involves the use of medical science to help in defining philosophical or ethical issues, such as when life begins and ends.

In a civil case, a private party, the plaintiff, files a complaint in court against another party, the defendant, requesting that a judge or a jury settle a dispute between the two parties. A party to a civil suit can be an individual, a corporation, an association, a government organization, or any other group. A civil suit differs from a criminal case in that neither party is claiming that a crime (such as theft, kidnapping, or murder) was committed and that someone should be put in jail. Instead, the plaintiff in a civil suit is asking that the defendant pay some amount of money to the plaintiff to compensate for damages that the plaintiff has suffered because of something the defendant did.

In a criminal case, however, the state or federal government, on behalf of "the people," files a complaint with the court claiming that the defendant committed a crime, and the government seeks to have a judge or a jury determine the guilt or innocence of that defendant. If the defendant is determined to be guilty, the judge has the authority to punish the defendant, usually by imposing a fine, by requiring community service, by setting a jail sentence, or ultimately, in some states, by having the defendant put to death.

In both civil and criminal cases, medical science is called upon to provide evidence that can be used to prove or disprove a party's case. In a civil case, the parties will often resort to medical experts to determine the extent of a plaintiff's mental and physical injuries. These experts are doctors who act as witnesses in their areas of expertise and testify in a court of law. For example, a plaintiff in a civil suit might claim that he or she was born with birth defects as a result of drugs that the mother had taken during pregnancy and may present evidence of that injury and its cause by the testimony of doctors and medical research experts specializing in those related areas of medicine. Such testimony would be presented to the jury to show that the plaintiff's claim of birth defects being caused by such a drug is supported by medical research.

As medical science reveals more about the causes of disease, injuries, and the workings of the body, more distinct specialties have been created. This trend is reflected in the increasing number of expert witnesses: At the beginning of the twentieth century, a general practitioner was considered qualified to testify on most areas of medicine; today, the courts require expert witnesses to be specifically qualified in the area of medicine about which they testify.

The practice of using highly qualified and specialized doctors as expert witnesses has long been accepted by courts as an effective way to educate a jury regarding the extent, cause, and treatment of the injury in question, but there are some limitations on the use

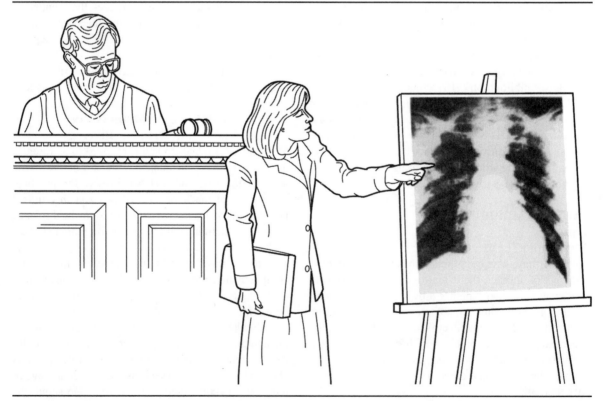

Physicians are often called to act as expert witnesses in the courtroom when medical matters are relevant to the trial and may sometimes testify in their own defense in malpractice cases.

of such testimony. In order for the court to allow a medical expert to testify as to specific facts from which conclusions are to be drawn, the facts must be outside what is considered to be the general or common knowledge of a lay jury. For example, a court may not allow a party to use a medical expert to explain sprained ankles. The court would, however, allow a medical expert to explain toxic shock syndrome, because the existence, causes, and effects of that impairment are not common knowledge. The reasoning behind this limitation is that the jury members are supposed to form their own opinions when such opinions do not involve or require specialized knowledge. Only when it is necessary or helpful to the jury to be educated in a specialized area of knowledge is expert testimony usually allowed.

The court also recognizes a distinction between testimony from a medical expert and testimony from the plaintiff's treating doctor. Whereas the former educates the jury regarding an area of medicine that is relevant to the case, the latter does not. Instead, the treating doctor is called to testify to actual events or facts of the case that the doctor personally witnessed: that the plaintiff was examined on a certain date, the extent of his or her injuries, and so on. Thus, although an expert witness may not be allowed by the court to educate the jury on the subject of a sprained ankle or other topic of common knowledge, the fact that the plaintiff sustained a sprained ankle and was treated for it may be testified to by the treating doctor.

In a civil suit, the plaintiff must prove that he or she was injured by some act of the defendant. That injury can be economic (the loss of property or money), physical (such as a torn muscle or broken leg), or mental (stress or anxiety). Over the years, more and more types of injuries have become recognized as compensable injuries in civil cases. The term "pain and suffering" has been used to describe physical and emotional symptoms that a plaintiff may claim were caused by the defendant. Medical facts can help determine the existence and extent of all these types of injury.

Sometimes the expert will testify only hypothetically (that is, based on the doctor's expertise). The expert may be asked to render an opinion based on certain assumptions concerning the plaintiff's condition. Sometimes, however, a medical expert will need to examine a plaintiff. It is not unusual for such examinations to take place years after the injury occurred, and the doctor will have to determine whether the injury exists, the extent of the injury, the cause of the injury, what (if any) limitations are caused by the injury, the treatment that is indicated, and the probable duration of the injury (perhaps based on the average rate of recovery for such an injury).

In the criminal justice system, medical experts may testify on a variety of scientific and medical issues. In the case of a murder, for example, it may be necessary to identify blood, tissue, bone, or some other human remains and to determine the source of those remains—namely, whether the remains belong to the alleged victim or perpetrator of the crime. Doctors who specialize in forensic medicine are often called upon to conduct special tests, such as DNA testing, to identify whose blood or tissue was found at the scene of a crime or on a murder weapon. Forensic experts can also determine the approximate time and cause of death. Testimony on these issues helps a jury determine the guilt or innocence of the accused.

Criminal cases occasionally also require the testimony of a forensic psychiatrist, who is an expert in mental and emotional disorders as they relate to legal principles. Testimony from such an expert assists in determining whether the defendant is "insane." According to section 4.01 of the Modern Penal Code, a person is insane if he or she "lacks substantial capacity either to appreciate the criminality [wrongfulness] of his conduct or to conform his conduct to the requirements of the law." Psychiatric evaluations of the accused are performed to determine whether the defendant fit this definition at the time the crime was committed. Testimony regarding the defendant's insanity would significantly affect the case's outcome and sentencing.

A separate issue, unrelated to the defendant's mental condition at the time of the crime, is the defendant's "competency" to stand trial. According to *Black's Law Dictionary* (5th ed., 1979), a defendant "lacks competency to stand trial if he or she lacks capacity to understand the nature and object of the proceedings, to consult with counsel, and to assist in preparing his or her defense." The law ensures that an accused person's rights are protected by requiring that the defendant be capable of understanding these proceedings and their implications before he or she is allowed to stand trial. If either of the attorneys, or the judge, asserts that the defendant is not competent to stand trial, the court will hold a competency hearing to decide whether the defendant is "competent." In determining the competency of the defendant, the court will hear the testimony of psychiatric experts. If the defendant is determined to be incompetent at the time of the trial, the defendant will not be tried but may instead be sent to a mental institution until such time as he or she is competent to stand trial.

In addition to being used in civil cases and criminal cases, medical science is used to provide scientific information to support or disprove wholly nonscientific determinations. Such philosophical and ethical issues include abortion and euthanasia. In the long-running debate over the legality of abortion, for example, many issues and circumstances come into play, including rape and the possibility that pregnancy may endanger the woman's life. One central and hotly contested question, however, is "When does life begin?" This question may also involve an equally difficult and controversial one: "What is life?" The courts and various state legislatures have turned to medical science to address these profound, and possibly unanswerable, questions. Medical science has identified two key concepts to answer these questions: the concept of "viability" (that is, the ability of the fetus to survive outside the womb) and the distinction between the first, second, and third trimesters of a pregnancy. The distinction of trimesters was originally based on the concept of viability: A fetus generally could not survive outside the womb during the first trimester (that is, was not viable), while a fetus was generally considered viable during the third trimester. Thus, the courts and legislature would often use the concept of trimesters in determining a cutoff date after which an abortion could not be performed.

These concepts have been used as the basis for legislation to regulate and authorize abortions. Medical science is, however, a rapidly evolving field. Because it is now possible for a human egg, once fertilized, to become viable outside the womb, the legal foundation upon which abortions are based is becoming more unstable.

THE APPLICATIONS OF MEDICAL TESTIMONY
Medical experts in almost every field of medicine have played a part in civil cases, criminal cases, and controversies involving philosophical and ethical issues. Sometimes, the interaction between medicine and the law has spawned new medical or legal subspecialties. In fact, medical expert testimony has become a field and an occupation in itself, supporting an entire group of medical professionals to the exclusion of medical practice. This phenomenon has in large part occurred in response to the greater acceptance by the courts of medical expert testimony and the increased reliability of recent medical testing.

Personal injury cases afford a good example of all the different types of testimony that come into play in civil suits. A physical injury case, as the name suggests, is based on a physical (or mental) injury, as opposed to a purely financial injury, suffered by the plaintiff. A physical injury case may involve an automobile accident and its resulting injuries. In such a case, doctors who are experts in the field of muscle damage, neurology (for head and nerve injuries), orthopedic surgery, and countless other areas could be called as experts, depending on the extent of the injuries.

Another type of case, called a product liability case, will often use expert medical testimony. A product liability case is one in which a person has been injured by a specific product on the market and sues the manufacturer, and often the seller, claiming that the product was defective. Famous examples of product liability cases include claims filed against manufacturers of asbestos products, certain tampons (for causing toxic shock syndrome), contraceptive devices such as the Dalkon Shield, and some generic or prescription drugs, such as thalidomide and Halcion. All these cases required medical experts in recently developed fields of medicine. Prior to the product liability suits filed against some tampon manufacturers, no one had heard of toxic shock syndrome. The testimony of medical experts was required to prove a link between an allegedly defective product and the resulting injury that was claimed. Without expert medical testimony in these cases, it would be impossible to prove that the defective products caused the injuries of which the defendants complained.

Another example of the medical profession developing to suit the law is in the area of workers' compensation. The California legislature, like the legislatures of many states, has established by statute (Labor Code section 3600 and following) a method by which to compensate any employee who has suffered a job-related injury. An employer is required by law to carry workers' compensation insurance, which will compensate an injured employee. If an employee is injured on the job in any manner, that employee is supposed to file a claim notifying his or her employer of the injury. The claim is then submitted to the workers' compensation insurance carrier. If the employer and the carrier accept liability, necessary treatment is provided to the employee. If the carrier denies further treatment or denies that an employee is disabled, the employee may file a claim with the Workers' Compensation Appeal Board. Once such a claim is filed, a judge will review all the medical reports of the injured worker. Additional medical evidence and testimony may be introduced to prove or disprove the employee's claim of injury or disability. The award of the Workers' Compensation Appeal Board is determined by the medical condition of the person claiming the injury. The growing popularity of workers' compensation has spawned an entire field of medicine, that of work-related injuries.

California courts routinely allow damages for "mental distress" in almost every type of tort action. Accordingly, psychiatrists and psychologists are routinely called upon to testify regarding whether a plaintiff has suffered such an injury. Emotional distress is not a specific medical condition, but rather a general emotional state, which may include anger, fear, frustration, anxiety, depression, and similar symptoms. Although psychiatric or psychological testimony is not required by the court for the plaintiff to recover damages for mental distress, it can be very effective in explaining to the jury the extent of the injuries and the effect of those injuries on the plaintiff's future life.

If a jury determines that the plaintiff suffered a physical or mental injury caused by the defendant, then, based on the medical testimony—of either the medical witness or the treating doctor—the jury may award any medical fees incurred, as well as anticipated medical fees and costs and compensation for the pain and suffering of the defendant. The jury may also award further damages not related to the medical condition of the plaintiff, if the case warrants such damages.

In criminal cases, particularly cases of homicide, forensic medicine often provides the key and fundamental evidence upon which the entire case is based. During the investigations of the assassination of President John F. Kennedy in the 1960's, the forensic evidence played a vital, although controversial, role. The testimony presented by the doctors who examined the president's body was used to reconstruct the crime. Forensic science was used to interpret the angle of entry of the bullets that killed Kennedy and thereby to extrapolate the source of the shots. Furthermore, forensic science was called upon to demonstrate how many shots were fired and the paths of the bullets upon entering the bodies of the president and Gover-

nor John Connally. Using medical evidence, along with other evidence, the Warren Commission concluded that the bullets all came from the book depository building behind the presidential caravan. Also using medical evidence and experts, critics of the Warren Commission's findings have alleged that the injuries suffered by the president could have been caused only by a bullet entering from the front of the president's neck and exiting the rear of the skull.

In another case, forensic evidence was able to reach a conclusive determination that certain bones were those of the Nazi war criminal Dr. Josef Mengele, known as the Angel of Death. In 1992, forensics experts discovered, using a method known as DNA testing, that some bones retrieved from a grave in Brazil were those of Mengele. In order to make this determination, doctors compared the DNA found in the blood of Mengele's son with DNA from the bones found in the grave. They found that the DNA from both sources was identical. Because DNA constitutes a "genetic fingerprint" that remains the same from parent to offspring, the doctors were able to conclude that the remains found in Brazil were those of Mengele.

DNA testing is now also commonly used in suits to determine the father of an infant. According to the Genetics Institute, DNA testing is at least 99.8 percent accurate. Medical science has so refined its ability to chart DNA "fingerprints" that the chance of coming upon two identical DNA patterns is approximately one in six billion. Prior to DNA testing, a blood testing method called human leukocyte antigen (HLA) typing was used to determine paternity, but this typing was only 95 percent accurate.

Some medical or scientific tests, while accepted by the courts, remain subject to much controversy. The Breathalyzer test, used to determine blood alcohol levels, is one such test. While the courts regularly accept the results of such tests to determine whether a suspect was intoxicated, the test is based on several assumptions and averages. Based on the alcohol content in the suspect's breath, the test extrapolates a probable amount of alcohol in the suspect's blood. The reliability of this test depends on the correct calibration of the equipment and the care of the person taking the readings. Since the tests are taken by nonmedical or nonscientific personnel in the field, mistaken readings are not uncommon. Furthermore, if the suspect used a spray breath freshener just before the test, the readings may be skewed, since such breath fresheners are usually alcohol-based.

PERSPECTIVE AND PROSPECTS

Medicine has always played some role in the outcome of court cases, but this relationship did not come into full flower until relatively recently. In the early twentieth century, courts placed strict limitations on the type and amount of medical testimony allowed into evidence. Often, certain types of medical evidence were not admissible because the science was not deemed reliable—there was too much room for error. The polygraph (lie detector), for example, could not be relied upon to reveal consistently whether a person was telling the truth, since it simply measured galvanic skin response, respiration rate, and other factors that only tend to be correlated with the subject's feelings of guilt. Most other evidence presented by medical experts concerned the likelihood of events or outcomes and therefore usually constituted opinion, rather than fact.

With the advent of new technologies in the later part of the twentieth century, medical science began to present "hard" (more precise) data that became more frequently accepted by the courts as reliable and relevant evidence. Even so, it took some time before medical scientists were able to present enough data to persuade the courts that the evidence of such methods as DNA "fingerprinting" was truly reliable. The acceptance of DNA testing, for example, was a long and hard-fought battle among legions of medical experts on both sides of the issue. Finally, DNA testing was accepted by the courts as a reliable source of evidence. As forensic medicine advances, no doubt its contribution to the law will also advance. The ability of the medical and other scientific professions to determine reliable conclusions relating to court cases is progressing rapidly with increases in scientific knowledge, methods, and technology.

In an ironic twist, however, this progress has clouded other areas of the law, including the constitutional rights of accused persons. In the early twentieth century, for example, no one could have dreamed of the technology that makes life support possible. With the advent of kidney dialysis machines, pacemakers, respirators, and other life support devices, medical science has achieved the ability to prolong an individual's bodily functioning. Whether this functioning alone is sufficient to define "life," however, remains a question that cannot be addressed by medical science alone but must be considered in the light of philosophical, ethical, and other values. Medicine is therefore becoming as much an area with which the law must contend as it is a tool for aiding existing law. Issues concerning abortion and the point at which life begins, euthanasia, the individual's right not to have life extended by extraordinary means if there is no hope of recovery, the right to reveal an individual's genetic predisposition toward disease, egg implantation, and genetic engineering have all challenged the existing, and inadequate, laws. Medical science not only has propagated these dilemmas but also has been called upon to solve them.

—Larry M. Roberts

See also Abortion; Animal rights vs. research; Autopsy; Blood testing; Cloning; Environmental health; Ethics; Euthanasia; Forensic pathology; Genetic engineering; In vitro fertilization; Malpractice; Occupational health; Screening.

FOR FURTHER INFORMATION:

Black, Henry Campbell. *Black's Law Dictionary.* 7th ed. St. Paul, Minn.: West, 1999. The fundamental legal dictionary, containing definitions and examples of how the terms have been interpreted by courts.

Loring, Charles A., ed. *California Jury Instructions, Civil: Book of Approved Jury Instructions.* 7th ed. 2 vols. St. Paul, Minn.: West, 1986. Sets forth the standard jury instructions, covering various aspects of civil duties and liabilities.

Tarantino, John A., and Patricia K. Rocha. *Estimating and Proving Personal Injury Damages.* Santa Ana, Calif.: James, 1988. A brief, step-by-step approach to pursuing personal injury damages. Generally geared for the attorney, but written in simple English. Contains helpful information on quantifying medical injuries for purposes of determining money damages in a personal injury lawsuit.

Witkin, B. E. *Summary of California Law.* 9th ed. 13 vols. San Francisco: Bancroft-Whitney, 1987-1990. This multivolume set (with a supplemental volume published in 1991) contains a brief explanation and analysis of almost every aspect of California civil law. The author has not only analyzed the law but also provided numerous examples of how the courts use and interpret the law.

LEAD POISONING
DISEASE/DISORDER

ANATOMY OR SYSTEM AFFECTED: Brain, circulatory system, endocrine system, musculoskeletal system, nervous system, reproductive system

SPECIALTIES AND RELATED FIELDS: Environmental health, pediatrics, preventive medicine, toxicology

DEFINITION: A major preventable environmental health problem in children.

KEY TERMS:

arthralgia: severe joint pain, especially when inflammation is not present

chelation: the taking up or release of a metallic ion by an organic molecule

encephalopathy: any disease of the brain

lead: a limited naturally occurring element widely distributed throughout the environment by industrial uses and pollution

paresis: partial paralysis

paresthesia: an abnormal sensation, such as burning, tingling, tickling, or pricking

CAUSES AND SYMPTOMS

Childhood lead poisoning is a major, preventable environmental health problem. Blood lead levels as low as 10 micrograms per deciliter are associated with harmful effects on children's ability to learn. Very high blood lead levels of 70 micrograms per deciliter can cause devastating health consequences, including seizures and other neurological symptoms, abdominal pain, developmental delays, attention deficit, hyperactivity, behavior disorders, hearing loss, anemia, coma, and death.

Children can be exposed to lead in many ways. Sources of exposure include automobile exhaust, lead-based paint, and environmental contaminates released by industrial processes that use or produce lead-containing materials. Contributors to childhood lead exposure also include lead-contaminated containers, food, dust, soil, air, and water; lead-containing ceramics and hobby supplies; substance abuse such as gasoline sniffing; parental transfer from lead-rich occupational environments; and traditional medicines such as azarcon and greta. Deteriorating lead-based paint in older homes is the most important source of lead exposure in children. Swallowing lead-based paint dust through normal hand-to-mouth activity or chewing directly on painted surfaces are major methods of lead ingestion. Children are often attracted to lead paint because of its sweet taste.

Upon entering the human body, inorganic lead is not metabolized but is directly absorbed, distributed, and excreted. The rate at which lead is absorbed depends on its chemical and physical form and on the physiologic characteristics of the exposed person.

Once in the blood, lead is distributed among three compartments: the blood; soft tissue zones such as the kidneys, bone marrow, liver, and brain; and mineralizing tissues such as bones and teeth. For lead poisoning to take place, major acute exposures to lead need not occur. The body accumulates lead and releases it slowly; therefore, even small doses over time can be toxic. It is the total body accumulation of lead that is related to the risk of adverse effects. Whether lead enters the body through inhalation or ingestion, the biologic effects are the same—interference with normal cell function and with certain physiologic processes.

By and large, children show a greater sensitivity to the effects of lead than do adults. Parents working in lead-related industries not only may inhale lead dust and lead oxide fumes but also may eat, drink, and smoke in or near contaminated areas, increasing the probability of lead ingestion and subsequent transfer to their children. Since lead readily crosses the placenta, the fetus is at risk. Fetal exposure can cause potentially adverse neurological effects in utero and during postnatal development. The incomplete development of the blood-brain barrier in very young children, up to thirty-six months of age, increases the risk of the entry of lead into the developing nervous system, which can result in prolonged neurobehavioral disorders. Children absorb and retain more lead in proportion to their weight than do adults. Young children also show a greater prevalence of iron deficiency, a condition that can increase the gastrointestinal absorption of lead.

Symptoms of lead poisoning and lead intoxication vary because of differences in individual susceptibility, and the severity of symptoms increases with increased exposure. Symptoms of mild lead toxicity include abdominal discomfort, fatigue, muscle pain, or paresthesia. Moderate toxicity is indicated by arthralgia, tremor, fatigue, difficulty concentrating, headache, abdominal pain, vomiting, weight loss, and constipation. Severe toxicity symptoms include paresis or paralysis, encephalopathy, seizures, severe abdominal cramps, hearing loss, changes in consciousness, and coma.

TREATMENT AND THERAPY

If a child is suspected of having lead poisoning, laboratory tests are necessary to evaluate lead intoxication levels. Laboratory techniques defining lead toxicity include blood lead level screening, erythrocyte protoporphyrin (EP) and zinc proporphyrin (ZPP) screening, creatinine, urinalysis, and hematocrit and hemoglobin tests with peripheral smear.

The physical examination for suspected lead poisoning cases includes special attention to hematologic, cardiovascular, gastrointestinal, and renal systems. Any neurological or behavioral changes are considered significant indicators. In addition, severe and prolonged lead poisoning may be indicated by a purplish line on the gums. A complete interview and medical evaluation of a suspected lead poisoning patient includes a full workup and medical history. Clues to potential exposure vectors can be obtained by discussing family and occupational history, use of traditional medicines, remodeling activities, hobbies, table and cookware, drinking water source, nutrition, proximity to industry or waste sites, and the physical condition and age of the patient's residence, school, and/or day care facility.

The treatment and management of lead poisoning first involves the separation of the patient from the source of lead. After a diagnosis of lead poisoning is made, local environmental health officials should be contacted to determine the lead source and what remediation action is necessary for its control.

The Centers for Disease Control recommends that children with blood lead levels of 45 micrograms per deciliter or greater should be referred for chelation therapy immediately. Several drugs are capable of binding or chelating lead, depleting both soft and hard (skeletal) tissues of lead and reducing its acute toxicity. All these drugs have potential side effects and must be used with caution. The most commonly used chelating agent is calcium disodium edetic acid, although several other agents are available.

—*Randall L. Milstein, Ph.D.*

See also Environmental diseases; Environmental health; Learning disabilities; Mental retardation; Occupational health; Poisoning; Safety issues for children; Screening; Toxicology.

FOR FURTHER INFORMATION:

Centers for Disease Control. *Preventing Lead Poisoning in Young Children: A Statement by the CDC.* 4th ed. Atlanta: Author, 1991. A study by the Centers for Disease Control on pediatric toxicology. Includes bibliographical references.

Cushing, N. Dolbeare, et al. *Putting the Pieces Together: Controlling Lead Hazards in the Nation's Housing.* Washington, D.C.: U.S. Department of Housing and Urban Development, 1995. This report envisions a system that will protect children from developing elevated blood lead levels, preserve the stock of affordable housing, and wisely invest scarce resources, both public and private. Includes charts and tables.

Gergely, Rita M., et al. *Screening Young Children for Lead Poisoning: Guidance for State and Local Public Health Officials.* Atlanta: Centers for Disease Control and Prevention, 1997. A study of the environmental exposure of children to lead, including information on medical screening for lead poisoning.

How to Prevent Lead Poisoning on Your Job! A Worker's Guide to Lead Safety in General Industry. Oakland, Calif.: The Program, 2000. A handbook for avoiding lead poisoning, this guide offers hints on industrial safety.

Kessel, Irene, and John T. O'Connor. *Getting the Lead Out: The Complete Resource on How to Prevent and Cope with Lead Poisoning.* New York: Plenum Press, 1997. A comprehensive resource for parents and homeowners describing the major sources of lead in the home and environment, as well as medical concerns, prevention strategies, and techniques for controlling lead hazards.

Millstone, Erik. *Lead and Public Health.* Washington, D.C.: Taylor & Francis, 1997. This book gives the background to the scientific debate about the toxicology of lead and examines the impacts on human health. The regulatory regimes of the United States and Great Britain are assessed, and further steps are suggested.

LEARNING DISABILITIES

DISEASE/DISORDER

ANATOMY OR SYSTEM AFFECTED: Brain, nervous system, psychic-emotional system

SPECIALTIES AND RELATED FIELDS: Neurology, pediatrics, psychology

DEFINITION: A variety of disorders involving the failure to learn an academic skill despite normal levels of intelligence, maturation, and cultural and educational opportunity; estimates of the prevalence of learning disabilities in the general population range between 2 and 20 percent.

KEY TERMS:

achievement test: a measure of an individual's degree of learning in an academic subject, such as reading, mathematics, and written language *dyslexia:* difficulty in reading, with an implied neurological cause

intelligence test: a psychological test designed to measure an individual's ability to think logically, act purposefully, and react successfully to the environment; yields intelligence quotient (IQ) scores

neurological dysfunction: problems associated with the way in which different sections and structures of the brain perform tasks, such as verbal and spatial reasoning and language production

neurology: the study of the central nervous system, which is composed of the brain and spinal cord

perceptual deficits: problems in processing information from the environment, which may involve distractibility, impulsivity, and figure-ground distortions (difficulty distinguishing foreground from background)

standardized test: an instrument used to assess skill development in comparison to others of the same age or grade

CAUSES AND SYMPTOMS

An understanding of learning disabilities must begin with the knowledge that the definition, diagnosis, and treatment of these disorders have historically generated considerable disagreement and controversy. This is primarily attributable to the fact that people with learning disabilities are a highly diverse group of individuals with a wide variety of characteristics. Consequently, differences of opinion among professionals remain to such an extent that presenting a single universally accepted definition of learning disabilities is not possible. Definitional differences most frequently center on the relative emphases that alternative groups place on characteristics of these disorders. For example, experts in medical fields typically describe these disorders from a disease model and view them primarily as neurological dysfunctions. Conversely, educators usually place more emphasis on the academic problems that result from learning disabilities. Despite these differences, the most commonly accepted definitions, those developed by the United States Office of Education in 1977, the Board of the Association for Children and Adults with Learning Disabilities in 1985, and the National Joint Committee for Learning Disabilities in 1981, do include some areas of commonality.

Difficulty in academic functioning is included in the three definitions, and virtually all descriptions of learning disabilities include this characteristic. Academic deficits may be in one or more formal scholastic subjects, such as reading or mathematics. Often the deficits will involve a component skill of the academic area, such as problems with comprehension or word knowledge in reading or difficulty in calculating or applying arithmetical reasoning in mathematics. The academic difficulty may also be associated with more basic skills of learning that influence functioning across academic areas; these may involve deficits in listening, speaking, and thinking. Dyslexia, a term for reading problems, is the most common academic problem associated with learning disabilities. Because reading skills are required in most academic activities to some degree, many view dyslexia as the most serious form of learning disability.

The presumption of a neurological dysfunction as the cause of these disorders is included, either directly or indirectly, in each of the three definitions. Despite this presumption, unless an individual has a known history of brain trauma, the neurological basis for learning disabilities will not be identified in most cases because current assessment technology does not allow for such precise diagnoses. Rather, at least minimal neurological dysfunction is simply assumed to be present in anyone who exhibits characteristics of a learning disorder.

The three definitions all state that individuals with learning disabilities experience learning problems despite possessing normal intelligence. This condition is referred to as a discrepancy between achievement and ability or potential.

Finally, each of the three definitions incorporates the idea that learning disabilities cannot be attributed to another handicapping condition such as mental retardation, vision or hearing problems, emotional or psychiatric disturbance, or social, cultural, or educational disadvantage. Consequently, these conditions must be excluded as primary contributors to academic difficulties.

Reports on the prevalence of learning disabilities differ according to the definitions and identification methods employed. Consequently, statistics on prevalence range between 2 and 20 percent of the population. Many of the higher reported percentages are actually estimates of prevalence that include individuals who are presumed to have a learning disorder but who have not been formally diagnosed. Males are believed to constitute the majority of individuals with learning disabilities, and estimated sex ratios range from 6:1 to 8:1. Some experts believe that this difference in incidence may reveal one of the causes of these disorders.

A number of causes of learning disabilities have been proposed, with none being universally accepted. Some of the most plausible causal theories include neurological deficits, genetic and hereditary influences, and exposure to toxins during fetal gestation or early childhood.

Evidence to support the assumption of a link between neurological dysfunction and learning disabilities has been provided by studies using sophisticated brain imaging techniques such as positron emission tomography (PET) and computed tomography (CT) scanning and magnetic resonance imaging (MRI). Studies using these techniques have, among other findings, indicated subtle abnormalities in the structure and electrical activity in the brains of individuals with learning disabilities. The use of such techniques has typically been confined to research; however, the continuing advancement of brain imaging technology holds promise not only in contributing greater understanding of the nature and causes of learning disabilities but also in treating the disorder.

Genetic and hereditary influences also have been proposed as causes. Supportive evidence comes from research indicating that identical twins are more likely to be concordant for learning disabilities than fraternal twins and that these disorders are more common in certain families.

A genetic cause of learning disabilities may be associated with extra X or Y chromosomes in certain individuals. The type and degree of impairment associated with these conditions vary according to many genetic and environmental factors, but they can involve problems with language development, visual perception, memory, and problem solving. Despite evidence to link chromosome abnormalities to those with learning disabilities, most experts agree that such genetic conditions account for only a portion of these individuals.

Exposure to toxins or poisons during fetal gestation and early childhood can also cause learning disabilities. During pregnancy nearly all substances the mother takes in are transferred to the fetus. Research has shown that mothers who smoke, drink alcohol, or use certain drugs or medications during pregnancy are more likely to have children with developmental problems, including learning disabilities. Yet not all children exposed to toxins during gestation will have such problems, and the consequences of exposure will vary according to the period when it occurred, the amount of toxin introduced, and the general health and nutrition of the mother and fetus.

Though not precisely involving toxins, two other conditions associated with gestation and childbirth have been linked to learning disabilities. The first, anoxia or oxygen deprivation, occurring for a critical period of time during the birthing process has been tied to both mental retardation and learning disabilities. The second, and more speculative, involves exposure of the fetus to an abnormally large amount of testosterone during gestation. Differences in brain development are proposed to result from the exposure causing learning disorders, among other abnormalities. Known as the embryological theory, it may account for the large number of males with these disabilities, since they have greater amounts of testosterone than females.

The exposure of the immature brain during early childhood to insecticides, household cleaning fluids, alcohol, narcotics, and carbon monoxide, among other toxic substances, may also cause learning disabilities. Lead poisoning resulting from ingesting lead from paint, plaster, and other sources has been found in epidemic numbers in some sections of the country. Lead poisoning can damage the brain and cause learning disabilities, as well as a number of other serious problems.

The number and variety of proposed causes not only reflect differences in experts' training and consequent perspectives but also suggest the likelihood that these disorders can be caused by multiple conditions. This diversity of views also carries to methods for assessing and providing treatment and services to individuals with learning disabilities.

Treatment and Therapy

In 1975, the U.S. Congress adopted the Education for All Handicapped Children Act, which, along with other requirements, mandated that students with disabilities, including those with learning disabilities, be identified and provided appropriate educational services. Since that time, much effort has been devoted to developing adequate assessment practices for diagnosis and effective treatment strategies.

In the school setting, assessment of students suspected of having learning disabilities is conducted by a variety of professionals, including teachers specially trained in assessing learning disabilities, school nurses, classroom teachers, school psychologists, and school administrators. Collectively, these professionals are known as a multidisciplinary team. An additional requirement of this educational legislation is that parents must be given the opportunity to participate in the assessment process. Professionals outside the school setting, such as clinical psychologists and independent educational specialists, also conduct assessments to identify learning disabilities.

Because the definition of learning disabilities in the 1975 act includes a discrepancy between achievement and ability as a characteristic of the disorder, students suspected of having learning disabilities are usually administered a variety of formal and informal tests. Standardized tests of intelligence, such as the third edition of the Wechsler Intelligence Scale for Children, are administered to determine ability. Standardized tests of academic achievement, such as the Woodcock-Johnson Psychoeducational Battery and the Wide Range Achievement Test, also are administered to determine levels of academic skill.

Whether a discrepancy between ability and achievement exists to such a degree to warrant diagnosis of a learning disability is determined by various formulas comparing the scores derived from the intelligence and achievement tests. The precise methods and criteria used to determine a discrepancy vary according to differences among state regulations and school district practices. Consequently, a student diagnosed with a learning disability in one part of the United States may not be viewed as such in another area using different diagnostic criteria. This possibility has been raised in criticism of the use of the discrepancy criteria to identify these disorders. Other criticisms of the method include the use of intelligence quotient (IQ) scores (which are not as stable or accurate as many assume), the inconsistency of students' scores when using alternative achievement tests, and the lack of correspondence between what students are taught and what is tested on achievement tests.

In partial consequence of these and other problems with standardized tests, alternative informal assessment methods have been developed. One such method that is frequently employed is termed curriculum-based assessment (CBA). The CBA method uses materials and tasks taken directly from students' classroom curriculum. For example, in reading, CBA might involve determining the rate of words read per minute from a student's textbook. CBA has been demonstrated to be effective in distinguishing among some students with learning disabilities, those with other academic difficulties, and those without learning problems. Nevertheless, many professionals remain skeptical of CBA as a valid alternative to traditional standardized tests.

Other assessment techniques include vision and hearing tests, measures of language development, and tests examining motor coordination and sensory perception and processing. Observations and analyses of the classroom environment may also be conducted to determine how instructional practices and a student's behavior contribute to learning difficulties.

Based on the information gathered by the multidisciplinary team, a decision is made regarding the diagnosis of a learning disability. If a student is identified with one of these disorders, the team then develops an individual education plan to address identified educational needs. An important guideline in developing the plan is that students with these disorders should be educated to the greatest extent possible with their nonhandicapped peers, while still being provided with appropriate services. Considerable debate has occurred regarding how best to adhere to this guideline.

Programs for students with learning disabilities typically are implemented in self-contained classrooms, resource rooms, or regular classrooms. Self-contained classrooms usually contain ten to twenty students and one or more teachers specially trained to work with these disorders. Typically, these classrooms focus on teaching fundamental skills in basic academic subjects such as reading, writing, and mathematics. Depending on the teacher's training, efforts may also be directed toward developing perceptual, language, or social skills. Students in these programs usually spend some portion of their day with their peers in regular education meetings, but the majority of the day is spent in the self-contained classroom.

The popularity of self-contained classrooms has decreased significantly since the 1960's, when they were the primary setting in which students with learning disabilities were educated. This decrease is largely attributable to the stigmatizing effects of placing students in special settings and the lack of clear evidence to support the effectiveness of this approach.

Students receiving services in resource rooms typically spend a portion of their day in a class where they receive instruction and assistance from specially trained teachers. Students often spend one or two periods in the resource room with a small group of other students who may have similar learning problems or function at a comparable academic level. In the elementary grades, resource rooms usually focus on developing basic academic skills, whereas at the secondary level time is more typically spent in assisting students with their assignments from regular education classes.

Resource room programs are viewed as less restrictive than self-contained classrooms; however, they too have been criticized for segregating children with learning problems. Other criticisms center on scheduling difficulties inherent in the program and the potential for inconsistent instructional approaches and confusion over teaching responsibilities between the regular classroom and resource room teachers. Research on the effectiveness of resource room programs also has been mixed; nevertheless, they are found in most public schools across the United States.

Though they remain a minority, increasing numbers of students have their individual education plans implemented exclusively in a regular classroom. In most schools where such programs exist, teachers are given assistance by a consulting teacher with expertise in learning disabilities. Supporters of this approach point to the lack of stigma associated with segregating students and the absence of definitive research supporting other service models. Detractors are concerned about the potential for inadequate support for the classroom teacher, resulting in students receiving poor quality or insufficient services. The movement to provide services to educationally handicapped students in regular education settings, termed the Regular Education Initiative, has stirred much debate among professionals and parents. Resolution of the debate will greatly affect how individuals with learning disabilities are provided services.

No one specific method of teaching these students has been demonstrated to be superior to others. A variety of strategies have been developed, including perceptual training, multisensory teaching, modality matching, and direct instruction. Advocates of perceptual training believe that academic problems stem from underlying deficits in perceptual skills. They use various techniques aimed at developing perceptual abilities before trying to remedy or teach specific academic skills. Multisensory teaching involves presenting information to students through several senses. Instruction using this method may be conducted using tactile, auditory, visual, and kinesthetic exercises. Instruction involving modality matching begins with identifying the best learning style for a student, such as visual or auditory processing. Learning tasks are then presented via that mode. Direct instruction is based on the principles of behavioral psychology. The method involves developing precise educational goals, focusing on teaching the exact skill of concern, and providing frequent opportunities to perform the skill until it is mastered.

With the exception of direct instruction, research has generally failed to demonstrate that these strategies are uniquely effective with students with learning disabilities. Direct instruction, on the other hand, has been demonstrated effective but has also been criticized for focusing on isolated skills without dealing with the broader processing problems associated with these disorders. More promisingly, students with learning disabilities appear to benefit from teaching approaches that have been found effective with students without learning problems when instruction is geared to ability level and rate of learning.

PERSPECTIVE AND PROSPECTS

Interest in disorders of learning can be identified throughout the history of medicine. The specific study of learning disabilities, however, can be traced to the efforts of a number of physicians working in the first quarter of the twentieth century who studied the brain and its associated pathology. One such researcher, Kurt Goldstein, identified a number of unusual characteristics, collectively termed perceptual deficits, which were associated with head injury.

Goldstein's work influenced a number of researchers affiliated with the Wayne County Training School, including Alfred Strauss, Laura Lehtinen, Newell Kephart, and William Cruickshank. These individuals worked with children with learning problems who exhibited many of the characteristics of brain injury identified by Goldstein. Consequently, they presumed that neurological dysfunction, whether it could specifically be identified or not, caused the learning difficulties. They also developed a set of instructional practices involving reduced environmental stimuli and exercises to develop perceptual skills. The work and writings of these individuals through the 1940's, 1950's, and 1960's were highly influential, and many programs for students with learning disabilities were based on their theoretical and instructional principles.

Samuel Orton, working in the 1920's and 1930's, also was influenced by research into brain injury in his conceptualization of children with reading problems. He observed that many of these children were left-handed or ambidextrous, reversed letters or words when reading or writing, and had coordination problems. Consequently, he proposed that reading disabilities resulted from abnormal brain development and an associated mixing of brain functions. Based on the work of Orton and his students, including Anna Gilmore and Bessie Stillman, a variety of teaching strategies were developed which focused on teaching phonics and using multisensory aids. In the 1960's, Elizabeth Slingerland applied Orton's concepts in the classroom setting and they have been included in many programs for students with learning disabilities.

A number of other researchers have developed theories for the cause and treatment of learning disabilities. Some of the most influential include Helmer Mykelbust and Samuel Kirk, who emphasized gearing instruction to a student's strongest learning modality, and Norris Haring, Ogden Lindsley, and Joseph Jenkins, who applied principles of behavioral psychology to teaching.

The work of these and other researchers and educators raised professional and public awareness of learning disabilities and the special needs of individuals with the disorder. Consequently, the number of special education classrooms and programs increased dramatically in public schools across the United States in the 1960's and 1970's. Legislation on both the state and federal level, primarily resulting from litigation by parents to establish the educational rights of their children, also has had a profound impact on the availability of services for those with learning disabilities. The passage of the Education for All Handicapped Children Act in 1975 not only mandated appropriate educational services for students with learning disabilities but also generated funding, interest, and research in the field. The Regular Education Initiative has since prompted increased efforts to identify more effective assessment and treatment strategies and generated debates among professionals and the consumers of these services. Decisions resulting from these continuing debates will have a significant impact on future services for individuals with learning disabilities.

—*Paul F. Bell, Ph.D.*

See also Aphasia and dysphasia; Attention-deficit disorder; Autism; Brain; Brain disorders; Down syndrome; Dyslexia; Mental retardation; Neuralgia, neuritis, and neuropathy; Neurology; Neurology, pediatric; Psychiatry; Psychiatry, child and adolescent; Speech disorders.

FOR FURTHER INFORMATION:

Cordoni, Barbara. *Living with a Learning Disability.* Rev. ed. Carbondale: Southern Illinois University Press, 1990. Written by a professor of special education and the mother of two children with learning disabilities, this book focuses on the social skill problems associated with these disorders.

Hallahan, Daniel P., James M. Kauffman, and John Wills Lloyd. *Introduction to Learning Disabilities.* 2d ed. Boston: Allyn & Bacon, 1999. This text addresses different learning disabilities and the education of the learning disabled. Includes a bibliography and indexes.

Lovitt, Thomas. *Introduction to Learning Disabilities.* Needham Heights, Mass.: Allyn & Bacon, 1989. This book is exceptionally well written and comprehensive in its review of topics associated with learning disabilities, including assessment and treatment issues, the history of these disorders, and recommendations for future efforts in the field.

Snowling, M. J., and M. E. Thomson, eds. *Dyslexia: Integrating Theory and Practice.* London: Whurr, 1991. This publication includes selected papers from the second International Conference of the British Dyslexia Association, held in 1991. Chapters include detailed descriptions of theoretical and practical aspects of reading disabilities and reviews of treatment strategies for individuals from early childhood to adulthood.

LEGIONNAIRES' DISEASE
DISEASE/DISORDER

ANATOMY OR SYSTEM AFFECTED: Chest, lungs, respiratory system

SPECIALTIES AND RELATED FIELDS: Bacteriology, environmental health, epidemiology, internal medicine, public health

DEFINITION: A rapidly progressing bacterial pneumonia caused by infection with an organism of the genus *Legionella* and characterized by influenza-like illness, with high fever, chills, headache, and muscle aches.

KEY TERMS:

alveolus: an outpouching of lung tissue in which gas exchange takes place between air in the lungs and blood capillaries

legionellosis: another name for any infection caused by a member of the genus *Legionella;* generally denotes Legionnaires' disease

macrophage: any of a variety of phagocytic cells;

macrophages are found in highest numbers in tissue; alveolar macrophages are found in lungs and function to remove respiratory pathogens

phagocytes: white cells capable of ingesting and digesting microbes, a process referred to as phagocytosis; primarily refers to neutrophils and macrophages

Pontiac fever: a self-limiting, nonpneumonic disease caused by *Legionella* bacteria; clinically and epidemiologically distinct from Legionnaires' disease

virulence factor: a bacterial factor that enhances the pathogenic potential of the organism; includes products such as toxins and capsules

CAUSES AND SYMPTOMS

Legionnaires' disease, or legionellosis, is an acute bacterial pneumonia that was unknown prior to 1976. In July and August of that year, an outbreak of pneumonia occurred among persons who had either attended an American Legion convention in Philadelphia or had been in the vicinity of the Bellevue-Stratford Hotel in the downtown area. The likely source of the epidemic was a contaminated air-conditioning unit in the hotel. Though speculation among the media and general public suggested all sorts of causes for the epidemic, the specific etiological agent was isolated by January, 1977. It turned out to be a somewhat common bacterium, which was subsequently given the genus and species names *Legionella pneumophila*; the genus name reflected the first known victims, while the species name meant "lung-loving."

Within several years, additional strains of *Legionella* bacteria were isolated from patients suffering from bacterial pneumonia. By 1992, thirty-two known species had been identified either as human pathogens or as microflora in environmental water sources. Most cases of Legionnaires' disease have been linked to infection by *L. pneumophila* or, to a lesser degree, *L. micdadei.*

Genetic evidence confirmed that *Legionella* was indeed a newly isolated bacterium. Several factors contributed to its previous invisibility. First, Legionnaires' disease is similar in its characteristics to other forms of nonbacterial pneumonia, such as that caused by viruses. Since no bacteria were readily isolated, there was no immediate reason to suspect a bacterium as the infectious agent. The second reason related to the initial difficulty of growing *Legionella* bacteria in the laboratory. Aspirates from pneumonia victims were inoculated onto routine laboratory media; most com-

mon bacteria grow quite readily on such media. No growth was observed, however, in the case of *Legionella.* Many nutrient supplements were tried. *Legionella* bacteria grew only on media that were supplemented with iron and the amino acid cysteine. Since the early 1980's, the medium of choice has been agar containing buffered charcoal yeast extract. Nutrients such as amino acids, vitamins, and iron are included in the medium while the charcoal removes potentially toxic materials.

Legionellosis actually constitutes two separate clinical entities: Legionnaires' disease and Pontiac fever. Legionnaires' disease is potentially the more serious of the two. The victim is initially infected through a respiratory route. In general, the source of the infection is an aerosol generated by contaminated water supplies such as those found in the cooling units of building air-conditioning systems. Rarely, if at all, does the disease pass from person to person. Most infections are unapparent, with either mild disease or none at all. The estimate is that less than 5 percent of exposed individuals actually contract Legionnaires' disease. Certain factors seem to increase the chances that the infection will progress toward pneumonia. Often, the lungs of the victim have suffered from previous trauma, such as that caused by emphysema or smoking. The person is generally, though not always, middle-aged or older. These observations suggest that, in most instances, the person's immune system is quite capable of handling the infection.

The disease begins with a dry cough, muscle aches, and rising fever—symptoms that resemble the flu. The person may also suffer from vomiting and diarrhea. In serious cases, the disease becomes progressively more severe over the next three to six days. The alveoli, or air sacs, of the lung become necrotized, increasing the difficulty in breathing. Small abscesses may also form in the lungs, as phagocytes infiltrate the area. The mortality rate has ranged from 15 to 60 percent in various outbreaks, although with early treatment, these numbers can be significantly lowered. Patients with other underlying lung problems, or who may be immunosuppressed, are at particular risk.

Pontiac fever is a much less serious form of disease. Named for the Michigan city in which a 1968 outbreak occurred in the Public Health Department building, the disease is self-limiting, nonpneumonic, and not life-threatening. Pontiac fever also seems to follow the inhalation of the etiological agent. Though the attack rate in exposed individuals appears to approach 100 percent, there is no infiltration of lung tissue and no abscess formation. A febrile period occurs one to two days following infection, with the individual progressing to recovery after several days. The difference between the two forms of disease remains obscure. There appears to be no obvious difference between the organisms associated with the two diseases, though strains associated with Pontiac fever may not replicate as readily inside human cells.

The mechanism by which infection by *Legionella* bacteria results in pneumonia is not altogether clear. Research into this area has centered on forms of virulence factors produced by the organism and their relationships to disease. Following their infiltration into the lung, *Legionella* bacteria are phagocytized by alveolar macrophages or other leukocytes (white blood cells). Unlike other ingested microbes, however, *Legionella* bacteria often survive the process and begin a process of intracellular replication. In this intracellular state, *Legionella* bacteria are shielded from many of the host's immune defenses.

Certain questions lend themselves to understanding this approach in elucidating the mechanisms of Legionnaires' disease. First, are intracellular survival and multiplication necessary factors in the development of the disease? Second, if these factors are indeed relevant, exactly how does the organism manage to evade the killing mechanisms that exist inside the cell?

The first question has been dealt with by various animal studies. Guinea pigs were exposed to a *Legionella* aerosol, and lung aspirates were prepared after forty-eight hours. Large numbers of viable organisms were found inside alveolar macrophages. Few live *Legionella* bacteria, however, were observed outside cells. In addition, mutant *Legionella* bacteria that were incapable of intracellular growth showed reduced virulence in guinea pigs. Therefore, initial intracellular infection and multiplication does appear to be necessary to initiate the disease process.

The mechanism of intracellular survival is less clear. Macrophages are professional phagocytes that have a wide variety of means for killing ingested microorganisms. These mechanisms range from the production of reactive oxygen molecules to the synthesis of oxidizing agents such as peroxides. In addition, after a foreign microbe has been phagocytized within the membrane-bound vessel called a phagosome, a cell organelle, the lysosome, will fuse with the phagosome. Contained within the lysosome are large numbers of digestive enzymes that proceed to digest the target. Under normal circumstances, foreign microbes are ingested and digested, eliminating the threat of infection.

Somehow, *Legionella* bacteria evade these defense mechanisms. Different strains of *Legionella* bacteria appear to have evolved a variety of mechanisms for survival. In particular, there are two types of molecules, a phosphatase and a cytoxin, whose presence is correlated with intracellular survival. Both appear to act by preventing the phagocytes from producing potentially lethal oxidation molecules such as hydrogen peroxide.

Another virulence factor that appears to be important for infectivity is a surface protein known as the macrophage infectivity potentiator, or MIP. The MIP proteins are apparently unique to *Legionella* bacteria; mutants that lack the MIP gene are significantly less virulent than wild-type strains. The MIP protein appears to be necessary for the internalization of *Legionella* bacteria by the macrophage, and for survival against the array of bacteriocidal activities.

A variety of other mechanisms may also exist that allow *Legionella* bacteria to escape the killing mechanisms of the macrophage. For example, in addition to the phosphatase, which removes phosphate molecules from host proteins or lipids, *Legionella* bacteria also produce protein kinases, which can add phosphate molecules to host cell proteins. In this manner, *Legionella* bacteria can potentially regulate the metabolism of the cells in which they find themselves by adding or subtracting phosphates from various sites or metabolic pathways.

Though a precise sequence of events that leads to the development of Legionnaires' disease remains to be worked out, certain steps appear to be necessary. Following the inhalation of a *Legionella* aerosol, probably from a contaminated water source, the organism lodges in the alveoli of the lung. Resident macrophages phagocytize the microbe, resulting in its internalization. Through a variety of virulence factors, *Legionella* survives, and multiplies within the macrophage. Death of the host cells along with the concomitant infiltration of other white cells results in the inflammation and lung damage recognized as Legionnaires' disease.

TREATMENT AND THERAPY

Despite the hysteria associated with the Philadelphia outbreak of Legionnaires' disease and the difficulty associated with the initial isolation of the etiological agent, there is nothing particularly unusual about the organism. The *Legionella* bacterium is a small, thin microbe some 2 to 10 micrometers in length, about the size of most average bacteria. Because of its characteristic staining pattern, it is classified as a gram-negative organism. This results from the molecular nature of its cell wall, which has a high lipopoly-saccharide (LPS) content.

Since legionellosis can resemble other forms of pneumonia, improper diagnosis can be a problem. Though the prognosis of the disease is generally favorable with early intervention, improper or delayed treatment can prove fatal. In general, legionellosis is suspected in a patient with a progressive pneumonia for which other organisms do not appear to be a factor. *Legionella* bacteria may be observed from lung aspirates using immunofluorescent examination. In this technique, a sample of aspirate is treated with a fluorescent-labeled antibody molecule that is capable of binding to the surface of the microorganism. The microbe will then fluoresce, or glow, when observed with a microscope containing ultraviolet optics. The advantage of this method is its speed. Often, however, there are too few bacteria in the lung to be identified.

A firm diagnosis is made by culturing the bacteria on artificial media. Generally, a buffered charcoal yeast extract medium is used that contains a variety of amino acids and vitamins necessary for the organisms to grow. *Legionella* bacteria will not grow on the more conventional media used to culture other types of bacteria, which caused problems in the early attempts to isolate the organism associated with the Legionnaires' disease outbreak. Diagnosis may also be carried out by measuring the level of anti-*Legionella* antibody in the serum of the suspected patient. A rising level of antibody is indicative of active infection by the organism.

There are several aspects of the clinical significance of the gram-negative character of the organism, one of which is that this type of bacteria responds poorly to penicillin or penicillin derivatives. This serves to limit the type of antimicrobial therapy available for treatment of severe cases of legionellosis. Other antibiotics exist, of course, that exhibit antibacterial characteristics similar to those of penicillin— for example, the cephalosporins. And, indeed, penicillin derivatives have been used to treat at least some types of gram-negative infections. Legionellosis patients did not respond well, however, to treatment with any of these agents. It was subsequently found that the basis for the resistance by *Legionella* bacteria to these antibiotics lay in a type of extracellular enzyme produced by these bacteria—a beta-lactamase.

The lack of pharmacologic activity associated with the penicillins, the cephalosporins, and certain other antibiotics is thus easy to explain. The activity of these antibiotics is associated with the presence of a structure in the molecule called a beta-lactam ring. The beta-lactamase produced by the *Legionella* bacterium causes a break in the ring, rendering the antibiotic harmless to the microbe, and thus useless as a form of treatment. Such resistance has become increasingly common among bacteria, since the genes encoding the beta-lactamase are passed from organism to organism.

Fortunately, other antibiotics did prove to be useful in the treatment of legionellosis. To a certain extent, the determination of the antibiotics of choice was fortuitous. During the Philadelphia outbreak, the nature of the illness was unknown. The primary assumption was that an infectious agent was at fault, but determination of the nature of that agent lay months beyond the extent of the epidemic. Therefore, as would be true in the treatment of any illness of unknown origin, various treatments were carried out. Two antibiotics in particular proved to be useful: erythromycin and rifampin. Erythromycin, which specifically inhibits bacterial protein synthesis, has continued to be useful. Though long-term use can result in liver damage and some individuals are hypersensitive to the drug, the intravenous administration of erythromycin remains the treatment of choice for legionellosis. Rifampin is used on occasion in association with other methods of treatment, but the high frequency of bacterial resistance to the drug precludes its use as a treatment of first choice.

Since the virulent properties of the *Legionella* bacterium depend on its intracellular presence in the macrophage, those antimicrobial agents that exhibit intracellular penetration would be expected to be most effective. Erythromycin fits this requirement, as do a number of other antibiotics. Not surprisingly, these agents have proved to be most efficacious in the treatment of the disease. Thus, alternative sources of treatment exist in the event that erythromycin proves ineffective.

Other aspects of treatment center on maintaining the comfort of the individual. This may include the use of analgesics for relief of pain.

Prevention of the disease is obviously preferable to dealing with the sequelae of infection. Epidemiological studies have demonstrated that the *Legionella* bacterium is a common soil organism that is often found in bodies of water contaminated by soil. The organism has been found in lakes and pond water, and it can survive for long periods in unchlorinated tap water. In fact, contaminated water appears to have been the source of infection for most outbreaks of the illness. Problems have often been associated with cooling towers, evaporative condensers, and other water supplies found with air-conditioning units of buildings. Infectious aerosols may be generated from these units, allowing for a respiratory route of infection. Though the disease is thus spread in an airborne manner, there is no evidence that it can be passed from person to person.

The epidemiological evidence for the disease supports an airborne hypothesis. Most outbreaks have occurred in regions of soil disruption, such as that occurring during construction. Subsequent isolation of *Legionella* bacteria from the cooling towers confirmed such contamination. Though the air-conditioning unit of the Bellevue-Stratford Hotel in Philadelphia was replaced prior to isolation of the organism, the assumption is that the unit was contaminated. The outbreaks of the disease during the summer, when air-conditioning use has peaked, are consistent with the role of air-conditioning units in the spread of *Legionella* bacteria.

The method by which the *Legionella* bacterium survives in the environment has not been completely determined. The organism is somewhat resistant both to chlorine treatment and to heat as high as 65 degrees Celsius. It appears to grow best in the presence of biological factors secreted by other microflora in the environment; growth stimulation may also be enhanced by the presence of physical factors such as sediment, silicone, and rubber compounds. Its ability to survive, and indeed be transmitted, may also be related to its tendency to penetrate and multiply intracellularly within environmental protozoa or amoeba.

Prevention of disease transmission must take into account these problems. Contamination of water supplies must be minimized. The resistance of the *Legionella* bacterium to standard methods of decontamination has made the process more difficult, and methods of choice remain controversial. Chlorination at relatively high levels remains the preferred method,

with subsequent treatment at lower concentrations over the long term. The disadvantages of this method include the cost of constant treatment and the eventual corrosion of the units. Continuous or intermittent heating of the water has also proved effective in decontamination.

PERSPECTIVE AND PROSPECTS

Prior to August, 1976, Legionnaires' disease was unknown. From July 21 to 24 of that year, however, the Pennsylvania branch of the American Legion held its annual convention at the Bellevue-Stratford Hotel in Philadelphia. Some 4,000 delegates and their families attended the festivities. Following the convention, as delegates returned to their homes, a mysterious illness began to appear among the attendees. A total of 149 conventioneers and 72 others became ill. Characterized by a severe respiratory infection that progressed into pneumonia, and high fever, the illness proved fatal to 34 of the victims.

By August, it became clear to the Pennsylvania Department of Health that an epidemic was at hand. The cause of the outbreak was not clear, and rumors began to circulate. At various times, the news media explained the outbreak as a Communist plot against former military men, a Central Intelligence Agency test gone awry, and even an infectious agent arriving from space. The truth was less dramatic. By the beginning of 1977, David Fraser, Joseph McDade, and their colleagues from the Centers for Disease Control isolated the etiological agent: a bacterium subsequently named *Legionella pneumophila*.

With the isolation and identification of the organism, it became possible to explain earlier outbreaks of unusual illness. For example, during July and August of 1965, an outbreak of pneumonia at a chronic-care facility at St. Elizabeth's Hospital in Washington, D.C., resulted in 81 cases and 14 deaths. An outbreak among personnel at the Oakland County Health Department in Pontiac, Michigan, during July and August of 1968 of a disease that was subsequently called Pontiac fever was also traced to the same organism. In this case, however, though 144 persons were affected, none died. In fact, illness associated with the *Legionella* bacterium has been traced as far back as 1947. The 1976 outbreak was not new; it was merely the first time that medical personnel were able to isolate the organism that caused the disease.

The precise prevalence of the *Legionella* bacterium remains murky, but it is clearly more common than was at first realized. Despite the public's fear of the disease, in most instances it probably remains a mild respiratory infection, resembling nothing worse than a bad cold. Most cases remain undetected. Estimates have suggested that as many as 25,000 persons in the United States develop infection. Based on seroconversions—the production of anti-*Legionella* antibody in the sera of persons—it has been estimated that more than 20 percent of the population of Michigan has been exposed to the organism. There is no reason to doubt that the same situation exists in many other states.

The basis for the difference in severity between Legionnaires' disease and Pontiac fever is also unclear. There is no obvious difference between the two diseases that accounts for the differences in virulence. It also remains to be seen whether *Legionella* bacteria are associated with other illnesses.

The final lesson of Legionnaires' disease is as subtle as its initial appearance. Humans exist in an environment replete with infectious agents. Despite the battery of modern methods of treatment for illness, there always remains the potential for new outbreaks of previously unknown disease.

—*Richard Adler, Ph.D.*

See also Bacterial infections; Epidemiology; Lungs; Pneumonia; Pulmonary diseases; Pulmonary medicine; Pulmonary medicine, pediatric; Respiration.

FOR FURTHER INFORMATION:

Biddle, Wayne. *Field Guide to Germs*. New York: Henry Holt, 1995. This comprehensive book is easily accessible to the nonspecialist and includes a discussion of nearly every virus, bacterium, and fungus known to cause human and nonhuman animal disease. The history of the microbe and the treatment of diseases are included.

Brock, Thomas D., ed. *Microorganisms: From Smallpox to Lyme Disease*. New York: W. H. Freeman, 1990. A collection of readings from *Scientific American*. The book includes a collection of accounts of the history of major infectious diseases. Divided into sections dealing with medical histories, methods of prevention, and means of transmission.

Dowling, John N., Asish K. Saha, and Robert H. Glew. "Virulence Factors of the Family *Legionellaceae*." *Microbiological Reviews* 56 (March 1, 1992): 32. A thorough discussion of the roles played by various virulence factors related to intra-cellular survival of the bacterium. A review article for which basic knowledge of microbiology would be helpful. Nevertheless, the article contains a wealth of information on the subject.

Hoebe, Christian J. P. A., and Jacob L. Kool. "Control of Legionella in Drinking-Water Systems." *The Lancet* 355, no. 9221 (June 17, 2000): 2093-2094. This article discusses the process of copper-silver ionization for the control of legionella. This process has reduced legionella counts when used simultaneously with continuous chlorine injection.

Ryan, Kenneth J., ed. *Sherris Medical Microbiology: An Introduction to Infectious Diseases*. Rev. 3d ed. Norwalk, Conn.: Appleton and Lange, 1994. A textbook dealing with major pathogenic organisms. The section on *Legionella* is a concise outline of what is known about the disease.

Springston, John. "Legionella Bacteria in Building Environments." *Occupational Hazards* 61, no. 8 (August, 1999): 51-56. Legionella bacteria tend to be unwanted occupants of the building environment. Their ability to contaminate domestic water systems, coupled with their potential to cause severe health complications, presents a very real concern to building owners and managers.

LEISHMANIASIS

DISEASE/DISORDER

ANATOMY OR SYSTEM AFFECTED: Skin

SPECIALTIES AND RELATED FIELDS: Dermatology, public health

DEFINITION: The term "leishmaniasis" refers to several diseases associated with the single-celled protozoan species *Leishmania*. Transmitted by the bite of a sand fly, the parasites cause ulcers in the skin or internal organs. There are four main types: visceral leishmaniasis, or kala-azar; and Old World cutaneous, New World cutaneous, and mucocutaneous leishmaniasis. Kala-azar is the most serious form because it affects the bone marrow and organs and may cause anemia and other disorders; it is found in Asia, Africa, and parts of South America. The cutaneous types occur either in Central and South America (New World) or in the Middle East, North Africa, and parts of the Mediterranean (Old World); a persistent skin ulcer forms and eventually heals, although disfigurement may result. Medications are available to treat all types of infection.

—*Jason Georges and Tracy Irons-Georges*

See also Arthropod-borne diseases; Bites and stings; Parasitic diseases; Protozoan diseases; Tropical medicine; Ulcers.

FOR FURTHER INFORMATION:

Busvine, James R. *Disease Transmission by Insects: Its Discovery and Ninety Years of Effort to Prevent It.* New York: Springer-Verlag, 1993.

_____. *Insects, Hygiene, and History.* 3d ed. London: Athlone Press, 1983.

James, Maurice T., and Robert F. Harwood. *Herm's Medical Entomology.* 6th ed. New York: Macmillan, 1969.

Snow, Keith R. *Insects and Disease.* New York: John Wiley & Sons, 1974.

LEPROSY

DISEASE/DISORDER

ANATOMY OR SYSTEM AFFECTED: Immune system, nerves, nervous system, skin

SPECIALTIES AND RELATED FIELDS: Bacteriology, epidemiology, immunology, internal medicine, public health

DEFINITION: A bacterial infection that affects skin and nerves, causing symptoms ranging from mild numbness to gross disfiguration.

KEY TERMS:

acid-fast: the ability of a bacterium to retain a pink stain in the presence of a mixture of acid and alcohol

antibody: a protein found in the blood and produced by the immune system in response to bodily contact with an antigen

antigen: a foreign substance (such as a bacterium, toxin, or virus) to which the body makes an immune response

bacillus Calmette-Guérin (BCG): a vaccine for tuberculosis made from a harmless strain of *Mycobacterium bovis*

bacterium: microscopic single-celled organism that multiplies by simple division; bacteria are found everywhere; most are beneficial, but a few species cause disease

cellular immune response: the reaction of the body that produces active white blood cells that can destroy antigens associated with other body cells

humoral immune response: the reaction of the body that produces antibodies that can destroy antigens present in body fluids

hypersensitivity: an overreaction by the immune system to the presence of certain antigens; this overreaction often results in some damage to the person as well as the antigen

immune response: the working of the body's immune system to prevent or combat an infectious disease

CAUSES AND SYMPTOMS

Leprosy, also known as Hansen's disease, is caused by the bacterium *Mycobacterium leprae (M. leprae).* Humans are the only natural host for this bacterium; it can be found only in leprosy victims. Most people who are exposed to this bacterium are unaffected by it; in the remainder, the bacterium grows inside skin and nerve cells, causing a wide range of symptoms that depend upon the person's immune response to the growth of the bacteria.

M. leprae is an obligate intracellular parasite, which means that it can grow only inside other cells. *M. leprae* has a unique waxy coating that helps to protect it while it is growing inside human skin and nerve cells. The bacterium grows very slowly, dividing once every twelve days, whereas the average bacterium will divide every twenty to sixty minutes. *M. leprae* grows best at temperatures slightly below body temperature (37 degrees Celsius). The leprosy bacterium is the only bacterium known to destroy peripheral nerve tissue (nerves that are not a part of the central nervous system) and will also destroy skin and mucous membranes. This bacterium is closely related to the bacterium that causes tuberculosis: *Mycobacterium tuberculosis.*

Leprosy is not very contagious. Several attempts to infect human volunteers with the bacteria have been unsuccessful. It is believed that acquiring leprosy from an infected person requires prolonged intimate contact with that person, such as living in the same house for a long time. Although the precise mode of transmission of *M. leprae* bacteria is unclear, it is highly probable that the bacteria are transferred from the nasal or respiratory secretions of the victim to the nasal passages or a skin wound of the recipient.

Once inside a person, *M. leprae* will grow and reproduce inside skin and nerve cells and destroy tissue. The exact mechanism of tissue destruction is not understood, but it probably results from a combination of nerve damage, massive accumulation of bacteria, and immunological reactions. Because the bacteria grow so slowly, the length of time from infection to appearance of the symptoms (the incubation period) is quite long. The average incubation period is two

Lepromatous Leprosy

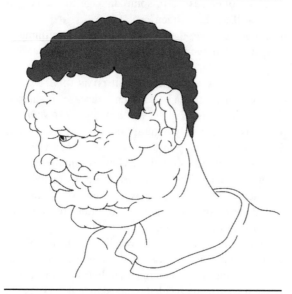

This more severe form of leprosy occurs in the absence of a strong immune response and results in lepromas, or tumor-like growths.

to seven years, but incubation can range from three months to forty years. Since the bacteria prefer temperatures slightly lower that normal body temperature, symptoms appear first in the cooler parts of the body, such as the hands, fingers, feet, face, nose, and earlobes. In severe cases, symptoms also appear in the eyes and the respiratory tract.

The symptoms associated with leprosy can range from very mild to quite severe, and the symptoms that a person gets depend heavily on that person's ability to mount a cellular immune response against the bacteria. In a normal infection, the human body is capable of defending itself through two processes of the immune system; the humoral immune response and the cellular immune response. The humoral response produces chemicals called antibodies that can attack and destroy infectious agents that are present in body fluids such as the blood. The cellular response produces white blood cells that can destroy infectious agents that are associated with cells. Since *M. leprae* hides and grows inside human cells, a cellular response is the only type of immune response that can be of any help in fighting the infection. The ability to generate a cellular immune response against *M. leprae* is dependent upon the genetic makeup and overall health of the victim, as well as the number of

infecting bacteria and their ability to invade the body and cause disease. A quick and strong cellular response by a person infected with *M. leprae* will result in no symptoms or in the mild form of the disease: tuberculoid leprosy. A slow or weak cellular response by a person exposed to leprosy may result in the more severe form of the disease: lepromatous leprosy.

Only one in two hundred people exposed to leprosy will get some form of the disease. The earliest symptom is a slightly bleached, flat lesion several centimeters in diameter that is usually found on the upper body or on the arms or legs. About three-fourths of all patients with an early solitary lesion heal spontaneously; the rest progress to tuberculoid or lepromatous leprosy or to one of the many forms that fall between these two extremes.

Tuberculoid leprosy is characterized by flat skin lesions 5 to 20 centimeters in diameter. The lesions are lighter in color than the surrounding skin and are sometimes surrounded by nodules (lumps). The lesions contain only a few bacteria, and they, along with the surrounding tissue, are numb. These lesions are caused by a hypersensitive cellular immune response to the bacteria in the nerves and skin. In an attempt to destroy the bacteria, the immune system overreacts, and some of the surrounding nerve and skin tissue is damaged while the bacteria are being killed. This causes the areas of the skin to lose pigment as well as sensation. Often, tuberculoid leprosy patients can experience more extensive physical damage if the numbness around the lesions leads to accidental loss of digits, skin, and so forth. Leprosy victims may burn and cut themselves unknowingly, since they have no feeling in certain areas of their bodies.

In lepromatous leprosy, the bacteria grow unchecked because of the weak cellular immune response. Often, there are more than 100 million bacterial cells present per square centimeter of tissue. These bacteria cause the formation of tumorlike growths called lepromas as well as tissue destruction of the skin and mucous membranes. Also, the presence of so many bacteria causes large numbers of antibacterial antibodies to be produced, but these antibodies are of no benefit in fighting off the infection. Instead, they can contribute to the formation of lesions and tissue damage both internally and on the skin through a process called immune complex hypersensitivity. This is a process whereby the large number of antibodies bind to the large number of bacteria in the body and form immune complexes. These complexes can be deposited in various parts of the body and trigger a chemical reaction that destroys the surrounding tissue. The large number of bacteria puts pressure on the nerves and destroys nerve tissue, which causes loss of sensation and tissue death.

The initial symptoms of lepromatous leprosy are skin lesions that can be spread out or nodular and are found on the cooler parts of the body, such as the inside of the nose, the front part of the eye, the face, the earlobes, the hands, and the feet. Often, the victim loses all facial features because the nodules enlarge the face, and the eyebrows and nose deteriorate, giving the victim a characteristic lionlike appearance. Severe lepromatous leprosy erodes bones; thus, fingers and toes become needlelike, pits form in the skull, nasal bones are destroyed, and teeth fall out. Also, the limbs become twisted and the hands become clawed. The destruction of the nerves leads to the inability to move the hands or feet, deformity of the feet, and chronic ulceration of the limbs. In addition, as is the case with tuberculoid leprosy, destruction of the small peripheral nerves leads to self-inflicted trauma and secondary infection (infection by another bacterium or virus). As the disease progresses, the growth of bacteria in the respiratory tract causes larynx problems and difficult breathing. Deterioration of the optic nerve leads to blindness. Bacteria can invade the bloodstream and spread infection throughout the whole body except the central nervous system. Death associated with leprosy usually results from respiratory obstruction, kidney failure, or secondary infection.

TREATMENT AND THERAPY

A physician can tell whether a person has leprosy by looking for characteristic symptoms (light-colored and numb lesions, nodules, and so forth) and by determining whether the patient may have been exposed to someone with leprosy. In addition, samples of scrapings from skin lesions, nasal secretions, fluid from nodules, or other tissue secretions can be examined for the presence of *M. leprae*. Samples are treated with a procedure called the acid-fast technique. Because of *M. leprae*'s waxy coating, these bacteria retain a pink stain after being washed in an acid-alcohol mixture, whereas all other bacteria lose the pink stain. Therefore, pink, rod-shaped bacteria observed in samples treated with the acid-fast technique indicate the presence of *M. leprae*. It is easy to find the acid-fast *M. leprae* in lepromatous leprosy patients because

they have so many bacteria in their lesions, but the bacteria are more difficult to find in the lesions of tuberculoid leprosy patients. The lepromin test was originally developed to be used as a diagnostic tool for leprosy, in the same way that the tuberculin test is used as a diagnostic tool for tuberculosis. Lepromin, which is heat-killed *M. leprae* taken from nodules, is injected under the skin in the lepromin test. Two reactions are possible: an early reaction that appears twenty-four to forty-eight hours later and a late reaction that appears three to four weeks later. In both reactions, a hard red lump at the injection site indicates a positive lepromin test. This test is not specific for leprosy, however, because a person who has been exposed to *M. leprae*, *M. tuberculosis*, or the tuberculosis vaccine, bacillus Calmette-Guérin (BCG), will show a positive early reaction. Even though this test is not useful as a diagnostic tool, it is useful in determining whether a patient has a strong or a weak cellular immune response to *M. leprae*. Tuberculoid leprosy patients show both the early and late reactions, while lepromatous leprosy patients show no reaction at all.

Leprosy can be treated with antibiotics. The antibiotic dapsone began to be used on a wide scale in the treatment of leprosy in 1950. Since that time, however, many dapsone-resistant strains of *M. leprae* have appeared. This means that, for some victims, this drug is no longer helpful in fighting the disease. In 1981, in response to the problem of dapsone-resistant strains, the World Health Organization recommended a multidrug regimen for leprosy victims. For lepromatous leprosy patients, dapsone, rifampin, and clofazimine are recommended, whereas tuberculoid leprosy patients need take only dapsone and rifampin. Treatment is expected to continue until skin smears are free from acid-fast bacteria, which can last from two years up to the lifetime of the patient. Since 1989, the U.S. recommendations for tuberculoid leprosy are six months of rifampin and dapsone daily, then dapsone alone for three years. For lepromatous leprosy, the recommendation is to use rifampin and dapsone daily for three years, then dapsone only for the rest of the person's life. Often, antibiotics are given to family members of leprosy patients in order to prevent them from contracting the disease. Antibiotic therapy can make a leprosy victim noncontagious, stop the progress of the disease, and in some cases cause a reversal of some of the symptoms. Until treatment is complete, however, it is recommended that patients sleep in separate bedrooms, use their own linens and utensils, and not live in a house with children. Thus, leprosy victims can lead nearly normal lives without fear of infecting others in the community.

The best ways to keep from getting leprosy are to avoid exposure to leprosy bacteria and to receive antibiotic therapy following exposure. It should be possible to control and, eventually, eliminate leprosy. If every case of leprosy were treated, the disease could not spread and the bacteria would die out with the last leprosy victim. Progress in this direction is slow, however, because of ignorance, superstition, poverty, and overpopulation in areas with many leprosy cases. The first strategy in controlling leprosy is to treat all leprosy cases with antibiotics. As of 1991, about 50 percent of all leprosy victims were not receiving drug therapy. Second, the early detection and rigid isolation of lepromatous leprosy patients are important, as is preventive antibiotic therapy for individuals in close contact with those patients. Finally, as of the early 1990's, too many countries lacked adequate basic health resources, and too many patients disabled by leprosy were not receiving adequate care. The development of a vaccine for leprosy would aid control efforts.

A global effort for the production of a vaccine for leprosy is being made under the auspices of the World Health Organization. The first problem with vaccine development is that, until recently, it was not possible to grow *M. leprae* bacteria outside of a leprosy victim; therefore, not much is known about the nature of the bacteria. Even though this bacterium was the first to be associated with a disease, it cannot be grown on an artificial laboratory medium, whereas nearly all other bacteria known can be grown artificially. It was not until 1960 that scientists at the Centers for Disease Control discovered that the bacterium could be grown in the footpads of mice. Finally, in 1969, scientists at the National Hansen's Disease Center in Carville, Louisiana, found that the bacteria would grow in the tissues of the nine-banded armadillo. Several potential vaccines for leprosy have been tested since that

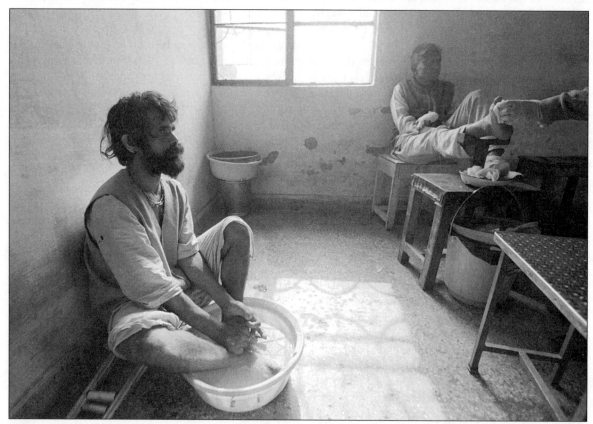

Leprosy patients in India wait to have their wounds cleaned. In 1999, India had 60 percent of the world's leprosy patients. (AP/Wide World Photos)

time. One vaccine being tested is BCG, a live bacterial vaccine of the bacteria *Mycobacterium bovis*, which is a close relative of *M. leprae*. In four major trials with BCG, a range of 20 to 80 percent protection from leprosy was obtained. It is not known why there was such a wide variation in results. As of the early 1990's, 250,000 persons in Venezuela, Malawi, and India were undergoing a preventive vaccine trial using a combination of BCG and *M. leprae* from armadillos. Because it takes so long for the disease to appear, however, five to ten years must pass before it can be determined whether this vaccine is effective in preventing leprosy. Other strategies for vaccine development include making a modified BCG that contains *M. leprae* cell wall antigens. It is more advantageous to use BCG than *M. leprae* in a vaccine because BCG is much easier to grow. In addition, scientists are trying to find a way to grow *M. leprae* artificially so that larger quantities will be available to be used for a vaccine.

PERSPECTIVE AND PROSPECTS

Leprosy is one of the oldest known diseases. References to leprosy are contained in Indian writings that are more than three thousand years old. The Bible refers to leprosy and the isolation of lepers, although the term refers to other skin diseases as well. The examination of ancient skeletons has provided insights into how leprosy spread in past centuries. Early evidence suggests that the disease was highly contagious and that leprosy was widespread in Europe during the Middle Ages. Leprosy was so prevalent, in fact, that both governments and churches moved to deal with the problem. At that time, the cause of leprosy was unknown, and the disease was generally believed to be a punishment for some personal sin. Lepers were treated as outcasts and required to shout "unclean." They were required to wear gloves and distinctive clothes and carry a bell or clapper to warn people of their approach. They were forbidden to drink from public fountains, speak loudly, eat with healthy people, or attend church. Some lepers were even pronounced legally dead, burned at the stake, or buried alive. Later, they were isolated in asylums called leprosaria, and at one time about nineteen thousand leprosaria existed—mostly in France. There was a sharp decrease in the number of leprosy cases in the sixteenth century. Several factors may have contributed to this decline, including the isolation of lepers, a better diet, warmer clothes, the plague epidemic, and the increase in tu-

berculosis, which may have provided resistance to leprosy. Leprosy is no longer as deadly or contagious as it once was, yet the stigma attached to this disease has remained. In an effort to alleviate the social stigma, the Fifth International Congress on Leprosy in 1948 banned the use of the word "leper" and encouraged the use of the term "Hansen's disease" instead of leprosy. *M. leprae*, the causative agent of leprosy, was first identified in the tissues of leprosy patients by the Norwegian physician Gerhard Armauer Hansen in 1873—hence the alternate name, Hansen's disease. Today, victims of leprosy are referred to as Hansenites or Hansenotic.

From the 1960's to the 1980's, estimates of the number of cases of leprosy worldwide ranged from 10 to 12 million. In 1992, the World Health Organization revised its estimate to 5.5 million cases. Efforts to promote multidrug therapy are believed to have caused the decline in the number of cases of leprosy. Leprosy is prevalent in tropical areas such as Africa, Southeast Asia, and South America. In the United States, most cases occur in Hawaii and small parts of Texas, California, Louisiana, and Florida. In 1987, the Centers for Disease Control reported approximately thirty new cases in the United States annually—mostly in foreign-born immigrants from leprosy-prone areas.

—Vicki J. Isola, Ph.D.

See also Antibiotics; Bacterial infections; Immune system; Immunology; Nervous system; Numbness and tingling; Thalidomide; Tropical medicine; Tuberculosis; World Health Organization.

FOR FURTHER INFORMATION:

Biddle, Wayne. *Field Guide to Germs*. New York: Henry Holt, 1995. This comprehensive book is easily accessible to the nonspecialist and includes a discussion of nearly every virus, bacterium, and fungus known to cause human and nonhuman animal disease. The history of the microbe and the treatment of diseases are included.

Bloom, B. R. "Learning from Leprosy: A Perspective on Immunology and the Third World." *Journal of Immunology* 137 (July, 1986): i-x. This article discusses leprosy as a disease, the immune response to leprosy, possible leprosy vaccines, and the problems of administering vaccines in the Third World.

Hastings, Robert C., ed. *Leprosy*. 2d ed. New York: Churchill Livingstone, 1994. This book contains a series of articles describing all aspects of leprosy, from the characteristics of the organism to the disease process to treatment.

Mandell, Gerald L., John E. Bennett, and Raphael Dolin, eds. *Mandell, Douglas, and Bennett's Principles and Practice of Infectious Diseases*. 5th ed. New York: Churchill Livingstone, 2000. Describes leprosy, discussing the organism, epidemiology, symptoms, complications, and diagnosis; an expanded section on therapy is included.

Zinsser, Hans. *Zinsser Microbiology*. Edited by Wolfgang K. Joklik et al. 20th ed. Norwalk, Conn.: Appleton and Lange, 1992. An excellent textbook describing all infectious diseases. The information presented is thorough and logical, and it is supplemented by interesting diagrams, photographs, and charts. Discusses all diseases caused by species of mycobacteria, including leprosy and tuberculosis.

LEPTIN
BIOLOGY

ANATOMY OR SYSTEM AFFECTED: All

SPECIALTIES AND RELATED FIELDS: Biochemistry, cardiology, endocrinology, genetics, gynecology, nutrition

DEFINITION: A protein hormone involved in regulation of food intake and obesity, with secondary effects on immunity, reproduction, and heart disease.

STRUCTURE AND FUNCTIONS

Leptin (from the Greek *leptos*, meaning "thin") is a protein hormone with important effects in regulating body weight, metabolism, and reproductive function. It is the product of the obese (ob) gene occurring on chromosome 7 in the human. Leptin is produced primarily by adipocytes (white fat cells). It is also produced by cells of the epithelium of the stomach and in the placenta. It appears that as adipocytes increase in size because of accumulation of triglycerides (fat molecules), they synthesize more and more leptin. However, the mechanism by which leptin production is controlled is largely unknown. It is likely that a number of hormones modulate leptin output, including corticosteroids and insulin.

DISORDERS AND DISEASES

At first leptin was assumed to be simply a signaling molecule involved in limiting food intake and increasing energy expenditure. Studies published as early as 1994 showed a remarkable difference in weight gain in mice deficient in leptin (mice with a nonfunctional

ob gene). Daily injections of leptin into these animals resulted in a reduction of food intake within a few days and a 50 percent decrease in body weight within a month.

More recent studies in the human have not been as promising. It appears that leptin's effects on body weight are mediated through effects on hypothalamic (brain) centers that control feeding behavior and hunger, body temperature, and energy expenditure. If leptin levels are low, appetite is stimulated and use of energy limited. If leptin levels are high, appetite is reduced and energy use stimulated. The most likely target of leptin in the hypothalamus is inhibition of neuropeptide Y, a potent stimulator of food intake. However, this inhibition alone could not account for the effects seen, and studies looking at other hormones are underway.

Leptin also affects reproductive function in humans. It has long been known that very low body fat in human females is associated with cessation of menstrual cycles, and the onset of puberty is known to correlate with body composition (fat levels) as well as age. Several studies have suggested that leptin stimulates hypothalamic output of gonadotropin-releasing hormone, which in turn causes increases of luteinizing and follicle-stimulating hormones from the anterior pituitary gland. These hormones stimulate the onset of puberty. Prepubertal mice treated with leptin become thin and reach reproductive maturity earlier than control mice. One report has also indicated that humans with mutations in the ob gene that prevent them from producing leptin not only become obese but also fail to achieve puberty.

Leptin has been identified in placental tissues; newborn babies show higher levels those found in their mothers. Leptin has also been found in human breast milk. Together, these findings suggest that leptin aids in intrauterine and neonatal growth and development, as well as in regulation of neonatal food intake.

Finally, leptin appears to have a role in immune system function. Studies have suggested a role for leptin in production of white blood cells and in the control of macrophage function. Mice that lack leptin have depressed immune systems, but the mechanisms for this remain unclear.

PERSPECTIVE AND PROSPECTS

Although early reports claimed that leptin could be useful in treating human obesity, clinical reports to date have not looked promising. It appears that deficiencies in leptin production are a rare cause of human obesity. However, since most obese individuals have plenty of leptin available, additional leptin will have no effect. In those individuals with a genetic deficiency of leptin, clinical use would require either daily injections of leptin or gene therapy. At this point neither of these options looks particularly promising.

—*Kerry L. Cheesman, Ph.D.*

See also Endocrinology; Endocrinology, pediatric; Hormones; Immune system; Obesity; Puberty and adolescence; Reproductive system; Weight loss and gain.

FOR FURTHER INFORMATION:

Barinaga, Marcia. "Obesity: Leptin Receptor Weighs In." *Science* 271 (January 5, 1996): 29. This article presents a summary of leptin receptor research accessible to the nonspecialist, as well as prospects for obesity drug research.

Rink, Timothy J. "In Search of a Satiety Factor." *Nature* 372 (December 1, 1994): 372-373. A history of the research into weight regulation and how leptin supports prior theories is presented in a general news format. References are provided for further reading.

LEUKEMIA

DISEASE/DISORDER

ANATOMY OR SYSTEM AFFECTED: Blood

SPECIALTIES AND RELATED FIELDS: Hematology, internal medicine, serology, toxicology

DEFINITION: A family of cancers that affect the blood, characterized by an increase in the number of white blood cells.

KEY TERMS:

bone marrow: the tissue within bones that produces blood cells; in children, all bones have active marrow, but in adults, blood cell production occurs only in the trunk

bone marrow transplant: the removal of bone marrow from an immunologically matched individual for infusion into a patient whose bone marrow has been destroyed

chemotherapy: the use of drugs to kill rapidly growing cancer cells; this treatment will also kill some normal cells, producing undesirable side effects

granulocytes: white blood cells that generally help to fight bacterial infection; they are capable of passing from the blood capillaries into damaged tissues

hematopoiesis: the process by which blood cells develop in the bone marrow; this maturation is regu-

lated by specific molecules called growth factors

immune system: the cells and organs of the body that fight infection; destruction of these cells leaves the body vulnerable to numerous diseases

lymphocytes: white blood cells that specifically target a foreign organism for destruction; the two classes of lymphocytes are B cells, which produce antibodies, and T cells, which kill infected cells

oncogenes: genes found in every cell which are capable of causing cancer if activated or mutated

CAUSES AND SYMPTOMS

The blood is essential for all the physiological processes of the body. It is composed of red cells called erythrocytes, white cells called leukocytes, and platelets, each of which has distinct functions. Erythrocytes, which contain hemoglobin, are essential for the transport of oxygen from the lungs to all the cells and organs of the body. Leukocytes are important for protecting the body against infection by bacteria, viruses, and other parasites. Platelets play a role in the formation of blood clots; therefore, these cells are critical in the process of wound healing. Blood cell development, or hematopoiesis, begins in the bone marrow with immature stem cells that can produce all three types of blood cells. Under the influence of special molecules called growth factors, these stem cells divide rapidly and form blast cells that become one of the three blood cell types. After several further divisions, these blast cells ultimately mature into fully functional erythrocytes, leukocytes, and platelets. In a healthy individual, the number of each type of blood cell remains relatively constant. Thus, the rate of new cell production is approximately equivalent to the rate of old cell destruction and removal.

Mature leukocytes are the key players in defending the body against infection. There are three types of leukocytes: monocytes, granulocytes, and lymphocytes. In leukemia, leukocytes multiply at an increased rate, resulting in an abnormally high number of white cells. All forms of leukemia are characterized by this abnormally regulated growth; therefore, leukemia is a cancer, even though tumor masses do not form. The cancerous cells live longer than the normal leukocytes and accumulate first in the bone marrow and then in the blood. Since these abnormal cells crowd the bone marrow, normal hematopoiesis cannot be maintained in a person with leukemia. The patient will usually become weak as a result of the lack of oxygen-carrying red cells and susceptible to bleeding because of a lack of platelets. The abnormal leukocytes do not function effectively in defending the body against infection, and they prevent normal leukocytes from developing; therefore, the patient is immunologically compromised. In addition, once the abnormal cells accumulate in the blood, they may hinder the functioning of other organs, such as the liver, kidney, lungs, and spleen.

It has become clear that leukemia, which was first recognized in 1845, is actually a pathology that comprises more than one disease. Leukemia has been divided into four main types, based on the type of leukocyte that is affected and the maturity of the leukocytes observed in the blood and the bone marrow. Both lymphocytes and granulocytes can be affected. When the cells are mainly immature blasts, the leukemia is termed acute, and when the cells are mostly mature, the leukemia is termed chronic. Therefore, the four types of leukemia are acute lymphocytic (ALL), acute granulocytic (AGL), chronic lymphocytic (CLL), and chronic granulocytic (CGL). The granulocytic leukemias are also known as myologenous leukemias (AML, CML) or nonlymphoid leukemias (ANLL, CNLL). These are the main types of leukemia, although there are additional rarer forms. These four forms of leukemia account for 5 percent of the cancer cases in the United States. The incidence of acute and chronic forms is approximately equivalent, but specific forms are more common at different stages of life. The major form in children is ALL; after puberty, there is a higher incidence of AGL. The chronic forms of leukemia occur in the adult population after the fourth or fifth decade of life, and men are twice as likely to be affected as women.

The causes of leukemia are still not completely understood, but scientists have put together many pieces of the puzzle. It is known that several environmental factors increase the risk of developing leukemia. Among these are exposure to radiation, chemicals such as chloramphenicol and benzene, and possibly viruses. In addition, there is a significant genetic component to this disease. Siblings of patients with leukemia have a higher risk of developing the disease, and chromosomal changes have been found in the cells of most patients, although they disappear when the patient is in remission. These different "causes" can be linked by understanding how oncogenes function. Every person, as part of his or her genetic makeup, has several oncogenes that are capable of causing cancer. In the healthy person, these oncogenes function in a carefully regulated manner to control cell growth. After exposure to an environmental or genetic influence that causes chromosome abnormalities, however, these oncogenes may become activated or deregulated so that uncontrolled cell growth occurs, resulting in the abnormally high number of cells seen in leukemia.

Leukemia is often difficult to diagnose in the early stages because the symptoms are similar to more common or less serious diseases. Cold symptoms, sometimes accompanied by fever, may be the earliest evidence of acute leukemia, and often in children the first symptoms may be less pronounced. The symptoms quickly become more pronounced as white cells accumulate in the lymph nodes, spleen, and liver, causing these organs to become enlarged. Fatigue, paleness, weight loss, repeated infections, and an increased susceptibility to bleeding and bruising are associated with leukemia. As the disease progresses, the fatigue and bleeding increase, various skin disorders develop, and the joints become painfully swollen. If untreated, the afflicted individual will die within a few months. Chronic leukemia has a more gradual progression and may be present for years before symptoms develop. When symptoms are present, they may be vague feelings of fatigue, fever, or loss of energy.

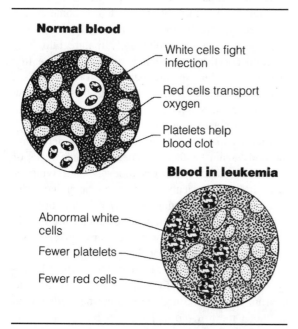

Normal blood

White cells fight infection

Red cells transport oxygen

Platelets help blood clot

Blood in leukemia

Abnormal white cells

Fewer platelets

Fewer red cells

Leukemia is characterized by a high number of white blood cells and a reduced number of red blood cells and platelets; also, abnormal cells may be visible.

There may be enlarged lymph nodes in the neck and armpits and a feeling of fullness in the abdomen because of an increase in the size of the spleen as much as tenfold. Loss of appetite and sweating at night may be initial symptoms. Often, chronic leukemia eventually leads to a syndrome resembling acute leukemia, which is ultimately fatal.

If these symptoms are present, a doctor will diagnose the presence of leukemia in two stages. First, blood will be drawn and a blood smear will be analyzed microscopically. This may indicate that there are fewer erythrocytes, leukocytes, and platelets than normal, and abnormal cells may be visible. A blood smear, however, may show only slight abnormalities, and the number of leukemic cells in the blood may not correspond to the extent of the disease in the bone marrow. This requires that the bone marrow itself be examined by means of a bone marrow biopsy. Bone marrow tissue can be obtained by inserting a needle into a bone such as the hip and aspirating a small sample of cells. This bone marrow biopsy, which is done under local anesthetic on an outpatient basis, is the definitive test for leukemia. Visual examination of the marrow usually reveals the presence of many abnormal cells, and this finding is often confirmed with biochemical and immunological tests. After a positive diagnosis, a doctor will also examine the cerebrospinal fluid to see if leukemic cells have invaded the central nervous system.

TREATMENT AND THERAPY

The treatment and life expectancy for leukemic patients varies significantly for each of the four types of leukemia. Treatment is designed to destroy all the abnormal cells and produce a complete remission, which is defined as the phase of recovery when the symptoms of the disease disappear and no abnormal cells can be observed in the blood or bone marrow. Unfortunately, a complete remission may be only temporary, since a small number of abnormal cells may still exist even though they are not observed under the microscope. These can, with time, multiply and repopulate the marrow, causing a relapse of the disease. With repeated relapses, the response to therapy becomes poorer and the durations of the remissions that follow become shorter. It is generally believed, however, that a remission that lasts five years in ALL, eight years in AGL, or twelve years in CGL may be permanent. Therefore, the goal of leukemia research is to develop ways to prolong remission.

By the time acute leukemia has been diagnosed, abnormal cells have often spread throughout the bone marrow and into several organs; therefore, surgery and radiation are usually not effective. Treatment programs include chemotherapy or bone marrow transplants or both. These treatments are aggressive and hazardous and are available only at specialized hospitals.

Chemotherapy is usually divided into several phases. In the first, or induction, phase, combinations of drugs are given to destroy all detectable abnormal cells and therefore induce a clinical remission. Vincristine, methotrexate, 6-mercaptopurine, L-asparaginase, daunorubicin, prednisone, and cytosine arabinoside are among the drugs that are used. Combinations that selectively kill more leukemic cells than they do normal cells are available for the treatment of ALL; however, in AGL no selective agents are available, resulting in the destruction of equal numbers of diseased and healthy cells. An alternative strategy does not rely on destroying the abnormal cells but instead seeks to induce immature leukemic cells to develop further. Once the cells are mature, they will no longer divide and will eventually die in the same way that a normal leukocyte does. Drugs such as cytarabine and retinoic acid have been tested, but the results are inconclusive.

Although the induction phase achieves clinical remission in more than 80 percent of patients, a second phase, called consolidation therapy, is essential to prevent relapse. Different combinations of anticancer drugs are used to kill any remaining cancer cells that were resistant to the drugs in the induction phase. Once the patient is in remission, higher doses of chemotherapy can be tolerated, and sometimes additional intensive treatments are given to reduce further the number of leukemic cells so that they will be unable to repopulate the tissues. During these phases of treatment, patients must be hospitalized. The destruction of their normal leukocytes along with the leukemic cells makes them very susceptible to infection. Their low numbers of surviving erythrocytes and platelets increase the probability of internal bleeding, and transfusions are often necessary. The dosages of chemotherapeutic agents must be carefully calculated to kill as many leukemic cells as possible without destroying so many normal cells that they cannot repopulate the marrow. In general, children handle intensive chemotherapy better than adults.

Following the induction and consolidation phases, maintenance therapy is sometimes used. In ALL, maintenance therapy is given for two to three years; however, its benefit in other forms of leukemia is a matter of controversy.

A second form of therapy is sometimes indicated for patients who have not responded to chemotherapy or are likely to relapse. Bone marrow transplantation has been increasingly used in leukemic patients to replace diseased marrow with normally functioning stem cells. In this procedure, the patient is treated with intensive chemotherapy and whole-body irradiation to destroy all leukemic and normal cells. Then a small amount of marrow from a normal donor is infused. The donor can be the patient himself, if the marrow was removed during a previous remission, or an immunologically matched donor, who is usually a sibling. If a sibling is not available, it may be possible to find a matched donor from the National Marrow Donor Program, which has on file approximately 350,000 people who have consented to be donors. Marrow is removed from the donor, broken up into small pieces, and given to the patient intravenously. The stem cells from the transplanted marrow circulate in the blood, enter the bones, and multiply. The first signs that the transplant is functioning normally occur in two to four weeks as the numbers of circulating granulocytes and platelets in the patient's blood increase. Eventually, in a successful transplant, the bone marrow cavity will be repopulated with normal cells.

Bone marrow transplantation is a dangerous procedure that requires highly trained caregivers. During this process, the patient is completely vulnerable to infection, since there is no functional immune system. The patient is placed in an isolation unit with special food-handling procedures. There is little chance that the patient will reject the transplanted marrow, because the immune system of the patient is suppressed. A larger problem remains, however, because it is possible for immune cells that existed in the donor's marrow to reject the tissues and organs of the patient. This graft-versus-host disease (GVHD) affects between 50 and 70 percent of bone marrow transplant patients. Even though the donor is immunologically matched, the match is not perfect, and the recently transplanted cells regard the cells in their new host as a "foreign" threat. Twenty percent of the patients who develop GVHD will die; therefore, drugs such as cyclophosphamide and cyclosporine, which suppress the immune system, are usually given to minimize this response. GVHD is not a problem if the donor is the patient. It is imperative, however, that marrow from the leukemic patient that has been removed during an earlier remission and frozen be treated to remove all leukemic cells before it is transplanted back into the patient.

Aggressive chemotherapy and bone marrow transplantation have dramatically increased the number of long-lasting remissions. For those who survive the therapy, it appears that, in ALL, approximately 60 percent of children and 35 percent of adults may be cured of the leukemia. The outlook for permanent remission is 10 to 20 percent in AGL and 65 percent for CGL patients. Statistics for chronic lymphocytic leukemia have been difficult to predict, because individual cases that have been similarly treated have had very different outcomes. The average lifespan after a diagnosis of CLL is three to four years; however, some patients live longer than fifteen years.

PERSPECTIVE AND PROSPECTS

As the number of deaths from infectious disease has decreased, cancer has become the second most common cause of disease-related death. It is estimated that one of three people in the United States will develop a form of cancer and that the disease will kill one of five people. The search for causes and treatments of various cancers is perhaps the most active area of biological research today. Multiple lines of experimentation are being pursued, and significant advances have been made.

Leukemia is one of the cancers that scientists understand fairly well, but many unanswered questions remain. Leukemia research can be divided into two broad approaches. In the first, the researcher seeks to modify and improve the current methods for treatment: chemotherapy and bone marrow transplantation. In the second, an effort is being made to understand more about the disease itself, with the hope that completely different strategies for treatment might present themselves.

The risks involved in current therapy for leukemia have been discussed in the previous section. Treatment schedules, individually designed for each patient, will add to the understanding of how other physiological characteristics affect treatment outcome. Significant advances in reducing the risk of GVHD are likely to come quickly. In marrow transplants in which the donor is the patient, research is in progress to improve ways to screen out abnormal cells, even if they are present at very low levels, before they are infused back into the patient. In addition, for transplants in which the donor is not the patient, techniques that remove the harmful components of the bone marrow are being developed. Bone marrow cells can be partially purified, resulting in an enriched population of stem cells. Administering these to the leukemic patient should greatly reduce the risk of GVHD. Since bone marrow can be stored easily, the day may come when healthy people will store a bone marrow stem cell sample in case they contract a disease that would require a transplant.

Basic research in leukemia focuses on a simple question, "Why are leukemic cells different from normal cells?" This question is asked from a variety of perspectives in the fields of immunology, cell biology, and genetics. Immunologists are looking for markers on the surfaces of leukemic cells that would distinguish them from their normal counterparts. If such markers are found, it should be possible to target leukemic cells for destruction by using monoclonal antibodies attached to drugs. These "smart drugs" would be able to home in on the diseased cells, leaving normal cells untouched or only slightly affected. This would be a great advance for leukemia treatment, since much of the risk for the leukemic patient following chemotherapy or bone marrow transplant involves susceptibility to infection because the normal immune cells have been destroyed. Similarly, it may be possible to "teach" the patient's immune system to destroy abnormal cells that it had previously ignored.

Cell biologists are seeking to understand the normal hematopoietic process so that they can determine which steps of the process go awry in leukemia. Some of the growth factors involved in hematopoiesis have been identified, but it appears that the process is quite complex, and as yet scientists do not have a clear picture of normal hematopoiesis. When the understanding of the normal process becomes more complete, it may be possible to localize the defect in a leukemic patient and provide the missing growth factors. This might allow abnormal immature cells to complete the developmental process and relieve the symptoms of disease.

Geneticists are studying the chromosomal changes that underlie the onset of leukemia. As the oncogenes that are involved are identified, the reasons for their activation will also be determined. Once the effects of these genetic abnormalities are understood, it may be possible to intervene by genetically engineering stem cells so that they can develop normally.

These areas of research will likely converge to provide the leukemia treatments of the future. Leukemia is a cancer for which there is already a significant cure rate. It is not unreasonable to expect that this rate will approach 100 percent in the near future.

—*Katherine B. Frederich, Ph.D.*

See also Blood and blood disorders; Bone marrow transplantation; Cancer; Chemotherapy; Malignancy and metastasis; Oncology; Radiation sickness.

FOR FURTHER INFORMATION:

Cook, Alan R., ed. *The New Cancer Sourcebook: Basic Information About Major Forms and Stages of Cancer.* Detroit: Omnigraphics, 1996. This well-written volume provides the reader with a background against which to understand leukemia. Describes each of the four main types of leukemia in a straightforward and practical manner.

Lackritz, Barb. *Adult Leukemia: A Comprehensive Guide for Patients and Families.* Cambridge, Mass.: O'Reilly, 2001. This guide is designed for the patient who has been diagnosed with leukemia. Includes bibliographical references and an index.

Murphy, G., L. Morris, and D. Lange. *Informed Decisions: The Complete Book of Cancer Diagnosis, Treatment, and Recovery.* New York: Viking Press, 1997. This text from the American Cancer Society is intended for the layperson. It is exemplary in its discussion of cancer.

Westcott, Patsy. *Living with Leukemia.* Austin, Tex.: Raintree-Steck-Vaughn, 1999. Designed for students in grades three through five, this book discusses a condition or disease through the stories of children experiencing it. Includes clear and easy-to-understand diagrams and full-color photographs.

LICE, MITES, AND TICKS
DISEASE/DISORDER

ANATOMY OR SYSTEM AFFECTED: Ears, genitals, hair, skin

SPECIALTIES AND RELATED FIELDS: Dermatology, pediatrics, public health

DEFINITION: Parasites that live on the human body, causing severe itching, skin rashes, and sometimes more serious diseases.

KEY TERMS:

*louse (*pl. *lice):* a wingless insect that sucks blood and that can be involved in transmitting diseases

mite: a very small spider that is parasitic to humans and can carry disease *molt:* to shed all or part of the skin or outer covering

parasite: an organism that lives off of another organism while contributing nothing to the survival of the host

tick: a wingless insect that sucks blood and can spread disease

CAUSES AND SYMPTOMS

Lice, mites, and ticks are parasites that live on human beings. Two species of lice survive on human blood: body lice and crab lice. Body lice are divided into two subspecies, the head louse (*Pediculus humanus capitis*) and the body louse (*Pediculus humanus corporis*). Head lice live on the scalp among the hairs of the head. Body lice actually live in and on clothing. They move off clothes and attach themselves to human skin to feed on blood frequently during the day. It is very difficult to tell the difference between these types of lice. They are both flat, wingless, grayish in color, and very small. The body louse is about .08 to .16 inch long, slightly larger than the head louse, which measures only .04 to .08 inch. Body lice are a slightly lighter shade of gray than are head lice.

Both subspecies of body lice live by sucking blood from their victims. These insects of the order *Anoplura* have three pointed tubes on their bodies called stylets that can jab into the skin and draw out blood. When not in use, the stylets are tucked away in a pouch. Body lice begin their lives as eggs dropped into the folds of clothing by mature adult females. Head lice eggs are glued to the base of a strand of hair on top of the head. The eggs, called nits, are about one-fourth the size of a mature female. After about seven to ten days, the nits hatch into young nymphs. Because hair grows about 0.3 millimeter a day, the nits hatch about 3 millimeters away from the scalp. After the nymph emerges, it leaves behind an empty egg shell still tightly cemented to the hair. Nymphs begin sucking blood as soon as they hatch. Within nine days, the nymph molts three times before a full adult louse is formed. Adults then live about two weeks, with females laying about ten eggs every day.

Lice are passed from head to head only by direct contact. This usually happens at school, often on the playground or in the gym. Head lice have different effects on different people. Some experience only slight itching, while others are terribly irritated and develop a swollen and inflamed scalp. An itching scalp is the most obvious symptom of head lice. Nits are visible upon inspection of hair near the scalp. On

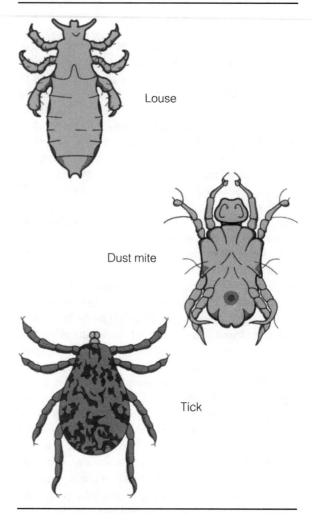

Magnified representations of a louse, a mite (normally microscopic), and a tick.

girls, they are usually found behind the ears, while on boys, they are most likely to be found attached near the top of the head. Parents should be very careful in treating head lice; they too can be infected. Head lice can be the transmitters of several dangerous infectious diseases, such as epidemic typhus, relapsing fever, and trench fever.

Body lice are less often found on children than are head lice. They thrive in clothing and bodies that are unclean for long periods of time. Body lice are especially troublesome and numerous on homeless people, prisoners of war, and others living in dirty conditions. (Cleanliness, however, is not a factor with head lice; they can thrive in clean or dirty hair.) Body lice have helped spread a number of contagious diseases, the most deadly of which is typhus. This disease starts with flulike symptoms, followed by a high fever and rash. During World War II, more than three million Russian prisoners of war died from louse-spread typhus. In recent years, however, typhus has been rare.

Crab lice (*Phthirus pubis*) are usually found living in pubic hair and are most likely to infect adults. Like all lice, they are very small, .083 inch in length when fully grown, but they cause great discomfort. As adults, they firmly grab pubic hair with their crablike legs (six per louse), insert their barbed tongue into the skin, and suck blood. The female lays its eggs about .08 inch from the skin. When the eggs hatch, the nymphs begin to feed and stop only while molting. Feeding causes intense itching and a rash. Rarely, but occasionally, the lice spread to the chest, eyebrows, or armpits. They can be passed on only by human carriers through direct contact. Crab lice cannot live on any other species except humans, and about 3 percent of people have them. Crab lice do not carry sexually transmitted diseases but are often associated with them.

Ticks are members of a blood-sucking family of insects called *Ixodidae*. Several different species suck blood from warm-blooded vertebrates, such as human beings, cows, and dogs. Common species in the United States and Canada include hard ticks and the American dog tick. Ticks have a hard, shieldlike plate on their backs called a scutum that makes them very difficult to crush. A female tick can swell up to the size of a pea when ingesting blood and can lay from four thousand to six thousand eggs within four to ten days.

The eggs hatch after about a month, and six-legged larvae, called seed ticks, emerge. A seed tick waits on the tip of a leaf of grass or other low-growing plant until a suitable animal walks by. The seed tick grabs onto its meal and, after sucking enough blood, molts into its next stage, an eight-legged nymph called a yearling tick. It finds another host, sucks more blood, and then molts one more time into an adult. After another week of feeding, adults mate, the female produces its eggs, and the three-stage cycle begins all over again.

Ticks are very good survivors: Eight-legged nymphs can live more than a year without food, while adults can go without a meal of blood for more than two years. Ticks carry many dangerous diseases, including Rocky Mountain spotted fever, Colorado tick fever, tularemia, anaplasmosis, and Lyme disease.

Mites are actually related to spiders, rather than insects. Dust mites (*Dermatophagiodes pteronyssinus*), the chief living forms found in house dust, are among the most numerous inhabitants of human environments. One study of 150 houses in Holland found mites in every one of them. Dust mites measure about .01 inch in diameter. They have eight legs, like all spiders, and are closely related to ear mites found in dogs and cats and scab mites found in sheep. House dust mites spend all of their life stages, from birth to death, in dust. There can be as many as five hundred mites in every gram of house dust. This measures out to about fourteen thousand mites per ounce of dust. They survive by eating human skin that is shed daily, scabs that fall off, and dandruff, which is about 10 percent fat and which they digest with the help of a fungus also found in house dust. Dust mites are responsible for some allergies and asthma attacks. They can also invade the skin and cause allergic reactions such as dermatitis. Although dust mites cannot penetrate the surface of the skin, they can live in ulcers, fungal infections, scabs, and other skin openings.

The scabies mite (*Sarcoptes scabei*) does burrow into the skin in search of its preferred food, skin cells and intestinal fluids. Female scabies mites are about .016 inch long, while males are only about half as big. The female lays its eggs only a few hours after mating and can lay two to three eggs a day for up to four weeks. The eggs hatch after only three to four days. The larvae often move about on the skin surface until they find a suitable space, usually between the fingers or at the bend in the knee, elbow, or wrist. The underarms, breasts, and genitals can also be invaded by these travelers. Frequently, they travel all the way down to the ankles or between the toes. Sometimes it takes up to six weeks before the pests are noticed by the person acting as their host.

Children are especially sensitive to the feces and eggs of scabies mites, which can cause an agonizing itch that is particularly irritating at night. Scabies mites are most active in the fall and winter, but they are transmissible at any time. They can be spread by shaking hands, by touching the infected areas of another person, and even by having contact with the clothes or bedsheets of the infected individual. Scabies mites do not carry any major diseases, but they do cause a good deal of itching and discomfort.

TREATMENT AND THERAPY

Treatments for lice, mites, and ticks vary according to the type and severity of infestation. The only way to protect a child against head lice is through regular inspection of the head. The hair should be combed and brushed every night; this will injure the lice, which will not be able to survive. Treatment involves an insecticidal shampoo such as Proderm, which contains malathion, or Kwell, which contains lindane or gamma benzene hexachlorine. These shampoos kill both the lice and the nits. Removing lice by hand or crushing them is a difficult and usually impossible task. The force required to remove a nit from a hair is greater than most parents can provide. Crushing a louse requires direct pressure of about five hundred thousand times the weight of a louse. The crushed body of a louse can also cause infection. The best treatment for body lice is washing clothes and infected areas with soap. Soap and hot water usually kill body lice. If an infection of either head or body lice is discovered, all members of a family should be checked, and a doctor should be consulted. If a child has head lice, his or her school should always be notified. If crab lice are discovered, a physician should be contacted immediately. Pubic lice can be treated with insecticides such as pyrethrin pediculicide. Pyrethrins are available over-the-counter in drugstores. Stronger treatments require a prescription. Crab lice can be controlled by washing clothing and bedding and drying them in a very hot dryer.

Ticks are very difficult to remove from the body. A tick should not be pulled or yanked out because its head, filled with jagged teeth, can remain in the wound and cause an infection. Ticks have to be removed so that their mouthparts do not break off. Unattached ticks can be brushed off with a hand, but an attached tick should not be removed with bare fingers. To remove a tick, the hands should be covered with a tissue or gloves. Then, the tick is grabbed with a pair of tweezers as close to its head as possible. Gentle, steady pressure is applied until the tick comes out. The tick should not be twisted or crushed until it is fully out. Body fluids from the tick can carry Lyme disease organisms, which can enter the body through broken skin. The safest way to kill the tick is to drown it in soapy water or crush it with thetweezers, avoiding contact with the hands. The site of the bite should be washed and checked carefully to see if any part of the head is still embedded. Anything that remains should be removed with tweezers, which will help prevent infection. If all parts cannot be removed, the spot should be rubbed with an antiseptic. A doctor should be consulted if the site becomes inflamed or filled with pus.

Scabies mites can be controlled by insecticidal lotions containing lindane or sulfur. The pesticide lindane is the one most commonly used for scabies mites, but it has been linked to cancer in some tests. Sulfur is preferred by most physicians because it is safer and more widely available. Sulfur requires three applications over three days, however, and frequently leaves stains on bedding and clothes. The fastest-acting miticide is permethrim. It usually requires only one application to be effective, but it is more toxic than sulfur. Scabies mites can be controlled by washing the clothing, bedding, and towels used by the infected person. If scabies mites are found, other people with whom the child has had contact should be told so that they can seek treatment, even though they might not have started to itch. Scabies mites cannot live long if detached from their hosts, usually no more than two to three days. Sealing infected clothes in a plastic bag for a week or so will also kill most of the mites.

Dust mites can be controlled by reducing their sources of food. This can be accomplished by covering mattresses in plastic, keeping pets away from beds and sleeping areas, reducing humidity in the house, and vacuuming once a week. Killing dust mites requires vacuuming with a water vacuum or one with special dust filters, washing sheets and pillowcases in hot soapy water, freezing or heating blankets, or using pesticides such as mosquito repellents containing diethyl-m-toluamide (DEET) or products containing boric acid.

PERSPECTIVE AND PROSPECTS

New chemicals have proven very effective in the treatment of diseases spread by lice, mites, and ticks. Louse-spread typhus, once responsible for millions of deaths, is no longer a great danger. Improved standards of cleanliness have done much to eliminate the problem of body lice in all but the poorest populations in the United States. Unfortunately, head lice cannot be controlled simply by keeping things clean, so they continue to cause itching and scratching when contracted even by the cleanest children. Lice, mites, and ticks will always be with humans, but the diseases that these parasites spread, with a few exceptions such as Rocky Mountain spotted fever and Lyme disease, are now much less deadly because of new medicines and drug treatments.

—Leslie V. Tischauser, Ph.D.

See also Allergies; Arthropod-borne diseases; Asthma; Bites and stings; Dermatitis; Dermatology; Dermatology, pediatric; Itching; Lyme disease; Parasitic diseases; Rashes; Scabies; Skin; Skin disorders; Typhoid fever and typhus.

FOR FURTHER INFORMATION:

Around People: Friends, Pests, Parasites, and Freeloaders. Danbury, Conn.: Grolier Educational, 2000. Discusses such topics as insect behavior and the rearing of insects. Includes an index.

Beaver, Paul Chester, Rodney Clifton Jung, and Eddie Wayne Cupp. *Clinical Parasitology*. 9th ed. Philadelphia: Lea & Febiger, 1984. Considered to be the authority on the subject. Includes a summary of information about dust mites.

Berenbaum, May R. *Ninety-nine Gnats, Nits, and Nibblers*. Urbana: University of Illinois Press, 1989. A scientist describes how insects affect human lives. Offers an informative description of the life cycles and habits of lice, mites, ticks, and other troublemakers.

Newman, Lisa S. *Parasites*. Freedom, Calif.: Crossing Press, 1999. This text is aimed at the veterinary professional and discusses such topics as dog and cat parasites and gives an overview of veterinary parasitology.

Olkowski, William, Sheila Daar, and Helga Olkowski. *Common-Sense Pest Control*. Newton, Conn.: Taunton Press, 1991. A very useful book by a biologist that describes the best methods of dealing with all kinds of insect problems, including lice, mites, and ticks. Offers detailed descriptions of how to remove these pests from your children and the environment safely.

Robinson, William H. *Urban Entomology: Insect and Mite Pests in the Human Environment*. London: Chapman & Hall, 1996. Discusses household pests in urban areas, including how to control them. Provides a bibliography and an index.

LIGHT THERAPY
PROCEDURE

ANATOMY OR SYSTEM AFFECTED: Brain, nervous system, psychic-emotional system, skin

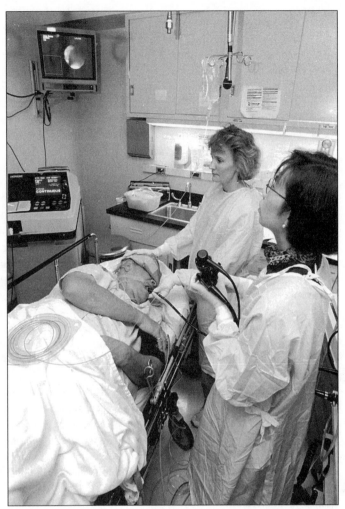

Photodynamic therapy is used on a cancer patient. (AP/Wide World Photos)

SPECIALTIES AND RELATED FIELDS: Dermatology, psychiatry, psychology

DEFINITION: A noninvasive procedure using exposure to light as the mechanism for clinical treatment.

INDICATIONS AND PROCEDURES

Light therapy, or phototherapy, treats a variety of disorders. By exposing individuals to different kinds of light (for example, monochromatic, polychromatic, ultraviolet), symptoms can often be delayed, reduced, and eradicated. Immunological and neuroendocrine systems are thought to play key roles in response to this type of treatment.

Best known in psychiatry, light therapy has been used to treat seasonal affective disorder (SAD), or winter depression; bulimia nervosa; sleep disorders; and "sundowner's syndrome," the late afternoon confusion and agitation sometimes accompanying Alzheimer's disease. Reduced environmental light is thought to be a factor in the etiology, onset, or maintenance of these disorders. Thus, treatment involves exposing individuals to bright, full-spectrum light for fixed periods of time. Duration of exposure and light intensity vary by the disorder and individual treated.

In dermatology and oncology, light therapy has been used to treat psoriasis, skin ulcers, tumors, and esophageal cancers. The type of light and the intensities used, however, vary considerably from those applied for the treatment of psychiatric disorders.

USES AND COMPLICATIONS

The side effects of light therapy are best documented in psychiatry: Insomnia, mania, and (less frequently) morning hot flashes have been noted. Careful monitoring by medical providers of the patient's response to treatment is necessary. Additionally, morning administrations of light therapy are advised in order to avoid these effects.

Light therapy is not effective universally; some patients may experience no improvement. For seasonal affective disorder, evidence suggests that younger individuals whose depression involves weight gain and increased sleep may be most likely to respond to treatment. For psoriasis, complementary treatments, such as psychotherapy, may be needed to facilitate a response to treatment.

PERSPECTIVE AND PROSPECTS

Light and dark cycles are a biological reality; thus, it is no surprise that light affects physical, emotional, and mental well-being. As the interest in noninvasive interventions increases, the attention given to environmental treatments such as light therapy is likely to increase as well. Recent developments in the use of light therapy for sleep and behavioral disorders are also likely to fuel interest in this procedure.

—*Nancy A. Piotrowski, Ph.D.*

See also Alternative medicine; Alzheimer's disease; Bulimia; Chronobiology; Depression; Dermatology; Psoriasis; Psychiatry; Skin disorders; Sleep disorders.

FOR FURTHER INFORMATION:

Goldberg, Burton, comp. *Alternative Medicine: The Definitive Guide.* Puyallup, Wash.: Future Medicine, 1993.

Jacobs, Jennifer, ed. *The Encyclopedia of Alternative Medicine: A Complete Family Guide to Complementary Therapies.* Rev. ed. Boston: Journey Edition, 1997.

Kastner, Mark, and Hugh Burroughs. *Alternative Healing: The Complete A-Z Guide to over 160 Different Alternative Therapies.* New York: Henry Holt, 1996.

Mills, Simon, and Steven J. Finando. *Alternatives in Healing.* London: Grange Books, 1995.

LIPIDS

BIOLOGY

ANATOMY OR SYSTEM AFFECTED: Cells, gastrointestinal system

SPECIALTIES AND RELATED FIELDS: Biochemistry, cytology, nutrition, vascular medicine

DEFINITION: Organic compounds found in the tissues of plants and animals that serve as energy-storage molecules, function as solvents for water-insoluble vitamins, provide insulation against the loss of body heat, act as a protective cushion for vital organs, and are structural components of cell membranes.

KEY TERMS:

alcohol: an organic compound containing a hydroxyl (–OH) group attached to a carbon atom

carboxylic acid: an organic compound that contains the carboxyl (–CO_2H) group

ester: the relatively non-water-soluble compound formed when an alcohol reacts with a carboxylic acid

fatty acid: an organic compound that is composed of a long hydrocarbon chain with a carboxyl group at one end

glycerol: a three-carbon alcohol that has one hydroxyl compound on each carbon atom

hydrocarbon: an organic compound composed of only hydrogen and carbon atoms that does not dissolve in water (water-insoluble)

hydrophilic: "water-loving" or "water-attracting"; a term given to molecules or regions of molecules that interact favorably with water

hydrophobic: "water-hating" or "water-repelling"; a term given to molecules or regions of molecules that do not interact favorably with water

saponification: a reaction in which a strong basic solution splits a molecule into a carboxylic acid unit and an alcohol unit

STRUCTURE AND FUNCTIONS

Lipids are a class of bio-organic compounds that are typically insoluble in water and relatively soluble in organic solvents such as alcohols, ethers, and hydrocarbons. Unlike the other classes of organic molecules found in biological systems (carbohydrates, proteins, and nucleic acids), lipids possess a unifying physical property—solubility behavior—rather than a unifying structural feature. Fats, oils, some vitamins and hormones, and most of the nonprotein components of cell membranes are lipids.

There are two categories of lipids—those that undergo saponification and those that are nonsaponifiable. The saponifiable lipids can be divided into simple and complex lipids. Simple lipids, which are composed of carbon, hydrogen, and oxygen, yield fatty acids and an alcohol upon saponification. Complex lipids contain one or more additional elements, such as phosphorus, nitrogen, and sulfur, yielding fatty acids, alcohol, and other compounds on saponification.

The fatty acid building blocks of saponifiable lipids may be either saturated, which means that as many hydrogen atoms as possible are attached to the carbon chain, or unsaturated, which means that at least two hydrogen atoms are missing. Saturated fatty acids are white solids at room temperature, while unsaturated ones are liquids at room temperature, because of a geometrical difference in the long carbon chains. The carbon atoms of a saturated fatty acid are arranged in a zigzag or accordion configuration. These chains are stacked on top of one another in a very orderly and efficient fashion, making it difficult to separate the chains from one another. When carbons in the chain are missing hydrogen atoms, the regular zigzag of the chain is disrupted, leading to less efficient packing, which allows the chains to be separated more easily. Saturated fatty acids have a higher melting temperature because they require more energy to separate their chains than do unsaturated fatty acids. Unsaturated fatty acids can be converted into saturated ones by adding hydrogen atoms through a process called hydrogenation.

Simple lipids can be divided into triglycerides and waxes. Waxes such as beeswax, lanolin (from lamb's wool), and carnauba wax (from a palm tree) are esters formed from an alcohol with a long carbon chain and a fatty acid. These compounds, which are solids at room temperature, serve as protective coatings. Most plant leaves are coated with a wax film to prevent attack by microorganisms and loss of water through evaporation. Animal fur and bird feathers have a wax coating. For example, the wax coating on their feathers is what allows ducks to stay afloat.

Edible fats and oils such as lard (pig fat), tallow (beef fat), corn oil, and butter are triglycerides. Triglyceride molecules are fatty acid esters in which three fatty acids (all saturated, all unsaturated, or mixed) combine with one molecule of the alcohol glycerol. Oils are triglycerides that are liquid at room temperature, while fats are solid at room temperature. The fluidity of a triglyceride is dependent on the nature of its fatty acid chains; the more unsaturated the triglyceride, the more fluid its structure. The triglycerides found in animals tend to have more saturated fatty acids than do those found in plants. Vegetable oils and fish oils are frequently polyunsaturated.

Complex lipids are classified as phospholipids or glycolipids. Structurally, phospholipids are composed of fatty acids, and a phosphate group. Glycerol-based lipids called phosphoglycerides contain glycerol, two fatty acids, and a phosphate group. The phosphoglyceride structure contains a hydrophilic (polar) head, the phosphate unit, and two hydrophobic (nonpolar) fatty acid tails. The polar head can interact strongly with water, while the nonpolar tails interact strongly with organic solvents and avoid water. Egg yolks contain a large amount of the phosphoglyceride phosphatidylcholine (also called lecithin). This lipid is used to form the emulsion mayonnaise from oil and vinegar. Normally, oil and water do not mix. The hydrophobic oil forms a separate layer on top of the water. Since lecithin's structure contains both a hydrophobic and a hydrophilic region, it can attach to the water with its polar head and the oil with its nonpolar tail, preventing the two materials from separating. Lipids derived from the alcohol sphingosine are called sphingolipids. They contain one fatty acid, one long hydrocarbon chain and a phosphate group. Like the phosphoglycerides, sphingolipids have a head-and-two-tail structure. Sphingolipids are important components in the protective and insulating coating that surrounds nerves.

Glycolipids differ from phospholipids in that they possess a sugar group in place of the phosphate group. Their structure is again the polar head and dual tail arrangement in which the sugar is the hydrophilic unit. Cerebrosides, which are sphingosine-based glycolipids containing a simple sugar such as galactose or glucose, are found in large amounts in the white matter of the brain and in the myelin sheath. Gangliosides, which are found in the gray matter of the brain, in neural tissue, and in the receptor sites for neurotransmitters, contain a more complex sugar component.

Nonsaponifiable lipids do not contain esters of fatty acids as their basic structural feature. Steroids are an important class of nonsaponifiable lipids. All steroids possess an identical four-ring framework called the steroid nucleus, but they differ in the groups that are attached to their ring systems. Examples of steroids are sterols such as cholesterol, the bile acids secreted by the liver, the sex hormones, corticosteroids secreted by the adrenal cortex, and digitoxin from the digitalis plant, which is used to treat heart disease.

Lipids constitute about 50 percent of the mass of most animal cell membranes. Biological membranes control the chemical environment of the space they enclose. They are selective filters controlling what substances enter and exit the cell, since they constitute a relatively impermeable barrier against most water-soluble molecules. The three types of lipids involved are phospholipids (most abundant), glycolipids, and cholesterol. Phospholipids, when surrounded by an aqueous environment, tend to organize into a double layer of lipid molecules, a bilayer, allowing their hydrophobic tails to be buried internally and their hydrophilic heads to be exposed to the water. These phospholipids have one saturated and one unsaturated tail. Differences in tail length and saturation influence the packing efficiency of the molecules and affect the fluidity of the membrane. Short, unsaturated tails increase the fluidity of the membrane. Cholesterol is important in maintaining the mechanical stability of the lipid bilayer, thereby preventing a change from the fluid state to a rigid crystalline state. It also decreases the permeability of small water-soluble molecules.

The lipid bilayer provides the basic structure of the membrane and serves as a two-dimensional solvent for protein molecules. Protein molecules are responsible for most membrane functions; for example, they can provide receptor sites, catalyze reactions, or transport molecules across the membrane. These proteins may extend across the bilayer (transmembrane proteins) or be associated with only one face of the bilayer. Cell membranes also have carbohydrates attached to the outer face of the bilayer. These carbohydrates are bound to membrane proteins or part of a glycolipid. Typically, 2 to 10 percent of a membrane's total weight is carbohydrate. Evidence exists that cell-surface carbohydrates are used as recognition sites for chemical processes.

Lipids play an important role in health and well-being. The body acquires lipids directly from dietary lipids and indirectly by converting other nutrients into lipids. There are two fatty acids, linoleic and linolenic acids, which are called essential fatty acids. Since these fatty acids cannot be synthesized in the body in sufficient amounts, their supply must come directly from dietary sources. Fortunately, these acids are widely found in foodstuffs, so deficiency is rarely observed in adults.

About 95 percent of the lipids in foods are triglycerides, which provide 30 to 50 percent of the calories in an average diet. Triglycerides produce 4,000 calories of energy per pound, compared to the 1,800 calories per pound produced by carbohydrates or proteins. Since the triglyceride is such an efficient energy source, the body converts carbohydrates and proteins into adipose (reserve fatty) tissue for storage to be used when extra fuel is required.

While carbohydrates and proteins undergo major degradation in the stomach, triglycerides remain intact, forming large globules that float to the top of the mixture. Fats spend a longer time than other nutrients in the stomach, slowing molecular activity before continuing into the intestines. Thus, a fat-laden meal gives longer satiety than a low-fat one.

In the small intestine, bile salts split fat globules into smaller droplets, allowing enzymes called lipases to saponify the triglycerides. In some instances, the fatty acids at the two ends are removed, leaving one attached as a monoglyceride. About 97 percent of dietary triglycerides are absorbed into the bloodstream; the remainder are excreted. Although glycerol and fatty acids with short carbon chains are water-soluble enough to dissolve in the blood, the long-chain fatty acids and monoglycerides are not. These insoluble materials recombine to form new triglycerides. Since these hydrophobic triglycerides would form large globules if they were dumped directly into the blood, small triglyceride droplets are surrounded with a protective protein coat that can dissolve in water, taking the encapsulated triglyceride with it. This structure is an example of a lipoprotein.

Cholesterol is found in relatively small (milligram) quantities in foods, compared to triglycerides. Cholesterol supplies raw materials for the production of bile salts and to be used as a structural constituent of brain and nerve tissue. Since these functions are important to animals but serve no purpose in plants, cholesterol is found only in animals. Only about 50 percent of dietary cholesterol is absorbed into the blood; the rest is excreted. Much of the body's supply of cholesterol is produced in the liver. For most individuals, the amount of cholesterol synthesized in the body is larger than the amount absorbed directly from the diet.

Digested lipids released from the intestine and those synthesized in the liver compose the lipid content of the blood. The fatty acids required by the liver are obtained directly from the bloodstream or by synthesis from sources such as glucose, amino acids, and alcohol. Liver-synthesized triglycerides are incorporated into lipoprotein packages before entering the bloodstream. There are three types of lipoprotein packages that transport lipids to and from the liver. Very-low-density lipoproteins (VLDLs) transport triglycerides to tissues; low-density lipoproteins (LDLs) transport the cholesterol from the liver to other cells; and high-density lipoproteins (HDLs) transport cholesterol from other tissues to the liver for destruction.

DISORDERS AND DISEASES

Lipid consumption is an important dietary concern. Lipid deficiency is rarely observed in adults but can occur in infants who are fed nonfat formulas. Since fatty acids are essential for growth, lipid consumption should not be restricted in individuals under two years of age. Excess lipid consumption is associated with health problems such as obesity and cardiovascular disease. Although excess calories from any dietary source can lead to obesity, the body must expend less energy to store dietary fat than to store dietary carbohydrate as body fat. Thus, high-fat diets produce more body fat than do high-carbohydrate, low-fat diets.

Atherosclerosis, or "hardening of the arteries," is the leading cause of cardiovascular disease. A strong correlation exists between diets high in saturated fats and the incidence of atherosclerosis. In this condition, deposits called plaques, which have a high cholesterol content, form on artery walls. Over time, these deposits narrow the artery and decrease its elasticity, resulting in reduced blood flow. Blockages can occur, resulting in heart attack or stroke. High serum cholesterol levels (total blood cholesterol content) often result in increased plaque formation. Since dietary cholesterol is not efficiently absorbed into the bloodstream and the serum cholesterol level is largely determined by the amount of cholesterol synthesized in

the liver, high serum cholesterol levels are frequently related to high saturated fat intake.

Since the measurement of the serum cholesterol level gives the total cholesterol concentration of the blood, it can be a somewhat misleading predictor of atherosclerosis risk; cholesterol is not free in blood, but is encapsulated in lipoproteins. Since the cholesterol packaged in the LDL, cholesterol that can be deposited in plaques ("bad" cholesterol), has a very different fate from that in the HDL, which is transporting cholesterol for destruction ("good" cholesterol), measuring the ratio of LDL cholesterol to HDL cholesterol has been found to be a better indicator of atherosclerosis risk. Decreasing dietary intake of cholesterol and saturated fats, increasing water-soluble fibers in the diet, removing excess body weight, and increasing the amount of aerobic exercise will all serve to improve the LDL-C/HDL-C ratio.

A number of hereditary diseases are known that result from abnormal accumulation of the complex lipids utilized in membranes. These diseases are called lipid-storage diseases, or lipidoses. In normal individuals, the amount of each complex lipid present in the body is relatively constant; in other words, the rate of formation equals the rate of destruction. The lipids are broken down by enzymes that attack specific bonds in the lipid structure. Lipid-storage diseases occur when a lipid-degrading enzyme is defective or absent. In these cases, the lipid synthesis proceeds normally, but the degradation is impaired, causing the lipid or a partial degradation product to accumulate, with consequences such as an enlarged liver and spleen, mental retardation, blindness, and death.

Niemann-Pick, Gaucher's, and Tay-Sachs diseases are examples of lipidoses. Niemann-Pick disease is caused by a defect in an enzyme that breaks down sphingomyelin. The disease becomes apparent in infancy, causing mental retardation and death normally by age four. Gaucher's disease, a more common disease involving the accumulation of a glycolipid, produces two different syndromes. The acute cerebral form affects infants, causing severe nervous system abnormalities, retardation, and death before age one. The chronic form, which may become evident at any age, causes enlargement of the spleen, anemia, and erosion of the bones. In Tay-Sachs disease, a partially degraded lipid accumulates in the tissues of the central nervous system. Symptoms include progressive loss of vision, paralysis, and death at three or four years of age. Although Tay-Sachs disease is relatively rare (1 in 300,000 births), it has a high incidence in individuals of Eastern European Jewish descent (1 in 3,600 births). This defect is a recessive genetic trait that is found in one of every twenty-eight members of this population. For two parents who are both carriers of this trait, there is a one in four chance that their child will develop Tay-Sachs disease. Tests have been developed to detect the presence of the defective gene in the parent, and the amniotic fluid of a developing fetus can be sampled using a technique called amniocentesis to detect Tay-Sachs disease. Lipid-storage diseases have no known cures; however, they can be prevented through genetic counseling.

PERSPECTIVE AND PROSPECTS

The ability of a cell to discriminate in its chemical exchanges with the environment is fundamental to life. How the cell membrane accomplishes this feat has been an intense subject of biochemical research since the beginning of the twentieth century.

In 1895, C. Overton observed that substances that are lipid-soluble enter cells more quickly than those that are lipid-insoluble. He reasoned that the membrane must be composed of lipids. About twenty years later, chemical analysis showed that membranes also contain proteins. Irwin Langmuir prepared the first artificial membrane in 1917 by mixing a phospholipid-containing hydrocarbon solution with water. Evaporation of the hydrocarbon left a phospholipid film on the surface of the water, which showed that only the hydrophilic heads contacted the water. When the Dutch biologists E. Gorter and F. Grendel deposited the lipids from red blood cell membranes on a water surface and decreased the occupied surface area with a movable barrier, a continuous film resulted that occupied an area approximately twice the surface area of the original red blood cells. In 1935, all these observations, along with the fact that the surfaces of artificial membranes containing only phospholipids are less water-absorbent than the surfaces of true biological membranes, were combined by H. Davison and J. Danielli into a membrane model in which a phospholipid bilayer was sandwiched between two water-absorbent protein layers.

The technological advances of the 1950's in X-ray diffraction and electron microscopy allowed the structures of membranes to be probed directly. Such studies revealed that membranes are indeed composed of two parallel orderly arrays of lipids; although many of the proteins are attached to one of the faces of the bilayer, however, the Danielli-Davison model was too simplistic. The freeze-fracture technique of preparing cells for electron microscopy has provided the most information about the nature of membrane proteins. In this technique, the two layers are separated so that the inner topography can be studied. Instead of the smooth surface predicted by the Danielli-Davison model, a cobblestone-like surface was observed that resulted from proteins penetrating into the interior of the membrane. All experimental evidence supports the fluid mosaic model for biological membranes, in which proteins are dispersed and embedded in a phospholipid bilayer that is in a fluid state. How membranes function was the next question to be considered.

Although most of the small molecules needed by cells cross the barrier via protein channels, some essential nutrients, such as cholesterol in its LDL package, are too large to pass through a small channel. In 1986, Michael Brown and Joseph Goldstein received the Nobel Prize for their discovery of specific protein receptors on the membranes of liver cells to which LDL molecules attach. These receptors move across the surface until they encounter a shallow indentation or pit. As the pit deepens, the membrane closes behind the LDL, forming a coating allowing transport across the hydrophobic membrane interior. The presence of insufficient numbers of these receptors causes abnormal LDL-cholesterol buildup in the blood.

Many questions remain unanswered concerning the roles of proteins and glycolipids in membranes. Membranes are involved in the movement, growth, and development of cells. How the membrane is involved in the uncontrolled multiplication and migration in cancer is one medically important question. Experiments that will answer questions about how membrane structure affects functioning should lead to the development of new medical treatments.

—Arlene R. Courtney, Ph.D.

See also Arteriosclerosis; Cholesterol; Digestion; Fluids and electrolytes; Food biochemistry; Heart disease; Hypercholesterolemia; Hyperlipidemia; Metabolism; Obesity; Steroids; Tay-Sachs disease.

FOR FURTHER INFORMATION:

Bettleheim, F. A., and J. March. *Introduction to General, Organic, and Biochemistry.* 6th ed. Fort Worth, Tex.: Harcourt Brace College, 2001. A text designed for students with little previous chemistry background. Chapter 17 discusses the structure and function of lipids, chapter 21 discusses the conversion of biological molecules into energy, and chapter 22 gives details of the synthesis of lipids in the body.

Bloomfield, Molly M. *Chemistry and the Living Organism*. 6th ed. New York: John Wiley & Sons, 1996. A text written for allied health students that has a well-written chapter on lipids. Other chapters provide good elementary coverage on organic compounds such as alcohols, carboxylic acids, and esters.

Brown, Michael S., and Joseph L. Goldstein. "How LDL Receptors Influence Cholesterol and Atherosclerosis." *Scientific American* 251 (November, 1984): 58-66. An article in which the Nobel laureates describe their work on LDL membrane receptors. This article is of an intermediate technical nature.

Christian, Janet L., and Janet L. Greger. *Nutrition for Living*. 4th ed. Redwood City, Calif.: Benjamin/Cummings, 1994. A human nutrition text written at a level requiring little or no technical knowledge. This book provides an elementary discussion of the nutritional aspects of fats and cholesterol.

Cornatzer, W. E. *Role of Nutrition in Health and Diseases*. Springfield, Ill.: Charles C Thomas, 1989. Gives a comprehensive description of medical conditions in which lipids are involved.

Liposuction
Procedure
Anatomy or system affected: Abdomen, arms, hips, knees, legs

Specialties and related fields: General surgery, plastic surgery

Definition: The removal of fat deposits with a cannula and a suction pump in order to recontour body areas.

Key terms:

abdomen: the area of the body between the diaphragm and the pelvis; it contains the visceral organs

adipose tissue: the tissue that stores fat

cannula: a tube used to drain body fluids or to administer medications

general anesthesia: anesthesia that induces unconsciousness

local anesthesia: anesthesia that numbs the feeling in a body part; administered by injection or direct application to the skin

subcutaneous: under the skin

Indications and Procedures

The fat contained in adipose tissue makes up 15 to 20 percent of the body weights of most healthy individuals. Much adipose tissue is found inside the abdominal cavity, but significant amounts are located under the skin of the abdomen, arms, breasts, hips, knees, legs, and throat. The quantity of this subcutaneous fat at any such site is based on individual heredity, age, and eating habits. When excessive eating greatly elevates body fat, a patient becomes obese, a condition that can be life-threatening. Until recently, the sole means for decreasing fat content resulting from obesity was time-consuming dieting, which requires much patience and will power. In addition, the positive consequences of long diets can be easily obliterated if dieters begin to overeat again. Recurrent overeating is common and often followed by the rapid regaining of the fat.

Persons who have undesired, unattractive fat deposits as a result of age, heredity, or obesity may undergo cosmetic surgery, such as so-called tummy tucks, to remove them. Such major procedures, however, often remove muscle along with fat and cause considerable scarring. Liposuction is a relatively easy way to lose unattractive body fat; it also is seen as a fast way to reverse obesity and is touted as more permanent than dieting. A cannula connected to a suction pump is inserted under the skin in the desired area. Then a chosen amount of fat is sucked out, the cannula is withdrawn, and the incision is closed. The result is a recontouring of the body part. Hence, liposuction has become a very popular cosmetic surgery procedure for the abdomen, arms, breasts, hips, knees, legs, and throat; many pounds can be removed from large areas such as the abdomen.

Liposuction begins with the administration of antibiotics and the anesthesia of the area to be recontoured. Local anesthesia is safer, but general anesthesia is used when necessary. The process usually begins after a 1.3-centimeter (0.5-inch) incision is made in a fold of the treated body region, so that the scar will not be noticeable after healing. At this time, a sterile cannula is introduced under the skin of the treatment area. Next, the surgeon uses suction through the cannula to remove the fat deposits. Liposuction produces temporary tunnels in adipose tissue. Upon completion of the procedure, the incision is closed and the surgical area is wrapped with tight bandages or covered with support garments. This final stage of recontouring helps the tissue to collapse back into the desired shape during healing. In most patients, the skin around the area soon shrinks into the new contours. When this does not happen easily, because of old age or other factors, liposuction is accompanied by surgical skin removal.

USES AND COMPLICATIONS

Liposuction can be used for body recontouring only when undesired contours are attributable to fat deposits; those attributable to anatomical features such as bone structure cannot be treated in this manner.

A major principle on which liposuction is based is the supposition that the body contains a fixed number of fat cells and that, as people become fatter, the cells fill with droplets of fat and expand. The removal of fat cells by liposuction is deemed to decrease the future ability of the treated body part to become fat because fewer cells are available to be filled. Dieting and exercise are less successful than liposuction because they do not diminish the number of fat cells in adipose tissue, only decreasing fat cell size. Hence, when dieters return to eating excess food again or exercise stops, the fat cells expand again.

Another aspect of liposuction which is becoming popular is the ability to remove undesired fat from

The Use of Liposuction

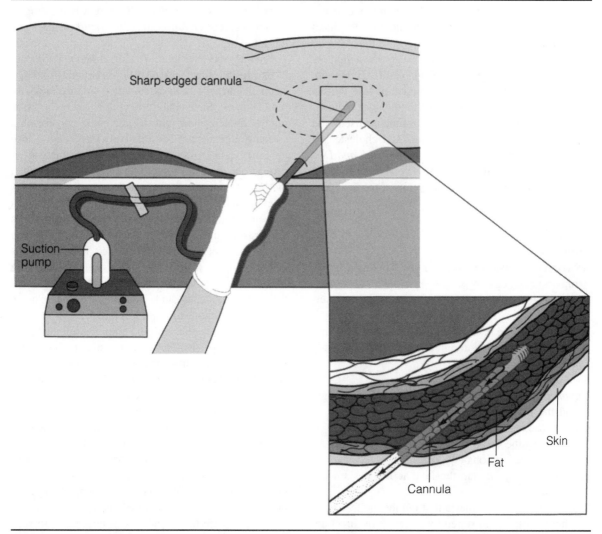

Sharp-edged cannula

Suction pump

Skin

Fat

Cannula

When unwanted areas of fat seem resistant to dieting and exercise, some patients turn to liposuction, the physical removal of fat deposits with a tube and a suction pump. The cosmetic results of this procedure may vary considerably.

some body sites and insert it where the fat is wanted for recontouring. Most often, this transfer involves enlarging women's breasts or correcting cases in which the two breasts are of markedly different size. Liposuction also can be used to repair asymmetry in other body parts as a result of accidents.

Liposuction, as with any other surgery, has associated risks and complications. According to reputable practitioners, however, they are temporary and relatively minor, such as black-and-blue marks and the accumulation of blood and serum under the skin of treated areas. These complications are minimized by fluid removal during surgery and by the application of tight bandages or garments after the operation. Another related complication is that subcutaneous fat removal leads to fluid loss from the body. When large amounts of fat are removed, shock occurs if the fluid is not replaced quickly. Therefore, another component of successful liposuction is timely fluid replacement.

The more extensive and complex the liposuction procedure attempted, the more likely it is to cause complications. Particularly prone to problems are liposuction procedures in which major skin removal is required. Hence, surgeons who perform liposuction suggest that potential patients be realistic about the goals of the surgery. It is also recommended that patients choose reputable practitioners.

PERSPECTIVE AND PROSPECTS

Liposuction, currently viewed as relatively safe cosmetic surgery, originated in Europe in the late 1960's. In 1982, it reached the United States. Since that time, its use has burgeoned, and about a half million liposuction surgeries are carried out yearly. Although its first use was as a purely cosmetic procedure, liposuction is now done for noncosmetic reasons, including repairing injuries sustained in accidents. Women were once the sole liposuction patients. Now, men make up about one-quarter of treated individuals.

In the United States, liposuction is not presently accepted by insurance companies or considered tax deductible. This situation may change because several studies have found that obese people have a greater chance of developing cardiovascular disease and cancer. It must be noted, however, that liposuction offers only temporary relief from body fat. Although it does decrease fat deposition in a treated region, lack of proper calorie intake and exercise will deposit fat elsewhere in the body.

—*Sanford S. Singer, Ph.D.*

See also Dermatology; Lipids; Nutrition; Obesity; Plastic surgery; Skin; Weight loss and gain.

FOR FURTHER INFORMATION:

Grazer, Frederick M., ed. *Atlas of Suction-Assisted Lipectomy in Body Contouring.* New York: Churchill Livingstone, 1992. This helpful atlas covers liposuction and lipectomy. Includes bibliographical references and an index.

Schein, Jeffery R. "The Truth About Liposuction." *Consumers Digest* 30 (January/February, 1991): 71-74. Liposuction is the most popular type of cosmetic surgery, and that means that many people are assuming that liposuction can do more than it really can. Some facts about liposuction and physicians' certification are given.

Sizer, Frances Sienkiewicz, and Eleanor Noss Whitney. "Lipids: Fats and Oils." In *Nutrition: Concepts and Controversies.* 8th ed. Belmont, Calif.: Wadsworth, 2000. Discusses all aspects of nutrition. Includes bibliographical references and an index.

Tcheupdjian, Leon. *Liposuction: New Hope for a New Figure Through the Art of Body Contouring.* Chicago: Liposuction Institute, 1988. This is one of the few comprehensive books on the latest state-of-the-art methods. It is written by a pioneer in the field.

LISPING

DISEASE/DISORDER

ANATOMY OR SYSTEM AFFECTED: Mouth, teeth

SPECIALTIES AND RELATED FIELDS: Dentistry, speech pathology

DEFINITION: The defective pronunciation of the sibilants "s" and "z," usually substituted with a "th" sound.

CAUSES AND SYMPTOMS

A central or frontal lisp is caused by a child pushing the tongue past the teeth while speaking, which tends to occur in cases of an open bite. This produces the familiar lisp in which "s" and "z" sounds are pronounced like "th." Sometimes, the child tries to correct the protrusion of the tongue by pulling it in, but lisping still occurs because the correct position of the tongue has not been learned.

A lateral lisp involves the escape of air on both sides of the tongue, yielding an unpleasant "blubbering" sound. A possible cause is missing teeth, particularly the two upper front teeth.

A recessive lisp is caused by holding the tongue too far back in the mouth. The "s" and "z" sounds come out sounding more like "sh." This mild lisp is often associated in the popular media with the speech of an intoxicated person.

TREATMENT AND THERAPY

Speech therapists work with lisping children in two ways. In the phonetic placement method, the child is asked to pronounce the "t" sound and then prolong it. Once this is learned, the bite is closed and the child then practices moving the lips in a slightly protracted position; the tongue is moved back and forth until the "s" sound is achieved. This same process is used in learning to pronounce "z"; the "d" sound, however, is used in practice instead of a "t." In some cases, asking the child to pronounce "sh" first and then move the tongue forward along the roof of the mouth will produce an "s" sound.

In the auditory stimulation method, the speech therapist pronounces the correct sound repeatedly and compares it to the incorrect articulation. This method is very successful in young children with lisps.

After a sound has been practiced by itself, the child attaches it to nonsense syllables and practices pronouncing them. Gradually, the sound is introduced in familiar words, followed by sentences. The final test is the use of the newly acquired sound in spontaneous conversation.

—*Rose Secrest*

See also Developmental stages; Motor skill development; Speech disorders; Stuttering; Voice and vocal cord disorders.

FOR FURTHER INFORMATION:

Cole, Patricia R. *Language Disorders in Preschool Children*. Englewood Cliffs, N.J.: Prentice Hall, 1982.

Egland, George O. *Speech and Language Problems*. Englewood Cliffs, N.J.: Prentice Hall, 1970.

Eisenson, Jon, and Mardel Ogilvie. *Speech Correction in the Schools*. 4th ed. New York: Macmillan, 1977.

Winitz, Harris, ed. *Human Communication and Its Disorders: A Review, 1987*. Norwood, N.J.: Abex, 1987.

LITHOTRIPSY

PROCEDURE

ANATOMY OR SYSTEM AFFECTED: Abdomen, bladder, kidneys, urinary system

Methods of Lithotripsy

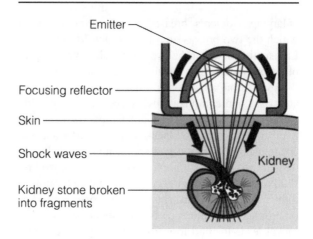

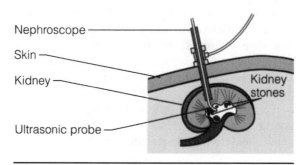

Kidney stones can be removed or broken into fragments using lithotripsy. In extracorporeal shock-wave lithotripsy (top), an emitter sends shock waves into tissues above the kidney stones, breaking the stones into very small fragments that can then be passed through the urine. In percutaneous lithotripsy (bottom), a nephroscope is inserted through the skin and into the kidney, where an ultrasonic probe breaks up and removes the stones.

SPECIALTIES AND RELATED FIELDS: Nephrology, urology

DEFINITION: A method of breaking up stones in the kidneys, ureters, and urinary bladder using shock waves or high-frequency sound waves.

INDICATIONS AND PROCEDURES

Stone fragmentation using shock waves or ultrasonic waves is less invasive, less painful, and less time consuming than conventional open surgery to remove stones or the organs that contain them. With lithotripsy, blood loss is minimal and recovery is quick, with a low morbidity (injury rate).

In extracorporeal shock-wave lithotripsy, the patient is given either local or general anesthesia. A machine called a lithotripter is placed on the abdomen over the site of the stones. An emitter in the lithotripter sends out shock waves that break the stones into fine fragments that can pass through the urinary tract without harm to the patient, who is encouraged to drink copious amounts of fluid following the procedure.

In ultrasonic lithotripsy, an incision is made in the skin. The stone is approached and visualized with an endoscope, a hollow instrument with a telescope at one end for visualization. The other end of the instrument is introduced via the urethra into the bladder or ureter or via a small skin hole into the kidney. For kidney stones, a small needle is introduced into the kidney through the back under X-ray control, and a nephrostomy tract is established between the skin and the kidney. The ultrasonographic lithotripsy probe is introduced through the endoscope and brought in contact with the stone.

A piezoceramic crystal is electrically stimulated, which generates ultrasonic waves that will fragment the stone. The design of the probe allows it to suction out the broken stone particles simultaneously. Larger stones can be fragmented into smaller pieces, which can then be grasped with forceps and pulled out. When a ureteral stone is treated by this method, a plastic tube (a double-J stent) is left in the ureter to prevent postoperative blockage and future scar formation. When a kidney stone is treated by this method, a large-caliber tube is left in the kidney (a nephrostomy tube) to drain the kidney and secure a tract for future X-ray studies and reinspection of the kidney for possible residual stone fragments.

USES AND COMPLICATIONS

The main morbidity associated with this procedure occurs during the establishment of the nephrostomy tract to gain access to the kidney, which can lead to bleeding, or during the introduction of the endoscope into the ureter, which can lead to perforation and future scarring. During stone fragmentation, it is imperative that the probe be in direct contact with the stone at all times, or it may cause ureteral perforation and bleeding. Overall, however, ultrasonographic lithotripsy is a safe and effective method of stone treatment, with few injuries and a quick recovery.

As with ultrasonic lithotripsy, few serious complications are associated with shock-wave lithotripsy. The presence of blood in the urine (hematuria) may be noted but is usually only temporary, as the stone fragments pass through the ureters, bladder, and urethra. Abdominal bruising may also occur, but this complication is minor in comparison to more invasive techniques.

—*Saeed Akhter, M.D.*

See also Cholecystectomy; Gallbladder diseases; Kidney disorders; Kidneys; Nephrology; Stone removal; Stones; Ultrasonography; Urinary disorders; Urinary system; Urology.

FOR FURTHER INFORMATION:

Clayman, Charles B., ed. *The American Medical Association Encyclopedia of Medicine*. Rev. 3d ed. New York: Random House, 1994.

Fredman, Lawrence S. "Liver, Biliary Tract, and Pancreas." In *Current Medical Diagnosis and Treatment: 2001*, edited by Lawrence M. Tierney, Jr., et al., eds. 39th ed. New York: McGraw-Hill, 2000.

Novick, Andrew C., and Stevan B. Streem. "Surgery of the Kidney." In *Campbell's Urology*, edited by Patrick C. Walsh, et al. 7th ed. Philadelphia: W. B. Saunders, 1998.

Presti, Joseph C., Marshall L. Stoller, and Peter R. Carroll. "Urology." In *Current Medical Diagnosis and Treatment*, edited by Lawrence M. Tierney, Jr., et al. 39th ed. New York: McGraw-Hill, 2000.

LIVER

ANATOMY

ANATOMY OR SYSTEM AFFECTED: Abdomen, blood, circulatory system, endocrine system, gastrointestinal system, glands

SPECIALTIES AND RELATED FIELDS: Endocrinology, gastroenterology, hematology, internal medicine, toxicology

DEFINITION: A vital organ that controls blood sugar levels; metabolizes carbohydrates, lipids, and proteins; stores blood, iron, and some vitamins; degrades steroid hormones; and inactivates and/or excretes certain drugs and toxins.

KEY TERMS:

cirrhosis: a condition of the liver in which injured or dead cells are replaced with scar tissue

endoplasmic reticulum: a component of cells which in the liver is responsible for, among other things, the metabolism of xenobiotics

hepatitis: an infectious disease of the liver that is caused by a virus; at least three different types of hepatitis exist

hepatocyte: the functional cell of the liver; the liver contains only one type of functional cell

plasma proteins: any proteins found in the plasma of blood, which include those proteins necessary for blood clotting and some necessary for the transport of other molecules; most are produced by the liver

subclinical: referring to an infection in which the patient has no symptoms of disease; the infection is detected by other indicators, such as the presence of antibodies

virus: a subcellular particle that enters cells and causes cellular damage; it uses the cells' mechanisms to reproduce itself

xenobiotic: a nonbiological chemical that can enter a biological system; it could be a prescribed drug, a pollutant, or another substance

STRUCTURE AND FUNCTIONS

The liver, an accessory gland of the digestive system, is the largest organ in the human body. Located in the upper-right quadrant of the abdominal cavity, it abuts the diaphragm on the anterior surface. The liver is composed of two lobes of unequal size; with the large right lobe further divided into two smaller lobes. The organ is protected by the ribs, which cover nearly the entire surface. The liver contains only one type of functional cell, known as a hepatocyte. Closely associated with the organ is the gallbladder, a saclike structure which holds bile, a product of the hepatocytes. Bile is continually produced by the hepatocytes but is stored in the gallbladder until it is required for digestive products.

The liver is unique in that it receives blood from two different sources. The hepatic artery delivers blood to the liver from the systemic circulation. The liver also receives blood via the portal vein, which collects blood that has previously passed through the small intestine and has absorbed nutrients from the digestive system. As the blood enters the liver, it flows into dilated capillaries called sinusoids. Blood flow through sinusoids is much slower than through capillaries, and the exchange of materials between hepatocytes and the bloodstream is accomplished with little difficulty. This slower process also allows the liver to serve as a storage organ for blood, which gives the organ its characteristic dark red appearance.

The liver is essential to the normal functioning of the body. Its activities are many and varied: It regulates the metabolism of carbohydrates, lipids, and proteins; synthesizes proteins, particularly those of blood plasma that control clotting; serves as a storage site for some vitamins and iron; degrades steroid hormones; and inactivates and/or excretes certain drugs and toxins.

The liver plays a major role in carbohydrate metabolism. As carbohydrates are absorbed from the small intestine, they are transported to the liver through the portal vein. The liver regulates blood sugar levels by removing excess quantities. If the diet includes too much glucose, this substance is stored in the liver or skeletal muscle as glycogen. If the blood sugar levels are low, the glycogen is broken down into glucose and released to the bloodstream. The liver is also capable of converting amino acids, lipids, or simple carbohydrates into glucose.

The principal functions of the liver in lipid metabolism are twofold. First, it is responsible for the breakdown of large fat molecules into small compounds that can be used for energy. Second, it synthesizes triglycerides, cholesterol, and phospholipids from other fats. All three of these compounds play important roles in cellular function.

The synthesis of proteins by the liver is of major importance for the body. The liver is capable of synthesizing not only a variety of proteins but also the

The Anatomy of the Liver

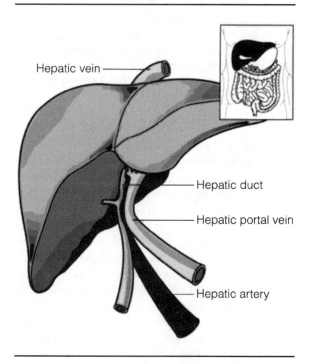

Hepatic vein

Hepatic duct

Hepatic portal vein

Hepatic artery

nonessential amino acids that are the building blocks of proteins. Many of the proteins that the liver synthesizes are found in blood plasma, including those factors responsible for blood clotting. In order to protect the body against deficiencies in these substances, the liver stores vitamins A, D, and B_{12}. It is also capable of storing iron, the mineral necessary for the production of hemoglobin.

Located in the smooth endoplasmic reticulum of hepatocytes are nonspecific enzymes called the mixed-function oxidases. They are capable of metabolizing a wide variety of hormones, including some polypeptide hormones and the steroid hormones, such as cortisol, estrogen, and testosterone. These same enzymes are responsible for the degradation of many foreign substances that enter the body, such as prescription medications, illegal drugs, and toxins. Most of the materials metabolized are made more water-soluble, and therefore more easily excreted, by the kidney. Others are removed from the hepatocytes in the bile that the cells produce.

Production of bile by the hepatocytes is of utmost importance to the digestive system. Bile is composed of lecithin, cholesterol, bile pigments, proteins, and bile acids, along with an isotonic solution similar to blood plasma. Bile is produced continually and stored in the gallbladder. Several minutes after a meal begins, the gallbladder releases bile to the duodenum of the small intestine. The highest rate of bile release occurs during the duodenal digestion of food and is controlled by the hormone cholecystokinin. In the duodenum, bile acts as an emulsifier of fat in the diet. It breaks large lipid droplets into many small lipid droplets, which can more easily be digested by enzymes in the small intestine. About 95 percent of the bile is reabsorbed and returned to the liver, and the other 5 percent is excreted with the feces. This provides one mechanism for the body to use the digestive system for the removal of waste products. One important product that is excreted in this manner is bilirubin, a by-product of the normal destruction of old red blood cells.

DISORDERS AND DISEASES

The liver is unique among body organs because it has the ability to regenerate in cases of injury or disease. It is estimated that in a young, healthy individual a liver which has suffered a physical injury could regenerate as much as 80 percent of the total organ. Many important organs are paired, such as the lungs

and kidneys. Though the liver is a single organ, its ability to regenerate ensures normal function even in cases of severe injury.

The presence of liver disease is detectable in many ways. With some diseases, the liver becomes enlarged and can be felt below the ribs. This swelling may be associated with localized discomfort or pain in the region. In more severe cases of liver disease, the organ may actually shrink and recede further under the ribs, a condition easily detected by a physician.

The pathophysiology of the liver is characterized by certain physiologic events that occur regardless of the underlying cause. Within the liver, disease may result in portal hypertension, blockage of bile ducts, and cellular injury or death. Cellular injury may be manifest by fatty infiltration and by interference with cellular functions, including the synthesis of proteins necessary for blood clotting, the metabolism of drugs or toxins, the regulation of glucose, and the production of bile. Any or all of these physiologic changes can lead to effects in other parts of the body.

Disease of the liver is often detectable by routine blood tests that include liver function tests. The patient may show decreased levels in the blood serum of proteins that are normally produced by the liver, anincreased blood-clotting time, or increased serum levels of enzymes that are normally found only in the liver. A yellow skin tone known as jaundice has been associated with liver disease. This discoloration of skin and the cornea of the eye is a result of excessively high levels of bilirubin in the blood. Bilirubin is a by-product of the breakdown of red blood cells that are near the end of their 120-day life cycle.

The injury or death of liver cells may present a pathology unique to the liver, the disease cirrhosis. When hepatocytes are injured or diseased, they begin to accumulate lipids in vacuoles, giving the liver a whitish appearance. Associated with the development of a fatty liver, the cells may divide to produce more cells that will ensure normal function. Sometimes, however, this stimulation of cell division leads to an excess of hepatocytes, a condition that may result in abnormal patterns of blood flow through the liver. In addition, this phenomenon may include the production of large nodules of connective tissue to replace dead or dying cells, a condition comparable to scarring. The development of scars may cause increased blood pressure in the portal veins and may block bile ducts. Cirrhosis may be caused by a variety of conditions, including alcoholism, exposure to toxic substances, or infection. It is irreversible and ultimately causes the death of the patient.

Diseases of the liver can be classified according to the following scheme: congenital liver disorders, viral and nonviral infections, drug-induced and toxin-induced disease, vascular disorders, metabolic disorders, iron accumulation, alcoholic liver disease, and tumors.

The most common types of congenital diseases of the liver involve abnormalities of the bile ducts or of the portal vein, which may be associated with portal hypertension. More important, however, are those diseases that lead to the formation of cysts, such as polycystic liver disease or hepatic fibrosis. Jaundice of the newborn, a discoloration of the skin at birth, usually clears within a week or so with no long-term effects.

Viral infections of the liver may be associated with the hepatitis viruses or other viruses less specific for the liver. The four most common hepatitis viruses are hepatitis A; hepatitis B; non-A, non-B hepatitis; and hepatitis D. Hepatitis can also be associated with yellow fever, infectious mononucleosis, cytomegalovirus infection, and herpes simplex.

Hepatitis A is also known as infectious hepatitis. It is generally transmitted via fecal contamination of milk, water, or seafood. It is most common in the areas of the world where untreated sewage may come into contact with the water supply or food sources. It has a short incubation period and is usually not fatal; it does not lead to chronic hepatitis. Hepatitis B, also known as serum hepatitis, is transmitted from persons with an active form of the disease or from carriers via contaminated blood or blood products. It is particularly prevalent among drug users who share needles. The threat of contraction of hepatitis B from a transfusion has been greatly reduced by the screening of blood products. Hepatitis B has a long incubation period, up to six months. The severity of the disease varies greatly from subclinical hepatitis (showing no symptoms) to chronic hepatitis and in some cases may result in death. The virus (or viruses) that causes non-A, non-B hepatitis has not yet been identified. The course of the disease resembles hepatitis B and may lead to chronic hepatitis. Hepatitis D is believed to be a defective virus that is found only in the presence of hepatitis B. It is transmitted via the same route and can result in chronic hepatitis. It occurs more commonly in Europe than in the United States.

Hepatitis from any cause may show subclinical or mild, influenza-like symptoms. Acute hepatitis may cause loss of appetite, vomiting, fever, jaundice, and enlargement of the liver. The viruses that cause hepatitis replicate within the liver cells, which could be the cause of the injury to these cells. Hepatocyte injury could also be a result of the immune system's attempt to fight the virus, which may injure the cells of the liver in the process. In either case, the damaged cells swell before they die. The liver can also be infected by bacterial cells, which usually reach the liver as a result of a systemic infection.

Many toxins or drugs can injure the liver, in a general pattern that is similar to the effects of infectious agents. The assault on the cell often leads to fatty infiltration, followed by swelling and finally by the death of the hepatocyte. Even in less severe cases of injury, those that do not lead to death of the hepatocyte, there is often impairment of the metabolic activities of the liver that can lead to diverse systemic effects. One of these effects is the ability to metabolize foreign compounds or naturally occurring steroids; the accumulation of these compounds throughout the body can have wide-ranging consequences.

The liver is adversely effected by the constant intake of excessive quantities of ethyl alcohol. In the early stages of alcoholism, the physiologic changes may be a result of improper nutrition or of vitamin deficiencies. During the more advanced stages of alcoholism, the patient is likely to suffer from a fatty liver and, ultimately, from cirrhosis. While those who stop drinking may slow down the advancement of cirrhosis, the disease appears to be irreversible.

There are more than five thousand metabolic enzymes in the liver, each of which is controlled genetically. Important in the treatment of metabolic disease is early diagnosis, which may prevent damage to other organs or to the liver. Dietary control may be used to minimize the effects of such conditions, leading to a near-normal life. Examples of treatable metabolic diseases are galactosemia, a condition which prevents the conversion of galactose to glucose; fructosemia, a condition that leads to the accumulation of fructose-1-phosphate; and Wilson's disease, an accumulation of copper in vital organs as a result of a defect in copper metabolism. In each case, the accumulation of a certain substance can lead to cellular damage, but dietary control of the substance can minimize the effects. Hemochromatosis is a similar disease which leads to accumulation of iron in the liver. As with Wilson's disease, the deposition of this element is not limited to the liver and can accumulate in other vital tissues of the body as well.

Cancer of the liver is usually caused by its spread from another site. Primary liver cancers are rare and usually do not occur until late in life. Risk factors may include exposure to hepatotoxins, chronic liver disease, or hepatitis B. There are two types of primary carcinomas of the liver: hepatocellular carcinoma, which develops in hepatocytes, and cholangiocellular carcinoma, which develops in bile ducts.

PERSPECTIVE AND PROSPECTS

The liver is a vital organ that plays a major role in the homeostasis of the body. Any condition that adversely influences the liver will have wide-ranging effects on other organs and the patient as a whole.

Because one of its functions is the metabolism of pollutants, drugs (including alcohol), and hormones, the liver is often exposed to substances that are toxic to its hepatocytes. When these compounds are encountered, the liver efficiently alters them for excretion. Sometimes, however, these substances may do damage to the cells before the liver can metabolize them.

When a liver cell is injured, the end result may be the death of the cell. Fortunately, liver cells are efficient at cell division and can replace those cells that have been injured or that have died. With continued damage to liver cells, however, the body can no longer replace them, and the resulting decrease in liver function leads to extensive complications throughout the body. A decrease in liver function will not only have an effect on the digestive system but will have wide-ranging effects on glucose and lipid metabolism (normal functions of the blood whose proteins are synthesized by the liver) and on the ability to remove certain foreign substances or toxins from the blood. For example, if the ability to metabolize medication is impaired by liver disease, the patient's body may accumulate high, even toxic, levels of drugs. These substances can have pronounced effects, particularly on the nervous system. With liver injury, the once-simple act of determining a medication dosage can become a critical problem.

Because there is only one liver and because the liver cells are genetically programmed to divide a limited number of times, any liver injury or disease can have permanent effects. There is little that medicine can do to cure liver disease. For example, there is no treatment for the hepatitis viruses; the body's own defense mechanisms must ultimately rid itself of the disease. The medical community can treat the symptoms of hepatitis.

Cancer of the liver is also difficult to treat. Because it is not easily detected, the diagnosis is rarely early. Unless the cancer is restricted to one lobe that can be removed, surgery is rarely the answer. Treatment is further complicated by the fact that the liver cells are particularly sensitive to radiation and that the doses needed to treat the cancer would be deadly to hepatocytes. Chemotherapy remains the primary hope for a cure.

With the discovery of immunosuppressive drugs, liver transplantation has become a positive procedure in the treatment of liver disease, and the results are promising. The availability of healthy livers for transplant, however, makes this an option limited to a small percentage of patients.

—*Annette O'Connor, Ph.D.*

See also Abdomen; Abdominal disorders; Alcoholism; Anatomy; Blood and blood disorders; Circulation; Cirrhosis; Gastroenterology; Gastroenterology, pediatric; Gastrointestinal disorders; Gastrointestinal system; Hematology; Hematology, pediatric; Hepatitis; Internal medicine; Jaundice; Liver cancer; Liver disorders; Liver transplantation; Metabolism; Systems and organs; Transplantation.

FOR FURTHER INFORMATION:

Chandrasoma, Parakrama, and Clive R. Taylor. *Concise Pathology*. 3d ed. Norwalk, Conn.: Appleton and Lange, 1998. A pathology book written for health care personnel. It is well designed, and most laypeople will be able to understand the clearly organized and simple explanations that are presented.

Dollinger, Malin, Ernest H. Rosenbaum, and Greg Cable. *Everyone's Guide to Cancer Therapy*. 3d ed. Kansas City: Andrews & McMeel, 1997. A well-organized book on therapy for various cancers, including a special section on liver cancers. Clearly describes the methods of treatment that are available and the treatment of choice. Written for the layperson and easily understood.

Guyton, Arthur C., and John E. Hall. *Textbook of Medical Physiology*. 10th ed. Philadelphia: W. B. Saunders, 2000. Although this is a text for medical students, the material is presented so well and with such a useful background that general readers will be able to understand the information that it contains. Offers good illustrations and tables that help to put everything in context.

McCance, Kathryn L., and Sue E. Huether. *Pathophysiology: The Biologic Basis for Disease in Adults and Children*. 3d ed. St. Louis: C. V. Mosby, 1998. A very well written book on pathophysiology which not only presents the facts regarding certain diseases but also explains their physiological bases. Designed for student nurses, but its description of the physiology of the organ provides an extensive background for the less informed reader.

LIVER CANCER
DISEASE/DISORDER
ANATOMY OR SYSTEM AFFECTED: Liver
SPECIALTIES AND RELATED FIELDS: Gastroenterology, immunology, oncology, radiology
DEFINITION: Malignancies of the liver, which may be primary (arising in the organ itself) but are more likely to be secondary (metastasizing from another site).

CAUSES AND SYMPTOMS

The liver filters the blood supply, removing and breaking down (metabolizing) toxins and delivering them through the biliary tract to the intestines for elimination with other wastes. Because of the large volume of blood flowing through the liver (about a quarter of the body's supply), blood-borne toxins or cancer cells migrating from tumors elsewhere (the process called metastasis) pose a constant threat. In fact, in the United States most liver cancers are metastatic; only about 1 percent actually originate in the liver. In Southeast Asia and sub-Saharan Africa, primary liver cancer is the most common type, accounting for as much as 30 percent of all cancers.

Two major types of cancer affect the liver: those involving liver cells (hepatocellular carcinomas) and those involving the bile ducts (cholangiocarcinomas). The first is by far the more common, although tumors may contain a mixture of both, and their development is similar. Tumors may arise in one location, forming a large mass; arise in several locations, forming nodes; or spread throughout the liver in a diffuse form. Liver cancers occur in men about four to eight times more frequently than in women and in blacks slightly more than in whites, although the proportions

vary widely among different regions of the world. In the United States, most cancers arise in people fifty years old or older; in other areas, people older than forty are at risk.

Primary liver cancer has so much regional and gender variation because causative agents are more or less common in different areas and men are more often exposed. A leading risk factor in the United States and Europe is cirrhosis, a scarring of liver tissue following destruction by viruses, toxins, or interrupted blood flow. In the United States, long-term alcohol consumption is the most common cause of cirrhosis, and men have long been more likely than women to become alcoholics. Likewise, hemochromatosis, a hereditary disease leading to the toxic buildup of iron, is a cancer precursor and more common in men than in women. In Africa and Southeast Asia, the hepatitis B and C viruses are leading precancer diseases because hepatitis has long been endemic in those areas, whereas in the United States it is not widespread (although the number of infected people began to rise in the 1980's).

Diet and medical therapies have also been implicated as liver carcinogens. Food toxins, especially aflatoxin from mold growing on peanuts (which are a staple in parts of Africa and Asia); oral contraceptives; anabolic steroids; and the high levels of sex hormones used in some treatments are thought to increase the likelihood of hepatobiliary tumors. Genetic factors, radiation, and occupational exposure to volatile chemicals may also play a minor role.

Although researchers generally agree about which agents are liver cancer precursors, the exact mechanism leading to tumor development is not thoroughly understood. Nevertheless, one factor may be universal. Viruses and toxins injure or destroy liver and bile duct cells; the body reacts to repair the damage with inflammation and an increased rate of new cell growth, a condition called regenerative hyperplasia. If the toxin damage continues, triggering ever more hyperplasia, as is the case with hepatitis and alcoholic cirrhosis, formation of a tumor becomes almost inevitable.

Like lymph nodes, the liver collects migrating cancer cells, so the cancers that physicians detect there often are metastases from cancers arising elsewhere in the body. In fact, liver involvement may be found before the primary cancer has been recognized. Colorectal cancer is especially given to metastasizing to the liver, since the digestive tract's blood supply is directly linked to the liver through the portal vein; similarly, lung and breast cancer may spread to the liver. Such metastases indicate advanced cancers that do not bode well for the patient's survival.

Symptoms may be ambiguous. Two common symptoms are jaundice and enlargement of the liver, with accompanying tenderness. Jaundice, a yellowing of the skin and eyes, is caused by an accumulation of bilirubin. Bilirubin builds up because a tumor has blocked the bile duct that normally empties it into the small intestine. (Both symptoms may also occur as a result of either gallstones or cirrhosis.) Patients with liver cancer may also have a fever and retain fluid in the abdominal cavities.

Liver Cancer

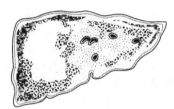

Solitary large tumor

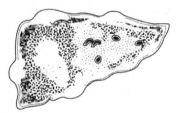

Nodular form

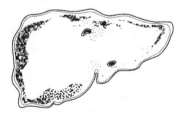

Diffuse growth

The liver is a frequent site of cancer, most commonly from malignancies that have spread from their original site. The particular form the cancer takes depends on several factors, notably the primary source and its possible cause.

TREATMENT AND THERAPY

Doctors suspecting liver cancer conduct tests designed to distinguish this disease from other disorders. Palpation of the liver may reveal that the organ is enlarged or contains an unusual tissue mass, which is likely to be a tumor. A rubbing sound heard through the stethoscope may also come from a tumor. Hepatocellular carcinoma often elevates the alpha-fetoprotein level in blood. Abdominal ultrasound or computed tomography (CT) scans can provide good evidence of a tumor in the liver, and a biopsy will supply a tissue sample capable of proving the presence of cancer, especially if the biopsy is done with CT scan or ultrasound guidance. A tumor can also disrupt normal biochemical action in the body, which doctors may detect in blood tests. Liver function blood tests may be abnormal with both primary and secondary liver cancer.

Under even the most favorable circumstances, the outlook for patients with liver cancer is still not good. If a primary cancer is found while still fairly small, surgical removal is the surest and fastest treatment, although it is a difficult, risky procedure because of the liver's complex, delicate structure. Radiation and chemotherapy have not succeeded in shrinking tumors effectively. Because symptoms usually appear late in the development of primary liver cancer, it seldom is found early enough for surgical cure; patients usually live only one to two months after detection. Those found with small, removable cancers live an average of twenty-nine months. Most liver cancers are metastases, however, and removal of the liver tumor will not rid the patient of cancer. In general, hepatobiliary cancer patients have a 5 percent chance of living five years after diagnosis.

Liver cancer screening tests can locate tumors while they are still treatable, although routine physical examinations in Western nations seldom include such tests. Usually only patients with cirrhosis or chronic hepatitis are screened. The best ways to ward off liver cancer are to avoid viral infection and to abstain from alcohol. For those at risk for infection, such as health care workers, the most effective primary prevention is vaccination for hepatitis B.

—Roger Smith, Ph.D.

See also Alcoholism; Cancer; Chemotherapy; Cirrhosis; Hepatitis; Jaundice; Liver; Liver disorders; Liver transplantation; Malignancy and metastasis; Oncology; Radiation therapy; Tumor removal; Tumors.

FOR FURTHER INFORMATION:

Curley, Steven A. *Liver Cancer.* New York: Springer, 1998. Provides the general surgeon, surgical oncologist, radiation oncologist, and medical oncologist with current information regarding diagnosis and multimodality treatment approaches for patients with primary or metastatic hepatobiliary cancer.

Murphy, G., L. Morris, and D. Lange. *Informed Decisions: The Complete Book of Cancer Diagnosis, Treatment, and Recovery.* New York: Viking Press, 1997. The American Cancer Society endorses this excellent book, which provides a complete consumer reference for cancer diagnosis, treatment, and recovery.

Sachar,k David B., Jerome D. Waye, and Blair S. Lewis. *Pocket Guide to Gastroenterology.* Rev. ed. Baltimore: Williams & Wilkins, 1991. Discusses such topics as gastroenterology, the digestive organs, and digestive system diseases. Includes bibliographical references and an index.

Shannon, Joyce Brennfleck. *Liver Disorders Sourcebook.* Detroit: Omnigraphics, 2000. This book includes basic consumer health information about the liver and how it works; liver diseases, including cancer, cirrhosis, hepatitis, and toxic and drug-related diseases; tips for maintaining a healthy liver; laboratory tests; radiology tests and facts about liver transplantation; and a section on support groups, a glossary, and resources listing.

Steen, R. Grant. *A Conspiracy of Cells: The Basic Science of Cancer.* New York: Plenum Press, 1993. Thorough, lucid explanations of all physiological aspects of cancer make this book instructive for readers willing to slog through the subject's complexity and terminology.

LIVER DISORDERS

DISEASE/DISORDER

ANATOMY OR SYSTEM AFFECTED: Liver

SPECIALTIES AND RELATED FIELDS: Gastroenterology, internal medicine

DEFINITION: As one of the most complex organs in the body, the liver is the target of a wide variety of toxins, infectious agents, and cancers that lead to hepatitis, cirrhosis, abscesses, and liver failure.

KEY TERMS:

abscess: a localized collection of pus and infectious microorganisms

ascites: the presence of free fluid in the abdominal cavity

bilirubin: a major component of bile, derived from the breakdown products of red blood cells

cirrhosis: the fibrous scar tissue that replaces the normally soft liver after repeated damage by viruses, chemicals, and/or alcohol

hepatitis: inflammation of the liver, such as that caused by viruses or toxins

jaundice: a yellow discoloration of the skin, eyes, and membranes caused by excess bilirubin in the blood

portal hypertension: elevated pressures in the portal veins caused by resistance to blood flow through a diseased liver; produces many regional problems, including ascites

portal system: a system of veins, unique to the liver, that carry nutrient-rich blood from the digestive organs to the liver

CAUSES AND SYMPTOMS

The liver is the largest internal organ, lying in the upper-right abdominal cavity. Intricately attached to it by a system of ducts on its lower surface is the pear-shaped gallbladder. Unique to the liver is a blood supply that derives from two separate sources: the hepatic artery, carrying freshly oxygenated blood from the heart, and the portal vein, carrying blood rich in the products of digestion from the digestive organs. The liver cells, or hepatocytes, are arranged in thin sheets that are separated by large pores, blood vessels, and ducts. The result is a very soft, spongy organ filled with a large volume of blood.

The liver performs a wide variety of complex and diverse functions, more so than any other organ. Most commonly known is the production of bile, which is formed from the breakdown of red blood cells, cholesterol, and salts; stored in the gallbladder; and used in the small intestine to digest fats. The liver also serves that all-important purpose of detoxification by chemically altering harmful substances such as alcohol, drugs, and ammonia from protein digestion. Additionally, the liver is involved in the formation of such essential materials as blood proteins, blood-clotting factors, and sugar and fat storage compounds.

Because of the liver's many responsibilities and unique position as an intermediary between the digestive process and the blood (via the portal vein), it easily falls prey to many disease-causing agents. Chemicals, illegal drugs, alcohol, viruses, parasites, hormones, and even medical drugs can damage the liver and have widespread effects on the rest of the

Liver Disorders

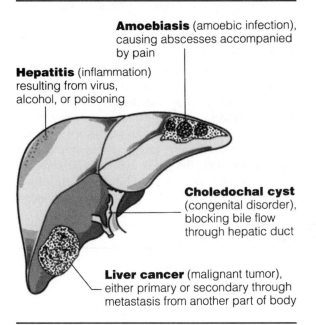

Amoebiasis (amoebic infection), causing abscesses accompanied by pain

Hepatitis (inflammation) resulting from virus, alcohol, or poisoning

Choledochal cyst (congenital disorder), blocking bile flow through hepatic duct

Liver cancer (malignant tumor), either primary or secondary through metastasis from another part of body

The liver's unique structure and functions leave it vulnerable to a wide range of diseases.

body. The liver is also the most frequent target of cancer cells that have spread beyond their primary site. In the United States and other industrialized countries, liver disease is usually related to alcoholism and cancer, while in Third World countries it is often the result of infectious contamination by viruses and parasites.

There are two simplified methods of classifying liver disorders: The first is based on cause: infections (viruses and parasites), injury (alcohol and other toxins), inheritance (inability to perform certain functions), infiltration (iron and copper deposits), and tumors (both benign and malignant). The second method of classification is based on the result: hepatitis (infections), cirrhosis (injury from alcohol or other toxins), and cancer, for example.

Each of these liver diseases produces a particular set of signs and symptoms depending on the length of time and the specific disruption of structure and function. Pain and swelling rarely occur alone and are usually associated with one or more of the following: nausea and vomiting, jaundice, ascites, blood-clotting defects, and encephalopathy. Indeed, in some cases liver failure ensues, leading to coma and death.

Jaundice, a yellow discoloration of the skin and whites (sclera) of the eyes, is caused by the secretion of bile precursors (bilirubin) from the damaged liver cells directly into the blood rather than into the ducts leading to the gallbladder. Consequently, bilirubin accumulates in the body's tissues, including the skin and eyes. Ascites, the collection of fluid beneath the liver in the abdomen, is an important sign of liver disease. This fluid comes primarily from the portal vein system, which lies between the liver and the digestive organs. As the liver becomes congested and enlarged in response to injury or infection, blood flow becomes difficult and pressure begins to build, causing liquid to leak from the blood vessels into the abdominal cavity. Easy bruising, excessive bleeding, and other problems with blood clotting are important signs that reflect the failure of the liver to produce essential blood proteins. Neuropsychiatric symptoms such as a flapping hand tremor and encephalopathy (a state of mental confusion and disorientation that can quickly progress to coma) are not well understood, but it is likely that they result from an accumulation of toxic substances that would normally be cleared from the blood by the liver. Several other problems, such as the enlargement of male breasts, atrophy of the testicles, and other sexual changes, derive from the inability of the liver to clear the blood of hormones.

Hepatitis, an inflammation of the liver generally caused by viruses, is one of the most common diseases in the world. Hepatitis A and B, Epstein-Barr virus (the causative agent of mononucleosis), and herpes are a few of the organisms that can infect the liver. Hepatitis A, transmitted through contaminated food, water, and shellfish, is usually a self-limited disease that resolves itself. Hepatitis B, transmitted through contact with infected blood and body secretions, is much more serious, with a carrier state, progressive organ damage, cancer, and death as possible sequelae. Noninfectious causes of hepatitis in susceptible people include such frequently used substances as acetaminophen (Tylenol), halothane (general anesthesia), and oral contraceptives.

Cirrhosis is the result of continuous toxic exposure that injures the liver beyond repair. Fibrous scar tissue replaces the normally soft, spongy organ, making it small and firm, with few hepatocytes capable of functioning normally. Chronic alcohol abuse is by far the most frequent factor in the development of cirrhosis. Severe ascites, bleeding disorders, encephalopathy, and sex organ changes often herald imminent liver failure and death from this disease.

Liver cancer is most often secondary to malignancies that have spread from other sites. In Asia and Africa, primary tumors of the liver itself are much more common, in part because of several factors: a high incidence of hepatitis B infection, food toxins, and parasite infestation. Chronic injury appears to play the critical role in liver cancer; hence the risk factors that have been established are cirrhosis, hepatitis B, and long-term exposure to a variety of chemicals, hormones, and drugs. Benign tumors may occur in young women who use oral contraceptives, but they are relatively infrequent.

Several other hepatic diseases warrant mention. Liver abscesses, encapsulated areas filled with infectious material, can be caused by bacteria, fungi, and parasites. These organisms enter the bloodstream through ingestion, skin puncture, or even intestinal rupture (as occurs in appendicitis and diverticulitis), and travel to the liver. Two unusual but notable disorders of iron and copper metabolism—hemochromatosis and Wilson's disease, respectively—have prominent liver involvement. While the disease mechanisms are not well understood, these essential metals are retained in excess and deposited in body tissues in toxic levels, causing damage. Finally, several genetic disorders of bile production run the gamut from mere nuisances to death in infancy. Disruption in bilirubin metabolism, the handling of red blood cell waste products by incor-

Signs and Symptoms of Liver Disease

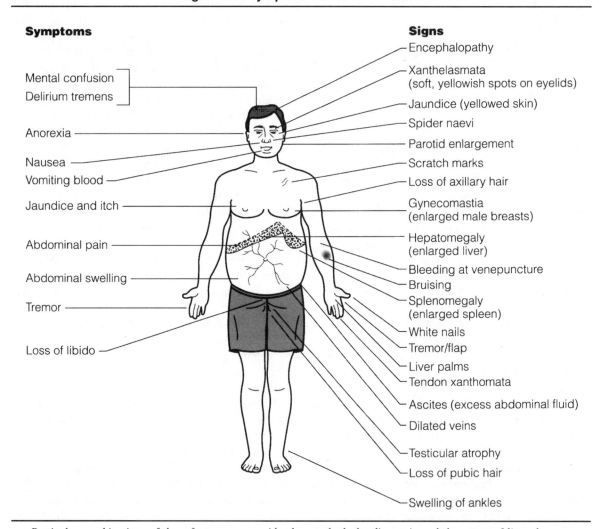

Symptoms

- Mental confusion
- Delirium tremens
- Anorexia
- Nausea
- Vomiting blood
- Jaundice and itch
- Abdominal pain
- Abdominal swelling
- Tremor
- Loss of libido

Signs

- Encephalopathy
- Xanthelasmata (soft, yellowish spots on eyelids)
- Jaundice (yellowed skin)
- Spider naevi
- Parotid enlargement
- Scratch marks
- Loss of axillary hair
- Gynecomastia (enlarged male breasts)
- Hepatomegaly (enlarged liver)
- Bleeding at venepuncture
- Bruising
- Splenomegaly (enlarged spleen)
- White nails
- Tremor/flap
- Liver palms
- Tendon xanthomata
- Ascites (excess abdominal fluid)
- Dilated veins
- Testicular atrophy
- Loss of pubic hair
- Swelling of ankles

Particular combinations of these factors can provide clues to both the diagnosis and the extent of liver damage.

poration into bile, is affected to varying degrees. Severe jaundice reflects the accumulation of toxic levels of bilirubin in all body tissues, including the brain.

TREATMENT AND THERAPY

The diagnosis of a patient with suspected liver disease occurs in an orderly process that begins with a thorough history and physical examination, supported by a number of valuable blood tests and imaging techniques. Liver biopsy, the obtaining of a tissue sample for microscopic analysis, is often a final and definitive procedure if the disorder remains ambiguous. Both the cause and the chronology or state of the disease (whether of recent onset or advanced) determine treatment and outcome. While many signs and symptoms are nonspecific—nausea, vomiting, pain, hepatic enlargement, and jaundice—others such as ascites, encephalopathy, blood-clotting defects, and sex organ changes reflect significant organ damage and an advanced stage of disease. Careful questioning of the recent and past history of a patient can elicit facts that point to a diagnosis: exposure to known liver toxins such as alcohol, anesthetics, certain medications, and occupational chemicals; travel to countries with known contaminated water supplies (hepatitis A); blood transfusions, kidney dialysis, sexual promiscuity, or intravenous drug abuse (hepatitis B); weight loss that is unexplained (cancer); or even a history of gallstones (blocked bile ducts between the liver and gallbladder). Armed with suspicions from the history, the physician uses the physical examination to note signs that confirm or reject the possibilities. A small and firm liver with ascites, tremor, enlarged male breasts, and small, shrunken testicles all point to an advanced stage of cirrhosis, for example. An enlarged painful liver, with vomiting, jaundice, fever, and recent raw shellfish ingestion, would likely suggest hepatitis A.

Blood tests play the second critical role in evaluating liver disease. An elevated bilirubin level would correlate with the severity of jaundice. Blood protein levels (albumin) and blood-clotting factors (prothrombin) may be dangerously low, revealing a near inability of the hepatocytes to synthesize these vital substances. Special chemicals that exist primarily in liver cells (hepatic enzymes and the aminotransferases) may be quite high, because the cells die and release their contents into the blood. Finally, elevated white blood cell counts and special tests for individual infections (viruses, bacteria, fungi, and parasites) can positively establish the diagnosis.

Depending on the suspected disease, confirmation may be needed from various imaging techniques, chosen specifically for a particular diagnosis. Plain X rays do little to visualize the liver, although they can reveal air in the abdomen, a consequence of a perforated intestine, appendix, or ulcer. A much more advanced method, the computed tomography (CT) scan, combines computer-generated views of multiple cross-sectional X rays, providing a highly detailed examination of the liver and thereby establishing a diagnosis in the majority of cases. Two other techniques that have more specific uses are ultrasound, which uses sound wave transmission, and magnetic resonance imaging (MRI), which uses magnetic fields to create an image. Ultrasound can readily distinguish solid masses from those that are fluid-filled (tumors versus abscesses) and can view the bile ducts. MRI is quite helpful in determining blood flow problems such as portal hypertension.

Finally, if a precise diagnosis remains ambiguous, a biopsy is performed. A sample of liver tissue is obtained using a large needle inserted through the skin, under the guidance of an ultrasound image. The sample is then viewed microscopically, and both the cause and the extent of liver damage are readily apparent.

Treatment options for the majority of liver diseases are few, and often little can be done beyond symptomatic relief and supportive care. For example, if drug toxicity is suspected, especially from alcohol, immediate withdrawal of the agent can prevent further damage, as has been shown in cirrhosis. Obstructing gallstones can be surgically removed to relieve pressure in the bile ducts. Combinations of surgery, radiation, and chemotherapy are used in liver cancer, but the prognosis is poor. Little can be done for the inherited diseases of bilirubin metabolism, while some success has been achieved in treating the iron and copper storage diseases. Infections of viral origin have no effective antibiotic treatment, but the prevention of hepatitis A and B is possible if pooled serum immunoglobulin is given immediately after exposure. This substance is a concentrated form of antibodies obtained from infected individuals whose diseases have completely resolved; essentially, it is a method of giving passive immunity. One area in which effective treatment does exist is in bacterial, fungal, and parasitic infections and abscesses. Appropriate antibiotics and surgical drainage yield dramatic improvement in most cases.

In the majority of cases of liver disease, symptom

relief and nutritional support, often carried out in the hospital, are the only options. Pain relief and the administration of intravenous fluid and nutrients to counteract vomiting and dehydration are the first steps. Ascites is relieved through bed rest, salt restriction, and paracentesis, a procedure that uses ultrasound to guide a needle into the abdomen and withdraw fluid. Attempts to correct encephalopathy by removing toxins such as ammonia from the blood are generally ineffective, and mental changes, along with other intractable symptoms, often herald complete liver failure and imminent death.

Clearly, preventive measures are the most important factor in liver disease. One effective measure that is widely available is the hepatitis B vaccine, which is recommended for anyone at high risk of contracting the virus. A three-injection series is suggested for health care personnel, kidney dialysis patients, sexually promiscuous people, and anyone else who is frequently in contact with blood and body secretions.

Perspective and Prospects

Little in the field of hepatology is as exciting or hopeful as liver transplantation, the replacement of the diseased organ by a normal, donated one. Begun experimentally in the early 1960's after decades of low success rates (less than 20 percent), it has finally been accepted as a lifesaving operation, with survival rates exceeding 60 percent at five years. Technical improvements, especially intraoperative blood circulation and cadaver organ preservation, have been combined with advances in immunosuppressive therapy that counteracts rejection and refined patient selection and timing. The result is that liver transplantation has become the method of choice for patients whose liver disease is life-threatening, progressive, and unresponsive to other treatments.

Specific guidelines exist for both children and adults to be considered candidates for the procedure. It is imperative that the person is otherwise healthy and that the heart, lungs, kidneys, and brain are functioning well. Malignancy, human immunodeficiency virus (HIV) infection, incorrectable congenital defects, and continuing drug or alcohol abuse are obvious contraindications. However, infants with inherited, inevitably fatal liver disorders are good candidates, as are adults with end-stage liver failure from chronic hepatitis, for example. Controversial indications, requiring case-by-case evaluation, include advanced viral hepatitis (as recurrent infection in the donated organ often

occurs) and alcohol-induced cirrhosis (because of the likelihood of damage to other organs and the high relapse rate after surgery). Relapse is also very common if the transplantation is done for a primary liver cancer.

Careful donor selection is equally important. The principal source of cadaver organs is victims of head trauma who are declared brain-dead. Organs are accepted from those sixty years of age or younger who had no viral, bacterial, or fungal infections and who were otherwise healthy up to the time of death. In the United States, recipient-donor matches are made through a nationwide organ transplantation registry, with highest priority going to those most critically ill. Only twelve to eighteen hours can elapse between organ retrieval and implantation—beyond that, liver tissue begins to degenerate.

The use of immunosuppressive therapy, drugs that keep the recipient's immune system in check, has contributed significantly to success and survival. Rejection of the transplanted organ remains one of the most feared postoperative complications, along with hemorrhaging. Because the body recognizes the organ as foreign tissue, the immune system's white blood cells attack and damage the implanted donor liver. The use of drugs to counteract this process allows the new liver to heal and the body to adapt to the presence of foreign tissue. Despite the use of these potent drugs, which themselves have serious side effects, rejection continues to be a problem. Nevertheless, one-year survival rates approach 85 percent, and at five years, nearly 60 percent of transplant patients are alive.

—Connie Rizzo, M.D.

See also Abdomen; Abdominal disorders; Alcoholism; Cirrhosis; Hepatitis; Jaundice; Liver; Liver cancer; Liver transplantation.

For Further Information:

Bennett, J. Claude, et al., eds. *Cecil Textbook of Medicine*. 21st ed. Philadelphia: W. B. Saunders, 2000. This bible of internal medicine has a superb section on liver diseases that is somewhat difficult but so well written and thorough that it is worth the effort. The text is well supplemented with diagrams and photographs.

Fishman, Mark, et al. *Medicine*. 4th ed. Philadelphia: J. B. Lippincott, 1996. This excellent soft cover text is the perfect place to start. Used by medical students and other health professionals, it is clear and understandable, exploring normal biology and the process of disease.

Yamada, Todataka, et al. *Textbook of Gastroenterology.* 3d ed. Philadelphia: J. B. Lippincott, 1999. The reference text used by specialists in the field, covering all aspects of the digestive system. A large section is devoted to the liver and gallbladder.

Zakim, David, and Thomas D. Boyer. *Hepatology: A Textbook of Liver Disease.* 3d ed. Philadelphia: W. B. Saunders, 1996. This extraordinary book is devoted entirely to the liver, with wonderful photographic atlases accompanying each disease. The text is difficult, because it is highly detailed, and should be read only after other, more comprehensive books have been used.

LIVER TRANSPLANTATION

PROCEDURE

ANATOMY OR SYSTEM AFFECTED: Abdomen, gallbladder, liver

SPECIALTIES AND RELATED FIELDS: Gastroenterology, general surgery

DEFINITION: Surgery performed to replace a diseased, nonfunctional liver with one that is healthy and capable of carrying out normal liver functions.

KEY TERMS:

bile: fluid produced by the liver and stored in the gallbladder to be secreted into the intestine; contains salts, bile pigments (bilirubin), cholesterol, and other waste products

cirrhosis: a severe degenerative condition in which healthy liver tissue is replaced with nonfunctional scar tissue; alcohol and drug abuse are the most common causes

hepatic: of or referring to the liver

hepatitis: inflammation of the liver

jaundice: a yellowish coloration of the skin and mucous membranes caused by high levels of bilirubin in the blood; the result of liver malfunction

INDICATIONS AND PROCEDURES

Liver transplantation is performed on individuals whose livers are severely diseased and unable to carry out normal liver functions. The most common cause of liver failure in adults is cirrhosis, which results from alcohol and/or drug abuse. In this condition, the liver becomes filled with tough, nonfunctional scar tissue. Symptoms of cirrhosis, as well as other liver diseases, include abnormal levels of liver enzymes in the blood, jaundice, a lack of blood-clotting factors, the inability to dispose of bile, and the failure to detoxify metabolic by-products and other poisons, which

can lead to coma and death. Other conditions that can lead to liver disease include hepatic cancer, long-term hepatitis B infection, and obstruction of the bile passages in the liver.

The donor liver may be obtained from a recently deceased individual, or a section of the liver can be obtained from a living donor. In either case, the donated organ must be a close immunological match to reduce the chance of transplant rejection. A preoperative injection is given to the recipient to dry up internal fluids and promote drowsiness. A vertical incision is made from just below the breastbone to the navel. Muscles are moved aside, and a second incision is made through the outer membranous lining of the body cavity, revealing the internal organs. Bypass tubes are inserted into the hepatic veins and connected to veins in the arm to divert the flow of blood from the liver. When this is completed, the hepatic veins are cut, and the liver and gallbladder are removed from the body cavity. The veins of the donor liver are connected to the recipient veins, and the bypass tubes are removed. The new liver is then connected to the intestine, and the incisions are closed.

USES AND COMPLICATIONS

Liver transplantation is performed only when the individual has no other chance for survival. Typically, there is a long waiting list for available organs. Certain factors such as blood type and protein markers on cell surfaces must be matched as closely as possible in order to avoid rejection by the recipient's immune system. A liver from a recently deceased donor may be kept functioning only for five hours with specific cooling fluid, thus limiting its ability to be transported long distances. Because of the lack of available transplant organs and the necessity of compatibility, many people die before an appropriate organ becomes available. It is possible to transplant a segment of liver from a close relative; the liver can grow considerably and regenerate itself. This is a preferable situation and eliminates the pressure of transporting a donor liver between hospitals while attempting to keep it functioning.

After liver transplantation, the patient is kept in an intensive care unit for several days and in bed for at least a week. Pain from the incisions is alleviated with drugs. Rejection is the major danger, even with closely matched donor organs. Drugs such as cyclosporine are administered to suppress the immune system and, in most cases, must be taken for life. These immunosuppressive drugs inhibit the normal functioning of the immune system, thus making the individual much more susceptible to frequent—and more severe—infections, including bacterial, fungal, and viral infections. Other possible complications of the long-term use of immunosuppressive drugs include cataracts, impaired wound healing, peptic ulcers, and steroid-induced diabetes mellitus. About 20 percent of patients suffer graft rejection, obstruction of the arteries, or infection. In the case of serious complications, another transplantation may be the patient's only hope for survival. In successful surgeries, patients are able to return to normal, active lives within a few weeks of the surgery.

PERSPECTIVE AND PROSPECTS

The first successful liver transplantation procedure was performed in 1967. Nevertheless, this surgery was considered an experimental procedure until 1983, when a National Institutes of Health (NIH) conference on liver transplantation accepted it as a routine procedure. In 1984, more than 250 liver transplantations were performed in the United States. Within five years, that number increased dramatically, to 2,188 transplantation procedures performed in 1989 and up to 3,442 in 1993. Long-term results are steadily improving; currently, more than half of recipients survive for five years or more. Improvements in survival rates are attributable to improved methods of preserving donor livers, the advent of living donor transplantation, better methods to prevent graft rejection, more suitable selection of recipients (for example, hepatic cancer patients typically have a high rate of recurrence of the disease in their transplanted liver), and improved surgical techniques.

Future prospects include further improvements in surgical techniques and advanced drug therapy to prevent graft rejection but not totally compromise the disease-fighting ability of the patient's immune system. Efforts at public education regarding the need for donor organs may cause more individuals to contact donor organ societies, family, and friends regarding their wishes to donate organs in the event of untimely death. In addition, improved treatments for the diseases that lead to liver failure may help to decrease the need for this surgical procedure.

—*Karen E. Kalumuck, Ph.D.*

See also Abdomen; Abdominal disorders; Alcoholism; Circulation; Cirrhosis; Gastroenterology; Gastroenterology, pediatric; Gastrointestinal disorders; Gastrointestinal system; Hepatitis; Internal medicine; Jaundice; Liver; Liver disorders; Transplantation.

FOR FURTHER INFORMATION:

Ahmed, Moustafa. *Surviving Liver Diseases: Life with a Liver Transplant*. London: MegaZette, 1999. Designed for the layperson, this resource offers guidance on the prevention of liver disease and offers personal narrative regarding liver transplantation.

Belzer, Folkert O., and Hans W. Sollinger. "Immunology and Transplantation." In *Basic Surgery*, edited by Hiram C. Polk, Jr., H. Harlan Stone, and Bernard Gardner. 5th ed. St. Louis: Quality Medical, 1995. A chapter in a text discussing such topics as operative and diagnostical surgery.

Youngson, Robert M. *The Surgery Book: An Illustrated Guide to Seventy-three of the Most Common Operations*. New York: St. Martin's Press, 1993. In a clear, easy-to-follow format, this dependable, comprehensive sourcebook answers questions about and gives information on a wealth of operations, including mastectomy, vasectomy, prostatectomy, cesarean section, hernia repair, hip replacement, heart bypass, and dozens more.

LOCKJAW. *See* TETANUS.

LOU GEHRIG'S DISEASE. *See* AMYOTROPHIC LATERAL SCLEROSIS.

LOWER EXTREMITIES

ANATOMY

ANATOMY OR SYSTEM AFFECTED: Bones, feet, hips, knees, legs, lymphatic system, musculoskeletal system, nerves, nervous system, skin

SPECIALTIES AND RELATED FIELDS: Neurology, orthopedics, physical therapy, podiatry

DEFINITION: The thighs, lower legs, and feet; the lower extremities are attached to the pelvis at the hip joint and consist of muscles, bones, blood vessels, lymph vessels, nerves, skin, and toenails.

KEY TERMS:

distal: farther away from the base or attached end

femur: the thigh bone

fibula: the smaller of the two bones in the lower leg, on the lateral side

knee: the joint between the thigh and the lower leg

lateral: on the outer side; toward the little toe when in reference to the leg

leg: the lower extremity, excluding the foot; the lower leg runs from the knee to the ankle

medial: on the side toward the midline; toward the big toe when in reference to the leg

proximal: closer to the base or attached end

tarsus: the ankle

thigh: the upper segment of the leg, from the hip joint to the knee

tibia: the larger of the two bones in the lower leg, on the medial side

STRUCTURE AND FUNCTIONS

The lower extremities consist of the thighs, lower legs, and feet. Each extremity attaches to the pelvis (innominate bone) at the hip joint. The lower extremity is made mostly of bones and muscles, but it also contains blood vessels, lymphatics, nerves, skin, toenails, and other structures. Important directional terms for the lower extremity include proximal (closer to the base or attached end), distal (further from the base or attached end), medial (on the same side as the tibia and big toe), and lateral (on the same side as the fibula and little toe). Along the foot, the lower surface is called plantar; the upper surface is called dorsal. The lower extremity is clothed in skin (or integument). The sole or plantar surface of the foot is unusual, along with the palm of the hand, in being completely hairless; it also contains the thickest outer skin layer (the stratum corneum) of any part of the body. Each toe has a hardened toenail on its dorsal surface.

The pelvic girdle that supports the lower extremity develops as three separate bones: the ilium, ischium, and pubis. All three help form the acetabulum, a socket into which the femur fits. Below the acetabulum, the ischium and pubis surround a large opening called the obturator foramen. The right and left pubis meet to form a pubic symphysis. The bones of the lower extremity include the femur, tibia, fibula, tarsals, metatarsals, and phalanges. The femur (thigh bone) is the largest bone in the body. Its rounded upper end, or head, fits into the acetabulum and is attached by a short neck. A rough-surfaced greater trochanter lies just beyond this neck and serves for the attachment of many muscles. The lesser trochanter, also for muscle attachments, lies just below the neck. The knee joint is covered and protected by the kneecap, or patella, the largest of the sesamoid bones formed within tendons at points of stress. The lower leg, from the knee to the ankle, contains two bones: the tibia on the medial side and the more slender fibula on the lateral

side. The tarsus, or ankle, includes the talus, calcaneus, and five smaller bones. The talus (or astragalus) has a pulleylike facet for the tibia and other curved surfaces for articulation with the calcaneus and navicular. The calcaneus, or heel bone, is vertically enlarged in humans; the Achilles tendon attaches to its roughened lower tuberosity. Smaller tarsal bones include the navicular, the medial (or inner) cuneiform, the intermediate cuneiform, the lateral (or outer) cuneiform, and the cuboid. Beyond the tarsal bones, the foot is supported by five metatarsal bones. The big toe, or hallux, contains two phalanges; each of the remaining toes contains three phalanges.

The muscles of the lower extremity include extensors, which straighten joints, and flexors, which bend joints. Abductor muscles move the limbs sideways, away from the midline, while adductors pull the limbs back, toward the midline. The muscles of the iliac region attach the lower extremity to the body. The psoas major runs from the lumbar vertebrae to the lesser trochanter of the femur. The iliacus runs from the ilium and part of the sacrum to the femur, including the lesser trochanter. The anterior muscles of the thigh include the sartorius, the quadriceps femoris, and the articularis genus. The sartorius, the longest muscle in the body, flexes both hip and knee joints. It runs obliquely from the anterior border of the ilium across the front of the thigh to insert onto the medial side of the knee at the upper end of the tibia. The quadriceps femoris consists of the rectus femoris and the three vastus muscles; all four are strong extensors of the knee. The rectus femoris originates from the region surrounding the acetabulum. The vastus lateralis, vastus medialis, and vastus intermedius muscles all originate along the shaft of the femur. All four quadriceps muscles insert onto a common tendon which runs over the knee and inserts onto the top of the tibia. The patella is a sesamoid bone enclosed within this tendon where it runs over the front of the knee. The smaller articularis genus muscle originates on the anterior side of the shaft of the femur; it inserts onto the kneecap.

The extensor muscles of the hip and thigh help to maintain upright posture. The gluteus maximus, the largest of these muscles, originates from the posterior portion of the ilium and inserts high on the femur, especially onto the greater trochanter. The gluteus medius and gluteus minimis both originate from the outer surface of the ilium and insert onto the greater trochanter. The tensor fasciae latae originates along the iliac crest; it inserts onto a broad, sheetlike tendon (the fascia lata) which covers much of the lateral surface of the thigh. The piriformis runs from the sacrum to the greater trochanter of the femur. The obturator internus runs from the inner surface of the pelvis through the obturator foramen to the greater trochanter of the femur. The gemellus superior and the gemellus inferior originate from the rear margin of the ischium; they both insert onto the greater trochanter. The quadratus femoris originates from the lateral surface of the ischium; it inserts between the greater and lesser trochanters of the femur. The obturator externus originates along the outer surface of the pelvis below the obturator foramen and inserts near the greater trochanter.

The muscles on the medial (or inner) side of the thigh are all abductors of the thigh. The gracilis is a long, thin muscle that originates from the pubis, runs along the medial side of the thigh, and inserts high on the tibia. The pectineus originates anteriorly on the pubis and inserts onto the shaft of the femur below the lesser trochanter. The adductor longus originates from the pubis and inserts onto the posterior edge of the femur. The adductor brevis originates from the pubis and inserts onto the posterior edge of the femur. The adductor magnus is a large, triangular muscle that originates from the lower portion of the ischium and pubis; it expands to a long, thin insertion along the posterior edge of the femur.

The hamstring muscles run along the posterior side of the femur; they flex the knee and extend the hip joint. The biceps femoris originates from the posterior portion (the tuberosity) of the ischium and separately from the posterior edge of the femur. Both portions converge onto a common tendon which inserts primarily onto the top of the fibula. The semitendinosus originates from the posterior end of the ischium; it inserts by a long tendon onto the medial side of the tibia. The semimembranosus runs from the ischium to the posterior surface of the tibia.

The muscles on the front (anterior) side of the lower leg raise the foot by flexing it dorsally. At the ankle, their tendons are all held in place by two transverse bands, the extensor retinacula. The tibialis anterior originates along the anterior edge of the tibia; it inserts by a tendon onto the medial cuneiform and the base of the first metatarsal. The extensor hallucis longus originates from the anterior surface of the fibula; its tendon passes beneath the extensor retinacula to insert onto the distal phalanx of the big toe. The extensor

digitorum longus originates near the top of the tibia and along the anterior side of the fibula. Its tendon passes beneath the extensor retinacula and splits into four tendons, inserted onto the second and third phalanges of the second through fifth digits. The peroneus tertius originates along the anterior edge of the fibula and runs alongside the extensor digitorum longus. It inserts onto the base of the fifth metatarsal bone.

The muscles on the posterior surface of the lower leg are mostly extensors of the foot; some also flex the knee. The gastrocnemius originates in two heads from opposite sides of the femur. It inserts onto the Achilles tendon, which attaches to the calcaneus. The soleus originates from the posterior surface of the fibula; it inserts onto the Achilles tendon. The plantaris originates from the posterior surface of the femur and inserts onto the posterior portion of the calcaneus. The popliteus runs from the lateral side of the femur across the back of the knee to insert onto the tibia. The flexor hallucis longus originates along the posterior surface of the fibula; its tendon runs around to the medial side of the ankle and inserts onto the base of the big toe. The flexor digitorum longus originates from the posterior surface of the tibia; its tendon crosses the sole of the foot obliquely and divides into four tendons which insert onto the distal phalanges of the second through fifth toes. The tibialis posterior originates from the posterior surfaces of the tibia, the fibula, and the interosseous membrane that joins them; its tendon passes around to insert onto the navicular bone. The peroneus longus originates along the lateral surface of the fibula; its tendon runs along a groove on the bottom of the cuboid to insert obliquely onto the base of the first metatarsal. The peroneus brevis originates along the lateral margin of the fibula; its tendon inserts onto the fifth metatarsal. The extensor digitorum brevis originates from the calcaneus and runs obliquely across the dorsal side of the foot, dividing into four tendons. One tendon inserts onto the base of the big toe; the remaining tendons insert onto the tendons of the extensor digitorum longus.

Several flexor muscles of the foot are attached to the plantar aponeurosis, a flat ligament which runs from the calcaneus along the sole of the foot to the bases of the toes and to several flexor tendons. The abductor hallucis originates from the calcaneus and the plantar aponeurosis; it inserts onto the base of the big toe. The flexor digitorum brevis originates from the plantar aponeurosis and the calcaneus; it divides into four portions, each of which gives rise to a tendon. These tendons run into the second through fifth toes, each splitting in half to insert onto opposite sides of the second phalanx, separated by the tendons of the flexor digitorum longus, which emerge between them. The abductor digiti quinti originates from the calcaneus and the plantar aponeurosis; it inserts onto the base of the fifth toe. The quadratus plantae originates from the calcaneus and inserts onto the tendons of the flexor digitorum longus. The four small lumbricales run from the tendons of the flexor digitorum longus to the corresponding tendons of the extensor digitorum longus. The flexor hallucis brevis originates from the cuboid and lateral cuneiform bones; its two portions insert onto the big toe from opposite sides. The adductor hallucis originates from the second through fourth metatarsals and also from the bases of the third through fifth toes. Its tendon inserts onto the base of the big toe. The flexor digiti quinti originates from the base of the fifth metatarsal and inserts onto the base of the fifth toe. The four dorsal interossei originate from the bases of the metatarsal bones; they insert onto the bases of the second through fourth toes. The three plantar interossei originate from the third through fifth metatarsals and run beneath these bones to insert onto the bases of the corresponding toes.

Blood vessels of the lower extremity include both arteries and veins. The common iliac arteries arise from the dorsal aorta; each divides into an internal and an external iliac. The internal iliac artery supplies many muscles of the thigh region and pelvis. The external iliac artery branches into an inferior epigastric artery and a deep iliac circumflex artery; it then continues along the femur as the femoral artery. The femoral artery gives rise to a deep femoral artery running to the medial and posterior regions of the thigh; the base of this artery also gives rise to two circumflex arteries that send branches upward into many thigh muscles. Near the knee, the femoral artery branches into a descending geniculate artery to the knee, then continues as the popliteal artery, forming several branches to the thigh muscles and other small branches to the knee before splitting into anterior and posterior tibial arteries.

The anterior tibial artery descends along the front of the tibia, forming several small branches. It then continues into the foot as the dorsalis pedis artery, giving rise to a lateral tarsal artery and an arcuate artery, both of which form arches by joining with branches of the peroneal artery. The deep plantar artery and hallucis dorsalis artery also branch from the dorsalis pedis artery, while individual arteries to the second through fourth metatarsals arise from the arcuate artery. Arterial branches to all the toes arise from the individual metatarsal arteries, including the hallucis dorsalis, forming a system of collateral circulation in which multiple alternate routes permit blood flow even if one of the routes is temporarily blocked.

The posterior tibial artery gives rise to a peroneal artery; the two arteries then run down the posterior side of the lower leg, forming small branches to the muscles of the lower leg and nutrient arteries to the tibia and fibula. The posterior tibial artery branches to the calcaneus before it splits into a medial plantar artery, which runs along the medial margin of the foot into the big toe, and a much larger lateral plantar artery. The lateral plantar artery runs across the foot obliquely to the lateral side, then turns and runs obliquely in the other direction to the base of the big toe, where it runs into the deep plantar artery to form a loop. From this loop arise a series of plantar metatarsal arteries to all five toes. Blood can reach each toe from either side, and the arch that supplies this blood can receive its blood either by way of the posterior tibial and lateral plantar arteries or by way of the anterior tibial and deep plantar arteries, providing another example of collateral circulation.

There are several important veins draining the lower extremity. The deep veins originate from a series of plantar digital veins draining the individual toes into a deep plantar venous arch. This arch is drained to either direction by a lateral plantar vein and a medial plantar vein, which later unite to form a posterior tibial vein; this vein and the peroneal vein run parallel to the corresponding arteries along the posterior side of the lower leg. An anterior tibial vein drains the anterior side of the lower leg and the dorsal side of the foot. Near the knee, the peroneal vein and the anterior and posterior tibial veins unite to form the popliteal vein, which continues into the thigh as the femoral vein. The femoral vein receives the deep femoral vein as a tributary, then the saphenous vein. The femoral vein then continues as the external iliac vein.

The lower extremity is also covered with a network of superficial veins that lie just beneath the skin. The vessels of this network are drained along the medial side of the lower leg and thigh by the great saphenous vein, which runs into the femoral vein just below the groin. The lateral side of the foot and the posterior surface of the lower leg are drained by the small saphenous vein, which drains into the popliteal vein.

The nerves to the lower extremity arise from two series of complex branchings, the lumbar plexus and sacral plexus. The largest nerve formed from the lumbar plexus is the femoral nerve, supplying muscles on the anterior side of the thigh and part of the lower leg. Other branches to the muscles include the obturator nerve to the adductor muscles and separate muscular branches to the psoas and iliacus muscles. Cutaneous sensory nerves to the skin include the lateral femoral cutaneous nerve to the lateral side of the thigh, the anterior cutaneous branches of the femoral nerve to the medial side of the thigh, and the saphenous nerve, a branch of the femoral nerve to the medial side of the lower leg.

The sacral plexus gives rise to the very large sciatic nerve and to several smaller nerves, including the superior gluteal and inferior gluteal nerves to the gluteal muscles, and separate muscular branches to the piriformis, quadratus femoris, obturator internus, and gemelli. Cutaneous branches such as the posterior femoral cutaneous nerve supply sensory fibers to the skin on the posterior surface of the thigh. The sciatic nerve, the largest nerve in the body, branches off to the hamstring muscles before splitting into tibial and peroneal nerves. The tibial nerve supplies the muscles on the posterior side of the lower leg and then runs onto the sole of the foot, where it splits into the medial and lateral plantar nerves, which together supply both cutaneous sensation and muscular innervation to the sole of the foot. The peroneal nerve divides into deep and superficial portions. The deep peroneal nerve supplies the muscles on the anterior side of the lower leg and the dorsal surface of the foot. The superficial peroneal nerve supplies cutaneous sensation to the lateral surface of the lower leg and the dorsal surface of the foot.

DISORDERS AND DISEASES

Many medical conditions and disorders affect the lower extremity; these include animal bites (including snakebites), injuries, fungus infections such as athlete's foot, contact dermatitis (including poison ivy), and an assortment of neuromuscular disorders, including nerve paralyses, muscular atrophies, and muscular dystrophies. Nerve paralyses of the lower extremities usually arise from traumatic injury.

Muscular atrophies are diseases in which muscle tissues become progressively weaker and smaller, usu-

ally beginning after the age of forty. Spastic movements sometimes occur. The small muscles of the hands and feet are usually affected sooner and more severely in comparison to the larger muscles of the legs and thighs. Amyotrophic lateral sclerosis (ALS), commonly known as Lou Gehrig's disease, is one such disease that usually begins with weakness and deterioration of the distal muscles. The disease proceeds to affect the rest of the extremities, then other parts of the body; it is usually fatal within three to five years after onset. A more rare type of atrophy, myelopathic muscular atrophy (or Aran-Duchenne atrophy), affects both upper and lower extremities and eventually spreads to the trunk. A degenerative lesion of the gray matter in the cervical region of the spinal cord is usually responsible.

Muscular dystrophy is a series of inherited diseases that begin in early childhood, affecting males more often than females. The most common type, Duchenne muscular dystrophy, is caused by a sex-linked recessive trait which impairs the body's ability to synthesize a large protein called dystrophin. Muscular dystrophy primarily affects the large muscles of the thigh and lower leg, impairing the ability to stand unassisted or to walk. The affected muscles become very weak but remain approximately normal in size and may even increase as muscle tissue is replaced by fatty and fibrous tissue. Progressive weakening makes walking and similar motor functions impossible, but, with proper care, patients can live for decades.

Sports injuries often occur in the lower extremities and are generally treated by orthopedic specialists. Fractured bones are generally set in casts and kept immobile until they heal. Injured or ruptured ligaments often require surgical treatment. Snakebites and other animal bites occur more often to the lower extremities than to other parts of the body. The bites of poisonous snakes must be treated quickly, before the venom reaches the heart. The patient must be kept calm and quiet, and experienced medical attention should be sought as soon as possible.

PERSPECTIVE AND PROSPECTS

The major muscles and bones of the lower extremities were studied in ancient societies by such individuals as Galen (or Caius Galenus), the physician to the Roman army in the second century. Ironically, the science of anatomy took many great strides because of the efforts of artists, who studied the human body in order to create realistic sculptures and paintings.

During the Renaissance, Leonardo da Vinci (1452-1519) and Michelangelo (1475-1564) dissected human corpses illegally in their quest for this knowledge. Andreas Vesalius (1514-1564) produced the first well-illustrated anatomical texts, containing information that corrected many of the errors made by Galen.

Injuries to the leg are generally treated surgically. Whenever possible, broken bones are set in place, immobilized in a cast, and then allowed to heal. Muscles (or their tendons) must be sewn together. Nerve endings must be matched with their former locations if they are to grow back correctly. Gangrene, or tissue death from lack of circulation, occurs more often in the lower extremities than in the upper extremities. When the lower extremity is gangrenous or is injured beyond repair, an amputation is often performed. Artificial legs or partial legs are sometimes attached to the lower extremity.

—Eli C. Minkoff, Ph.D.

See also Amputation; Arthritis; Arthroplasty; Arthroscopy; Bone cancer; Bone disorders; Bone grafting; Bones and the skeleton; Bowlegs; Bunions; Bursitis; Feet; Flat feet; Foot disorders; Fracture and dislocation; Fracture repair; Frostbite; Grafts and grafting; Hammertoe correction; Hammertoes; Heel spur removal; Hemiplegia; Hip fracture repair; Hip replacement; Kneecap removal; Knock-knees; Liposuction; Motor skill development; Muscle sprains, spasms, and disorders; Muscles; Nail removal; Nails; Orthopedic surgery; Orthopedics; Orthopedics, pediatric; Osgood-Schlatter disease; Osteoarthritis; Osteochondritis juvenilis; Osteogenesis imperfecta; Osteopathic medicine; Paralysis; Paraplegia; Physical rehabilitation; Podiatry; Poliomyelitis; Quadriplegia; Pigeon toes; Rheumatoid arthritis; Rheumatology; Rickets; Tendon disorders; Tendon repair; Upper extremities; Varicose vein removal.

FOR FURTHER INFORMATION:

Agur, Anne M. R., and Ming J. Lee. *Grant's Atlas of Anatomy.* 10th ed. Baltimore: Williams & Wilkins, 1999. Excellent, detailed illustrations can be found in this standard reference work.

Crouch, James E. *Functional Human Anatomy.* 4th ed. Philadelphia: Lea & Febiger, 1985. A good beginning reference for an introduction to anatomy. This easy-to-read book provides clear explanations.

Gray, Henry. *Gray's Anatomy.* Edited by Peter L. Williams et al. 38th ed. New York: Churchill Livingstone, 1995. This work stands as a classic in the field of anatomy. Thorough descriptions and excellent color illustrations are provided.

Rosse, Cornelius, and Penelope Gaddum-Rosse. *Hollinshead's Textbook of Anatomy.* 5th ed. Philadelphia: Lippincott-Raven, 1997. Helpful descriptions and illustrations mark this thorough, detailed reference source.

LUMBAR PUNCTURE

PROCEDURE

ANATOMY OR SYSTEM AFFECTED: Back, spine

SPECIALTIES AND RELATED FIELDS: Emergency medicine, neurology

DEFINITION: The insertion of a needle into the lower spine to reach the cerebrospinal fluid.

INDICATIONS AND PROCEDURES

The central nervous system, which consists of the brain and the spinal cord, has three layers of protection: bone (skull and spine), circulating cerebrospinal fluid, and membranous sheaths (the meninges). Lumbar puncture (also known as a spinal tap) is used to gain access to the spinal fluid, either to withdraw a sample for diagnosis or to infuse substances for therapeutic purposes.

Lumbar Puncture

A lumbar puncture, commonly known as a spinal tap, is a diagnostic procedure in which cerebrospinal fluid is extracted from the meninges of the spine and analyzed for the presence of infection.

Infections and injury to the central nervous system are common indications for lumbar puncture. Laboratory analysis of the sample can be critical for proper treatment. Antibiotics, anticancer agents, anesthetics, and dyes are examples of substances that can be administered directly into the spinal fluid.

In order for the procedure to be safe and comfortable, the patient must be properly positioned. The lower back is thoroughly cleaned, and the area is anesthetized. With the patient lying on his or her side with knees at the chest, the vertebral bones of the spine separate somewhat, allowing the insertion of a needle through the layers of skin, ligaments, and finally, the fluid-filled space around the lowest part of the cord.

USES AND COMPLICATIONS

When infections of the brain and spinal cord (encephalomyelitis) or of the meningeal covering (meningitis) are suspected, the withdrawal of cerebrospinal fluid samples is required to determine the exact cause. In cases of head or spinal injury, which have not fractured bone but which show evidence of neurologic impairment (a concussion, for example), lumbar puncture may be used to complement radiologic studies if bleeding is suspected.

The infusion of substances through lumbar puncture access has several therapeutic functions. Antibiotics can be given to combat severe, life-threatening infections, such as meningitis. Anticancer agents can be used for brain and spinal cord tumors. Spinal anesthesia is used frequently in obstetrics and surgical procedures. Excellent visualization of the central nervous system can be achieved with the injection of dyes into the spinal fluid to enhance conventional X rays.

Lumbar puncture is a relatively safe procedure. Headache is its most common complication: Thought to be caused by fluid loss, it is relieved by lying still in a darkened room for several hours after the procedure.

—*Connie Rizzo, M.D.*

See also Anesthesia; Anesthesiology; Antibiotics; Bacterial infections; Bacteriology; Biopsy; Fluids and electrolytes; Infection; Meningitis; Nervous system; Neurology; Neurology, pediatric; Neurosurgery; Spine, vertebrae, and disks; Viral infections.

FOR FURTHER INFORMATION:

Adams, Raymond, Maurice Victor, and Allan H. Ropper. *Adams and Victor's Principles of Neurol-*

ogy. 7th ed. New York: McGraw-Hill, 2000. This classic "teaching text" in neurology is completely revised and features a new art program and the latest advances in diagnosis and treatment. Each chapter is rigorously reviewed and updated.

Lee, J. A., R. S. Atkinson, and M. J. Watt. *Sir Robert Macintosh's Lumbar Puncture and Spinal Analgesia: Intradural and Extradural.* 5th ed. New York: Churchill Livingstone, 1985. A classic text on spinal and epidural anesthesia, updated periodically to reflect advances in the field. Contains chapters devoted to the anatomy, physiology, pharmacology, techniques, and management of, and the complications associated with, spinal and epidural anesthesia.

LUMPECTOMY. *See* MASTECTOMY AND LUMPECTOMY.

LUMPS, BREAST. *See* BREAST CANCER; BREAST DISORDERS; BREASTS, FEMALE.

LUNG CANCER

DISEASE/DISORDER

ANATOMY OR SYSTEM AFFECTED: Chest, lungs, lymphatic system, respiratory system

SPECIALTIES AND RELATED FIELDS: Environmental health, immunology, occupational health, oncology, pulmonary medicine, radiology

DEFINITION: The appearance of malignant tumors in the lungs, which is usually associated with cigarette smoking.

CAUSES AND SYMPTOMS

Most forms of lung cancer fall within one of four categories: squamous cell (or epidermoid) carcinomas and adenocarcinomas (each of which accounts for approximately 30 percent of all pulmonary cancers), small or oat cell carcinomas (accounting for about 25 percent of lung cancers), and large cell carcinomas (which represent about 15 percent of lung cancers). Each of these forms can be further categorized on the basis of cell differentiation within the tumor: either well differentiated (resembling the original cell type) or moderately or poorly differentiated. Upon biopsy, stage groupings are also determined on the basis of size, invasiveness, and possible extent of metastasis.

Oat or small cell carcinomas usually consist of small, tightly packed, spindle-shaped cells, with a high nucleus-to-cytoplasm ratio within the cell. Oat cell carcinomas tend to metastasize early and widely, often to the bone marrow or brain. As a result, by the time that symptoms become apparent, the disease is generally widely disseminated within the body. Coupled with a resistance to most common forms of radiation and chemotherapy, oat cell carcinomas present a particularly poor prognosis. In general, patients diagnosed with this form of cancer have a survival period measured, at most, in months.

Adenocarcinomas are tumors of glandlike structure, presenting as nodules within peripheral tissue such as the bronchioles. Often these forms of tumors may arise from previously damaged or scarred tissue, such as has occurred among smokers. The development of adenocarcinoma of the lung is not as dependent upon smoke inhalation, however, as are other forms of lung cancer.

Squamous cell, also called epidermoid, carcinomas tend to be slower-growing malignancies which form among the flat epithelial cells on the surface of a variety of tissues, including the bladder, cervix, or skin, in addition to the lung. The cells are often polygonal in shape, with keratin nodes on the surface of lesions. Squamous cell carcinomas tend to metastasize less frequently than other forms of lung cancer, allowing for a more optimistic prognosis.

Large cell carcinomas are actually a more general form of cancer in which the cells are relatively large in size, with the cell nucleus being particularly enlarged. Often these carcinomas have arisen as either squamous cell carcinomas or adenocarcinomas. Metastasis, when it occurs, is frequently within the gastrointestinal tract.

There is no question that the single leading cause or factor resulting in lung cancer is smoking. Persons who do not smoke, and indeed even smokers who smoke fewer than five cigarettes per day, are at relatively low risk of developing any form of lung cancer. Those who smoke more than five cigarettes per day run an increased risk of developing lung cancer at rates approaching two hundred times that of the nonsmoker. This risk is greatest for oat cell carcinomas and least for adenocarcinomas (but still approximately a tenfold risk over that for nonsmokers). The relative risk is related to the number of cigarettes smoked: The more cigarettes, the greater the risk. In addition, though other environmental hazards can be related to the development of lung cancers, the risk associated with those hazards is without exception amplified by cigarette smoke.

Exposure to other specific environmental factors has also been associated with the formation of certain forms of pulmonary cancers. Individuals chronically exposed to materials such as asbestos, hydrocarbon products (coal tars or roofing materials), nickel, vinyl chloride, or radiochemicals (uranium and pitchblende) are at increased risk. Chronically damaged lungs, for whatever reason, are at significantly increased risk for development of cancer.

The symptoms of lung cancer may represent the damage caused by the primary tumor or may be the result of metastasis to other organs. The most common symptom is a persistent cough, sometimes accompanied by blood in the sputum or difficulty breathing. Chest pain may be present, especially upon inhalation. There may also be repeated attacks of bronchitis or pneumonia that tend to persist for abnormal periods of time.

Treatment and Therapy

Diagnosis of a tumor in the lung generally includes a chest X ray, along with use of a variety of diagnostic tests: bronchography (X-ray observation of the bronchioles following application of an opaque material), tomography (cross-sectional observation of tissue), and cytologic examination of sputum or bronchiole washings. Confirmation of the diagnosis, in addition to determination of the specific type of tumor and its clinical stage, generally requires a needle biopsy of material from the lung.

The treatment of the tumor is dependent on the form of the disease and on the extent of its spread. Surgery remains the preferred method of treatment, but because of the nature of the disease, less than half the cases are operable at the time of diagnosis. Of these, a large proportion are beyond the point at which the surgical removal of the cancer and resection of remaining tissue are possible. A variety of chemotherapeutic measures are available and along with the use of radiation therapy can be used to produce a small number of cures or at least temporary alleviation of symptoms. Nevertheless, only a small proportion of lung cancers, perhaps 10 percent, respond with a permanent remission or cure.

Lung cancer represents the leading cause of cancer deaths among American men and the second leading cause of cancer deaths among American women. By the 1990's, however, lung cancer was gaining among women and was poised to surpass breast cancer as the major cause of cancer deaths for this group. Each year, between 150,000 and 175,000 new cases of lung cancer are diagnosed in the United States, with about 50,000 deaths. The prognosis for most forms of lung cancer remains poor.

—*Richard Adler, Ph.D.*

See also Addiction; Bronchitis; Cancer; Carcinoma; Chemotherapy; Lungs; Malignancy and metastasis; National Cancer Institute (NCI); Occupational health; Oncology; Pneumonia; Pulmonary diseases; Pulmonary medicine; Radiation therapy; Respiration; Smoking; Tumor removal; Tumors.

FOR FURTHER INFORMATION:

Murphy, G., L. Morris, and D. Lange. *Informed Decisions: The Complete Book of Cancer Diagnosis, Treatment, and Recovery.* New York: Viking Press, 1997. This text from the American Cancer Society is intended for the layperson. It is exemplary in its discussion of cancer.

Pass, Harvey I., et al. *Lung Cancer: Principles and Practice.* Reprint. Philadelphia: Lippincott, Williams & Wilkins, 1996. This illustrated text addresses neoplasms of the lungs. Includes a bibliography and an index.

Steen, R. Grant. *A Conspiracy of Cells: The Basic Science of Cancer.* New York: Plenum Press, 1993. Provides a fine discussion of a variety of factors which cause cancers to develop.

Williams, C. J. *Lung Cancer: The Facts.* 2d ed. Oxford, England: Oxford University Press, 1992. A work that deals specifically with pulmonary cancer.

LUNG DISEASES. *See* PULMONARY DISEASES.

LUNG SURGERY

PROCEDURE

ANATOMY OR SYSTEM AFFECTED: Lungs, respiratory system

SPECIALTIES AND RELATED FIELDS: Emergency medicine, general surgery, pulmonary medicine

DEFINITION: The correction and treatment of such lung problems as bronchiectasis, cancer, emphysema, and pneumothorax.

KEY TERMS:

catheter: a flexible tube inserted into a body cavity to distend it or maintain an opening

diaphragm: the muscular partition that separates the abdomen and the thorax

expiration: the act of breathing out, which partly collapses the lungs

inspiration: the act of breathing in, which expands the lungs

trachea: a cartilaginous, air-carrying tube that runs from the larynx to the bronchi of the lungs

INDICATIONS AND PROCEDURES

Located in the chest (or thoracic) cavity, the lungs rest on the diaphragm. Each lung is connected to the trachea, which brings air in on inspiration and carries it away on expiration. Prior to its entry into the lungs, the trachea forms two bronchi. Each enters a lung near its middle and subdivides into smaller and smaller passages called bronchioles. The smallest tubes open into tiny air sacs called alveoli. Each alveolus contains blood vessels called capillaries which take up oxygen and release carbon dioxide into the lungs to be expelled as waste. Alveoli are arranged into lobules, which are united into lung lobes. The left lung contains two such lobes, and there are three in the larger right lung. Appropriate alveolar function is essential to life. To optimize their action, the lungs are surrounded by a double membrane, the pleura, and supplied by nerves that control expansion on inspiration and contraction on expiration. This size change, accomplished by muscular action, normally occurs eighteen times per minute throughout life. It slows during sleep and accelerates during exercise.

Good health requires adequate lung operation, which can be compromised in many ways. The best-known lung disorders are abscesses, asthma, bronchiectasis, bronchitis, cancer, emphysema, pneumonia, pneumothorax, and tuberculosis. Of these, lung cancer, abscesses, bronchiectasis, and pneumothorax can be corrected surgically.

Lung cancer is a leading cause of cancer death among both men and women. The disease has been attributed primarily to smoking, although causative agents such as asbestos, radioactive substances, and other air pollutants also have been implicated. The development of lung cancer is slow until severe symptoms appear. An early warning is a persistent cough unassociated with asthma or emphysema, chest pain, shortness of breath, fatigue, and general listlessness. The detection of lung cancer in its beginning stages requires regular chest X rays. Early detection greatly enhances long-term survival.

Lung cancer is best treated by surgery. This requires the removal of a small wedge of lung tissue, a lobectomy (lobe removal), or a pneumonectomy (lung removal), depending on the stage of the cancer. During surgery, general anesthesia is followed by an incision around the rib cage on the affected side, along a lower rib. The rib is then detached to produce a gap, and the tumor and/or section of the lung is removed. Postsurgical patients are kept in an intensive care unit for several days, where they are fed and given therapeutic drugs intravenously. Chest drainage tubes are used to drain the incision site. Convalescence takes several months after leaving the hospital. Complications can include infection at the site of the incision and lung collapse.

Lung abscesses most often result from the inhalation of food or tooth fragments. The symptoms are chills, fever, chest pain, and a severe cough that brings up phlegm containing blood and pus. Abscesses are often located using X rays. In many cases, antibiotics are curative. Severe and/or large lung abscesses, however, require surgical drainage or—in extreme cases—the surgical removal of affected lung tissue. For lung abscesses to require surgery, the affected tissue must be thick-walled and antibiotic-resistant. The simplest such cases involve the placement of a catheter in the abscess to act as a drain. In very severe cases, the affected lung portion (usually a wedge) is removed surgically, as with lung cancer.

Bronchiectasis, the distortion of air tubes, is often the result of childhood lung infections and takes years to develop. In most cases, it causes the production of large amounts of foul-smelling phlegm and predisposes the patient to repeated severe lung infections following colds. Diagnosis is by X ray, and treatment is often the use of antibiotics at the first sign of any cold. In some cases, the problem is severe enough to require lung surgery. Bronchiectasis that is severe enough to cause recurrent pneumonia in the same lung segment is treated by surgery when the air tube involved can be removed as well. The potential dangers of this procedure are infection and lung collapse, but they are uncommon.

Pneumothorax occurs when air enters the space between the pleura layers around a lung, causing the afflicted lung parts to collapse. It may be attributable to chest injury (such as knife wounds) or to air from ruptured blisters on the surface of the lungs. The symptoms of pneumothorax are breathlessness, chest pain, and chest tightness. Minor pneumothorax often cures itself, but severe pneumothorax can be fatal if left untreated. Surgery to correct major pneumo-

thorax, although rare, must be carried out quickly. Minor pneumothorax cases that require surgical intervention usually involve the insertion of a catheter to remove the intrapleural air. Patients are then monitored for several days to ensure proper healing. In cases in which the leakage of air persists or a pleural tear is responsible for the pneumothorax, surgical repair of the pleura is required.

Uses and Complications

Lung surgery is straightforward but potentially dangerous because it can lead to death as a result of respiratory failure. After major operations, it is important for patients to convalesce slowly and to comply with the physician's instructions. It is particularly important for the patient to ensure that infection does not occur, to report pain and other danger signs, and to convalesce carefully. The resumption of work and physical activity should be as directed by a physician.

Major advances in treating problems associated with lung surgery include better diagnosis of their extent via computed tomography (CT) scanning and magnetic resonance imaging (MRI). Furthermore, the use of cytotoxic drugs and radiotherapy to treat cancer, including lung cancer, seems to minimize the severity of the surgical treatment of these lesions.

—*Sanford S. Singer, Ph.D.*

See also Abscess drainage; Abscesses; Cancer; Chest; Edema; Embolism; Heart transplantation; Internal medicine; Lung cancer; Lungs; Pleurisy; Pulmonary diseases; Pulmonary medicine; Pulmonary medicine, pediatric; Respiration; Resuscitation; Thoracic surgery; Thrombosis and thrombus; Transplantation; Tumor removal; Tumors.

For Further Information:

Berkow, Robert, and Andrew J. Fletcher, eds. *The Merck Manual of Diagnosis and Therapy*. 17th ed. Rahway, N.J.: Merck Sharp & Dohme Research Laboratories, 1999. Contains a useful exposition of the characteristics, etiology, diagnosis, and treatment of lung disease. Designed for physicians, the material is also useful for less specialized readers.

Professional Guide to Diseases. 7th ed. Springhouse, Pa.: Springhouse, 2001. A comprehensive yet concise medical reference covering more than six hundred disorders, this book includes information about the latest AIDS treatments, new parameters for defining diabetes, current information on cancers, updates on Alzheimer's disease, and more.

Tierney, Lawrence M., Jr., et al., eds. *Current Medical Diagnosis and Treatment: 2001.* 39th ed. New York: McGraw-Hill, 2000. This text, updated yearly, is the point of reference for physicians and other health care practitioners. It incorporates each year's biomedical research discoveries that have immediate, relevant, and applicable use for the patient.

LUNGS
ANATOMY

ANATOMY OR SYSTEM AFFECTED: Chest, respiratory system

SPECIALTIES AND RELATED FIELDS: Environmental health, exercise physiology, oncology, pulmonary medicine, vascular medicine

DEFINITION: Vital organs that allow gas exchange between an organism and its environment.

KEY TERMS:

aerobic respiration: the chemical reactions that use oxygen to produce energy; some small organisms do not use oxygen and are called anaerobic

alveoli: small, thin-walled sacs at the end of the airways; most gas exchange with the blood occurs here

cellular respiration: the chemical reactions that produce energy in the cell; these reactions can be aerobic or anaerobic

cilia: hairlike structures on cells that sweep mucus containing bacteria and foreign particles out of the airways

diffusion: the constant motion of molecules that tends to spread them from places of high concentration to those of lower concentration; gases move across the alveoli by diffusion

gas exchange: the movement of oxygen and carbon dioxide across the membrane of the lungs; other gases, such as nitrogen, may also cross the membrane

mucus: a thick, clear, slimy fluid produced in many parts of the body; in the lungs, mucus catches foreign material and provides lubrication to allow smooth airflow

respiration: the exchange of gases in breathing or the cellular chemistry that involves the same gases in the cell and produces energy

STRUCTURE AND FUNCTIONS

Efficient gas exchange with the environment is critical for larger organisms because oxygen is required for the last step in a series of cellular chemical reactions which processes nutrients from food. These reactions, called aerobic respiration, provide most of the energy that maintains life. Furthermore, as these reactions proceed, parts of larger carbon molecules are removed. Carbon dioxide is produced as a by-product and must be removed from the body. Hence, oxygen and carbon dioxide must be exchanged.

Small aerobic organisms can simply absorb the oxygen from air or water across their moist membranes or skins. The oxygen travels from where it is more concentrated to where it is less concentrated, a process called diffusion. The carbon dioxide inside the cells also diffuses across the membrane in the opposite direction to the environment. Larger organisms, however, have relatively less outside surface area and require special structures for their gas exchange. Various types of gills, swim bladders, and lungs are all examples of ways to absorb more oxygen and release more carbon dioxide.

This article focuses on one of these specialized structures: the lung. The lung is found in air-breathing land creatures. It allows oxygen to enter the blood and carbon dioxide to be removed. Form reflects function: The lung provides large amounts of moist surface area, close to many small blood vessels for gas exchange. Humans have a joined pair of lungs suspended in the chest cavity. The two lungs are somewhat different in size: The left lung is divided into two lobes, while the right has three lobes. This difference reflects the fact that the left side of the chest cavity has less room because of the position and shape of the heart.

The pathway to the lungs begins with the nose. The air entering each nostril is temporarily divided among three pathways (nasal conchae) and then warmed and moisturized by contact with a mucous membrane containing many blood vessels. Bacteria and particles get caught on the sticky mucus on this membrane. If objects pass this point they can be trapped by mucus lower in the tract and be swept out by waving cilia, hairlike fibers extending from cells of the airway that move in unison to push particles backward. Large particles that irritate the mucous membranes can cause a sneeze, which may eject the offending particle at speeds up to 169 kilometers per hour.

The air then continues to the pharynx (throat), where the nasal passageways and the mouth meet, and moves into the larynx, the organ that produces the voice. Swallowing pulls the larynx upward, allowing the epiglottis to flip over the opening and prevent food from entering this part of the airway. This movement of the larynx during swallowing can be felt by light touch with the fingers.

The trachea, or windpipe, follows. It is 11 centimeters long and made rigid by rings of cartilage. The inside of the trachea has cilia and also produces mucus. As the trachea approaches the lungs, it branches into two bronchi, which enter sides of the lungs at a midpoint between top and bottom. The walls of the bronchi contain cartilage rings and smooth muscles. Irritation in the larynx, the trachea, or the bronchi may cause coughing. Coughing is a reflex, like sneezing, that attempts to cast out impurities.

The bronchi continue to branch until they contain only smooth muscle; at this point, they are called bronchioles. The smooth muscle can contract or relax to allow the diameter of the bronchioles to adjust. Hence, the airflow can be changed according to the needs of the body. The pathways inside the lungs resemble an upside-down tree. Millions of cilia line the bronchial "tree" and constantly beat to remove particles. Each bronchial tube branches into several alveolar ducts. Each duct ends with a grapelike cluster of sacs called alveoli. The irregular branching that has led to this point ranges from eight to twenty-five divisions, with an average of twenty-three. Each alveolus has walls that are only one cell thick. Because of the large number of these air sacs, the lungs are very light in weight.

Gas exchange occurs in the alveoli. These structures are closely associated with the body's smallest blood vessels, the capillaries. Oxygen dissolves into the moisture on the vast surface of the alveoli. It then crosses the thin tissue of the lungs and moves into the capillaries to enter the blood. Carbon dioxide moves in the other direction to the lungs. Direction is maintained by the principle of diffusion: Flow is always from a higher to a lower concentration. The surface tension of the watery film inside the alveoli can cause a problem in gas exchange. Water molecules have a strong attraction for one another and can cause the alveoli to collapse to a smaller volume, reducing the surface area available for gas exchange. Fortunately, among the regular cells of the lining of the alveoli is found a second type of cell, called the type II cell. Type II cells produce surfactant, a mixture of chemicals that lowers the overall surface tension in the alveoli by separating the water molecules. Therefore, the alveoli stay fully inflated.

Roaming white blood cells called macrophages are a final defense against foreign objects at the alveolar level. Macrophages protect the lungs by attacking and eating bacteria and particles. They can be found elsewhere in the body performing the same function.

The pleural membrane is a double covering, one layer lining the outside of the lungs and the other lining the inside of the chest cavity. These two layers, which are really the same membrane, move over each other as breathing occurs, reducing friction. If air enters the space between the double membrane, however, the lung will collapse, a condition known as pneumothorax.

Air enters the entire airway by expansion of the chest cavity, or thorax. The cavity can be thought of as a box in which the top cannot be moved upward but the bottom and the sides may move outward. The arched diaphragm muscle at the base of the cavity contracts to lower the bottom of the box. Muscles between the ribs, called intercostals, contract to elevate the chest. The ribs, which slant downward when relaxed, move outward. This expansion pushes the walls out, increases the volume of the chest cavity, and lowers its internal pressure, causing air to be pushed into the lungs. Exhalation results when the muscles relax and allow the natural recoil of the lungs to expel the air.

Young children breathe differently than do older children or adults. Babies and toddlers have ribs that are nearly horizontal. They depend mainly on the descent of the diaphragm muscle for breathing. By two years of age, the ribs have moved to the adult position and rib muscles increase in importance. In addition, a sexual difference in breathing has been observed. Females tend to rely mainly on rib movement, while males tend to use both rib and diaphragm movement, with an emphasis on the diaphragm.

The rate of breathing is controlled by the medulla of the brain, which checks the carbon dioxide content of the blood. Activity produces more carbon dioxide and affects the rate. The normal relaxed breathing rate is about twelve times a minute. A person resting in bed may inhale 8 liters of air per minute, while a runner may reach 50 liters per minute. If a person relaxes and falls into a very shallow rhythm, a yawn attempts to break the pattern. A yawn is a deeper breath that causes more gas exchange.

DISORDERS AND DISEASES

The lungs are the only major internal organs exposed to the outside environment, and they tend to show the effects of both age and type of use. A child's lungs are pink, but with age this color becomes darker and mottled because of particles that are trapped inside the macrophages of the lung. The lungs of city dwellers and coal miners show the greatest effects because of the poor quality of the air being inhaled. Understanding the pathologies of the lungs is linked to understanding the function of the lung itself.

For example, smoking and air pollution are known to cause chronic bronchitis. The repeated irritation of the bronchi by pollutants causes the linings of the air tubules to thicken, closing down the airways. Muscles contract, and the secretion of mucus increases. Poor drainage may lead to pneumonia. Smoking tobacco can also lead to cancer of the lung, mouth, pharynx, and esophagus. Tobacco smoke may contain as many as forty-three carcinogenic (cancer-causing) chemicals. Lung cancer usually begins with changes in the lining of the bronchi among the cells with cilia and those that produce mucus. The long-term irritation of smoking eventually destroys these cells faster than the bronchi can replace them. Abnormal cells, without cilia or the ability to produce mucus, begin to take their place. These cells offer less protection and, as irritation and replacement continues, may become cancerous. In the United States, lung cancer is the leading cause of cancer deaths in both men and women, and evidence has revealed the danger of inhaling smoke from someone else's cigarette. Smoking also leads to greater risk of various other lung diseases.

Pneumonia is a general term for any inflammation that produces a fluid buildup in the lungs. The excess fluid makes breathing difficult by blocking the alveoli. The cause of the inflammation can be bacterial, viral, fungal, or chemical. For example, Legionnaires' disease is a type of pneumonia caused by a bacterium that lives in air conditioners, humidifiers, and other water-storage devices. Because it causes a lack of oxygen in the body, pneumonia can be fatal if it is not controlled: More than 70,000 deaths attributed to pneumonia occur in the United States each year. The very young and the very old are in the most danger, especially if they have already been weakened by other illnesses. Since the discovery of antibiotics, however, the majority of those infected recover.

Bronchitis is an inflammation of the mucous membrane of the bronchi that often follows a cold. A telltale symptom is a deep cough that eventually brings up gray or greenish phlegm. Bronchitis may be viral or bacterial; if the cause is bacterial, antibiotics can help in recovery. Chronic bronchitis can result from repeated attacks of bronchitis and is aggravated by smoking and air pollution.

Another lung disease is emphysema, which is usually caused by smoking. This condition is often seen in advanced cases of chronic bronchitis. In emphysema, the alveoli overinflate and break. Nearby alveoli are damaged and merge into larger units, leaving less surface area for gas exchange. Therefore, less of the air coming into the lungs comes into contact with the membrane. The increase in dead air space requires deeper breaths to obtain oxygen, and the lungs suffer further damage. Because the air sacs are permanently broken down, the damage is irreversible.

Tuberculosis is a highly contagious bacterial infection that damages the lungs and can spread to the kidneys and the bones. Immunization, screening for exposure, and antibiotics have controlled the number of cases found in countries with modern medical care systems. Worldwide, however, tuberculosis remains a major danger, and millions of lives are still lost to this disease every year.

According to the Mayo Clinic, cases of asthma appear to be increasing in the United States population. Asthma involves a hyperactive response of the airways. During an attack, the smooth muscles of the bronchi and bronchioles contract, and excess mucus is produced. In other cases, the airways may become inflamed and swollen. The cause may be allergies or other stimuli. Asthma is rarely fatal but interferes with normal functioning, as breathing becomes difficult. The blockage of breathing can be reversed with proper medications. Asthma does not lead to emphysema.

Respiratory distress syndrome occurs in about 50,000 premature infants every year. These infants have not yet developed the ability to produce sufficient surfactant in their alveoli to prevent collapse. The importance of surfactant can be illustrated by the difficulty of a baby's first breath. To inflate the alveoli requires up to twenty times the force of a normal breath. Without surfactant, the alveoli would collapse again and the next breath would be just as difficult. In 1990, a surfactant treatment derived from calf lungs became available. Treatment of premature babies with this surfactant before symptoms develop has resulted in an 88 percent survival rate.

Cystic fibrosis is a severe genetic problem in which the mucus produced in the airways (and the gastrointestinal tract) is abnormally thick. This thick mucus interferes with gas exchange, causing the heart to work harder and the valves to be damaged. As a result, the lung may collapse. Serious infections are more likely to occur. While about 50 percent of those with cystic fibrosis live only until their late teens and twenties, an increasing number of children and young adults with this disease are living into adult life. Progress on curing cystic fibrosis is being made: Researchers working in this area have located the gene that causes the condition.

If air is allowed to enter between the pleural membrane, the lungs will instantly collapse. The two lungs are independent enough so that one lung can be collapsed for healing while the other performs the gas exchange for the body. Furthermore, each lung subdivides into its lobes and then into ten bronchopulmonary segments. Each of these segments is a structural unit that can be removed surgically if diseased.

PERSPECTIVE AND PROSPECTS

The ancient Greeks established the first understandings of lung function. They rightly accepted that life depended on air but overgeneralized that air carried all disease. Empedocles of Agrigentum (c. 500-430 B.C.E.) demonstrated that air was a real substance by filling a wineskin with it. Empedocles erred, however, in explaining the mechanism of breathing. He compared the body to a pipe and thought that the movement of air in and out of the lungs caused vital air to move in and out of pores in the body's skin.

The writings of Galen of Pergamum (129-c. 199 C.E.) came to dominate Western medicine until the Renaissance. In his physiology, Galen attempted to connect the function of the lungs with the blood. He believed, however, that the liver produced a "vegetative" blood which traveled to the vena cava and then took different pathways. Some then flowed to other veins to nourish the whole body for growth. The rest entered the right side of the heart. Some of this substance entered the pulmonary artery into the lungs to allow impurities to be exhaled. The rest filtered to the left side of the heart through imagined pores in the septum.

In Galen's complicated scheme, the lungs were not only for exhaust: Vital air was inhaled there to be modified. The heart then pumped the modified air through the pulmonary vein to its left side. Here the air joined the blood to become "vital spirit," which traveled by arteries to warm the whole body. The brain converted this vital spirit into "animal spirit,"

distributing it by the nerves to cause movement and sensation. Galen did not know that blood traveled from one side of the heart to the other by moving through the lungs. He believed that the lungs acted as a reservoir of air for the heart. Galen also thought that breathing cooled the heart.

William Harvey (1578-1657) studied the position of valves in the veins and realized that Galen's vegetative blood traveled backward. Harvey then argued for a single blood that must go through the lungs to reach the other side of the heart. Blood travels in a circle, he bravely suggested. He was supported when the new microscopes discovered the necessary small vessels that connect arteries to veins.

Antoine-Laurent Lavoisier (1743-1794) noted that the lungs take in oxygen and that carbon dioxide is exhaled. He concluded that a slow combustion must occur in the lungs to warm the blood, while opponents noted that the lungs are not warmer than other parts of the body. By the 1790's, the idea was accepted that the lungs exchange Lavoisier's gases with the blood. Many believed that blood was the essence of life. In the 1850's, however, Georg Liebig and Hermann von Helmholtz showed that muscle tissue uses oxygen and releases carbon dioxide and heat. It was finally realized that the cells are the location of Lavoisier's slow fire of respiration and that the blood is the carrier of gases between the cells and the lungs.

—Paul R. Boehlke, Ph.D.

See also Abscess drainage; Abscesses; Allergies; Altitude sickness; Anatomy; Apnea; Asphyxiation; Asthma; Bacterial infections; Bronchiolitis; Bronchitis; Cancer; Chest; Childhood infectious diseases; Choking; Common cold; Coughing; Croup; Cystic fibrosis; Diphtheria; Edema; Embolism; Emphysema; Environmental diseases; Environmental health; Exercise physiology; Heart transplantation; Influenza; Internal medicine; Interstitial pulmonary fibrosis (IPF); Kinesiology; Legionnaires' disease; Lung cancer; Lung surgery; Measles; Multiple chemical sensitivity syndrome; Occupational health; Oxygen therapy; Physiology; Plague; Pleurisy; Pneumonia; Pulmonary diseases; Pulmonary medicine; Pulmonary medicine, pediatric; Respiration; Respiratory distress syndrome; Resuscitation; Smoking; Systems and organs; Thoracic surgery; Thrombolytic therapy and TPA; Thrombosis and thrombus; Toxoplasmosis; Transplantation; Tuberculosis; Tumor removal; Tumors; Whooping cough.

FOR FURTHER INFORMATION:

Corrin, Bryan. *Pathology of the Lungs*. London: Churchill Livingstone, 2000. This volume discusses such topics as lung development, infectious diseases, vascular disease, tumors, and transplantation.

Guinness, Alma, ed. *ABC's of the Human Body*. Pleasantville, N.Y.: Reader's Digest, 1987. This well-illustrated book is both informative and entertaining. Using a question-and-answer format, the writers tend to deal with the subjects about which most people wonder. The chapter on the respiratory system is excellent. Some sample questions in this section are "What is mountain sickness?" and "Can your house be dangerous?"

Sarosi, George A., and Scott F. Davies. *Fungal Diseases of the Lung*. Philadelphia: Lippincott, Williams & Wilkins, 2000. This resource covers a wide range of topics, including blastomycosis, coccidioidomycosis, cryptococcosis, and sporotrichosis.

Tapley, Donald F., et al., eds. *The Columbia University College of Physicians and Surgeons Complete Home Medical Guide*. Rev. 3d ed. New York: Crown, 1995. A comprehensive, practical health guide explaining all aspects of illness and treatment in common language. The section on respiratory diseases and lung health covers both the causes and the prevention of various diseases and problems.

LUPUS ERYTHEMATOSUS

DISEASE/DISORDER

ANATOMY OR SYSTEM AFFECTED: Immune system, joints, musculoskeletal system, skin

SPECIALTIES AND RELATED FIELDS: Dermatology, immunology, internal medicine

DEFINITION: A chronic inflammation of connective tissue that may prove fatal if it becomes systemic and spreads to the kidneys. Known popularly as lupus, but not to be confused with a variety of unrelated diseases with this name—especially lupus vulgaris, a form of tuberculosis; these diseases share only the symptoms of red or purple lesions appearing on the face.

KEY TERMS:

antigen: a protein in the blood serum which represents foreign material detrimental to the body; the presence of antigens results in the manufacture of other serum proteins (antibodies) that attack the foreign material in an attempt to protect the system

autoimmunity: sensitivity to one's own body in which antibodies may attack some of the body's cells

edema: the collection of serous fluid in the spaces between cell structures or body cavities

etiology: the physical basis of a disease, especially its medical study

L.E. cell: a white blood cell that has destroyed the nucleus of another white blood cell and shows particular staining characteristics

leukocyte: a white blood cell; these cells are vital in the body's defenses against disease

nucleic acids: very large molecules that control the synthesis of proteins and carry basic information determining heredity

phagocytosis: the process in which white blood cells destroy bacteria and other unwanted components of body fluids

tuberculosis: a large family of diseases which may affect virtually any of the tissues of the body

CAUSES AND SYMPTOMS

It is essential that a careful distinction be made among several diseases known by the same popular name of lupus. For example, lupus erythematosus and lupus vulgaris are radically different from each other yet share one highly visible symptom—a red rash often limited to the face. In the nineteenth century, it was observed that the rash leads to extensive, ragged deterioration of structures beneath the skin of the face in the vulgaris form. This early diagnostic confusion and the similarity of its manifestation on the face to an attack by a hungry animal produced the alarming designation of "lupus" (meaning "wolf").

The most striking difference between these two most common forms of lupus is their relationship to sunlight. This subject is of significance in a discussion of their treatment and management. A second important distinction is the frequency of occurrence. Lupus vulgaris is essentially of historical interest because it is actually a well-described form of tuberculosis that can now be cured. Lupus erythematosus, however, has no known etiology and remains a significant area of research.

A fascinating, and maddening, aspect of lupus erythematosus lies in its huge array of manifestations. Typically, the physician sees a patient who complains of aches and pains in the joints. Often this symptom is accompanied by swollen and inflamed joints. The joints of the hands are the usual site, but sometimes the elbows, wrists, hips, knees, or ankles are affected; other joints are not. Bones too are rarely involved in cases eventually diagnosed as lupus. Along with fatigue and low-grade fever, these symptoms are found in approximately 90 percent of lupus patients. Sensitivity to sunlight is often reported.

Efforts to understand the disease, and especially to facilitate correct and early diagnosis, have produced well documented lists of typical symptoms together with their frequency of occurrence. The characteristic "butterfly rash" that led to the earliest description of lupus erythematosus is found in less than half of the cases studied. In the 1970's and 1980's, the American Rheumatism Association compiled a list of common symptoms as a result of a massive survey of experts in the diagnosis of lupus. The original list of about sixty signs was studied for specificity in differentiating this condition from others with similar symptoms. The number of criteria was reduced to fourteen, and it was concluded by the committee of physicians that a patient must show at least four to establish lupus as the condition under treatment.

While such studies are of immense importance in diagnosis and in directing further study of the disease, they also point out how inadequate understanding remains. For example, it is not known why women are afflicted more than ten times as often as men, why African American women are three or perhaps more times as frequently diagnosed, or why several studies have shown higher incidence of mortality rates among Asians. These unsolved pieces of the puzzle remain intriguing clues, but they lack solid ties to the root causes of lupus erythematosus.

In 1948, Malcolm M. Hargraves and his colleagues at the Mayo Clinic made an important discovery related to lupus. Microscopic study of properly stained bone marrow material revealed a particular type of white blood cell called a polymorphonuclear leukocyte. This imposing name denotes one of the most important advances in lupus research. In plain language, Hargraves found cells with more than one collection of nuclear substance because one cell has, in essence, destroyed the nucleus of another. They designated this process with the elegant term "aberrant phagocytosis."

From this key observation came a blood test which, while not foolproof, is of significance in diagnosing lupus. The new direction suggested was even more important, proven by the fact that present research continues to progress along the same lines. It is well established that the body protects itself against disease-causing organisms through a system of antigen-antibody reactions. An example can be seen in the

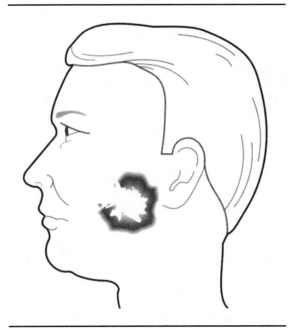

Lupus erythematosus and lupus vulgaris are radically different from each other yet often share the symptom of a red rash on the face; however, this rash does not occur in all cases. In lupus erythematosus, the rash may be a circular, thickened, reddened area with white scar tissue in the center. More typically, those suffering from lupus erythematosus complain of aches and pains in the joints, fatigue, and low-grade fever.

immunity of the body after a case of measles or vaccination against that virus.

In the late 1950's, a class of antibodies that act against the nuclear material of cells in general, rather than specific disease-causing antigens, was found in essentially all lupus patients. A condition in which antibodies act against the body's own cells is called autoimmunity. These antinuclear antibodies do not enter living cells but react with the nucleic acids that control protein synthesis and transmit heredity information. It is quite possible that these antibodies are activated by liberated proteins and lead to the formation of L.E. cells, which subsequently destroy the nuclei of other cells.

Although these studies and many others reveal much about the causes of lupus, there is still much to be explained. One especially fortunate finding was that a particular strain of mice native to New Zealand spontaneously develop an autoimmune hemolytic anemia. The breeding of hybrids produced a mouse that developed an ailment bearing a striking resemblance to lupus. Much of the research accomplished since 1960 is directly related to the development of these laboratory animals.

A most promising line of research into the cause of lupus erythematosus lies among the viruses. Several types of known viral organisms have been discounted. Among these are the arboviruses, which are transmitted by ticks or mosquitoes, and the myxoviruses or influenza viruses. However, large quantities of antibodies that fight the paramyxoviruses (including measles, mumps, and perhaps rubella) are reported in all lupus studies. While the actual virus has not been located, these data show an important future direction.

The other major condition known as lupus, lupus vulgaris, is rare to the point of extinction. It is a form of tuberculosis, and the tireless efforts of Niels Ryberg Finsen, the third Nobel laureate in physiology or medicine (1903), account for its disappearance. Finsen was so ill that he was unable to write or deliver the traditional Nobel lecture, but his book *La Photothérapie* (1899) provides a full discussion of his thoughts and the technical progress that he achieved. The following remarks are based on *Phototherapy*, the English translation of that work published in 1901.

Finsen begins his treatise with a review of earlier applications of light to medical problems. In evaluating these studies, he accepts the hypothesis that light is bactericidal. He attributes the absence of positive clinical results in his predecessors' work to their use of weak sources and short treatment times. He concludes that a systematic scientific study is needed. Experimenting with pure bacterial cultures and a variety of filtering apparatuses on the ear, Finsen was able to offer convincing evidence that concentrated rays were more effective. In the course of these studies, he also discovered that the radiant energy was even more effective when the ear was partially deprived of blood. From these carefully considered experiments, Finsen was prepared to make the intellectual leap to the treatment of lupus vulgaris.

TREATMENT AND THERAPY

Few medical conditions have been more fully described in terms of patient-physician relationships than has lupus erythematosus. Because of the terrifying nature of the name itself—coupled with its unknown cause, its difficulty of diagnosis, and its uncertain prognosis—the sufferer will probably need careful counseling and reassurance. The physician too is faced with a substantial emotional investment in trying to deal with a condition which is so unpredictable.

The most important fact for the patient to understand is that lupus is a manageable malady. In fact, the great majority of people afflicted with lupus have only some of its symptoms, and the most serious and fatal forms involving kidney failure are rare indeed. Sir William Osler, who at the beginning of the twentieth century described the involvement of the kidneys in lupus, made the most penetrating observation concerning medical conditions such as lupus: "If you want to live a long life, get a chronic disease and learn how to take care of it."

The lupus sufferer, as well as the physician, must be content with treating symptoms; no cause or cure has yet been discovered. In spite of this sobering reality, much has been learned that makes such treatment useful. As Osler's comment suggests, a basic premise lies in the recognition of the importance of adequate rest and the avoidance of tension. These two ingredients of a balanced life are crucial to the well-being of the lupus patient.

One of the most common complaints of the patient is fatigue. Many find that doing their normal, daily chores demands most or all of their strength. Some physicians treating lupus cases believe that reduced work schedules, greater-than-average time for sleep, and strict rest periods are essential for good control. Others advocate a more active program during the characteristic periods of remission.

Closely related to the need for rest is another truism of good living—the demand to avoid stress. A number of chronic ills respond to either physical or emotional stress; among the most widely known of these conditions are peptic ulcers, migraine headaches, and heart disease. Lupus too has such a connection, and in relation to other factors specific to this disease, it is of even greater concern.

There are several erratic aspects of lupus, all of which contribute directly to feelings of stress. Most important are the variable periods of remission and activity and the shifting symptoms within an individual. There is evidence that infections, injuries, cold, sunlight, and ultraviolet radiation all may set in motion active phases of lupus. Avoiding such situations is important to all who desire a healthy life; for the lupus patient, such a sensible lifestyle becomes a necessity.

There is clear evidence of the patient's vital role in the successful management of lupus. Several excellent books and articles have described in detail the nature of the team effort of patients and doctors and the benefits to be obtained from it. A specific example is found in the need to seek the advice of one's physician before using any over-the-counter drugs. Even the most innocent of these materials might cause allergic reactions, which seem to be much more common in lupus sufferers. There is also the distinct possibility that such medications might interfere with the utility of a drug that has been prescribed.

Perhaps the most common of all materials on the medical scene, aspirin, continues to be the treatment of choice for the very common painful inflammation of arthritis that comes with lupus. This utility is obviously related to aspirin's cost and effectiveness. Of greater significance is the ability of many patients to take large quantities of the drug over long periods of time with very limited side effects. A number of other drugs are available to combat pain and inflammation, and in specific cases they may be used to great benefit.

Many lupus patients require more aggressive treatment for inflammation than the nonsteroidal drugs described above. Traditionally, the alternative has been cortisone and an array of related steroid hormones. So much has been written concerning the adverse effects associated with the misuse of steroids, especially by athletes, that it is easy to lose sight of their benefits. While careful supervision of their use, by both patient and physician, is essential, these materials can relieve much suffering.

While some kidney malfunction occurs in 50 percent of lupus patients, most of these cases are mild and produce no symptoms. In the much rarer circumstance, when kidney functions drop to less than 25 percent of normal, symptoms of nausea, fatigue, or edema are found. In all cases, careful attention must be paid to blood and urine tests, and any observed abnormalities must be treated to prevent further damage. The only treatments for life-threatening kidney dysfunction currently available are dialysis or transplant surgery. Both of these alternatives make clear how far medical science is from a cure for lupus.

The treatment of lupus vulgaris differs greatly from that of lupus erythematosus. Finsen's life work in the study of radiant energy and its bactericidal properties was focused largely on this condition. The sensitivity to sunlight in lupus erythematosus offers a marked contrast to the cure he achieved using high-powered radiation.

In introducing Finsen as the winner of the 1903 Nobel Prize in Physiology or Medicine, Count K. A. H.

Mörner, the rector of the Royal Caroline Institute, proclaimed that Finsen's work would never be forgotten in the history of medicine. His contribution to the treatment of skin diseases through the advancement of knowledge of phototherapy was such an "immense step forward" that he "deserves the eternal gratitude of suffering humanity." The great success of these treatments with light (or "photothérapie") caused Mörner to concur with Finsen in proclaiming that the disease would soon be permanently eradicated.

From Finsen's first treatments in November, 1895, until the summary report of November, 1901, eight hundred cases of lupus vulgaris were treated. A complete cure was achieved in 50 percent of these, and marked improvement resulted in an additional 45 percent of cases, even among those patients who had been afflicted for as long as fifty years. That early diagnosis and treatment enhanced the likelihood of a complete cure was shown with the treatment of three hundred additional cases during the period following this report up to the time of the Nobel Prize presentation. The symptoms in the majority of these cases were in the early stages, and Finsen stated that here the cure was almost certain. Finsen had crossed a major hurdle, for Denmark could henceforth consider this disease conquered.

X rays have also been studied as a treatment for lupus vulgaris, and some reports of cure have been published. Like phototherapy, these more powerful energies ultimately were replaced by the use of drugs. Today, sulfa drugs are used to some extent, but isoniazid provides the most effective treatment by inhibiting certain key enzymes.

PERSPECTIVE AND PROSPECTS

The family of conditions known as lupus has an ancient pedigree. Hippocrates may have been referring to it when he wrote in the fourth century B.C.E. of "an erosive, disfiguring malady, eating away at the skin and flesh of the face." In the sixteenth century, the great iatrochemist Paracelsus, along with several of his contemporaries and successors, recognized similar maladies. It was in the mid-nineteenth century that the term "lupus" was first used, and shortly afterward, the distinction between the two rather different conditions of lupus erythematosus and lupus vulgaris was made. These two forms of lupus present a vivid contrast in terms of their importance to medical science as a whole, their present significance, and probable future development.

Lupus erythematosus represents a significant field of research and has for many years. There is an extensive literature of original author research, textbook chapters, and reports of international conferences all dealing with the study of the causes and treatment of this disease. As more sensitive diagnostic methods become available, researchers come to understand that what was once thought to be a rare and certainly fatal condition is neither. Of greater importance is the appreciation gained of the suffering of its victims. Much of this suffering is the direct result of ignorance and misunderstanding on the part of the patient, the physician, and the general public.

In a general way, the study of this complicated disease is likely to contribute significantly to the development of methodology useful in the study of other important conditions. For example, since there is significant evidence of viral involvement in lupus, its study seems virtually certain to enhance medical science's ability to deal effectively with a range of totally unrelated viral conditions. In a similar fashion, the need to produce and assess new drugs in the treatment of lupus makes it likely that an increase in medical knowledge will follow.

While lupus vulgaris might now be considered of mere historical interest, one ought to be careful of something being "merely historical." Examples of "extinct" diseases that return to catch the scientific community unaware are not unknown. One of the most pressing problems of modern pharmaceutical research and productivity is the emergence of strains of organisms resistant to the available drugs.

—*K. Thomas Finley, Ph.D.*

See also Arthritis; Fatigue; Kidney disorders; Light therapy; Rashes; Stress; Tuberculosis.

For Further Information:

Aladjem, Henrietta. *Understanding Lupus.* Rev. ed. New York: Charles Scribner's Sons, 1985. Written by a patient with lupus, working with a team of physicians experienced in treating the disease. Offers extensive background concerning the problem. Also contains supplementary materials, such as a glossary and a bibliography.

Aladjem, Henrietta, and Peter H. Schur. *In Search of the Sun.* Rev. ed. New York: Charles Scribner's Sons, 1988. A collaboration between a patient and physician, with alternating chapters describing their complementary views of their joint problems with lupus. Contains an extensive glossary, a bibliography, and support group data.

Horowitz, Mark, and Marietta Abrams Brill. *Living with Lupus.* New York: Plume Books, 1994. This succinct and easy-to-read book provides detailed information about lupus, its causes and diagnosis. Practical advice for lifestyle improvement and information on therapy are included. Contains a useful glossary and resource lists.

Stehlin, Dori. "Living with Lupus." *FDA Consumer* 23 (December, 1989): 8-12. An excellent example of the literature of personal stories of the courage of lupus sufferers. Especially strong on the problems of pregnancy for those with lupus.

Wallace, Daniel J. *The Lupus Book: A Guide for Patients and Their Families.* Rev. ed. New York: Oxford University Press, 2000. Wallace's real-life case studies are based on his experience of having treated more than one thousand lupus patients. This book is highly relevant, since nearly one million people suffer from lupus in the United States, more than from leukemia, multiple sclerosis, cystic fibrosis, and muscular dystrophy combined.

Lyme disease

Disease/disorder

Anatomy or system affected: Heart, joints, nervous system, skin

Specialties and related fields: Bacteriology, environmental health, internal medicine, public health, rheumatology

Definition: Lyme disease involves a mild-to-serious infection caused by the bacteria *Borrelia burgdorferi*, which is spread by the bite of infected ticks of the genus Ixodes.

Key terms:

Borrelia burgdorferi: a member of the family of spirochete (corkscrew-shaped) bacteria

erythema migrans: a red, circular patch that generally appears at the site of a tick bite a few days to one month after infection, and later expands

Causes and Symptoms

Lyme disease is a multistage, multisystem, bacterial infection caused by the spirochete *Borrelia burgdorferi* spread exclusively through bites from infected ticks (not insects). The infected deer tick is much smaller than common dog or cattle ticks and feeds on the white-footed mouse, the white-tailed deer, other mammals, and birds. Ticks transmit Lyme disease during their nymph stage, going unnoticed during this point in their development because of their small size (less than 2 millimeters) and dark brown color. Ticks most likely transmit infection following several days of feeding, which involves inserting their mouth into hidden, often-hairy body areas such as the groin, armpits, and scalp. The tick's body remains outside the host's skin and slowly fills with blood. Ticks do not jump or fly; they crawl from grasses and shrubs (not trees) onto hosts that come into physical contact with the vegetation. Outdoor recreationalists and workers building new homes in wooded, brush-filled areas are most commonly exposed.

The early stages of Lyme disease are marked by one or more of the following: fatigue, malaise, chills and fever, headache, muscle and joint pain, swollen lymph nodes, and a warm, nonpainful skin rash called erythema migrans. This characteristic rash is seen in 75 percent of cases and varies in size and shape; the rash center often clears as it enlarges, resulting in a bulls'-eye appearance.

Signs and symptoms of the later stages of Lyme disease may not appear for years following infection. These include arthritis (brief bouts of pain and swelling in large joints such as the knees), nervous system abnormalities such as numbness, pain, Bell's palsy (paralysis of the muscles on one side of the face), lymphocytic meningitis (fever, stiff neck, and severe headache), and conduction disturbances between the atria and ventricles of the heart.

TREATMENT AND THERAPY

Lyme disease can be deceptive to diagnosis because its characteristic symptoms mimic other diseases or never develop at all. Fever, muscle aches, and fatigue can be mistaken for viral infections such as influenza or infectious mononucleosis. Joint pain can be confused with other types of arthritis, such as rheumatoid arthritis, and neurologic signs can mimic conditions such as multiple sclerosis. Allergic reactions to tick saliva that occur hours to days after a tick bite, do not expand, and disappear rapidly are often mistaken for Lyme disease. Occasionally, erythema migrans never develops, and the first and only sign of Lyme disease is migratory arthritis or nerve impairment. A diagnosis of Lyme diseases always includes a history of possible exposure to ticks and blood testing to determine if antibodies to *Borrelia burgdorferi* bacteria have been produced.

Early treatment of Lyme disease with oral antibiotics such as tetracycline or penicillin for ten to twenty days generally enables a rapid and complete recovery. Although patients nearly always respond to antibiotics, untreated Lyme disease can progress to arthritic, neurologic, and cardiac problems. About 10 percent of chronic cases require hospitalization, 40 to 60 percent involve joint disease, 15 to 20 percent involve neurologic disease, and about 8 percent involve carditis. Patients not treated until advanced disease progression may require intravenous antibiotics for one month or longer, but they still often respond well. Persisting infections rarely continue or recur, but they do have the potential to cause permanent damage and even death.

Tick prevention measures include clearing tall brush and leaves away from houses and gardens, managing high deer traffic areas, and regularly checking domestic animals. Acaricide chemicals are toxic to ticks and are often applied under supervision by a pest control professional, but their effectiveness and environmental safety remain controversial. Personal protection from tick bites involves avoiding tick-infested areas, wearing a hat and long-sleeved light-colored clothing to enable better visibility of ticks, and tucking pantlegs into socks or footwear and shirts into pants and taping these areas to discourage ticks from crawling underneath. Spraying repellent containing DEET on clothes and exposed skin other than the face and applying permethrin, which kills ticks on contact, are also effective. After outdoor activities, clothing should be removed immediately and then washed and dried at high temperatures. After showering, one should inspect the body carefully. Any ticks must be removed using tweezers, grasping the tick close to the skin surface and pulling straight back with a slow, steady force without crushing the tick's body against the skin. All ticks suspected of *Borrelia burgdorferi* infection should be submitted in a sealed container of alcohol to local health department officials.

PERSPECTIVE AND PROSPECTS

Lyme disease was classified in 1975 after a mysterious juvenile arthritis outbreak in the region surrounding Lyme, Connecticut. It has since accounted for more than 90 percent of vector-borne illnesses reported in North America. The annual total of reported cases increased thirty-two-fold between 1982 and 1996, with a cumulative total of more than 99,000 cases during this period. In 1996, more than 16,000 cases were reported in the United States in forty-eight states. In most states, only 2 percent of ticks are thought to be infected, but figures up to 50 percent in highly infected areas have been recorded. Lyme disease is most prevalent in northern temperate regions with a constant high relative humidity. The United States experiences the highest incidence of Lyme disease in the Northeast (from Massachusetts to Maryland), in the north-central states (especially Wisconsin and Minnesota), and on the West coast (particularly in northern California).

Ongoing research will continue to explore the habitats where infected ticks thrive, what measures provide optimal protection, and which chemicals are most effective in various kinds of habitats. Improved reliability and validity of diagnostic tests and antibiotic regimens, vaccine development, the influence of maternal infection on the developing fetus, and the mechanisms by which Lyme disease infects the joints and nervous system are also under investigation.

—*Daniel G. Graetzer, Ph.D.*

See also Antibiotics; Arthritis; Arthropod-borne diseases; Bacterial infections; Bites and stings; Epidemiology; Lice, mites, and ticks.

FOR FURTHER INFORMATION:

Brock, Thomas D., ed. *Microorganisms: From Smallpox to Lyme Disease*. New York: W. H. Freeman, 1990. A collection of readings from *Scientific American*. The book includes a collection of accounts of the history of major infectious diseases. Divided into sections dealing with medical histories, methods of prevention, and means of transmission.

Fell, Elizabeth. "An Update on Lyme Disease and Other Tick-Borne Illnesses." *Nurse Practitioner* 25, no. 10 (October, 2000): 38. Lyme disease, the most common vector-borne illness in North America, is a multisystem, multistage infectious disease caused by the tick-transmitted spirochete *Borrelia burgdorferi*.

France, David. "The War over Lyme Disease." *Newsweek*, November 13, 2000, 72. Discusses the dispute over how best to treat Lyme disease. One side, which includes academics and insurance companies, says Lyme can be cured with just four weeks of antibiotics. The other side, mostly doctors and their patients, says that in rare, intractable cases the infection will require repeated or prolonged courses of antibiotics.

Rahn, Daniel W., and Janine Evans, eds. *Lyme Disease*. Philadelphia: American College of Physicians, 1998. Intended as a single and all-encompassing source of information for readers interested in Lyme disease, this is an outstanding monograph produced by a diverse group of physicians with expertise in the field.

Silverstein, Alvin, Virginia Silverstein, and Laura Silverstein Nunn. *Lyme Disease*. New York: Franklin Watts, 2000. A concise volume aimed at the lay reader. Includes bibliographical references and an index.

Vanderhoof-Forschner, Karen. *Everything You Need to Know About Lyme Disease and Other Tick-Borne Disorders*. New York: Rosen, 2000. Basically a consumer guide to Lyme disease, this book aims to provide concerned parents with basic knowledge and useful insights into the prevention and management of disease.

LYMPHADENOPATHY AND LYMPHOMA
DISEASE/DISORDER

ANATOMY OR SYSTEM AFFECTED: Lymphatic system

SPECIALTIES AND RELATED FIELDS: Hematology, internal medicine, oncology, vascular medicine

DEFINITION: Lymphadenopathy, or enlarged lymph nodes, refers to any disorder related to the lymphatic vessels of lymph nodes; lymphoma is a group of cancers consisting of unchecked multiplication of lymphatic tissue cells.

KEY TERMS:

B lymphocyte: a blood and lymphatic cell that plays a role in the secretion of antibodies

Hodgkin's disease: a malignant disorder of lymphoid tissue, generally first appearing in cervical lymph nodes, which is characterized by the presence of the Reed-Sternberg cell

lymphoma staging: a classification of lymphomas based upon the stage of the disease; used in the determination of treatment

non-Hodgkin's lymphoma: any malignant lymphoproliferative disorder other than Hodgkin's disease

Reed-Sternberg cell: a large atypical macrophage with multiple nuclei; found in patients with Hodgkin's disease

T lymphocyte: a blood and lymphatic cell that functions in cell-mediated immunity, which involves the direct attack of diseased tissues; subclasses of T cells aid B lymphocytes in the production of antibodies

CAUSES AND SYMPTOMS

The lymphatic system consists of a large complex of lymph vessels and groups of lymph nodes ("lymph glands"). The lymph vessels include a vast number of capillaries that collect fluid and dissolved proteins, carbohydrates, and fats from tissue fluids. The lacteals of the intestinal villi are lymph vessels that serve to absorb fats from the intestine and transport them to the bloodstream.

Lymph nodes are found throughout the body but are concentrated most heavily in regions of the head, neck, armpits, abdomen, and groin. Nodes function to filter out foreign materials, such as bacteria or viruses, which make their way into lymphatic vessels.

The sizes of lymph nodes vary: Some are as small as a pinhead, some as large as a bean. In general, they are shaped much like kidney beans, with an outer covering. Internally, they consist of a compartmentalized mass of tissue that contains large numbers of B and T lymphocytes as well as antigen-presenting cells (APC). The lymphatic circulation into the lymph nodes consists of a series of entering, or afferent, vessels, which empty into internal spaces, or sinuses. A network of connective tissue, the reticulum, regulates the lymph flow and serves as a site of attachment for lymphocytes and macrophages. The lymphatic circulation leaves the node through efferent, or exiting, vessels in the lower portion of the organ, the hilum.

Among the functions of lymph nodes are those of the immune response. B and T lymphocytes tend to congregate in specialized areas of the lymph nodes: B cells in the outer region, or cortex, and T cells in the underlying paracortex. When antigen is presented by an APC, T- and B-cell interaction triggers B-cell maturation and proliferation within the germinal centers of the cortex. The result may be a significant enlargement of the germinal centers and subsequently of the lymph node itself.

Lymphadenopathy, or enlarged lymph nodes, may signify a lymphoma, or cancer of the lymphatic system. More commonly, however, the enlarged node is secondary to other phenomena, usually local infections. For example, an ear infection may result in the entrance of bacteria into local lymphatic vessels. These vessels drain into regional nodes of the neck. The result is an enlargement of the nodes in this area, as an immune response is carried out.

Enlarged nodes caused by infections can, in general, be easily differentiated from those caused by malignancies. Infectious nodes are generally smaller than 2 centimeters in diameter, soft, and tender. They usually occur in areas where common infections occur, such as the ears or the throat. Malignant lymph nodes are often large and occur in groups. They are generally firm and hard, and they often appear in unusual areas of the body (for example, along the diaphragm). In order to confirm a malignancy, a biopsy of material may be necessary.

Infectious nodes can also be caused by diseases such as infectious mononucleosis, tuberculosis, and acquired immunodeficiency syndrome (AIDS). Lymphadenopathy syndrome (LAS), a generalized enlargement of the lymph nodes, is a common feature of the prodromal AIDS-related complex (ARC).

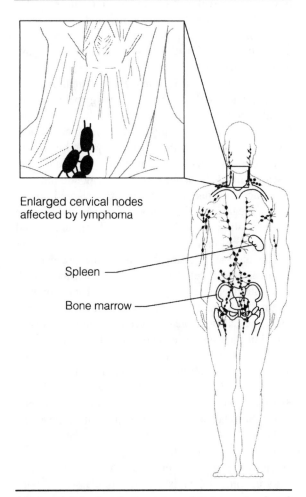

Enlarged cervical nodes affected by lymphoma

Spleen

Bone marrow

Anatomy of the lymphatic system, showing major lymph nodes; enlarged lymph nodes may occur for a wide variety of reasons, including but not limited to lymphoma (cancer).

Since lymphadenopathy can be caused by any immune proliferation in the germinal centers, allergy-related illnesses may also cause enlargement of the lymph nodes. Consequently, immune disorders such as rheumatoid arthritis, systemic lupus erythematosus, and even hay fever allergies may show enlarged nodes as part of their syndromes.

As is the case for any cell in the body, cells constituting the lymphatic system may undergo a malignant transformation. The broadest definition of these lymphoproliferative diseases, or lymphomas, can include both Hodgkin's disease and non-Hodgkin's lymphomas, in addition to acute and chronic lymphocytic leukemias (ALL and CLL). With the understanding of, and ability to detect, specific cell markers, it is possible to classify many of these lymphomas on the basis of their cellular origin. Such is the case for ALL, CLL, Burkitt's lymphoma, and many other forms of non-Hodgkin's lymphomas. The cell type that ultimately forms the basis for Hodgkin's disease remains uncertain.

Hodgkin's disease is a malignant lymphoma that first presents itself as a painless enlargement of lymphoid tissue. Often, this is initially observed in the form of swollen lymph nodes in the neck or cervical region. Occasionally, the victim may exhibit a mild fever, night sweats, and weight loss. Untreated, the disease spreads from one lymphatic region to another, resulting in diffuse adenopathy. An enlarged spleen (splenomegaly) is a common result. As the disease spreads, other organs such as the liver, lungs, and bone marrow may be involved.

The disease is characterized by the presence of a characteristic cell type—the Reed-Sternberg cell. Reed-Sternberg cells appear to be of macrophage origin, with multilobed nuclei or multiple nuclei. They may also be present in other lymphatic disorders, but their presence is considered to be indicative of all cases of Hodgkin's disease. The precise relationship of the cell to the lymphoma is unclear, but some researchers in the field believe that the Reed-Sternberg cell is the actual malignant cell of the disease. The other infiltrative cells present in the node, including many B and T lymphocytes, may simply represent the reaction to the neoplasm. This interpretation, however, has been disputed.

Lymphoma staging is a system of classifying lymphomas according to the stage of development of the disease. Staging is important in that the prognosis and basis for treatment are in part determined by the stage of disease. Characterizing the form of Hodgkin's disease, therefore, involves two forms of classification. The first is a four-part classification based on the histology or cell type (Rye Conference classification). This scheme is based upon the proportion of Reed-Sternberg cells, ranging from their being "hard to find" to their being the predominant type. The prognosis becomes less favorable as the proportion of these cells increases.

Clinical staging, like that based on histology, is a four-part classification scheme (it is actually six parts, since stage III can be divided into subclasses). In this system, classification is based upon the extent of spread or extralymphatic involvement. For example, stage I features the involvement of a single lymph node region or a single extralymphatic site. Stage IV involves multiple disseminated foci. Early-stage disease is more easily treated and has a better prognosis than late-stage disease.

Non-Hodgkin's lymphomas (NHLs) represent a multitude of malignant disorders. Unlike Hodgkin's disease, they frequently arise in lymphatic tissue that is not easily observed; for example, in the gastrointestinal tract, tonsils, bone, and central nervous system. They have a tendency to spread rapidly, with malignant cells being released into the bloodstream early in the disease. Consequently, by the time diagnosis of NHL is made, the disease has often spread and the prognosis may be poor.

Though the etiology of most forms of NHL remains unknown, certain characteristics are evident in some forms of these diseases. For example, a portion of chromosome 14 is elongated in about 60 percent of NHL patients. Nearly one-third of patients with NHLs of B-cell origin demonstrate a chromosomal translocation, often involving a piece of chromosome 14 being translocated to chromosome 18. Though the relationship of these changes to disease is unclear, one can surmise that chromosomal defects play at least some role in the development of some forms of these disorders.

At least two forms of NHL are either caused by viruses or related to their presence: Burkitt's lymphoma and adult T-cell lymphoma/leukemia. Burkitt's lymphoma, which was first described by Denis Burkitt in central Africa, is a B-cell tumor that occurs primarily in children. It is generally presented as a large tumor of the jaw. This type of lymphoma is associated with early infection by the Epstein-Barr virus, or EBV (also the etiological agent of infectious mononucleosis).

The relationship of the disorder to the virus remains unclear, and EBV may be either a specific cause or a necessary cofactor.

Specific chromosomal abnormalities are also associated with Burkitt's lymphoma. In 75 percent of cases, a translocation from chromosome 8 to chromosome 14 is evident, while in most other cases, a portion of chromosome 8 is translocated to either chromosome 2 or chromosome 22. Each of these translocations involves the transfer of the same gene from chromosome 8, the c-myc gene. The site to which the c-myc is translocated is in each instance a region that encodes protein chains for antibody production, proteins that are produced in large quantities. The c-myc gene product normally plays a role in committing a cell to divide. By being translocated into these specific regions, the c-myc gene product is overproduced, and the B cell undergoes continual replication.

Approximately 80 percent of NHL tumors are of B-cell origin; the remainder are primarily of T-cell origin. Those lymphomas that arise within the thymus, the organ of T-cell maturation, are called lymphoblastic lymphomas. Those that originate as more differentiated and mature T cells outside the thymus include a heterogeneous group of diseases (for example, peripheral T-cell lymphomas and Sézary syndrome). Often, by the time of diagnosis, these disorders have spread beyond the early stage of classification and have become difficult to treat.

TREATMENT AND THERAPY

Treatment and other means of dealing with lymphadenopathy depend on the specific cause. In the case of lymph node enlargement that is secondary to infections, treatment of the primary cause is sufficient to restore the normal appearance of the node. For example, in a situation in which nodes in the neck region are enlarged as the result of a throat infection, antibiotic treatment of the primary cause—that is, the bacterial infection—is sufficient. The nodes will resume their normal size after a short time.

Dealing with lymph node enlargement caused by lymphoma requires a much more aggressive form of treatment. There are many kinds of lymphomas, which differ in type of cell involvement and stage of differentiation of the involved cells. The manifestations of most lymphomas, however, are similar. In general, these disorders first present themselves as painless, enlarged nodes. Often, this occurs in the neck region,

but in many forms of NHL, the lymphadenopathy may manifest itself elsewhere in the lymphatic system. As the disease progresses, splenomegaly (enlarged spleen) and hepatomegaly (enlarged liver) may manifest themselves. Frequently, the bone marrow becomes involved. If the enlarged node compresses a vital organ or vessel in the body, immediate surgery may be necessary. For example, if one of the veins of the heart is compressed, the patient may be in immediate, life-threatening danger. Treatment generally includes radiation therapy and/or chemotherapy.

As is true for lymphomas in general, Hodgkin's disease is found more commonly in males than in females. In the United States, it occurs at a rate of 2 per 100,000 population per year, resulting in more than 6,000 cases being diagnosed each year. Approximately 1,500 persons die of the disease each year. The cause of the disease is unknown, though attempts have been made to assign the Epstein-Barr virus to this role.

Hodgkin's disease has an unusual age incidence. The age-specific incidence exhibits a bimodal curve. The disease shows an initial peak among young adults between 15 and 30 years of age. The incidence drops after age 30, only to show an additional increase in frequency after age 50. This is in contrast to NHL, which shows a sharp increase in incidence only after age 45. The reasons for this are unknown.

As noted earlier, the staging of Hodgkin's disease is important in determining methods of treatment; the earlier the stage, the better the prognosis. Patients in stage I (single node or site of involvement) or stage II (two or more nodes on the same side of the diaphragm involved, or limited extralymphatic involvement) have a much better prognosis than patients in stages III and IV (splenic or disseminated disease). Prior to the mid-1960's, a diagnosis of Hodgkin's disease was almost a death sentence. The development of radiation therapy and chemotherapy has dramatically increased the chances for survival; long-term remission can be achieved in nearly 70 percent of patients, and the "cure" rate may be higher than 90 percent with early detection. In part, this has been the result of understanding the progression of the disease (reflected in the process of staging) and utilizing a therapeutic approach to eradicate the disease both at its current site and at likely sites of spreading.

Radiation therapy is the treatment of choice for patients in stages I and II; spreading beyond local nodes is still unlikely in these stages. The body is divided into three regions to which radiation may be delivered: the mantle field covers the upper chest and arm-pits, the para-aortic field is the region of the dia-phragm and spleen, and the third field is the pelvic area. For example, a patient presenting lymphadenop-athy in a single node in the neck region may undergo only "mantle" irradiation. As noted above, with early detection, such treatment is effective 90 percent of the time (based on five-year disease-free survival).

Beyond stage II, a combination of radiation ther-apy and chemotherapy treatment is warranted. A vari-ety of chemotherapy programs have been developed, the most common of which is known by the acro-nym MOPP (nitrogen mustard/Oncovin/procarbazine/prednisone). With combined radiation therapy and chemotherapy, even stage III disease may go into re-mission 60 to 70 percent of the time, while 40 to 50 percent of stage IV patients may enter remission. In general, therapy takes six to twelve months.

Non-Hodgkin's lymphomas represent a heteroge-neous group of malignancies. Eighty percent are of B-lymphocyte origin. The wide variety of types has made classification difficult. The most useful method of classification for clinical purposes is based on the relative aggressiveness of the disease, low-grade be-ing the slowest growing, followed by intermediate-grade and high-grade, which is the most aggressive.

NHLs often arise in lymphoid areas outside the mainstream. For example, the first sign of disease may be an abdominal mass or pain. Fever and night sweats are uncommon, at least in the early stages. Consequently, once the disease is presented, it is of-ten deep and widespread. Because the disorder is no longer localized by this stage, radiation therapy by it-self is of limited use. For comparison, nearly half of Hodgkin's disease patients are in stage I at presenta-tion; not quite 15 percent of NHL patients are in stages I and II. Consequently, treatment almost always in-volves extensive chemotherapy.

A variety of aggressive forms of chemotherapy may be applied. These may include either single drugs such as alkaloids (vincristine sulfate) and alkylating agents (chlorambucil) or combination programs such as that of MOPP. Low-grade types of NHL are frequently slow growing and respond well to less aggressive forms of therapy. Low-grade NHL patients often en-ter remission for years. Unfortunately, the disorder of-ten recurs with time and may become resistant to treatment; remission may occur in 50 percent of the patients, but only about 10 percent survive disease-free after ten years. High-grade lymphomas are rap-idly growing, and the prognosis for most patients in the short term is not good. Those patients who do achieve remission with aggressive therapy, however, often show no recurrence of disease. As many as 50 percent of these persons may be "cured." The differ-ence in prognosis between low-grade and high-grade disease may relate to the characteristics of the malig-nant cell. A rapidly growing cancer cell may be more susceptible to aggressive therapy than a slow-growing cancer and more likely to die as a result. Thus, if a patient enters remission following therapy, there is greater likelihood that the cancer has been eradicated.

PERSPECTIVE AND PROSPECTS

What was likely Hodgkin's disease was first described in 1666 as an illness in which lymphoid tissues and the spleen had the appearance of a "cluster of grapes." The disorder was invariably fatal. In 1832, Thomas Hodgkin published a thorough description of the dis-ease, including its progression from the cervical region of the body to other lymphatic regions and organs. The unusual histological appearance of the cellular mixture characteristic of Hodgkin's disease was noted during the nineteenth century. It was early in the twen-tieth century, however, that Dorothy Reed and Karl Sternberg described the cell that is characteristic of the disorder: the Reed-Sternberg cell. As noted earlier, the number and proportion of such cells are the bases for the classification of the disease.

Two forms of non-Hodgkin's lymphoma are known to be associated with specific viruses: Burkitt's lym-phoma (BL) and adult T-cell leukemia (ATL). BL was described by Denis Burkitt, who studied the pattern of certain forms of lymphomas among Ugandan children during the late 1950's. He noted that nearly all cases were found in children between the ages of 2 and 14, and noted that most cases in Africa were found in the malarial belt. Burkitt suspected that a mosquito might be involved in the transmissions of BL. Though no link has been found with arthropod transmission, the idea that BL might be associated with a viral agent bore fruit. In 1964, Michael Epstein and Yvonne Barr reported the presence of a particle in BL tissue that resembled the herpes virus. The Epstein-Barr virus was eventually linked to BL, though the specific role played by the virus remains elusive.

Adult T-cell leukemia was first noted in Japan dur-ing the 1970's. Japanese scientists observed that the majority of NHLs there were of T-cell origin and ex-hibited a similar clinical spectrum. The disease was later observed in the Caribbean basin, the southeastern United States, South America, and central Africa. In 1980, Robert Gallo isolated the etiological agent, the human T-cell lymphophic type I virus (HTLV-I).

The treatment of Hodgkin's disease represents one of the few success stories in dealing with cancers. In addition, some forms of NHL—notably, Burkitt's lymphoma—respond well to treatment. The prognosis for most patients with NHL, however, is less than optimal. In addition, the specific causes of most NHL syndromes are not known. Those with which a virus is linked may, in theory, be prevented by means of vaccination. The etiological agents or factors associated with the development of other forms of lymphomas remain elusive.

—Richard Adler, Ph.D.

See also Cancer; Chemotherapy; Hodgkin's disease; Infection; Lymphatic system; Malignancy and metastasis; Oncology; Radiation therapy.

FOR FURTHER INFORMATION:

Beck, William S., ed. *Hematology*. 5th ed. Cambridge, Mass.: MIT Press, 1991. A series of lectures dealing with hematology. Though the text was written for medical students, the material is not excessively detailed. The book is appropriate for anybody with a basic knowledge of biology, and the section on lymphomas is easy to follow. Numerous tables and photographs.

Bruning, Nancy. *Coping with Chemotherapy*. Rev. ed. New York: Ballantine Books, 1993. Written by a woman who survived breast cancer and its aftermath, this book provides a vivid description of chemotherapy. The author discusses methods of treatment and her own experiences.

Cerroni, Lorenzo, Helmut Kerl, and Kevin Gatter. *An Illustrated Guide to Skin Lymphoma*. Malden, Mass.: Blackwell Science, 1998. This book is an extremely practical guide to diagnosis that will help any pathologist spot skin lymphoma. It combines stunning pictures of histopathology (tissue specimens) with the clinical features making it attractive and useful to pathologists and clinicians.

Franks, L. M., and N. M. Teich, eds. *Introduction to the Cellular and Molecular Biology of Cancer*. 3d ed. New York: Oxford University Press, 1997. A general description of cancer and areas of research. The text discusses features of cancer and its possible origins. The possible role of oncogenes in the disease is also included. Though not intended for the layperson, the book does present a good overview of the subject.

Jandl, James H. *Blood: Textbook of Hematology*. 2d ed. Boston: Little, Brown, 1996. A textbook on hematology. The book is quite detailed but is recommended for anyone who is seriously interested in the subject. Though the lymphatic system is not specifically covered, blood and lymphatic cells are extensively covered.

Levine, Arnold. *Viruses*. New York: W. H. Freeman, 1992. A discussion of viruses and the diseases with which they are associated. Included are sections that deal with viruses and human cancers. The book is vividly illustrated and is intended for a general audience with some basic knowledge of biology.

National Cancer Institute. *What You Need to Know About Non-Hodgkin's Lymphoma*. Rev. ed. Bethesda, Md.: U.S. Department of Health and Human Services, Public Health Service, National Institutes of Health, 1999. Aimed at the patient who has been diagnosed with non-Hodgkin's lymphoma, this publication offers the latest advice.

Roitt, Ivan. *Roitt's Essential Immunology*. 9th ed. Boston: Blackwell Scientific, 1997. An outstanding textbook on immunology written by a leading researcher in the field. The early chapters on the lymphatic system, lymph nodes, and the immune response provide an excellent background for the subject.

Varmus, Harold, and Robert Weinberg. *Genes and the Biology of Cancer*. New York: W. H. Freeman, 1993. The authors provide an excellent discussion of the role played by genetic factors in development of cancers. Several chapters deal with chromosome translocation as a possible cause of certain cancers, including Burkitt's lymphoma.

LYMPHATIC DISORDERS. *See* LYMPHADENOPATHY AND LYMPHOMA.

LYMPHATIC SYSTEM

ANATOMY

ANATOMY OR SYSTEM AFFECTED: Circulatory system, immune system, spleen

SPECIALTIES AND RELATED FIELDS: Hematology, immunology, vascular medicine

DEFINITION: A network of vessels, paralleling those of the circulatory system, and nodules that collect extravascular materials and fluids from tissue in order to return them to the bloodstream.

KEY TERMS:

antigen-presenting cell (APC): a type of macrophage or interstitial cell that initiates the immune response by "presenting" processed antigen to B and T lymphocytes

edema: an abnormal accumulation of fluids around tissues

lacteals: lymphatic capillaries in the villi of the small intestine that absorb fat, producing a milky substance called chyle

lymph: the straw-colored fluid of the lymphatic system; as much as 1 to 2 liters is collected from tissue each day and returned to the bloodstream

lymph node: a small, oval structure that filters tissue fluids; lymph nodes are found in areas such as the armpits, groin, mouth, and neck, and serve as sites of immune response

lymphocytes: cells of the lymphatic system; B lymphocytes function in antibody production, while T lymphocytes function in cellular immunity

Peyer's patches: lymphatic nodules in the ileum of the intestine; Peyer's patches are one kind of mucosal associated lymphoid tissue (MALT), which, unlike lymph nodes, are not enclosed by tissue capsules

spleen: a lymphatic organ found between the stomach and the diaphragm; destroys old blood cells and filters foreign material from the blood

thoracic duct: the largest lymphatic vessel, which collects lymphatic fluid and returns it to the bloodstream at the left subclavian vein in the region of the neck

thymus: the lymphatic gland in which T lymphocytes mature; located in humans just below the thyroid

STRUCTURE AND FUNCTIONS

The lymphatic system is a complex of capillaries, ducts, nodes, and organs that filters and maintains interstitial fluid—that is, fluid from body tissues. Fluid is collected from body tissues and returned to the bloodstream. In addition, the system functions as a site of the immune response, primarily in the spleen and the lymph nodes, and transports fat and protein to the bloodstream.

The organs of the lymphatic system are divided into primary lymphoid organs and secondary organs. The primary organs include the thymus and the bone marrow, which are sites where lymphocytes are produced and mature. Secondary lymphoid organs are those in which the immune response is carried out.

These include both encapsulated organs such as the spleen and lymph nodes and unencapsulated organs such as the mucosal associated lymphoid tissue, which includes Peyer's patches in the intestine and Waldemeyer's ring in the throat (the tonsils and adenoids), which encircles the pharnyx. Lymph nodes are found throughout the body, but they occur in large numbers in the head, neck, armpits (the axial nodes), and abdomen and groin (the inguinal nodes).

The lymphatic vessels essentially parallel those of the bloodstream. The system originates in peripheral tissue as small openings, or sinuses, within the tissue. Fluid that drains from the tissue collects in these sinuses and forms lymph. In addition, a significant amount of liquid (1 to 2 liters) that is lost from blood capillaries each day also collects in the interstitial fluid. The lymph is physiologically similar to blood plasma in that it is a balanced solution of electrolytes containing some carbohydrates, lipids, and proteins. In general, the protein level is about half that found in blood, since most blood proteins are too large to pass through the endothelial walls of blood capillaries. Arguably, the major function of the lymphatic system is the return of this fluid, and its constituent materials, to the blood. The buildup of abnormal amounts of fluid in tissue results in swelling, or edema. Approximately 60 percent of lost fluid is returned to the blood through the lymphatics, and the remainder is collected directly into small blood capillaries.

Generally speaking, the peripheral portion of the lymphatic system is completely separate from that of the blood. Once the interstitial fluid is collected, it begins to move toward the thoracic duct. Since the duct is found in the neck region, this movement is primarily in an upward direction. The fluid moves through regional lymph nodes, such as those found in the groin or armpits, and gradually collects in the larger ducts of the major lymphatics. Though an extensive system of valves is found in the lymphatic system to prevent the movement of lymph in the wrong direction, no internal pumping mechanism analogous to the heart exists. The movement of the lymph is mediated by the musculature of the body: respiratory pressure, muscular movement, and the pulsing or motion of nearby organs. Lymphatic fluids from all portions of the body, except for the upper-right quadrant, eventually collect in the thoracic duct. Lymph from the upper-right quadrant of the body collects in the right lymphatic duct. The endothelia of these major lymphatic ducts are contiguous with those of the veins in the neck, and it is here that the fluid is returned to the bloodstream. Valves present in the lymphatic ducts serve to prevent the backup of blood from the bloodstream into the lymphatic system.

In addition to the electrolytes and proteins that collect in lymph, foreign materials such as infectious agents may also penetrate the skin or internal surfaces of the body. These materials pass into tissue fluids and also collect in the lymphatic system. From here, they travel to regional lymph nodes, where they are filtered out by phagocytic cells such as macrophages. In addition, antigen-collecting cells in the skin, including dendritic cells, may transport foreign materials such as bacteria to these regional nodes. These cells may intercalate, or interdigitate, among the lympho-

Major Sites of Lymph Nodes

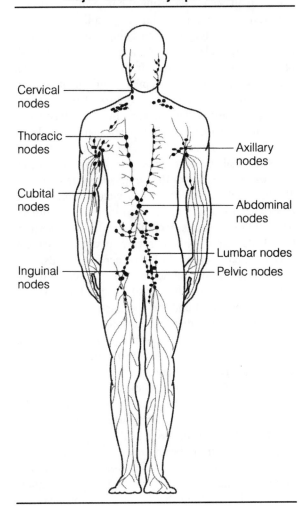

Cervical nodes

Thoracic nodes

Cubital nodes

Inguinal nodes

Axillary nodes

Abdominal nodes

Lumbar nodes

Pelvic nodes

cytes of the lymph nodes and, along with the macrophages, "present" antigen to B and T cells. In this manner, the immune response is initiated.

An analogous situation exists in the blood system. In this case, however, it is the macrophages of the spleen that serve to filter foreign material, such as infectious agents, from the blood. Damaged or old red blood cells are removed in a similar manner. The macrophages then degrade the foreign material and "present" it to B and T lymphocytes in the spleen.

Most of the immune response occurs in the lymph nodes and the spleen. Once the interaction has occurred between the APCs and the lymphocytes, differentiation of the B and T cells begins. The B cells develop into plasma cells, which are essentially antibody-producing factories, while T cells may undergo proliferation. Within the nodes, B and T cells are generally confined to specific areas: the outer cortex for B cells and the underlying paracortex for T cells. Embedded within the cortex are collections of primary nodules, which consist primarily of B cells. Once antigenic stimulation occurs, the cells within the nodules enlarge and proliferate, forming secondary follicles that surround germinal centers. These germinal centers enlarge as B lymphocytes mature and proliferate, and they account for the enlargement of regional lymph nodes in the event of infection. In addition, blood vessels within the node may become enlarged, increasing blood flow. Though some of the activated lymphocytes eventually find their way to the bloodstream, most remain within the lymphatic system. Antibodies produced in response to an infection, however, are transported to the blood.

Since lymph nodes serve as regions of drainage for local tissue, they also represent a route through the body for cancer cells that break away from a tumor. For example, cells from a breast cancer may lodge in regional lymph nodes of the neck or armpit and travel from there to other areas of the body. Although specialized types of lymphocytes capable of killing tumor cells are found in the nodes, some cancer cells may survive. It is for this reason that, during the removal of tumors, localized nodes are examined for evidence of metastasis. If no cancer cells are observed in the nodes, the chances are high that the cancer has not spread.

Mucosal associated lymphatic tissue (MALT) is found along mucosal membranes in regions of the intestines (Peyer's patches and the appendix) and the throat (tonsils). The tonsils actually consist of a network of three groups of tissues that are located at the base of the tongue, at the back of the throat, and at the roof of the nasopharynx (adenoids). Like the spleen and the lymph nodes, MALT tissues may be sites of germinal centers. Unlike the spleen and lymph nodes, however, these tissues are not enclosed by defined capsules of connective tissue. They may be loosely organized, like the mucosa of the intestinal villi, or they may form organized regions like those of the tonsils and adenoids.

MALT appears to function to protect the body against respiratory or gastrointestinal agents. For example, agents such as bacteria or viruses that enter through the oral or respiratory route may stimulate an immune response by the tonsils. The swelling of the tonsils, tonsillitis, is the result of a localized immune response much like that found in the spleen or the lymph nodes. Germinal centers within the tissue represent areas of B cell maturation and proliferation. In the same way, the Peyer's patches consist of approximately 30 to 40 nodules along the wall of the intestines. Gastrointestinal antigens that penetrate the intestinal wall stimulate germinal centers in these regions.

Digestion products of carbohydrates and proteins are actively transported into the villi of the small intestine and enter the bloodstream directly. Fats, however, enter the blood in a more roundabout way through the lymphatic system. Fats are digested in the small intestine and diffuse into underlying cells. There they are assembled into triglycerides and, along with cholesterol, are enclosed in protein envelopes; the resulting bodies are called chylomicrons. Once these bodies pass into the lacteals of the lymphatic system, the whitish fluid, chyle, is transported to a region at the beginning of the thoracic duct called the cisterna chyli. It is here that the fat enters the bloodstream.

DISORDERS AND DISEASES

If the interstitial fluid—that is, the fluid in the tissues—increases beyond the capacity of the lymphatic system to handle the situation, an abnormal accumulation of fluid will build up in the tissue. This creates a situation known as edema. A variety of etiological factors can cause edema. For example, burns, inflammation, and certain allergic reactions may increase the level of capillary permeability. This is particularly true if a large amount of protein is lost as the result of a serious burn.

An increase in capillary hydrostatic pressure may also increase the rate of fluid buildup in the tissues. This may be a by-product of several conditions: congestive heart failure, renal failure, or the use of a variety of drugs (estrogen, phenylbutazone). For example, an increase in the sodium concentration of the blood caused by retention resulting from renal failure or simply an excess of salt in the diet may cause water retention and increased blood volume. The sequelae include increased fluid leakage and edema. It is for this reason that a reduction in sodium intake is often recommended for those who suffer from this problem. Diuretics may be prescribed to promote the excretion of sodium and water. Similarly, venous obstruction as serious as phlebitis or as minor as the pressure from a tight bandage or clothing may increase hydrostatic pressure and lead to edema.

A buildup of fluid in the lungs, or pulmonary edema, may occur as a result of congestive heart failure. Hydrostatic pressure in the capillaries of the lungs is relatively low when compared with that of the circulation elsewhere. As a result, the "wetness" of lung tissue is minimal. In patients with serious congestive heart disease, capillary fluid is backed up into the lung (and, indeed, in tissues of the extremities). The result is fluid leakage into the alveoli and bronchioles. Though the lymphatics are capable of removing small amounts of excess fluids, at some point the leakage of plasma and dissolved proteins exceeds the capacity of the lymphatic system to handle the problem. The result is a vicious circle. Since less oxygen is taken up through the lungs, capillary permeability increases. More fluid and protein are then lost. Unless intervention is carried out, the patient may eventually drown in his or her own fluids.

Intervention for pulmonary edema generally involves elevating the head and knees of the patient (Fowler's position) and the administration of diuretics. A low-sodium diet, allowing for decreased fluid retention, may also relieve some of the stress on the lymphatic system. With time, the number of lymphatic vessels in the lungs may increase, allowing for a greater capacity to remove fluids.

A variety of disorders may directly involve the lymphatic system itself. Lymphedema, or the accumulation of lymph in tissue with subsequent swelling, may result from the absence of lymphatic vessels or from obstructions within the vessels. The symptoms of lymphedema, particularly in the lower extremities, include mild swelling that becomes increasingly severe with time. The problem may be exacerbated by menstruation or pregnancy. In some instances, lymphatic vessels may be absent, either congenitally or because of surgical removal. Diagnosis of the problem often requires the use of lymphangiography (lymphography). In this procedure, a contrast medium is injected, and the lymphatic vessels are examined by means of X rays.

The etiologic factors associated with lymphatic obstruction may be either congenital or have external causes. Milroy's disease is a hereditary lymphedema characterized by chronic obstructions. The obstruction of lymphatic vessels may also be caused by the presence of tumor cells or the infiltration of parasites. For example, elephantiasis is caused by an infestation of a parasitic worm that obstructs the flow of fluid. The affected limb or region of the body may swell to an astounding degree.

The treatment of most of these disorders is essentially symptomatic. An obstruction may be treated or removed. Often, lymphedema may be treated by having the patient sleep with the feet elevated. A low-salt diet or diuretics may be indicated, and a light massage in the direction of lymph flow may also be helpful.

As is true for all tissues in the body, the cells and organs of the lymphatic system may also undergo malignant transformation. Any neoplasm of lymphoid tissue is referred to as a lymphoma. In general, these are malignant. Though lymphomas may be of different forms and involve different types of cells, they are characterized by enlarged lymph nodes (generally in the neck), fever, and weight loss. Among the more common forms of lymphomas are Hodgkin's disease and non-Hodgkin's lymphomas, a mixed collection of malignant solid tumors originating among the secondary lymphoid tissues of the lymph nodes. Hodgkin's disease generally appears first among the cervical or axillary lymph nodes. Its manner of presentation usually allows for early diagnosis and treatment. As a result, the prognosis with early intervention has significantly improved since the 1960's.

Non-Hodgkin's lymphomas often develop in less obvious areas of the lymphatic system, such as the gastrointestinal tract, the central nervous system, and the oral and nasal pharynx. The result is that diagnosis is often delayed until the disease has spread, and therefore the prognosis is less optimistic. More than 80 percent of non-Hodgkin's lymphomas are of B-lymphocyte origin, and they often arise within the follicles of the lymph node. There is some evidence that neoplastic transformation may be related to antigen exposure. In some instances, molecular defects of the cell DNA may result in the neoplastic event. Non-Hodgkin's lymphomas may also be of T-lymphocyte or, less commonly, macrophage origin. Most treatments of lymphomas include both radiation therapy and chemotherapy.

PERSPECTIVE AND PROSPECTS

The first description of the lymphatic system was made by the Italian anatomist Gasparo Aselli in 1622. Aselli observed the lacteals in the intestinal walls of dogs that he had dissected, and he included diagrams of the lacteals in his text *De Lactibus* (1627), the first anatomical medical text with color plates.

The role of the lymphatic system in maintaining the fluid dynamics of the body was understood by the beginning of the twentieth century. Much of this knowledge resulted from the early work of the British physiologist Ernest Henry Starling.

Beginning about 1900, Starling's research centered on the secretion and circulation of lymph. It was known that the lymphatic system as a parallel to blood circulation was found only among the higher vertebrates. This indicated that it had developed relatively late during the course of evolution. There occurred, along with the increasing development of the body's circulatory system as organisms evolved, an increase in the hydrostatic pressure within the system—that is, as the circulatory system became more complex, blood vessels branched into smaller and thinner capillaries. The pressure within those capillaries became higher. Starling pointed out the significance of the hydrostatic pressures within the capillaries: Fluids and dissolved materials leak out of the capillaries into the tissues.

Starling did not believe, however, that protein was able to leak through the capillary walls. In the 1930's, Cecil Drinker demonstrated that protein is a major constituent of dissolved material in lymph and suggested that an important role of the lymphatic system is the return of this protein to the bloodstream. Drinker was unable to prove definitively that the protein in lymph originated with the blood, and it remained for H. S. Mayerson to confirm this point in the 1940's.

Lymphocytes had been observed in the blood as early as the nineteenth century. Their role in the immune process was not readily apparent, however, and various functions were assigned to them. In 1948,

Astrid Fagraeus demonstrated that lymphocytes mature into antibody-producing plasma cells. It remained unclear whether this was the sole purpose of these cells.

In 1956, Bruce Glick and Timothy Chang, working with chickens, discovered that an organ called the bursa, found near the cloaca in the region of the tail, was the site of the production of antibody-producing cells. Their discovery, along with those of Robert Good and Jacques Miller some years later, showed that lymphocytes are not all identical; at least two distinct populations exist. It remained for Henry Claman and his coworkers, in 1966, to demonstrate that these two populations of lymphocytes act cooperatively in the production of antibodies.

In 1969, Ivan Roitt called those lymphocytes that mature in the thymus gland T cells. The lymphocytes that mature in the bursa, an organ found only in birds, were called B cells. Since mammals lack the bursa, B cells in these organisms mature within the bone marrow (considered a bursa equivalent). Once the cells are released from the marrow, they migrate into both the lymphatic system and the bloodstream.

—*Richard Adler, Ph.D.*

See also Angiography; Bacterial infections; Blood and blood disorders; Breast cancer; Breast disorders; Cancer; Cervical, ovarian, and uterine cancers; Chemotherapy; Circulation; Colon cancer; Edema; Elephantiasis; Histology; Hodgkin's disease; Immune system; Immunology; Immunopathology; Liver cancer; Lower extremities; Lung cancer; Lymphadenopathy and lymphoma; Lymphatic system; Malignancy and metastasis; Mononucleosis; Oncology; Prostate cancer; Skin cancer; Sleeping sickness; Splenectomy; Stomach, intestinal, and pancreatic cancers; Systems and organs; Tonsillectomy and adenoid removal; Tonsillitis; Tumors; Upper extremities; Vascular medicine; Vascular system.

FOR FURTHER INFORMATION:
Asimov, Isaac. *The Human Body: Its Structure and Operation.* Rev. ed. New York: Penguin Books, 1992. A basic text on the human body by an outstanding science writer. Asimov had a unique style in which information was laid out in a manner easily understood by the general public. Sections on the structure and operation of the immune and lymphatic systems are included.

Dwyer, John M. *The Body at War: The Story of Our Immune System.* 2d ed. London: J. M. Dent, 1993. Provides a good general description of the immune system. The immune function of the lymphatic system, the roles of lymph nodes in the immune response, and the functions of lymphatic cells are described in a basic manner for the nonscientist.

Kuby, Janis. *Immunology.* 4th ed. New York: W. H. Freeman, 2000. An excellent textbook on the subject of immunology. The section on the cells and organs of the immune system is well organized and includes the latest information on lymphatic circulation. The immune function of the lymphatic system is the major emphasis.

Roitt, Ivan. *Roitt's Essential Immunology.* 9th ed. Boston: Blackwell Scientific, 1997. A standard immunology text written by a leading researcher in the field. Though the lymphatic system is not singled out in any particular section of the book, its role in the immune response is an underlying theme throughout the text.

LYMPHOMA. *See* **LYMPHADENOPATHY AND LYMPHOMA.**

MACULAR DEGENERATION

DISEASE/DISORDER

ANATOMY OR SYSTEM AFFECTED: Eyes

SPECIALTIES AND RELATED FIELDS: Ophthalmology

DEFINITION: A degenerative condition of the macula or central retina.

CAUSES AND SYMPTOMS

The macula is the tiny central region of the retina in the eye. It is made up of millions of light-sensing cells that help to produce central vision and provide maximum visual acuity. When the macula is damaged, a blind spot called drusen, made up of tiny yellow drops, develops in the central field of vision, and central vision becomes blurred or distorted. Central vision is needed to see clearly and to perform everyday activities such as reading, writing, driving, and recognizing people and things. Macular degeneration does not cause complete blindness since peripheral (side) vision is not affected.

There are two forms of age-related macular degeneration (ARMD): dry and wet. The dry form involves thinning of the macular tissues and disturbances in its pigmentation. About 70 percent of patients have the dry form. The remaining 30 percent have the wet form, which can involve bleeding within and beneath the retina, opaque deposits, and eventually scar tissue. The wet form accounts for 90 percent of all cases of legal blindness in macular degeneration patients.

Neither dry nor wet macular degeneration causes pain. The most common early sign of dry macular degeneration is blurring vision that prevents people from seeing details clearly that are in front of them, such as faces or words in a book. In the early stages of wet macular degeneration, straight lines appear wavy or crooked. This is the result of fluid leaking from blood vessels and lifting the macula, distorting vision.

The root causes of macular degeneration are still unknown, but medical authorities consider a number of factors as probable factors. Aging is the leading cause, with genetics, nutrition, smoking, and sunlight exposure all playing a role.

Age is the most important risk factor for macular degeneration. The older the patient, the higher the risk. Studies have shown that having a family with a history of macular degeneration raises the risk factor. Because macular degeneration affects most patients later in life, however, it has proven difficult to study cases in successive generations of a family.

Heavy smoking, at least a pack of cigarettes a day, can double a person's risk of developing ARMD. The more a person smokes, the higher the risk of macular degeneration. Moreover, the adverse effects of smoking persist, even fifteen to twenty years after quitting.

Poor dietary habits contribute as well. A diet high in saturated fats may clog the vessels leading to the eyes, thus reducing the flow of nutrient-rich blood. Excess fat may deposit itself directly in the mem-

---

In the News: Proton Beam Therapy for Wet Macular Degeneration

While use for the control of macular degeneration is still in the experimental stage, proton beam therapy may retard the development of wet macular degeneration. Proton beam therapy was developed in 1946, but its use in a clinical setting began in the 1980's. In 1990, Loma Linda University Medical Center (LLUMC) was established as the first proton beam treatment center. Generally used for the treatment of cancer, proton beam therapy uses energized protons (charged particles) to deliver a localized, uniform dose of energy to the target site. Proton beam therapy can be delivered with greater precision than can conventional radiation therapy, thus avoiding unnecessary damage to surrounding tissue.

In March, 1994, LLUMC researchers began to study the use of this therapy in the treatment of wet macular degeneration by inhibiting blood vessel growth. Researchers there reported that 90 percent of patients treated showed improvement with no further loss of vision during the twenty-one months of follow-up study. In 1999, the results of a later study of fifty patients showed that vision improved or remained stable in 65 percent of them eighteen months after treatment. Control of lesions was seen in 89 percent of the patients, including those who could not be treated by lasers because of lesion location and size. Other researchers emphasize, however, that long-term studies are still needed to ascertain the potential for later damage.

—Betty Richardson, Ph.D.

brane behind the retina. In this case, nutrients might not be able to pass through the "fat wall" to reach the cells that nourish the retina. There is evidence that eating fresh fruits and dark green leafy vegetables (such as spinach and collard greens) may delay or reduce the severity of age-related macular degeneration.

Some studies indicate that the mineral zinc might affect the development of macular degeneration. Zinc is important to chemical reactions in the retina. It is highly concentrated in the eye, particularly in the retina and the tissues surrounding the macula. Older people may have low levels of zinc because of poor diet or poor absorption from food. Some doctors believe that zinc supplements may slow down the progress of macular degeneration. Studies are not complete, however, and there are some adverse side effects of zinc supplements. They might interfere with other important trace metals such as copper, and in some people, the long-term use of zinc can cause digestive problems and anemia.

Strong sunlight seems to accelerate macular degeneration. Wearing special sunglasses may decrease the progress of the disease.

An effective test to determine if a person has wet macular degeneration is fluorescent angiography. A special dye is injected into a vein in the patient's arm and then flows to the blood vessels in the eye. Photographs are taken of the retina. The dye highlights any problems in the blood vessels and allows the doctor to determine if they can be treated. Annual eye examinations that include dilation of the pupils are also useful in early detection. Early detection is important because a person destined to develop macular degeneration can sometimes be treated before symptoms appear, which may delay or reduce the severity of the disease. Anyone who notices a change in vision should contact an ophthalmologist immediately.

TREATMENT AND THERAPY

People with macular degeneration learn to make use of the areas just outside the macula to see details. This ability to look slightly off center usually improves with time, though vision is never as good as it was before the macula was damaged.

A number of aids can help people with ARMD make the most of their remaining vision. Some low-vision aids include magnifying glasses, special lenses, electronic systems, and large-print books and newspapers. Sound aids include books on audiotape

and products equipped with voice synthesizers such as calculators and computers. Using lamps that provide direct lighting for reading or tasks that require close vision, keeping curtains open, and painting walls and ceilings white make it easier for macular degeneration patients to see in the home.

There is no proven medical treatment for dry macular degeneration. In some cases of wet macular degeneration, laser photocoagulation is effective in sealing leaking or bleeding vessels. Laser photocoagulation usually does not restore vision but does prevent further loss. The surgery can be performed in a doctor's office or in an eye clinic on an outpatient basis.

Three other treatments have shown promise. One is surgery to reposition the retina. The doctor cuts through the outer layer of the eye to gain access to the retina, which can then be detached and repositioned without cutting. This technique enables the surgeon to maneuver the center of the macula away from the leaking blood vessels and place it next to healthier eye tissue.

Low-level radiation can also be used to stop blood vessel proliferation. The radiation is carefully measured to be high enough to stop the growth but low enough so that the retina is not damaged.

The third treatment is to inject photosensitive chemicals into the bloodstream of people with macular degeneration and to use lasers to stimulate those chemicals in the eye. When activated, the substances halt the proliferation of blood vessels. If blood vessels begin to grow again, repeat doses can be administered without adverse side effects.

PERSPECTIVE AND PROSPECTS

Age-related macular degeneration (ARMD) affects about 15 percent of the U.S. population by age fifty-five and over 30 percent by age seventy-five. It is the leading cause of legal blindness in people over the age of sixty-five.

A radical and controversial treatment was made by a team of doctors from the University of Chicago Medical Center in 1997. They took cells from the retina of an aborted fetus and surgically transplanted them into the severely impaired left eye of an eighty-four-year-old patient. The transplanted cells proliferated, forming minute projections that stretched toward the patient's macula.

Fetal cells can divide and thus increase in number. Also they are likely to continue functioning for a number of years. Because the fetal cells are immature, they provoke little or no response from a transplant recipient's immune system. In the short term, the transplant appeared successful, but long-term results were not yet available. Because of the radical nature of the operation, the patient selected was severely impaired and had no other hope for improvement. Moreover, some people protested the use of cells from an aborted fetus. The need for severely impaired patients and ethical concerns virtually stopped research into this surgical procedure.

—*Billie M. Taylor, M.A.*

See also Aging; Blindness; Blurred vision; Cataracts; Eye surgery; Eyes; Fetal tissue transplantation; Laser use in surgery; Myopia; Ophthalmology; Smoking; Visual disorders.

FOR FURTHER INFORMATION:

D'Amato, Robert, and Joan Snyder. *Macular Degeneration: The Latest Scientific Discoveries and Treatments for Preserving Your Sight*. New York: Walker, 2000. Ophthalmologist and noted researcher D'Amato here teams up with macular degeneration patient Snyder to write a reassuring, hopeful, and informative book providing the facts sufferers need to understand the disorder, handle treatment options, and live successfully with low vision.

Munson, Marty, and Yun Lee. "See Better Days." *Prevention* 48, no. 9 (September, 1996): 32-34. New research suggests that certain compounds in fruits and vegetables may be able to keep people seeing clearly even if their eyes have fallen prey to macular degeneration. It seems more clear that age-related macular degeneration is a nutrition-responsive disease.

Munson, Marty, Therese Walsh, and Yun Lee. "Please Pass the Butter: Skipping the Fat May Save Your Sight." *Prevention* 448, no. 1 (January, 1996). Preliminary research links fatty foods to early age-related macular degeneration (ARMD). Fat can clog the vessels leading to the eyes, reducing the flow of nutrient-rich blood.

Pennisi, Elizabeth. "Gene Found for the Fading Eyesight of Old Age." *Science* 277, no. 5333 (September 19, 1997). Macular degeneration is a disease that destroys the macula, the part of the retina that sees fine details, and is the most common cause of uncorrectable vision loss in the elderly. New research has discovered that mutations in a gene called ATP-binding cassette transporter-retina (ABCR) may account for 16 percent of the age-related cases.

Ross, Linda M., ed. *Ophthalmic Disorders Sourcebook*. Detroit: Omnigraphics, 1997. This book makes reliable information available to those afflicted with ophthalmic diseases and disorders. This comprehensive collection of authoritative information presents material in a nontechnical, humanitarian style for patients, their families, and caregivers.

Seppa, Nathan. "New Treatments for Macular Degeneration." *Science News* 152, no. 13 (September 27, 1997). Three new treatments are showing promise in the treatment of wet macular degeneration: surgery to reposition the retina, low-level radiation to stanch blood flow, and photochemical dyes that assail the offending blood vessels.

Wolfe, Yun Lee. "'Rays' Your Eyesight: Radiation May Stabilize Age-Related Blindness." *Prevention* 49, no. 4 (April, 1997). Recent studies show that X-rays may hold the brightest hope for treating macular degeneration. Radiation therapy can improve the "wet" type of age-related macular degeneration.

MAGNETIC FIELD THERAPY
PROCEDURE

ANATOMY OR SYSTEM AFFECTED: Cells, immune system

SPECIALTIES AND RELATED FIELDS: Alternative medicine

DEFINITION: A practical and inexpensive modality that uses magnets to relieve chronic and acute pain incurred through overuse or trauma.

INDICATIONS AND PROCEDURES

In this treatment method, which is based on physics principles called the Hall effect and Faraday's law, magnetic pads are placed on or near the site of injury or soreness in order to stimulate local circulation by attracting positive and negatively charged ions in the blood and lymph. This biomagnetic attraction of electrolytes utilizes an alternating pattern of polarities that penetrate 5 to 20 centimeters into the body's tissues, depending on field strength (which is normally between 300 and 950 gauss). A common magnet will not produce this effect because only the ions and fluid in vessels that are precisely in line with the north-south poles will be attracted. Many advocates claim that magnetic therapy works faster than diathermies such as ultrasound. A warm tingling sensation is often felt minutes after application because of the increase of microcirculation, which brings more oxygen, nutrients, white blood cells, and antibodies to the damaged tissues and which removes metabolic waste products.

USES AND COMPLICATIONS

Several forms of magnetic field therapy (including pulsed electromagnetic therapy) have been used for years in Japan, Germany, and other countries, and double-blind studies are being conducted in the United States to determine the validity of numerous testimonials. Disorders that are regularly treated with magnetic therapy in other countries include carpal tunnel syndrome, osteoarthritis, tendinitis, bursitis, migraine headaches, and energy problems such as chronic fatigue syndrome and malaise. Magnetic deficiency syndrome is now documented in Japanese medical literature, and many American physicians agree that proper magnetic balance in the tissues is an overlooked ingredient to health.

Magnetic pads come in several sizes and shapes to allow for comfortable attachment to any area of the body, including silver dollar-sized pads that are one-eighth of an inch thick, for concentrated force, and 5-by-7-inch pads for larger areas such as the back. Magnetic massage balls, mattress pads, pillows, seat cushions, and orthotic insoles are also sold. The magnets are permanently charged and have no harmful side effects, although they are not recommended for pregnant women or patients wearing pacemakers.

—*Daniel G. Graetzer, Ph.D.*

See also Alternative medicine; Bursitis; Carpal tunnel syndrome; Chronic fatigue syndrome; Circulation; Fatigue; Migraine headaches; Osteoarthritis; Pain management; Tendon disorders.

FOR FURTHER INFORMATION:

Goldberg, Burton, comp. *Alternative Medicine: The Definitive Guide.* Puyallup, Wash.: Future Medicine, 1993.

Jacobs, Jennifer, ed. *The Encyclopedia of Alternative Medicine: A Complete Family Guide to Complementary Therapies.* Rev. ed. Boston: Journey Edition, 1997.

Kastner, Mark, and Hugh Burroughs. *Alternative Healing: The Complete A-Z Guide to over 160 Different Alternative Therapies.* New York: Henry Holt, 1996.

MAGNETIC RESONANCE IMAGING (MRI)

PROCEDURE

ANATOMY OR SYSTEM AFFECTED: All

SPECIALTIES AND RELATED FIELDS: Biotechnology, nuclear medicine, radiology

DEFINITION: A noninvasive, nonradiological method of obtaining detailed information concerning normal and diseased tissue.

KEY TERMS:

electromagnetic waves: a convenient way of understanding energy as a wave; visible light, X rays, and radiowaves, which have the longest wavelength and lowest energy, are the most familiar examples

Fourier-transform: a mathematical method which allows MRI to utilize one radiofrequency pulse and thereby examine all wavelengths, as opposed to examining each wavelength individually with a continuous wave

nucleus: the dense, positively charged, central core of an atom, containing its massive protons and neutrons

zeugmatography: a name applied to MRI characterizing the close relationship of nuclear magnetic

---

MRI Scanning

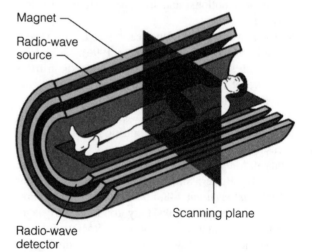

Magnet

Radio-wave source

Scanning plane

Radio-wave detector

This diagnostic imaging technique employs a powerful magnet to generate a magnetic field that is capable of aligning the protons in the body's hydrogen atoms, which are then knocked out of alignment by radio-wave pulses; as the protons realign, they emit radio signals that can be detected and used to create a cross-sectional image of the body.

forces and electromagnetic waves (from the Greek *zeugma*, meaning "to yoke together")

INDICATIONS AND PROCEDURES

In 1901, Wilhelm Conrad Röntgen won the first Nobel Prize in Physics for his discovery of X rays. Twentieth century applications of this radiation have produced medical miracles. Magnetic resonance imaging (MRI), often called nuclear magnetic resonance (NMR or nmr) imaging, differs in fundamental ways from X rays and other imaging methods. It is capable of producing a far richer array of three-dimensional images without the dangers attendant on ionizing radiation or the introduction of radioactive chemicals. MRI allows both safe diagnosis and study in healthy subjects. Furthermore, the method can be used to examine flowing matter, such as in the circulatory system.

The nuclei of hydrogen atoms behave like tiny magnets when they are placed in a magnetic field. When radiowaves are superimposed on the magnetic waves, hydrogen atoms can be made to change their alignment with the magnetic field. The time required for the atoms to return to their original orientation, after the radiowaves cease, varies with the nature of the tissue in which the hydrogen atoms reside. This combination of natural circumstances together with the marvels of modern electronics have made it possible to obtain detailed images of brain tumors, spinal fluid, and blood vessels.

The discovery, in the mid-1940's, by Edward M. Purcell and Felix Bloch of the basic techniques of nuclear magnetic resonance won for them the 1952 Nobel Prize in Physics. Their innovation changed dramatically the practice of chemistry, biochemistry, and biology. Following new theoretical and practical contributions, diagnostic medicine is participating fully in this revolution.

Both permanent magnets and electromagnets are used, and each has advantages, but the superconducting magnet is rapidly becoming the standard. The essential factors in producing detailed images are constant field strength and a highly uniform field. A transmit-

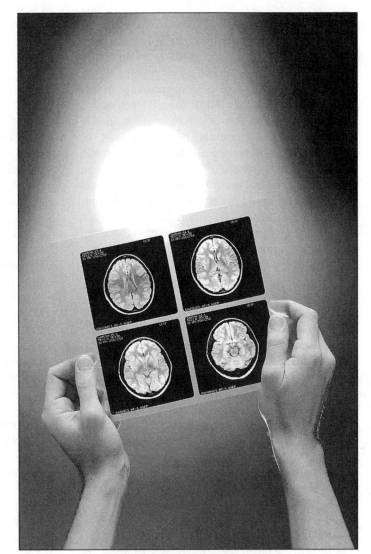

MRI scans of the head. (Digital Stock)

ter, connected to a radiofrequency transmitter-receiver, is used to broadcast the signal and to receive the signal returned from the patient. A short but intense pulse of radiofrequency power is required, and its duration is critical to control electronic noise, which obscures the signal required to form the final image. These signals must be processed by complex computer methods to allow the final image to be displayed.

During the 1970's, several innovations were introduced allowing broad application of the MRI technique. Paul Lauterbur demonstrated the generation of spatial maps by rotating the object to obtain a series of projections from which an image can be reconstructed. His method, called nmr zeugmatography, introduced a radically new approach to MRI. By superimposing a magnetic field gradient on the main magnetic field, it is possible to make the resonance frequency a function of the spatial origin of the signal. Later, Richard R. Ernst built on his earlier introduction of Fourier-transform NMR to develop methods of "two-dimensional nmr." Such techniques provide detailed information concerning the local structure of large molecules of biological importance. He was awarded the 1991 Nobel Prize in Chemistry because this same method laid the groundwork for the clinical use of MRI. Methods are now available for the creation of three- and four-dimensional MRI, which are important in protein studies and which promise future applications in nonchemical research.

Uses and Complications

MRI has been used in the evaluation of a wide variety of medical situations. The earliest uses involved the brain and the spinal cord, where it is absolutely necessary to avoid high-energy radiation or radioactivity. Since MRI is capable of providing excellent soft-tissue images and of penetrating bony and air-filled structures, it is also well suited to examination of the chest and abdomen. In these applications, it was first necessary to overcome problems associated with motion. A further important modification, the flow imaging technique, allows the use of MRI in studies of the vascular system and has led to magnetic resonance angiography. This latter approach has clear advantages over the invasive X-ray procedure. Additional modifications allow the direct study of tissues of living organisms under physiological conditions.

In spite of the broad applicability of MRI, there are limitations. Patients on life support systems or with unstable physiological conditions must be evaluated with other imaging techniques. The presence of a magnetic metal apparatus in the body is another limitation. There have also been discussions concerning effects that might be related to the electrical currents induced by magnetic gradient fields.

—*K. Thomas Finley, Ph.D.*

See also Computed tomography (CT) scanning; Imaging and radiology; Noninvasive tests; Nuclear medicine; Positron emission tomography (PET) scanning; Radiopharmaceuticals; Ultrasonography.

For Further Information:

Buxton, Richard B. *An Introduction to Functional Magnetic Resonance Imaging: Principles and Techniques*. New York: Cambridge University Press, 2001. Designed for the medical professional, this guide covers all aspects of magnetic resonance imaging.

Cahill, Donald R., Matthew J. Orland, and Gary M. Miller. *Atlas of Human Cross-sectional Anatomy: With CT and MR Images*. 3d ed. New York: Wiley-Liss, 1995. Discusses such topics as X-ray computed tomography and magnetic resonance imaging. Includes bibliographical references and an index.

Smith, Michael B., K. Kirk Shung, and Timothy J. Mosher. "Magnetic Resonance Imaging." In *Principles of Medical Imaging*, edited by Shung, Smith, and Benjamin M. W. Tsui. San Diego, Calif.: Academic Press, 1992. A chapter in a text devoted to biophysics and diagnostic imaging. Includes bibliographical references and an index.

Wehrli, Felix W. "The Origins and Future of Nuclear Magnetic Resonance Imaging." *Physics Today* 45 (June, 1992): 34-42. Although nuclear magnetic resonance began as a curiosity of physics, magnetic resonance imaging (MRI) has become the preeminent method of medical imaging. A look at how MRI works is presented.

Malabsorption

Disease/disorder

Anatomy or system affected: Gallbladder, gastrointestinal system, intestines, liver, pancreas, stomach

Specialties and related fields: Biochemistry, biotechnology, family practice, gastroenterology, genetics, neonatology, nutrition, pediatrics

Definition: The impaired absorption of nutrients from food into the bloodstream.

Causes and Symptoms

The nutritive components of food—carbohydrates, protein, fats, vitamins, and minerals—must be digested in the gastrointestinal tract and absorbed into the circulatory system to be of use to the body. Malabsorption of these nutrients is caused by specific defects in any one of the many separate processes involved in the digestion and absorption of food. It is also the result of general impairment of the structure or function of the gastrointestinal tract.

Malabsorption leads to poor growth when it affects the uptake of any essential nutrient, which is one that must be obtained from the diet. It may cause diarrhea if one of the more abundant constituents of food is not absorbed; carbohydrate malabsorption will usually lead to a watery diarrhea, while protein and fat malabsorption will cause a foul-smelling diarrhea that is dark or whitish, respectively. Diarrhea itself may reduce the absorption of nutrients.

Cystic fibrosis is one the most common causes of malabsorption in children. The mucus accompanying this disease is secreted into the gastrointestinal tract; it is largely indigestible and can obstruct the passage of nutrients.

TREATMENT AND THERAPY

Treatment for malabsorption depends entirely on its cause. In the case of bacterial infections that affect intestinal function, treatment with appropriate antibiotics will return this function to normal. In celiac sprue, an intolerance to the gluten found in wheat and other grains that alters the absorptive surface of the intestines, the removal of gluten from the diet restores normal activity. Some specific defects can be cured by the elimination or replacement of the dietary constituent that is not well digested or absorbed. In other cases, no curative treatment is known, as with cystic fibrosis.

PERSPECTIVE AND PROSPECTS

In 1825, William Beaumont, a U.S. Army surgeon, was the first to study human digestion in the stomach. Since then, the processes of digestion and absorption have become well understood, as have many of the causes of acquired and inherited malabsorption. Effective treatment has been developed in all but the most intractable cases. It is hoped that progress in understanding the genetic basis for inherited malabsorption will lead to earlier and definitive identification of affected individuals and eventually to suitable therapies.

—James L. Robinson, Ph.D.

See also Allergies; Celiac sprue; Cystic fibrosis; Diarrhea and dysentery; Digestion; Gastroenterology; Gastroenterology, pediatric; Gastrointestinal system; Malnutrition; Nutrition.

FOR FURTHER INFORMATION:

Christian, Janet L., and Janet L. Greger. *Nutrition for Living.* 4th ed. Redwood City, Calif.: Benjamin/ Cummings, 1994.

Jackson, Gordon, and Philip Whitfield. *Digestion: Fueling the System.* New York: Torstar Books, 1984.

Janowitz, Henry D. *Indigestion: Living Better with Upper Intestinal Problems.* New York: Oxford University Press, 1992.

MALARIA

DISEASE/DISORDER

ANATOMY OR SYSTEM AFFECTED: Blood, brain, liver, nervous system

SPECIALTIES AND RELATED FIELDS: Epidemiology, hematology, public health, serology

DEFINITION: A serious parasitic infection borne by mosquitoes in tropical and subtropical regions and characterized by recurrent bouts of severe fever, chills, sweating, vomiting, and damage to kidneys, blood, brain, and liver.

KEY TERMS:

Anopheles: the genus of mosquito that transmits malaria parasites to human hosts

falciparum, ovale, malariae, vivax: the species or kinds of *Plasmodium* parasites that cause malaria in humans

merozoite: the stage of the malaria parasite's residence in the human host at which the red blood cells are infected

oocyst: the encysted or encapsulated ookinete in the wall of an infected mosquito's stomach

ookinete: the fertilized form of the malaria parasite in the mosquito's body

Plasmodium: the genus of the protozoan parasite that contains the different species of malaria parasites that infect humans

pulmonary edema: accumulation of fluid in the lungs, which may lead to death

schizogony: the process in which sporozoites develop into merozoites within the liver of a human host

schizont: a multinucleate parasite that reproduces by schizogony

vector: an organism (such as a mosquito) that transmits a pathogen (such as the malaria parasite), especially from one human to another

CAUSES AND SYMPTOMS

Malaria in humans is caused by one of four species of protozoan parasites of the genus *Plasmodium*: *P. falciparum*, *P. vivax*, *P. ovale*, and *P. malariae*. The most severe form of malaria is caused by *P. falciparum*; the symptoms of this type include fever and chills occurring at irregular intervals. *P. vivax* is the most widespread parasite, causing most of the malaria infections in the world; this type of malaria results in recurrent periods of fever known as relapses. *P. malariae* is also widespread but has a patchier distribution than *P. falciparum* or *P. vivax*. *P. malariae* is common in many parts of Central Africa. It also occurs in India, Malaya, the East Indies, New Guinea, North Africa, and South America. *P. ovale* is found primarily in tropical Africa. These parasites belong to the subphylum Sporoza and the family Plasmodiidae. Malaria parasites also infect birds, lizards, and monkeys; the *Culex* mosquito carries parasites that infect birds. These other forms of malaria do not infect humans.

People may carry the malaria parasite but not develop the disease. Many variables determine whether the disease develops from *Plasmodium* infection. A person's age and genetic makeup, the species of the parasite, the density of the infection, and duration of exposure to mosquitoes carrying the parasites may influence the severity of the disease.

The clinical aspects of malaria are varied. Often a person with malaria has shaking chills to drenching sweats to intense fevers. Severe, complicated malaria is most often caused by *P. falciparum*; about 80 percent of the deaths from this parasite are caused by cerebral malaria, which is characterized by altered consciousness and often coma. Renal failure, hypoglycemia, severe anemia, pulmonary edema, and shock may also play a role in fatal malaria cases. Pregnant women that contract malaria may miscarry. They may also suffer severe anemia. If they survive childhood, people in areas of endemic malaria may have a moderate level of resistance to the disease. They often suffer recurrent but nonfatal fevers.

A definitive diagnosis of malaria is made by microscopic examination of stained blood smears for the presence of parasites. Because the parasite may disappear from the blood during the process of

Cycle of Malaria Infection

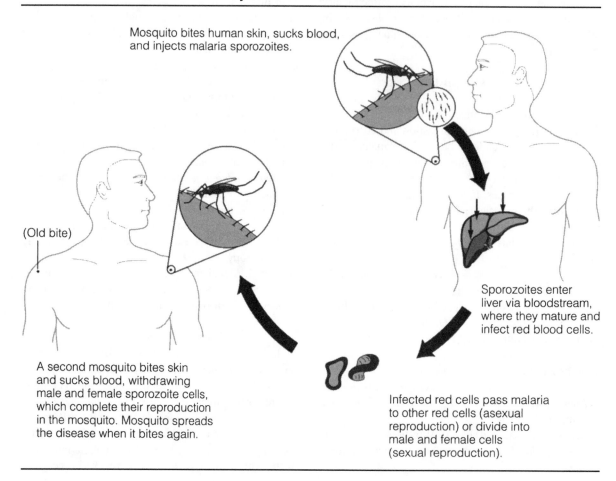

Mosquito bites human skin, sucks blood, and injects malaria sporozoites.

(Old bite)

A second mosquito bites skin and sucks blood, withdrawing male and female sporozoite cells, which complete their reproduction in the mosquito. Mosquito spreads the disease when it bites again.

Sporozoites enter liver via bloodstream, where they mature and infect red blood cells.

Infected red cells pass malaria to other red cells (asexual reproduction) or divide into male and female cells (sexual reproduction).

schizogony or not be visible in its early stages, blood smears must be taken at frequent intervals to diagnose the disease properly.

Of the twenty-five hundred known species of mosquitoes worldwide, only fifty to sixty species of the genus *Anopheles* transmit malarial parasites to humans by their bite. *Anopheles* mosquitoes are both a host and a vector of the malaria parasite. The females need blood meals to reproduce; it is during this biting and sucking of blood that the malaria parasite is passed to the human or the protozoan parasite is introduced into the mosquito's own system. During feeding, the mosquito injects a small amount of saliva into the host to increase blood flow to the area. Sporozoites are transmitted to the human host by this salivary fluid.

Anopheles mosquitoes can be identified from other genera of mosquitoes by their characteristic stance; they appear to be standing on their heads. (Other mosquitoes hold their bodies parallel to the surface on which they are resting.) The mosquito has four stages of growth: egg, larva, pupa, and adult. It is the bite of the adult *Anopheles* mosquito that transmits the malaria parasite to the human host. An adult mosquito will emerge from an egg in seven to twenty days. Females live at least a month.

The life cycle of the malaria parasite is complex. It has three phases in the mosquito and two in the human host; twelve different life history stages exist. The parasite is transmitted to humans as the sporozoite forms in the saliva of infected female *Anopheles* mosquitoes.

After entering the human host, the sporozoites invade liver cells, where during the next five to fifteen days, they develop into schizonts. Each schizont contains between ten thousand and thirty thousand daughter parasites called merozoites. The merozoites are released from the liver cells and invade the red blood cells. Once inside a red blood cell, the merozoite matures into a schizont containing eight to thirty-two new merozoites. The red blood cell ruptures and releases these merozoites so that they can invade additional red blood cells. The rupturing of the red blood cells is associated with fever and signals the clinical onset of malaria. Some merozoites differentiate into sexual forms, gametocytes, which are ingested by a mosquito during its next blood meal. Once in the mosquito, the sexual forms leave the blood cells, and male and female gametes fuse to form a zygote. In twelve to forty-eight hours, the zygote elongates to form an ookinete, which penetrates the wall of the mosquito's stomach and becomes an oocyst. During the next seven days or more, depending on the species of *Plasmodium* and the temperature in the gut of the mosquito, the oocyst enlarges, forming more than ten thousand sporozoites. The oocyst ruptures, and its sporozoites immigrate to the mosquito's salivary glands. The sporozoites are then injected into the next human host that the female mosquito bites.

Mosquitoes seek their hosts in response to a combination of chemical and physical stimuli, including carbon dioxide plumes, body odors, color, warmth, and movement of the host. Anopheline mosquitoes feed most frequently at night or in heavily shaded or dark areas during the early morning hours.

TREATMENT AND THERAPY

It is still not understood why some people develop the disease malaria after being infected by the *Plasmodium* parasite from an *Anopheles* mosquito's bite while others do not. *P. falciparum* causes almost all the cases of severe and complicated malaria. Cerebral malaria, hypoglycemia, and malarial anemia are all serious diseases caused by this parasite. Fluid concentration in the lungs, kidney failure, and enlargement of the spleen also may occur with this disease.

Even without complications, malaria has a variety of symptoms: fever, headache, malaise, cough, nausea, vomiting, and diarrhea. Visitors to areas where malaria is found benefit from preventive drug therapy. Chloroquine is effective and safe, but chloroquine-resistant *P. falciparum* and *P. vivax* require alternative drugs for malaria prevention, such as mefloquine. While residents in malaria zones have no optimal treatment alternatives, the drugs dapsone and pyrimethamine, used to protect pregnant women from malaria, have been effective in Gambia.

Microscopic examination of blood smears provides definitive proof of infection by malaria parasites. Two drops of blood, usually from the tip of a finger pricked by a lancet, are placed on a glass microscope slide. One is smeared to a thin film, and both are air-dried. Chemicals are then added that fix and stain the parasites so that they are visible through a microscope. The quantitative buffy coat (QBC) technique, based on fluorescence microscopy, is also used to detect the presence of the malaria parasite; however, it is more expensive than usual microscopic screening and requires more technical equipment. Immunoassays are also possible diagnostic tools for malaria detection.

Controlling malaria is focused on destroying the *Anopheles* mosquito. If the females bearing the malarial parasite do not bite a human host, the vector chain is broken and the disease will be prevented. Once a female mosquito is infected, however, it remains so for life. Spraying of insecticides to kill adult mosquitoes is the best antivector method in malaria control. Long-lasting or residual insecticides are preferred. The use of chemicals to kill the larvae of *Anopheles* mosquitoes in aquatic habitats has only limited application. Other ways to destroy mosquito larvae include intermittent flushing of ponds with fresh water; aquatic plant control; use of larvae-eating fishes, such as mosquito fish (*Gambusia affinis*); and covering or draining hatching sites such as wells, small ponds, or water barrels.

There are many simple ways that individuals may protect themselves from mosquitoes bearing the malaria parasite. Repellents, such as skin lotions or those applied or built into clothing, may work well. Mosquito coils, material that releases insecticide when burned, may be used. Netting impregnated with insecticide around beds and screens on the windows and doors of homes will often prevent mosquitoes from entering and biting human hosts.

The economic cost of malaria is high, but precise estimates of its exact economic impact are difficult to make. Premature death, loss of productivity as a result of illness, and the failure to grow certain crops or to use new lands productively occur because of the presence of malaria. The costs of medical treatment for the disease may also be high, especially for those in poor countries. Migration to find work or to avoid malaria often spreads the disease to other areas.

About 40 percent of the world's population lives where malaria may occur. This is primarily in the tropics, but malaria can also be found in temperate regions, including the Middle East and Asia. Malaria is present in 102 countries and causes millions of clinical cases and several million deaths each year. Control of this disease was partially successful in the 1950's and 1960's, but by the 1970's and 1980's, cases of malaria were increasing worldwide.

Drug-resistant strains of *P. falciparum* and *P. vivax* reduce the effectiveness of drugs used to treat the disease. The mosquitoes that carry malaria to humans are now resistant to some chemicals that were once able to kill them. Some of the vector mosquitoes avoid insecticide-treated surfaces, making control of *Anopheles* mosquitoes less effective.

People who travel to many different parts of the world may expose themselves to the threat of malaria. The lack of adequate health care facilities and the often-critical economic conditions in malaria-infected areas of the world prevent effective malaria control and its eradication. In fact, although considered a single disease, malaria is more correctly viewed as many diseases, each different because of biological, ecological, sociological, and economic conditions that interact to determine its final morbidity (rate of incidence) and mortality (fatality rate) within a population. While malariologists do not agree on how best to treat and control this disease, it is agreed that malaria must be attacked on the local, regional, and global levels for any control to be effective.

Effective treatment of malaria requires trained personnel and the efforts and resources of health care organizations. More funds are needed for research on the development of a malaria vaccine. Long-term, guaranteed support for malaria research must be provided by funding agencies. Malaria surveillance should monitor high-risk groups and detect potential malaria epidemics early in their development. Drug discovery and development must also continue so that drug-resistant strains of malaria can be treated with new medicines. Better vector control methods should be developed.

The most basic priority in malaria control is to prevent infected individuals from becoming severely ill and dying. Effective clinical treatment involves diagnostic and referral actions that provide treatment for infected patients in the early stages of the disease. Personal protection measures, such as insecticide-treated netting, screens, and mosquito coils, reduce the risk of infection for individuals living in endemic areas. Draining or filling small bodies of water where mosquito larvae develop and widespread use of residue insecticides are needed to reduce vector mosquito populations. Malaria control is in crisis in many areas of the world; it represents one of the greatest challenges for health professionals.

PERSPECTIVE AND PROSPECTS

European colonization of the New World probably spread malaria to the Americas; it is unclear if the disease existed there before that time. Malaria became one of the most widespread and dehabilitating diseases of early North America. *P. vivax* and *P. malariae* were introduced by the English in 1607 when they settled Jamestown, Virginia. The importation of African slaves in 1620 brought the virulent *P. falciparum* to North America. Boston was hard hit by malaria-related illness and death in the seventeenth century, and in the eighteenth and nineteenth centuries, malaria was endemic in the southern and western portions of the Colonies. During the Civil War, eight thousand soldiers died from malaria and 1.2 million cases of the disease were recorded. As recently as the early 1900's, 500,000 cases of malaria were reported each year in the United States, most occurring in the South.

European explorers found South Americans using cinchona tree bark to combat fevers. In 1639, Jesuit missionaries brought some of the bark to Europe, where it became a popular treatment. It was not until 1820, however, that French chemists Pierre-Joseph Pelletier and Joseph-Bienaimé Caventou identified quinine as the active ingredient in cinchona bark that effectively fought these fevers.

In 1846, the Italian physician Giovanni Rasori theorized that a parasite caused malaria. In 1880, Charles-Louis-Alphonse Laveran, a French army medical officer, observed live parasites in blood taken from a feverish soldier in Algeria. In 1898, Giovanni Battista Grassi, Amico Bignami, and Guiseppe Bastianelli documented the transmission of human malaria parasites by *Anopheles* mosquito bites. Sir Ronald Ross, a British military doctor, did research on malaria transmission at the same time as the Italian team. Sir Patrick Manson was the first scientist to speculate that mosquitoes spread malaria, but Ross was the first to demonstrate the complete cycle of malaria in mosquitoes. Ross was awarded the Nobel Prize in Physiology or Medicine in 1902 for his work on malaria.

The first efforts to control malaria were made by the Greeks and Romans in the sixth century B.C.E. when they drained many marshy areas. Malaria control by drainage had minimal success, however, until the twentieth century. General William C. Gorgas directed a complex malaria control program during the construction of the Panama Canal from 1904 to 1914. This program included drainage, application of chemicals to kill the larval stage of the mosquitoes, and treatment of workers in the malaria zone of the Panama Canal with quinine. Malaria was eliminated from the Canal Zone by 1910.

From the mid-1940's through the mid-1950's, public health officials tried to eradicate malaria throughout the world. The development of the powerful insecticide DDT during World War II made this erad-

ication seem possible. DDT was sprayed widely to kill *Anopheles* mosquitoes. The World Health Organization (WHO) directed this effort, and by the mid-1960's malaria was essentially controlled in North America and Europe. It had become evident, however, that eradication was not technically or economically feasible in many areas of the world. In 1969, WHO malaria control efforts shifted from eradication to control. Because of the environmental problems that it caused, DDT was banned from use in the United States in 1972 and its production in the United States stopped in 1982. More toxic and expensive insecticides, such as dieldrin and malathion, were used to replace DDT in mosquito control actions.

Beginning in the early 1970's, resistance by the *Plasmodium* parasite to antimalarial drugs became prevalent. In many areas of the world, no effective drugs exist to control malaria. Chloroquine, once the treatment of choice for *P. falciparum*, is of limited effectiveness. Research using irradiated sporozoites, however, indicates that development of a vaccine for malaria may be possible. In addition, the antimalarial drugs mefloquine and halofantrine are useful in fighting the disease. Yet political and social instability has increased the incidence of this disease by limiting or preventing its eradication and treatment. A shortage of malariologists also complicates fighting this disease. In 1986, 2.3 million deaths and 489 million clinical cases of malaria were reported.

Many governmental and private organizations around the world support malaria prevention, research, and control efforts. The World Bank, the European Commission, and WHO contribute extensively to solving this disease problem. In the United States, the U.S. Agency for International Development (USAID), the Centers for Disease Control (CDC), the Department of Defense (DOD), and the National Institute of Allergy and Infectious Diseases (NIAD) of the National Institutes of Health (NIH) all work to reduce the effects of malaria.

—*David L. Chesemore, Ph.D.*

See also Arthropod-borne diseases; Bites and stings; Centers for Disease Control and Prevention (CDC); Epidemiology; National Insitutes of Health (NIH); Parasitic diseases; Protozoan diseases; Tropical medicine.

FOR FURTHER INFORMATION:

Biddle, Wayne. *Field Guide to Germs*. New York: Henry Holt, 1995. This comprehensive book is easily accessible to the nonspecialist and includes a discussion of nearly every virus, bacterium, and fungus known to cause human and nonhuman animal disease.

Butcher, G. A. *Malaria: The Intelligent Traveller's Guide*. Canberra, Australia: ANUTECH, 1990. This popular work offers helpful advice for travelers who seek to avoid malaria.

Litsios, Socrates. *The Tomorrow of Malaria*. Karori, New Zealand: Pacific Press, 1996. An account of the history of malaria. Includes a bibliography and an index.

Oaks, Stanley C., Jr., Violaine S. Mitchell, Greg W. Pearson, and Charles C. J. Carpenter, eds. *Malaria: Obstacles and Opportunities*. Washington, D.C.: National Academy Press, 1991. One of the best books available, with information about malaria all over the world.

Poser, Charles M., G. W. Bruyn. *An Illustrated History of Malaria*. New York: Parthenon, 1999. Accessible to the lay reader, this text includes bibliographical references and an index.

MALIGNANCY AND METASTASIS
DISEASE/DISORDER

ANATOMY OR SYSTEM AFFECTED: All

SPECIALTIES AND RELATED FIELDS: Internal medicine, oncology, pathology, plastic surgery

DEFINITION: "Malignancy" is the uncontrolled growth of tumor cells that invade and compress surrounding tissues and break through the skin or barriers within the body; "metastasis" describes the tendency of malignant cells to break loose from their tumor of origin to travel to other locations within the body.

KEY TERMS:

benign tumors: tumors that grow relatively slowly, do not interfere with normal body functions, and do not metastasize

carcinogen: a natural or artificial substance inducing the transformation of cells toward the malignant state

chemotherapy: the use of chemicals to kill or inhibit the growth of cancer cells

multistep progression: the typical pathway of induction of cancer, beginning with an initial alteration to a gene and progressing to the fully malignant state

oncogene: a gene directly or indirectly inducing the transformation of cells from the normal to the malignant state; most oncogenes have normal counterparts in body cells

retrovirus: a virus infecting mammalian and other cells that sometimes carries and introduces oncogenes into host cells

transfection: a technique used to introduce genes into cells by exposing the cells to fragmented deoxyribonucleic acid (DNA) under conditions that promote the uptake and incorporation of DNA

tumor suppressor gene: a gene that, in its normal form, inhibits cell division

CAUSES AND SYMPTOMS

Cancer cells are characterized by two primary features. One of these is uncontrolled cell division: Cells enter an unregulated, rapid growth phase by losing the controls that normally limit division rates to the amount required for normal growth and maintenance of body tissues. The second feature is metastasis, in which tumor cells lose the connections that normally hold them in place in body tissues, break loose, and spread from their original sites to lodge and grow in other body locations. Tumor cells with these characteristics are described as malignant.

The detrimental effects of solid malignant tumors result from the interference of rapidly growing masses of cancer cells with the activities of normal tissues and organs, or from the loss of vital functions because of the conversion of cells with essential functions to nonfunctional forms. Some malignant tumors of glandular tissue upset bodily functions by producing and secreting excessive quantities of hormones.

Solid malignant tumors, as they grow, compress surrounding normal tissues; they destroy normal structures by cutting off blood supplies and interrupting nerve function. They may also break through barriers that separate major body regions, such as internal membranes and epithelia or the gut wall. They may also break through the skin. Such breakthroughs cause internal or external bleeding and infection, and they destroy the organization and separation of body regions necessary for normal function. Both compression and breakthroughs can cause pain that, in advanced cases, may become extreme.

Malignant tumors of blood tissues involve cell lines that normally divide to supply the body's requirements for red and white blood cells. Cancer in these cell lines crowds the bloodstream with immature, nonfunctional cells that are unable to accomplish required activities, such as the delivery of oxygen to tissues or the activation of the immune response.

When the total mass of actively growing and dividing malignant cells becomes large, their demands for nutrients may deprive normal cells, tissues, and organs of their needed supplies, leading to generally impaired functions, fatigue, weakness, and weight loss.

Not all unregulated tissue growths are malignant. Some tumors, such as common skin warts, are benign—they do not usually interfere with normal body functions. They grow relatively slowly and do not metastasize. Often, benign tumors are surrounded by a closed capsule of connective tissue that prevents or retards expansion and breakup. Some initially benign tumors, however, including even common skin warts, may change to malignant forms.

Individual cells of a malignant tumor exhibit differences from normal cells in activity, biochemistry, physiology, and structure. First and foremost is the characteristic of uncontrolled division. Cancer cells typically move through the division cycle much more rapidly than normal cells. The rapid division is accompanied by biochemical changes characteristic of dividing cells such as high metabolic rates; increases in the rate of transport of substances across the plasma membrane; increases in protein phosphorylation; raised cytoplasmic concentrations of sodium, potassium, and calcium ions; and an elevated pH. Often chromosomal abnormalities are present, including extra or missing chromosomes, exchanges of segments between chromosomes, and breakage.

Cancer cells also typically fail to develop all the characteristics and structures of fully mature cells of their type. They may also lose mature characteristics if these were attained before conversion to the malignant state. Frequently, loss of mature characteristics involves disorganization or disappearance of the cytoskeleton. Alterations are also noted in the structure and density of surface carbohydrate groups. Cancer cells lose tight attachments to their neighbors or to supportive extracellular materials such as collagen; some cancer cells secrete enzymes that break cell connections and destroy elements of the extracellular material, aiding their movement into and through surrounding tissues. If removed from the body and placed in test-tube cultures, most cancer cells have the capacity to divide indefinitely. In contrast, most normal body cells placed in a culture medium eventually stop dividing.

The conversion of normal cells to malignant types usually involves multiple causes inducing a series of changes that occur in stages over a considerable length of time. This characteristic is known as the multistep progression of cancer. In most cases, the complete sequence of steps leading from an initiating alteration to full malignancy is unknown.

The initial event in a multistep progression usually involves the alteration of a gene from a normal to an aberrant form known as an oncogene. The gene involved is typically one that regulates cell growth and division or that takes part in biochemical sequences with this effect. The alteration may involve substitutions or the loss of DNA sequences, the movement of the gene to a new location in the chromosomes, or the movement of another gene or its controlling elements to the vicinity of the gene. In some cases, the alteration involves a gene that in normal form suppresses cell division in cells in which it is active. Loss or alteration of function of such genes, known as tumor suppressor genes, can directly or indirectly increase growth and division rates.

An initiating genetic alteration may be induced by a long list of factors, including exposure to radiation or certain chemicals, the insertion of viral DNA into the chromosomes, or the generation of random mutations during the duplication of genetic material. In a few cancers, the initiating event involves the insertion of an oncogene into the DNA by an infecting virus that carries the oncogene as a part of its genetic makeup.

In some cases, about 5 percent in humans, an initiating oncogene or faulty tumor suppressor gene is inherited, producing a strong predisposition to the development of malignancy. Among these strongly predisposed cancers are familial retinoblastoma, familial adenomatous polyps of the colon, and multiple endocrine neoplasia, in which tumors develop in the thyroid, adrenal medulla, and parathyroid glands. In addition to the strongly predisposed cancers, some, including breast, ovarian, and colon cancers other than familial adenomatous polyps, show some degree of disposition in family lines—members of these families show a greater tendency to develop the cancer than individuals in other families.

Subsequent steps from the initiating change to the fully malignant state usually include the conversion of additional genes to oncogenic form or the loss of function of tumor suppressor genes. Also important during intermediate stages are further alterations to the initial and succeeding oncogenes that increase their activation. The initial conversion of a normal gene to oncogenic form by its movement to a new location in the chromosomes may be compounded at successive steps, for example, by sequence changes or the multiplication of the oncogene into extra copies. The subsequent steps in progression to the malignant state are driven by many of the sources of change responsible for the initiating step. Because genetic alterations often occur during the duplication and division of the genetic material, an increase in the cell division rate by the initiating change may increase the chance that further alterations leading to full malignancy will occur.

A change advancing the progression toward full malignancy may take place soon after a previous change or only after a long delay. Moreover, further changes may not occur, leaving the progression at an intermediate stage, without the development of full malignancy, for the lifetime of the individual. The avoidance of environmental factors inducing genetic alterations—such as overexposure to radiation sources such as sunlight, X rays, and radon gas and chemicals such as those in cigarette smoke—increases the chance that progressions toward malignancy will remain incomplete.

The last stage in progression to full malignancy is often metastasis. After the loss of normal adhesions to neighboring cells or to elements of the extracellular matrix, the separation and movement of cancer cells from a primary tumor to secondary locations may occur through the development of active motility or from breakage into elements of the circulatory system.

Relatively few of the cells breaking loose from a tumor survive the rigors of passage through the body. Most are destroyed by various factors, including deformation by passage through narrow capillaries and destruction by blood turbulence around the heart valves and vessel junctions. Furthermore, tumor cells often develop changes in their surface groups that permit detection and elimination by the immune system as they move through the body. Unfortunately, the rigors of travel through the body may act as a sort of natural selection for the cells that are most malignant—that is, those most able to resist destruction—and that can grow uncontrollably and spread by metastasis.

Many natural and artificial agents trigger the initial step in the progression to the malignant state or push cells through intermediate stages. Most of these agents, collectively called carcinogens, are chemicals or forms of radiation capable of inducing chemical changes in DNA. Some, however, may initiate or further this progression by modifying ribonucleic acids (RNAs) or proteins, or they may act by increasing the rate of DNA replication and cell division.

TREATMENT AND THERAPY

Cancer is treated most frequently by one or a combination of three primary techniques: surgical removal of tumors, radiation therapy, and chemotherapy. Surgical removal is most effective if the growth has remained localized so that the entire tumor can be detected and removed. Often, surgery is combined with radiation or chemotherapy in an attempt to eliminate malignant cells that have broken loose from a primary tumor and lodged in other parts of the body. Surgical removal followed by chemotherapy is presently the most effective treatment for most forms of cancer, especially if the tumor is detected and removed before extensive metastasis has taken place. Most responsive to surgical treatments have been skin cancers, many of which are easily detected and remain localized and accessible.

Radiation therapy may be directed toward the destruction of a tumor in a specific body location. Alternatively, it may be used in whole-body exposure to kill cancer cells that have metastasized and lodged in many body regions. In either case, the method takes advantage of the destructive effects of radiation on DNA, particularly during periods when the DNA is under duplication. Because cancer cells undergo replication at higher rates than most other body cells, the technique is more selective for tumors than for normal tissues. The selection is only partial, however, so that body cells that divide rapidly, such as those of the blood, hair follicles, and intestinal lining, are also affected. As a consequence, radiation therapy often has side effects ranging from unpleasant to serious, including hair loss, nausea and vomiting, anemia, and suppression of the immune system. Because radiation is mutagenic, radiation therapy carries the additional disadvantage of being carcinogenic—the treatment, while effective in the destruction or inhibition of a malignant growth, may also initiate new cancers or push cells through intermediate stages in progression toward malignancy.

When possible, radiation is directed only toward the body regions containing a tumor in order to minimize the destruction of normal tissues. This may be accomplished by focusing a radiation source on the tumor or by shielding body regions outside the tumor with a radiation barrier such as a lead sheet.

Chemotherapy involves the use of chemicals that retard cell division or kill tumor cells more readily than normal body cells. Most of the chemicals used in chemotherapy have been discovered by routine screening of substances for their effects on cancer cells in cultures and test animals. Several hundred thousand chemicals were tested in the screening effort that produced the thirty or so chemotherapeutic agents available for cancer treatment.

Many of the chemicals most effective in cancer chemotherapy alter the chemical structure of DNA, produce breaks in DNA molecules, slow or stop DNA duplication, or interfere with the natural systems repairing chemical lesions in DNA. The effects inhibit cell division or interfere with cell functions sufficiently to kill the cancer cells. Because DNA is most susceptible to chemical alteration during duplication and cancer cells duplicate their DNA and divide more rapidly than most normal tissue cells, the effects of these chemicals are most pronounced in malignant types. Normal cells, however, are also affected to some extent, particularly those in tissues that divide more rapidly. As a result, chemotherapeutic chemicals can produce essentially the same detrimental side effects as radiation therapy. The side effects of chemotherapy are serious enough to be fatal in 2 to 5 percent of persons treated. Because they alter DNA, many chemotherapeutic agents are carcinogens and carry the additional risk, as with radiation, of inducing the formation of new cancers.

Not all chemicals used in chemotherapy alter DNA. Some act by interfering with cell division or other cell processes rather than directly modifying DNA. Two chemotherapeutic agents often used in cancer treatment, vinblastine and taxol, for example, slow or stop cell division through their ability to interfere with the spindle structure that divides chromosomes. The drugs can slow or stop tumor growth as well as the division of normal cells.

Tumors frequently develop resistance to some of the chemicals used in chemotherapy, so that the treatment gradually becomes less effective. Development of resistance is often associated with random duplication of DNA segments, commonly noted in tumor cells. In some, the random duplication happens to include genes that provide resistance to the chemicals

employed in chemotherapy. The genes providing resistance usually encode enzymes that break down the applied chemical or its metabolic derivatives, or transport proteins of the plasma membrane capable of rapidly excreting the chemical from the cell. One gene in particular, the multidrug resistance gene (MDR), is frequently found to be duplicated or highly activated in resistant cells. This gene, which is normally active in cells of the liver, kidney, adrenal glands, and parts of the digestive system, encodes a transport pump that can expel a large number of substances from cells, including many of those used in chemotherapy. Overactivity of the MDR pump can effectively keep chemotherapy drugs below toxic levels in cancer cells. Cells developing resistance are more likely to survive chemotherapy and give rise to malignant cell lines with resistance. The chemotherapeutic agents involved may thus have the unfortunate effect of selecting cells with resistance, thereby ensuring that they will become the dominant types in the tumor.

Success rates with chemotherapy vary from negligible to about 80 percent, depending on the cancer type. For most, success rates do not range above 50 to 60 percent. Some cancer types, including lung, breast, ovarian, and colorectal tumors, respond poorly or not at all to chemotherapy. The overall cure rate for surgery, radiation, and chemotherapy combined, as judged by no recurrence of the cancer for a period of five years, is about 50 percent.

Full success in the treatment of cancer hopefully will come from the continued study of the genes controlling cell division and the regulatory mechanisms that modify the activity of these genes in the cell cycle. An understanding of the molecular activities of these genes and their modifying controls may bring with it a molecular means to reach specifically into cancer cells and halt their growth and metastasis.

PERSPECTIVE AND PROSPECTS

Indications that malignancy and metastasis might have a basis in altered gene activity began to appear in the nineteenth century. In 1820, a British physician, Sir William Norris, noted that melanoma, a cancer involving pigmented skin cells, was especially prevalent in one family under study. More than forty kinds of cancer, including common types such as cancer of the breast and colon, have since been noticed to occur more frequently in some families than in others. Another indication that cancer has a basis in altered gene activity was the fact that the chromosomes of many tumor cells show abnormalities in the chromosomes, such as extra chromosomes, broken chromosomes, or rearrangements of one kind or another. These abnormalities suggested that cancer might be induced by altered genes with activities related to cell division.

These indications were put on a firm basis by research with tumors caused by viruses infecting animal cells, most notably those caused by a group of viruses infecting mammals and other animals, the retroviruses. Many retroviral infections cause little or no damage to their hosts. Some, however, are associated with induction of cancer. (Another type of pathogenic retrovirus is responsible for acquired immunodeficiency syndrome, or AIDS.) The cancer-inducing types among the retroviruses were found to carry genes capable of transforming normal cells to the malignant state. The transforming genes were at first thought to be purely viral in origin, but DNA sequencing and other molecular approaches revealed that the viral oncogenes had normal counterparts among the genes directly or indirectly regulating cell division in cells of the infected host. Among the most productive of the investigators using this approach were J. Michael Bishop and Harold E. Varmus, who received the 1989 Nobel Prize in Medicine for their research establishing the relationship between retroviral oncogenes and their normal cellular counterparts.

The discovery of altered host genes in cancer-inducing retroviruses prompted a search for similar genes in nonviral cancers. Much of this work was accomplished by transfection experiments, in which the DNA of cancer cells is extracted and introduced into cultured mouse cells. Frequently, the mouse cells are transformed into types that grow much more rapidly than normal cells. The human oncogene responsible for the transformation is then identified in the altered cells. Many of the oncogenes identified by transfection turned out to be among those already carried by retroviruses, confirming by a different route that these genes are capable of contributing to the transformation of cells to a cancerous state. The transfection experiments also identified some additional oncogenes not previously found in retroviruses.

In spite of impressive advances in treatment, cancer remains among the most dreaded of human diseases. Recognized as a major threat to health since the earliest days of recorded history, cancer still counts as one of the most frequent causes of human fatality. In technically advanced countries, it accounts for about 15 to 20 percent of deaths each year. In a typical year, more persons die from cancer in the United States than the total number of Americans killed in World War II and the Vietnam War combined. Smoking, the most frequent single cause of cancer, is estimated to be responsible for about one-third of these deaths.

—*Stephen L. Wolfe, Ph.D.*

See also Biopsy; Cancer; Carcinoma; Cytology; Cytopathology; Imaging and radiology; Laboratory tests; Lymphadenopathy and lymphoma; Mammography; Oncology; Pathology; Radiation therapy; Tumor removal; Tumors.

FOR FURTHER INFORMATION:

Alberts, Bruce, et al. *Molecular Biology of the Cell.* 3d ed. New York: Garland, 1994. Chapter 21 describes the development and characteristics of malignance and metastasis. The text is clearly written at the college level and is illustrated by numerous diagrams and photographs.

Darnell, James, Harvey Lodish, and David Baltimore. *Molecular Cell Biology.* 2d ed. New York: Scientific American Books, 1990. An excellent textbook written at the college level. Chapter 24 provides an unusually complete discussion of the characteristics and causes of malignancy and metastasis. Many highly illustrative diagrams and photographs are included.

Lackie, J. M., J. A. T. Dow, and S. E. Blackshaw. *The Dictionary of Cell and Molecular Biology.* San Diego, Calif.: Academic Press, 1999. Encompasses cytology and molecular biology. Includes bibliographical references.

Murphy, G., L. Morris, and D. Lange. *Informed Decisions: The Complete Book of Cancer Diagnosis, Treatment, and Recovery.* New York: Viking Press, 1997. This text from the American Cancer Society is intended for the layperson. It is exemplary in its discussion of cancer.

Weinberg, Robert A. "Finding the Anti-Oncogene." *Scientific American* 259 (September, 1988): 44-51. A lucidly written description of tumor suppressor genes and their possible use as a means to inhibit tumor growth. Many innovative and informative illustrations are included with the article.

Wolfe, Stephen L. *Molecular and Cellular Biology.* Belmont, Calif.: Wadsworth, 1993. Chapter 22,

"The Cell Cycle, Cell Cycle Regulation, and Cancer," describes the cellular factors and processes regulating the growth and division of both normal and malignant cells. Written at the college level, the book is readable and illustrated with many useful and informative diagrams and photographs.

MALIGNANT MELANOMA REMOVAL
PROCEDURE

ANATOMY OR SYSTEM AFFECTED: Skin

SPECIALTIES AND RELATED FIELDS: Cytology, dermatology, general surgery, histology, oncology, plastic surgery

DEFINITION: The excision of any of several neoplasms (cancers) composed primarily of melanocytes that usually develop on the skin.

INDICATIONS AND PROCEDURES

Melanomas compose the most serious form of skin cancers. They originate among the melanocytes, cells which produce the dark pigment melanin. Most commonly, this form of cancer develops among light-skinned individuals on areas of the body frequently exposed to the sun.

Symptoms or signs of melanomas include black or brown blemishes with irregular borders, moles that suddenly change size or shape, or a nodule which becomes hard or lumpy, particularly if it is itchy or painful. Diagnosis is based on histological observation of biopsy material. Types of melanomas include superficial spreading melanomas, nodular forms, lentigo maligna melanomas, and amelanotic melanomas.

Treatment depends on the type and stage (size or penetration) of the disease. Chemotherapy and radiation therapy may be used if the disease has spread, but the most common form of treatment involves surgical removal. If the disease is considered stage 1 (according to Clark's classification system) and is confined to the superficial layers of skin, without having spread past underlying tissue or lymph nodes, the melanoma may be removed through a simple excision. If the cancer has begun to spread through dermal tissue (stage 2), it may be necessary to remove wider areas of skin in order to eliminate any remaining cancerous cells. Once the disease has spread into underlying lymph nodes or beyond (stages 3 through 5), surgical removal may be supplemented with chemotherapy or radiation therapy of the neoplasm.

USES AND COMPLICATIONS

Because of their rapid progression, malignant melanomas are among the more difficult forms of cancer to eliminate. If the disease is caught early, surgical excision may be sufficient for a cure. Once the disease has extended beyond stage 3, however, the prognosis becomes less optimistic.

The surgery itself usually produces only superficial scarring, though the removal of wider areas of skin may require a graft using skin taken from another area of the body. If chemotherapy is included with treatment, side effects such as hair loss or nausea are common.

—*Richard Adler, Ph.D.*

See also Cancer; Chemotherapy; Dermatology; Dermatopathology; Grafts and grafting; Laser use in surgery; Malignancy and metastasis; Oncology; Plastic surgery; Radiation therapy; Skin; Skin cancer; Skin disorders; Skin lesion removal.

FOR FURTHER INFORMATION:

Levitt, Paul M., et al. *The Cancer Reference Book: Direct and Clear Answers to Everyone's Questions*. New York: Facts on File, 1983.

Murphy, G., L. Morris, and D. Lange. *Informed Decisions: The Complete Book of Cancer Diagnosis, Treatment, and Recovery*. New York: Viking Press, 1997.

Siegel, Mary-Ellen. *The Cancer Patient's Handbook: Everything You Need to Know About Today's Care and Treatment*. New York: Walker, 1986.

MALNUTRITION
DISEASE/DISORDER

ANATOMY OR SYSTEM AFFECTED: Gastrointestinal system, intestines, nails, stomach, all bodily systems

SPECIALTIES AND RELATED FIELDS: Gastroenterology, nutrition, pediatrics, public health

DEFINITION: Impaired health caused by an imbalance, either through deficiency or excess, in nutrients.

KEY TERMS:

anemia: a condition in which there is a lower-than-normal concentration of the iron-containing protein in red blood cells, which carry oxygen

famine: a lack of access to food, the cause of which can be a natural disaster, such as a drought, or a situation created by humans, such as a civil war

kwashiorkor: the condition that results from consuming a diet that is sufficient in energy (kilocalories) but inadequate in protein content

marasmus: the condition that results from consuming a diet that is deficient in both energy and protein

osteoporosis: a bone disorder in which the bone's mineral content is decreased over time, resulting in a weakening of the skeleton and susceptibility to bone fractures

protein energy malnutrition (PEM): a deficient intake of energy (kilocalories) and/or protein, the most common type of undernutrition in developing countries; the two major types of PEM are kwashiorkor and marasmus

undernutrition: continued ill health caused by a long-standing dietary deficiency of the energy (kilocalories) and the nutrients that are required to maintain health and provide protection from disease

CAUSES AND SYMPTOMS

Malnutrition literally means "bad nutrition." It can be used broadly to mean an excess or deficiency of the nutrients that are necessary for good health. In industrialized societies, malnutrition typically represents the excess consumption characterized by a diet containing too much energy (kilocalories), fat, and sodium. Malnutrition is most commonly thought, however, to be undernutrition or deficient intake, the consumption of inadequate amounts of nutrients to promote health or to support growth in children. The most severe form of undernutrition is called protein energy malnutrition, or PEM. It commonly affects children, who require nutrients not only to help maintain the body but also to grow. Two types of PEM occur: kwashiorkor and marasmus.

Kwashiorkor is a condition in which a person consumes adequate energy but not enough protein. It usually is seen in children between one and four who are weaned so that the next baby can be breast-fed. The weaning diet consists of gruels made from starchy foods that do not contain an adequate supply of amino acids, the building blocks of protein. These diets do, however, provide enough energy.

Diets in many developing countries are high in bulk, making it nearly impossible for a child to consume a sufficient volume of foods such as rice and grain to obtain an adequate amount of protein for growth. The outward signs of kwashiorkor are a potbelly, dry unpigmented skin, coarse reddish hair, and edema in the legs. Edema results from a lack of certain proteins in the blood that help to maintain a nor-

mal fluid balance in the body. The potbelly and swollen limbs often are misinterpreted as signs of being "fat" among the developing world cultures. Other signs requiring further medical testing include fat deposits in the liver and decreased production of digestive enzymes. The mental and physical growth of the child are impaired. Children with kwashiorkor are apathetic, listless, and withdrawn. Ironically, these children lose their appetites. They become very susceptible to upper-respiratory infection and diarrhea. Children with kwashiorkor also are deficient in vitamins and minerals that are found in protein-rich foods. There are symptoms caused by these specific nutrient deficiencies as well.

Marasmus literally means "to waste away." It is caused by a deficiency of both Calories (kilocalories) and protein in the diet. This is the most severe form of childhood malnutrition. Body fat stores are used up to provide energy, and eventually muscle tissue is broken down for body fuel. Victims appear as skin and bones, gazing with large eyes from a bald head with an aged, gaunt appearance. Once severe muscle wasting occurs, death is imminent. Body temperature is below normal. The immune system does not operate normally, making these children extremely susceptible to respiratory and gastrointestinal infections.

A vicious cycle develops once the child succumbs to infection. Infection increases the body's need for protein, yet the PEM child is so protein deficient that recovery from even minor respiratory infections is prolonged. Pneumonia and measles become fatal diseases for PEM victims. Severe diarrhea compounds the problem. The child is often dehydrated, and any nourishment that might be consumed will not be adequately absorbed.

The long-term prognosis for these PEM children is poor. If the child survives infections and is refed, PEM returns once the child goes home to the same environment that caused it. Children with repeated episodes of kwashiorkor have high mortality rates.

Children with PEM are most likely victims of famine. Typically, these children either were not breast-fed or were breast-fed for only a few months. If a weaning formula is used, it has not been prepared properly; in many cases, it is mixed with unsanitary water or watered down because the parents cannot afford to buy enough to use it at full strength.

It is difficult to distinguish between the cause of kwashiorkor and that of marasmus. One child ingesting the same diet as another may develop kwashiorkor, while the other may develop marasmus. Some scientists think this may be a result of the different ways in which individuals adapt to nutritional deprivation. Others propose that kwashiorkor is caused by eating moldy grains, since it appears only in rainy, tropical areas.

Another type of malnutrition involves a deficiency of vitamins or minerals. Vitamin A is necessary for the maintenance of healthy skin, and even a mild deficiency causes susceptibility to diarrhea and upper respiratory infection. Diarrhea reinforces the vicious cycle of malnutrition, since it prevents nutrients from being absorbed. With a more severe vitamin A deficiency, changes in the eye and, eventually, blindness result. Night blindness is usually the first detectable symptom of vitamin A deficiency. The blood that bathes the eye cannot regenerate the visual pigments needed to see in the dark. Eventually, the tissues of the eye become infected and total blindness results. Vitamin A deficiency, the primary cause of childhood blindness, can result from the lack of either vitamin A or the protein that transports it in the blood. If the deficiency of vitamin A occurs during pregnancy or at birth, the skull does not develop normally and the brain is crowded. An older child deficient in vitamin A will suffer growth impairment.

Diseases resulting from B-vitamin deficiencies are rare. Strict vegetarians, called vegans, who consume no animal products, are at risk for vitamin B_{12} deficiency resulting in an anemia in which the red blood cells are large and immature. Too little folate (folic acid) in the diet can cause this same anemia. Beriberi is the deficiency disease of thiamine (vitamin B_1) in which the heart and nervous systems are damaged and muscle wasting occurs. Ariboflavinosis (lack of riboflavin) describes a collection of symptoms such as cracks and redness of the eyes and lips; inflamed, sensitive eyelids; and a purple-red tongue. Pellagra is the deficiency disease of niacin (vitamin B_3). It is characterized by "the Four Ds of pellagra": dermatitis, diarrhea, dementia, and death. Isolated deficiency of a B vitamin is rare, since many B vitamins work in concert. Therefore, a lack of one hinders the function of the rest.

Scurvy is the deficiency disease of vitamin C. Early signs of scurvy are bleeding gums and pinpoint hemorrhages under the skin. As the deficiency becomes more severe, the skin becomes rough, brown, and scaly, eventually resulting in impaired wound healing, soft bones, painful joints, and loose teeth.

Finally, hardening of the arteries or massive bleeding results in death.

Rickets is the childhood deficiency disease of vitamin D. Bone formation is impaired, which is reflected in a bowlegged or knock-kneed appearance. In adults, a brittle bone condition called osteomalacia results from vitamin D deficiency.

Malnutrition of minerals is more prevalent in the world, since deficiencies are observed in both industrialized and developing countries. Calcium malnutrition in young children results in stunted growth. Osteoporosis occurs when calcium reserves are drawn upon to supply the other body parts with calcium. This occurs in later adulthood, leaving bones weak and fragile. General loss of stature and fractures of the hip, pelvis, and wrist are common, and a humpback appears. Caucasian and Asian women of small stature are at greatest risk for osteoporosis.

Iron-deficiency anemia is the most common form of malnutrition in developing societies. Lack of consumption of iron-rich foods is common among the poor, especially in women who menstruate. This deficiency, which is characterized by small, pale red blood cells, causes weakness, fatigue, and sensitivity to cold temperatures. Anemia in children can cause reduced ability to learn and impaired ability to think and to concentrate.

Deficiencies of other minerals are less common. Although these deficiencies are usually seen among people in developing nations, they may occur among the poor, pregnant women, children, and the elderly in industrialized societies. Severe growth retardation and arrested sexual maturation are characteristics of zinc deficiency. With iodine deficiency, the cells in the thyroid gland enlarge to try to trap as much iodine as possible. This enlargement of the thyroid gland is called simple or endemic goiter. A more severe iodine deficiency results from a lack of iodine that leads to a deficiency of thyroid hormone during pregnancy. The child of a mother with such a deficiency is born with severe mental and/or physical retardation, a condition known as cretinism.

The causes of malnutrition, therefore, can be difficult to isolate, because nutrients work together in the body. In addition, the underlying causes of malnutrition (poverty, famine, and war) often are untreatable.

TREATMENT AND THERAPY

Treatment for PEM involves refeeding with a diet adequate in protein, Calories, and other essential nutrients. Response to treatment is influenced by many factors, such as the person's age, the stage of development in which the deprivation began, the severity of the deficiency, the duration of the deficiency, and the presence of other illnesses, particularly infections. Total recovery is possible only if the underlying cause that led to PEM can be eliminated.

PEM can result from illnesses such as cancer and acquired immunodeficiency syndrome (AIDS). Victims of these diseases cannot consume diets with enough energy and protein to meet their body needs, which are higher than normal because of the illness. Infections also increase the need for many nutrients. The first step in treatment must be to cure the underlying infection. People from cultures in which PEM is prevalent believe that food should not be given to an ill person.

Prevention of PEM is the preferred therapy. In areas with unsafe water supplies and high rates of poverty, women should be encouraged to breast-feed. Education about proper weaning foods provides further defense against PEM. Other preventive efforts involve combining plant proteins into a mixture of high-quality protein, adding nutrients to cereal products, and using genetic engineering to produce grains with a better protein mix. The prevention of underlying causes such as famine and drought may not be feasible.

Prekwashiorkor can be identified by regular plotting of the child's growth. If treatment begins at this stage, patient response is rapid and the prognosis is good. Treatment must begin by correcting the body's fluid imbalance. Low potassium levels must be corrected. Restoration of fluid is followed by adequate provision of Calories, with gradual additions of protein that the patient can use to repair damaged immune and digestive systems. Treatment must happen rapidly yet allow the digestive system to recover—thus the term "hurry slowly." Once edema is corrected and blood potassium levels are restored, a diluted milk with added sugar can be given. Gradually, vegetable oil is added to increase the intake of Calories. Vitamin and mineral supplements are given. Final diet therapy includes a diet of skim milk and other animal protein sources, coupled with the addition of vegetables and fat.

The residual effects of PEM may be great if malnutrition has come at a critical period in development or has been of long duration. In prolonged cases, damage to growth and the digestive system may be irreversible. Mortality is very high in such cases. Normally, the digestive tract undergoes rapid cell replacement; therefore, this system is one of the first to suffer in PEM. Absorptive surfaces shrink, and digestive enzymes and protein carriers that transport nutrients are lacking.

Another critical factor in the treatment of PEM is the stage of development in which the deprivation occurs. Most PEM victims are children. If nutritional deprivation occurs during pregnancy, the consequence is increased risk of infant death. If the child is carried to term, it is of low birth weight, placing it at high risk for death. Malnutrition during lactation decreases the quantity, but not always the nutritional quality, of milk. Thus, fewer Calories are consumed by the baby. Growth of the child is slowed. These babies are short for their age and continue to be shorter later in life, even if their diet improves.

During the first two years of life, the brain continues to grow. Nutritional deprivation can impair mental development and cognitive function. For only minimal damage to occur, malnutrition must be treated in early stages. Adults experiencing malnutrition are more adaptive to it, since their protein energy needs are not as great. Weight loss, muscle wasting, and impaired immune function occur, and malnourished women stop menstruating.

Successful treatment of a specific nutrient deficiency depends on the duration of the deficiency and the stage in a person's development at which it occurs. Vitamin A is a fat-soluble vitamin that is stored in the body. Thus, oral supplements or injections of vitamin A can provide long-term protection from this deficiency. If vitamin A is given early enough, the deficiency can be rapidly reversed. By the time the child is blind, sight cannot be restored, and frequently the child dies because of other illnesses. Treatment also is dependent upon adequate protein to provide carriers in the blood to transport these vitamins. Treatment of the B-vitamin deficiencies involves oral and intramuscular injections. The crucial step in treatment is to initiate therapy before irreversible damage has occurred. Scurvy (vitamin C deficiency) can be eliminated in five days by administering the amount of vitamin C found in approximately three cups of orange juice. Treatment of vitamin D deficiency in children and adults involves an oral dose of two to twelve times the recommended daily allowance of the vitamin. Halibut and cod liver oils are frequently given as vitamin D supplements.

Successful treatment of a mineral deficiency depends on the timing and duration of the deficiency. Once the bones are fully grown, restoring calcium to optimal levels will not correct short stature. To prevent osteoporosis, bones must have been filled to the maximum with calcium during early adulthood. Estrogen replacement therapy and weight-bearing exercise retard calcium loss in later years and do more than calcium supplements can.

Iron supplementation is necessary to correct iron-deficiency anemia. Iron supplements are routinely prescribed for pregnant women to prevent anemia during pregnancy. Treatment also includes a diet with adequate meat, fish, and poultry to provide not only iron but also a factor that enhances absorption. Iron absorption is also enhanced by vitamin C. Anemias caused by lack of folate and vitamin B_{12} will not respond to iron therapy. These anemias must be treated by adding the appropriate vitamin to the diet.

Zinc supplementation can correct arrested sexual maturation and impaired growth if it is begun in time. In areas where the soil does not contain iodine, iodine is added to salt or injections of iodized oil are given to prevent goiter. Cretinism cannot be cured—only prevented.

In general, malnutrition is caused by a diet of limited variety and quantity. The underlying causes of malnutrition—poverty, famine, and war—are often untreatable. Overall treatment lies in prevention by providing all people with a diet that is adequate in all nutrients, including vitamins, minerals, and Calories. Sharing the world's wealth and ending political strife and greed are essential elements of the struggle to end malnutrition.

PERSPECTIVE AND PROSPECTS

Over the years, the study of malnutrition has shifted to include the excessive intake of nutrients. In developing countries, the primary causes of death are infectious diseases, and undernutrition is a risk factor. In industrialized societies, however, the primary causes of death are chronic diseases, and overnutrition is a risk factor. The excessive consumption of sugar is linked to tooth decay. Also, overnutrition in terms of too much fat and Calories in the diet leads to obesity, high blood pressure, stroke, heart disease, some cancers, liver disease, and one type of diabetes.

Historically, the focus of malnutrition studies was deficiencies in the diet. In the 1930's, classic kwashiorkor was described by Cicely Williams. Not until after World War II was it known that kwashiorkor was caused by a lack of protein in the diet. In 1959, Derrick B. Jelliffe introduced the term "protein-calorie malnutrition" to describe the nutritional disorders of marasmus, marasmic kwashiorkor, and kwashiorkor.

PEM remains the most important public health problem in developing countries. Few cases are seen in Western societies. Historically, the root causes have been urbanization, periods of famine, and the failure to breast-feed or early cessation of breast-feeding. Marasmus is prevalent in urban areas among infants under one year old, while kwashiorkor is prevalent in rural areas during the second year of life.

Deficiencies of specific nutrients have been documented throughout history. Vitamin A deficiency and its cure were documented by Egyptians and Chinese around 1500 B.C.E. In occupied Denmark during World War I, vitamin A deficiency, caused by dairy product deprivation, was common in Danish children. Beriberi, first documented in the Far East, was caused by diets of polished rice that were deficient in thiamine. Pellagra was seen in epidemic proportions in the southern United States, where corn was the staple grain, during World War I.

Zinc deficiency was first reported in the 1960's. The growth and maturation of boys in the Middle East were studied. Their diets were low in zinc and high in substances that prevented zinc absorption. Consequently, the World Health Organization recommended increased zinc intake for populations whose staple is unleavened whole grain bread. Goiter was documented during Julius Caesar's reign. Simply adding iodine to salt has virtually eliminated goiter in the United States.

If classic malnutrition is observed in industrialized societies, it usually is secondary to other diseases, such as AIDS and cancer. Hunger and poverty are problems that contribute to malnutrition; however, the malnutrition that results is less severe than that found in developing countries.

Specific nutrients may be lacking in the diets of the poor. Iron-deficiency anemia is prevalent among the poor, and this anemia may impair learning ability. Other deficiencies may be subclinical, which means that no detectable signs are observed, yet normal nutrient pools in the body are depleted. Homelessness, poverty, and drug or alcohol abuse are the major contributing factors to these conditions. In addition, malnutrition as a result of poverty is exacerbated by lack of nutritional knowledge and/or poor food choices.

—*Wendy L. Stuhldreher, Ph.D, R.D.*

See also Anemia; Anorexia nervosa; Beriberi; Breast-feeding; Bulimia; Celiac sprue; Cholesterol; Eating disorders; Failure to thrive; Food biochemistry; Galactosemia; Goiter; Growth; Hirschsprung's disease; Hypercholesterolemia; Hyperlipidemia; Kwashiorkor; Lactose intolerance; Lead poisoning; Malabsorption; Metabolism; Nutrition; Osteoporosis; Scurvy; Supplements; Thyroid disorders; Vitamins and minerals; Weaning; Weight loss and gain; Weight loss medications.

FOR FURTHER INFORMATION:

Christian, Janet L., and Janet L. Greger. *Nutrition for Living*. 4th ed. Redwood City, Calif.: Benjamin/Cummings, 1994. This introductory textbook of nutrition is easy to understand. It provides brief explanations of various vitamin and mineral deficiencies, as well as of PEM. Photographs showing symptoms are included.

Garrow, J. S., and W. P. T. James, eds. *Human Nutrition and Dietetics*. 10th ed. New York: Churchill Livingstone, 2000. Several chapters in this book provide information on malnutrition, from PEM to specific nutrient deficiencies. History, causes, symptoms, and treatments of the disorders are covered. An excellent list of references is provided.

Kreutler, Patricia A., and Dorice M. Czajka-Narins. *Nutrition in Perspective*. 2d ed. Englewood Cliffs, N.J.: Prentice Hall, 1987. This textbook provides a chapter on the food supply, including issues for meeting the problem of undernutrition. It also describes the deficiency diseases for vitamins and minerals and PEM in various chapters.

Wardlaw, Gordon M., Paul M. Insel, and Marcia F. Seyler. *Contemporary Nutrition*. St. Louis: Mosby Year Book, 1991. Chapter 18 of this text covers undernutrition. This chapter emphasizes the types of undernutrition and hunger found in America.

Whitney, Eleanor Noss, and Sharon Rady Rolfes. *Understanding Nutrition*. 8th ed. St. Paul, Minn.: West, 1999. This is an introductory nutrition textbook. Various chapters have information about the different nutrient deficiencies and malnutrition.

MALPRACTICE
ETHICS
DEFINITION: The failure to care for patients in accordance with professional standards, for which injured patients are allowed to sue for compensation.

KEY TERMS:
common law: the accumulation of court decisions that serves as a basis for deciding legal principles
damages: compensation awarded to a plaintiff for an injury incurred because of a defendant's action or lack of action
defendant: a person or corporation alleged in a lawsuit to have committed a wrong
liability: responsibility for a wrongdoing
plaintiff: a person or corporation that brings legal action against another person or corporation
tort: an action or the result of an action that is defined by law to be a wrong or injury

CONTROVERSIES SURROUNDING MALPRACTICE LITIGATION
In the United States, few medical topics arouse more anger in physicians, more debate in state legislatures, or more confusion in the public than malpractice. In part, the media encourages this attention when it reports multimillion-dollar jury awards for damages, sensational stories that often make all the parties involved—lawyers, the defendant doctor, the plaintiff patient, and juries—look somehow reprehensible. In part, the rise in malpractice insurance, which has contributed to the increasing cost of medical care, has upset both doctors and the public. Yet inflation and the rare spectacular settlement obscure the value of a system that since the late eighteenth century has given patients legal redress for injury, has helped maintain professional standards of medical care, and has allowed state governments some control over the local health care industry.

As the word's elements imply, "malpractice" simply means the poor execution of duties. The definition bears close examination, however, on one key feature: what "poor" entails. The first recourse of a patient who feels inadequately cared for is to discuss the complaint with the doctor (or dentist, chiropractor, or other health care provider). This measure clears up many complaints, since most are based on simple misunderstandings. A patient receiving no satisfaction from the doctor may file a complaint with the state board of medical examiners, which is each state's official government body, staffed by doctors, that issues medical licenses and disciplines physicians and surgeons. In both cases, the doctor or a panel of peers will decide if the patient's complaint meets the professional standards of "poor." A patient who is not pleased with this decision may bring suit in civil court. No patient, however, can press a lawsuit for malpractice simply because he or she feels wronged. For legal action to have any chance of succeeding, the doctor must have injured the patient because of negligent care. Even then, lawyers for the patient must rely on expert testimony from other doctors to establish that the physician gave the patient poor care. All official avenues of redress therefore depend on the medical profession's own standards.

Four basic standards guide doctors in ethically performing their professional duties, and failure in any one of them may constitute malpractice. First, doctors must inform their patients about treatments for an ailment and receive their explicit consent. The patient must understand the doctor's plan of treatment and any procedure's potential risks and benefits; if a patient cannot understand because of age or mental condition, a guardian must consent, except in some emergency situations. The consent may be verbal unless an invasive technique, such as surgery, is involved, in which case the law requires a signed consent form. Without the patient's consent, a physician performing a medical procedure not only may be subject to a malpractice lawsuit but also can be charged with assault under criminal law. Second, a doctor must treat a patient with reasonable skill, as defined by accepted medical practice. This point is crucial. Doctors do not have to render the best aid possible, or even the best aid of which they are capable; they must only meet professional guidelines for any specific diagnostic, palliative, or corrective measure. Both the key terms in this standard—"reasonable" and "accepted medical practice"—have been notoriously hard to define in court because they vary from region to region and from school of medicine to school of medicine. Rural physicians, for example, cannot be expected to give the level of care available in cities, since cities have more specialists available and support technology; nor are general practitioners expected to have the skill of a specialist, such as a cardiologist. Third, physicians are responsible for what other health care workers under their charge do to patients. If other doctors (such as medical residents), nurses, physical therapists, or medical technicians act on a doctor's orders, that doctor is ultimately responsible for supervising their performance. Fourth, a doctor accepting responsibility for a patient enters a contractual obligation and may not abandon that obligation without either finding another physician to take his or her place or notifying the patient

well in advance so the patient can engage another doctor. At the same time, however, the patient's obligation is to follow the doctor's medical advice.

Doctors are not the only health care workers who can be charged with malpractice. If other medical personnel act as a team with a doctor or surgeon, they may also be held liable. For example, during surgery a surgeon is assisted by an anesthesiologist and various nurses, any of whom may separately fail in his or her duties and be sued as a result. Thus, whenever a patient suffers at the hands of a medical team, the trend has been to sue each member. Furthermore, if the facilities or personnel employed by a hospital prove substandard, the hospital itself may be liable.

Tort liability and contractual responsibility govern the legal treatment of malpractice, both of which fall under civil law. (This classification assumes that doctors inadvertently cause harm; if they intentionally injure a patient, they are subject to charges under criminal law.) A patient may sue for breach of contract if his or her doctor has broken that contract—usually by abandoning the patient without proper notice. This sort of lawsuit is by far the least common. Tort liability means that the doctor is responsible for any injury (tort) caused to the patient through negligence. The patient may seek compensation for a tort by suing the doctor for damages. The presumption is that money, which is almost always the form of compensation sought, can make up for the harm done. Damages can be awarded for two types of injury. Concrete physical injury is the most typical, and damages may include money to cover medical bills, lost wages, convalescent care, and other expenses relating directly to the disability. A jury may also grant damages for pain and suffering, a difficult type of injury on which to place a price; such damages account for some of the largest monetary awards.

Because damages may amount to millions of dollars, most doctors who lose a malpractice suit cannot hope to pay them without help. Insurance provides that help, which usually takes one of three forms. First, for monthly payments (premiums), traditional insurance companies offer policies to doctors that will guarantee money up to a certain amount to pay damages. Also, if its client is sued, the insurance company assigns attorneys who handle the legal negotiations and the defense in court. Second, hospitals or other large organizations may pay for malpractice damages from a pool of money reserved for that purpose alone. Third, doctors and other health care providers may set up an insurance company of their own for mutual coverage, often called "bedpan mutuals."

Malpractice litigation in the United States is a ponderous, expensive business. In the mid-1970's, malpractice insurance began to rise sharply; between 1983 and 1985 alone, the cost increased 100 percent. Doctors pass on some or all of these costs to patients by charging higher fees. If a patient sues, however, the insurance cannot cover every type of loss. The amount of time that doctor must spend with lawyers, the time in court, and the overall distraction from practicing mean reduced earnings. Yet the cost is not only to the doctor. The plaintiff pays attorneys by contingency fee, which means that the attorney receives a percentage (usually 20 to 30 percent) of money from any settlement. A patient losing a suit still must pay the lawyer's expenses, which can quickly amount to thousands of dollars. Finally, when suits reach court, public funds contribute to the court's expenses, and those expenses climb if a decision is appealed or retried, as is sometimes the case.

Patients and doctors alike complain that soaring malpractice litigation in the United States since 1960 has been destructive, introducing suspicion into the doctor-patient relationship. In addition to its emotional impact, the suspicion concretely affects medical practice, most medical economists claim. Because physicians fear lawsuits, they perform more diagnostic tests than are called for by medical protocols. Often the chances are remote that these tests will reveal any useful information, yet doctors order them to show that they have done everything possible for the patient if they are sued. The extra tests cost money, which either the patient or the insurance company must pay. In either case, the expenditures inflate the cost of medicine. The practice of such "defensive medicine" has also led some doctors to refuse to perform high-risk procedures except in hospitals that have extensive facilities. Obstetricians provide a signal case in point. Fearing lawsuits for any complications that may arise, many obstetricians will not deliver babies at home or in small hospitals, forcing rural patients to rush long distances to the nearest big-city hospital for delivery.

One scholar of the malpractice system has remarked that it seems designed to protect the interests of everyone except the person who most needs help: the injured patient. While this is surely a rhetorical exaggeration, all studies have found that only a fraction of injuries are ever compensated. Moreover, the

system, based on adversarial disputation, seems hostile and dauntingly complex to both patient and physician. Yet, although no one thinks it perfect, the system evolved in accordance with two widely held American attitudes toward regulation in general: It limits abuses, and it preserves professional autonomy.

TRIAL PROCEDURES IN MALPRACTICE CASES

Few malpractice claims actually end in jury awards for damages. Only about 10 percent of patients injured by doctors file lawsuits, of which about 20 percent end in payment to the plaintiff. Overwhelmingly the payments come from out-of-court settlements that win the plaintiff only a part of the money sought in the suit. Taking a suit all the way to a jury settlement is risky for plaintiffs; they win only about two in ten cases.

From the outset, then, the chances are against the injured patient, and for this reason malpractice litigation is not popular among lawyers. To have a reasonable chance to win a case in court, or at least to force the doctor's insurance company to offer a settlement out of court, the lawyer must first be sure that a causal connection can be made between the patient's injury and physician negligence. In other words, patients cannot sue simply on the hope of winning damages; courts try to reject such "frivolous" suits before they come to trial.

A lawyer believing that a reasonable causal link can be established will write up a summons and complaint on the client's behalf and send them to the doctor. The summons warns the doctor that the patient is filing a lawsuit. The complaint explains the patient's allegation of harm and the amount of damages that the patient demands in compensation. The doctor must answer in a specific time—about a month in most states—and the answer, issued through the doctor's lawyers or those of his or her insurance company, almost always denies responsibility for any injury. The legal battle is then joined.

During a pretrial period known as discovery, each side investigates the other, hoping to find facts that will support arguments in court. Lawyers rely on three investigative methods. The first is documentary disclosure. The plaintiff's lawyer will demand records, especially the patient's medical record, and the doctor must furnish them in a reasonable time. In the second method, written interrogatories, the plaintiff's lawyer sends the doctor a list of questions that must be answered in writing. Third is the deposition, a formal legal proceeding. Lawyers from both sides meet and together question, in separate sessions, the defendant, plaintiff, and key witnesses, all of whom answer the questions under oath, so that they are guilty of perjury if they lie. Many suits are dropped during discovery, with or without monetary settlement. If the suit continues but one side has little evidence on which to base arguments, the other side will probably file a motion for summary judgment, which essentially asks a judge to end the litigation by disqualifying the weak case. Discovery and pretrial motions may take years to complete.

Trials follow a pattern, with some variations, designed to allow each side to present claims and counterclaims systematically. A trial starts with opening statements in which the lawyers describe the general plan for their cases; no actual arguments are made. Next, to clarify matters for the jury, the judge may summarize the applicable legal principles for the case. Then witnesses are called and questioned, first by the plaintiff's lawyer. After he or she finishes with each witness, the defendant's lawyer may also ask questions, a procedure called cross-examination. When the plaintiff's side is done calling witnesses, then the defense lawyer calls and questions more, which the lawyer for the plaintiff may also cross-examine.

During the questioning, two types of evidence are admitted: testimony, the oral or written statements of what people have seen or heard, and "real" or "demonstrative" evidence, physical objects such as an X ray or a needle that have a bearing on the case. The testimony is crucial for the plaintiff, because at this point an expert witness must swear that the defendant was negligent to a "medical certainty" by failing to adhere to one or more medical standards of practice. Since only a doctor is qualified to make this judgment, expert witnesses are always physicians. Finally, the lawyers make closing statements, each insisting that the evidence supports the position of his or her client, and the jury retires to decide on a verdict. If the jurors decide in favor of the plaintiff, they can also lower or raise the amount of requested damages. If they decide for the defendant, the doctor, then the case ends without a monetary settlement. A victorious plaintiff cannot expect immediate payment. Appeals to higher courts may last years, and the appellate courts, after examining the trial records, can reverse a verdict, change the amount of damages, or order a new trial.

Even if a trial does get under way, however, it may not end in a verdict. At any point in the proceedings, one side or the other may give up. Insurance companies regularly send observers to malpractice trials who assess the progress of arguments objectively. An observer detecting a weakness in the defense or noticing that the jury favors the plaintiff for any reason will offer a settlement to the plaintiff's lawyer, because such a settlement will save court costs and probably involve less money than a jury award for damages. Likewise, the plaintiff's lawyer, recognizing that the chances of winning are slim, may try to make a deal with the insurance company. Such dickering may even continue after a verdict is announced, if it is appealed. Also, at any point in the trial the judge may end the case if he or she thinks that one side cannot possibly win; similarly, the judge may reverse a verdict or change the amount of damages if the jury's decision shocks his or her professional conscience.

PERSPECTIVE AND PROSPECTS

By the mid-1970's, the entire American health care system, in the view of most health care observers, was in a state of crisis. Costs had risen, and facilities, especially in urban areas, were strained, while rural areas were often underserved. Critics have blamed the problems on increasingly costly technology and drugs, government regulation, professional salaries, and inadequate preventive medicine. Few doubt that malpractice litigation has contributed significantly as well.

Estimates in 1993 claimed that defensive medicine alone had increased the annual cost of American health care from $10 billion to $36 billion. Combined with increasing fees for medical services and other costs, defensive medicine has helped drive up the cost of medical insurance. Because of these financing problems, legislatures around the country have tried to control the increasing numbers of malpractice suits with tort reform, arbitration or review panels, and legal fee limits.

Tort reforms include a number of measures that modify the procedures or awards of malpractice litigation. Two reforms are designed to shorten the process. One method is to reduce the statute of limitations for malpractice claims— the period after injury when a lawsuit can be started. The second involves limiting the rules governing the discovery phase of pretrial action. Two further reforms restrict the amount of damages. The most popular of these is to impose maximum amounts for types of injury, especially pain and suffering. In the second reform, jury damages must be reduced by the amount of money from other sources, such as health insurance, that a patient receives for the injury.

Several states have instituted review panels or required arbitration before a suit can proceed to court. Laypeople and judges, as well as doctors, make up the review panels, which try to identify and disallow frivolous suits. Arbitration panels actually decide on the amount of damages, if any, to be made, and their decisions cannot be appealed.

Finally, some states, and the federal government, have limited the percentage of a settlement that lawyers can claim in contingency fees. The limits are intended to discourage lawyers from filing marginal suits.

These reforms have only slowed the rate of lawsuits and the rise in the amount of money spent on paying damages and fees. Whatever its defects, the tort system has succeeded in making doctors wary of negligence. Critics insist, however, that the system for addressing malpractice has punished all physicians, not simply the incompetent, and has contributed to the increasingly litigious tenor of American society.

—*Roger Smith, Ph.D.*

See also American Medical Association; Autopsy; Critical care; Critical care, pediatric; Emergency medicine; Ethics; Euthanasia; Forensic pathology; Health maintenance organizations (HMOs); Hippocratic oath; Hospitals; Law and medicine; Obstetrics; Pathology; Resuscitation.

FOR FURTHER INFORMATION:

Edwards, Frank John. *Medical Malpractice: Solving the Crisis*. New York: Henry Holt, 1989. Edwards is a physician who began writing about malpractice after a suit was initiated against him. His approach is an intensely personal physician's view of malpractice litigation—both its rationale and its effects on medicine. His writing is readable, often dramatic, and ruminative.

Groopman, Jerome E. *Second Opinions: Stories of Intuition and Choice in the Changing World of Medicine*. New York: Viking, 2000. Among other examples, Groopman describes the case of a woman with leukemia wrongly diagnosed as having asthma, a patient with melanoma who became the object of professional infighting about the availability and advisability of interferon treatment, and a young physicist told that he had fewer than six months to live and the ensuing tussle between specialists about the usefulness of bone marrow transplant.

Isaacs, Stephen L., and Ava C. Swartz. *The Consumer's Legal Guide to Today's Health Care: Your Medical Rights and How to Assert Them*. Boston: Houghton Mifflin, 1992. Only the last chapter of this handbook pertains to malpractice; it contains a sensibly cautionary explanation of the basic procedures and concepts by Isaacs, a lawyer, and an example of physicians' negligence suffered by Swartz, a journalist.

Rosenthal, Marilynn M. *Dealing with Medical Malpractice: The British and Swedish Experience*. Durham, N.C.: Duke University Press, 1988. A scholarly sociological study, this book contains a detailed introduction to the malpractice system in the United States that serves to define its inadequacies in protecting patients and in quality control of medical practice.

Sloan, Frank A., Randall R. Bovbjerg, and Penny B. Githens. *Insuring Medical Malpractice*. New York: Oxford University Press, 1991. Evaluates objectively the methods for providing malpractice insurance and the industry's share in the crises of the 1970's and 1980's in a presentation designed for policymakers who must decide how to control the system.

Zobel, Hiller B., and Stephen N. Rous. *Doctors and the Law: Defendants and Expert Witnesses*. New York: W. W. Norton, 1993. Hiller, a judge, and Rous, a physician, give advice to physicians on how best to endure a malpractice suit. The step-by-step account of the legal proceedings, evidential requirements, and possible psychological effects on the physician make insightful reading for nonphysicians as well.

MAMMOGRAPHY

PROCEDURE

ANATOMY OR SYSTEM AFFECTED: Breasts

SPECIALTIES AND RELATED FIELDS: Gynecology, oncology, preventive medicine, radiology

DEFINITION: A method of imaging that has become routine in the screening and diagnosis of breast cancer; the fundamental objective of mammography is the early detection of abnormalities in breast tissue.

INDICATIONS AND PROCEDURES

A variety of sophisticated modalities for diagnostic imaging of the breast have been developed. Mammography, however, has repeatedly proved to be the most effective procedure for the early detection of breast cancer. As with any medical imaging method, the objective of the examination is to provide optimal image quality for visualizing pathology, at the minimum possible risk to the patient. Mammography requires high-quality images to detect small breast cancers. It also requires greater sharpness and contrast than does general radiographic imaging.

Mammography is an X-ray examination of the breast that produces a picture of breast structures on film. The image of the breast results from differential absorption of X rays by breast tissues, based on their density and thickness. With film-screen mammography, a light-intensifying screen is used to produce results with a low dosage of radiation. This is called a low-dose examination. The screen generates light when exposed to X rays; thus, it is principally the light that exposes the film. As a result, a relatively small number of X rays are required.

Recent advances in X-ray film and light-intensifying screen technology have resulted in further reduction in the radiation dose to the breast. These developments permit the high resolution necessary for quality images. Film-screen mammography has the advantage of broad area contrast, which aids in the visualization of mass lesions in the breast. There are fewer technical failures with the film-screen imaging technique, reducing the need to retake images. Because of the narrow exposure latitude of the film-screen combination, the breast must be tautly compressed between rigid plates in an effort to reduce the thickness variations from front to back. This compression is also important in reducing the dosage of X rays needed for optimal imaging.

Since the relationship of the breast and the thoracic wall is complex, some areas of breast tissue may be difficult to image. To avoid the overlap of the breast with chest structures and to provide the high level of detail desired, the breast must be held away from the chest by rigid plates. This allows the projection of the breast onto the film surface. Taut compression reduces the lack of sharpness that results from motion and improves geometric sharpness by pushing the structures of the breast closer to the detector system. This degree of compression feels tight and may be uncomfortable, but it should not be painful.

In general, film-screen mammography offers higher image contrast, requires a lower dose of radiation, and endures less equipment downtime. In comparison with earlier models, the modern dedicated units for film-screen mammography have smaller focal spots and longer distance between the X-ray source and the breast, resulting in better image resolution. They also

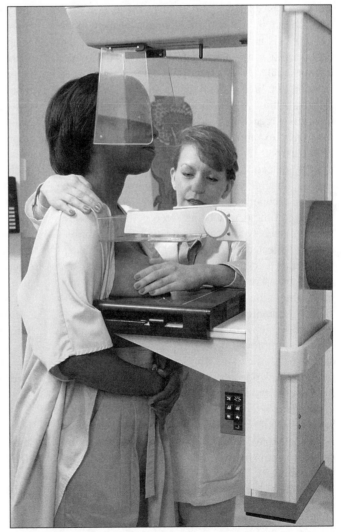

A woman has a mammogram. It is recommended that regular screenings take place beginning in middle age. (PhotoDisc)

have more effective compression devices, configurations that allow easy and rapid positioning of the patient, and a microfocal spot X-ray target for magnification images. Used with the newest film-screen combinations, these X-ray systems provide greater image contrast and detail.

A screening mammography examination should consist of at least two views of each breast: a side view (also called lateral or oblique) and a top-down view (more technically referred to as craniocaudal). For film-screen mammography, the mediolateral-oblique is the most efficient single projection. This is a side view that is taken at a slight angle in an attempt to capture the advantages of both views with a single exposure to X rays. It depicts the greatest amount of breast tissue and includes the deeper structures found in the portion of breast nearest to the armpit. This is where the highest percentage of cancers occurs. A direct side view in conjunction with a craniocaudal view is essential to determine the exact location of a breast lesion that cannot be felt with the fingers. Although the chest wall is not included on the film-screen image, a properly performed mammography examination includes most or all of the breast tissue.

Early detection of breast cancer depends on high-quality imaging techniques. Paramount among the imaging techniques for breast cancer detection is positioning of the person being screened. Optimal positioning is achieved by understanding the capabilities of the dedicated mammography equipment and applying this understanding to take full advantage of natural breast mobility in overcoming various anatomic limitations.

Breast compression is one of the critical aspects of positioning in a mammography. Appropriate compression improves resolution by bringing breast structures closer to the film and by preventing breast motion. It also decreases the required radiation dose by reducing the thickness of the breast. Compression separates overlapping structures and aids in the differentiation of cystic and solid masses. Most patients accept the taut compression requirement for film-screen mammography when they understand its importance.

Additional views may be needed when a suspicious finding is identified. Modified craniocaudal views are needed when a lesion is identified on one but not both of two views. The abnormality can usually be imaged in the craniocaudal projection by turning the patient so as to move either the outer or the inner aspect of the breast directly over the detector system.

Magnification views can be used to enhance the clarity of microcalcifications, masses, and equivocal findings. Because the magnification image requires considerably more radiation, however, its major role is to supplement standard mammography when the latter discloses equivocal findings.

In 2000, the Food and Drug Administration (FDA) approved the first digital mammography system which, in contrast to film-screen mammography, displays X-ray images on a high-resolution computer screen. In this system, breast X rays are captured with a detector; the X rays are then measured and assigned tones on a gray scale from black to white before a computer uses the tones to generate an image. The difference between film-screen mammography and digital mammography is in how the image is produced and processed, not in the X-ray technology itself. Most researchers agree that the potential benefits of digital mammography remain to be evaluated. It is hoped that digital mammography will improve the detection of breast abnormalities and small, early cancers, especially for women with dense breasts. Other advantages of digital mammography include improved enhancement of the image, lower doses of radiation exposure to the patient, fewer callbacks for false positives or unclear results, electronic storage of images, easy transmittal of images by telephone lines, and a faster review process since digital mammography takes only ten seconds of exposure.

The biggest disadvantage of digital mammography is cost; the equipment needed to perform the procedure was, at least on the eve of the FDA's approval, too expensive for most clinics and hospitals to procure. Digital mammography is not, therefore, widely used in the United States.

USES AND COMPLICATIONS

The first significant study to demonstrate the value of screening mammography was started in 1963 by the Health Insurance Plan of Greater New York. In this study, 31,000 women were screened annually using both mammography and physical examination and then compared to a control group of 31,000 women who sought medical attention only as the need arose. By 1975, the experimental group showed a 30 percent decrease in the rate of breast cancer mortality. A

1982 follow-up study continued to demonstrate a 23 percent decrease in death from breast cancer.

A similar large-scale project was launched in Europe. The ongoing Two County Swedish Study evaluated more than 130,000 women, who were randomly assigned to either a mammography group or a control group. In the absence of a physical examination, the mammography group showed a 25 percent decrease in the rate of breast cancers that are stage II and beyond, as well as a 31 percent reduction in breast cancer mortality. As the number describing the stage of cancer increases, the chances for long-term survival decrease.

The benefits of a lower stage at the time of detection and reduced mortality result from screening mammography alone. This study obtained only one image for each mammogram to accomplish this benefit. Other investigations have shown that single-view mammography misses 8 to 11 percent of cancers. Thus, even greater benefit would probably have been achieved in the Swedish study had two-view mammography been utilized.

Several large studies report the sensitivity of mammography in detecting breast cancer to be 86 to 95 percent. Of even greater consequence is that these studies demonstrate between 20 and 49 percent of breast cancers were detected solely by mammography. One should not conclude that physical examination is not necessary. Although mammography can detect the majority of breast cancers, there are some that elude X-ray detection yet may be detected by palpation with the fingers.

Any screening test will have both false positives and false negatives. A false-positive conclusion is when a test result indicates the presence of a disease or cancer when, in fact, none exists. A false-negative conclusion is when a test indicates that no disease or cancer is present when one actually exists. A false-negative mammogram can lead to a delay in biopsy that may reduce the chances for a full recovery. Dense breast tissue is the major reason for false-negative interpretations. Other causes for a false-negative mammogram include faulty radiographic techniques and errors in interpretation.

The American Cancer Society recognizes the complementary nature of mammography and physical examination. It thus recommends clinical breast examination by a physician every three years between the ages of twenty and thirty-nine and annual examinations after the age of forty. The Cancer Society also encourages women to perform monthly breast self-examinations after age twenty, despite the fact that mortality reduction from this method has not been shown objectively.

A major risk factor for breast cancer is aging. Multiple medical organizations—including the National Cancer Institute, American Medical Association, American College of Radiology, American College of Obstetricians and Gynecologists, American Academy of Family Physicians, and College of American Pathologists—have compiled specific recommendations, which differ slightly, for the screening of asymptomatic women. They have all endorsed and accepted various parts of the recommendations put forth by the American Cancer Society, which currently recommends annual or biannual screening mammography between the ages of forty and forty-nine and annual mammograms after the age of fifty. This is an area of ongoing change and controversy. Individuals are best advised to consult with their own physicians.

Over the years, the ability of mammography to detect breast cancers has significantly increased, while radiation doses to patients have decreased. The relatively high radiation exposures of the 1960's have now been drastically reduced. This diminished radiation exposure, coupled with increased understanding of radiation effects based on studies of women exposed to repeated chest fluoroscopy in tuberculosis sanatoriums and exposed at the Hiroshima and Nagasaki atomic explosions, has led to the conclusion that the benefit-risk ratio of screening mammography is overwhelmingly favorable. With modern dedicated mammography equipment, the radiation dose of a two-view screening mammogram is extremely low, about the same as a dental X ray. In 1985, the World Health Organization Committee on Technology Assessment stated that there is negligible risk when dedicated equipment for the screening mammography of women over the age of forty is used.

Mammography is often utilized as a screening technique in asymptomatic women for the detection of breast cancer. It can also serve as a diagnostic tool in patients with breast problems. Diagnostic mammography is performed when breast cancer is suspected. This is the case, for example, when a palpable mass or bloody nipple discharge has been noted. Ideally, mammography should be done before and after a surgical biopsy so that the postoperative changes within the breast tissue do not interfere with the interpretation of later mammograms.

Occasionally, mammography determines that a palpable mass, such as a calcified fibroadenoma, is clearly benign and therefore biopsy is not necessary. Because false-negative mammograms do occur, however, the function of mammography should not be to defer biopsy of a suspicious mass. Diagnostic mammography is also performed in a prebiopsy setting to detect hidden or multicentric cancer in either breast. Multicentricity has been reported in 20 to 75 percent of breast cancers.

Breast augmentation has become a popular surgery in contemporary society. Silicone implants do not place a woman at a higher risk than normal for breast cancer, but they may be associated with the development of several complications. The complications that can be observed on a mammogram include irregularities of the prosthesis and leakage of silicone into the surrounding tissues. The usefulness of mammography in patients with augmentation mammoplasty depends on the size of the implants and the quantity of breast tissue. It is important that both physician and patient are aware of the limitations. Recent improvements in mammography and positioning have made the imaging of implants more effective.

The features of breast cancer depicted on mammography can be primary, secondary, or indirect. The primary signs of malignancy include an ill-defined mass and clustered microcalcifications. Secondary signs include skin thickening with or without dimpling, nipple retraction, or axillary node enlargement. Indirect signs include architectural distortion, unilateral asymmetry, or a new density. An early cancer is defined as being asymptomatic, too small to be palpated, and without regional or distant metastases. Mammography signs of early breast cancer may be subtle.

One of the common features of benign breast disease seen on a mammogram are masses less than 1.5 centimeters in size with smooth margins and containing no microcalcifications. Repeated mammography in six months and then annually for a total of two and a half to three years may be sufficient to establish the stability of such masses. If a mass is circumscribed, ultrasound examination should be performed to determine if it is a cyst. If sonography shows that the mass is solid, then it must be biopsied. If the mass is not palpable, excision may be performed with prebiopsy needle localization.

Preoperative localization, performed by a radiologist, has become an important technique for the re-moval or biopsy of nonpalpable breast lesions. This method is extensively used to minimize the amount of breast tissue excised at biopsy. These localization techniques have simplified breast biopsy to the extent that it is usually conducted on an outpatient basis. This decreases the risk associated with general anesthesia and can be highly cost-effective. Fine needle aspiration has been used successfully for many types of breast abnormalities, often eliminating the need for surgical biopsy.

Because of the gloomy statistics on the high incidence of breast cancer, the well-publicized guidelines for periodic screening mammography, the overwhelming evidence that mammography can help detect breast cancer even before a physician or a woman feels a lump, and the national programs offering free or low-cost mammograms to the uninsured and poor, a high percentage of women do undergo screening mammography. This high compliance contrasts with the number of women in the 1980's who avoided mammograms because of cost, fear of radiation exposure, doubts about the sensitivity of mammograms, and inconvenience. In 2000, for example, 70 percent of women over fifty had a mammogram in the past two years compared with 27 percent in 1987.

As with any other medical procedure, it is essential that mammography be of high quality. To ensure this, the American College of Radiology Mammography Accreditation Program was begun in 1987. The program evaluates mammography equipment, radiation dose, and the qualifications of radiologists, radiologic technologists, and radiologic physicists. The goals of the program are to establish standards of quality for mammography and to provide a mechanism for radiologists to compare their own performance with national standards. Further, the program seeks to collect and disseminate data on the current practice of mammography, to encourage quality assurance practices in mammography, and to ensure reproducible high-quality images at a low radiation dose to the patient. The program has been designed to make the accreditation process instructive, encouraging compliance while pointing out potential deficiencies in mammography practice. A successful review of the facility results in accreditation for a period of three years, after which reevaluation is necessary.

If there are no accredited facilities nearby, the American College of Radiology advises women to choose one that possesses all the following qualities and credentials, because such a facility is likely to produce good images with minimal radiation exposure. The radiologist should be certified by the American Board of Radiology. Technologists should be certified by either the American Registry of Radiological Technologists or their state licensing board. Equipment used to produce mammograms should be specifically designed for breast imaging and should be calibrated, at least once a year, by a certified radiologic physicist. Both radiologists and technologists should have taken special courses or additional training in mammography. Finally, the radiologist who performs the mammography procedure should do so often as a regular part of practice.

Perspective and Prospects

It was not until the early 1950's that mammography began to gain recognition as a useful diagnostic procedure. At that time, surgeons and primary care physicians were only vaguely aware that it was possible to perform a radiographic examination of the breast. Albert Salomon, a German surgeon, performed the first radiographic studies of the breast on mastectomy specimens. He correlated the radiographic, gross, and microscopic anatomy of three thousand specimens and was the first to recognize and report nonpalpable breast cancer on specimen radiography.

In the United States, Stafford Warren pioneered the clinical use of breast radiography in 1930. He reported the appearance of normal breasts, identified fatty and glandular types, and illustrated the changes of pregnancy, mastitis, and benign and malignant tumors. Warren also emphasized the importance of comparing images of the right and left breasts by viewing them side by side. In 1938, Jacob Gershon-Cohen and Albert Strickler published a report signifying the amount of variations in the normal mammogram. During the 1940's, the literature emphasized only the technical difficulties and limitations of mammography.

In the 1950's, Raul Leborgne revitalized interest in mammography and helped to advance the morphologic principles, many of which remain relevant today. Gershon-Cohen and his associates published extensively on the characteristic findings of a mammogram. They noted the incidence of benign and malignant disease and were therefore able to establish reliable diagnostic criteria for carcinoma. Parallel work in Europe, particularly in France by Charles M. Gros, confirmed and amplified these findings. By the late 1950's, however, mammography was employed by only a few radiologists, and use of this procedure was hampered by a lack of studies showing its reliability and reproducibility.

The widespread adoption of mammography is attributable primarily to the work of Robert Egan and his colleagues. In 1960, Egan described a reproducible technique and reported successful results in imaging the breasts of his first thousand patients. This exciting news overcame the technical barrier to the widespread use of mammography and led to the training of radiologists and technologists across the United States in the performance and interpretation of mammograms.

The first significant screening project was undertaken in the 1960's by the Health Insurance Plan of Greater New York. In 1973, it was followed by a large-scale study, the Breast Cancer Detection Demonstration Project, sponsored by the American Cancer Society and National Cancer Institute, that involved the screening of 280,000 women by physical examination and mammography in twenty-seven centers across the United States. Mammography came under fire following concerns raised by John Bailar in 1976 that the doses used in the 1960's might induce the formation of breast carcinoma. This assessment generated public fear and halted much of the routine mammography. While this was a setback for screening, it did serve to stimulate the development of improved equipment to permit low-dose studies.

Modern mammography equipment is capable of detecting early, curable cancer with markedly reduced radiation doses. This advancement has enabled radiologists to conclude that the benefits of mammography far outweigh the theoretical risks. The challenges that continue to face mammography are both difficult and fascinating. They include working toward the goal of universal screening for all women and training an adequate number of qualified personnel to perform and interpret mammograms.

—*Stan Liu, M.D., and Lawrence W. Bassett, M.D.;*
updated by L. Fleming Fallon, Jr.,
M.D., Ph.D., M.P.H.,
and Cassandra Kircher, Ph.D.

See also Breast biopsy; Breast cancer; Breast disorders; Breast surgery; Breasts, female; Cancer; Cyst removal; Cysts; Glands; Gynecology; Imaging and radiology; Mastectomy and lumpectomy; Mastitis; Noninvasive tests; Oncology; Pathology; Screening; Tumor removal; Tumors.

FOR FURTHER INFORMATION:

Bassett, Lawrence W., ed. *The Radiologic Clinics of North America: Breast Imaging, Current Status and Future Directions*. Philadelphia: W. B. Saunders, 1992. This exceptional monograph, contributed by multiple preeminent physicians and researchers in the field of breast imaging, offers its readers definitive work on mammography and its related issues.

Bassett, Lawrence W., Reza Jahanshahi, Richard H. Gold, and Yao S. Fu. *Film-Screen Mammography: An Atlas of Instructional Cases*. London: Martin Dunitz, 1991. This teaching atlas is an anthology of high-quality mammograms with a wide variety of pathologically proved cases. These cases offer a significant diversity of mammographic manifestations with emphasis on the often-subtle features of carcinoma.

Gamagami, Parvis. *Atlas of Mammography: New Early Signs in Breast Cancer*. London: Blackwell Science, 1996. This interesting book provides many examples of mammogram images that will help laypeople to understand a mammogram.

Homer, Marc J. *Mammographic Interpretation: A Practical Approach*. 2d ed. New York: McGraw-Hill, 1997. This book is not intended to be a scholarly text. Rather, it is designed as an easy-to-follow guide and directly focuses on the day-to-day needs of the working radiologist.

Jatoi, Ismail. *Breast Cancer Screening*. New York: Chapman & Hall, 1997. The controversial area of mammographic screening of women under the age of fifty is addressed by Dr. Kopans, who argues in favor of screening, and by Dr. Jatoi, who argues against screening.

Kinne, David W., ed. *Multidisciplinary Atlas of Breast Surgery*. Philadelphia: Lippincott-Raven, 1997. Both professional and general readers will find this text to be useful. Five breast surgeons, two radiologists, four plastic surgeons, two pathologists, and one radiation oncologist have joined forces to present their primary techniques for breast surgery pertaining to cancer and subsequent reconstruction.

Kopans, Daniel B., ed. *Breast Imaging*. Philadelphia: Lippincott-Raven, 1998. This volume is well written and comprehensive as well as being an important reference in the field. Each chapter includes extensive scientific documentation with references to the literature, both classic and up-to-date.

MANIC-DEPRESSIVE DISORDER. *See* BIPOLAR DISORDER.

MARFAN SYNDROME
DISEASE/DISORDER

ANATOMY OR SYSTEM AFFECTED: Bones, eyes, heart, musculoskeletal system, spine

SPECIALTIES AND RELATED FIELDS: Cardiology, genetics, ophthalmology, orthopedics

DEFINITION: A condition in which the connective tissue does not form correctly and tends to be too flexible. The abnormal chemical composition, especially of the skeleton and heart, leads to major medical characteristics that are sometimes in evidence only at puberty.

CAUSES AND SYMPTOMS

Recent studies have located the gene that causes the inherited form of Marfan syndrome. About 25 percent of Marfan syndrome cases result from spontaneous mutation. While this knowledge promises better future recognition of the condition, the range and severity of the condition is so variable that diagnosis remains difficult.

Usually, Marfan syndrome is discovered through a detailed family history. The observation that a person is tall and slender and has unusually long fingers or arms is often an early clue. The presence of loose joints with great suppleness is characteristic of the disease. Manifestations of this condition may occur in any part of the body, but the heart, eyes, and spinal column are the most common.

TREATMENT AND THERAPY

Because a variety of organs may be involved in Marfan syndrome, it is essential that several specialists form a team to evaluate and monitor the patient during his or her lifetime. The most serious, and most common, problem area is the heart. Mitral valve problems may lead to leakage or regurgitation of blood. The aortic valve can develop a backflow into the heart.

In the eyes, a characteristic sign is the dislocation of the lens. This symptom is difficult to detect and, like many others, can vary widely in intensity. Cataracts are also associated with this condition.

Other characteristics are found in the skeleton. Spinal curvature, or scoliosis, and a breastbone that either protrudes or indents are observed. Crowded teeth and an arched palate are not uncommon.

Any of these symptoms can lead to serious consequences and should be discovered as early as possible. Regular examinations by specialists in cardiology, ophthalmology, and orthopedics are essential. Most of the possible progressive aspects of the condition can be treated effectively.

—K. Thomas Finley, Ph.D.

See also Bones and the skeleton; Cardiology; Cardiology, pediatric; Eyes; Genetic diseases; Growth; Heart; Mitral valve prolapse; Optometry; Optometry, pediatric; Orthopedics; Orthopedics, pediatric; Scoliosis; Visual disorders.

FOR FURTHER INFORMATION:

Fox, Elizabeth Lieber. *An Overview of the Marfan Syndrome.* Bossier, City, La.: Everett, 1989.

Hetzer, R., P. Gehle, and J. Ennker. *Cardiovascular Aspects of Marfan Syndrome.* New York: Springer-Verlag, 1994

Kaplan, Paul E., and Ellen D. Tanner. *Musculoskeletal Pain and Disability.* Norwalk, Conn.: Appleton and Lange, 1989.

Reed, E. Pyeritz, and Cheryll Gasner. *Marfan Syndrome.* 4th ed. Port Washington, N.Y.: National Marfan Foundation, 1994.

MASSAGE

TREATMENT

ANATOMY OR SYSTEM AFFECTED: All

SPECIALTIES AND RELATED FIELDS: Alternative medicine, exercise physiology, geriatrics and gerontology, oncology, pediatrics, physical therapy, preventive medicine, sports medicine

DEFINITION: The intentional and systematic manipulation of the soft tissues of the body to promote health and healing.

INDICATIONS AND PROCEDURES

Massage is used in both wellness and treatment models of health care. Wellness implies the achievement of an optimal state of well-being. The health enhancing effects of massage such as relaxation, stress reduction, increased body conditioning or awareness contribute to general wellness. In the treatment model, massage is considered a modality indicated to alleviate the symptoms and/or pain of a specific condition. A particular massage technique can be more or less effective for each illness or injury. The treatment model includes the subspecialty of sports massage, a beneficial intervention for athletes and people engaged in strenuous physical activity.

Two men were instrumental in the development of classic Western massage: Per Henrik Ling (1776-1839) and Johann Mezger (1838-1909). Ling developed an approach for treating medical conditions called the Swedish movement cure in the nineteenth century. Mezger defined four categories of massage using French terminology: *effleurage*, *petrissage*, *tapotement*, and *frictions*. The work of these men was further developed by their students and was incorporated into both regular and alternative medicine.

The physical effects of massage include healthy skin, relaxation, increased blood circulation and immune system functioning, metabolic balance in the muscles, connective tissue pliability, increased joint mobility and flexibility, and pain reduction. The mental and emotional benefits include increased mental clarity, reduced anxiety, and emotional release.

USES AND COMPLICATIONS

Massage has proven benefits for mind and body health. Research in the twentieth century showed a positive relationship between the reduction of pain and stress after massage. Other studies revealed that massage promoted weight gain in premature infants and reduced anxiety in adolescents hospitalized for psychiatric conditions. It can help slow the aging process among older adults and bring comfort to the terminally ill.

A basic tenet of massage practice is "Do no harm." Massage practitioners are trained to identify "endangerment sites." These are areas of the body which are less protected and more vulnerable to damage. "Contraindications" are conditions under which receiving massages are not advisable, such as when it could worsen a condition or spread infection. Health history information is essential for a safe massage session.

As of the year 2000, twenty-five states and the District of Columbia had licensing requirements for massage therapists. The American Massage Therapy Association (AMTA) had thirty thousand members who had to have a minimum of five hundred hours of training from a recognized school. Every practitioner must adhere to a code of ethics and standards of practice.

PERSPECTIVE AND PROSPECTS

Massage has been used for centuries in native and folk cultures all over the world. It has periodically lost and regained popularity in the Western world.

After a decline in the 1950's, it experienced a revival of credibility and value during the human potential movement of the late 1960's. Since then, it has been increasingly incorporated into medical treatment and prevention programs. The Office of Alternative Medicine was established by the National Institutes of Health to explore alternative medical practices. Massage therapy was included in the comprehensive 1994 report.

—Susan L. Sandel, Ph.D.

See also Acupressure; Alternative medicine; Headaches; Muscle sprains, spasms, and disorders; Muscles; Pain; Pain management; Physical rehabilitation; Stress; Stress reduction.

FOR FURTHER INFORMATION:

Alternative Medicine: Expanding Medical Horizons, a Report to the National Institutes of Health on Alternative Medicine Systems and Practices in the United States. Rockville, Md.: Office of Alternative Medicine, National Institutes of Health, 1994.

Fritz, Sandy, Kathleen Maison Paholsky, and M. James Grosenbach. *Mosby's Fundamentals of Therapeutic Massage.* 2d ed. St. Louis: Mosby Year Book, 1999.

Salvo, Susan G., and Maureen Pfeiffer, eds. *Massage Therapy: Principles and Practice.* Philadelphia: W. B. Saunders, 1999.

MASTECTOMY AND LUMPECTOMY

PROCEDURE

ANATOMY OR SYSTEM AFFECTED: Breasts (female), glands, muscles, musculoskeletal system

SPECIALTIES AND RELATED FIELDS: General surgery, gynecology, oncology

DEFINITION: Two surgical procedures for the treatment of breast cancer, which are equally effective in treating most patients with the disease.

KEY TERMS:

biopsy: a surgical procedure in which a lump or an abnormality is removed

breast preservation therapy: lumpectomy, followed by radiation therapy to the affected breast, with or without lymph node removal

chemotherapy: drugs, usually given by vein, that are used to kill cancer cells that have or may have spread to parts of the body beyond the breast and lymph nodes

clinical trial: a research study to compare standard treatment against potentially better treatment

in situ (noninvasive) breast cancer: cancer that is contained within the breast structure from which it arose

invasive breast cancer: cancer that has spread beyond the structure of the breast in which it arose and into surrounding breast tissue

lumpectomy: a breast biopsy which removes a rim of normal breast tissue around the abnormality

lymph nodes: structures that drain tissue fluid, bacteria, and tumor cells; the "glands" which, in breast cancer, are located under the arms and near the collarbone

mammography: an X ray of the breasts

mastectomy: removal of the breast

radiation therapy: X-ray treatment that is given after lumpectomy to decrease the chances of the cancer recurring in the treated breast

recurrence: the appearance of cancer after initial treatment has been completed

TREATMENT OPTIONS

Few Americans have traveled through their lives without being touched by breast cancer. More than 180,000 women, and about 1,400 men, are diagnosed with this disease every year in the United States. Breast cancer affects women so much more often than men that it is considered primarily a disease of women, and this discussion will be therefore restricted to the disease as it affects women. Women diagnosed with breast cancer are mothers, grandmothers, sisters, aunts, cousins, coworkers, and friends of many other people. When breast cancer is diagnosed, it affects all these people in important ways. Although the mass media have done an excellent job of trying to keep the public informed about breast cancer, especially in recent years, the anxiety that is precipitated when breast cancer is diagnosed results in confusion and often in a tendency to follow recommendations without much personal input. The treatment for breast cancer has changed so much since the mid-1980's, though, that the more educated a woman can become about current treatment options, the more ability that woman will have to participate in her own health care. This participation ultimately can lead to a sense of well-being and control over her own destiny.

The type of breast cancer with which a woman is diagnosed can have a major influence on treatment choices. Essentially, breast cancer exists in two major forms, corresponding to the two basic functional units of the breast: the lobules and the ducts. The lobules represent the cells that produce milk, and the ducts are the structures that carry the milk to the nipples. The two major forms of breast cancer are therefore referred to as lobular and ductal. Under each of these categories, there are two major subdivisions: invasive and in-situ (also called noninvasive). Thus, the basic classification is lobular, either invasive or noninvasive (in situ), and ductal, either invasive or noninvasive (in situ).

As a general rule, noninvasive breast cancer is unlikely to spread, whereas the invasive type is made up of cells that are often able to spread to local lymph nodes and/or to other parts of the body. Because of this, as well as many other factors, noninvasive breast cancer is treated differently from invasive breast cancer.

During the 1970's and 1980's, research studies were conducted throughout the world that changed scientists' understanding of the disease and its treatment. The largest was conducted in the United States and was called the National Surgical Adjuvant Breast and Bowel Project (NSABP) Trial B-06. The NSABP consists of a large group of cancer specialists interested in research. It was founded by Bernard Fisher, a surgeon from the University of Pittsburgh who believed that it was not necessary to remove the entire breast to treat breast cancer effectively. The B-06 trial began in the mid-1970's and represented a radical departure from the belief of most surgeons that breast cancer spread systematically from the breast to the lymph nodes to other parts of the body, and that if the breast and lymph nodes were removed quickly enough, the patient could be potentially cured of the disease. Fisher believed that breast cancer cells were unique in their ability to spread and that if the cancer had the biological characteristics to do so, it could spread to other parts of the body without necessarily being present in the lymph nodes. He further theorized that as long as the tumor was removed from the breast, the patients would do just as well as if they had their entire breast removed. To test his theories, women and their doctors were asked to participate in the B-06 study.

This research study started out by identifying patients who had been diagnosed with invasive breast cancer but had not yet been treated for the disease. To participate, all women had to have been diagnosed within thirty days of entry into the trial. More than eighteen hundred women throughout the United States agreed to participate in the B-06 research study. The participants agreed to accept, by chance, one of three treatments for their disease: lumpectomy, lumpectomy with radiation treatment to the breast, or mastectomy. A lumpectomy refers to the removal of a lump with a rim of normal breast tissue around it; oftentimes, this is accomplished at the time of the biopsy to diagnose the cancer. All women had the lymph nodes under their arm removed. Radiation therapy was given five days a week for about six weeks if a woman was assigned to the radiation therapy group. Any woman in any group who had positive lymph nodes (nodes to which the tumor had spread) had chemotherapy to kill tumor cells that may have spread beyond the lymph nodes to other parts of the body. The patients were then followed closely by their doctors to monitor for tumor recurrence, just as any breast cancer patient would be. At the end of five years, the percentage of women who were alive and who had no sign of the tumor returning to parts of the body separate from the breast was checked in each group. The percentages were the same in each group, proving that Fisher's theory was correct for at least a five-year follow-up. These results were made known to the medical world in 1985.

In 1988, eight-year follow-up results showed that, again, the percentage of women in each group who were alive with no sign of the tumor returning in parts of the body separate from the breast was the same. An important finding, however, was that women in the group that had lumpectomy alone had breast cancer recur in the breast almost half of the time; treatment for this recurrence meant a mastectomy in most cases. In the group that had a lumpectomy with the addition of radiation therapy, only 10 percent of the patients had cancer come back in the breast after eight years of follow-up. The women who had a mastectomy obviously could not have breast cancer recurrence, but about 8 percent had tumor recurrence in the mastectomy incision or on the chest wall. Many women are surprised to learn that breast cancer can recur at the surgical site even if they choose a mastectomy. In summary, the NSABP B-06 trial demonstrated that equal results could be achieved with breast preservation techniques (lumpectomy plus radiation therapy) as compared with mastectomy.

In March, 1994, *The Chicago Tribune* published a series of news articles about research fraud within the NSABP. It had been discovered that a researcher in

Montreal had falsified data submitted to the NSABP in several studies, one of which was the B-06 trial. This revelation caused an understandable amount of concern among women who had chosen breast preservation therapy, as well as their doctors. To address this concern, the trial results were reanalyzed without the fraudulent data by an independent group of statisticians hired by the National Cancer Institute. In addition, original medical charts of trial participants were audited to make sure that the data submitted to the NSABP by other investigators were correct. The outcome of the audits and data reanalysis confirmed the original conclusions. In addition, several other trials had been conducted by this time comparing breast preservation therapy with mastectomy. All have concluded that lumpectomy with radiation therapy and mastectomy are equivalent in the local treatment of breast cancer.

TYPES OF BREAST CANCER

Lobular carcinoma in situ (noninvasive lobular carcinoma). Lobular carcinoma in situ (LCIS) is viewed by most pathologists and breast cancer specialists as a "marker" for the development of breast cancer in the future, rather than as a true cancer that needs to be treated aggressively. Most of the time, LCIS does not form a lump in the breast, nor does it appear as an abnormality on a mammogram. Instead, it is usually found incidentally when a woman has a breast biopsy for any one of a number of different reasons. Although the number of studies about this disease is low, almost all that exist demonstrate that about 30 percent of women diagnosed with LCIS will develop this cancer in the breast that had the original diagnosis of LCIS, the rest in the opposite breast. In addition, about half of the women develop the lobular form of breast cancer, the other half the ductal form. If a woman is examined by a health care provider every four or six months and is willing to undergo yearly mammography, many breast specialists will suggest that the woman needs no treatment for LCIS but does need close follow-up. The only other logical treatment, if a woman either cannot be followed closely or if she chooses to have treatment, is bilateral mastectomies, meaning the removal of both breasts. Some patients find this confusing. Why would one treat LCIS, if it is only a marker for breast cancer, with bilateral mastectomy? The answer is that since both breasts are at risk, both need to be treated. The treatment is purely preventive.

One way to think about this approach is that if a woman's mother or sister was diagnosed with breast cancer, especially if the diagnosis was premenopausal, then the woman's risk for developing breast cancer at some point in the future is about 20 to 30 percent; this is very close to the same percent risk as if a woman was diagnosed with LCIS herself. Under these circumstances, one could choose close follow-up—which most women do—or preventive mastectomies. If the latter were chosen, it would not make sense to have only one breast removed—the one on the same side as the family member's diagnosis—as both breasts would be at risk for developing cancer. The same is true for LCIS.

Ductal carcinoma in situ (noninvasive ductal carcinoma; intraductal carcinoma). The terminology for this type of breast cancer can be confusing; "intraductal carcinoma" is not the same as "invasive ductal carcinoma." Ductal carcinoma in situ (DCIS), intraductal carcinoma, and noninvasive ductal carcinoma all refer to the same process: cancer that arises from the duct but that has not spread outside it. Whenever the term "invasive" precedes a classification for cancer, it means that the cancer cells have spread beyond the structure from which they arose.

DCIS is being increasingly diagnosed. Unfortunately, it is a much more serious kind of cancer than LCIS. It is not, however, nearly as serious as invasive breast cancer. DCIS can present as a lump in the breast, but more commonly it presents as a mammographic abnormality exclusively. DCIS is considered an early form of breast cancer, but there are many subtypes of it, and some behave more aggressively than others. DCIS behaves much differently from LCIS, for reasons that are not well understood. Although, again, research studies about this disease are few, the studies that do exist reveal some interesting facts. In the past, most women who were diagnosed with DCIS had the involved breast removed. The only way, then, to do research to determine what would happen to women who were diagnosed with DCIS who did not have mastectomy was to review thousands of slides of benign biopsy results and find cases where the proper diagnosis was actually DCIS. Predictably, only a few cases could be found that would fall into that category. Those women were then contacted to establish what had happened to them. The studies show that an average of about 40 percent of women had breast cancer recur in the breast; of those who did, almost all represented the ductal type of breast cancer, and almost all recurred not only in the same breast but also in the same part of the breast as the original diagnosis. Because of these findings, the treatment recommendations for DCIS are totally different than those for LCIS.

One of the biggest problems with DCIS is that the optimum treatment is currently unknown. For many years, breast removal was considered curative, and in the great majority of women, it was, and still is. Many surgeons seriously question, though, whether removal of the entire breast is necessary in cases of DCIS, especially because the NSABP B-06 data revealed breast preservation to be equivalent to mastectomy for most patients with a much more aggressive type of breast cancer—the invasive type. Currently, clinical trials are under way to try to help sort out the treatment dilemmas faced by patients and their surgeons regarding the best treatment for DCIS.

Invasive breast cancer; lobular or ductal. Invasive breast cancer is the most common type of breast cancer diagnosed, and the ductal variety is by far the type that affects most of these women. From what has been learned about noninvasive breast cancer, one might predict big differences in the way that invasive lobular and invasive ductal carcinoma behave. Actually, however, the behavior of the two varieties, as well as the treatment, is similar. One pathologist compared the two major types of invasive breast cancer as similar to the difference between Indian and African elephants—not much difference to the majority of observers.

In contrast to the treatment of the noninvasive types of breast cancer, much is known about the optimal treatment of the invasive disease. This situation has proven to have advantages and disadvantages for women newly diagnosed with invasive breast cancer, who face a bewildering array of issues, often for the first time. Under these circumstances, it is often emotionally easier to simply tell the doctor to "do whatever has to be done" and to accept the recommendation willingly. When there are no treatment options of equal benefit, this is obviously appropriate. In the case of breast cancer, however, treatment options do exist. Although these may be initially confusing, when sorted out these choices provide women with a sense of control over their lives that can be of enormous emotional benefit to them. The basic surgical decision to be made is whether an individual woman is eligible for breast preservation; almost all women are eligible for the mastectomy option. Actually,

about 75 percent (or more) of women are candidates for breast preservation; the National Cancer Institute has issued a statement that breast preservation is the preferred treatment in most women with breast cancer, whether it has spread to the lymph nodes or not. Factors that may disqualify a patient from breast preservation therapy include pregnancy, previous radiation therapy to the breast, no radiation treatment center available, more than one cancer in the breast, or a tumor size in relation to breast size that would make the cosmetic results undesirable. For those who require or desire mastectomy, immediate or delayed reconstruction is an option that many women choose. Many also choose a mastectomy alone. It is not the treatment that seems to matter, but the woman's ability to exercise her options and make choices that are right for her. Health providers can and should help guide the decision by answering questions, but if a woman is eligible for either breast preservation or mastectomy, the ultimate treatment decision is hers. Some women worry about the idea of radiation therapy. Actually, the most common side effect from radiation therapy to the breast is a skin reaction similar to a sunburn. This is usually easily treated with creams. The side effects that cause the most worries, such as nausea, vomiting, and hair loss, do not occur from radiation therapy to the breast. Another common area of confusion is the difference between radiation therapy and chemotherapy. It is important to know that breast cancer treatment usually involves two major concerns: treatment to the breast itself, and treatment to the rest of the body, as breast cancer cells sometimes spread even before the diagnosis can be made. Chemotherapy is medicine that treats the whole body, but it is not very effective by itself in treating the breast tissue. It is important, therefore, for a woman who needs chemotherapy to have radiation therapy to the breast as well, if she chooses breast preservation treatment.

To find out the best treatment options available, women are advised to consult with surgeons experienced in breast preservation therapy, as well as with one or more radiation oncologists, physicians who administer radiation therapy. It is especially helpful to seek the opinion of the entire team of treating physicians prior to making a final decision about what treatment choice is preferred. This team includes a surgical oncologist or general surgeon, a radiation oncologist, a medical oncologist, and often a plastic surgeon. These physicians will work together to provide recommendations most optimal for an individual patient. Second opinions are to be encouraged.

Perspective and Prospects

Until the mid-1980's, most women who were diagnosed with breast cancer presented to their doctors with a self-discovered breast lump or were found to have a mass in the breast on a routine breast examination. Thinking that this situation represented a true medical emergency, women were often advised to have surgery within one to two days, so that the cancer would have minimal opportunity to spread. The routine at that time was to perform almost all surgical procedures as inpatient procedures under general anesthesia. The women were almost always asked to sign a consent form that read similar to "breast biopsy possible modified radical mastectomy." With this consent, the woman gave her permission to have her breast removed if the lump proved to represent cancer. In the 1970's, a journalist by the name of Rose Kushner questioned the practice of signing for a breast biopsy and allowing a surgeon to remove the diseased breast in the same operation. She became the voice for thousands of women with breast problems in encouraging doctors to consider a different way of doing things, one which involved more active participation on the part of the woman.

Since that time, much has been learned about the biology of breast cancer—how it grows, when it might spread, and how quickly it does so. This knowledge has changed the approach to the diagnosis and treatment of the disease. At the same time, the American Cancer Society began an active campaign to promote screening mammography as a method to detect breast cancer earlier than it might be felt as a lump in the breast. In one large study, called the Breast Cancer Detection and Demonstration Project (BCDDP), 40 percent of women diagnosed with breast cancer were diagnosed solely on the basis of mammography, 45 percent of the women had both an abnormal physical exam and an abnormal mammogram, and 15 percent of the women with breast cancer had an abnormal physical examination but a normal mammogram. This latter fact is very important: Mammograms are great tools for helping to detect breast cancer in early stages, but they are not fool-proof. Any woman with a breast lump needs to have it evaluated, even if the mammogram result is "normal." As mammography came into more widespread use, and tumors were diagnosed that were smaller in size, it became more difficult for pathologists (doctors who view slides under the microscope) to tell surgeons whether the small abnormality removed really represented cancer while the patient was still in the operating room. This change contributed to the trend toward diagnosing the lump or abnormal mammogram during one operation, and treating the cancer in a separate operation. Consequently, a woman was given some time to think about the fact that she had cancer, to learn about the disease and to ask questions about it, and to learn about her treatment options. It also allowed her time to make arrangements for an upcoming hospitalization for breast cancer treatment. Concurrent with this trend was the increased understanding that breast cancer grows much more slowly than was originally thought. Most breast cancer experts agree that the first cancerous cell that appears in the breast is probably present about eight to ten years before it can be detected, even by mammography. This knowledge has contributed to the understanding that it is perfectly safe to treat breast cancer within a few days or weeks after the diagnosis, after the patient and family have had time to absorb the diagnosis and get answers to their questions.

Research findings continue to challenge the assumptions and beliefs of medicine regarding the diagnosis and treatment of breast cancer. As much has changed since the mid-twentieth century, so too are research advances expected to change the medical profession's approach to the disease in the future. The ultimate goal is to eradicate the disease entirely for future generations of women.

—*Janet Rose Osuch, M.D.*

See also Breast biopsy; Breast cancer; Breast disorders; Breast surgery; Breasts, female; Cancer; Chemotherapy; Gynecology; Malignancy and metastasis; Mammography; Oncology; Plastic surgery; Radiation therapy; Sex change surgery; Tumor removal; Tumors.

For Further Information:

"Doctor Main Variable in Mastectomy Choice." *The New York Times*, November 28, 2000, 12. A recent study has found that the specialist a patient chooses and the surgeon's preference for either radical breast surgery (mastectomy) or surgery to remove the tumor only (lumpectomy) may determine a woman's course of treatment.

Gottlieb, Scott. "Lumpectomy as Good as Mastectomy for Tumors up to 5 cm Across." *Western Journal of*

Medicine 173, no. 4. According to a new study, in women with breast cancers up to 5 cm across, the rates of long-term survival and metastasis-free survival are similar for mastectomy and breast-conserving treatment.

Love, Susan M. *Dr. Susan Love's Breast Book*. Reading, Mass.: Addison-Wesley, 2000. This easy-to-read paperback is one of the most influential books in women's health written for a general audience. The splendidly well written guide explains with exceptional clarity and detail breast development, changes with age, and breast cancer detection and treatment.

"Lumpectomy Possible for Bigger Breast Tumors." *Nursing Standard* 15, no. 1 (September 20-September 26, 2000): 10. While lumpectomy is widely used in women with tumors smaller than two centimeters, its suitability for larger tumors was unknown. The first study of its kind has determined that metastatic spread was no more common in women who had a lumpectomy than in those who had a mastectomy.

MASTITIS

DISEASE/DISORDER

ANATOMY OR SYSTEM AFFECTED: Breasts

SPECIALTIES AND RELATED FIELDS: Bacteriology, gynecology

DEFINITION: Mastitis is an infection of the female breast resulting in inflammation, tenderness, swelling, and pain. The condition often occurs with breast-feeding, when bacteria enter through the nipple. The infection does not spread rapidly, generally remaining localized, because the breast is composed of much fatty tissue and has a widely dispersed system of blood vessels. An abscess may form, in which the infected tissue hardens and becomes walled off from healthy tissue. Antibiotics usually destroy the bacteria; if not, a needle biopsy, mammogram, or surgical biopsy may be indicated to rule out cancer. Mastitis can also be caused by changes in sex hormones in newborns and at puberty, and chronic mastitis, which is characterized by lumps in the breasts, may be attributable to hormone changes as well.

—*Jason Georges and Tracy Irons-Georges*
See also Abscess drainage; Abscesses; Antibiotics; Bacterial infections; Breast biopsy; Breast disorders; Breast-feeding; Breasts, female; Hormones; Mammography.

FOR FURTHER INFORMATION:

Boston Women's Health Book Collective. *Our Bodies, Ourselves for the New Century*. New York: Simon & Schuster, 1998.

Epps, R., and the American Medical Women's Association, eds. *The Women's Complete Handbook*. New York: Dell Books, 1995.

Kinne, David W., ed. *Multidisciplinary Atlas of Breast Surgery*. Philadelphia: Lippincott-Raven, 1997.

Love, Susan M., and Karen Lindsey. *Dr. Susan Love's Breast Book*. 2d ed. Reading, Mass.: Addison-Wesley, 1995.

MASTURBATION

DEVELOPMENT

ANATOMY OR SYSTEM AFFECTED: Genitals

SPECIALTIES AND RELATED FIELDS: Psychiatry

DEFINITION: A manual stimulation of one's own or another person's genital organs usually resulting in orgasm without engaging in sexual intercourse.

PHYSICAL AND PSYCHOLOGICAL FACTORS

Masturbation is the first sexual experience among a great majority of people. Some young people inadvertently stumble on sexual arousal and orgasm in the course of engaging in some other physical activity. Others purposefully stimulate themselves, aroused by curiosity after reading erotic literature, watching sexually explicit films, or listening to imaginary or real sexual adventures of their peers.

Most men and women practice masturbation to relieve sexual tension, achieve sexual pleasure, enjoy sexual stimulation in the absence of an available partner, and experience relaxation. When masturbating, men tend to focus on the stimulation of penis. Stimulation of the clitoral shaft and clitoral area with a hand or an object is the method that women most commonly employ. Some women masturbate by using a vibrator. Mutual masturbation provides a satisfying and pleasurable form of sexual intimacy and release for many couples. It is also one of the most common techniques that gay and lesbian couples use during sexual intimacy.

DISORDERS AND EFFECTS

Under certain circumstances, masturbation may result in some undesirable consequences. If a child masturbates constantly, it may be an indication of excessive anxiety and tension. Compulsive and frenzied masturbation may reflect abuse or maltreatment in a child's home life. Frequent masturbation may be a child's way of relieving tension or unconsciously re-enacting past or present traumatic sexual episodes. Among adults, excessive masturbation may point toward a person's lack of self-esteem and the resultant fear and inability to develop healthy interpersonal relationships with persons of the opposite sex. Psychiatry, psychotherapy, and sex therapy have proven helpful in successfully alleviating these problems.

PERSPECTIVE AND PROSPECTS

Throughout history, attitudes toward the practice of masturbation have been riddled with misconceptions, guilt, and fear. Fear of masturbation and its supposed harmful effects, such as loss of memory and intelligence, was widespread in the nineteenth century. Semen was considered a vital fluid important for bodily functioning, and wasting it through masturbation was considered as contributing to weakening of the body and production of illness. Medical authorities today do not find any evidence of physical damage from masturbation. In fact, many modern sex therapists encourage self-stimulation as part of healthy sexuality. In modern sex therapy, masturbation has become part of the therapeutics used in treating certain sexual dysfunctions. Patients with difficulties or inability to have orgasm are encouraged by their therapists to engage in masturbation. It is widely believed that orgasm once achieved through masturbation will eventually generalize and transfer to satisfactory sexual intercourse.

—*Tulsi Saral, Ph.D.*

See also Domestic violence; Puberty and adolescence; Reproductive system; Sexual dysfunction; Sexuality.

FOR FURTHER INFORMATION:

Dodson, Betty. *Sex for One: The Joy of Selfloving.* New York: Crown, 1996.

Marcus, Irwin. *Masturbation: From Infancy to Senescence.* Madison, Conn.: International Universities Press, 1975.

Rowan, Edward L. *The Joy of Self-Pleasuring: Why Feel Guilty About Feeling Good.* Amherst, Mass.: Prometheus Books, 2000.

Sarnoff, Suzanne, and Irving Sarnoff. *Masturbation and Adult Sexuality.* Bridgewater, N.J.: Replica Books, 2000.

MEASLES

DISEASE/DISORDER

ALSO KNOWN AS: Morbilli, rubeola

ANATOMY OR SYSTEM AFFECTED: Ears, lungs, mouth, nervous system, respiratory system, skin

SPECIALTIES AND RELATED FIELDS: Family practice, internal medicine, pediatrics, public health, virology

DEFINITION: A highly contagious disease contracted through a virus transmitted in respiratory secretions and characterized by a spreading skin rash.

KEY TERMS:

buccal mucosa: the tissue of the mouth and cheeks

desquamation: the sloughing off of the outer layers of skin

Koplik's spots: small red spots with white centers generally found in the mouth during early stages of measles

maculopapular rash: reddish skin eruptions characterized by small, flat discolorations that may progress into small pimples

otitis media: infection or inflammation of the middle ear, an occasional complication of measles infection

paramyxoviruses: a group of ribonucleic acid (RNA) viruses that includes the etiological agents for measles, mumps, and a variety of respiratory infections

pharyngitis: infection or inflammation of the pharynx, or throat

photophobia: abnormal sensitivity of the eyes to light, a condition common to a variety of illnesses including measles

prodromal stage: the early stage of a disease during which symptoms first appear

viremia: a condition characterized by the presence of a virus in the bloodstream

CAUSES AND SYMPTOMS

Measles is a highly contagious viral disease characterized by a maculopapular (pimply) rash that develops on the skin and spreads rapidly over much of the cutaneous surface of the body. Measles virus is classified with the paramyxoviruses, a class of viruses in which ribonucleic acid (RNA) serves as the genetic material. Closely related viruses in the same group include rinderpest and distemper virus, agents associated with disease in ruminants such as cows and in dogs or cats, respectively. It is likely that measles originated when one of these other animal viruses became adapted to humans several thousand years ago.

In modern times but before the advent of measles vaccination, measles was a common disease of childhood, usually appearing between the ages of five and ten. The illness is among the most contagious of infections, and the virus was generally spread among children in schools. Widespread immunization of children, begun in the 1960's, tended to push the age of exposure into the teenage years. Most outbreaks since the 1980's have occurred among college students. Since recovery from the disease confers lifelong immunity, infection among older adults is infrequent. In developing or Third World nations, places where vaccination may be haphazard, measles is still a disease of early childhood; malnutrition and related problems of poverty have resulted in a significant level of mortality among infected children.

Exposure generally follows an oral-oral means of transmission, as the person inhales contaminated droplets from an infected individual. The incubation period for active measles ranges from seven to fourteen days. During this early stage, the infected individual becomes increasingly contagious. The lack of any obvious symptoms during these early stages lends itself to the spread of the disease.

Contact by the virus with the surface cells of the respiratory passages, or sometimes the conjunctiva (the inner surface of the eye), allows the infectious agent to enter the body. The virus spreads through the local lymph nodes into the blood, producing a primary viremia. During this period, the virus replicates both in the lymph nodes and in the respiratory sites through which the virus entered the body. The virus returns to the bloodstream, resulting in a secondary viremia and widespread passage of the virus throughout the body by the fifth to seventh day after the initial exposure. Viral levels in the blood reach their peak toward the end of the incubation period, some fourteen days after infection. Once symptoms begin, the virus is widely disseminated throughout the body, including sites in small blood vessels, lymph nodes, and even the central nervous system.

The initial incubation period is followed by a prodromal stage, in which active symptoms appear. This stage is characterized by a fever that may reach as high as 103 degrees Fahrenheit, coughing, sensitivity of the eyes to light (photophobia), and malaise. Koplik's spots appear on the buccal mucosa in the mouth one to two days prior to development of the characteristic measles rash.

The maculopapular rash first appears on the head and behind the ears and gradually spreads over the rest of the body during the course of twenty-four to forty-eight hours. Clear signs of respiratory infection appear, including a cough, pharyngitis, and occasional involvement of the bronchioles or even pneumonia. While malaise and anorexia (appetite loss) are common during the fever period, diarrhea and vomiting generally do not occur. Over time, the rash becomes increasingly dense, exhibiting a blotchy character. Desquamation is common in many affected areas of the skin. Gradually, over a period of three to five days, the rash begins to fade, usually following the sequence by which it first appeared. The rash fades first on the forehead, then on the extremities.

Complications, while they do occur, are unusual in otherwise healthy individuals. Most result from secondary bacterial infections. Occasionally, these complications may manifest themselves as infections of the ear. Pulmonary infections are common among cases of measles and account for most of the rare deaths that follow development of the disease. Photophobia is also common, accounting for the former belief that measles patients had to be kept in a dark room; as long as the patient is comfortable, this step is unnecessary.

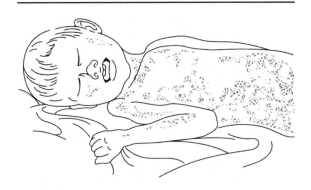

Red measles most often affects children; its calling card is the rash that appears on the face and spreads downward.

The obvious manifestations of measles infection make the isolation of the virus unnecessary for diagnosis. Ironically, the near disappearance of measles in the United States has made most physicians unfamiliar with the disease; it is not unusual for an attending physician to mistake the rash for another illness. For this reason, laboratory diagnosis is often useful. Laboratory confirmation is generally based on a serological assay for measles antibodies in the blood of infected persons.

A rare sequela to measles infection is the development of subacute sclerosing panencephalitis, a disease characterized by progressive neurological deterioration. The specific mechanism by which measles infection may develop into this disease remains unclear, but it may be the result of a rare combination of events in the victim. Since spread of the virus into the central nervous system is common during measles infection while the development of subacute sclerosing panencephalitis is rare (approximately one case per 100,000 measles infections), it is likely that some form of immune impairment is at the root of this disease. Diagnosis of subacute sclerosing panencephalitis is difficult and is based on developing dementia accompanied by unusual levels of measles antibodies in cerebrospinal fluid.

TREATMENT AND THERAPY

No specific treatment for measles is available; therapy consists of symptomatic intervention. Bed rest is recommended, and the patient should not come into contact with persons not previously exposed to the virus through either natural infection or immunization.

Itching of the rash is common and may be treated with cool water or the standard regimen of cornstarch or baking soda applications. The most common complications result from secondary bacterial infections, which generally take the form of otitis media (middle-ear infection), pharyngitis, or pneumonia. Appropriate use of antibiotics is usually sufficient to prevent or treat such complications.

Immunization with the measles virus may be either passive or active. Children less than one year of age and patients who are immunocompromised or chronically ill may be protected if human immunoglobulin is administered within a week after exposure. While effective immunity is short term, it is capable of protecting these individuals during this period. Since no active disease or infection develops, however, immunity to future infection remains minimal in these cases.

During the early 1960's, an effective vaccine was developed to immunize children against measles. The vaccine consists of an attenuated form of the virus. Although early forms of the vaccine were inconsistent in producing a lifelong immunity, they were effective in decreasing the prevalence of the disease. Later generations of the attenuated vaccine proved more effective in developing long-term immunity among the recipients.

Since maternal antibodies are present in newborns, it is recommended that measles immunization begin between twelve and fifteen months of age. Often, this program is part of a combination MMR vaccine, for measles, mumps, and rubella (German measles). A second booster is given following elementary school. The American Academy of Pediatrics does not consider a third vaccination to be necessary if the approved routine has been followed. It is recommended that children who were first immunized prior to their first birthday should receive boosters at fifteen months of age and again at age twelve. Indications are that immunity from vaccination is long term, if not lifelong. Recovery from natural infection results in a lifelong immunity to measles.

Inconsistency of the first generation of vaccine resulted in ineffective immunity among some individuals vaccinated during the 1960's. A number of small outbreaks during the 1980's were the result. Most cases of measles, however, have occurred in individuals who failed to be immunized.

PERSPECTIVE AND PROSPECTS

The origin and early history of measles is uncertain, as the first authentic description of measles as a specific entity was that by the Arab physician al-Razi (Rhazes) in a 910 treatise on smallpox and measles. Rhazes quoted earlier work by the Hebrew physician El Yehudi, so it is likely that familiarity with these respective illnesses had existed for some time.

Measles is entirely a human disease, with no known animal reservoir. Consequently, the paucity of human populations of sufficient size to maintain transmission means that the spread of such an epidemic disease would have been unlikely before 2500 B.C.E. It is probable that the disease entered the human species through adaptation of the similar animal viruses of rinderpest or distemper. The absence of any description of a disease like measles in the writings of Hippocrates (c. fourth century B.C.E.) likewise renders it unlikely that the disease was widespread before that date.

Epidemic disease with a rash characteristic of measles is known to have spread through the Roman Empire during the early centuries of the common era. The difficulty in differentiating measles from smallpox by the physicians of the time contributes to the difficulty in understanding the history of the illness. It is certain that by the time of Rhazes, measles had become common in the population.

The terminology of measles lent further confusion during the Middle Ages. Measles was often referred to as *morbilli*, a Latin term meaning "little disease," to distinguish it from *il morbo*, or plague. The word "measles" first appeared in the fourteenth century treatise *Rosa Anglica*, by John of Gaddesden. The term may have been applied initially to the sores on the legs of lepers (*mesles*), and it was only later that illnesses characterized by similar rashes (measles, smallpox, and rubella) were clearly differentiated by European physicians. The significance of a rash with white centers in the mouth was probably recognized by John Quier in Jamaica and Richard Haxeltine in New England during the latter portion of the eighteenth century, but it was in 1896 that the American pediatrician Henry Koplik firmly reported their role in early stages of the disease.

Measles followed the path of European explorers to the Americas during the sixteenth century. Repeated outbreaks of measles devastated the native populations, which had minimal immunity to the newly introduced disease. The most thorough epidemiological investigation of measles newly introduced into a population was that by Peter Panum in his study *Observations Made During the Epidemic of Measles on the Faroe Islands in the Year 1846* (1940). In the population of 7,864 persons, 6,100 of them became ill, with 102 deaths. Mortality rates as high as 25 percent were not unusual in previously unexposed populations. In Hawaii in 1848, 40,000 deaths occurred among the population of 150,000 persons following the introduction of measles. Even higher mortality rates probably occurred among the populations of Peru and Mexico in 1530-1531, following their exposure to infected Spanish explorers.

The earliest attempt at immunization was probably that of Francis Home of Edinburgh in 1758. Home soaked cotton in the blood of measles patients and placed it on the small cuts on the skin of children. The viral nature of measles was first demonstrated by John Anderson and Joseph Goldberger of the United States Public Health Service, who in 1911 induced the disease in monkeys using filtered extracts from human tissue. In 1954, the virus itself was isolated by John Enders, who grew the agent in human and monkey tissue in a laboratory.

The first effective vaccine was developed by Enders in 1958 using an attenuated (live) form of the virus. The vaccine was tested and then licensed in 1963. Several variations of the vaccine that proved superior in producing long-term immunity were developed in the decades that followed. In 1974, the World Health Organization introduced a widespread vaccination program within developing countries.

The absence of any natural reservoir for measles other than humans has made the eradication of the disease possible. Active immunization of children in the United States reduced the annual incidence of the disease from 482,000 reported cases in 1962 to fewer than 1,000 in the late 1990's. Widespread vaccination and worldwide surveillance has made global eradication of the disease a realistic possibility.

—Richard Adler, Ph.D.

See also Childhood infectious diseases; Fever; Immunization and vaccination; Mumps; Rashes; Rubella; Viral infections.

FOR FURTHER INFORMATION:

Bernstein, David, and Gilbert Schiff. "Viral Exanthems and Localized Skin Infections." In *Atlas of Infectious Diseases*, edited by Sherwood L. Gorbach et al. Philadelphia: W. B. Saunders, 2000. This book contains extensive discussions of bacterial and viral illnesses. The section addressing measles contains much information about the symptoms and progression of the disease.

Clayman, Charles B., ed. *The American Medical Association Family Medical Guide*. New York: Random House, 1994. An excellent general source for information about illnesses and questions about medical problems.

Evans, Alfred S. *Causation and Disease: A Chronological Journey*. New York: Plenum Press, 1993. The author provides a thorough discussion of the nature of infectious disease and factors associated with its spread. The science of epidemiology is emphasized.

Kiple, Kenneth F., ed. *The Cambridge World History of Human Disease*. New York: Cambridge University Press, 1993. In addition to being an encyclopedia describing human diseases, this book provides an epidemiological history of disease and discusses possible origins and treatments. The authors target a general population.

McGrew, Roderick E., with Margaret P. McGrew. *Encyclopedia of Medical History*. New York:

McGraw-Hill, 1985. As an encyclopedia, the text provides at best an abbreviated discussion of the topic of measles, but it does provide a useful history of the subject.

Madigan, Michael, et al. *Brock Biology of Microorganisms*. 9th ed. Upper Saddle River, N.J.: Prentice Hall, 2000. A college textbook on the subject of microbiology. An extensive section on microbial diseases provides a concise description of measles and its prevention.

MEDICARE
HEALTH CARE SYSTEM

DEFINITION: A U.S. federal program that covers many of the hospital costs and doctor bills for elderly and disabled persons and those with end-stage renal (kidney) disease.

KEY TERMS:

cost sharing: the contribution required from a Medicare beneficiary toward the cost of health services; usually figured in terms of coinsurance (a share of the bill) and deductibles (the amount that beneficiaries must pay before coverage kicks in at all)

Medicare part A: the part of the Medicare program that covers hospital, skilled nursing, and home health services; sometimes simply referred to as hospital insurance (HI)

Medicare part B: the part of the Medicare program that covers physician services, outpatient care, and other ambulatory services; also called supplementary medical insurance (SMI)

RULES AND PROVISIONS

The Medicare program was established in the United States in 1965 as Title XVIII of the Social Security Act and first went into effect on July 1, 1966. This federal government program is divided into two basic parts: part A, or hospital insurance (HI); and part B, or supplementary medical insurance (SMI).

In 1992, this constantly changing program covered three groups of individuals: persons aged sixty-five or older who are also eligible for any type of Social Security benefit; persons who have been receiving Social Security disability benefits for two years; and insured workers and their spouses or children with end-stage renal disease (ESRD). Disability coverage is limited to the covered worker or an adult disabled child of a covered worker. Eligible persons are enrolled in Medicare part A at no charge.

Almost all Americans over the age of sixty-five are eligible and participate in Medicare—31 million people in 1992. Anyone over the age of sixty-five not otherwise eligible may enroll in Medicare by paying a monthly premium of $192. In 1992, nearly 20,000 persons elected such enrollment. These are generally individuals who have had little or no labor force attachment or who immigrated to the United States from abroad.

A two-year waiting period for Medicare coverage existed in 1992 for the disabled. Coupled with a five-month waiting period for eligibility for Social Security, this meant that individuals with disabilities did not receive Medicare coverage until twenty-nine months after the onset of the disability. In 1991, 3.4 million disabled Americans were covered by Medicare. Dependents of disabled beneficiaries are not eligible for Medicare unless they are aged sixty-five or older.

ESRD patients are covered once they file for benefits and if they are entitled to monthly Social Security benefits or are children or spouses of covered workers. In 1990, there were 144,000 ESRD beneficiaries of HI.

All persons enrolled in part A of Medicare and all Americans over the age of sixty-five could, in 1992, join part B, which requires a monthly premium contribution to pay some of the costs of these additional benefits. If an eligible individual elects to delay joining part B, a penalty (of 10 percent for each year of delay) is added to the premium to discourage individuals from joining only when they become sicker.

The relative generosity of the Medicare subsidy means that most (although not all) people who are eligible to join part B do so. Most elderly beneficiaries elect this portion, but a smaller percentage of the disabled join. In 1991, more than 98 percent of elderly and 91 percent of disabled part A beneficiaries elected part B coverage.

Medicare coverage is limited to acute care services, particularly physician services and acute hospital care. The basic benefit package has changed little since Medicare's inception in 1966, although the costs borne by the beneficiary have increased.

Hospital coverage is limited to ninety days within a "spell of illness," plus a onetime supply of sixty "lifetime reserve days" that can be used to extend the covered period within one or more spells of illness. The first sixty days of the spell of illness are fully covered after payment of a deductible. After that, the beneficiary is liable for coinsurance for the next thirty days. Coinsurance is a charge assessed against the user of a service defined as a percentage of the cost of that care. The term "cost sharing" normally refers to coinsurance and deductibles—the costs of care that beneficiaries are required to share.

A spell of illness begins when the patient receives hospital or extended care services and ends when sixty days have elapsed between such periods of treatment. Thus, a spell of illness is not actually related to a particular illness but rather refers to a period of time elapsing before the next spell begins. Inpatient psychiatric services are limited to 190 days over a patient's lifetime.

In 1992, part B of Medicare paid 80 percent of physicians' "reasonable" charges (also called allowed charges) for surgery, consultation, and home, office, and institutional visits after the enrollee meets a $100 deductible. Restrictions are placed, however, on certain nonphysician providers of care such as dentists, chiropractors, and podiatrists. In 1992, mental health services were limited to the lesser of $562.50 per year or 62.5 percent of actual service costs. Covered services include X-ray and radiation therapy, ambulance services, physical and speech therapy, and rural health clinic services. Physicians are also permitted, within limits, to charge beneficiaries over and above the reasonable amounts established by Medicare—a practice referred to as "balance billing."

In 1992, part B also covered 80 percent of the reasonable charges for laboratory and other diagnostic tests, home dialysis supplies, durable medical equipment and artificial devices, and biennial mammography screening coverage.

Normally, the Medicare premium is automatically deducted from the beneficiary's Social Security check. Each January, both the Social Security cost-of-living allowance (COLA) adjustment and the premium increase go into effect. An additional protection for beneficiaries with small monthly payment amounts is that for each enrollee, the part B premium is not allowed to rise (in dollars) by an amount greater than the Social Security COLA adjustment. Consequently, while a few enrollees effectively have their COLA adjustment each year eliminated by the increase in part B premiums, no one actually receives less in nominal dollars from one year to the next because of Medicare premium increases.

Medicare providers (such as hospitals and doctors) must generally be certified for meeting certain stan-dards. They then bill Medicare on a fee-for-service basis. Hospitals and other major providers do not, however, file each claim separately. Rather, they are paid periodically, with adjustments to reconcile the actual amounts that they are owed. These periodic interim payments were originally established to smooth the cash flow for hospitals.

Physicians may ask patients to pay in full at the time of service rather than seeking reimbursement from Medicare. Even after the requirement that physicians must file claims for their patients, they can ask for payment directly from the beneficiary rather than being paid by Medicare. Physicians who bill Medicare directly are said to "accept assignment." If they accept assignment for all their Medicare patients, they are termed "participating providers" and are eligible for somewhat higher payments (allowed charges) for services. This distinction was made to encourage physicians to take assignment.

If physicians decline to take Medicare assignment, they deal directly with the patient, who then must be reimbursed by Medicare. When such physicians bill their patients for more than the allowed charges, they are said to "balance bill" the patients, effectively asking patients to pay more than the formal coinsurance of 20 percent of allowed charges.

The Health Care Financing Administration (HCFA) is in charge of overseeing the Medicare program. The HCFA promulgates rules and regulations that govern the operations of the program. The administrative costs of the program are quite low overall—about 2.5 percent of program outlays in 1992. The HCFA has contracts with "fiscal intermediaries" to process part A claims and "carriers" to process part B claims. These groups, usually insurance companies, deal directly with hospitals and physicians, respectively, to determine the appropriate levels of payment and then pay those providers. These entities also check claims for accuracy and fraud and provide summary records of health care use to the HCFA.

PROBLEMS ASSOCIATED WITH THE PROGRAM

In actual practice, Medicare is confusing and constantly changing. Interpretation of its regulations contributes to the complexity of the program. For example, for home health care, the care must be "intermittent," usually defined as less than daily, but more recent guidelines permit a period of daily visits of up to eight hours per day. Further, the patient must be confined to the home—a requirement somewhat at odds with the requirement that the care received be intermittent. The dual, and essentially conflicting, requirements of intermittency and confinement to the home were criticized in the 1980's by elderly advocates as providing a Catch-22 that precluded eligibility for many Medicare enrollees.

For the Medicare user, frustration has come from the fact that insurance companies, hospitals, and other intermediaries have always had considerable latitude in interpreting the HCFA's instructions, often resulting in inconsistent enforcement of regulations. In turn, these actions affect whether beneficiaries have access to certain benefits. In addition to the home health regulation cited above, the skilled nursing benefits are also severely limited by rigid application of the eligibility rules.

The rules governing payment for hospital outpatient services are extremely complicated. Through the 1980's, reforms were promised but always delayed. Consequently, outpatient services continued to be paid in a variety of ways, depending on whether the facility was part of a hospital or some other organization. Moreover, while Medicare pays hospital outpatient departments on the basis of costs, coinsurance is calculated on the basis of charges, which are generally higher. As a result, most beneficiaries pay more than 20 percent coinsurance for hospital outpatient facility services.

A revised Medicare fee schedule, issued in 1992 to determine payments to physicians, still uses more than seven thousand codes, makes geographic adjustments, and distinguishes between doctors who accept fees as payment in full and those who do not. Hospital payment is equally complicated and depends on the diagnosis of the patient, the type of hospital, and the location of the hospital. Hospital payment reform in 1983 caused many disruptions for patients and facilities alike because hospitals generally began to receive a fixed amount for the patient, whether he or she stays for two days or twenty days. The practice of medicine in the hospital certainly was changed significantly in the 1980's because of this reform in Medicare.

Periodic changes and revisions also make the Medicare program confusing. For example, in 1983 hospice care was added to part A as a Medicare benefit. Hospice includes nursing care, physical and occupational therapy, medical social services, home health aide services, continuous home care if necessary, medical supplies, physicians' services, short-term inpatient

care, and counseling. Persons electing hospice benefits, however, face limitations on what other Medicare services related to the terminal illness are covered.

For example, if a person elects to be in the hospice program, only inpatient care for the alleviation of pain, respite care, or acute symptom management is permitted. Aggressive treatment for the terminal illness would not be covered. A physician must certify that the patient is terminally ill and expected to die within six months. After an initial period of 210 days, benefits may be extended for a second 210-day period if patients are recertified by their doctors. Services must be performed by a certified hospice program and reflect a written plan of care.

Yet another dimension of changing and confusing eligibility came with the 1988 creation of "qualified Medicare beneficiaries" (QMBs) under the Medicare Catastrophic Coverage Act. These special beneficiaries, whose incomes must be below 100 percent of the federal poverty level and whose resources are under the amount specified for supplemental security income (SSI), are entitled to have the Medicaid program pick up the costs of Medicare's premium, deductibles, and coinsurance.

To protect Medicare recipients, the HCFA has contracts with peer review organizations (PROs) for further oversight of the use of services and quality control, particularly for hospital care. These organizations assess the appropriateness of care delivered, determine whether hospitalization was required, and, to a much lesser degree, assess the quality of that care. The HCFA defines the mix of these activities in its scope of work for contractors, and these descriptions have changed over time. In the period from 1988 to 1990, more attention was directed to assessing the quality of care.

The tools for quality oversight are limited. For example, when hospitals or physicians are found to be at fault, the main penalty available is exclusion from the Medicare program. This option leaves little room for intermediate remedies for less serious offenses. Further, many of the activities of PROs still center on cost containment efforts. For example, retrospective reviews of a sample of inpatient hospital cases include generic quality screening, discharge review, admission review, review of invasive procedures, coverage review, and determination of the application of the waiver of liability provision.

Controversy grew in the 1980's when enrollees were required to share more and more of the costs of their own care—both through a higher premium for coverage under part B and through payment of a greater portion of the costs of services received in the form of deductibles and coinsurance. All enrollees are liable for these payments, although Medicare pays for certain low-income enrollees and others may receive or purchase private insurance to cover these liabilities.

Under part B, the deductible is a set amount—in 1992, it was $100 per year—that does not rise automatically over time. It had been increased three times by legislation from an initial level of $50 per year, however, and more increases should be expected.

For physician and certain other services, the coinsurance is set at 20 percent of the amount that Medicare establishes as its allowed charge. A major exception is laboratory services, for which Medicare usually reimburses 100 percent of the fee schedule. Since physician fees generally rise each year, the amount that Medicare beneficiaries pay in cost sharing consequently goes up even when the same level of services is used from year to year.

The part B premium is also tied to the costs of part B services. Enrollees must pay 25 percent of the costs of care for an elderly enrollee. That amount was first introduced as a temporary change in 1982 and has periodically been extended since then. The original share that enrollees paid had been higher, set at 50 percent in the enacting legislation. Over time, however, the premium grew much faster than Social Security payments, resulting in a part B premium deduction from Social Security that was consuming an ever-increasing portion of monthly Social Security checks.

Calculations, at times, can become gruesome. For example, in addition to the hospital deductible, there is a deductible charge equal to the cost of the first three pints of whole blood received by a beneficiary as part of covered inpatient services. This deductible is also calculated on the basis of a spell of illness. The patient can avoid this deductible only by arranging for replacement of the blood by donors.

In the end, the most fundamental problem with Medicare has been the double-digit growth of the cost of the program—a problem facing all health care in the United States.

PERSPECTIVE AND PROSPECTS

Medicare provided one of the most important changes in medical coverage in the history of the United States.

In its first three decades, Medicare contributed significantly to the public health of Americans, and it has become one of the largest federal programs.

The Medicare program passed in 1965 initially covered everyone over the age of sixty-five. Consequently, by 1993 all persons aged ninety and over in 1992 had Medicare coverage regardless of their Social Security status. Subsequently, only those over the age of sixty-five who were eligible for some type of Social Security benefit were eligible for Medicare.

Medicare part A is financed almost entirely by a 1.45 percent tax on the first $125,000 of earnings, assessed of both employees and employers. This tax is part of the Federal Insurance Contributions Act (FICA) tax that most individuals see as a deduction in their paychecks each pay period. It is assessed regardless of wage level (up to a cap) on persons of all ages but is paid mostly by persons under the age of sixty-five since most Medicare recipients have retired. The upper limit on earnings was increased as part of the budget summit in 1990, a change that more than doubled the amount subject to tax. The 1992 Medicare limit of $130,200 compares to a limit of $55,500 applicable to the other parts of the FICA tax.

Many expect this upper limit to rise steadily as it did through the first decades of the program. In 1992, together the earnings limit and the combined employer/employee tax rate yielded a maximum contribution of $3,775.80 on behalf of a worker, which compared to an initial tax rate of 0.7 percent (combined) against a base of $6,600.00 in 1966—for a maximum payment of $46.20. Converted to an average over twenty-six years, this represents an annual growth rate of 18.5 percent, reflecting not only the increasing tax rate but also an expanded tax base as well.

This payroll tax generates the bulk of the revenues for part A. These revenues are combined with premiums (paid by those elderly not otherwise eligible), small general revenue transfers to cover beneficiaries such as railroad retirees, and interest from previous balances to form the part A trust fund. Under the law, payments are made only as long as there is a positive balance in the trust fund.

Despite the rapid growth in tax contributions over time, Medicare's benefits were growing even faster. While on strong footing in 1992, the Medicare program in the 1990's faced crisis after crisis. For example, the Trustee's Report for 1992 indicated total exhaustion of the trust fund within a decade.

Through the 1980's, the Medicare program was subjected to a broad range of attempts by Republican administrations to contain costs, including higher charges on beneficiaries as described above. Cuts in payments to doctors and particularly to hospitals, however, were even more severe in this decade. For example, the hospital payment system was reformed in 1983 and led to substantial reductions in payments to those institutions.

Since part B's funding comes from the premium contributions of beneficiaries and general revenue contributions by the federal government, its growth has been even more controversial. Although there is a trust fund for part B as well as for part A, it is much less important since, by law, the Treasury must make up the difference between premium contributions and part B spending. Thus, while general revenue contributions may be large, there is no crisis in funding requiring legislation (as is the case with part A) as long as the general public is willing to subsidize the beneficiaries of Medicare.

—Douglas Gomery, Ph.D.

See also Aging: Extended care; American Medical Association; Geriatrics and gerontology; Hospitals; Terminally ill: Extended care.

FOR FURTHER INFORMATION:

Callahan, Daniel. *Setting Limits: Medical Goals in an Aging Society.* New York: Simon & Schuster, 1987. The archconservative Callahan has forcefully argued for cutting back on Medicare for the elderly in general and limiting Medicare in particular. His analysis is flawed, but he does raise crucial and important concerns.

Kronick, Richard, and Joy de Beyer. *Medicare HMOs: Making Them Work for the Chronically Ill.* Chicago: Health Administration Press, 1999. This volume offers a history of the Medicare program, detailing its structure in its early years, and recounts the developments that have been made since its inception in 1965.

Marmor, Theodore. *The Politics of Medicare.* 2d ed. New York: Aldine, 1993. This history of the program stands as the basic primer of how Medicare came into existence.

Moon, Marilyn. *Medicare Now and in the Future.* Washington, D.C.: Urban Institute Press, 1993. This important book examines the state of the Medicare program and offers prescriptions for making it better. Moon writes clearly and presents the general reader and the policy analyst with the central book in Medicare literature.

Russell, Louise B. *Medicare's New Hospital Payment System: Is It Working?* Washington, D.C.: Brookings Institution Press, 1989. As the Medicare system was reviewed and cost-cutting measures instituted during the 1980's, public policy analysts examined the implications of these changes. Most come only in the form of hard-to-find and equally hard-to-read reports and articles.

MEDITATION

PROCEDURE

ANATOMY OR SYSTEM AFFECTED: All

SPECIALTIES AND RELATED FIELDS: Alternative medicine, preventive medicine, psychology

DEFINITION: A mental exercise to enhance personal understanding of the self and the universe.

INDICATIONS AND PROCEDURES

A wide variety of methods are employed in the different schools of meditation (as varied as Anglican and Zen). All these methods aim toward the concentration of the mind and the mastery of both external and internal distractions. A certain bodily posture may be employed, such as kneeling or sitting. A particular activity may be used, such as speaking (chanting a hymn or mantra, repeating a specific syllable), gazing (staring at an object to focus attention, such as a candle, a cross, a circle, or a spot), and breathing (rhythmically exhaling and inhaling). These exercises can be done either privately or publicly with a tutor or master. Meditation experts suggest that it occur daily, at set times (usually morning, noon, and evening) and for a duration of at least ten to twenty minutes per session. A conducive environment, free of audible and visual distractions, is preferred.

USES AND COMPLICATIONS

Although meditation has been an integral part of the Western spiritual tradition, it was regarded with indifference by the medical profession until the birth of modern psychology. Scholars such as William James (1842-1910), an American physician and psychologist, suggested that it might be worth study. Recent empirical studies have indicated that meditation does have a regenerative impact on the body, reducing tension, the heart rate, blood pressure, and the consumption of oxygen while increasing the production of alpha waves in the brain. With the increased interest in stress reduction and anxiety control, meditation will have a more important role in health care in the future.

PERSPECTIVE AND PROSPECTS

The practice of meditation had its origins within the religions of Hinduism, Buddhism, Christianity, and Islam. Within those traditions, its primary purposes are the comprehension of truth, the appropriation of power and a sense of peace, the transcendence of self-centeredness, and the experience of a unification with God and/or the universe. St. Ignatius of Loyola (1491-1556), one of the masters of Western meditation, described it as an exercise for the soul comparable to the training of the body in gymnastics.

Though long connected with religion as a preparation for contemplation (deep reflection on a theological issue) and prayer (personal conversation with God), meditation can be practiced for its psychological benefits apart from involvement within a faith tradition. By the 1960's, the Maharishi Mahesh Yogi had popularized Transcendental Meditation (TM) in the Western world as a means of reducing stress, enhancing the quality of life, and fulfilling one's potential.
—*C. George Fry, Ph.D.*

See also Alternative medicine; Anxiety; Biofeedback; Hypnosis; Stress; Stress reduction; Tai Chi Chuan; Yoga.

FOR FURTHER INFORMATION:

Davis, Martha, Elizabeth Robbins Eshelman, and Matthew McKay. *The Relaxation and Stress Reduction Workbook.* 3d ed. Oakland, Calif.: New Harbinger, 1988.

Hadley, Josie, and Carol Staudacher. *Hypnosis for Change.* 3d ed. New York: Ballantine Books, 1996.

Schultz, J. H., and Wolfgang Luthe. *Autogenic Methods.* Vol. 1 in *Autogenic Therapy.* New York: Grune & Stratton, 1969.

MELANOMA. *See* MALIGNANT MELANOMA REMOVAL; SKIN CANCER.

MELATONIN
BIOLOGY

ANATOMY OR SYSTEM AFFECTED: Brain, endocrine system, glands

SPECIALTIES AND RELATED FIELDS: Alternative medicine, endocrinology, neurology, pharmacology, preventive medicine

DEFINITION: A substance produced by the pineal gland that has been used as a controversial therapeutic agent.

KEY TERMS:

endocrine system: the glands that produce hormones

hormone: a substance produced in one part of the body that has effects in other parts of the body

melatonin: the hormone produced by the pineal gland

pineal gland: a small organ inside the brain that produces melatonin

STRUCTURE AND FUNCTIONS

Melatonin, also known as N-acetyl-5-methoxytryptamine, is a hormone found in a wide variety of living organisms. In vertebrates (animals with backbones), including humans, it is produced by the pineal gland. The pineal gland is located deep within the center of the brain. Although it is inside the brain, it is considered part of the endocrine system rather than the nervous system. In humans, the pineal gland is a gray or white organ less than 1 centimeter long and shaped like a pinecone.

The pineal gland produces varying amounts of melatonin in response to changes in light. Light inhibits the production of melatonin, and darkness stimulates it. In some small animals, light reaches the pineal gland directly through the skull. In larger animals, including humans, information about light and darkness is transmitted by the nervous system from the eyes to the suprachiasmatic nucleus, a cluster of nerve cells in a region of the brain known as the hypothalamus. The suprachiasmatic nucleus regulates the secretion of melatonin by the pineal gland.

Melatonin is believed to be involved in regulating the sleep cycle in response to changes in light. Because the amount of melatonin produced by the pineal gland declines sharply at puberty, it is believed to be involved in the development of the reproductive system. Because melatonin production continues to decline with age, some researchers believe that it is associated with the process of aging.

DISORDERS AND DISEASES

Disorders of melatonin production other than its normal decline with age are rare. Tumors of the pineal gland may reduce melatonin production. Some evidence suggests that this may lead to premature aging. Children with tumors of the pineal gland may reach puberty at a very early age.

Some researchers suggest that the normal decline in melatonin production with age is associated with diseases of the elderly. Animal studies suggest that loss of melatonin is associated with increased cell damage. Melatonin is believed to act as an antioxidant, a substance that protects cells from free radicals, which are produced when cells use oxygen. Cell damage has been linked to a large number of diseases of the elderly, including various forms of cancer, heart disease, and Alzheimer's disease.

Based on this evidence, melatonin has been used to treat and prevent a wide variety of illnesses. In the 1990's, melatonin became widely used in the United States. Because it was classified as a dietary supplement rather than as a drug, it was available without a prescription and with little government regulation. While some researchers suggested caution until more was known about melatonin, others suggested taking small daily doses of the hormone to slow down the aging process. Popular books such as *The Melatonin Miracle* (1995), by Walter Pierpaoli, William Regelson, and Carol Colman, claim that melatonin can stimulate the immune system, prevent cancer and heart disease, improve sexual relations, reduce the effects of stress, act as a contraceptive, and add years to the human life span. Critics argue that these claims are greatly exaggerated.

The least controversial suggested use for melatonin is as a sleeping aid. Human studies have indicated that melatonin is safe and effective for this use. Unlike many other sleeping pills, melatonin seems to have no effect on normal sleep patterns and few side effects. Melatonin has also been shown to be effective in treating jet lag, the difficulty that travelers have adjusting to a new time zone.

Critics of routine melatonin use point out that little is known about its long-term effects. They also point to evidence that some people may experience short-term side effects such as nightmares, headaches, daytime sleepiness, and mild depression. A major concern is the lack of regulation of melatonin products, leading to the possibility that other, unknown substances may be present.

Even the most optimistic proponents of melatonin suggest certain precautions. Many products contain more melatonin than researchers believe is necessary, leading to the possibility of a greater risk of side effects with no increase in benefit. Melatonin should only be taken at bedtime to avoid unwanted sleepiness. It should not be used by children, who already produce high levels of melatonin. It should not be used by pregnant women because its effect on the fe-

tus is unknown. Because it is believed to stimulate the immune system, melatonin should be avoided in people with severe allergies, autoimmune disorders, or cancer of the immune system.

PERSPECTIVE AND PROSPECTS

The pineal gland was known to exist in ancient times. It was first described scientifically by the Greek physician Galen in the second century. The French philosopher René Descartes (1596-1650) suggested that it was the location of the human soul. The true function of the pineal gland remained unknown until the middle of the twentieth century.

Melatonin was discovered in 1958 and first described as a hormone in 1963. Research into its effects began in the 1970's and 1980's. Interest in this hormone increased dramatically in 1995, with the publication of several books and articles publicizing its possible benefits. Research on melatonin is expected to continue for many years, particularly in regard to its long-term effects.

—*Rose Secrest*

See also Aging; Antioxidants; Brain; Chronobiology; Endocrine disorders; Endocrinology; Endocrinology, pediatric; Glands; Hormone replacement therapy; Hormones; Light therapy; Pharmacology; Sleep disorders.

FOR FURTHER INFORMATION:

Brzezinski, Amnon. "Melatonin in Humans." *New England Journal of Medicine* 336, no. 3 (January 16, 1997): 186-195. Evidence has been found that melatonin may have a role in the biologic regulation of circadian rhythms, sleep, and mood and perhaps reproduction, tumor growth, and aging.

Cowley, Geoffrey. "Melatonin." *Newsweek* 126, no. 6 (August 7, 1995): 46-49. The potential cure-all drug melatonin is described. The drug is slowly gaining acceptance as a way to lengthen human lives, bolster immune systems, slow the growth of tumors and cataracts, ward off heart disease, and help ease insomnia.

"Melatonin: Questions, Facts, Mysteries." *University of California, Berkeley, Wellness Letter* 16, no. 8 (May, 2000): 1-2. Melatonin is a human hormone produced by the pineal gland in the brain. The bottom line on this supplement is that too little is known about its dosage and health effects.

Raloff, Janet. "Drug of Darkness." *Science News* 147, no. 19 (May 13, 1995): 300-301. A host of medical laboratories around the world are addressing health problems with a new class of drugs they hope to introduce within the next decade. Each drug would rely on a synthetic form of melatonin.

Memory loss
Disease/disorder

Anatomy or system affected: Brain, nervous system, psychic-emotional system

Specialties and related fields: Geriatrics and gerontology, neurology, psychiatry, psychology

Definition: An impairment of memory which may be total or limited, sudden or gradual.

Causes and Symptoms

Memory impairment is a common problem, especially among older people. It occurs in various degrees and may be associated with other evidence of brain dysfunction. Amnesia is complete memory loss.

Benign forgetfulness. In this condition, the memory deficit affects mostly recent events, and although a source of frustration, it seldom interferes with the individual's professional activities or social life. An important feature of benign forgetfulness is that it is selective and affects only trivial, unimportant facts. For example, one may misplace the car keys or forget to return a phone call, respond to a letter, or pay a bill. Cashing a check or telephoning someone with whom one is particularly keen to talk, however, will not be forgotten. The person is aware of the memory deficit, and written notes often are used as reminders. Patients with benign forgetfulness have no other evidence of brain dysfunction and maintain their ability to make valid judgments.

Dementia. In dementia, the memory impairment is global, does not discriminate between important and trivial facts, and interferes with the person's ability to pursue professional or social activities. Patients with dementia find it difficult to adapt to changes in the workplace, such as the introduction of computers. They also find it difficult to continue with their hobbies and interests.

The hallmark of dementia is no awareness of the memory deficit, except in the very early stages of the disease. This is an important difference between dementia and benign forgetfulness. Although patients with early dementia may write themselves notes, they usually forget to check these reminders or may misinterpret them. For example, a man with dementia who is invited for dinner at a friend's house may write a note to that effect and leave it in a prominent place. He may then go to his host's home several evenings in succession because he has forgotten that he already has fulfilled this social engagement. As the disease progresses, patients are no longer aware of their memory deficit.

In dementia, the memory deficit does not occur in isolation but is accompanied by other evidence of brain dysfunction, which in very early stages can be detected only by specialized neuropsychological tests. As the condition progresses, these deficits become readily apparent. The patient is often disoriented regarding time and may telephone relatives or friends very late at night. As the disease progresses, the disorientation affects the patient's environment: A woman with dementia may wander outside her house and be unable to find her way back, or she may repeatedly ask to be taken back home when she is already there. In later stages, patients may not be able to recognize people whom they should know: A man may think that his son is his father or that his wife is his mother. This stage is particularly distressing to the caregivers. Patients with dementia may often exhibit impaired judgment. They may go outside the house inappropriately dressed or at inappropriate times, or they may purchase the same item repeatedly or make donations that are disproportional to their funds. Alzheimer's disease is one of the most common causes of dementia in older people.

Multiple infarct dementia. Multiple infarct dementia is caused by the destruction of brain cells by repeated strokes. Sometimes these strokes are so small that neither the patient nor the relatives are aware of their occurrence. When many strokes occur and significant brain tissue is destroyed, the patient may exhibit symptoms of dementia. Usually, however, most of these strokes are quite obvious because they are associated with weakness or paralysis in a part of the body. One of the characteristic features of multiple infarct dementia is that its onset is sudden and itsprogression is by steps. Every time a stroke occurs, the patient's condition deteriorates. This is followed by a period during which little or no deterioration develops until another stroke occurs, at which time the patient's condition deteriorates further. Very rarely, the stroke affects only the memory center, in which case the patient's sole problem is amnesia. Multiple-infarct dementia and dementia resulting from Alzheimer's disease should be differentiated from other treatable conditions which also may cause memory impairment, disorientation, and poor judgment.

Depression. Depression, particularly in older patients, may cause memory impairment. This condition is quite common and at times is so difficult to differentiate from dementia that the term "pseudodementia" is used to describe it. One of the main differences between depression that presents the symptoms of dementia and dementia itself is insight into the memory deficit. Whereas patients with dementia are usually oblivious of their deficit and not distressed (except those in the early stages), those with depression are nearly always aware of their deficit and are quite distressed. Patients with depression tend to be withdrawn and apathetic, given a marked disturbance of affect, whereas those with dementia demonstrate emotional blandness and some degree of lability. One of the problems characteristic of depressed patients is their difficulty in concentrating. This is typified by poor cooperation and effort in carrying out tasks with a variable degree of achievement, coupled with considerable anxiety.

Head trauma. Amnesia is sometimes seen in patients who have sustained a head injury. The extent of the amnesia is usually proportional to the severity of the injury. In most cases, the complete recovery of the patient's memory occurs, except for the events just preceding and following the injury.

PERSPECTIVE AND PROSPECTS

Memory impairment is a serious condition which can interfere with one's ability to function independently. Every attempt should be made to identify the underlying condition because, in some cases, a treatable cause can be found and the memory loss reversed. Furthermore, it may soon be possible to arrest the progress of amnesia and memory loss and even to treat the dementias which now are considered as irreversible, such as Alzheimer's disease and multiple infarct dementia.

—*Ronald C. Hamdy, M.D.,*
and Louis A. Cancellaro, M.D.

See also Aging; Alzheimer's disease; Amnesia; Anxiety; Brain; Brain disorders; Concussion; Dementias; Depression; Geriatrics and gerontology; Head and neck disorders; Psychiatry; Psychiatry, geriatric; Strokes.

FOR FURTHER INFORMATION:

Cummings, Jeffrey L., and D. Frank Benson. *Dementia: A Clinical Approach.* 2d ed. Boston:

Butterworth-Heinemann, 1992. This is a standard textbook, comprehensively presenting the clinical, diagnostic, therapeutic, and basic science aspects of the dementias. This edition has been revised and updated with nearly one thousand new references and revised descriptions of all major dementia syndromes.

Cummings, Jeffrey L., and Bruce L. Miller, eds. *Alzheimer's Disease: Treatment and Long-term Management.* New York: Marcel Dekker, 1990. Presents helpful therapeutic treatments for this debilitating disease. Includes bibliographical references and an index.

Hamdy, Ronald C., et al., eds. *Alzheimer's Disease: A Handbook for Caregivers.* 3d ed. St. Louis: Mosby Year Book, 1998. This handbook offers nursing tips for people caring for Alzheimer's patients. Includes bibliographical references and an index.

Terry, Robert D., ed. *Aging and the Brain.* New York: Raven Press, 1988. The structure and function of the brains of both normal elderly people and those with various types of dementias (including Alzheimer's disease) are compared. Reviews the neurobiological and technological concepts developed in the 1980's in this field of study.

West, Robin L., and Jan D. Sinnott, eds. *Everyday Memory and Aging.* New York: Springer-Verlag, 1992. This work discusses the methodology of research into the human memory. Focuses on the changes in memory that occur naturally with age, as well as those that are brought about by various forms of dementia in the older individual.

MÉNIÈRE'S DISEASE
DISEASE/DISORDER

ANATOMY OR SYSTEM AFFECTED: Ears
SPECIALTIES AND RELATED FIELDS: Audiology, neurology, otorhinolaryngology
DEFINITION: Ménière's disease is a dysfunction of the inner ear, or labyrinth; it is thought to result from a buildup of fluid in the labyrinth, which creates pressure. Consequently, hearing and balance are affected, with severe vertigo, tinnitus (ringing or buzzing in the ears), and progressive hearing loss. In addition, acute attacks of vertigo can occur, lasting from ten minutes to several hours. These attacks may cause nausea, vomiting, and sweating. Periods of remission may increase along with hearing loss, and attacks may stop completely with to-

tal loss of hearing. At this point, in order to restore balance, surgery may be used to destroy the inner ear, since hearing can no longer be affected.

—Jason Georges and Tracy Irons-Georges
See also Audiology; Dizziness and fainting; Ear infections and disorders; Ears; Hearing loss; Nausea and vomiting; Otorhinolaryngology.

FOR FURTHER INFORMATION:

Clayman, Charles B., ed. *The American Medical Association Family Medical Guide.* 3d rev. ed. New York: Random House, 1994.

Kitahara, M., ed. *Ménière's Disease.* New York: Springer-Verlag, 1990.

Oosterveld, W. J., ed. *Ménière's Disease: A Comprehensive Appraisal.* New York: Wiley, 1983.

Pender, Daniel J. *Practical Otology.* Philadelphia: J. B. Lippincott, 1992.

Roland, Peter S., Bradley F. Marple, and William L. Meyerhoff, eds. *Hearing Loss.* New York: Thieme, 1997.

MENINGITIS

DISEASE/DISORDER

ANATOMY OR SYSTEM AFFECTED: Brain, head, nervous system, spine

SPECIALTIES AND RELATED FIELDS: Emergency medicine, neurology, public health

DEFINITION: An inflammation of the meninges of the brain and spinal cord.

CAUSES AND SYMPTOMS

The meninges is the three-layered covering of the spinal cord and brain. The layers are the outer dura mater, inner pia mater, and middle arachnoid. Meningitis is the inflammation or infection of the arachnoid and pia mater. It is characterized by severe headaches, vomiting, and pain and stiffness in the neck. These symptoms may be preceded by an upper-respiratory infection. The age of the patient may affect which signs and symptoms are displayed. Newborns may exhibit either fever or hypothermia, along with lethargy or irritability, disinterest in feeding, and abdominal distension. In infants, examination may find bulging of the fontanelles (the soft areas between the bones of the skull found in newborns). The elderly may show lethargy, confusion, or disorientation. As pressure in the skull increases, nausea and vomiting may occur. With meningococcal meningitis, a rash of pinpoint-sized or larger dots appears.

Most cases of meningitis are the result of bacterial infection. These cases are sometimes referred to as septic meningitis. The bacteria invade the subarachnoid space and may have traveled from another site of infection, having caused pneumonia, cellulitis, or an ear infection. It is unclear if the bacteria make their way from the original area of infection to the meninges by the bloodstream or the lymphatic system. Once they have entered the subarachnoid space, they divide without inhibition since there is no impediment posed by defensive cells. In other words, the cerebrospinal fluid (CSF) contains very few white blood cells to inactivate the bacteria. More rarely, some bacteria may be introduced into the area by neurological damage or surgical invasion.

The most common cause of bacterial meningitis in adults and older children is meningococcus (*Neisseria meningitidis*). It is a diplococcus that typically does its damage inside the cell. The incidence of meningococcal meningitis is 2 to 3 cases per 100,000 people per year, and it most often affects schoolchildren and military recruits. *Haemophilus influenzae* is the most common culprit infecting babies between two months and one year of age. Complications or residual effects often follow bacterial meningitis. These may include deafness, delayed-onset epilepsy, hydrocephalus, cerebritis, and brain abscess. In addition, for several weeks after resolution of the disease the patient may experience headaches, dizziness, and lethargy.

Aseptic meningitis is meningitis attributable to causes other than bacteria. These causes include neurotropic viruses, such as those that cause poliomyelitis or encephalitis; other viruses such as those that cause mumps, herpes, mononucleosis, hepatitis, chickenpox, and measles; spirochetes; bacterial products from brain abscesses or previous cases of bacterial meningitis; and foreign bodies, such as those found in the air or chemicals, in the CSF. Most cases of aseptic meningitis are viral in origin. The signs and symptoms are similar to those of bacterial meningitis. Onset is usually gradual, with symptoms starting mildly. The slight headache becomes worse over the course of several days, the neck becomes characteristically stiff, and photophobia (dislike of bright light) occurs.

Tuberculous meningitis is different from most other forms of meningitis because it lasts longer, has a higher mortality rate, and affects the CSF less. It mostly strikes children and is usually the result of a

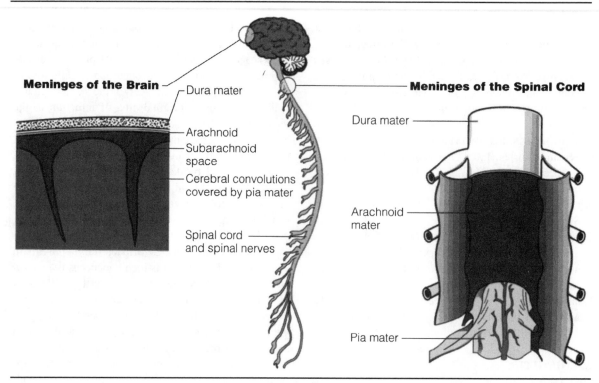

Meninges of the Brain

Dura mater

Arachnoid

Subarachnoid space

Cerebral convolutions covered by pia mater

Spinal cord and spinal nerves

Meninges of the Spinal Cord

Dura mater

Arachnoid mater

Pia mater

Meningitis attacks the meninges of the brain or the spinal cord or both.

bacillus infection from the respiratory tract or the lymphatic system that has relocated to the meninges. When the bacilli are translocated to the central nervous system, they form tubercles that release an exudate. If tuberculous meningitis is left untreated, death may occur within three weeks. Even with treatment, it may result in neurologic abnormalities.

TREATMENT AND THERAPY

If meningitis is suspected, the first testing procedure is an examination of the CSF. To obtain CSF, a lumbar puncture, sometimes called a spinal tap, is made. Opening pressure, protein and glucose concentrations, total cell count, and cultures of microbes are determined. In cases of meningitis, the CSF is almost always cloudy and generally comes out under higher-than-normal pressure. An elevated white blood cell count in the CSF would be one indication that the patient has bacterial meningitis; another would be lowered serum glucose but slightly raised protein concentration, especially albumin. About 90 percent of bacterial meningitis cases show gram-positive staining. The examination of this slightly atypical fluid, along with presenting symptoms and signs, gives the

diagnostician some confidence in diagnosing meningitis accurately. Further cultures and a repeat puncture are necessary to pinpoint the kind of meningitis and to check the effect of the treatment.

Bacterial meningitis should be promptly treated with antibiotics specific for the causative bacteria. The success of treatment is contingent on the magnitude of the bacterial count and the quickness with which the bacteria can be controlled. Virtually all bacterial cases are treated with ampicillin or penicillin. Cases aggressively treated with very large doses of antibiotics are the most successful. If antibiotics do not destroy the areas of infection, surgery should be considered. Surgery is especially effective if meningitis is recurrent or persistent. Viral meningitis may be treated with adenine arabinoside if the cause is herpes simplex. No medication will kill other viruses causing the infection. The condition usually resolves itself in a few days, even without treatment. When necessary, supportive therapy should be employed, including blood transfusions. Young children with open fontanelles often undergo subdural taps to relieve pressure caused by CSF buildup.

Mortality rates in meningitis vary with age and

the pathogen responsible. Those suffering from meningococcal meningitis (without overwhelming bacterial numbers) have a fatality rate of only 3 percent. Newborns suffering from gram-negative meningitis, however, have a 70 percent mortality rate. In addition, the younger the patient, the more likely the incidence of lasting neurological damage.

There are two basic ways to prevent meningitis: chemoprophylaxis for likely candidates of the disease and active immunization. Those exposed to a known case are usually treated with rifampin for four days; rifampin is especially useful in inactivating *H. influenzae*. Active immunization is suggested for toddlers eighteen to twenty-four months of age, especially for those in situations where there is a high risk of exposure (such as day care centers).

—*Iona C. Baldridge*

See also Abscesses; Bacterial infections; Brain; Brain disorders; Chickenpox; Encephalitis; Hepatitis; Herpes; Immunization and vaccination; Lumbar puncture; Measles; Mononucleosis; Mumps; Nervous system; Neurology; Neurology, pediatric; Poliomyelitis; Spinal cord disorders; Spine, vertebrae, and disks; Viral infections.

FOR FURTHER INFORMATION:

Biddle, Wayne. *Field Guide to Germs*. New York: Henry Holt, 1995.

Clayman, Charles B., ed. *The American Medical Association Family Medical Guide*. 3d rev. ed. New York: Random House, 1994.

Coe, R. P. K. "Primary Mumps Orchitis with Meningitis." *The Lancet* 1, no. 6333 (January 13, 1945): 49-50.

Schiefer, W., M. Klinger, and M. Brock. *Brain Abscess and Meningitis: Subarachnoid Hemorrhage*. New York: Springer-Verlag, 1981.

Shaw, Michael, ed. *Everything You Need to Know About Diseases*. Springhouse, Pa.: Springhouse Press, 1996.

MENOPAUSE

BIOLOGY

ANATOMY OR SYSTEM AFFECTED: Psychic-emotional system, reproductive system, uterus

SPECIALTIES AND RELATED FIELDS: Endocrinology, gynecology

DEFINITION: The time during a woman's life when her ability to conceive and bear children ends, marked by irregular, and eventually complete cessation of, menstruation, accompanied by hormonal changes such as the dramatic reduction in the body's production of estrogen.

KEY TERMS:

climacteric: that phase in the aging process of women marking the transition from the reproductive stage of life to the nonreproductive stage

estrogen: the female hormones estradiol and estrone, produced by the ovary and responsible for the development of secondary sex characteristics

exogenous: originating outside an organ or part

osteoporosis: a condition characterized by a loss of bone density and an increased susceptibility to fractures

progesterone: a hormone, released by the corpus luteum and placenta, responsible for changes in the uterine endometrium

PROCESS AND EFFECTS

The word "menopause" comes from two Greek words meaning "month" and "cessation." It is used medically to mean a cessation of, not a "pause" in, menstrual periods. Technically, the menopause begins the moment a woman has had her final menstrual period; until then, her menstrual periods may have shown a wide variety of irregularities, including missed periods.

Medical experts refer to the time when the body is noticeably preparing for the menopause as the perimenopause, which can begin anywhere from five to ten years before the menopause. While estrogen levels begin to decrease gradually, periods are normal but memory may be less sharp and mood swings may occur. During that time, a woman still experiences menstrual periods, but they are erratic. Some women stop menstruating suddenly, without irregularities; however, they are in the minority. For some women, signs of the menopause, such as hot flashes, may begin during the perimenopause. For even more women, such signs begin, or at least increase in intensity, at the menopause.

The term "climacteric" covers a longer span and includes all the years of diminishing estrogen production, both before and after a woman's last menstrual period. Some experts believe that women may undergo declines in their levels of estrogen even when they are in their late twenties; almost all experts believe that estrogen levels drop at least by a woman's mid-thirties, and the process accelerates in the late forties.

The average age at which the menopause occurs in women from the United States is 51.4 years, with the usual range between ages forty-five and fifty-five. For some it occurs much earlier, for others much later. Only 8 percent of women reach the menopause before age forty, and only 5 percent continue to menstruate after age fifty-three. A very few have menstrual periods until they are sixty.

Even after the menopause, the climacteric continues. Declining hormonal levels bring more changes, until the situation stabilizes. A decade or more of noticeable changes can take place before the climacteric is completed. Unlike the climacteric, the menopause itself is usually considered completed after one full year without a period. After two years, a woman can be reasonably certain that her periods have ceased permanently. The signs and symptoms of the menopause, however, can linger for years longer.

Starting in her mid-forties, a woman's ovaries gradually lose their ability to respond to the follicle-stimulating hormone (FSH), which is released by the pituitary into the blood, triggering the release of estrogen from the ovaries. A few eggs do remain even after menstrual flows have ceased, and the production of estrogen does not stop completely after the menopause; in much smaller amounts, it continues to be released by the adrenal glands, in fatty tissue, and in the brain. At the menopause, however, the blood levels of estrogen are drastically reduced—by about 75 percent. Many experts believe that the presence of some estrogen is important for a woman's total well-being, bone health, and skin suppleness and for the prevention of heart disease.

About two to four years before the menopause, many women stop ovulating or ovulate irregularly or only occasionally. Although almost all the follicles enclosing the eggs are depleted by this time, the ovaries continue to produce estrogen. Estrogen continues to build up the endometrium (the lining of the uterus), but without ovulation no progesterone is produced to shed the extra lining. Therefore, instead of regular periods, a woman may bleed at unexpected times as the extra lining is shed sporadically.

During the perimenopause, menstrual periods may be late or early, longer than usual or shorter, and lighter than before or heavier. They may disappear for several months, then reappear for several more. It has been noted that in 15 to 20 percent of women the typical menopausal symptoms, sometimes accompanied by noticeable mood swings similar to premenstrual tension, begin during the perimenopausal period.

According to the National Institutes of Health, about 80 percent of women experience mild or no signs of the menopause. The rest have symptoms troublesome enough to seek medical attention. The two most important factors in determining how a woman will fare are probably the rate of decline of her female hormones and the final degree of hormone depletion. A woman's genes, general health, lifetime quality of diet, level of activity, and psychological acceptance of aging are also major influences. The most severe symptoms occur in women who lose their ovaries through surgery or radiation when they are perimenopausal.

When only the uterus is removed (hysterectomy) and the ovaries remain intact, menstrual periods stop but all other aspects of the menopause occur in the same way and at the same age. When only one ovary is removed, the menopause occurs normally. If both ovaries are removed, a complete menopause takes place abruptly, sometimes with intense effects. Women who have had a tubal ligation to prevent pregnancy will experience a normal menopause because tubal ligation does not affect ovaries, the uterus, or hormonal secretions.

Although experts disagree about the causes of a variety of symptoms that may appear at the menopause, there is no disagreement about the fact that the majority of women experience hot flashes, or flushes.

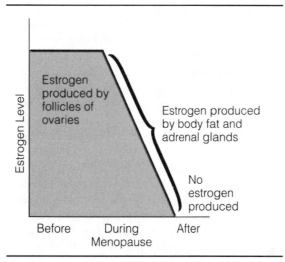

During the menopause, which may last for several years, estrogen production diminishes; after the menopause, estrogen is no longer produced by the body.

For two out of three women, hot flashes can start well before the last menstruation. Generally, however, hot flashes increase dramatically at menopause and continue to occur, with intermittent breaks (sometimes lasting several months), for five years or so.

While hot flashes are not dangerous, they are uncomfortable. Many women have only three or four episodes a day—or even a week—and hardly notice them. Others have as many as fifty severe flashes a day. The intense waves of heat generally last several minutes, but some unusual flashes have been reported to last as long as an hour. Usually there is some perspiration; with a severe flash, there is heavy perspiration. Because the blood vessels dilate (expand) and then contract, the hot flash is often followed by chills, even intense shivering. Since the flashes are usually worse at night, they can cause insomnia.

Other vasomotor symptoms can also appear with the menopause. Experts believe that they are the result of disruptions of the same mechanisms—vasomotor instability—that are manifested as hot flashes. Palpitations, which are distinct and rapid heartbeats, may also occur. A woman may experience dizziness or may feel faint or nauseated at times. She may have peculiar sensations in her arms and hands, especially her fingers. Some feel these sensations as tingling, or pins and needles, while others say that their fingers occasionally feel numb. One of the oddest, most frightening sensations associated with the menopause is formication, a feeling of insects crawling over the skin.

Headaches, depression, mood swings, insomnia, and weight gain often affect women at the menopause and may be related to the body's hormonal readjustments. Insomnia is second only to hot flashes as the symptom that causes women to seek out their doctors' help at the menopause. The hypothalamus controls sleep as well as temperature and hormone production; insomnia is caused by changes in sleep patterns and brain waves from the same hypothalamic disturbances that result in the hot flashes and an over-stimulated central nervous system.

COMPLICATIONS AND DISORDERS

One of the problems that women encounter with the menopause is calcium deficiency. Many experts believe that before the menopause a woman requires a minimum of 1,000 milligrams of calcium a day in food or supplements. At the menopause, however, a woman who is not taking estrogen needs 1,500 milli-grams of calcium a day. Since it is very difficult to obtain these daily allotments from food without consuming considerable amounts of milk or milk products, calcium supplements are often recommended for menopausal and postmenopausal women.

If the calcium deficiency is allowed to persist, osteoporosis, a loss of bone density that can lead to dangerous fractures, can result. Osteoporosis is known to have less of a damaging effect on women who are somewhat overweight because estrogen continues to be produced in fatty tissues after the menopause. Cigarettes, alcohol, and caffeine increase bone loss because they interfere with the body's ability to absorb calcium. A well-balanced diet, calcium supplements, and regular exercise—especially weight-bearing exercise—are effective ways of controlling osteoporosis. Hormone replacement therapy is another means of coping with osteoporosis brought on by the menopause. Since nearly half of all women do not develop osteoporosis, however, many physicians do not believe that administering estrogen therapy to combat this disease is worth the risks except in women at high risk for osteoporosis.

Although estrogen was isolated as a substance in the 1920's, the modern study of hormones—how they work, where they are produced, what their benefits are—began in the 1940's. Originally, estrogen was administered cautiously to women who had lost their ovaries through surgery and to those with severe distress after the menopause. It was not until the 1960's that estrogen replacement therapy became widespread, however, when books such as Robert A. Wilson's *Feminine Forever* (1966) promoted its use as the newfound fountain of youth for women. The replacement of estrogen was suddenly fashionable, with the hormone being viewed as a miracle drug that could keep women looking and feeling youthful well into their later years. Physicians began prescribing it for women well before the menopause, and it was recommended for use throughout life. Often, large doses were prescribed.

By the mid-1970's, twenty million American women were taking estrogen. A decade later, however, the number had fallen to four or five million. Beginning in 1975, research studies began documenting dramatic increases—sometimes as high as 500 percent—in cases of cancer of the lining of the endometrium among women taking estrogen, compared with those not taking it. Other studies at that time found higher rates of breast cancer as well as other problems, such as gallbladder conditions, among women taking estrogen.

Some studies found the overall risk of contracting uterine cancer increased 350 percent for women who took estrogen for a year or more. Some women who were on the therapy for long periods were judged to be as much as 100 percent more likely to contract uterine cancer. Furthermore, contrary to expectations, some studies claimed that the risk persisted even ten years after the estrogen use was discontinued. Other studies also found that the risk of cancer persisted, though for a shorter period.

All those studies were based on replacement therapy using estrogen only. Estrogen stimulates the growth of cells in the endometrium, which is one of the aspects of the development of cancer. Yet the researchers also reported that a newer treatment in which estrogen was combined with a form of progesterone appeared to reduce the risk of uterine cancer. Further studies have shown lower rates of both endometrial and breast cancer, as well as lower rates of heart disease among women using the two hormones, compared with nonusers.

The most widely recommended regimen in the early 1990's called for using estrogen in the lowest effective dose three weeks each month. During the last week to thirteen days of this therapy, a form of progesterone is added. Then both hormones are stopped. Uterine bleeding, similar to that of a menstrual period, may occur. This bleeding allows the progesterone to break down any excess buildup of cells in the endometrium.

During the menopause, the walls of the vagina become smooth and dry and produce less lubrication, producing a condition called atrophic vaginitis. It has been assumed that this condition is attributable to a lack of estrogen. Despite doubts concerning the relationship between circulating estrogen and objective measures of vaginal atrophy, estrogen (often topical) is frequently prescribed and effectively used in the alleviation or elimination of symptoms.

To help alleviate menopausal symptoms, many women require only short-term therapy; other women, such as those at risk for developing osteoporosis, may need the therapy for years or even for the rest of their lives. Some physicians believe that estrogen should not be taken during the perimenopause, when there may still be high levels of estrogen in the patient's system. Other physicians believe that the levels of estrogen should be checked using a vaginal smear test during the perimenopause and estrogen prescribed if necessary.

Some physicians prescribe estrogen therapy for women with severe symptoms after a surgical menopause. The therapy is usually continued for at least five years or until the time that the natural menopause would have occurred, unless the woman has an estrogen-dependent malignancy.

The most popular method for administering hormone replacement therapy is oral, but this method is relatively ineffective because of poor gastrointestinal absorption. One way of increasing the effectiveness of oral medication is to provide it in micronized form; micronization increases the total surface area of the medication by reducing the size of the particles and increasing their numbers, thereby facilitating dissolution and absorption. Estrone increases at a faster rate than does estradiol when hormone replacement therapy is administered orally because the intestines and the liver convert estradiol, the more active form of estrogen, to estrone. Other routes of administration, such as a transdermal patch, have been studied in order to discover a method that might bypass the gut and liver and avoid the rapid conversion of estradiol to estrone.

Another method of administering hormone replacement therapy is intravaginally, which also bypasses the gut and liver. When intravaginal administration was compared to oral administration at a variety of doses, it was found that at each dosage level, the vaginal route resulted in significantly lower blood estrogen values than did the oral route. Relief from vaginal symptoms was achieved in all cases, however, where the hormone was administered vaginally. Routes that bypass the liver and gut produce a more natural ratio of estrone to estradiol.

After a woman has gone through the menopause, she also experiences changes in her heart and blood vessels. After the age of fifty, a woman has an approximately 46 percent chance of developing heart disease. Estrogen replacement therapy can be effective in preventing the circulatory system changes that can lead to heart disease. Because the changes occur over the course of many years, women who have not chosen estrogen replacement therapy can still reap its benefits even ten to fifteen years after the menopause.

There is considerable evidence that exogenous estrogen treatment in menopausal women is associated with an increase in the probability of developing uterine cancer. Research results released in 1997 suggest essentially no association with breast cancer. Initially, hormone replacement therapy consisted of estrogen administered on a continual basis. Since the increased risk of uterine cancer was thought to be the result of the hyperplastic effects of unopposed estrogen on the endometrium, other forms of medication have been advocated. For example, estrogen is sometimes given on a cyclic basis, with twenty-five days of medication and five days off. The rationale for this form of treatment is that it more precisely conforms to premenopausal hormone levels and, more important, that it prevents hyperplasia (enlargement of the uterus).

Anecdotal evidence and some research studies suggest that stress reduction and exercise can relieve some of the symptoms of the menopause, including hot flashes and mood swings. In addition, a host of herbal remedies on the market claim to improve menopausal symptoms, although caution should be used in choosing these products. A double-blind pilot study of women using soy as a natural estrogen replacement therapy turned out positive; hot flashes decreased significantly in women taking soy powder for six weeks. The isoflavones in soy are chemically similar to estrogens. Vitamin E, which is structurally similar to estrogen at the molecular level, decreases hot flashes in some women, but the evidence so far is anecdotal and no large studies have been conducted. Black cohosh is the best documented of all the herbal remedies. Studies suggest that it can relieve menopause-related headaches, depression, anxiety, hot flashes, night sweats, heart palpitations, and vaginal dryness and thinning. Black cohosh suppresses the secretion of luteinizing hormone, a hormone that is believed to be at the root of many menopausal symptoms. One European study of eighty women found that black cohosh relieved menopausal symptoms more effectively than estrogen replacement therapy.

PERSPECTIVE AND PROSPECTS

The menopause, in various guises, was referred to in many early cultures and texts. Initially, an association was made between age and the loss of fertility. By the sixth century, written records on the cessation of menstruation were well documented. At that time, it was believed that menstruation did not cease before the age of thirty-five, nor did it usually continue after the age of fifty. It was thought that obese women ceased menstruation very early and that the periods remained normal or abnormal and increased in flow or became diminished depending on age, the season

of the year, the habits and peculiar traits of women, the types of food eaten, and complicating diseases. Similar descriptions of menstrual cessation and its age of onset continued for another thousand years. It was not until the late eighteenth and early nineteenth centuries, however, that much advancement in the knowledge of the topic took place.

John Leake, influenced by William Harvey's historic description of the circulatory system, made one of the first reasonable attempts to explain the etiology of the menopause in his 1777 book *Medical Instructions Towards the Prevention and Cure of Chronic or Slow Diseases Peculiar to Women*. He believed that as long as the "prime of life" continued, along with the circulating force of the blood being more than equal to the resistance of the uterine vessels, the menses would continue to flow. When these vessels became firm from the effect of age, however, the diminished current of blood would be insufficient to force the uterine vessels open, and then periodic discharge would cease.

A later development in the history of menstruation studies was to link menstruation with all sorts of other problems, both emotional and organic. Leake commented that at the time of cessation of menses, women were often afflicted by various chronic diseases. He added that some women were prone to pain and lightheadedness, others were plagued by an intolerable itching at the neck of the bladder, and some were affected by low spirits and melancholy. Leake thought, because it seemed extraordinary that so many disorders should result from such a natural occurrence in a woman's life, that these symptoms could be explained away by indulgence in excesses, luxury, and an "irregularity" in the passions. Laying the blame for complications with the menopause on societal (in particular, female) excesses continued for some time.

Specific disease associations were also made; in 1814, John Burns announced that the cessation of menses seemed to cause cancer of the breast in some women. Edward John Tilt, a British physician, wrote one of the first full-length books on *The Change of Life in Health and Disease* (1857). Some of his views were that women should adhere to a strict code of hygiene during menstruation because they are often afflicted with cancer, gout, rheumatism, and nervous disorders.

These beliefs reflect a tendency from the mid-nineteenth century onward for medical literature to associate the menopause with many negative sociological features. For example, Colombat de l'Isère, in his book *Traité des maladies des femmes et de l'hygiène spéciale de leur sexe* (1838; *A Treatise on the Diseases and Special Hygiene of Females*, 1845), believed that during the menopause women ceased to live for the species and lived only for themselves. He thought that it was prudent for men to avoid having erotic thoughts about women in whom these feelings ought to have become extinct; he believed that after the menopause sexual enjoyment for women was ended forever.

Not all physicians, however, took such a negative attitude. Some believed that examining this phase in a woman's life presented a challenge. They believed that the boundaries between the physiological and the pathological in this field of study were ill-defined and that it was in the interest of the male gender that more research into this stage of a woman's life be done. The narrow boundary between normal physiology and pathology was not fully defined nearly a hundred years later, nor did the many negative and unsubstantiated theories cease. Well into the 1960's, the menopause was still considered "abnormal" and a "negative" state by some physicians.

Three major milestones exist in the history of menopause research in the twentieth century. The first event was the achievement of Adolf Butenandt, a Nobel Prize winner in chemistry. He succeeded in 1929 in isolating and obtaining, in pure form, a hormone from the urine of pregnant women which was eventually called estrone. The second development was the publication of the book *Feminine Forever*, by Robert A. Wilson, in 1966. The book, which became an instant best-seller, popularized a theory called "estrogen replacement treatment" or "hormone replacement therapy." As a result of the book's publication, physicians were prompted to take sides in a heated and continuing debate. The third landmark was the publication of an editorial and two original articles in *The New England Journal of Medicine* of December 4, 1975, claiming an association between exogenous estrogens and endometrial cancer. This claim brought about legal action by initiating, at least in the United States, a series of health administration inquiries.

—Genevieve Slomski, Ph.D.;
updated by Karen E. Kalumuck, Ph.D.

See also Aging; Arteriosclerosis; Breast cancer; Cervical, ovarian, and uterine cancers; Endocrinology; Endometrial cancer; Estrogen replacement therapy; Gynecology; Heart disease; Herbal medicine; Hormone replacement therapy; Hormones; Hysterectomy; Infertility in females; Menstruation; Midlife crisis; Obesity; Osteoporosis; Ovarian cysts; Sterilization.

FOR FURTHER INFORMATION:
Doress-Worters, Paula B., and Diana Laskin Siegal. *The New Ourselves Growing Older*. New York: Touchstone, 1994. In this updated version of a classic work developed in collaboration with the Boston Women's Health Book Collective, a host of issues related to maturing in women are addressed, including the menopause, osteoporosis, and estrogen replacement therapy. The positive aspects of changes are emphasized, and the book is filled with practical advice and resource lists.

Greenwood, Sadja. *Menopause Naturally*. Volcano, Calif.: Volcano Press, 1996. This updated, classic book gives a clear description of the natural changes in the menopause and up-to-date holistic approaches to its management.

Hammond, Charles B., et al., eds. *Menopause*. New York: Liss, 1989. A series of essays on the evaluation and treatment of and the health concerns surrounding the menopause, stressing hormone replacement therapy in particular. Contains numerous charts and graphs.

Maas, Paula, Susan E. Brown, and Nancy Bruning. *Natural Medicine for Menopause and Beyond*. New York: Dell, 1997. After giving a concise and lucid description of the physiological changes that occur during the menopause, this concisely written text addresses a host of symptoms and dispenses the current wisdom from a host of alternative medical traditions, including ancient Chinese medicine, acupressure, herbal therapy, and homeopathy.

Sheehy, Gail. *The Silent Passage: Menopause*. Rev. ed. New York: Pocket Books, 1998. Expanding on an article that she published in the October, 1991, issue of *Vanity Fair*, Sheehy draws from more than one hundred interviews conducted with women experiencing various stages of the menopause, as well as interviews with dozens of experts in many disciplines.

Swartz, Donald P. *Hormone Replacement Therapy*. Baltimore: Williams & Wilkins, 1992. Discusses the physiological role of the sex hormones and the growing evidence for the pathology that results from a long-term deficiency in these hormones.

MENORRHAGIA
DISEASE/DISORDER

ANATOMY OR SYSTEM AFFECTED: Reproductive system, uterus

SPECIALTIES AND RELATED FIELDS: Gynecology

DEFINITION: Menorrhagia is excessive or prolonged bleeding during menstruation. Large amounts of blood (up to three times the normal amount) may be lost during the menstrual cycle each month, and iron-deficiency anemia may result. There are several possible causes of such abnormal bleeding, such as uterine tumors or polyps and endometriosis, in which uterine tissue grows in other locations in the body. Changes in the production and release of hormones may also be suspected. Hormone therapy may be used, and hysterectomy is required in some cases.

—*Jason Georges and Tracy Irons-Georges*
See also Anemia; Bleeding; Dysmenorrhea; Endometriosis; Genital disorders, female; Hysterectomy; Menstruation; Reproductive system.

FOR FURTHER INFORMATION:

Boston Women's Health Book Collective. *Our Bodies, Ourselves for the New Century.* New York: Simon & Schuster, 1998.

Lark, Susan M. *Anemia and Heavy Menstrual Flow.* Los Altos, Calif.: Westchester, 1993.

Quilligan, Edward J., and Frederick P. Zuspan, eds. *Current Therapy in Obstetrics and Gynecology.* 5th ed. Philadelphia: W. B. Saunders, 1994.

Yen, Samuel S. C., and Robert B. Jaffe. *Reproductive Endocrinology: Physiology, Pathophysiology, and Clinical Management.* 4th ed. Philadelphia: W. B. Saunders, 1999.

MENSTRUATION
BIOLOGY

ANATOMY OR SYSTEM AFFECTED: Reproductive system, uterus

SPECIALTIES AND RELATED FIELDS: Endocrinology, gynecology, pediatrics

DEFINITION: The monthly discharge of blood and tissue (menses) by women of childbearing age, caused by changes in hormonal levels.

KEY TERMS:

endometrium: the layer of cells lining the inner cavity of the uterus; the source of menstrual discharge

feedback: a system in which two parts of the body communicate and control each other, often through hormones; can be either negative (inhibitory) or positive (stimulatory)

follicle: a spherical structure within the ovary that contains a developing ovum and that produces hormones; each ovary contains thousands of follicles

hormone: a chemical signal produced in some part of the body that is carried in the blood to another body part, where it has some observable effect

menstrual cycle: the cycle of hormone production, ovulation, menstruation, and other changes that occurs on an approximately monthly schedule in women

ovary: the organ that produces ova and hormones; the two ovaries lie on either side of the uterus, within the abdominal cavity

ovulation: the process by which an ovum is released from its follicle in the ovary; occurs in the middle of each menstrual cycle

ovum (pl. ova): the egg or reproductive cell produced by the female, which when fertilized by a sperm from the male will develop into an embryo

prostaglandins: chemical signals that have local effects on the organ that produces them

uterus: the organ that nourishes and supports the developing embryo; also called the womb

PROCESS AND EFFECTS

Menstruation is the monthly discharge of bloody fluid from the uterus. It occurs in humans and in other primates (apes and monkeys), but not in all mammals; for example, horses, cats, and dogs do not menstruate. The menstrual fluid consists of blood, cells and debris from the endometrial lining of the uterus, and mucus and other fluids. The color of the discharge varies from dark brown to bright red during the period of flow. The menstrual discharge does not normally clot after leaving the uterus, but it may contain endometrial debris that resembles blood clots. The flow lasts from four to five days in most women, with spotting (the discharge of scant fluid) possibly continuing another day or two. The volume of fluid lost ranges from 10 to 80 milliliters, with a median of about 40 milliliters. The blood in the menstrual discharge amounts to only a small fraction of the body's total blood volume of about 5,000 milliliters, and so normal physiological functioning is not usually impaired by the blood loss that occurs during menstruation.

The first menstruation (menarche) begins when a girl goes through puberty at the age of twelve or thir-

Menstrual Cycle

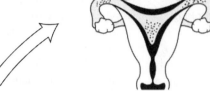

Days 1-6: Shedding of the endometrium; estrogen and progesterone low.

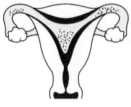

Days 24-28: Unfertilized egg passes through uterus; estrogen and progesterone levels drop.

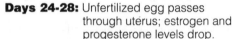

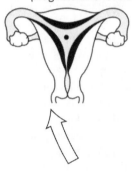

Days 7-12: Ripening of new egg; estrogen rising.

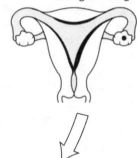

Days 19-23: Thickening of the endometrium.

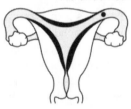

Days 13-18: Release of egg; estrogen and progesterone rising.

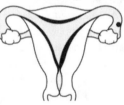

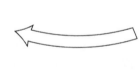

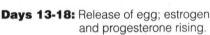

Exact timing varies from woman to woman; day 1 is defined as the day of onset of menstrual flow; ovulation occurs in mid-cycle (around day 14). Hormonal levels are rising and falling throughout the cycle.

teen; the last episodes of menstruation occur some forty years later at the time of menopause. Menstruation does not occur during the months of pregnancy or for the first few months after a woman has given birth.

Menstruation is the most visible event of the woman's monthly menstrual cycle. The average length of the menstrual cycle in the population is about 29.1 days, but it may vary from 16 to 35 days, with variation occurring between different individuals and in one individual from month to month. Girls who have just gone through puberty and women who are approaching the menopause tend to have more variation in their cycles than do women in the middle

of their reproductive years. There is also an age-related change in cycle length: Cycles tend to be relatively long in teenagers, then decrease in length until a woman is about forty years old, after which cycles tend to lengthen and become irregular.

Hormones cause menstruation to be coordinated with other events in the menstrual cycle. Uterine function is regulated by two hormones, estrogen and progesterone, that are produced in the ovaries. In turn, the production of estrogen and progesterone is controlled by follicle-stimulating hormone (FSH) and luteinizing hormone (LH), both of which are produced in the pituitary gland. The hormones from the ovaries and from the pituitary have mutual control over each other: They participate in a feedback relationship. The fact that females produce ova only once a month, in a cycle, rather than continuously, is the result of a change in the feedback relationships between the ovarian and pituitary hormones as the menstrual cycle proceeds.

In the first half of the cycle, the follicular phase, a predominant negative feedback effect keeps pituitary hormone levels low while allowing estrogen to increase. Day 1 of the menstrual cycle is defined as the day of the onset of the menstrual flow. During the days of menstrual bleeding, levels of estrogen and progesterone are low, but FSH levels are high enough to cause the growth of follicles in the ovary. As the follicles start to grow, they secrete estrogen, and increasing amounts are secreted as the follicles continue to enlarge over the next five to ten days. The estrogen exerts negative feedback control over the pituitary: FSH and LH production is inhibited by estrogen, so levels of these hormones remain low during the follicular phase. Besides producing estrogen, the growing follicles contain ova that are maturing and preparing for ovulation. Meanwhile, estrogen acts on the uterus to cause the growth of the endometrial lining. The lining becomes thicker and its blood supply increases; glands located in the lining also grow and mature. These uterine changes are known as endometrial proliferation.

As the woman nears the middle of her cycle, a dramatic change in hormonal feedback occurs. The increasing secretion of estrogen shifts the hormonal system into a positive feedback mode, whereby an increase in estrogen stimulates the release of LH and FSH from the pituitary instead of inhibiting it. Thus, at the middle of the cycle (around day 14), simultaneous peaks in levels of estrogen, LH, and FSH occur. The peak in LH triggers ovulation by causing changes in the wall of the follicle, allowing it to break open to release its ovum. Although a group of follicles had matured up to this point, usually only the largest one ovulates, and the remainder in the group die and cease hormone production.

Following ovulation, negative feedback is reestablished. The follicle that just ovulated remains as a functional part of the ovary; it becomes transformed into the corpus luteum, a structure which produces estrogen and progesterone throughout most of the second half of the cycle, the luteal phase. During this phase, the combined presence of estrogen and progesterone reestablishes negative feedback over the pi-

tuitary, and LH and FSH levels decline. A second ovulation is prevented because an LH peak is not possible at this time. The combined action of estrogen and progesterone causes the uterus to enter its secretory phase during the second half of the cycle: The glands in the thickened endometrium secrete nutrients that will support an embryo if the woman becomes pregnant, and the ample blood supply to the endometrium can supply the embryo with other nutrients and oxygen. If the woman does in fact become pregnant, the embryo will secrete a hormone that will ensure the continued production of estrogen and progesterone, and because of these hormones, the uterus will remain in the secretory condition throughout pregnancy. Menstruation does not occur during pregnancy because of the high levels of estrogen and progesterone, which continually support the uterus.

If the woman does not become pregnant, the corpus luteum automatically degenerates, starting at about the twenty-fourth day of the menstrual cycle. As the corpus luteum dies, it fails to produce estrogen and progesterone, so levels of these hormones decrease. As the amounts of estrogen and progesterone drop, the uterus begins to produce prostaglandins, chemicals that act as local signals within the uterus. The prostaglandins cause a number of changes in uterine function: Blood flow to the endometrium is temporarily cut off, causing the endometrial tissue to die, and the uterine muscle begins to contract, causing further changes in blood flow. The decreased blood flow and the muscle contractions contribute to the cramping pain that many women feel just before and at the time of menstrual bleeding. Menstrual bleeding starts when the blood flow to the endometrium is reestablished and the dead tissue is sloughed off and washed out of the uterus. This event signals the start of a new menstrual cycle.

COMPLICATIONS AND DISORDERS

Many disorders involving menstruation exist. Toxic shock syndrome is a disease that, while not caused directly by menstruation, sometimes occurs during menstruation in women who use tampons to absorb the menstrual flow. The symptoms of toxic shock syndrome—fever, rash, a drop in blood pressure, diarrhea, vomiting, and fainting—are caused by toxins produced by the bacterium *Staphylococcus aureus*. This bacterium is normally present in limited numbers within the vagina, but the use of high-absorbency tampons is associated with a higher-than-normal bacterial growth and toxin production. Toxic shock syndrome requires immediate medical attention, since it may be fatal if left untreated. Women can reduce the risk of toxic shock syndrome by changing tampons often, using lower-absorbency types, and by alternating the use of tampons and sanitary napkins.

Amenorrhea is defined as the absence of menstruation. It is usually, but not always, coincident with lack of ovulation. Amenorrhea may be primary (the woman has never menstruated) or secondary (menstrual cycles that were once normal have stopped). The condition is usually associated with abnormal patterns of hormone secretion, but the problem in hormone secretion may itself be merely the symptom of some other underlying disorder. One of the most common situations leading to both primary and secondary amenorrhea is low body weight, caused by malnutrition, eating disorders, or sustained exercise. Body fat has two roles in reproduction: It provides energy needed for tissue growth and cell functions, and it contributes to circulating estrogen levels. Loss of body fat may create a situation in which the reproductive system ceases to function because of low estrogen levels and because of lack of needed energy. The result is seen as amenorrhea. Emotional or physical stress may also cause amenorrhea, because stress results in the release of hormones that interfere with the reproductive hormones. Ideally, amenorrhea is treated by removing its cause; for example, a special diet or a change in an exercise program can bring about an increase in body fat stores, or stress level can be reduced through changes in lifestyle or with counseling. Ironically, sometimes birth control pills are prescribed for women with amenorrhea. The pills do not cure the amenorrhea, but they counteract some of the long-term problems associated with it, such as changes in the endometrial lining and loss of bone density.

Dysmenorrhea refers to abnormally intense uterine pain associated with menstruation. It is estimated that 5 to 10 percent of women experience pain intense enough to interfere with their school or work schedules. Dysmenorrhea may be primary (occurring in women with no known disease) or secondary (caused by a disease condition such as a tumor or infection). Studies have shown uterine prostaglandin levels to be correlated with the degree of pain perceived in primary dysmenorrhea, and drugs that interfere with prostaglandins offer an effective treatment for this condition. These drugs include aspirin, acetaminophen, ibuprofen, and naproxen; some formulas are available without a doctor's prescription, but the stronger drugs require one. Secondary dysmenorrhea is best managed by removing the underlying cause; if this is not possible, the antiprostaglandin drugs may be useful in controlling the pain.

Menorrhagia is excessive menstrual blood loss, usually defined as more than 80 milliliters of fluid lost per cycle. This condition can have serious health consequences because of the loss of red blood cells, which are essential for carrying oxygen to tissues. Women who have given birth to several children are more likely to suffer from menorrhagia, possibly because of enlargement of the uterine cavity and interference with the mechanisms that limit menstrual blood flow. Women who have diseases that interfere with blood clotting may also have menorrhagia. Although the menstrual discharge itself does not usually form clots after it leaves the uterus, clots do form within the uterine endometrium; these clots normally prevent excessive blood loss. Treatment for menorrhagia may begin with iron and vitamin supplements to induce increased red blood cell production, or transfusions may be used to replace the lost red blood cells. If this is unsuccessful, treatment with birth control pills, destruction of the endometrium by laser surgery, or a hysterectomy (surgical removal of the uterus) may be necessary.

Endometriosis is a condition in which endometrial cells from the uterus become misplaced within the abdominal cavity, adhering to and growing on the surface of internal organs. The outside of the uterus, the oviducts (Fallopian tubes), the surface of the ovaries, and the outer surface of the intestines can all support the growth of endometrial tissue. Endometriosis is thought to arise during menstruation, when endometrial tissue enters the oviducts instead of being carried outward through the cervix and vagina. Through the oviducts, the endometrial tissue has access to the abdominal cavity. Since the misplaced endometrial tissue responds to hormones in the same way that the normal endometrium does, it undergoes cyclic changes in thickness and attempts to shed at the time of menstruation. Endometriosis results in intense pain during menstruation and can cause infertility because of interference with ovulation, ovum or sperm transport, or uterine function. Endometriosis is treated with birth control pills or with drugs that suppress menstrual cycles, or the endometrial tissue may be removed surgically.

Premenstrual syndrome (PMS) is a set of symptoms that occurs in some women in the week before the start of menstruation, with the symptoms disappearing once menstruation begins. Researchers and physicians who study PMS have struggled to devise a standard definition for the disorder, but the list of possible symptoms is lengthy and varies from woman to woman and even within one woman from month to month. The possible symptoms include both psychological and physical changes: irritability, nervous tension, anxiety, moodiness, depression, lethargy, insomnia, confusion, crying, food cravings, fatigue, weight gain, swelling and bloating, breast tenderness, backache, headache, dizziness, muscle stiffness, and abdominal cramps. A diagnosis of PMS requires that the symptoms show a clear relation to the timing of menstruation and that they recur during most menstrual cycles. Researchers estimate that 3 to 5 percent of women have PMS symptoms that are so severe that they are incapacitating, but that milder symptoms occur in about 50 percent of all women. Because of the variability in symptoms between women, some researchers believe that there are several subtypes of PMS, each with its own cluster of symptoms. It is possible that each subtype has a unique cause. Suggested causes of PMS include an imbalance in the ratio of estrogen to progesterone following ovulation, changes in the hormones that control salt and water balance (the renin-angiotensin-aldosterone system), increased levels of prolactin (a hormone that acts on the breast), changes in amounts of brain chemicals, altered functioning of the biological clock that determines daily rhythms, poor diet or sensitivity to certain foods, and psychological factors such as attitude toward menstruation, stresses of family or professional life, and underlying personality disorders. Studies evaluating these theories have yielded contradictory results, so that no one cause of PMS has yet been found. Current treatments for PMS include dietary therapy, hormone administration, and psychological counseling, but no treatment has been found effective in all PMS patients.

An interesting phenomenon associated with menstruation is menstrual synchrony, also known as the "dormitory effect." Among women who live together, menstrual cycles gradually become synchronized, so that the women begin to menstruate within a few days of one another. Researchers have found that this phenomenon probably occurs because of pheromones, chemical signals that are produced by an individual and that have an effect on another individual. Pheromones act on the brain through the sense of smell, even though there may not be an odor that is consciously perceived.

PERSPECTIVE AND PROSPECTS

Early beliefs about menstruation were based on folk magic and superstition rather than on scientific evidence. Even today, some cultures persist in believing that menstruating women possess deleterious powers: that the presence of a menstruating woman can cause crops to fail, farm animals to die, or beer, bread, jam, and other foods to be spoiled. Some people believe that these incidents will occur even if the menstruating woman has no evil intention. Because of the possibility of these events, some cultures prohibit menstruating women from interacting with others. In the most rigorous example of such a taboo, some societies require that menstruating women live in special huts for the duration of the bleeding period.

Folk beliefs about menstruating women have been bolstered by religious views of menstruating women as "unclean" and in need of purification. In Orthodox Judaism, there are detailed proscriptions to be observed by a menstruating woman, including the avoidance of sexual intercourse. Seven days after her menstrual flow has stopped, the Orthodox Jewish woman undergoes a ritual purification, after which she may resume sexual relations with her husband. Early Christians absorbed the Jewish belief in the uncleanliness of a menstruating woman and prohibited her from entering church or receiving the sacraments. These injunctions were lifted by the seventh century, but the view of women as spiritually and bodily impure persists in some Christian groups to this day.

In the United States, most couples abstain from intercourse during the woman's menstrual period. There is no medical justification for this behavior; in fact, research has demonstrated that intercourse can alleviate menstrual cramping, at least temporarily. Still, surveys have shown that a majority of both men and women think that it is wrong for a woman to have intercourse while menstruating.

There are also persistent beliefs that women's physical and mental abilities suffer during menstruation. In fact, this was the predominant medical opinion up through the nineteenth and early twentieth centuries. Medical writings from this time are filled with injunctions for women to rest and refrain from exercise and intellectual strain while menstruating. It was a common belief that education could actually cause physical harm to women. Some men used this advice as justification for excluding women from equal opportunities in education and employment. Starting in the late 1800's, however, scientific studies clearly demonstrated that education has no harmful effects and that there is no diminution of intellectual or physical performance during menstruation. Nevertheless, the latter finding has been one that the general population finds difficult to accept.

The latest view of menstruation is that, far from being harmful, menstrual bleeding is directly beneficial to a woman's health. Margie Profet, an evolutionary biologist at the University of California, theorizes that menstruation evolved as a means of periodically removing disease-causing bacteria and viruses from the woman's uterus. These organisms might enter the uterus along with sperm after sexual activity. In Profet's view, the energetic cost of replacing the blood and tissue lost through menstruation is more than outweighed by the protective benefits of menstruation. Her theory implies that treatments which suppress menstruation, as birth control drugs sometimes do, are not always advantageous.

—*Marcia Watson-Whitmyre, Ph.D.*

See also Amenorrhea; Cervical, ovarian, and uterine cancers; Childbirth; Conception; Contraception; Dysmenorrhea; Endocrinology; Endometriosis; Genital disorders, female; Gynecology; Hormones; Infertility in females; Menopause; Menorrhagia; Ovarian cysts; Pregnancy and gestation; Premenstrual syndrome (PMS); Puberty and adolescence; Reproductive system.

FOR FURTHER INFORMATION:

Covington, Timothy R., and J. Frank McClendon. *Sex Care: The Complete Guide to Safe and Healthy Sex.* New York: Pocket Books, 1987. Parts 1 and 2 deal with contraception and sexually transmitted diseases, but part 3 covers some topics directly related to menstruation: premenstrual syndrome, toxic shock syndrome, feminine hygiene, and various myths.

Golub, Sharon. *Periods: From Menarche to Menopause.* Newbury Park, Calif.: Sage, 1992. An exceptionally complete book that presents information on all aspects of the menstrual cycle. The chapters dealing with scientific studies are accurate and easy to read. The author includes her thoughts on how society could make menstruation easier for women and on further research that needs to be done.

Laws, Sophie. *Issues of Blood: The Politics of Menstruation.* Basingstoke, England: Macmillan, 1990. Written by a sociologist, the text explores the results of the author's interviews with men about their attitudes toward menstruation. It is the premise of the author that the dominant group in a society determines the beliefs of the oppressed; thus, women's feelings about menstruation can be understood by referring to what men think.

Quilligan, Edward J., and Frederick P. Zuspan, eds. *Current Therapy in Obstetrics and Gynecology.* 5th ed. Philadelphia: W. B. Saunders, 1999. A standard medical reference on treatment for women's disorders, arranged in an encyclopedia format, with short articles on each topic. There is a particularly good description of premenstrual syndrome, written by Guy E. Abraham and Richard J. Taylor.

MENTAL ILLNESS. *See* PSYCHIATRIC DISORDERS; *specific diseases.*

MENTAL RETARDATION
DISEASE/DISORDER
ANATOMY OR SYSTEM AFFECTED: Brain, nervous system, psychic-emotional system

SPECIALTIES AND RELATED FIELDS: Genetics, psychiatry, psychology

DEFINITION: Significant subaverage intellectual development and deficient adaptive behavior accompanied by physical abnormalities.

KEY TERMS:

educable mentally retarded (EMR): individuals with mild-to-moderate retardation; they can be educated with some modifications of the regular education program and can achieve a minimal level of success

idiot: an expression which was formerly used to describe a person with profound mental retardation; such an individual requires custodial care

inborn metabolic disorder: an abnormality caused by a gene mutation which interferes with normal metabolism and often results in mental retardation

mental handicap: the condition of an individual classified as "educable mentally retarded"

mental impairment: the condition of an individual classified as "trainable mentally retarded" *neural tube defects:* birth defects resulting from the failure of the embryonic neural tube to close; usually results in some degree of mental retardation

trainable mentally retarded (TMR): individuals with moderate-to-severe retardation; only low levels of achievement may be reached by such persons

CAUSES AND SYMPTOMS

Mental retardation is a condition in which a person demonstrates significant subaverage development of intellectual function, along with poor adaptive behavior. Diagnosis can be made fairly easily at birth if physical abnormalities also accompany mental retardation. An infant with mild mental retardation, however, may not be diagnosed until problems arise in school. Estimates of the prevalence of mental retardation vary from 1 to 3 percent of the world's total population.

Diagnosis of mental retardation takes into consideration three factors: subaverage intellectual function, deficiency in adaptive behavior, and early-age onset (before the age of eighteen). Intellectual function is a measure of one's intelligence quotient (IQ). Four levels of retardation based on IQ are described by the American Psychiatric Association. An individual with an IQ between 50 and 70 is considered mildly retarded, one with an IQ between 35 and 49 is moderately retarded, one with an IQ between 21 and 34 is severely retarded, and an individual with an IQ of less than 20 is termed profoundly retarded.

A person's level of adaptive behavior is not as easily determined as an IQ, but it is generally defined as the ability to meet social expectations in the individual's own environment. Assessment is based on development of certain skills: sensory-motor, speech and language, self-help, and socialization skills. Tests have been developed to aid in these measurements.

To identify possible mental retardation in infants, the use of language milestones is a helpful tool. For example, parents and pediatricians will observe whether children begin to smile, coo, babble, and use words during the appropriate age ranges. Once children reach school age, poor school achievement may identify those who are mentally impaired. Psychometric tests appropriate to the age of the children will help with diagnosis.

Classification of the degree of mental retardation is never absolutely clear, and dividing lines are often arbitrary. There has been debate about the value of classifying or labeling persons in categories of men-

tal deficiency. On the one hand, it is important for professionals to understand the amount of deficiency and to determine what kind of education and treatment would be appropriate and helpful to each individual. On the other hand, such classification can lead to low self-esteem, rejection by peers, and low expectations from teachers and parents.

There has been a marked change in the terminology used in classifying mental retardation from the early days of its study. In the early twentieth century, the terms used for moderate, severe, and profound retardation were "moron," "imbecile," and "idiot." In Great Britain, the term "feeble-minded" was used to indicate moderate retardation. These terms are no longer used by professionals working with the mentally retarded. "Idiot" was the classification given to the most profoundly retarded until the middle of the twentieth century. Historically, the word has changed in meaning, from William Shakespeare's day when the court jester was called an idiot, to an indication of psychosis, and later to define the lowest grade of mental deficiency. The term "idiocy" has been replaced with the expression "profound mental retardation."

Determining the cause of mental retardation is much more difficult than might be expected. More than a thousand different disorders that can cause mental retardation have been reported. Some cases seem to be entirely hereditary, others to be caused by environmental stress, and others the result of a combination of the two. In a large number of cases, however, the cause cannot be established. The mildly retarded make up the largest proportion of the mentally retarded population, and their condition seems to be a recessive genetic trait with no accompanying physical abnormalities. From a medical standpoint, mental retardation is considered to be a result of disease or biological defect and is classified according to its cause. Some of these causes are infections, poisons, environmental trauma, metabolic and nutritional abnormalities, and brain malformation.

Infections are especially harmful to brain development if they occur in the first trimester of pregnancy. Rubella is a viral infection that often results in mental retardation. Syphilis is a sexually transmitted disease which affects adults and infants born to them, resulting in progressive mental degeneration.

Poisons such as lead, mercury, and alcohol have a very damaging effect on the developing brain. Lead-based paints linger in old houses and cause poisoning in children. Children tend to eat paint and plaster chips or put them in their mouths, causing possible mental retardation, cerebral palsy, and convulsive and behavioral disorders.

Traumatic environmental effects that can cause mental retardation include prenatal exposure to X rays, lack of oxygen to the brain, or a mother's fall during pregnancy. During birth itself, the use of forceps can cause brain damage, and labor that is too brief or too long can cause mental impairment. After the birth process, head trauma or high temperature can affect brain function.

Poor nutrition and inborn metabolic disorders may cause defective mental development because vital body processes are hindered. One of these conditions, for which every newborn is tested, is phenylketonuria (PKU), in which the body cannot process the amino acid phenylalanine. If PKU is detected in infancy, subsequent mental retardation can be avoided by placing the child on a carefully controlled diet, thus preventing buildup of toxic compounds that would be harmful to the brain.

The failure of the neural tube to close in the early development of an embryo may result in anencephaly (an incomplete brain or none at all), hydrocephalus (an excessive amount of cerebrospinal fluid), or spina bifida (an incomplete vertebra, which leaves the spinal cord exposed). Anencephalic infants will live only a few hours. About half of those with other neural tube disorders will survive, usually with some degree of mental retardation. Research has shown that if a mother's diet has sufficient quantities of folic acid, neural tube closure disorders will be rare or nonexistent.

Microcephaly is another physical defect associated with mental retardation. In this condition, the head is abnormally small because of inadequate brain growth. Microcephaly may be inherited or caused by maternal infection, drugs, irradiation, or lack of oxygen at birth.

Abnormal chromosome numbers are not uncommon in developing embryos and will cause spontaneous abortions in most cases. Those babies that survive usually demonstrate varying degrees of mental retardation, and incidence increases with maternal age. A well-known example of a chromosome disorder is Down syndrome (formerly called mongolism), in which there is an extra copy of the twenty-first chromosome. Gene products caused by the extra chromosome cause mental retardation and other physical problems. Other well-studied chromosomal abnormalities involve the sex chromosomes. Both males and females may be born with too many or too few sex chromosomes, which often results in mental retardation.

Mild retardation with no other noticeable problems has been found to run in certain families. It occurs more often in the lower economic strata of society and probably reflects only the lower end of the normal distribution of intelligence in a population. The condition is probably a result of genetic factors interacting with environmental ones. It has been found that culturally deprived children have a lower level of intellectual function because of decreased stimuli as the infant brain develops.

TREATMENT AND THERAPY

Diagnosis of the level of mental retardation is important in meeting the needs of the intellectually handicapped. It can open the way for effective measures to be taken to help these persons achieve the highest quality of life possible for them.

Individuals with an IQ of 50 to 70 have mild-to-moderate retardation and are classified as "educable mentally retarded" (EMR). They can profit from the regular education program when it is somewhat modified. The general purpose of all education is to allow for the development of knowledge, to provide a basis for vocational competence, and to allow opportunity for self-realization. The EMR can achieve some success in academic subjects, make satisfactory social adjustment, and achieve minimal occupational adequacy if given proper training. In Great Britain, these individuals are referred to as "educationally subnormal" (ESN).

Persons with moderate-to-severe retardation generally have IQs between 21 and 49 and are classified as "trainable mentally retarded" (TMR). These individuals are not educable in the traditional sense, but many can be trained in self-help skills, socialization into the family, and some degree of economic independence with supervision. They need a developmental curriculum which promotes personal development, independence, and social skills.

The profoundly retarded (formerly called idiots) are classified as "totally dependent" and have IQs of 20 or less. They cannot be trained to care for themselves, to socialize, or to be independent to any degree. They will need almost complete care and supervision throughout life. They may learn to understand a few simple commands, but they will only be able to speak a few words. Meaningful speech is not characteristic of this group.

EMR individuals need a modified curriculum, along with appropriately qualified and experienced teachers. Activities should include some within their special class and some in which they interact with students of other classes. The amount of time spent in regular classes and in special classes should be determined by individual needs in order to achieve the goals and objectives planned for each. Individual development must be the primary concern.

For TMR individuals, the differences will be in the areas of emphasis, level of attainment projected, and methods used. The programs should consist of small classes that may be held within the public schools or outside with the help of parents and other concerned groups. Persons trained in special education are needed to guide the physical, social, and emotional development experiences effectively.

A systematic approach in special education has proven to be the best teaching method to make clear to students what behaviors will result in the successful completion of goals. This approach has been designed so that children work with only one concept at a time. There are appropriate remedies planned for misconceptions along the way. Progress is charted for academic skills, home-living skills, and prevocational training. Decisions on the type of academic training appropriate for a TMR individual are not based on classification or labels, but on demonstrated ability.

One of the most important features of successful special education is the involvement of parents. Parents faced with rearing a retarded child may find the task overwhelming and have a great need of caring support and information about their child and the implications for their future. Parental involvement gives the parents the opportunity to learn by observing how the professionals facilitate effective learning experiences for their children at school.

Counselors help parents identify problems and implement plans of action. They can also help them determine whether goals are being reached. Counselors must know about the community resources that are available to families. They can help parents find emotional reconciliation with the problems presented by their special children. It is important for parents to be able to accept the child's limitations. They should not lavish special or different treatment on the retarded child, but rather treat this child like the other children.

Placing a child outside the home is indicated only when educational, behavioral, or medical controls are needed which cannot be provided in the home. Physicians and social workers should be able to do some counseling to supplement that of the trained counselors. Those who offer counseling should have basic counseling skills and relevant knowledge about the mentally retarded individual and the family.

EMR individuals will usually marry, have children, and often become self-supporting. The TMR will live in an institution or at home or in foster homes for their entire lives. They will probably never become self-sufficient. The presence of a TMR child has a great impact on families and may weaken family closeness. It creates additional expenses and limits family activities. Counseling for these families is very important.

Sheltered employment provides highly controlled working conditions, helping the mentally retarded to become contributing members of society. This arrangement benefits the individual, the family, and society as the individual experiences the satisfaction and dignity of work. The mildly retarded may need only a short period of time in the sheltered workshop. The greater the degree of mental retardation, the more likely shelter will be required on a permanent basis. For the workshop to be successful, those in charge of it must consider both the personal development of the handicapped worker and the business production and profit of the workshop. Failure to consider the business success of these ventures has led to failures of the programs.

There has been a trend toward deinstitutionalizing the mentally retarded, to relocate as many residents as possible into appropriate community homes. Success will depend on a suitable match between the individual and the type of home provided. This approach is most effective for the mentally retarded if the staff of a facility is well trained and there is a fair amount of satisfactory interaction between staff and residents. It is important that residents not be ignored, and they must be monitored for proper evaluation at each step along the way. Top priority must be given to preparation of the staff to work closely with the mentally impaired and handicapped.

In the past, there was no way to know before a child's birth if there would be abnormalities. With advances in technology, however, a variety of prenatal tests can be done and many fetal abnormalities can be detected. Genetic counseling is important for persons who have these tests conducted. Some may have previously had a retarded child, or have retarded family members. Others may have something in their backgrounds that would indicate a higher-than-average risk for physical and/or mental abnormalities. Some come for testing before a child is conceived, others do not come until afterward. Tests can be done on the fetal blood and tissues that will reveal chromosomal abnormalities or inborn metabolic errors.

Many parents do not seek testing or genetic counseling because of the stress and anxiety that may result. Though most prenatal tests result in normal findings, if problems are indicated the parents are faced with what may be a difficult decision: whether to continue the pregnancy. It is often impossible to predict the extent of an abnormality, and weighing the sanctity of life in relation to the quality of life may present an ethical and religious dilemma. Others prefer to know what problems lie ahead and what their options are.

PERSPECTIVE AND PROSPECTS

Down through history, the mentally retarded were first ignored, and then subjected to ridicule. The first attempts to educate the mentally retarded were initiated in France in the mid-nineteenth century. Shortly afterward, institutions for them began to spring up in Europe and the United States. These were often in remote rural areas, separated from the communities nearby, and were usually ill-equipped and understaffed. The institutions were quite regimented and harsh discipline was kept. Meaningful interactions usually did not occur between the patients and the staff.

The medical approach of the institutions was to treat the outward condition of the mentally retarded and ignore them as people. No concern for their social and emotional needs was shown. There were no provisions for children to play, nor was there concern for the needs of the family of those with mental handicaps.

Not until the end of the nineteenth century were the first classes set up in some U.S. public schools for education of the mentally retarded. The first half of the twentieth century brought about the expansion of the public school programs for individuals with both mild and moderate mental retardation. After World War II, perhaps in response to the slaughter of mentally handicapped persons in Nazi Germany, strong efforts were made to provide educational, medical, and recreational services for the mentally retarded.

Groundbreaking research in the 1950's led to the normalization of society's attitude about the mentally retarded in the United States. Plans to help these individuals live as normal a life as possible were made. The National Association for Retarded Citizens was founded in 1950 and had a very strong influence on public opinion. In 1961, President John F. Kennedy appointed the Panel on Mental Retardation and instructed it to prepare a plan for the nation, to help meet the complex problems of the mentally retarded. The panel presented ninety recommendations in the areas of research, prevention, medical services, education, law, and local and national organization. Further presidential commissions on the topic were appointed and have had far-reaching effects for the well-being of the mentally retarded.

A "Declaration of the Rights of Mentally Retarded Persons" was adopted by the General Assembly of the United Nations in 1971, and the Education for All Handicapped Children Act was passed in the United States in 1975, providing for the development of educational programs appropriate for all handicapped children and youth. These pieces of legislation were milestones in the struggle to improve learning opportunities for the mentally retarded.

Changes continue to take place in attitudes toward greater integration of the retarded into schools and the community, leading to significant improvements. The role of the family has increased in emphasis, for it has often been the families themselves that have worked to change old, outdated policies. The cooperation of the family is very important in improving the social and intellectual development of the mentally retarded child. Because so many new and innovative techniques have been used, it is very important that programs be evaluated and compared to one another to determine which methods provide the best training and education for the mentally retarded.

—Katherine H. Houp, Ph.D.

See also Birth defects; Cretinism; Down syndrome; Endocrine disorders; Fetal alcohol syndrome; Fragile X syndrome; Genetic diseases; Genetics and inheritance; Learning disabilities; Phenylketonuria (PKU); Pregnancy and gestation; Psychiatry; Psychiatry, child and adolescent.

FOR FURTHER INFORMATION:

Clarke, Ann M., Alan D. B. Clarke, and Joseph M. Berg. *Mental Deficiency: The Changing Outlook.* 4th ed. New York: Free Press, 1985. A classic text in the field of mental retardation which summarizes the tremendous amount of knowledge that has been amassed on the subject. Covers the genetic and environmental causes of mental retardation, prevention, help, intervention, and training.

Dudley, James R. *Confronting the Stigma in Their Lives: Helping People with a Mental Retardation Label.* Springfield, Ill.: Charles C Thomas, 1997. This book is written for anyone concerned about combating the negative effects of being labeled as having a mental disorder.

Jakab, Irene, ed. *Mental Retardation.* New York: Karger, 1982. A clearly written text for training health professionals who work with the mentally retarded. Contains useful, practical information and emphasizes those things which can be done to improve the quality of life for the mentally retarded.

Matson, Johnny L., and Rowland P. Barrett, eds. *Psychopathology in the Mentally Retarded.* 2d ed. Boston: Allyn & Bacon, 1993. This book addresses an often-neglected topic: the psychological problems that may be found in mentally retarded individuals. Discusses special emotional problems of various types of mentally retarded persons based on the causation of their deficiency.

METABOLISM

BIOLOGY

ANATOMY OR SYSTEM AFFECTED: Gastrointestinal system, intestines, kidneys, liver, pancreas, spleen, stomach

SPECIALTIES AND RELATED FIELDS: Biochemistry, cytology, exercise physiology, gastroenterology, nutrition, pharmacology

DEFINITION: The processes by which the substance of plants and animals incidental to life is built up and broken down.

KEY TERMS:

adipose tissue: tissue that stores fat; occurs in humans beneath the skin, usually in the abdomen or in the buttocks

anabolism: the metabolic activity through which complex substances are synthesized from simpler substances

basal metabolic rate (BMR): the standardized measure of metabolism in warm-blooded organisms

calorie: a measurement of heat, particularly in measuring the value of foods for producing energy and heat in an organism

catabolism: the complete breaking down of molecules by an organism for the purpose of obtaining chemical building blocks

essential nutrients: molecules that an organism needs for survival but cannot manufacture itself

standard metabolic rate (SMR): the standardized measure of metabolism in cold-blooded organisms

storage compounds: areas in the body that store nutrients not immediately required by an organism

STRUCTURE AND FUNCTIONS

Metabolism is an ongoing process in living organisms. It is fundamentally concerned with the chemistry of life. An organism's metabolic rate is the rate at which it consumes the energy it derives from the nutrients that sustain it. Organisms consume energy by converting chemical energy to heat and external work; most of the latter is converted to heat also, as external work, such as walking or moving in any way, overcomes friction. A workable measure of metabolic rate, therefore, is the rate at which an organism produces heat. The food that organisms ingest is measured in calories, each calorie being the measure of what is required to raise one kilogram of water by one degree Celsius.

Metabolism consists of two essential underlying processes, anabolism and catabolism. In vertebrates, the food ingested is immediately mixed with digestive enzymes in the mouth. These enzymes are produced by the salivary glands. As a ball of food, a bolus, passes through the digestive system, additional enzymes found in the stomach, the pancreas, and the small intestine work upon it, accelerating the digestive process.

Some nonenzymes are also vital to the digestive process. Most notable are hydrochloric acid, which, in the stomach, is a necessary ingredient for the efficient use of the stomach's pepsin, and bile salts in the small intestine, nonenzymes essential to the digestive process. The action of the digestive apparatus results in catabolism, or the breaking down of the components of food, notably lipids, carbohydrates, and proteins, into small molecules used to build and repair cells. Such molecules, through absorption, traverse the wall of the small intestine to enter the blood or the lymph so that they can be distributed throughout the body to meet its immediate requirements.

Amino acids break down protein, permitting it to enter the bloodstream, whereas glucose and other enzymes act to break down the large carbohydrates into

The Pathways of Metabolism

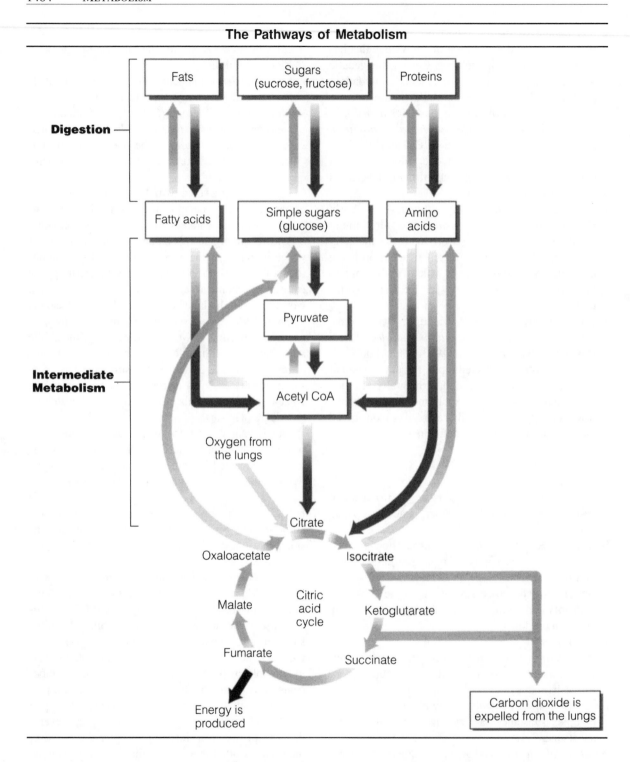

small molecules that are absorbed into the bloodstream. After they are catabolized into smaller molecules, the lipids or fats, unlike proteins and carbohydrates, enter the lymphatic system rather than the bloodstream, which they can enter only after they have passed through the lymphatic system.

Organisms typically cannot digest all the types of nutrients they ingest. Most vertebrates, for example, are incapable of digesting cellulose, the major carbohydrate component of most plants. This material, therefore, simply passes through the digestive system and is excreted. High-fiber foods, which pass through the digestive tract essentially undigested, perform a valuable function in keeping the colon clear and, over the long term, in preventing colon cancer.

A remarkably complex biochemical process occurs when the circulatory system delivers its absorbed sugars, lipids, and amino acids to the parts of the body where they are needed to build new cells and repair existing cells. Sometimes, this process requires the conversion of sugar molecules to fat molecules or animo acids. For a cell to construct a protein, it must connect in a specific, complex order the many animo acid molecules that the process requires. While some of the requisite amino acids result directly from ingesting nutrients, others are not available in this way and must be obtained through the synthesis of sugar molecules.

Molecules that an organism needs for survival but that it cannot manufacture itself are obtained through ingestion. Such molecules are called essential nutrients. It takes twenty different kinds of amino acids, for example, to manufacture protein, but the body is capable of producing only half of these. Because green plants can synthesize all twenty forms of amino acids, they become a major and ready source of the essential nutrients required to sustain life.

Also, as part of a nutritional chain, one can note that although neither humans nor chickens can synthesize valine, a vital amino acid, chickens obtain valine by eating grain that is rich in it. Humans, in turn, eat chickens, through which they obtain valine. This amino acid is also available to humans through the green vegetables they eat.

The food that organisms ingest is used both to provide the necessary building blocks for the synthesis of membranes, enzymes, and other parts of cells and to provide energy. If the nutrients ingested are greater than the body's requirements for such synthesis and for the production of energy, then food molecules may be husbanded for future use in storage compounds within the organism. The excess stored in this way is usually in the form of lipids. In humans, such excesses are stored essentially around the abdomen and buttocks, where they can accumulate in considerable quantity.

If a human's food supply is severely reduced or completely cut off, the body draws on these reserves, using the stored fat cells until they have been completely depleted. Afterward, nutrients, mostly proteins, will be drawn from muscle mass, the sudden reduction of which can quickly eventuate in death.

The survival of organisms is usually dependent upon the work that they perform. Energy to carry out this work is derived through the splitting of the chemical bonds of adenosine triphosphate (ATP) and the splitting of the bonds of food molecules. Highly sophisticated and refined series of biochemical reactions called cellular respiration and aerobic catabolism permit most animals to transfer energy from the chemical bonds of nutrient molecules to the bonds of ATP.

Every cell in the body has the enzymes and cellular equipment to carry out aerobic catabolism and to manufacture its own ATP. Oxygen, carried through the blood, is the essential ingredient in aerobic catabolism, which results in the oxidization of nutrient molecules and their being broken up into small molecules composed largely of carbon dioxide and water. In this process, energy is released, some of it lost as heat and some of it conserved in the bonds of ATP.

As amino acids, lipids, and carbohydrates are catabolized in humans, the lipids and carbohydrates are used by the muscles, whereas the brain gains its energy almost exclusively through the glucose that catabolized carbohydrates produce. Excess amino acids are converted by the liver and, to a smaller extent, by the kidneys to carbohydrates or lipids.

In a process called anaerobic glycolysis, which involves the creation of ATP without the presence of oxygen, energy is produced by converting glucose or glycogen into lactic acid. The body cannot excrete lactic acid, thereby making impossible its accumulation in its original form in the body. Lactic acid is released into the bloodstream after exercise and, now subjected to oxygen, is metabolized by the liver and either converted to glucose or oxidized aerobically in order to release additional energy.

As vertebrates age, their metabolic rate often decreases. In humans, a decreased metabolic rate, reduced activity in old age, and a failure to reduce caloric intake can result in substantial weight gain. Therefore, as humans age, their physicians usually encourage them to engage in physical activity and to reduce the overall number of calories that they consume. Physical activity generally helps to sustain the basal metabolism at levels higher than those found among the sedentary.

DISORDERS AND DISEASES

All metabolic disorders stem either from genetic or environmental origins, or from a combination of the two. For example, a person with a predisposition for diabetes, an inherited genetic disorder, may exacerbate this predisposition by indulging in a diet high in fats and carbohydrates, by overindulging in alcoholic beverages, and by engaging in little physical activity.

Environmental factors such as diet and exercise can hasten the onset of a disease of genetic origins that lurks in one's genes. On the other hand, people with this predisposition who control diet and alcohol consumption and who make strenuous exercise regular parts of their daily activity may forestall the onset of the disease, possibly keeping it at bay for their entire lifetimes.

Some environmental factors, such as urban air pollution, can lead to metabolic disorders such as lung cancer in large segments of a population. Even in such situations, however, not everyone exposed to the pollution will contract lung cancer, suggesting that those who do contract it probably have some genetic predisposition to it, however small that predisposition may be.

Significant advances were first made in the 1960's in tracing the genetic origins of diseases. The discovery that deoxyribonucleic acid (DNA), the molecular basis of heredity, exists in the nucleus of every cell of living organisms was a major biochemical discovery. It has led to vastly increased insights into heredity and into metabolic disorders of genetic origin, certainly the overwhelming majority of all such disorders.

Among the thousands of metabolic disorders attributable to inheritance are diabetes, arthritis, gout, mental retardation, hypothyroidism or hyperthyroidism and other glandular malfunctions, hemophilia, lupus, obesity, respiratory distress, congenital heart problems, Down syndrome, kidney dysfunction, baldness, the rapid acceleration of the aging process identified as progeria, melancholia, skeletal abnormalities, muscular weakness, cancer in its many forms, multiple sclerosis, muscular dystrophy, cerebral palsy, and countless other anomalies. Even such behavioral patterns as pedophilia, sexual orientation, disposition, and temperament are currently thought to be the result of genetic factors that predetermine what a person will inevitably become.

Microbiologists can detect a number of abnormalities in fetuses by analyzing the amniotic fluid that surrounds them in the womb. This process, known as amniocentesis, can identify more than twenty inherited metabolic disorders before an infant is born. Genetic manipulation in utero can alter some metabolic disorders, thereby bypassing or modifying faulty or abnormal genes. The genes of a person carrying a predisposition for a metabolic defect usually do not carry the information required for the synthesizing of a particular protein, usually an enzyme. This deficiency inhibits catalytic activity and blocks a metabolic pathway, resulting in a genetic abnormality.

In a minority of cases, the protein serves a role in transport or acts as a cell-surface receptor. Whatever role the protein in question serves, a delicate balance exists within the cells. When this balance is disturbed, metabolic problems ensue. For example, a gene may be responsible for producing an enzyme that converts one substance to another substance. If this gene is defective, the enzyme derived from it may be deficient and may fail to carry out the conversion or carry it out so slowly as to result in an inefficient conversion. While the first substance, a protein, accumulates in the cell, causing a surplus, it will be in short supply in the cell involved in the conversion, resulting in a deficiency. The surplus or the shortage may eventuate in a metabolic disorder, the genetic disbalance often revealing itself in overt symptoms.

Evidence of metabolic disorders can occur at any time in a person's life. They sometimes are detectable prenatally, but they may occur in early childhood, adolescence, adult life, or old age. In some cases, the onset of a serious metabolic disorder will be followed quickly by death. On the other hand, many people suffering from such disorders live long, active, full lives, many of them exceeding the average life span. Some metabolic disorders, such as diabetes, are manageable over long periods through diet and medication. Disorders such as lupus or hemophilia, while potentially fatal, have been managed successfully in many patients who, although they may eventually succumb to the disorder, live fruitful lives for many years.

Some types of metabolic disorders can be treated successfully with massive doses of vitamins. At least twenty fairly common disorders respond favorably to such treatment. For example, Wilson's disease, which results in excessive amounts of copper being accumulated in the tissues, is generally treated successfully with D-penicillamine, a compound that removes copper from the tissues and deposits it into the urinary system for excretion as urine.

Certain nutrients trigger metabolic disorders in

some organisms. The avoidance of these nutrients can prevent the triggering of the disorder on a permanent basis. Also, where the disorder results from a deficiency of an end product in a reaction, the disorder may be forestalled by replacing the end product. Such is the case, for example, among hemophiliacs, whose physical reaction to a cut is uncontrollable bleeding. If a clotting factor is introduced on a regular basis, the end product in this reaction is thwarted and clotting takes place.

PERSPECTIVE AND PROSPECTS

The metabolism was scarcely understood until the 1770's, when Joseph Priestley discovered oxygen and set other researchers on the path to understanding its role in the biochemical aspects of all life. In the next decade, Antoine-Laurent Lavoisier and Adair Crawford were the first researchers to measure the heat produced by animals and to suggest convincingly that animal catabolism is a form of combustion.

These early, tentative steps toward understanding how organisms derive energy and how they expend it led to further research that, in 1828, resulted in Friedrich Wohler's synthesis of an organic compound, urea, from inorganic substances, demonstrating that the compounds that living organisms produce can be converted from inorganic to organic through metabolism.

It was not until 1842 that Justus von Liebig categorized foods as falling into three essential types, carbohydrates, lipids, and proteins. He measured the caloric values of nutrients and advanced considerably what was known about nutrition and its role in metabolism. At about the same time, Julius Robert von Mayer and James Joule discovered that motion, heat, and electricity are all forms of the same thing, energy. It was not until the 1890's, however, that Max Rubner and Wilbur Atwater demonstrated conclusively through empirical data that animals release energy according to thermodynamic and biochemical principles established through studies of inanimate systems.

Landmark discoveries about metabolism proceeded into the twentieth century. In 1907, Walter Fletcher and Frederick Gowland Hopkins discovered that lactic acid results when glucose is subjected to the anaerobic contraction of muscles. Five years later, Hopkins discovered substances that are now recognized as vitamins, a term invented in 1912 by Casimir Funk. Ten years later, Frederick Banting and others

pinpointed insulin as a substance that could be synthesized and used to reduce levels of blood-sugar in humans, thereby making diabetes a manageable rather than a clearly fatal disorder.

A turning point in the understanding of metabolism and especially of metabolic disorders came in 1926 when James B. Sumner purified the first enzyme, showing it to be a protein, clearly leading to the realization that metabolic disorders result from a faulty protein in the genes. In 1941, Fritz Lipmann established the central role of ATP as a carrier of energy in living organisms, and the following year, Rudolf Schoenheimer demonstrated that the adult body's chemical constituents are in constant flux, suggesting that normal, healthy organisms are constantly renewing themselves.

As one surveys the future in terms of the rapidly increasing knowledge of metabolism and genetics, it is clear that genetic engineering offers daunting biological challenges. Birth defects can be detected well before birth and many of them, through genetic manipulation, can be prevented. It is now within the capability of genetic engineering to predetermine the sex of fetus and to control matters of gender. Amniocentesis can reveal abnormalities by the second trimester of pregnancy, revealing such conditions as Down syndrome.

The capabilities that currently lie within reach pose substantial ethical problems and challenges. For example, if a fetus clearly shows evidence of being afflicted with Down syndrome, what use should be made of this information? Some parents would elect to terminate the pregnancy, in effect serving as judge and jury in ending a life that has already begun. Given the challenges of raising a Down syndrome child, it is understandable that some parents might opt to avoid the situation through abortion. Others would argue, however, that to do so is to commit murder.

Other sorts of challenges have been raised. For example, homosexuality is currently thought to be of genetic origins in many people whose orientation is clearly and overtly homosexual. If genetic evidence of homosexuality is detected in a fetus, do parents have the right either to alter the genetic make-up of that fetus, which will soon be within the realm of possibility, or to destroy that fetus? To follow either course would be to imply that homosexuality is an undesirable trait. This, however, is a conclusion with which millions of people would disagree, pointing to the achievements of homosexuals throughout history who, but for their homosexuality, might never have achieved the eminence they did.

At present, the children of a parent suffering from lupus can be tested and told categorically whether they have inherited the gene that will inevitably cause them to suffer from the disease. Many people in this situation decline to be tested both because they do not want to know and because they do not want to run the risk that, through breaches in confidentiality, their employers might be made aware of their disease and might terminate their employment.

As society understands more about metabolism and its relation to the biochemical aspects of life, other possibilities present themselves. The cloning of complex organisms has already taken place. In 1996, Dolly, a sheep cloned from a single cell from a donor parent, was brought to full term and developed as any sheep conceived by conventional means develops. The potential for the cloning of humans exists, and the prospects are appealing to some people who argue that a human cloned from another human would provide a ready supply of compatible organs for the original cell donor were his or her organs to need replacement. The danger of rejection would, thereby, be virtually eliminated.

In such cases, ethical problems arise regarding the rights of a cloned being. In 1997, living frogs were cloned without heads. These frogs' bodies can be sustained indefinitely in a sort of limbo and their parts used as needed or desired. The frogs are brainless; therefore, it might be argued that they cannot be said to be living entities in any real sense, inasmuch as life is often defined as not existing in the absence of brain activity.

If such cloning can be done with frogs, the potential exists for it be done with higher forms of life, in which case a human might conceivably own a preserved body whose chief function is to provide spare parts for the cell donor as needed. The bioethical considerations in such instances are chilling.

Biochemically, humankind has reached the brave new world and must find equitable means of managing the changes that such processes as genetic engineering are bound to effect in the lives of everyone living today. The promise of genetic engineering made possible through a comprehensive understanding of metabolic processes is enormous, but the hazards associated with it are daunting.

—R. Baird Shuman, Ph.D.

See also Acid-base chemistry; Arthritis; Cancer; Cerebral palsy; Cholesterol; Cloning; Congenital heart disease; Diabetes mellitus; Digestion; Down syndrome; Endocrinology; Endocrinology, pediatric; Enzymes; Exercise physiology; Food biochemistry; Gastroenterology; Gastroenterology, pediatric; Gastrointestinal system; Genetic diseases; Glands; Glycolysis; Gout; Hair loss and baldness; Hemophilia; Hormones; Kidney disorders; Lipids; Lupus erythematosus; Mental retardation; Multiple sclerosis; Muscular dystrophy; Obesity; Thyroid disorders.

FOR FURTHER INFORMATION:
Becker, K., et al., eds. *Principles and Practices of Endocrinology and Metabolism.* 3d ed. Philadelphia: J. B. Lippincott, 2000. The treatment of metabolic disorders is extensive and accurate. The contributors are well informed and current in their information.
Edwards, Christopher R., and Dennis W. Lincoln, eds. *Recent Advances in Endocrinology and Metabolism.* New York: Churchill Livingstone, 1989. Particularly thorough in its treatment of such common metabolic disorders as diabetes, arthritis, and thyroid problems. The contributors also treat the less common metabolic disorders directly and clearly.
Feek, C. M., and C. R. Edwards. *Endocrine and Metabolic Disease.* New York: Springer-Verlag, 1988. This comprehensive volume presents information about every conceivable sort of metabolic disorder. The language is sometimes technical, but readers not specifically schooled in the field will be able to comprehend the salient points the authors make.
Whitehead, Roger G. *New Techniques in Nutritional Research.* San Diego, Calif.: Academic Press, 1990. This book provides the most thorough treatment of the nutritional aspects of metabolic disorders. It is especially strong in its presentation of disorders stemming from the accumulation of trace minerals, suggesting ways of treating such situations with vitamins or by other means.

METASTASIS. *See* **CANCER; MALIGNANCY AND METASTASIS.**

MICROBIOLOGY
SPECIALTY
ANATOMY OR SYSTEM AFFECTED: Cells, immune system

SPECIALTIES AND RELATED FIELDS: Bacteriology, environmental health, epidemiology, immunology, pathology, public health, virology

DEFINITION: The study of organisms too small to be seen by the unaided human eye, especially the identification, transmission, and control of microorganisms that cause disease.

KEY TERMS:

deoxyribonucleic acid (DNA): the genetic material of a cell that directs the synthesis of proteins; ribonucleic acid (RNA) is the intermediary needed to complete protein synthesis

flora: the microorganisms that are commonly found on or in the human body; also called microflora

infectious disease: an illness caused by a microorganism or its products, in contrast to diseases caused by factors such as heredity or poor nutrition

microorganism: an organism that is too small to be seen without a magnifying lens; also known as a microbe

pathogen: an organism that causes an infectious disease

SCIENCE AND PROFESSION

Microbiology is the field of science that focuses on microorganisms, living things that can only be studied by using microscopes and other special equipment. Microorganisms have an important place in the ecology of the planet. They form a basis for food chains and, as decomposers, recycle many materials in the environment. Because microbes are everywhere, humans come in contact with a wide variety every day; many live on or in the human body. Most of these organisms either are harmless or are prevented from multiplying by the immune system and other defenses. Others are able to penetrate these defenses and cause an illness. Medical microbiologists study microorganisms that cause these diseases. These pathogens come primarily from four groups: bacteria, fungi, protozoans, and viruses.

Bacteria, along with blue-green algae, belong to the Monera kingdom and are the simplest organisms that exist in cellular form. The bacterial chromosome consists of a loop of deoxyribonucleic acid (DNA) containing several hundred genes. Because it is unprotected by a nuclear membrane, bacterial DNA can be manipulated more easily than can DNA in plants and animals. Several traits are used to identify bacterial species. There are three basic shapes: coccus (round), bacillus (rod), and spirillum (spiral). Gram's

stain procedure divides bacteria into two main groups based on their cell wall content. Other staining procedures can identify the presence of such structures as flagella, capsules, and endospores, which may have implications for control measures. For example, endospores are resistant to many common disinfectants, and boiling them for up to four hours may not destroy them. In addition to staining, chemical and metabolic tests are used to differentiate bacterial species.

Although the fungi kingdom includes larger organisms such as mushrooms, the yeasts, molds, and related microorganisms are the ones of interest to medical microbiology. Like plants, they have cell walls. They cannot manufacture their own food by photosynthesis, however, and must either be saprophytes, living on dead organic material, or parasites, obtaining nutrients from another living organism. Fungi reproduce by means of spores that are released and carried by the air to a suitable medium. They thrive in a warm, moist environment with a carbohydrate source of food.

Protozoa, members of the Protista kingdom, are often referred to as one-celled animals. They have no cell walls and must ingest or absorb their food. Their ability to move enables them to spread more quickly than can nonmotile microbes. Four main categories exist. The amoebas move by means of projections called pseudopodia. The flagellates move by means of long hairlike structures (flagella) that whip back and forth. Ciliates are covered with short hairlike structures (cilia) that beat in a synchronized way to cause movement. Sporozoans must move by means of the circulation of blood and tissue fluids within a host. Of all the microorganisms, protozoa are the ones that most resemble human cells. Treatment for a protozoal disease must be monitored closely; most chemicals that are effective against protozoa are also toxic to humans.

Viruses are on the borderline between living and nonliving things. They are not cellular in form, unlike all other forms of life. Each virus particle, called a virion, is made up of a protein coat and a nucleic acid core of either DNA or RNA. Viruses are classified by size, shape, the type of nucleic acid in their core, and the type of cell they invade or disease they cause.

In order to reproduce, a virion attaches itself to a living cell and injects its core into the cell. The nucleic acid then takes over the cell's protein-manufacturing apparatus to make new virus particles. The host cell ruptures as these viruses are released to infect other cells. Some viral DNA can incorporate itself into the host DNA and remain dormant until some factor triggers a new reproductive cycle. Viruses usually can attack only one type of cell or species; however, mutations can occur that allow them to infect other species. For example, human immunodeficiency virus (HIV), the cause of acquired immunodeficiency syndrome (AIDS), is believed to have mutated from simian immunodeficiency virus (SIV) in monkeys.

DIAGNOSTIC AND TREATMENT TECHNIQUES

When the type of microorganism causing an infectious disease is unknown, a medical microbiologist follows a series of procedures known as Koch's postulates. Named for Robert Koch, who proposed them, these procedures identify and confirm that a particular microorganism is the cause of the disease. First, the microorganism must be present in the tissues of all individuals who have the disease. This means that all the microorganisms in a sample of diseased tissue must be identified and classified so that a possible pathogen may be differentiated from the normal flora. Second, the suspected pathogen must be isolated and grown in a pure culture. Many microorganisms can be grown on a simple medium called nutrient agar. Some microorganisms may need specific nutrients added to the medium or may be obligate parasites—that is, they can grow only on or in living cells. Anaerobic organisms cannot grow at all if oxygen is present. Since these special needs are not known in advance, the detection of some pathogens may be difficult.

The third step the researcher takes is to inoculate an animal with the organism in an effort to duplicate the disease. In the case of human diseases, mammals—such as rabbits, guinea pigs, and mice—are used. Finding the right animal subject may also pose a problem, since not all animals are susceptible to human diseases. For example, armadillos must be used to study leprosy, because the more common laboratory animals are not susceptible to it. In the last of Koch's procedures, the organism must be reisolated from the diseased animal. This step verifies the identity of the pathogen and confirms that it is the same as the original form. If the organism has been identified correctly as the cause of the disease, researchers can then proceed to learn more about the microorganism and its role in the disease process.

The identification of a pathogen as the cause of a specific disease and knowledge of its biological characteristics aid medical researchers in finding prevention and treatment strategies. In order to cause illness, a microorganism must meet several criteria. First, it must survive transfer to the new host. Some pathogens can form protective structures, such as endospores, that will keep them alive outside a host for a long period of time. A pathogen that cannot survive outside a host must be passed directly in some way from an infected person to a healthy one. Second, a pathogen must overcome the host's defenses. Some may enter through a wound, bypassing the skin barrier that protects the human body from many infections. Some produce chemicals that damage cells and weaken the body. Still others may be able to cause illness only if the person's defenses are weakened by some factor such as age, malnutrition, or another existing illness. Finally, the organism must cause some damage to the host, resulting in the symptoms and signs associated with that illness. The disease process can best be understood by examining several examples of pathogens, the diseases they cause, and the strategies used against them.

The members of the genus *Clostridium* are all anaerobic, form endospores, and produce toxins. Among the bacteria in this group are the pathogens that cause gangrene, tetanus, and botulism. Gangrene usually occurs when a wound has cut off the blood supply to an area of the body. *Clostridium perfringens* enters the body and is able to survive because the lack of blood has created an anaerobic condition. It produces a toxin that destroys surrounding tissue, allowing it to spread. Antibiotics may be effective in preventing the bacteria from spreading to healthy tissue but, because drugs are transported in the blood, may not be able to reach the infected site. Placing the patient in a chamber containing oxygen under high pressure is one strategy used to destroy anaerobic bacteria. *Clostridium tetani* also enters the body through a wound—sometimes a very small one. Since this organism is common and a small wound may go unnoticed, regular immunizations with tetanus vaccine are recommended. Once *C. tetani* bacteria enter the body, they produce a neurotoxin. This nerve poison causes the muscles to stiffen, resulting in a condition called tetanus, or lockjaw. In addition to antibiotics, an antitoxin must be given to neutralize the poison. *Clostridium botulinum* causes botulism, a type of food poisoning. If proper canning techniques are not used, the endospores will germinate. The food then provides a medium on which they can grow, and the sealed can provides the perfect anaerobic conditions. *C. botulinum* produces a neurotoxin that, if it is not destroyed by adequate cooking, will produce neurological symptoms such as double vision and dizziness. This disease must be treated by an appropriate antitoxin or death from respiratory failure can occur in a matter of days.

The human intestine contains large numbers of microorganisms. Some of them provide benefits to their host by producing vitamins and inhibiting the growth of other, potentially harmful, microorganisms. Disease can result if the balance is changed. *Escherichia coli*, part of the normal intestinal flora, can cause infections when it is transferred to another part of the body, such as the urinary bladder. In developing countries, *E. coli* bacteria contaminate drinking water in such large numbers that they result in infantile diarrhea, a common cause of death in those countries. A 1993 epidemic in the United States involved a particularly virulent strain of *E. coli* that had been ingested in improperly cooked ground beef. The characteristics of the strain, combined with the large number of bacteria in the meat, disrupted the intestinal balance of those who ingested it, caused hundreds of people to become ill, and resulted in the deaths of three young children.

The use of antibiotics can disrupt the natural balance by destroying beneficial bacteria as well as pathogens. *Candida albicans*, a yeastlike fungus, is part of the normal human flora. Its growth in the intestine is controlled by certain kinds of bacteria. When antibiotics are used, these beneficial bacteria are destroyed and the *Candida* begins to multiply. This may not only result in intestinal yeast infections but also contribute to yeast infections in the vagina and other areas where *Candida* can be found. Strategies used to restore the balance may involve eating yogurt or capsules containing *Acidophilus*, one of the beneficial bacteria. Sugars, an important source of food for yeast, should be eliminated from the diet. If these measures do not work, antifungal medication may have to be used.

Fungi that cause skin infections such as athlete's foot are called dermatophytes. When an infected person takes a shower, dermatophyte spores are left in the shower stall. The warm, moist environment then allows the spores to survive until a potential new host comes. Since feet are usually enclosed in shoes and socks, the dermatophytes are again provided with an ideal warm, moist environment. Prevention strategies involve using fungicidal disinfectants to kill the spores and wearing sandals in the shower to avoid coming in contact with the spores. Treatment includes antifungal medication and making the environment less suitable for fungi by keeping the feet dry.

Protozoa are also vulnerable to dry conditions. *Entamoeba histolytica*, the cause of amebic dysentery, is usually ingested in contaminated water. It can, however, form cysts, which allows it to resist drying and freezing. An individual can become ill after eating food rinsed in contaminated water or drinking a "safe" beverage that contained ice made from contaminated water.

Plasmodium species are responsible for malaria, which kills 2 million people in the world each year. Because this protozoan cannot live outside a host, it is dependent on the female *Anopheles* mosquito to transmit it from one person to another. When a mosquito "bites," it actually pierces the skin with a hypodermic-like mouth and injects a local anesthetic to prevent the host from feeling its presence. At the same time, if it is infected with *Plasmodium*, it will inject malarial parasites into the bloodstream. These parasites spend most of their life cycle inside red blood cells, where they are protected from normal immune defenses. When they have multiplied, they rupture the cells as they leave. Treatment involves maintaining sufficiently high levels of medicine, such as quinine, in the plasma that the parasites die. The most important public health strategy is to control the mosquito population and prevent transmission.

Other than bacteria, viruses are the most common pathogens. The mode of transmission of viruses from one host to another depends on the type of virus. Some can survive for a long period of time outside a host, others must be transferred quickly through the air or by contact, and others can survive only when passed directly into the host by body fluids or insect bites. The damage done to the host depends on the type of tissue that is infected by the virus. For example, the Epstein-Barr virus invades the lymphatic system. It causes the enlarged lymph nodes and abnormal lymphocytes that are characteristic of mononucleosis. It is also associated with Burkitt's lymphoma and Hodgkin's disease, both of which are cancers of the lymphatic system. The human immunodeficiency virus (HIV) invades the T lymphocytes, the white blood cells that are crucial to the functioning of the immune system. Damage to the immune system not only makes the individual vulnerable to disease organisms coming from outside the body but also disrupts the balance between the host and normal human flora. This allows other viruses, bacteria, protozoa, and fungi such as *Candida* to multiply and cause potentially fatal secondary infections.

PERSPECTIVE AND PROSPECTS

Infectious diseases have had devastating effects on human populations and societies. For example, during the eighty-year period starting in 1347, recurrent plague epidemics resulted in the deaths of 75 percent of the European population. For many centuries, some physicians and others hypothesized that invisible creatures were the cause of disease. In 1546, Girolamo Fracastoro suggested the presence of germs (seeds) of disease that could be passed from person to person. Because these creatures could not be seen, this "germ" theory was not widely accepted. Then, in 1673, Antoni van Leeuwenhoek began sending descriptions and pictures of what he called "animalcules" to the Royal Society of London. An amateur scientist, Leeuwenhoek made simple microscopes and systematically studied the objects and materials around him. His discoveries of what are now known to be protozoa and bacteria were verified, and they opened the field of microbiology as a science. Using their new knowledge of the microbial world, nineteenth century researchers began to reexamine the germ theory of disease. In 1857, Louis Pasteur, a chemist, discovered that certain bacteria caused wine to spoil. A few years later, he isolated a protozoan as a cause of a silkworm disease and predicted that microbes could cause human illness. In 1875, Robert Koch, a German physician, devised a procedure by which he demonstrated that anthrax was caused by a specific type of bacterium: *Bacillus anthracis*. His experiments led to widespread acceptance of the germ theory of disease, and his procedures provided a systematic method by which researchers could identify those germs. The twenty-five years that followed are referred to as the golden age of microbiology; one by one, nearly all the major bacterial pathogens were identified.

During this intense period of discovery, researchers soon found that, although fine porcelain filters were used to trap microorganisms, in some cases the liquid filtrate was capable of causing disease. The term "virus," meaning poison, was used because it was thought at first that the liquid contained a toxic substance. Pasteur hypothesized that there might be an organism too small to be seen using the light microscope. Later, this was verified, when researchers were able to remove the water from the filtrate, leaving crystals. After the invention of the electron microscope in 1933, individual virions could be seen.

The discovery of pathogens quickly led to research aimed at finding ways to prevent and treat infectious diseases. The contagious nature of disease was known in ancient times. This is illustrated by the practices of Greek physicians and Jewish hygiene laws. Prior to Koch's work, Ignaz Phillipp Semmelweis in the 1840's and Joseph Lister in the 1860's showed that antiseptic techniques could control transmission of diseases. In 1849, John Snow traced the source of a cholera epidemic to a water pump in London. The knowledge that a specific pathogen was involved made it possible for more specific means of prevention to be applied. Within ten years of Koch's report, Louis Pasteur developed vaccines for anthrax and rabies. Immunizations for many infectious diseases were developed, public sanitation measures were taken to reduce the contamination of food and water, and surgeons adopted techniques to control surgical and wound infection.

Although progress in disease prevention was being made, once a person became ill, treatment was still primarily a matter of keeping the patient alive until the disease ran its course. In the early 1900's, a German physician named Paul Ehrlich began to search for what he called a "magic bullet"—a chemical that would specifically treat a disease by killing the pathogens that caused it. After several years of work, compound 606, an arsenic derivative, was made available to treat syphilis. Sulfa drugs were developed in the 1920's. In 1929, Alexander Fleming discovered penicillin, a substance produced by the mold *Penicillium* that could destroy bacteria in cultures. In 1939, Ernst Chain and Howard Florey used penicillin successfully to treat bacterial infections. In 1944, Selman Waksman discovered streptomycin and used the term "antibiotic" to refer to a substance manufactured by a living organism that kills or inhibits the growth of a pathogen.

By the 1970's, it seemed that the end of infectious disease as a major medical problem was in sight. Several developments brought an end to this complacency. Strains of *Staphylococcus* appeared that were resistant to common antibiotics and caused an increase in postsurgical infections. Antibiotic-resistant strains of gonorrhea and syphilis also became widespread. Childhood diseases, once thought to be under control, reappeared as a result of neglected vaccination programs. Increased world travel also facilitated the spread of disease from country to country. Then, in 1981, AIDS was first described; within a few years, it became a worldwide health problem. As people with AIDS began to succumb to previously uncommon secondary diseases, these diseases had to be studied. A new antibiotic-resistant strain of tuberculosis also appeared as a direct result of the AIDS epidemic. These developments have reemphasized the study of microbiology and demonstrated its importance to human health.

—Edith K. Wallace, Ph.D.

See also Anthrax; Antibiotics; Bacterial infections; Bacteriology; Bionics and biotechnology; Botulism; Candidiasis; Cells; Creutzfeldt-Jakob disease and mad cow disease; Cytology; Cytopathology; Diarrhea and dysentery; DNA and RNA; Drug resistance; *E. coli* infection; Ebola virus; Epidemiology; Fungal infections; Gangrene; Gastroenterology; Gastroenterology, pediatric; Gastrointestinal disorders; Gastrointestinal system; Genetic engineering; Gram staining; Hodgkin's disease; Immune system; Immunization and vaccination; Immunology; Laboratory tests; Microscopy; Mutation; Pathology; Pharmacology; Pharmacy; Prion diseases; Protozoan diseases; Serology; Smallpox; Tetanus; Toxicology; Tropical medicine; Tuberculosis; Urinalysis; Urinary system; Urology; Urology, pediatric; Viral infections.

FOR FURTHER INFORMATION:

Alcarno, I. Edward, and Lawrence M. Elson. *Microbiology Coloring Book*. New York: HarperCollins, 1996. This volume is one in a series of "coloring books" that are excellent sources of information. Detailed instructions help the reader navigate the intricacies of the world of microbes through observation and reading.

Crook, William G. *The Yeast Connection: A Medical Breakthrough*. 3d ed. Jackson, Tenn.: Professional Books, 1994. Written for the general reader, this book explains the balance between the normal human flora and *Candida*, disrupting factors, and the correction of imbalances. Diagrams, recipes, questionnaires, and detailed references add to the value of this work.

Gallo, Robert. *Virus Hunting*. New York: Basic Books, 1991. Written for the general reader by one of the discoverers of the AIDS virus. It examines the field of virology and the methods used to study viruses, especially cancer-causing viruses. The search for the AIDS virus is detailed. Name and subject indexes are included.

Gladwin, Mark, and Bill Trattler. *Clinical Microbiology Made Ridiculously Simple*. Rev. 2d ed. Miami: Med Master, 1999. The authors explain the principles behind microbiology in easy-to-understand terms. Includes a bibliography and an index.

Jensen, Marcus M., and Donald N. Wright. *Introduction to Microbiology for the Health Sciences*. 4th ed. Englewood Cliffs, N.J.: Prentice Hall, 1997. An introductory college textbook that focuses on the field of medical microbiology. It reviews the general characteristics of microorganisms, but the emphasis is on pathogenic species, and the prevention and treatment of disease. Each chapter contains case histories illustrating the direct application of principles.

MICROSCOPY

PROCEDURE

ANATOMY OR SYSTEM AFFECTED: Cells

SPECIALTIES AND RELATED FIELDS: Bacteriology, cytology, histology, microbiology, pathology, virology

DEFINITION: The use of a microscope to enlarge extremely small objects to make them visible.

INDICATIONS AND PROCEDURES

Conventional microscopy uses a beam of light to illuminate a thin slice of material to be viewed. The material may be stained to provide contrast among its components. The visible light is aimed through the material and collected in a lens. Additional lenses magnify the image until it is visible to the eye of the viewer.

Electron microscopy is a procedure in which a beam of electrons, rather than visible light, is projected toward an object to be viewed. The object is prepared by coating it with a fine layer of metal, frequently gold, that is one or two atoms thick. The electrons reflect off the coated object and hit a screen. The image on the screen is magnified and becomes visible to the human eye. An alternative procedure involves a very thin section of material which is dried and put into a vacuum chamber. A beam of electrons is directed through the prepared specimen. A coated screen receives the electron beam and transforms the image into one visible to the human eye.

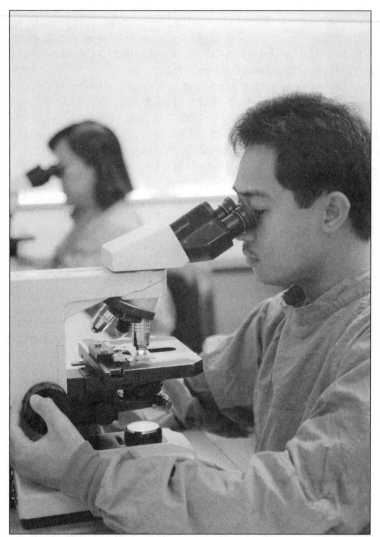

Microscopes are essential in the analysis of laboratory specimens. (Photo-Disc)

USES AND COMPLICATIONS

Microscopy has extended the range of understanding for physical objects. Intracellular organelles are routinely made visible. Microscopy has made possible the science of microbiology. Fluorescence allows immunoglobulins to be routinely assayed. Viruses are too small to be seen with a light microscope, but electron microscopy has enabled virologists to view and classify viruses.

The drawbacks of current microscopy techniques are primarily that only small samples of material can be viewed at a time. Usually, the material must be destroyed while it is being prepared. Living tissue may be viewed, but only at levels of magnification below those possible at the limits of normal microscopy and far below those possible with electron microscopy.

Electron microscopy allows the greatest amount of magnification for objects. Because the wavelength of electrons is thousands of times shorter than that of visible light, the resulting magnification is several thousand times greater than that possible with visible light. The use of subatomic particles theoretically increases the potential of magnification, but a continuous source of subatomic particles is difficult and quite expensive to supply.

—*L. Fleming Fallon, Jr., M.D., Ph.D., M.P.H.*

See also Antibiotics; Bacteriology; Cells; Cytology; Cytopathology; Gram staining; Laboratory tests; Microbiology; Pathology.

Fluorescence microscopy is a procedure that is based on the fact that fluorescent materials emit visible light when they are irradiated with ultraviolet light, which is outside the spectrum visible to the human eye. Some materials manifest this property naturally; others may have to be treated with fluorescent solutions in a process similar to staining. When the absorption of the specimen is in the relatively long ultraviolet range, two filters are also used. The first is placed over the light source to eliminate all but the desired long ultraviolet rays. The second is placed over the eyepiece. The result is a field that becomes dark and allows any red or yellow fluorescence to be visible.

FOR FURTHER INFORMATION:

Alcarno, I. Edward, and Lawrence M. Elson. *Microbiology Coloring Book.* New York: HarperCollins, 1996.

Madigan, Michael T., John M. Martinko, and Jack Parker. *Brock Biology of Microorganisms.* 9th ed. Upper Saddle River, N.J.: Prentice Hall, 2000.

Singleton, Paul. *Introduction to Bacteria.* 2d ed. New York: John Wiley & Sons, 1992.

MICROSCOPY, SLITLAMP
PROCEDURE

ANATOMY OR SYSTEM AFFECTED: Eyes

SPECIALTIES AND RELATED FIELDS: Ophthalmology

DEFINITION: The use of a special instrument to examine the tissues of the eye.

INDICATIONS AND PROCEDURES

The slitlamp microscope, or biomicroscope, is used to examine and evaluate tissues of the eye with both stereopsis and multiple values of optical magnification. The anterior segment of the eye is observed with several types of illumination: diffuse, direct (both broad and narrow beam, the latter allowing an almost slidelike examination of the clear corneal layers), indirect (side illumination), retroillumination (in which abnormalities are back-illuminated with light reflected from more internal structures), specular (in which light is reflected off various layers to show the detail of each surface), and sclerotic scatter (internal illumination). Various dyes (such as fluorescein or rose bengal) may be employed to help differentiate normal from abnormal tissues.

The instrument has two coaxial rotating arms controlled by a joystick level; one arm carries the adjustable slitlamp illumination system, with attendant filters and optical stops, and the other arm carries the observation optics (a binocular microscope). An adjustable chin and forehead rest positions the subject's head.

Auxiliary devices allow the measurement of intraocular pressure (tonometer) and corneal thickness (pacometer) and the evaluation of the angle between

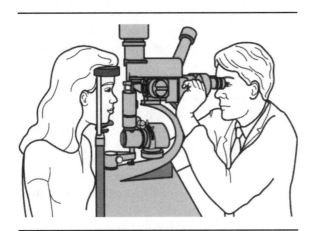

The slitlamp microscope, or biomicroscope, is used by ophthalmologists to examine the health of the eye.

the cornea and iris (gonioscope lens). Cameras, both still and video, may be attached at various sites. High-powered auxiliary optical lenses have also been developed, which allow the clinician to use the slitlamp microscope to observe the posterior pole of the eye (through the pharmacologically dilated pupil), including the optic nerve and most of the retina. Ophthalmic lasers can also be attached to this system in order to treat the various structures of the eye as they are observed directly through the same optics, using the principle of the reversibility of the path of light.

Allvar Gullstrand received a Nobel Prize in 1911 for his contributions to optics, and the same year he introduced his refinement of the slitlamp microscope. Modern instruments and techniques are largely based on his work.

—*Barry A. Weissman, O.D., Ph.D.*

See also Eye surgery; Eyes; Laser use in surgery; Ophthalmology; Optometry; Visual disorders.

FOR FURTHER INFORMATION:

Davson, Hugh. *Physiology of the Eye.* 5th ed. New York: Academic Press, 1990.

Miller, Stephen J. H. *Parsons' Diseases of the Eye.* 18th ed. New York: Churchill Livingstone, 1990.

Newell, Frank W. *Ophthalmology.* 8th ed. St. Louis: C. V. Mosby, 1996.

Vaughan, Daniel, Taylor Asbury, and Paul Riordan-Eva, eds. *General Ophthalmology.* 15th ed. Norwalk, Conn.: Appleton and Lange, 1999.

MIDLIFE CRISIS
DISEASE/DISORDER

ANATOMY OR SYSTEM AFFECTED: Psychic-emotional system

SPECIALTIES AND RELATED FIELDS: Psychiatry, psychology

DEFINITION: The emotional, psychological, physical, spiritual, and relationship crises that arise during the transition from early to later adulthood.

KEY TERMS:

development: a generally predictable process of physical, emotional, cognitive, and/or spiritual growth or differentiation

developmental stressors: the events or other characteristics associated with the developmental process, which may be experienced as causing subjective or objectively measurable discomfort

midlife crisis: a crisis resulting from stressors related

to the transition from early adulthood to later adulthood

situational stressors: the events or characteristics that may be experienced unpredictably during life and that may cause subjective or objectively measurable discomfort

Causes and Symptoms

Before the nature of the midlife crisis can be explored, it is first helpful to identify what is meant by "midlife." As the average life expectancy has changed throughout history, so has the period termed midlife. For example, by the 1990's, the human life expectancy in the United States had risen to approximately seventy-four years for men and seventy-eight years for women. These figures are more than twice as long as the average life expectancy during the time of the Massachusetts Bay Colony, and more than three and a half times as long as someone in ancient Greece could have expected to live.

Life expectancy changes as it is influenced by any number of factors, including nutrition, health care and prevention, stress and lifestyle issues, historical period, culture, race, individual variability, gender, and social context. Consequently, there is no precise age at which midlife can be said to commence. It is also difficult to state unequivocally when the possibility for a midlife crisis ends. Nevertheless, some developmental theorists, such as D. J. Levinson, suggest the period from forty to forty-five is the time of the midlife transition or "crisis." Others have indicated that this time period may last until the age of fifty-three. Yet the results of these studies, collected primarily from Caucasian males in the United States, may not be applicable to the general population.

Other researchers, Carol Gilligan among them, have engaged in a critique of the assumptions underlying previous comments on midlife crises and theories of how human beings develop, pointing out how this research may be based on outdated and/or incomplete studies of human development and experience. Gilligan's book *In a Different Voice* (1982) demonstrates, for example, how it may be that women have an experience of the aging process which is different from the one commonly experienced by men. As a result, the process of normal adult development and the nature of this crisis remain less than crystal clear.

Midlife crisis experiences seem to arise in response to a variety of precipitating factors, including both normal developmental changes and severe or numerous stressors. This variability raises another interesting challenge to the notion of a midlife crisis. Is experience of a midlife crisis a predictable event or an aberration? Some experts claim that the belief in a "midlife crisis" is one of the many myths about the aging process.

Richard Schulz and Robert B. Ewen, in their book *Adult Development and Aging* (1988), insist that many adults do not experience an unusually severe crisis at midlife. It is the perspective of these authors that those who do experience a significant midlife crisis tend to have suffered similar crises throughout their adulthood. The stresses involved in the transitions in midlife may be similar to, and not necessarily occurring more frequently than, those experienced by the same individual in any stage of life. If so, the adjective "midlife," as indicative of a qualitatively different kind of crisis, may be misleading.

On the other hand, Lois Tamir states that clinical studies reveal the male population in midlife to have a significant increase in mental health problems, including depression, alcoholism, and suicide. In *Men in Their Forties* (1982), Tamir insists that most studies of adulthood display something atypical among middle-aged men, whether dramatic or subtle.

Caution is necessary when making general statements about a phenomenon such as midlife crisis, but for the sake of this discussion, a more general perspective is taken. It is assumed that midlife crises, however varied in form, intensity, or duration, do commonly occur. In addition, they are best understood from a holistic and contextual perspective on the individual's life.

A developmental framework which describes the cycle that an individual experiences in life further clarifies an understanding of midlife crises. The life changes of an individual may be seen as summative and consecutive. During this life cycle, one stage, with its tasks and crises, is lived and resolved before another is reached. In *Adulthood* (1978), Erik Erikson developed one framework for understanding the individual life cycle and its tasks, crises, and stages. Life crises are attributable in large part to the stress of transitioning from one part of life to another. The stage relevant to a discussion of midlife crises is termed generativity versus stagnation; in other words, midlife is the period of time during which individuals strive to come to terms with whether they are and may continue to be productive, or whether they will stagnate.

Development is also a physical experience. Therefore, an individual's psychological and emotional responses are influenced by changing physiology and health. One common midlife example in women is menopause and its attendant hormonal changes. At few other times in a woman's life is there such a complex interaction between physical and psychological factors. Along with the physical stresses brought about by hormonal changes, the psychological and emotional reactions of each woman to this normal transition vary depending on her lifestyle, attitudes, self-image, and network of supportive relationships. This type of experience may contribute to crises in midlife.

In addition to the impact of changing physiology, the experience of midlife is emotional, cognitive, and spiritual. Midlife crises may be precipitated by an individual's reflection on or reevaluation of the meaning of life. Similarly, midlife may be a time during which people begin or intensify the process of spiritual evaluation and reckoning. It is a time during which people take stock of their lives and come to grips with their mortality.

A decline or change in physical functioning may trigger thoughts about mortality and death. A frequent phenomenon is evident in the change of one's perspective on time, from a focus on "time since birth" to one on "time left to live." Self-assessment may lead to greater emphasis on long-neglected aspects of the self or relationships with others.

All these issues are known as developmental issues or stressors, which are more or less predictable in life according to the person's stage of development. Situational stressors also contribute to the development of life crises. Situational stressors include such things as unexpected illness or injury, unemployment, and war—all those things which are not necessarily related to the person's chronological age or development through time. Consequently, it is reasonable to conclude that these factors may be potent in midlife as well.

Typically, individuals live not in isolation from one another but within the context of relationships. The most common network of relationships is the family. A discussion of issues that have biological, emotional, psychological, and social components, therefore, must include an examination of what is happening with other family members and the family as a group. These factors, including what is termed the family life cycle, may influence the development or

severity of the subjective experience of midlife crisis. In fact, the crises of midlife often arise from the interaction between individual and family factors.

Those experiencing midlife crisis are usually members of what has become known as the "sandwich generation": a generation sandwiched between, and with the responsibility for taking care of, those in two others. For example, a middle-aged woman may have responsibilities with aging parents on the one hand and with an adolescent son on the other. Any crisis experience that she might have then becomes much more than the psychological or emotional process of an individual. The coincidence of adolescence, with her son's focus on the development of an identity and his constant evaluation of his own and his parents' values, beliefs, and behaviors, may only exacerbate her similar search for meaning. She also may be reevaluating her accomplishments and striving to do more of what she believes has been meaningful so far in life. In contrast, the elder generation may be struggling to find some sense of integrity about a life which is coming to an end. Each individual in the family becomes a point of contact, contrast, or conflict with the other.

The various manifestations of a midlife crisis are much like the symptoms exhibited by people in response to stress. The symptoms include an anxious or depressed mood, loss of interest in normal activities, an intensified reevaluation of life (both past and future), sudden changes in relationships, difficulty with organic processes (such as sleeping, eating, and concentration), and a subjective feeling of the need for a change. Extreme reactions may be a function of the psychology and emotional makeup of a particular individual in the context of his or her life. In addition, people who have less social support or who are living a lifestyle which they have long been aware was unfulfilling are more likely to experience a more significant crisis.

Not only do people and family groups vary in their reactions to midlife stress, but different ethnic and cultural groups do as well. The meaning associated with life events is generated within the context of these various social groups. Each social group develops its own culture with its own rules and regulations regarding how to respond or behave. In other words, individuals understand and respond to stressors as they do because of their experience within larger social groups. For example, within the Caucasian culture in the United States, a certain mythology has developed around the midlife crisis. Midlife is sometimes seen as a time when a man will buy a red sports car and leave his middle-aged wife for a young blonde. Someone else might give up her booming career and begin working with the underprivileged. As a result, within the context of this particular culture, dramatic lifestyle changes are predicted, explained, and possibly even supported.

In summary, midlife crises are those crises that may arise during the developmental stage associated with midlife. Like crises or other stress reactions, midlife crises vary in timing, intensity, duration, and character from one person, family, and social group to another. Crises in midlife seem to be no more frequent than crises at other stages of development.

TREATMENT AND THERAPY

Medical science has contributed to the understanding of the concept of midlife crisis through research, theory building, and the development and testing of treatment strategies, including the use of medication and psychotherapeutic techniques. Yet there are no specific treatments for a midlife or any other kind of crisis because the needs of the individual and the family group vary considerably. The range of possible treatments or clinical applications of medical science to this area are largely in the form of supporting the preexisting resources and coping skills of the individual and his or her family and other social support systems.

As with other life skills, an individual's ability to cope with and manage crises depends on the nature of one's character and personality, past experiences in managing crises, and degree of social support. The more well developed the person's character and coping mechanisms, the more numerous his or her experiences in successfully resolving past crises, and the greater amount of perceived support from family and friends, the more likely he or she will be able to resolve conflicts and crises in the present and future successfully.

Since midlife crises can differ from those in other stages, because of the particular tasks to be negotiated at this stage, resolution may involve the need to address certain tasks constructively. An individual may be called on to reevaluate or reassess his or her life, putting into perspective what is hoped for relative to what has transpired. An individual struggling with crises associated with midlife should be encouraged to explore the contributing situational and de-

velopmental issues openly. This process may involve cognitive reevaluation, working through feelings, or spiritual and existential reassessment.

Tamir suggests several tasks that must be addressed in order to facilitate the successful resolution of a midlife crisis. The individual must reckon with his or her own mortality, go through a process of self-assessment, examine sex role obligations and expectations, and gain perspective on his or her generativity. Self-assessment involves taking stock and putting life into perspective. Life's polarities and contradictions must be examined and resolved in some manner.

One central polarity involves sex roles. The traditional differences between men and women often break down during the period of midlife. This process is facilitated by the life review accompanying a midlife crisis. For example, a woman may decide that she has devoted much of her life to the care and nurture of others while putting her own needs second. As a result, she may attempt to remedy the situation by developing the more stereotypical male characteristics of being assertive and goal-directed. Similarly, a male may turn away from his career as the primary source of self-esteem and gratification to developing richer interpersonal relationships.

Clinical and research evidence as reported by Richard Rahe and Thomas Holmes in *Life Change, Life Events, and Illness* (1989) demonstrates a solid link between life crisis and disease onset. Consequently, medical health professionals may be called on to assist individuals struggling with the effects of a midlife crisis. These professionals, as well as other concerned individuals, may intervene in a variety of ways.

In a preventive fashion, helpers may offer what is termed anticipatory guidance to the individual approaching midlife transitions. In other words, conversations can include predictive or educative content orienting the person toward what may be expected as he or she approaches or anticipates these changes. An individual in the midst of midlife review and crisis may also need assistance, support, and/or direction in resolving generativity issues. The individual needs to resolve how he or she will make a significant contribution to others rather than stagnate and become increasingly self-absorbed. Accomplishment of these tasks may involve repercussions in work, family, and social relationships.

Physicians occasionally are called on to treat an individual exhibiting physical and/or psychological symptoms. While the prescription of medication for symptoms of depression and anxiety is recommended only in relatively extreme circumstances, antidepressant and antianxiety medications are very effective with some conditions, normally those in which the symptoms are impairing the person's ability to function over an extended period of time.

These various forms of assistance may be offered in an office visit for brief counseling, within the process of psychotherapy for a longer term approach, or during an informal conversation. Regardless of the context, however, being able to anticipate or come to grips with the issues involved helps an individual to feel less out of control and to believe that the problems are being dealt with constructively.

Family and social support are very helpful in times of crisis. The degree to which these relationship contexts are flexible and supportive can either exacerbate problems or ameliorate struggles. A balance between permission and validation, with encouragement for the individual to continue managing daily functioning and obligations, is important. In the absence of an individual's ability to negotiate and resolve successfully the conflicts associated with the crisis, and perhaps without the presence of a supportive network of family and friends, individual and/or family therapy or a support group may be of help. These modes of therapy and support provide helpful perspective, normalization of the experience, and training or advice regarding constructive problem-solving and conflict resolution techniques.

PERSPECTIVE AND PROSPECTS

In many areas of medical science pertaining to human behavior and emotional experience, important ideas from different theories are often integrated to yield a more comprehensive understanding. Congruently, several theoretical frameworks shape approaches to and perspectives on the understanding of midlife crises. Rudolf H. Moos explains in *Coping with Life Crises* (1986) that these include evolutionary theory, human growth and development, theories about the life cycle, behavior theory, family systems theory, learning theory, and theories of stress and coping.

The theory of evolution proposed by Charles Darwin provides the understanding of human beings as living interdependently, as well as adapting to their changing environment. The development of effective coping strategies ensures survival and promotes human community. Midlife crises present the individual and his or her social context with an opportunity for testing the effectiveness of these strategies.

The work of psychologist Abraham Maslow emphasized the tendency of human beings to strive toward the maintenance of life and the promotion of growth. An individual negotiating transitions in life taps into this growth motivation in order to maximize and enrich personal experience. In the midst of crisis, basic necessities of life are the first priority. Once the fundamental needs for food, shelter, and physical survival are satisfied, an individual will strive toward fulfilling what Maslow termed higher-level goals, such as emotional security and spiritual enlightenment.

According to Moos, crisis theory deals with the impact of disruptions on established patterns of personal and social identity. This framework suggests that, in addition to seeking to maximize human growth and potential, each individual first struggles to maintain a state of social and psychological equilibrium. In crisis, the midlife adult will seek homeostasis or balance prior to exploring opportunities for productive change. Thus, the similarity between crisis theory and theories of human growth and development may be apparent. The crises involved in midlife are more often related to the higher-level goals defined within each of these frameworks.

The stage or developmental theories described previously provide a framework within which to understand some of these transitions and the emotional, psychological, and physical changes that are involved. In addition, the perspective of the individual as developing, growing, evolving, and coping within the context of a family system enriches the view of midlife crisis.

The resulting context for an understanding of midlife crisis, then, is one of an integration of ideas and theories. This integration supports an understanding of midlife crisis as a product of the normative development and transitions in life. An individual's reaction to the required transitions depends on his or her personal characteristics, coping skills, family and social relationships, aspects of the transition or crisis itself, and other features of the physical and social environments.

—Layne A. Prest, Ph.D.

See also Aging; Anxiety; Death and dying; Depression; Factitious disorders; Hypochondriasis; Menopause; Neurosis; Panic attacks; Psychiatric disorders; Psychiatry; Psychoanalysis; Psychosomatic disorders; Sexual dysfunction; Sexuality; Stress; Stress reduction.

FOR FURTHER INFORMATION:

Gilligan, Carol. "New Maps of Development: New Visions of Maturity." *American Journal of Orthopsychiatry* 52 (April, 1982): 199-212. In this article, Gilligan begins to map out her alternatives to previously accepted theories of adult development. These alternatives are based on comparative research that contrasts male and female experiences. The author suggests that a woman's development cannot be measured according to the same yardstick as a man's.

Holmes, Thomas H., and E. M. David, eds. *Life Change, Life Events, and Illness.* New York: Praeger, 1989. The editors of this book have compiled an important collection of research and clinical applications of stress and coping theories to practical and everyday experience. The authors of the various papers clarify the connection between life stressors and both psychological and physical illness.

Moos, Rudolf H., ed. *Coping with Life Crises.* New York: Plenum Press, 1986. Moos is a pioneer in the field of stress, families, and development. The book and its authors provide a view of midlife crises within the larger context of life development and transitions, as well as of crises in general. The authors emphasize the perspective that many crises are normal or normative.

Schulz, Richard, and Robert B. Ewen. *Adult Development and Aging.* 3d ed. New York: Macmillan, 1999. This textbook can be easily understood by the general reader and includes a comprehensive view of the development and aging processes.

MIGRAINE HEADACHES
DISEASE/DISORDER

ANATOMY OR SYSTEM AFFECTED: Brain, head, nervous system, psychic-emotional system

SPECIALTIES AND RELATED FIELDS: Neurology

DEFINITION: The cause of migraine headaches, which are characterized by intense, throbbing pain that may incapacitate the sufferer, is not known. Studies have shown, however, that they are linked to the constriction and dilation of arteries in the brain and scalp and that abnormalities in the body's biochemistry may occur during a migraine. The two main types of migraine headaches are common migraine and classic migraine. Common

migraines are preceded by fatigue, nausea, vomiting, and fluid imbalance; during an attack, extreme sensitivity to noise and light occurs. With classic migraines, visual, sensory, and motor disturbances, called auras, may foretell an attack, such as diagonal lines and bright spots in the field of vision, tingling in the face and hands, and a tendency to stagger. Certain drugs, when taken at the onset of an attack, can stop the migraine from proceeding.

—*Jason Georges and Tracy Irons-Georges*

See also Auras; Brain; Brain disorders; Cluster headaches; Fatigue; Headaches; Multiple chemical sensitivity syndrome; Nausea and vomiting; Pain; Pain management; Stress.

FOR FURTHER INFORMATION:

Blanchard, Edward B., and Frank Andrasik. *Management of Chronic Headaches: A Psychological Approach.* New York: Pergamon Press, 1985.

Diamond, Seymour. "Migraine Headaches." *The Medical Clinics of North America* 75, no. 3 (May 1, 1991): 545-566.

Saper, Joel R., et al., eds. *Headache Disorders: Current Concepts and Treatment Strategies.* Boston: John Wright/PSG, 1983.

MISCARRIAGE
DISEASE/DISORDER

ANATOMY OR SYSTEM AFFECTED: Reproductive system, psychic-emotional system, uterus

SPECIALTIES AND RELATED FIELDS: Embryology, obstetrics

DEFINITION: Miscarriage, sometimes called spontaneous abortion, is the death, breakdown, and/or expulsion of an embryo or fetus before it is viable outside the uterus. About 20 percent of all pregnancies end in miscarriage. Such a high percentage of these happen in the first trimester, however, that miscarriage often occurs before a woman even knows she is pregnant. The primary causes of miscarriage are abnormalities and structural defects in the fetus, as a result of genetic defects, syphilis, or drug use. Contributing factors may include the excessive ingestion of alcohol or caffeine, heavy smoking, poor nutrition, or hormone imbalance in the mother, perhaps as a result of severe stress. Most women who suffer a miscarriage will have no future problems in carrying a baby to term, but some women show a pattern of failed pregnancies.

—*Jason Georges and Tracy Irons-Georges*

See also Abortion; Addiction; Ectopic pregnancy; Fetal alcohol syndrome; Genetic diseases; Genetics and inheritance; Obstetrics; Pregnancy and gestation; Premature birth; Stillbirth.

FOR FURTHER INFORMATION:

Gabbe, Steven G., Jennifer R. Niebyl, and Joe Leigh Simpson, eds. *Obstetrics: Normal and Problem Pregnancies*. 3d ed. New York: Churchill Livingstone, 1996.

Hotchner, Tracie. *Pregnancy and Childbirth*. Rev. ed. New York: Avon Books, 1997.

Scher, Jonathan. *Preventing Miscarriage: The Good News*. New York: Harper & Row, 1990.

MITES. *See* BITES AND STINGS; LICE, MITES, AND TICKS; PARASITIC DISEASES.

MITRAL VALVE PROLAPSE
DISEASE/DISORDER

ANATOMY OR SYSTEM AFFECTED: Circulatory system, heart

SPECIALTIES AND RELATED FIELDS: Cardiology, family practice, internal medicine, vascular medicine

DEFINITION: The inability of the mitral valve in the heart to close properly.

Valves of the Heart

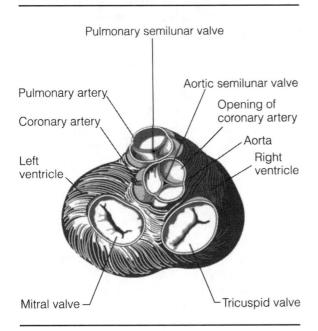

Pulmonary semilunar valve

Pulmonary artery

Coronary artery

Left ventricle

Aortic semilunar valve

Opening of coronary artery

Aorta

Right ventricle

Mitral valve

Tricuspid valve

CAUSES AND SYMPTOMS

The mitral valve connects the heart's left ventricle and left atrium. The oxygenated blood, having already passed through the right heart chambers and the lungs, arrives in the left atrium through the pulmonary veins and then passes through the mitral valve into the left ventricle. Compression of the left ventricle pumps the blood into the aorta and on to the rest of the body. A properly functioning mitral valve closes and prevents regurgitation or backflow into the left atrium. Mitral valve prolapse occurs when the two leaves of the mitral valve close imperfectly, allowing leakage. This condition, known also as mitral valve insufficiency prolapse, is the most common cardiac syndrome. Found in all segments of society, it is most common in young adult women.

Mitral valve prolapse has several possible causes including rheumatic fever, inflammation of the heart lining (endocarditis), cardiac tumors, or most often, genetic error. Its symptoms are undue fatigue after exercise, shortness of breath, and chest pain. Other common complaints are anxiety, depression, and panic, all related to stress. The number of diagnosed cases in Western countries is rising markedly and may be the result of more sophisticated diagnostic techniques or the increasing stress in modern society.

PERSPECTIVE AND PROSPECTS

Until the 1960's, the detection of mitral valve prolapse was through a characteristic "click" heard by the physician when the mitral leaves attempted to close. Now the use of echocardiograms, allowing ultrasound images of the beating heart and blood flow, is standard practice.

People with mitral valve prolapse lead a normal life, and many are unaware that they have the condition. Repeated irregularity in breathing or an inexplicable shortness of breath is a sign to see one's physician. Regular exercise and good eating habits are recommended for this mild condition. Fear and anxiety, however, can cause a disastrous situation: People should know that only in severe cases is mitral valve prolapse treated surgically or considered life-threatening.

—*K. Thomas Finley, Ph.D.*

See also Anxiety; Cardiology; Cardiology, pediatric; Circulation; Congenital heart disease; Endocarditis; Fatigue; Heart; Heart disease; Rheumatic fever; Stress.

FOR FURTHER INFORMATION:

Boudoulas, Harisios, and Charles F. Wooley. *Mitral Valve: Floppy Mitral Valve, Mitral Valve Prolapse, Mitral Valvular Regurgitation.* 2d ed. Armonk, New York: Futura, 2000. A thorough study of mitral valve insufficiency. Includes bibliographical references and an index.

Frederickson, Lyn. *Confronting Mitral Valve Prolapse Syndrome: The Mysterious Heart Condition of the Young and Healthy.* San Marcos, Calif.: Slawson Communications, 1988. Designed for the lay reader, this guide offers concise coverage of mitral valve prolapse. Includes bibliographical references and an index.

Hayes, Denise Drummond. "Mitral Valve Prolapse Revisited." *Nursing* 27, no. 10 (October, 1997): 34-40. Hayes discusses mitral valve prolapse (MVP), a condition in which the heart valve leaflets fail to close properly. The clinical signs and symptoms of the disorder and ways nurses can help MVP patients are examined.

MOLD AND MILDEW

DISEASE/DISORDER

ANATOMY OR SYSTEM AFFECTED: All

SPECIALTIES AND RELATED FIELDS: Environmental health, toxicology

DEFINITION: Growths of fungi that can be parasitic on plants and humans.

CAUSES AND SYMPTOMS

Mold is the common term used to describe a furry growth on the surface of plants, rocks, walls, or organic matter. Mildew is another term for a specific type of mold found on wet clothes, food, or in basements. Scientists use the terms to identify a variety of microscopic organisms, including fungi, algae, rusts, yeast, and bacteria. Fungi are simple-celled organisms that can live without light for energy or growth. Molds are types of fungi that reproduce by the formation of spores. The spores are single cells out of which mature molds grow. A single mold can produce millions of spores. They are dispersed through the air and if they land on food or plants they can grow, reproduce, and cause diseases. Molds can resist exposure to extreme heat and cold. They do not need water and are resistant to drying out. Mold of the genera *Aspergillus*, *Penicillium*, and *Rhizopus* cause food to spoil and also transfer many plant diseases, such as downy and powdery mildews. Powdery mildews are parasitic and attack the leaves of willow trees, grape vines, and flowers such as roses and lilacs. One downy mildew (*Plasmopara viticola*) is a major disease of grapes in the United States. It causes millions of dollars of losses every year by destroying leaves and killing the whole plant. Another powdery mildew (*Podosphaera leucotricha*) destroys millions of dollars worth of apples every year. Fortunately, both kinds of molds can be controlled by the use of fungicides.

For humans, mold and mildew are the source of many allergies and can trigger asthma attacks. Mold thrives in dark and damp conditions. In the modern world, because many new homes are tightly sealed, mold spores become much more concentrated through being trapped indoors by air conditioners and heating systems. Some molds and mildews are fond of the cellulose in wallpaper paste and in the paper backing of drywall and insulation. Other molds feast on the everyday dust and dirt that gathers in moist regions of houses, including bathroom ceilings and under sinks. Mold can turn walls white with spiderweblike growths that create the musty smell found in many basements. Molds usually do not cause major structural damage to homes but can make people ill simply from breathing in their spores.

Perhaps 10 percent of the population is severely allergic to molds and their spores. Spores are extremely small; twenty of them sitting side by side could fit in the period at the end of this sentence. Their smallness makes spores very difficult to filter out. Spores are also able to remain suspended in the air for many hours. When people sensitive to mold spores inhale them, they can cause headaches, runny noses, skin rashes, nausea, sinus problems, memory loss, and coughs. Victims may feel as though they have a perpetual case of the flu. Newborns, the elderly, the sick, and those without immunities can become very ill. Crawling babies who stick things in their mouths, often picked up from carpets infected with molds, are highly susceptible to diseases carried by fungi. Highly sensitive adults frequently must remove soft, textured drapes, vinyl-upholstered furniture, and metal window blinds.

The mold *Stachybotrys atra* grows in areas that are always wet. This slimy black mold is a true public health hazard that has been found in all areas of the United States and has caused dozens of infant deaths. It grows in areas subjected to leaking plumbing, sewer backups, and washing machines that frequently overflow. Studies show that when babies are exposed to both this mold and cigarette smoke, their lungs begin to bleed and they can die.

TREATMENT AND THERAPY

Experts suggest several ways to reduce mold and mildew in homes. Moldy or moist surfaces should be cleaned with household bleach, which kills such fungi. All leaks should be fixed, because mold flourishes in damp conditions. An air conditioner should be installed; it will dry out the air, making it more difficult for mold to live. Houseplant soil should be checked to make sure it is not always very wet; mold thrives on moist soil. Firewood should not be brought into the house; wet wood is another good environment for mold and mildew. Basements should be kept as dry as possible; this is the part of the home where mold is most likely to be found (the next most likely place is the shower stall or bathtub). Showers, floors, and walls should be cleaned frequently to ensure that mold does not accumulate. Refrigerators should be cleaned, both inside and underneath, with a fungicide such as bleach.

Air should be allowed to circulate. When the air outside is drier than that inside, ventilation allows the dry air to enter, take up excess moisture, and carry it outside. When natural circulation is not sufficient, a fan can be placed in a window. Poorly ventilated closets get damp and musty during wet weather, and articles in them can get mildew. One should either improve air circulation by opening the door or hang clothes loosely so that air can circulate around them.

All wet clothing should be dried before being put in closets. Musty odors on basement floor or tiled walls and floors can be eliminated by scrubbing them with a solution of a half-cup of liquid bleach to a gallon of water. They should then be rinsed with clear water and wiped as dry as possible. Windows should be kept open until walls and floors are thoroughly dry.

Not all molds are destructive; many are useful, such as those employed in the making of cheeses. Camembert and Roquefort cheeses get their flavor from molds, *Penicillium camemberti* and *P. roquerti* respectively. Penicillin, the great antibiotic drug discovered in 1929, is produced from the green mold *P. notatum*.

—*Leslie V. Tischauser, Ph.D.*

See also Allergies; Antibiotics; Asthma; Coughing; Environmental diseases; Fungal infections; Headaches; Immune system; Immunology; Lungs; Microbiology; Multiple chemical sensitivity syndrome; Nausea and vomiting; Parasitic diseases; Pulmonary diseases; Pulmonary medicine; Rashes; Respiration; Sinusitis; Skin; Skin disorders.

FOR FURTHER INFORMATION:

Margulis, Lynn, and Katherine V. Schwartz. *Five Kingdoms: An Illustrated Guide to the Phyla of Life on Earth.* 3d ed. New York: W. H. Freeman, 1999.

National Park Service. *Mold and Mildew: Prevention of Microorganism Growth.* Washington, D.C.: U.S. Government Printing Office, 1998.

Ritchie, D. F. *Disease and Insect Management in the Home Orchard.* Raleigh: North Carolina State University Cooperative Extension, 1997.

MOLES

DISEASE/DISORDER

ALSO KNOWN AS: Nevi pigmentosa

ANATOMY OR SYSTEM AFFECTED: Skin

SPECIALTIES AND RELATED FIELDS: Dermatology, family practice, plastic surgery

DEFINITION: Nonmalignant marks, pigmented spots, or growths on the skin.

CAUSES AND SYMPTOMS

The common mole, also known as a nevus pigmentosus, is a mark, spot, or growth found on the skin that is generally benign and may be either congenital (present at birth) or developmental. Moles may be various colors, shapes, and sizes, and they can be flat or raised. Caucasian adults usually have about twenty pigmented nevi, the majority of which are less than 0.5 inch in diameter, with fewer pigmented ones evident at birth.

A mole is primarily the result of an accumulation of melanocytes, cells that form the skin pigment melanin. The greater the number of melanocytes, the darker the brown color of the mole. When the melanocytes are located deep below the skin surface, the mole appears dark bluish in color. Melanocytes also form the relatively larger vascular nevi (birthmarks) that derive from abnormal vascular construction in the skin. Types of birthmarks include the strawberry hemangioma and the port-wine stain, which arise from poorly developed blood vessels, and the nevus anemicus, which is attributed to a reduced blood flow.

TREATMENT AND THERAPY

In most cases, moles are benign, but occasionally they develop into malignant melanoma, especially after puberty. This transformation may be indicated by the development of a flat, pigmented zone around the base of a mole or the progressive enlargement of an existing mole. Other evidence of skin cancer involves increased darkening and loss of the hair surrounding a mole, as well as ulceration and bleeding.

A newly formed mole is usually flat. If it arises between the dermis and the epidermis, then the mole is called a junction nevus; this type may become malignant. A dermatologist's care in a timely manner is usually recommended. The main treatment involves removal of the mole by cauterization or laser treatment.

Moles occasionally disappear with age. Generally, however, more nevi form with aging, such as freckles, and they are usually permanent. The growth of new moles and darkening or other changes in existing ones should be monitored. New moles are usually dome-shaped and elevated slightly above the surrounding skin. Plucking the hair associated with moles is not recommended, as this may damage the skin and lead to ulceration and bleeding.

—*Soraya Ghayourmanesh, Ph.D.*

See also Birthmarks; Dermatology; Dermatology, pediatric; Malignant melanoma removal; Skin; Skin cancer; Skin disorders; Warts.

FOR FURTHER INFORMATION:

Lookingbill, Donald P., and James G. Marks. *Principles of Dermatology*. Philadelphia: W. B. Saunders, 1986.

Mackie, Rona M. *Clinical Dermatology*. 4th ed. New York: Oxford University Press, 1997.

Pillsbury, Donald M. *A Manual of Dermatology*. Philadelphia: W. B. Saunders, 1971.

Rook, Arthur, et al., eds. *Textbook of Dermatology*. 4th ed. 3 vols. Oxford, England: Blackwell Scientific, 1986.

MONONUCLEOSIS

DISEASE/DISORDER

ALSO KNOWN AS: Infectious mononucleosis, the kissing disease

ANATOMY OR SYSTEM AFFECTED: Heart, lymphatic system, spleen, throat

SPECIALTIES AND RELATED FIELDS: Family practice, pediatrics, virology

DEFINITION: An acute viral infectious disease that produces lymph node enlargement (hyperplasia).

KEY TERMS:

anorexia: loss of appetite

dysphagia: difficulty in swallowing

lymph nodes: glandlike masses or knots of lymphatic tissue that are distributed along the lymphatic vessels to filter bacteria or foreign bodies from the body

periorbital: referring to the region around the eyes

spleen: a large lymphatic organ in the abdominal cavity that forms lymphocytes and other blood cells and stores blood

splenomegaly: enlargement of the spleen

CAUSES AND SYMPTOMS

Mononucleosis is caused by the Epstein-Barr virus, which is transmitted through infected saliva or by blood transfusions. It has an incubation period of four to six weeks. The saliva may remain infective for aslong as eighteen months, and after the primary infection, the virus may be present in the nasal secretions and shed periodically for the rest of the host's life. Many cases occur in adolescents—hence the popular name "the kissing disease." The virus can be cultured from the throat of 10 to 20 percent of most healthy adults. The incidence of mononucleosis varies seasonally among high school and college students but does not vary among the general population. The disease is fairly common in the United States, Canada, and Europe and occurs in both sexes.

Mononucleosis is characterized by fever, fatigue, anorexia, a sore throat, chills, a skin rash, bleeding gums, red spots on the tonsils, malaise, and periorbital edema. Lymph nodes in the neck enlarge, and splenomegaly develops in about half of patients. In a small number of patients, liver involvement with mild jaundice occurs.

The diagnosis is made by several different tests, such as the differential white blood count. In mononucleosis, lymphocytes and monocytes make up greater than 50 percent of the blood cells, with a figure of more than 10 percent being atypical. The leukocyte count is normal early in the disease but rises during the second week. Serology studies show an increase in the heterophile antibody titer, although the monospot test is more rapid and can detect the infection earlier and is widely used. Children under four years of age often test negative for heterophil antibodies, but the test will identify 90 percent of cases in older children, adolescents, and adults.

TREATMENT AND THERAPY

The treatment of mononucleosis is mainly supportive, since the disease is self-limiting. The patient is usually placed on bed rest during the acute stage of the disease, and activity is limited to prevent rupture of the enlarged spleen, usually for at least two months. Acetaminophen (Tylenol) is given for the fever, and saline gargles or lozenges may be used for the sore throat. Patients need to increase their fluid intake. Many doctors use corticosteriods such as prednisone during the course of the disease to lessen the severity of the symptoms. If rupture of the spleen occurs, emergency surgery is necessary to remove the organ.

Complications are uncommon but may include rupture of the spleen, secondary pneumonia, heart involvement, neurologic manifestations such as Guillain-Barré syndrome, meningitis, encephalitis, hemolytic anemia, and orchitis (inflammation of the testes).

PERSPECTIVE AND PROSPECTS

Viruses, such as the one responsible for mononucleosis, were first studied in the 1930's, and they remain a challenge to laboratory investigators. Most information about viruses has come from studying their effects, rather than the viruses themselves. The majority of methods for destroying or controlling viruses are ineffective. There is no prevention for many of the diseases caused by viruses, such as infectious mononucleosis. It may be reassuring to know that the disease seldom causes severe complications if the symptoms are treated and medical care is given to those infected with the Epstein-Barr virus.

—Mitzie L. Bryant, B.S.N., M.Ed.

See also Childhood infectious diseases; Chronic fatigue syndrome; Fatigue; Fever; Hodgkin's disease; Immune system; Jaundice; Lymphadenopathy and lymphoma; Lymphatic system; Otorhinolaryngology; Sore throat; Viral infections.

FOR FURTHER INFORMATION:

Berkow, Robert, and Andrew J. Fletcher, eds. "Infectious Mononucleosis." In *The Merck Manual of Diagnosis and Therapy.* 17th ed. Rahway, N.J.: Merck Sharp & Dohme Research Laboratories, 1999. Contains a useful exposition of the characteristics, etiology, diagnosis, and treatment of mononucleosis. Designed for physicians, the material is also useful for less specialized readers. Information on related topics is also included.

Dreher, Nancy. "What You Need to Know About Mono." *Current Health 2* 23, no. 7 (March, 1997): 28-29. Infectious mononucleosis is an illness that is most common among young people ages fifteen to twenty-five. The infection is caused by the Epstein-Barr virus. Facts about mono are presented.

Harkness, Gail, ed. *Medical-Surgical Nursing: Total Patient Care.* 10th ed. St. Louis: C. V. Mosby, 1999. This textbook briefly covers the cause, symptoms, diagnosis, and treatment of infectious mononucleosis. The clinical pathology and possible complications of the disease are discussed as well.

Long, Barbara C., Wilma J. Phipps, and Virginia L. Cassmeyer, eds. *Medical-Surgical Nursing: A Nursing Process Approach.* 3d ed. St. Louis: C. V. Mosby, 1993. This textbook briefly discusses the symptoms, treatment, and complications of mononucleosis.

Rosenbaum, Michael, and Murray Susser. *Solving the Puzzle of Chronic Fatigue Syndrome.* Tacoma, Wash.: Life Sciences Press, 1992. This book takes an immune-system approach to chronic fatigue syndrome, explaining the mechanisms of the disease and outlining conventional and alternative methods of treatment.

Scherer, Jeanne C., and Barbara K. Timby. *Introductory Medical-Surgical Nursing.* Philadelphia: J. B. Lippincott, 1995. This textbook stresses the pathology of mononucleosis as well as the diagnosis, symptoms, and treatments of this disease caused by the Epstein-Barr virus.

Thompson, June, et al., eds. *Mosby's Clinical Nursing.* 4th ed. St. Louis: C. V. Mosby, 1997. This book details what happens to lymphocytes when the Epstein-Barr virus attacks them and what causes the symptoms of mononucleosis.

MOSQUITO BITES. *See* ARTHROPOD-BORNE DISEASES; BITES AND STINGS.

MOTION SICKNESS

DISEASE/DISORDER

ALSO KNOWN AS: Carsickness, airsickness, seasickness

ANATOMY OR SYSTEM AFFECTED: Ears, gastrointestinal system, head, nervous system, stomach

SPECIALTIES AND RELATED FIELDS: Family practice, neurology, otorhinolaryngology

DEFINITION: A disorder characterized by nausea, vomiting, and vertigo and caused by a combination of repetitive back-and-forth and up-and-down movements.

KEY TERMS:

cranial: pertaining to the bones of the head

medulla oblongata: a continuation of the spinal cord that forms the lower portion of the brain stem; the site of many regulatory centers, as for cardiac rhythm, breathing, and the diameter of blood vessels

transdermal patch: a drug delivery system in which medication is slowly released from a patch and absorbed through the skin over a period of days

vertigo: a specific type of dizziness in which people feel as though either they themselves are spinning around or the room is spinning around them

CAUSES AND SYMPTOMS

Motion sickness appears to be caused by overstimulation of the balance centers of the inner ears by repeated back-and-forth and up-and-down movements. Messages are carried from this area of the inner ear, known as the vestibular apparatus, to the vomiting center in the medulla oblongata. The nerve pathways for this journey are not entirely known, but certainly the cranial nerve, which is responsible for hearing and balance, is involved. Responses in the medulla oblongata set into motion automatic motor reactions in the upper gastrointestinal tract, diaphragm, and abdominal muscles that lead to vomiting.

Individuals vary considerably in their susceptibility to motion sickness, and experts believe that there may be an inherited tendency toward the problem. Shifting visual input (such as watching waves on the horizon), a poorly ventilated environment, and fear and anxiety all seem to play a role in the development and severity of motion sickness.

The diagnosis of motion sickness is usually self-evident. Vertigo, nausea, and vomiting follow exposure to a repetitive and usually irregular rocking motion while in a moving vehicle or on an amusement park ride. The first indication of motion sickness may be yawning, excessive salivation, pale skin, and sweating. The person may begin to breathe deeply or complain of sleepiness. The patient may also develop a need for air, dizziness, or a headache. In most cases, nausea and vomiting occur sooner or later. On an extended trip, patients with motion sickness may eventually develop a tolerance to the motion and feel better, or they may continue to feel sick. If severe rocking motions develop once again, however, patients may also become sick again. Repeated vomiting may lead to dehydration and low blood pressure. Depression is another feature of prolonged motion sickness. As one patient with extreme motion sickness has described it, "First you are afraid you are going to die, and then you are afraid you *won't* die."

TREATMENT AND THERAPY

This malady is far easier to prevent than to treat. People who suffer from motion sickness should avoid drinking liquids just before and during short trips. On longer trips, they should limit liquids and have only small, easy-to-digest foods at regular intervals. Plenty of fresh air may also help prevent sickness. Those prone to motion sickness should not read in a car or other moving vehicle. Focusing the eyes well above the horizon while riding in a car or on a boat may help. People who are susceptible to motion sickness should also avoid amusement park rides that involve swinging and rocking.

Sufferers may be treated with over-the-counter or prescription medications an hour before travel begins. Medications used for this purpose include diphenhydramine, promethazine, scopolamine, dimenhydrinate, cyclizine, and meclizine. They are available in a variety of forms, including tablets, rectal suppositories, and transdermal patches. Many of these drugs cause sleepiness, which may be helpful during a trip but cause drowsiness or lack of alertness on arrival. Another common side effect of some of these drugs is dry mouth. In most cases, these medications are more effective when given before vomiting begins.

If the person has already begun vomiting, medications must be given by injection, rectal suppository, or a transdermal patch. In cases of prolonged vomiting, where dehydration is a concern, the patient may require intravenous fluids. Of particular concern is the individual who is already ill with another disease and also suffers from motion sickness. Such patients may have serious complications related to the vomiting and resulting dehydration.

PERSPECTIVE AND PROSPECTS

Motion sickness is a common problem in children and some adults. Drug companies are working on new drug delivery systems to make antinausea medications easier to take. Other advances include drug regimens that will provide antinausea effects without sleepiness.

—Rebecca Lovell Scott, Ph.D.

See also Acupressure; Acupuncture; Audiology; Balance disorders; Biofeedback; Dehydration; Dizziness and fainting; Ear infections and disorders; Ears; Gastrointestinal system; Nausea and vomiting; Nervous system; Neurology; Neurology, pediatric.

FOR FURTHER INFORMATION:

Berkow, Robert, ed. *The Merck Manual of Medical Information, Home Edition*. New York: Pocket, 2000. A team of nearly two hundred experts, consultants, and authors has assembled a body of information so vast that listing select items fails to do it justice. Provides reams of useful medical information, ranging from fundamentals, such as anatomy, to crisp, easily understood descriptions of complicated diseases.

Crampton, George H., ed. *Motion and Space Sickness*. Boca Raton, Fla.: CRC Press, 1990. This state-of-the-art compendium, written by active researchers in the field, encompasses anatomical and physiological subjects, such as analyses of stimulus characteristics, prediction of sickness, and consideration of human factors.

Schmitt, Barton D. *Your Child's Health: The Parents' Guide to Symptoms, Emergencies, Common Illnesses, Behavior, and School Problems*. Rev. ed. New York: Bantam Books, 1991. This book discusses such things as what to do in the event of an emergency, how to treat common illnesses, the best response to behavior problems, and health promotion from birth through adolescence.

Spock, Benjamin, and Steven J. Parker. *Dr. Spock's Baby and Child Care*. 7th ed. New York: Pocket Books, 1998. For more than a half a century, this book has been a virtual bible for parents seeking trustworthy information on child care. Informative, easy to use, and responsive to the changes in society, this revised and updated seventh edition makes a classic work more essential than ever.

MOTOR NEURON DISEASES
DISEASE/DISORDER

ANATOMY OR SYSTEM AFFECTED: Muscles, musculoskeletal system, nerves, nervous system, spine

SPECIALTIES AND RELATED FIELDS: Neurology

DEFINITION: Progressive, debilitating, and eventually fatal diseases affecting nerve cells in muscles.

KEY TERMS:

Babinski's sign: an abnormal response to a neurological test involving a brisk stroke with a sharp object on the bottom of the foot; the normal response is for the toes to bunch together and curve downward, while the abnormal response is for the big toe to pull upward and not in unison with the other toes

corticospinal tracts: neurological pathways descending from the brain to the spinal cord that control and allow voluntary movement

fasciculations: spontaneous electrical impulses from neurons that result in irregular, involuntary muscular contractions; in motor neuron disease, these contractions indicate nerve death

lower motor neuron: a nerve cell whose cell body resides either in the brain stem (to form a cranial nerve) or in the spinal cord (to form a spinal motor neuron)

motor neuron: a nerve that functions either directly or indirectly to control a target organ

muscular atrophy: a wasting of muscle mass; a greatly reduced size of muscle cells caused by the lost innervation (neuron death) or disuse of muscles

spasticity: an abnormal condition in which the limbs demonstrate resistance to passive movement as a result of damage to the corticospinal tracts; the reflexes are hyperactive

tropic factors: chemicals released from nerve cells that have a vital influence on muscle health; in the absence of tropic factors, muscles atrophy

upper motor neuron: a nerve whose cell body resides within the brain but whose axon descends the brain stem and spinal cord to form a corticospinal tract

CAUSES AND SYMPTOMS

In motor neuron diseases, certain nerves die, specifically those that allow any and all body movement. The actual cause of spontaneous motor neuron death is unknown, but genetic defects, neurotoxins, viruses, autoimmune disruptions, and metabolic disorders are contributing factors.

The predominant features of motor neuron disorders are muscular weakness, muscular wasting, and the presence of fasciculations. As a nerve dies, it can no longer effectively innervate its target muscle, but neighboring nerves may sprout to keep the muscle active. A consequence of nerve sprouting is the onset of brief, spontaneous contractions, or twitches. These visible twitches are called fasciculations. Eventually, as increasing numbers of nerves die, fewer healthy nerves are left to sprout until, finally, all muscles are denervated. Dead nerves cannot prompt muscle movement, nor can they release tropic factors as they do in health. This loss of tropic input from the neuron causes muscular atrophy and renders the muscle useless.

Motor neuron diseases are usually first noticed in the hands or upper limbs, where muscle weakness and decreased ability to use arms or hands cause problems. Unlike some disorders, motor neuron diseases fail to show stages of exacerbation or remission. Rather they progress—either rapidly or slowly, but relentlessly—until death, usually as a result of respiratory complications.

Although there are childhood forms of motor neuron diseases, they are more likely to strike between the ages of fifty and fifty-five, and they are seen in males more than females by a ratio of 1.5 to 1. Motor neuron diseases seem to occur rarely in the obese person and tend to afflict otherwise healthy, thin, and perhaps athletic persons. A famed person afflicted by the debilitating motor neuron disease amyotrophic lateral sclerosis (ALS) was baseball player Lou Gehrig, in whose honor it is often called Lou Gehrig's disease.

Motor neuron diseases are often subgrouped into three categories: ALS, progressive spinal muscular atrophy, and progressive bulbar (brain-stem) palsy. In the plural form, motor neuron diseases refer to all forms of the affliction, whereas the singular form, motor neuron disease, is synonymous with ALS.

Amyotrophic lateral sclerosis is the most familiar of the motor neuron diseases primarily because it accounts for a full 60 percent of all such disorders. The name has clinical meaning: "Amyotrophy" refers to the loss of muscle bulk as a result of missing tropic factors from dying or dead neurons; "lateral" refers to the locations within the spinal cord that are affected; and "sclerosis" refers to the hardened quality of the lateral regions of the diseased spinal cord, which otherwise would be soft tissue. The brain stem may also be sclerotic (hardened). ALS has an incidence of 1 or 2 persons per 100,000, although some Pacific islands, such as Guam, seem to have a higher incidence attributable to undetermined genetic factors. In addition, some populations show an autosomal dominant genetic component. ALS is fatal, and death generally occurs as a result of respiratory failure within three to five years after the onset of symptoms.

ALS is characterized by upper and lower motor neuron signs of neural death; thus the presence of both fasciculations and spasticity is required for a di-

agnosis. Spasticity is a medical term that describes a certain kind of muscular resistance (stiffness) to movement. In particular, spastic means a resistance that increases the more rapidly a muscle is extended; tendon reflexes are also hyperactive and Babinski's sign (abnormal reflexes of the toes) must be present. Babinski's sign reveals the death of neurons in the corticospinal tracts, which signals the occurrence of upper motor neuron death. The presence of fasciculations reveals lower motor neuron death.

Progressive spinal muscular atrophy (SMA) will show only lower motor neuron signs—namely, muscular weakness, fasciculations, and atrophy. Babinski's sign or spasticity is not found. The early symptoms may include increased clumsiness in using the fingers for fine movements (including writing or using kitchen utensils), stiffness of the fingers and hands, and cramping of the upper and lower limbs. Once the brain-stem nerves become involved, difficulty in speaking and swallowing occur. Of all persons afflicted with one of the motor neuron diseases, 7 to 15 percent will have lower motor neuron signs only and are presumed to have the progressive spinal muscular atrophy form.

Progressive bulbar palsy literally means progressive brain-stem paralysis. This form of motor neuron disease accounts for 20 to 25 percent of all cases. The tongue is usually the first place to show muscular wasting and fasciculations. As the nerves controlling the tongue die, the tongue shrivels and shrinks so that speaking, chewing, and moving solids or liquids to the back of the mouth for swallowing become difficult or impossible.

Children can be afflicted with spinal muscular atrophy. This disease is believed by many experts to be completely unique from the adult form. The childhood form seems to be more associated with environmental and genetic factors. (This concept is greatly debated, however, since the actual cause of any of the motor neuron diseases is unknown.) Three forms of childhood SMA have been identified: type 1, or acute infantile SMA (also known as Werdnig-Hoffman disease); type 2, or intermediate SMA; and type 3, or juvenile SMA (also known as Kugelberg-Welander disease).

Of children afflicted with SMA, 25 percent have type 1. This form of the disease is an autosomal recessive genetic disorder which occurs in 1 of 15,000 to 25,000 births. In an experienced mother, there may be awareness of minimal fetal movement in the last trimester of pregnancy; the fetus tends to stay still as a result of muscular weakness. Upon birth, the newborn may be a "floppy" baby of great weakness and may immediately have trouble with nursing and breathing. In other cases, it may take three to six months before symptoms begin. Because of the eventual weakening of the muscles of respiration, the child becomes prone to respiratory infections that cannot be cleared because of a lost cough reflex. Death usually occurs at two to three years of age.

When a child fails to stand or walk between six to twelve months of age, the physician considers the possibility that the child has type 2 SMA. An abnormal curvature of the spine to the forward and sideways position (kyphoscoliosis) is often seen, but rarely is there any problem with feeding or breathing. It is generally the case that very fine tremors of the child's hands can be noticed, and sometimes contractures of the hips and knees can occur. There is no delay in terms of mental health or intellect for these children.

Type 3 SMA is most often seen in the adolescent, but this disease can be observed in some children as early as five years of age. The predominant feature is weakness of the hip muscles. Since these children have been walking for some time, a change in their walking gait to a waddle can be seen over the course of years. Most people with type 3 SMA must use wheelchairs in their mid-thirties, but some may lose their ability to walk earlier. Type 3 SMA has been shown to be an autosomal recessive disorder in many cases, but there are also reported cases of sporadic occurrences within families that have previously been unaffected. Clearly, there are unanswered questions about this disease.

It should be noted that controversy abounds on the assigned classifications of motor neuron diseases. This controversy arises from the fact that the origins of the diseases are not known. Since cause has not been established for any form of motor neuron disease, physicians must use clusters of symptoms to sort the differences in disease manifestation. This sorting is used to plan the best possible treatment programs for the circumstances; nevertheless, these distinctions may seem arbitrary once more is known about the causes of motor neuron death.

TREATMENT AND THERAPY
Perhaps one of the most frustrating attributes of motor neuron diseases is that neither prevention nor effective treatment and cures are available. For a person living with motor neuron disease, physicians and health care professionals must work as a team to manage the symptoms of the diseases and offer palliative care.

In general, patients are encouraged to use and exercise their muscles cautiously in order to avoid disuse atrophy, but activity to the point of fatigue is forbidden since it is believed to aggravate the progression of muscular wasting. In addition, exposure to cold may worsen muscular contractures. Physical therapy facilitates a delay in the total loss of willed body movement by allowing the use of braces, walkers, and wheelchairs as modes of locomotion. Adults are encouraged to continue nonexertive work for as long as possible; it aids both the body and the mind to maintain independence and a sense of wholeness, well-being, and dignity.

As muscular control of the voice wanes, sketch pads, word boards, and computers can aid the ill person in communicating with loved ones, doctors, nurses, and colleagues. In addition, respiratory therapy aids in maintaining healthy breathing in spite of ever-weakening respiratory muscles. Prophylactic immunizations for influenza and pneumococci are given, especially to those who are wheelchair-dependent or bedridden. Forced deep breathing and coughing are needed at least once every four hours to bring up any congestion that may otherwise lead to grave consequences. Almost all persons with motor neuron diseases die from respiratory insufficiency. For this reason, it is imperative that the patient and physician discuss respiratory care early after diagnosis to determine whether the patient wants to be placed on mechanical ventilators in the later stages of the disease. Other issues such as tube feedings should be discussed while the patient is still able to voice an opinion and express any concerns about the dying process associated with the disease.

PERSPECTIVE AND PROSPECTS
Life can be socially difficult for people with motor neuron diseases. Others tend to assume that persons who must use wheelchairs and are unable to control mouth movements (so that speech and swallowing are lost and drooling may occur) are not intelligent, thinking, or aware. This is a sad misperception.

Many persons suffering from a motor neuron disease rise above its physical challenges to conquer in spirit that which the body cannot. For example, former United States senator Jacob Javits labored hard to improve the awareness of and funding for ALS in spite of being on a ventilator and completely immobile because of his battle with the disease. Another example of how well the intellect is preserved in this physically tragic disease can be seen in the life and work of the world-renowned astrophysicist Stephen Hawking.

Until there is an established cause or causes for these diseases effective treatments or cures are likely to remain hidden. The research continues in the hope of pinning down the ever-elusive motor neuron diseases.

—*Mary C. Fields, M.D.*

See also Amyotrophic lateral sclerosis; Aphasia and dysphasia; Muscle sprains, spasms, and disorders; Muscles; Nervous system; Neuralgia, neuritis, and neuropathy; Neurology; Neurology, pediatric; Palsy; Paralysis; Spinal cord disorders; Spine, vertebrae, and disks.

FOR FURTHER INFORMATION:

Bannister, Roger. *Brain and Bannister's Clinical Neurology*. 7th ed. Oxford, England: Oxford University Press, 1992. Although much of this text is advanced, chapter 27 ("Motor Neuron Disease") is more descriptive than technical. The black-and-white photographs provide memorable images of the destruction that these diseases cause.

Calne, Donald B. *Neurodegenerative Diseases*. Philadelphia: W. B. Saunders, 1994. An excellent book with a section devoted to amyotrophic lateral sclerosis and related motor neuron diseases.

Ferguson, Kitty. *Stephen Hawking: Quest for a Theory of Everything*. New York: Bantam Books, 1992. Ferguson describes Dr. Hawking's brilliant and complex theories in simple language, as well as how he and those around him cope with ALS.

Leigh, P. Nigel, and Michael Swash, eds. *Motor Neuron Disease: Biology and Management*. New York: Springer-Verlag, 1995. This text addresses motor neuron disease from the point of view of health care providers.

Parsons, Malcolm. *Color Atlas of Clinical Neurology*. 2d ed. St. Louis: Mosby Year Book, 1993. Impeccably assembled, this atlas shows the most distinguishing clinical features associated with motor neuron diseases, such as muscular wasting of the hands and tongue.

Thompson, C. E. *Raising a Child with a Neuromuscular Disorder: A Guide for Parents, Grandparents, Friends, and Professionals*. New York: Oxford University Press, 1999. Although the field of neuromuscular disorders has grown, many of the guideposts have remained the same. In this rich resource, the author has kept sight of these guideposts, describing them and capturing the most current resources, references, and medical help available.

MOTOR SKILL DEVELOPMENT

DEVELOPMENT

ANATOMY OR SYSTEM AFFECTED: Bones, circulatory system, eyes, joints, muscles, musculoskeletal system, nerves, nervous system, psychic-emotional system

SPECIALTIES AND RELATED FIELDS: Exercise physiology, genetics, neonatology, neurology, orthopedics, pathology, pediatrics, perinatology, physical therapy, psychology, sports medicine

DEFINITION: The process of change in motor behavior with advancing age and the numerous physiological and psychological processes that underlie these changes, which describe the adjustments in posture, movement, and skillful manipulation of objects achieved through the coordination of several neurologic control structures.

KEY TERMS:

central nervous system: the brain and spinal cord, which process incoming information from the peripheral nervous system and form the main network of coordination and control in advanced organisms

motor control: the nature and cause of movement, which focuses on stability and movement of the body, and the manipulation of objects, which is achieved through the coordination of many structures organized both hierarchically and in a parallel manner

motor learning: the acquisition and modification of movement as a result of practice and experience, which leads to relatively permanent intrinsic changes in the ability to perform skilled activities; not directly measurable, but inferred from measures of motor performance

motor performance: the directly measurable extent to which the objective of a motor task is met, the scientific study of which originated as a branch of experimental psychology

motor skills: skills in which both movement and the outcome of actions are emphasized

peripheral nervous system: the system of nerves that

link the central nervous system to the rest of the body; consists of twelve pairs of cranial nerves, thirty-one pairs of spinal nerves, and the autonomic nervous system

skeletal muscle: striated muscle that contracts voluntarily and involuntarily to carry out the functions of body support, posture, and locomotion

somatosensory system: the system by which muscle, joint, and cutaneous sensory receptors contribute to the perception and control of movement through ascending pathways

PHYSICAL AND PSYCHOLOGICAL FACTORS

Motor skill development, the process of change in motor behavior with increasing age, focuses on adjustments in posture, movement, and the skillful manipulation of objects. Early researchers attributed essentially all developmental changes to modifications occurring within the central nervous system, with increasing motor abilities reflecting increasing neural maturation. Contemporary researchers have determined that the central nervous system works in combination with other body systems (such as the musculoskeletal, cardiovascular, and respiratory systems) and the environment to influence motor development, with all systems interacting in an extremely complex fashion as the individual ages.

Prenatal development of motor behavior takes place between approximately seven weeks after conception and birth, as was first determined during the 1970's using technology to visualize the fetus in utero. Following approximately eight weeks of gestation, the fetus is able to exert reflex and reaction actions, as well as active spontaneous movement. It is currently believed that the ability to self-initiate movements within the womb is an integral part of development, as compared to the traditional view that the fetus is passive and reflexive.

Infancy, the period from birth until the child is able to stand and walk, lasts approximately twelve months. The neonate begins life essentially helpless against the force of gravity and gradually develops the ability to align body segments with respect both to other body segments and to the environment. The Bayley Scales of Infant Development measure the following milestones of motor skill development for the first year of life (with the average age of accomplishment listed in parentheses): erect and steady head holding (0.8 months), side to back turning (1.8 months), supported sitting (2.3 months), back to side turning (4.4 months), momentary independent sitting (5.3 months), rolling from back to stomach (6.4 months), steady independent sitting (6.6 months), early supported stepping movements (7.4 months), arm pull to standing position (8.1 months), assisted walking (9.6 months), independent standing (11.0 months), and independent walking (11.7 months). The transition from helplessness to physical independence during the first twelve months creates many changes for growing children and their caregivers. New areas of exploration open up for the baby as greater body control is gained, the force of gravity is conquered, and less dependence on holding and carrying by caregivers is required.

During the first three months after birth, the infant's motor skill development focuses on getting the head aligned from the predominating posture of flexion. Flexor tone, the tendency to maintain a flexed posture and to rebound back into flexion when the limbs are extended and released, probably results from a combination of the elasticity of soft tissues that were confined to a flexed position while in the womb and of central nervous system activity. As antigravity activity progresses, the infant develops the ability to lift the head. Movements during this period involve brief periods of stretching, kicking, and thrusting of the limbs, in addition to turning and twisting of the trunk and head. Infants tend to be the most active prior to feeding and more quiet and sleepy after feeding.

The third to sixth months after birth are marked by great strides in overcoming the force of gravity by both flexion and extension movements. The infant becomes more competent in head control with respect to symmetry and midline orientation with the rest of the body, is able to sit independently for brief periods, and can push up onto hands and knees. These major milestones enable considerably more independence and permit a much greater ability to interact with the rest of the world.

During the sixth to ninth months after birth, the infant is constantly moving and exploring the surrounding environment. As nine months is approached, most babies are able to pull themselves into a standing position using a support such as furniture. The child expends a great deal of energy to stand and often bounces up and down once standing is achieved. The up-and-down bouncing eventually leads to the shifting of body weight from side to side and the taking of first steps, with a caregiver assisting alongside the furniture; this is often called cruising.

The ninth to twelfth months involve forward creeping on hands and knees. This locomotor pattern requires more complicated alternating movements of the opposite arms and legs. Some infants have a preference for creeping even after they are able to walk independently, with many preferring plantigrade creeping (on extended arms and legs) to walking. The ease to which the child moves from sitting to creeping, kneeling, or standing is greatly improved and balance is developed to the point where the child can pivot around in circles while sitting, using the hands and feet for propulsion. The child begins to move efficiently from standing to floor sitting and can initiate rolling from the supine position using flexed legs. Unsupported sitting is accomplished with ease, and weight while sitting can be transferred easily from buttocks to hands.

The early childhood period lasts from infancy until about six years. It involves the child attaining new skills but not necessarily new patterns of movement, with the learning patterns that were acquired during the first year of life being put to use in more meaningful activities. The locomotor pattern of walking is refined, and new motor skills that require increased balance and control of force—such as running, hopping, jumping, and skipping—are mastered.

Running is usually begun between years two and four, as the child learns to master the flight phase and the anticipatory strategies necessary when there is temporarily no body contact with the ground. It is not until about age five or six that control during running with respect to starting, stopping, and changing directions is effectively mastered. Jumping develops at about age 2.5, as the ability and confidence to land after jumping from a height such as a stair is achieved. The ability to jump to reach an overhead object then emerges, with early jumpers revealing a shallow preparatory crouch that progresses to a deeper crouch. Hopping, an extension of the ability to balance while standing on one leg, begins at about age 2.5 but is not performed well until about age six, when a series of about ten hops can be performed consecutively and are incorporated into games such as hopscotch. Skipping, a step and a hop on one leg followed by a step and hop of the other leg, is generally not achieved until about six years, with the opportunity and encouragement for practice being a primary determining factor, as with other locomotor skills.

Throwing is typically acquired during the first year, but advanced throwing, striking (such as with a plastic baseball and bat), kicking (such as with a soccer ball), and catching are not developed until early childhood. Catching develops at approximately age three, with the child initially holding the arms in front of the body and later making anticipatory adjustments to account for the direction, speed, and size of the thrown object. Kicking, which requires balancing on one foot while transferring force to an object with the other foot, begins with little preparatory backswing and eventually develops to involve the knee, hip, and lean of the trunk at about age six.

Fine motor manipulation skills in the upper extremity that are important to normal activities of daily living such as feeding, dressing, grooming, and handwriting are greatly improved in early childhood. The key components include locating a target, which requires the coordination of eye-head movement; reaching, which requires the transportation of the hand and arm in space; and manipulation, which includes grip formation, grasp, and release.

During later childhood (the period from seven years to about eleven years), adolescence, and adult life throughout the remainder of the life span, changes in movement are influenced predominantly by age. Adolescence begins with the onset of the physical changes of puberty, at approximately eleven to twelve years of age in girls and twelve to thirteen years of age in boys, and ends when physical growth is curtailed. Most authorities believe that the growth spurt of adolescence leads to the emergence of new patterns of movement within the skills that have already been acquired. Most adolescents have strong drives to develop self-esteem and become socially acceptable with their peers in school and various recreational activities. Cooperation and competition become strong components of motor skill development, whereby many skills are stabilized prior to adolescence and preferences for various sports activities emerge. Boys typically demonstrate increased speed and strength as compared to girls, despite recent dramatic changes in available opportunities for girls in recreational and competitive sports activities. Even though age-related changes in motor behavior continue throughout adulthood, the physical skills that permit independence are primarily acquired during the first year of life.

Psychological factors that influence motor skill development include attention level, stimulus-response compatibility, arousal level, and motivation. The level of attention when attempting a motor task is critical, with humans displaying a relatively fixed capacity for concentration during different stages of development. Stimulus identification, response selection, and response programming stages—whereby an individual remembers or determines how to perform a task—affect skill development because the central nervous system takes longer to synthesize and respond to more complex skills. Also important are stimulus-response compatibility—the better the stimulus matches the response, the shorter the reaction time—and arousal, which is described as an "inverted U" by the Yerkes-Dodson model. The inverted U hypothesis implies that there exists an optimal level of psychological arousal to learn or perform a motor skill efficiently, with performance declining when the arousal level at a given moment in time is too great or too small. At a low level of arousal, the scope of perception is broad, and all stimuli (including irrelevant information) are being processed. As arousal level increases, perception narrows so that when the optimal level of arousal is reached and attention is sufficiently focused, concentration on only the stimuli relevant to successful skill learning and performance is enabled. If arousal level surpasses this optimal level, perception narrows to the point of tunnel vision, some relevant stimuli are missed, and learning and skill performance are reduced. The influence of personal motivation during motor skill development encompasses the child's perceived relevance of the activity and also the child's individual ability to recognize the goal of the activity and desire to achieve it.

Three main factors that affect motor skill development in early and later childhood include feedback, amount of practice, and practice conditions. Feedback can be intrinsic, arising from the somatosensory system and senses such as vision and hearing, as information is gathered about a movement and its consequences rather then the actual achievement of the goal. In pathological conditions such as cerebral palsy, intrinsic feedback is often greatly impaired. Feedback can also be extrinsic and is often divided by researchers into knowledge of results, or information about the success of the movement in accomplishing the goal that is available after the skill is completed, and knowledge of performance, or information about skill performance technique or strategy. Knowledge of results provides information about errors as well as successes. True learning occurs by a process of trial and error, with the nervous system serving to detect and correct inappropriate or inefficient movements.

DISORDERS AND EFFECTS

Physical therapists, psychologists, teachers, and other professionals who work with pediatric patients often plan their treatment interventions and instructional lessons based on the normal age-related progression of motor skill development. Motor skill development is often significantly decreased as a consequence of a neurological impairment, however, with the child's resulting movement patterns revealing primary impairments such as inadequate activation of muscle, secondary impairments such as contractures, and compensatory strategies that are adopted to overcome the impairment and achieve mobility. The categories for impairments that have an impact on motor development can generally be divided into musculoskeletal, neuromuscular, sensory, perceptual, and cognitive.

Damage to various nervous system structures somewhat predictably reduces the motor control of movement via both positive symptoms (the presence of abnormal behavior) and negative symptoms (the loss of normal behavior). Positive symptoms include the presence of exaggerated reflexes and abnormalities of muscle tone. Negative symptoms include the loss of muscular strength and the inappropriate selection of muscles during task performance. The broad spectrum of muscle tone abnormalities ranges from flaccidity to rigidity, with muscle spasticity defined as the velocity-dependent increase in tonic stretch reflexes (also called muscle tone), with exaggerated tendon jerks resulting from changes in the threshold of the stretch reflex.

Secondary effects of central nervous system lesions are not directly caused by the lesions themselves but develop as a consequence of the lesions. For example, children with cerebral palsy often exhibit the primary problem of spasticity in muscles of the lower extremities, which causes the secondary problem of muscular and tendon tightness in the ankles, knees, and hips. The secondary problem of limited range of motion in these important areas for movement often impairs motor skills more than the primary problem of spasticity, with the resulting movement strategies reflecting the growing child's best attempt to compensate.

Another common compensatory strategy seen in children with a motor development dysfunction involves standing with the knee hyperextended because of an inability to generate enough muscular force to keep the knee from collapsing. Standing with the knee in hyperextension keeps the line of gravity in front of the knee joint. Contractures of joints are frequent consequences of disordered postural and movement patterns. For example, a habitual crouched sitting posture results in chronic shortening of the hamstring, calf, and hip flexor muscles, and a backward-tipped pelvis accommodates the shortened hamstrings. Chronic shortening of the calf muscles often results in toe walking (in which the heel does not strike the ground) and a reduced walking speed and stride length, because of decreased balance and leg muscle strength. Changes in the availability of sensory information and cognitive factors such as fear of falling and inattention may also contribute strongly to motor skill development in some pediatric patients.

PERSPECTIVE AND PROSPECTS

Interest in the scientific study of motor development was greatly enhanced by Myrtle B. McGraw's *The Neuromuscular Maturation of the Human Infant* (1945). It described four stages of neural maturation: a period in which movement is governed by reflexes as a result of the dominance of lower centers within the central nervous system; a period in which reflex expression declines as a result of maturation of the cerebral cortex and the inhibitory effect of the cortex over lower centers; a period in which an increase in the voluntary quality of activity as a result of increased cortical control produces deliberate or voluntary movement; and a period in which integrative activity of the neural centers takes place, as shown by smooth and coordinated movements.

Arnold Gesell then used cinematography to conduct extensive observations of infants during various stages of growth. He described the maturation of infants based on four behavior categories: motor behavior, adaptive behavior, language development, and personal-social development. Gesell identified six principles of development. The principle of motor priority and fore-reference states that the neuromotor system is laid down before it is voluntarily utilized. The principle of developmental direction states that development proceeds in head-to-foot and proximal-to-distal directions. The principle of reciprocal interweaving states that opposing movements such as extension and flexion show a temporary dominance over one another until they become integrated into mature motor patterns. The principle of functional asymmetry states that humans have a preferred hand, a dominant eye, and a lead foot, with this unilateral dominance being subject to change during development. The principle of self-regulation states that periods of stability and instability culminate into more stable responses as maturity proceeds. The principle of optimal realization states that the human action system has strong growth potential toward normal development if environmental and cultural conditions are favorable and if compensatory and regeneration mechanisms come into play when damage occurs to facilitate attainment of the maximum possible growth.

Esther Thelen suggested the dynamic systems theory. This theory argues that the maturing nervous system interacts with other biomechanical, psychological, and social environment factors to create a dimensional system whereby behavior represents a compression of the degrees of freedom.

A more refined systems theory of motor control developed by Anne Shumway-Cook and Marjorie Woollacott claims that the three main factors that interact in the development of efficient locomotion are progression (ability to generate rhythmic muscular patterns to move the body in the desired direction), stability (the control of balance), and adaptation (the ability to adapt to changing task and environmental requirements). These three factors generally appear sequentially, with muscular patterns appearing first, followed by equilibrium control, and finally adaptive capabilities. Although research on the emergence of human motor skills has primarily concentrated on the developmental milestones of infants and children, it appears that important changes in motor behavior continue throughout the human life span.

—Daniel G. Graetzer, Ph.D.

See also Cerebral palsy; Cognitive development; Developmental stages; Growth; Muscle sprains, spasms, and disorders; Muscles; Muscular dystrophy; Nervous system; Physical examination; Reflexes, primitive; Speech disorders; Well-baby examinations.

FOR FURTHER INFORMATION:

Kalverboer, Alex F., Brian Hopkins, and Reint Geuze. *Motor Development in Early and Later Childhood: Longitudinal Approaches.* New York: Cambridge University Press, 1992. An excellent text that reviews motor development in early and later childhood in a longitudinal fashion.

Newell, K. M. "Motor Skill Acquisition." *Annual Review of Psychology* 42 (1991): 213-237. This review focuses on the general laws of motor learning and the specifics of what is learned through repetitive practice.

Shumway-Cook, Anne, and Marjorie Woollacott. *Motor Control: Theory and Practical Applications.* 2d ed. Baltimore: Williams & Wilkins, 2000. This excellent text provides a framework by which the various motor control theories can be incorporated into physical therapy clinical practice for a variety of patient populations.

Thelen, Esther, and Linda B. Smith. *A Dynamic Systems Approach to the Development of Cognition and Action.* Cambridge, Mass.: MIT Press, 1994. This 376-page text examines perceptual motor processes, motor abilities, and cognition in infants and children, in addition to describing various points of view of developmental psychobiology.

Whitall, Jill. "The Evolution of Research on Motor Development: New Approaches Bring New Insights." In *Exercise and Sport Science Reviews.* Baltimore: Williams & Wilkins, 1995. A description of how research into motor development evolved from 1980 to 1995, beginning with a central focus by kinesiologists and physical educators to include developmental psychologists, neurophysiologists, cognitive and perceptual psychologists, and physical therapists.

MRI. *See* MAGNETIC RESONANCE IMAGING (MRI).

MULTIPLE BIRTHS
BIOLOGY

ANATOMY OR SYSTEM AFFECTED: All

SPECIALTIES AND RELATED FIELDS: Embryology, genetics, neonatology, obstetrics, pediatrics

DEFINITION: The presence of two or more fetuses in the womb.

KEY TERMS:

chromosomes: the rod-shaped structures in the nucleus of a cell that carry genes

concordance: the condition among twins of having the same physical or psychological trait

dizygotes: fraternal twins; born from two ova separately fertilized by two sperm

embryo: the cells growing after conception until the eighth week of pregnancy

monozygotes: identical twins; born of a single ovum that divides after a single sperm fertilizes it

ovum: the egg cell released from the ovaries during ovulation

placenta: the membrane sac developed from the uterine wall that passes nutrients to the fetus through interconnected blood vessels

ultrasonography: an imaging technique that uses high-frequency sound waves to view fetuses in the womb, as well as other internal structures

zygote: a fertilized ovum before multicellular development begins

Multiple births are rare events. The most common are twins; this occurs in approximately one out of every eighty complete pregnancies. Twins can come from a single egg or from two different eggs. Triplets occur once in approximately eight hundred completed pregnancies. Quadruplets occur once in every eight thousand completed pregnancies. Quintuplets occur naturally in approximately one out of every eighty thousand completed pregnancies.

As the number of fetuses increases, the chances that all will survive decreases. Multiple births are most commonly combinations of twins and single eggs. By reviewing the mechanics of twin formation, greater multiples can be understood.

THE DIFFERENT TYPES OF TWINS

Two types of twins are well known: fraternal twins and identical twins. Behind these general terms, however, lies considerable variation. This variation is based on the many changes that a human ovum can undergo after it is released by the ovary, is fertilized, travels along the Fallopian tube to the uterus, and implants there to develop into an embryo.

Fraternal twins are also known as dizygotic or binovular twins. In a normal menstrual cycle, only a single egg is released. When a sperm penetrates an ovum, the fertilized egg releases a chemical that prevents other sperm from penetrating the same egg. If a second egg has been released, however, it can also be fertilized. A newly fertilized egg is called a zygote. If both zygotes succeed in attaching to the uterine walls, a twin pregnancy begins. Usually, this dual insemination occurs during a single release of semen in a single copulation, so that the embryos have the same father. Occasionally, the two eggs may be fertilized in separate copulations during the same ovulation, a phenomenon called superfecundation. It is then possible for dizygotic twins to have different fathers. This possibility seems to have long been recognized. The Greek myth of Leda and the Swan derives from such a pregnancy.

Very rarely, an impregnated woman continues her monthly ovulation cycle. If a second ovulation occurs in the three months following conception, theoretically she could be impregnated again. This phenomenon is called superfetation and would result in twins who are one, two, or three months different in age. No unquestionable example of human superfetation has been documented because distinguishing the relative ages of twin fetuses is extremely difficult.

Fraternal twins have separate placentas and membranes in the womb. The placenta comprises maternal and fetal tissues interconnected by blood vessels. Nutrients pass from mother to the fetus through the placenta. Waste products are removed from the fetus by a reverse process. Sometimes, the placentas press against each other in the womb and fuse. Having had separate placentas or one fused together, however, does not affect the nature of the twins after birth. Fra-

---

The Two Main Types of Twins

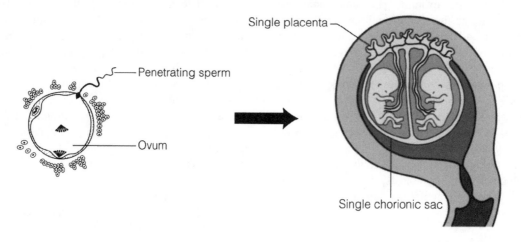

Identical twins

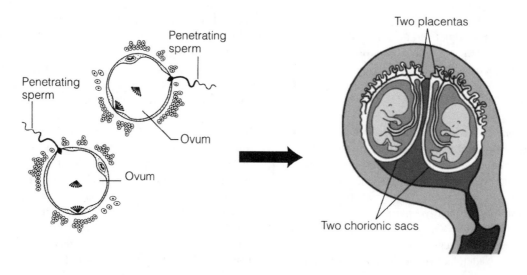

Nonidentical twins

---

ternal twins, even though they share the same birthday, are no more similar in appearance or manner than two siblings from separate births.

Identical twins are the result of different initial events. They are also called monozygotic or monovular twins. Identical or look-alike twins originate when a single egg spontaneously divides after penetration by a sperm cell. Each half develops separately. The reason for this division is not known. One theory holds that sometimes the fertilized ovum does not implant in the uterus right away as is normally the case. During the delay, the chromosomes double and the zygote halves, with each half then implanting and becoming a separate embryo.

Another theory suggests that early in the pregnancy, a genetic mutation occurs in one of the cells. Later, while the embryo is still no more than a few hundred cells, the unmutated cells recognize the genetic difference and reject the mutant cells, much as the immune system rejects substances foreign to it. The rejected group of cells develops separately. If this theory proves to be true, identical twins must not be completely identical after all. Cases in which one identical twin has a genetic disease and the other remains healthy appear to support this theory, although mutation in one twin may occur after splitting rather than causing the splitting.

Variation sometimes appears after birth in monozygotic siblings. Twins can vary in birth weight greatly (one may weigh twice as much), develop at different rates, and die from unrelated natural causes. As a rule, however, identical twins share an overwhelming majority of traits. When two (or more) siblings share a trait, they are considered to be concordant for that trait. Typically, body structures and coloration will be strikingly concordant. Features such as facial shape, hair texture and color, eye color, and height are typical examples of concordance. "Mirror" twins are an uncommon phenomenon. They show mirror image symmetry in some traits. For example, one may be left-handed while the other is right-handed. Whorls on the scalp may also occur as mirror images. In very rare cases, one mirror twin will have situs inversus: The placement of all internal organs is reversed. An individual with situs inverses will have the liver and appendix on the left side of the abdomen and the spleen on the right.

Genetic variation may account for the subtle variations in even the most concordant of twins. The internal environment of the womb also has an effect. Most

identical twin fetuses share the same placenta but have different inner or chorionic sacs. They may have separate placentas (and separate chorions) depending on when the initial splitting of the zygote took place. Usually, those sharing a single placenta have separate chorions. In the rarest variation, the fetuses also share the same amnion. The degree of separation or number of barriers can influence the amount of oxygen or nutrients that each twin receives. Relatively minor differences can affect development.

A third type of twin is theoretically possible. During maturation and before becoming fertilized, the mature ovum could divide into a secondary oocyte (the cell to be fertilized) and a much smaller polar body. It is possible for the ovum to divide into roughly equal portions, both of which are viable and contain the same genetic material. If separate sperm then fertilize these ova, they would become two zygotes. Such twins would have exactly the same maternal genes, but a portion of the paternal genes would differ. They would be less identical than monozygotes but more so than dizygotes. Although this type of twinning has been described in rats and mice, no human case has been indisputably identified and reported.

A fourth variant of twinning is conjoined twins, popularly called Siamese twins. Conjoined twins share some tissue. This can range from simple joining of skin on the head or shoulder to having one heart or kidney or two torsos and a single pair of legs. Conjoined twins are created by incomplete cell division during early fetal life. The portion of cells that divide normally continue to develop in a normal fashion. The cells that did not divide completely also develop normally. The result is a portion of the body that is duplicated and a portion that is not. If the incomplete division occurred early in fetal development, the amount of shared tissue is likely to be greater than with an incomplete division that occurred later in fetal development.

About one-third of all twin births result in identical twins. The proportion of males and females is approximately equal. The incidence of identical twins remains constant throughout the world's diverse ethnic populations. Fraternal twins, however, show different proportions and distributions. About half the pairs have the same gender (with a nearly equal number of male-male and female-female pairs); about half are male-female pairs. Fraternal twin births occur most frequently among rural Nigerians (45 pairs per 1,000 births) and least frequently among Chinese and Japanese parents (4 pairs per 1,000 births). European and American rates, for both blacks and whites, are approximately halfway between these extremes.

Evidence suggests that women inherit a tendency to conceive fraternal twins from their mothers. There is little scientific evidence to support the belief that fathers possess a gene for monozygotic twins. Physiological factors can increase the likelihood of a woman having fraternal twins. Women who are tall and heavy and who have previously given birth to children have more twins than small women or those who have not been pregnant before. Women between thirty-five and forty years of age are the most likely to have twins, but the chances decrease thereafter.

Multiple pregnancies (triplets and more) are usually combinations of twins. Identical triplets do rarely occur, but triplets consisting of two identical and one fraternal sibling are the norm. Multiple births of four or more infants are almost always combinations of twins. Physicians can ascertain the status of multiple birth siblings by examining placentas and chorionic sacs.

POSSIBLE COMPLICATIONS OF MULTIPLE BIRTHS
Multiple births create special problems for mothers. Specifically, they are more difficult to carry in the womb and to nurture through infancy than singletons. Multiples are smaller, so that vaginal deliveries are easier. Many physicians, however, recommend birth by Cesarean section to manage complications better. Most twins are born healthy, but they must be monitored carefully. As the number of fetuses increases, their size decreases. Because they are not fully mature, this increases the chances for medical problems.

Positively identifying multiple fetuses in the womb is not always an easy task, even though medical science has developed a variety of techniques. The traditional signs of considerable fetal movement, multiple heartbeats, and a large weight gain by the mother can be inaccurate and contradictory. Tests for the human chorionic gonadotropin hormone in the mother's blood or urine or alpha-fetoprotein in the blood may suggest the presence of multiple fetuses if the hormone or protein levels are unusually elevated. Nevertheless, imaging technologies provide the most reliable test. Ultrasonography has supplanted X rays, which declined in use because of the radiation hazard to fetuses. The images produced by ultrasonography can usually resolve multiple fetuses early in the pregnancy.

A multiple pregnancy itself strains the mother's body and is particularly subject to medical complications. Typically, a mother carrying multiple fetuses gains from 30 to 80 pounds, about twice the weight of a single pregnancy. The added weight can cause skeletal and muscular problems. The fetuses' demands on the mother's body may also worsen preexisting medical conditions, such as heart or kidney disease. As the multiple fetuses develop, their size stretches the uterus, which can initiate early labor. For this reason, the premature birth rate is higher for multiple fetuses than for single fetuses. Twins occasionally reach full term; triplets and greater multiples do not.

Similarly, multiple pregnancies miscarry at more than three times the rate of singletons. Occasionally, one fetus will develop at the expense of the other by drawing a disproportionate amount of nutrients from the mother, a condition called twin transfusion syndrome. In about two-thirds of these cases, the undernourished fetus dies in the womb. If one fetus dies for any reason, the mother's body may reabsorb it partially or completely, a phenomenon known as the vanishing twin. Some doctors believe that because of unobserved vanishing twins, miscarriages, and induced abortions, the number of twin conceptions has been underestimated.

Doctors carefully monitor the fetal development of multiple fetuses to ensure their health and, especially, to prepare for delivering them. Amniocentesis and genetic tests detect potential biochemical defects, genetic anomalies, and diseases. Ultrasonography allows doctors to identify defects in shape and the relative position of the fetuses in the womb. Their position is important during labor. Normally, babies are born headfirst. In multiples, one of the fetuses frequently lies crosswise or feet first. These positions greatly lengthen and complicate delivery, so that the second fetus runs a higher risk of dying during labor. Moreover, the mother's overdistended uterus, unable to contract properly after delivery, may begin to bleed. The fact that labor lasts too long may exhaust her dangerously. Because of such problems, many obstetricians recommend delivery by cesarean section—that is, by cutting a passage through the abdomen into the uterus—at the first sign of trouble to either mother or fetuses.

The prematurity and low birth weight common in multiple infants means that many are placed on life support. Studies have found that multiple infants suffer congenital defects as much as three times more often than singletons. Identical siblings are the most likely of all to have abnormalities. Heart malformations are most common. According to some studies, closed esophagus, clubfeet, excess fingers or toes, and forms of mental retardation such as Down syndrome occur at a slightly higher rate.

Conjoined twins are relatively rare, appearing approximately once in a hundred thousand pregnancies. Most are attached at the back or at the back of the head or neck. In an extreme rarity, one identical twin has a full set of chromosomes while the other has only the X chromosome from the mother and will be a female with a condition called Turner syndrome. Therefore, identical twins will be of opposite gender if the first twin has the XY chromosomes that defines a male and the other is a female with Turner syndrome.

That multiple birth siblings develop in the same environment and from a common origin allows researchers to trace the genetic and environmental influences on human development in general. Most of this research has been conducted on twins because of the relative rarity of triplets or larger groups of siblings. The reasoning is straightforward. In the case of identical twins, either their genetic heritage (nature) or the environment (nurture) dominates in determining how they grow mentally and physically. Researchers have tested the idea by tracking down identical twins that were separated while young, usually at birth, and reared separately. If genetics control development, the separated twins should still look and behave similarly. If environment predominates, then separated twins should show variations in appearance and temperament.

The reported research results have been mixed. Some separated twins do not look and act any more alike than siblings separately born. Others show an uncanny degree of similarity throughout their lives—dressing the same way, marrying in the same year, having the same number of children, and dying nearly at the same time of the same disease. Their intelligence, which many scientists believe is heavily influenced by environment, nevertheless shows high concordance.

PERSPECTIVE AND PROSPECTS

Worldwide, superstitions and a strong moral overtone have traditionally accompanied multiple births. Some societies viewed one twin as automatically good and the other evil and treated them accordingly as they matured. Others thought twins shameful, a sign of corruption or promiscuity in the mother. These babies might be killed at birth or separated because of it. An African curse reflects the deep suspicion that some societies have held for twins: "May you be the mother of twins." On the other hand, some nations believed that twins have divine origin or power over the elements or special talents for prophecy and telepathy.

Multiple siblings enjoy a special advantage: They are rarely lonely. Their common development means increased requirements of time and money for their families. It also provides continuous opportunities for sharing and relying on each other. The many national and international organizations created by and for twins and other multiple birth siblings reflect their pride in their status.

Triplets have historically had a reasonable chance for survival. Before the advent of support equipment for premature babies, lung immaturity was the factor that usually determined life or death. Surfactant is a chemical that is secreted in the seventh month of pregnancy. Without surfactant, lung tissues stick together and infants cannot breathe. Because of the combined size of all fetuses, many multiple infants are born before the seventh month of gestation. The Dionne quintuplets, who were born in the 1930's, were unusual in that for the first time in history, all five survived into adulthood. Modern support technology has helped several sets of sextuplets (six infants) to survive. In November, 1997, the same technology permitted all the McCaughey septuplets (seven infants) to survive. This was the first time such an event has occurred. (The chances of naturally conceiving septuplets are one in eight to ten million conceptions.)

Recent advances in the field of assisted reproduction have increased the odds of multiple pregnancies. Women who have difficulty conceiving are initially treated with drugs that cause more than one egg to be released during ovulation. This increases the chance of pregnancy but also increases the chance of carrying multiple fetuses. Couples who seek medical assistance to achieve pregnancy routinely use fertility drugs. A woman will have several eggs or zygotes implanted to improve the odds of successfully initiating a pregnancy. The result of this approach is an increased number of multiple births. In 1988, twelve fetuses, which were miscarried, resulted from a fertility drug. Artificially induced pregnancies have posed ethical dilemmas for many who believe that scientists should not manipulate human biological processes.

Multiple births raise other moral and ethical questions as well. Genetic tests can now identify potential fetal defects in the womb early enough that surgeons can remove a defective fetus without harming the healthy fetus, a procedure called selective birth, selective abortion, or selective fetocide. Those who hold abortions to be immoral have reservations about selective fetocide even when the defective fetus has little chance of surviving and may threaten the lives of the remaining healthy fetuses. That selective fetocide may be used simply because a mother does not want to rear more than one child has caused far greater concern. Since the procedure is tricky to perform and can result in the death of all fetuses, most doctors find selective fetocide for nonmedical reasons to be ethically indefensible.

Twin births bear witness to the successes of modern health care. In the United States, incidents of multiple births, both fraternal and identical, have increased slightly since the 1970's and more multiples are surviving to adulthood. Fertility drugs may account for part of the increase, as does the trend among American women to delay childbearing until their thirties. Nevertheless, prenatal care, better diet, improvements in neonatal intensive care, and education about pregnancy and birth are as important.

—Roger Smith, Ph.D.;
updated by L. Fleming Fallon, Jr.,
M.D., Ph.D., M.P.H.

See also Abortion; Amniocentesis; Birth defects; Cesarean section; Childbirth; Childbirth complications; Chorionic villus sampling; Conception; Embryology; Ethics; Genetics and inheritance; In vitro fertilization; Miscarriage; Neonatology; Obstetrics; Pregnancy and gestation; Premature birth; Reproductive system; Sibling rivalry; Ultrasonography.

FOR FURTHER INFORMATION:
Albi, Linda, Donna Florien, and Deborah Johnson. *Mothering Twins: From Hearing the News to Beyond the Terrible Twos.* New York: Simon & Schuster, 1993. Advice from the real experts— mothers of twins. Information and on-target anecdotes cover common problems, from the complications of multiple births to coping with nursing and caring for two or more infants to organizing support systems.

Malmstrom, Patricia Maxwell, and Janet Poland. *The Art of Parenting Twins.* New York: Random House International, 2000. Malmstrom and Poland cover the biology and causes of twinning; the emotional terrain of parenting multiples; the differences between twin and single pregnancies; twin development in babyhood, toddlerhood, the preschool and school-age years, and adolescence; and twins' relationships with each other from babyhood to adulthood.

Noble, Elizabeth. *Having Twins: A Parent's Guide to Pregnancy, Birth and Early Childhood.* 2d ed. New York: Houghton-Mifflin, 1991. This book is well written and easy to understand. The author is a professional with many years of experience with multiple births.

Novotny, Pamela P. *The Joy of Twins and Other Multiple Births: Having, Raising, and Loving Babies Who Arrive in Groups.* Avenel, N.J.: Crown Books, 1994. The author provides interesting information for parents of multiple infants.

Rothbart, Betty. *Multiple Blessings: From Pregnancy Through Childhood—A Guide for Parents of Twins, Triplets, or More.* San Francisco: Hearst Books, 1994. In a clear presentation of all the facts, the author helps parents through all stages of pregnancy, providing advice on feeding, home care, juggling hectic schedules, and other critical issues related to the raising of twins and triplets.

MULTIPLE CHEMICAL SENSITIVITY SYNDROME
DISEASE/DISORDER

ANATOMY OR SYSTEM AFFECTED: Eyes, immune system, lungs, muscles, nerves, nervous system, respiratory system, skin

SPECIALTIES AND RELATED FIELDS: Dermatology, environmental health, epidemiology, immunology, neurology, occupational health, public health, toxicology

DEFINITION: An increasing intolerance to commonly encountered chemicals at concentrations well tolerated by other people.

CAUSES AND SYMPTOMS
Multiple chemical sensitivity (MCS) syndrome, reactive airway dysfunctions, and the "sick building" syndromes are overlapping disorders caused by intolerance of environmental chemicals. Exactly how many people are affected by MCS is unknown. The onset is

often associated with initial acute chemical exposure; patients may report the onset of MCS after moving into a new home, after exposure to chemicals in the workplace, or following the use of pesticides in the home. Patients often describe an increasing intolerance to commonly encountered chemicals at concentrations well tolerated by other people.

Symptoms usually wax and wane with exposure and are more likely to occur in patients with preexisting histories of migraine or classical allergies. Idiosyncratic medication reactions (especially to preservative chemicals) are common in MCS patients, as are dysautonomic symptoms (such as vascular instability), poor temperature regulation, and food intolerance. It is thought that patients with MCS have organ abnormalities involving the liver, the nervous system (including the brain and the limbic, peripheral, and autonomic systems), the immune system, and perhaps porphyrin metabolism, probably reflecting chemical injury to these systems. There is often a substantial overlap of MCS symptoms with fibromyalgia and chronic fatigue syndrome.

The common clinical symptoms may include headaches (often migraine), chronic fatigue, musculoskeletal aching, chronic respiratory inflammation (rhinitis, sinusitis, laryngitis, asthma), attention-deficit disorder, and hyperactivity (affecting younger children). Less common complaints include tremor, seizure, and mitral valve prolapse. Agents associated with the onset of MCS include gasoline, kerosene, natural gas, pesticides (especially chlordane and chlorpyrifos), organic solvents, new carpet and other renovation materials, adhesives and glues, fiberglass, carbonless copy paper, fabric softener, formaldehyde and glutaraldehyde, carpet shampoo (lauryl sulfate) and other cleaning agents, isocyanates, combustion products (poorly vented gas heaters, overheated batteries), and medications (dinitrochlorobenzene for warts, intranasally packed neosynephrine, prolonged antibiotics, and general anesthesia with petrochemicals).

It is believed that the mechanisms that lead to MCS may be multifactorial and include neurogenic inflammation (respiratory, gastrointestinal, and genitourinary symptoms), kindling and time-dependent sensitization (neurologic symptoms), and immune activation or impaired porphyrin metabolism (multiple-organ symptoms). Pathological findings of MCS have rarely been examined. A preliminary study of nasal pathology in these patients indicates that they are characterized by defects in the junctions between cells, desquamation of the respiratory epithelium, glandular hyperplasia, lymphocytic infiltrates, and peripheral nerve fiber proliferation. A consistent physiologic abnormality in these patients has not been established.

Psychiatric, personality, cognitive/neurologic, immunologic, and olfactory studies have been conducted comparing MCS subjects with various control groups. Thus far, the most consistent finding is that patients with MCS have a higher rate of psychiatric disorders across studies and relative to diverse comparison groups. Since these studies are cross-sectional, however, causality cannot be implied. Various working groups have proposed several research questions addressing the relationship between neurogenic inflammation and toxicant-induced loss of tolerance with the development of MCS.

TREATMENT AND THERAPY

The management of patients with MCS at present involves symptomatic and supportive therapy. There is a general consensus among researchers and clinicians that in order to treat patients with MCS effectively, a double-blind, placebo-controlled study performed in an environmentally controlled facility, with rigorous documentation of both objective and subjective responses, is needed to help elucidate the nature and origin of MCS.

—*Shih-Wen Huang, M.D.*

See also Allergies; Asthma; Autoimmune disorders; Chronic fatigue syndrome; Dermatitis; Dermatology; Dizziness and fainting; Environmental diseases; Fatigue; Hay fever; Headaches; Host-defense mechanisms; Immune system; Immunology; Laryngitis; Lungs; Migraine headaches; Mold and mildew; Nasopharyngeal disorders; Nausea and vomiting; Occupational health; Pulmonary medicine; Rashes; Seizures; Sinusitis; Skin; Skin disorders; Sore throat.

FOR FURTHER INFORMATION:

Dwyer, John M. *The Body at War: The Miracle of the Immune System.* 2d ed. New York: Penguin Books, 1993.

Gaudin, Anthony J., and Kenneth C. Jones. *Human Anatomy and Physiology.* New York: Harcourt Brace Jovanovich, 1989.

Life, Death, and the Immune System. New York: W. H. Freeman, 1994.

Mazure, Carolyn, ed. *Does Stress Cause Psychiatric Illness?* Washington, D.C.: American Psychiatric Press, 1995.

Shaw, Michael, ed. *Everything You Need to Know About Diseases.* Springhouse, Pa.: Springhouse Press, 1996.

MULTIPLE SCLEROSIS
DISEASE/DISORDER

ANATOMY OR SYSTEM AFFECTED: Muscles, musculoskeletal system, nerves, nervous system, spine

SPECIALTIES AND RELATED FIELDS: Internal medicine, neurology, pediatrics

DEFINITION: A debilitating disease affecting the central nervous system.

CAUSES AND SYMPTOMS

Multiple sclerosis (MS) is a chronic and disabling disease of the nervous system. Symptoms can be mild, such as limb numbness, or severe, such as paralysis and loss of vision. How the disease will progress and its severity in specific individuals are difficult to predict because it progresses differently in each of its victims.

Multiple sclerosis is caused by degeneration of the nervous system. A fatty substance called myelin surrounds and protects many nerve fibers of the brain and spinal cord, the central nervous system. Myelin is important because it speeds up signals that move along the nerve fibers. In MS, the body attacks its own tissues, termed an autoimmune reaction, and a breakdown in the myelin layer along the nerves occurs. When any part of the myelin sheathing is destroyed, nerve impulses to and from the brain are slowed, distorted, or interrupted. The disease is called "multiple" because it affects many areas of the brain. Sclereids are hardened, scarred patches that form over the damaged areas of myelin.

The initial symptoms of MS may include tingling, numbness, slurred speech, blurred or double vision, loss of coordination, and muscle weakness. Later manifestations include unusual fatigue, muscle tightness, bowel and bladder control difficulties, sexual dysfunction, and paralysis. The most common cognitive functions influenced are short-term memory, abstract reasoning, verbal fluency, and speed of information processing. All the mental and physical symptoms listed may come or go in any combination. The symptoms may also vary from mild to severe in intensity throughout the course of the disease.

The symptoms of MS not only vary from person to person but also may periodically vary within the same person. This makes the prognosis of the disease difficult to foresee. Although the general course of the disease may be anticipated, the symptoms and their severity seem to be quite unpredictable in most individuals. In the "classic" course of MS, as time progresses, chronic problems gradually accumulate over many years, slowly worsening the sufferer's quality of life. The total level of disability will vary from patient to patient.

The typical pattern of MS is marked by active periods of the disease during which the nerves are being ravaged by the immune system. These periods are called attacks, relapses, or exacerbations. The active periods of the disease are followed by calm periods called remissions. The cycle of attack and remission will differ from sufferer to sufferer. Some people have few attacks, and their MS disabilities slowly accumulate over time; in these sufferers, it takes decades to become truly debilitated. Most people with MS have what is known as the relapsing-remitting form of the disease. They suffer many attacks over time, and these attacks occur unpredictably; the attacks are then followed by complete remission which may last months or years. Again, the injuries may take many years to accumulate to complete disability.

The most aggressive form of the disease is primary progressive MS. In this type of MS, the disease follows a rapid course that steadily worsens from its first onset. Although there are still attacks and partial remission, the attacks are quite severe and occur more regularly in time. Full paralysis may develop in primary progressive MS in three to five years. Secondary progressive MS occurs in patients who initially have the relapsing-remitting type and later develop the more aggressive form.

Both genetic and environmental factors have been implicated in inducing the onset of MS. Viral infection has been suggested as a cause, but no single virus has ever been shown to be associated with MS. Risk may be conferred by exposure to a specific environment during adolescence, but that environment and the genetic risk factors have not yet been characterized.

Researchers Sharon Lynch and John Rose suggested that certain racial and geographic populations are less susceptible than others to the disease. MS is uncommon in Japanese people as well as among American Indians. The disease is more common among Northern European Caucasians as well as among North Americans of higher latitudes. There is an additional sexual dimorphism in the epidemiology of MS; the disease is found more frequently in women, by a ratio of 2:1.

The disease usually begins its first manifestations in late adolescence (around age eighteen) to early middle age (around age thirty-five). It is not clear how the interaction between the genetics of the sufferer and the environment may trigger onset. The pro-gressive type of MS is more common over the age of forty, so those with late-onset MS often have the quickest deterioration of motor function. The reason that an older age predisposes someone to primary chronic progressive MS is still not clear.

Studies by Swiss researcher Avinoam Safran have shown that occasionally MS manifests after the age

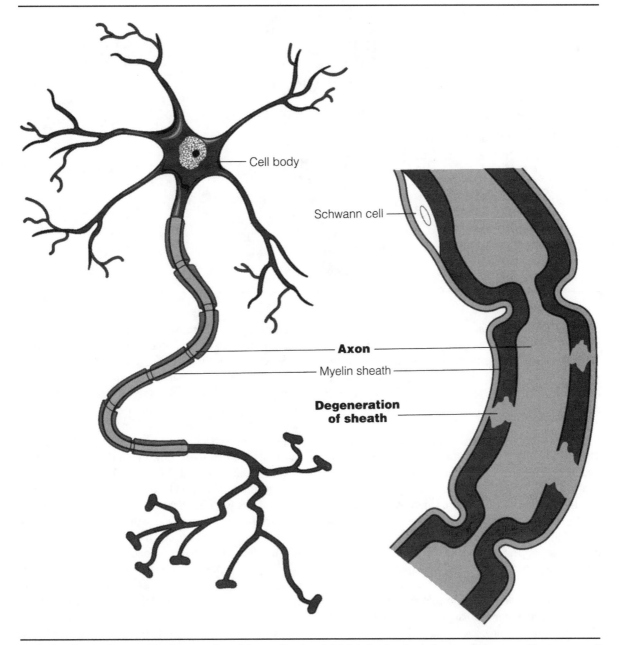

Cell body

Schwann cell

Axon

Myelin sheath

Degeneration of sheath

Multiple sclerosis is caused by degeneration of the myelin sheath (right) that insulates the axons of nerve cells; a nerve cell is shown on the left.

Effects of Multiple Sclerosis

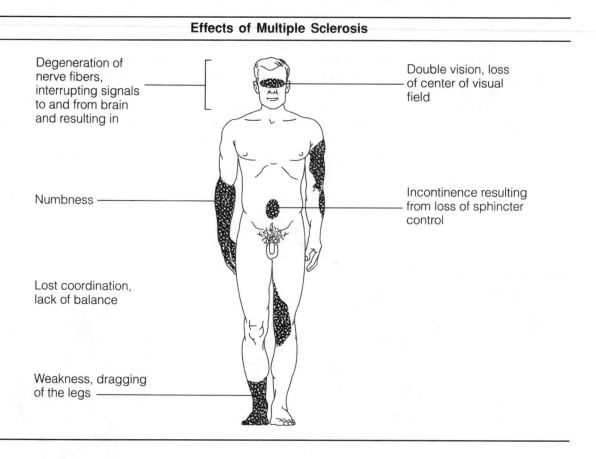

Degeneration of nerve fibers, interrupting signals to and from brain and resulting in

Double vision, loss of center of visual field

Numbness

Incontinence resulting from loss of sphincter control

Lost coordination, lack of balance

Weakness, dragging of the legs

of fifty. This condition has been named late-onset multiple sclerosis. Late-onset MS is not rare. Nearly 10 percent of MS patients demonstrate their first symptom after the age of fifty. This type of MS is often not recognized by physicians, who do not expect it in the aged.

TREATMENT AND THERAPY

There is no cure for MS, but there are many effective treatments. In most cases, steroidal drugs are used to treat relapses or attacks of the disease. Corticotropin was the first steroidal immunosuppressant to be used widely in MS treatment. The primary effect of the drug is to shorten the duration of an attack, although it does not appear to reduce the severity of the attack. Although it is still used with patients who respond well to it, corticotropin has been supplanted by other drugs. Methylprednisolone is an immunosuppressant and steroid that has replaced corticotropin. It has been shown to control the inflammation that accompanies demyelination. These steroids seem to work by sealing leaking blood vessels in the brain

and coating the white blood cells of the immune system so that they cannot attack the myelin as easily.

Several federally approved drugs can slow the rate of attacks: Avonex, Betaseron, and Copaxone. Although these drugs do not stop MS entirely, they actually limit the level of myelin destruction, as observed in magnetic resonance imaging (MRI) scans of the brain. Avonex slows down the rate of increased disability, and all three slow down the natural course of MS. University of Western Ontario researcher George Ebers performed experimental treatments on MS patients with interferons. Interferons are proteins produced by the immune system that enter cells and induce them to set up defenses against attack. The myelin sheath is actually produced by a special nerve cell called a schwann cell; presumably the schwann cells are stimulated to protect themselves by exposure to interferons. Patients treated with human interferons demonstrated a 34 percent reduction in frequency of attack; that reduction was sustained over five years of treatment. More impressive was the 80 percent reduction of MS activity detected in their brains. Steroid treatment was rarely required in these patients.

As additional therapy, patients with MS should participate in a regular exercise program. Exercise is vital to the maintenance of functional ability in MS sufferers. It strengthens muscles, benefits gait, and generally improves coordination. The best type of exercise is aquatic in nature. Sufferers are often heat-intolerant, and participation in a regular aerobic program would be unpleasant. Also, aquatic exercise is a low-impact activity that puts less stress on chronically sore muscles. Exercise programs also encourage socialization of patients and engender peer support.

PERSPECTIVE AND PROSPECTS

The first written report of MS was published in 1400 when the famed Dutch skater Lydwina of Schieden was diagnosed. It was recognized initially as a wasting disease of unknown origin. The disease was described clinically by Jean-Martin Charcot in 1877. Charcot initially characterized the clinical signs and symptoms of MS. He recognized that the disease affected the nervous system and tried many remedies, without success. In 1890, the cause of MS was thought to be suppression of sweat; the treatment was electrical stimulation and bed rest. At the time, life expectancy for a sufferer was five years after diagnosis. By 1910, MS was thought to be caused by toxins in the blood, and purgatives were alleged the best treatment. In the 1930's, poor circulation was believed to cause MS, and blood-thinning agents became the treatment of choice. In the 1950's through 1970's, MS was thought to be caused by severe allergies; treatments included antihistamines. Not until the 1980's was the basis of MS understood and effective treatment developed.

In the late 1990's, it was estimated that 400,000 Americans had this disorder of the brain and spinal cord, which causes disruption in the smooth flow of electrical messages from brain and nerves to the body. The progress of the disease is slow and may take decades to achieve complete nerve degeneration and paralysis. New, effective medical treatments are available to slow the advance of the disease. Although often considered a disease of youth, MS has the potential to become an increasing problem in aging populations. More cases of late-onset MS are coming to light in individuals over forty years of age, including such celebrities as comedian Richard Pryor, former Mouseketeer Annette Funicello, and talk-show host Montel Williams.

—*James J. Campanella, Ph.D.*

See also Amyotrophic lateral sclerosis; Muscle sprains, spasms, and disorders; Muscles; Nervous system; Neuralgia, neuritis, and neuropathy; Neurology; Paralysis; Spinal cord disorders; Spine, vertebrae, and disks.

In the News: Plasma Exchange Treatment

In a study supported by the National Institutes of Health, conducted at the Mayo Clinic and headed by Brian G. Weinshenker, M.D., plasma exchange was proven to be an effective new treatment for patients suffering from severe symptoms of multiple sclerosis (MS) who were not responsive to conventional methods of treatment. Plasma exchange involves the removal of the patient's blood, the separation of the plasma, which is then replaced by a fluid with similar properties, usually containing albumin, and its return to the patient. This procedure has been used for treatment of many other diseases in the past, but has never before been used as a treatment for MS. According to the Mayo Foundation for Medical Education and Research, "42 percent of people with MS and related conditions experienced moderate to marked improvement."

Though plasma exchange has been shown to be an effective new treatment for qualified patients, the exact reasons for its effectiveness are not known. However, researchers feel that further studies are warranted based on the idea that some people may have antibodies in their plasma that are instrumental in certain disease activities which allow disabilities to occur.

The results from Dr. Weinshenker's study of plasma exchange were presented at joint conference of the European and American Committees for Treatment and Research in MS on September 17, 1999, in Switzerland.

—*Chrissy Watkins and*
Massimo D. Bezoari, M.D.

FOR FURTHER INFORMATION:

Carroll, David L., and Jon D. Dorman. *Living Well with MS: A Guide for Patient, Caregiver, and Family*. New York: HarperPerennial Library, 1993. A book for any person affected by MS. Information ranges from how to buy a wheelchair to staying out of one.

Halbreich, Uriel. *Multiple Sclerosis: A Neuropsychiatric Disorder*. Boston: American Psychiatric Press, 1993. Describes the psychological conditions that often accompany multiple sclerosis.

Iams, Betty. *From MS to Wellness*. Chicago: Iams House, 1998. An autobiography of an MS sufferer who outlines treatments that have helped her overcome the disease.

Kalb, Rosalind, ed. *Multiple Sclerosis: The Questions You Have, the Answers You Need*. 2d ed. New York: Demos Vermande, 2000. A guide for everyone concerned about multiple sclerosis.

Larson, David E., ed. "Multiple Sclerosis." In *Mayo Clinic Family Health Book*. 2d ed. New York: William Morrow, 1996. A chapter in a text that discusses both muscles and bones, underscoring the intimate relationship between disorders in the two systems. The text and illustrations are complete and easy to understand.

Sibley, William. *Therapeutic Claims in Multiple Sclerosis: A Guide to Treatments*. 4th ed. New York: Demos Vermande, 1996. A guide to treatments available for MS and their effectiveness.

Taggart, Helen. "A Multiple Sclerosis Update." *Orthopaedic Nursing* 17, no. 2 (March/April, 1998). Provides a history of MS and its treatments from a nursing perspective.

Tapley, Donald T., et al., eds. *The Columbia University College of Physicians and Surgeons Complete Home Medical Guide*. Rev. 3d ed. New York: Crown, 1995. An outstanding reference guide organized by each organ system and its function. Written in easily understandable terms and avoids the use of medical jargon. Part 3 of the book provides in-depth information on how the body works and includes a full-color atlas showing major organ systems.

Tierney, Lawrence M., Jr., et al., eds. *Current Medical Diagnosis and Treatment: 2001*. 39th ed. New York: McGraw-Hill, 2000. This text, updated yearly, is the point of reference for physicians and other health care practitioners. It incorporates each year's biomedical research discoveries that have immediate, relevant, and applicable use for the patient.

MUMPS

DISEASE\DISORDER

ALSO KNOWN AS: Epidemic parotitis

ANATOMY OR SYSTEM AFFECTED: Genitals, glands, nervous system, pancreas

SPECIALTIES AND RELATED FIELDS: Family practice, pediatrics

DEFINITION: An acute, contagious childhood disease caused by a virus and characterized by swollen salivary glands.

KEY TERMS:

encephalitis: infection and inflammation of the brain

meningitis: infection and inflammation of the covering of the brain

orchitis: infection, inflammation, and swelling of a testicle or ovary; usually occurs only on one side and usually only in adults with mumps infection

parotitis: infection, inflammation, and swelling of the parotid gland, the major salivary gland, located near the angle of the jaw; this swelling will often push out the earlobe

CAUSES AND SYMPTOMS

Mumps infection is acquired after contact with infected respiratory secretions. An infected person can spread the disease from twelve to twenty-two days after infection. One case in a family generally means that every family member has been infected. Mumps is most commonly transmitted in the winter and early spring. During the sixteen- to eighteen-day incubation period, the virus grows first in the nose and throat, moves to the regional lymph nodes and then into the bloodstream, and spreads to multiple organs, including the central nervous system.

One-third of patients with mumps infection do not have symptoms or have very mild symptoms. Mumps is more severe after puberty. The first symptoms include fever, headache, stomach upset, loss of appetite, and a mildly congested nose. The most common finding is swelling of the salivary glands. This swelling usually starts on one side and then moves to both sides in three-quarters of cases. Salivary gland pain is most pronounced during the first few days and is associated with discomfort when eating or drinking acidic foods such as orange juice. Rarely, a thin red rash can occur. The fever usually resolves in three to five days, and the salivary gland swelling subsides within seven to ten days.

Between 1 and 10 percent of patients have clinical evidence of central nervous system infection, most commonly meningitis but very rarely encephalitis. Infection of the central nervous system is more common in males than in females. Central nervous system disease typically occurs one to three weeks after the onset of salivary gland swelling, but it can also precede or follow this swelling. Symptoms include headache, fever, lethargy, stiff neck, and vomiting. Seizures occur in 20 percent of hospitalized patients. Central nervous system infection is almost always limited, without any lasting effect or complications. Hearing loss occurs during mumps illness in 4 percent of patients but is not higher in those with central nervous system involvement. Higher-tone deficits are noted most frequently. Recovery from hearing loss usually occurs within a few weeks following onset. Persistent hearing loss is usually only one-sided.

Mumps

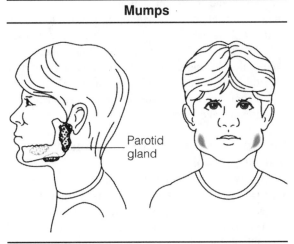

Mumps cause a characteristic swelling of the parotid (salivary) glands.

Orchitis, an infection of the testicles or ovaries, can also occur with mumps. The highest risk for this disease occurs after puberty, usually in males from fifteen to twenty-nine years of age. Between 14 and 35 percent of males with mumps infection develop orchitis. Fever, malaise, vomiting, and stomach pain are common symptoms. Testicular pain, swelling, and tenderness generally last for three to seven days. Involvement is one-sided in most cases. Symptoms usually began four to eight days following the onset of salivary gland swelling, but they can occur in the absence of gland swelling.

Mumps infection can cause other, less common complications. Infection of the kidney is almost al-

ways limited, but rare reports of kidney failure with mumps do exist. Multiple joint migratory arthritis with joint fluid has been described and is usually of short duration. Joint complaints are more common in males in their twenties. The usual signs of joint disease occur one to three weeks after the onset of salivary gland swelling. The large joints are more commonly affected.

Inflammation of the heart occurs in 4 to 15 percent of patients with mumps. It is most common in adults and generally resolves itself within two to four weeks. Infection and inflammation of the pancreas can occasionally occur. Pancreatitis can lead to fatty diarrhea and, very rarely, diabetes. Women who have mumps infection during pregnancy do not have an increased risk of delivering an infant with congenital malformation.

Very rarely, mumps will cause death. It is unclear why, prior to the advent of vaccination, mumps infection killed forty persons in the United States. More than 50 percent of deaths are of adults.

Not all patients with salivary gland swelling have mumps. Swelling in this area of the face may be attributable to another disease of the salivary gland or another disease affecting other tissues in the face such as lymph nodes or bones. Persistent or recurrent swelling of the parotid gland should be evaluated by a physician.

TREATMENT AND THERAPY

Conservative therapy is indicated for mumps infection. No antiviral therapy is available. Adequate fluids and nutrition are important. A patient's diet should avoid acidic foods and should be light and generous in fluids. Occasionally, mild pain medications may be necessary for severe headaches or salivary gland discomfort. Stronger pain medications may be needed with testicular involvement. In unusual cases where vomiting is severe, intravenous fluids may be required. A spinal tap (lumbar puncture) is rarely indicated, but patients who have this procedure frequently find that it relieves their headaches.

Exposure to mumps infection may cause anxiety in adult family members or day care employees. A child with mumps should be isolated for nine days after the start of salivary gland swelling. Vaccine administration will probably not prevent infection after exposure, and a history of family exposure to mumps probably indicates past infection. The physician will reassure any adult exposed family members and indicate that it is unlikely that the vaccine will prevent this disease. Nevertheless, exposure may dictate the need to administer the vaccine, as determining immune status is generally not practicable.

Mumps is a self-limited illness and does not require the administration of antiviral medications, antibiotics, or antibody preparations. Mumps vaccine should be given to children to prevent this disease. The combined vaccine containing measles, mumps, and rubella (MMR) vaccines should be given routinely to children from twelve months to eighteen months of age. About 98 percent of children will respond to this vaccine and not acquire mumps infection.

PERSPECTIVE AND PROSPECTS

The term "mumps" is derived from an English dialect meaning "grimace," attributed to the painful parotid gland swelling. The virus was first described in 1934, and a live vaccine was first licensed in 1967. Prior to 1980, the age group most affected by mumps was five to nine-year-olds. In the 1980's, this group shifted to children and adolescents aged ten to nineteen. In 1990's, most cases occurred in adults over twenty. This change was caused by the increased use of the mumps vaccine in children but not in adults.

Vaccination has been very successful, especially when combined with measles and rubella vaccine, given in the second year of life, and repeated prior to school. Side effects from mumps vaccine are extremely rare and can include anything that is seen in mumps infection. Recent research in the area has been directed toward determining whether the vaccine in its present form or in another form should be considered for administration both to decrease adverse reactions and to decrease its cost and improve its applicability to a broader population.

—Peter D. Reuman, M.D., M.P.H.

See also Childhood infectious diseases; Encephalitis; Fever; Glands; Immunization and vaccination; Infertility in males; Meningitis; Orchitis; Viral infections.

FOR FURTHER INFORMATION:

Bellenir, Karen, and Peter D. Dresser, eds. *Health Reference Series: Contagious and Noncontagious Infectious Diseases Sourcebook.* Detroit: Omnigraphics, 1997. A handy reference source on infectious diseases. Includes bibliographical references and an index.

Berkow, Robert, and Andrew J. Fletcher, eds. *The Merck Manual of Diagnosis and Therapy.* 17th ed. Rahway, N.J.: Merck, Sharpe & Dohme Research Laboratories, 1999. Contains a useful exposition of the characteristics, etiology, diagnosis, and treatment of mumps.

Clayman, Charles B., ed. *The American Medical Association Family Medical Guide.* New York: Random House, 1994. An excellent reference for the beginner. The scientific accuracy of the text is not compromised by its accessibility.

Rakel, Robert E., ed. *Conn's Current Therapy 2000.* Philadelphia: W. B. Saunders, 2000. Selecting a prominent team of physician authors for each standard category of medical illness, Rakel enables the attending physician reader to stay up-to-date on recent developments in disease etiology, workup, diagnosis, and treatment options.

Shaw, Michael, ed. *Everything You Need to Know About Diseases.* Springhouse, Pa.: Springhouse, 1996. This well-illustrated consumer reference, compiled by more than one hundred doctors and medical experts, describes five hundred illnesses and conditions, their causes, symptoms, diagnosis, treatment, and prevention.

MÜNCHAUSEN SYNDROME BY PROXY

DISEASE/DISORDER

ANATOMY OR SYSTEM AFFECTED: All

SPECIALTIES AND RELATED FIELDS: Ethics, family practice, pediatrics, psychiatry, psychology

DEFINITION: A disorder in which a parent fabricates, simulates, or induces a medical condition in a child in order to receive attention and acknowledgment as the source of information about the child's health.

KEY TERMS:

covert video surveillance: the monitoring of a child using video equipment in which the parent is unaware of the taping

narcissistic personality disorder: a disorder characterized by maladaptive patterns of behavior that are used to deal with common life situations

CAUSES AND SYMPTOMS

Münchausen syndrome by proxy may occur in different forms. In its least invasive form, this syndrome involves lying about a child's medical problems. For example, a father may claim that his child stopped breathing or had a seizure. The harm to the child comes from the medical studies that are ordered by the physician in an attempt to evaluate and diagnose the condition. A second situation involves the simulation of symptoms in the child. For example, a mother may maintain that her child is experiencing hematuria, and examination of the urine reveals the presence of blood. The blood comes not from the child but from some external source, such as the mother's menstrual blood or animal blood from packaged meat. Again, the child is subjected to needless diagnostic tests, some of which can be invasive.

The most injurious form of Münchausen syndrome by proxy comes when a parent induces the symptoms in the child. This can be done in many ways: The parent can administer syrup of ipecac to induce vomiting, administer substances such as diphtheria-pertussis-tetanus (DPT) vaccine to cause a fever, or inject fecal materials into already existing intravenous lines to induce a bacterial bloodstream infection. Parental induction of an apparent life-threatening event (ALTE) has been documented through the use of covert video surveillance. Parents have been observed placing their hands or other objects over the infant's face. Many of these children demonstrated bleeding from the mouth or gums, a finding not reported in any of the control infants who were experiencing an ALTE.

In addition to being subjected to multiple and invasive diagnostic procedures, some children die as a direct result of their parents' actions. Some families have a history of sudden or unexplained deaths of siblings that may be attributable to Münchausen syndrome by proxy or other types of child abuse.

TREATMENT AND THERAPY

A physician should become concerned about the possibility of Münchausen syndrome by proxy in a child with multiple health care visits in whom an explanation for the problems is elusive. The most common complaints include bleeding, vomiting, apnea, seizures, and fever. In each case, the chronic nature of the problems and the constant switching of health care providers should be clues. Statements by experienced physicians such as "I've never seen anything like this" should also signal that the child may be the victim of Münchausen syndrome by proxy. Some physicians become trapped in the process of ordering multiple studies for fear of missing an exotic disease.

On the other hand, some parents represent the "worried well." These people bring their children in for many minor complaints: every runny nose, low-grade temperature, or nonapparent skin rash. Their motivation is not personal attention. Rather, they are fearful and view their children as vulnerable.

The psychologic profile of the parent helps to distinguish the overly concerned mother from the one with Münchausen syndrome by proxy. The usual perpetrator is the child's mother. The father is often detached, distant, and not involved in the child's care, although cases in which the father is the perpetrator have been documented. Most perpetrators are believed to have borderline personalities and narcissistic personality disorders. They enjoy the attention that they receive in a medical setting. Medical staff members often characterize these individuals as excellent parents because they are knowledgeable about their child's health, attentive to their needs, and cooperative with the staff. Many of the mothers have some type of medical or science background, which facilitates their understanding medical conditions. Some have worked in physicians' offices, making them knowledgeable about medical terminology or procedures. Psychological assessment is needed to help define parental pathology. Members of the medical staff may be disbelieving of the diagnosis, since they often find the parent to be nice and helpful. Many parents deny the accusations and are resistant to psychiatric intervention.

The task of the medical team is to entertain the diagnosis, obtain evidence, and protect the child. In some institutions, covert video surveillance is used to catch the parent in the act of inflicting the symptoms. Although there is concern about issues of privacy, legal counsel at most institutions has supported the use of covert video surveillance because it assesses the situation of the child.

PERSPECTIVE AND PROSPECTS

Münchausen syndrome by proxy was initially described by Roy Meadow in 1977. In the twenty years after his initial report, more than three hundred cases were reported in the literature. The diversity of ways in which this syndrome is inflicted on children has expanded with each case report. In many cases, the prognosis for affected children is somewhat guarded because of the complexity of establishing the diagnosis on a legal level.

Once the child and the parent are separated, the symptoms resolve. Cases may be difficult to substantiate in court, without the presence of concrete evidence. Some children suffer from long-term sequelae, sometimes behaving like invalids because of the role in which they have been cast since childhood. There are reports of self-destructive behavior and Münchausen syndrome in some survivors. Psychological counseling is critical to ensure the well-being of these children. In most cases, the children cannot be returned to the parental perpetrator because of the intractable nature of the parent's problem.

—*Carol D. Berkowitz, M.D.*

See also Bacterial infections; Critical care; Critical care, pediatric; Domestic violence; Emergency medicine; Emergency medicine, pediatric; Fever; Hypochondriasis; Nausea and vomiting; Physical examination; Psychiatric disorders; Psychiatry; Psychiatry, child and adolescent; Psychosomatic illness.

FOR FURTHER INFORMATION:

Eminson, Mary, and R. J. Postlethwaite, eds. *Münchausen Syndrome by Proxy Abuse: A Practical Approach.* Boston: Butterworth-Heinmann, 2000. Aimed at the health professional, this book brings together a collection of essays discussing different aspects of this syndrome. Chapters deal with confirming factitious illness and the child protection process.

Rosenberg, D. A. "Munchausen Syndrome by Proxy." In *Child Abuse*, edited by Robert M. Reece. Philadelphia: Lea & Febiger, 1994. A discussion of the diagnosis and treatment of this abusive syndrome, in a text that includes bibliographical references and an index.

Southall, D. P., M. C. Plunkett, and M. W. Banks, et al. "Covert Video Recordings of Life-Threatening Child Abuse: Lessons for Child Protection." *Pediatrics* 100, no. 5 (November, 1997): 735-760. A descriptive, retrospective, partially controlled case study involving a total of thirty-nine children in whom hospital recordings were used to investigate suspicions of induced illness.

MUSCLE SPRAINS, SPASMS, AND DISORDERS

DISEASE/DISORDER

ANATOMY OR SYSTEM AFFECTED: Legs, ligaments, muscles, musculoskeletal system

SPECIALTIES AND RELATED FIELDS: Exercise physiology, family practice, osteopathic medicine, physical therapy, sports medicine

DEFINITION: Injuries, defects, or disorders of the muscles of the body.

CAUSES AND SYMPTOMS

There are three kinds of muscle tissue in the human body: smooth muscle, cardiac muscle, and striated muscle. Smooth muscle tissue is found around the intestines, blood vessels, bronchioles in the lung, and in other areas. These muscles are controlled by the autonomic nervous system, which means that their movement is not subject to voluntary action. They have many functions: They maintain the airway in the lungs, regulate the tone of blood vessels, and move foods and other substances through the digestive tract. Cardiac muscle is found only in the heart. Striated muscles are those that move body parts. They are also called voluntary muscles because they must receive a conscious command from the brain in order to work. They supply the force for physical activity, and they also prevent movement and stabilize body parts.

Muscles are subject to many disorders: Muscle sprains, strains, and spasms are common events in everyone's life and, for the most part, they are harmless, if painful, results of overexercise, accidents, falls, bumps, or countless other events. Yet these symptoms can also signal serious myopathies, or disorders within muscle tissue.

Myopathies constitute a wide range of diseases. They are classified as inflammatory myopathies or metabolic myopathies. Inflammatory myopathies include infections by bacteria, viruses, or other microorganisms, as well as other diseases that are possibly autoimmune in origin (that is, resulting from and directed against the body's own tissues). In metabolic myopathies, there is some failure or disturbance in the body's ability to maintain a proper metabolic balance or electrolyte distribution. These conditions include glycogen storage diseases, in which there are errors in glucose processing; disorders of fatty acid metabolism, in which there are derangements in fatty acid oxidation; mitochondrial myopathies, in which there are biochemical and other abnormalities in the mitochondria of muscle cells; endocrine myopathies, in which an endocrine disorder underlies muscular symptoms; and the periodic paralyses, which can be the result of inherited or acquired illnesses. This is only a partial list of the myopathies, the symptoms of which include weakness and pain.

Muscular dystrophies are a group of inherited disorders in which muscle tissue fails to receive nourishment. The results are progressive muscular weakness and the degeneration and destruction of muscle fibers. The symptoms include weakness, loss of coordination, impaired gait, and impaired muscle extensibility. Over the years, muscle mass decreases and the arms, legs, and spine become deformed.

Neuromuscular disorders include a wide variety of conditions in which muscle function is impaired by faulty transmission of nerve impulses to muscle tissue. These conditions may be inherited; they may be attributable to toxins, such as in food poisoning (for example, botulism) or by pesticide poisoning; or they may be side effects of certain drugs. The most commonly seen neuromuscular disorder is myasthenia gravis.

The muscular disorders most often seen are those that result from overexertion, exercise, athletics, accidents, and trauma. As a matter of fact, injuries sustained during sports and games have become so significant that sports medicine has become a recognized medical subspecialty. Besides the muscles, the parts of the body involved in these disorders include tendons (tough, stringy tissue that attaches muscles to bones), ligaments (tissue that attaches bone to bone), synovia (membranes enclosing a joint or other bony structure), and cartilage (soft, resilient tissue between bones). A sprain is an injury in which ligaments are stretched or torn. In a strain, muscles or tendons are stretched or torn. A contusion is a bruise that occurs when the body is subjected to trauma; the skin is not broken, but the capillaries underneath are, causing discoloration. A spasm is a short, abnormal contraction in a muscle or group of muscles. A cramp is a prolonged, painful contraction of one or more muscles.

Sprains can be caused by twisting the joint violently or by forcing it beyond its range of movement. The ligaments that connect the bones of the joint stretch or tear. Sprains occur most often in the knees, ankles, and arches of the feet. There is pain and swelling, and at least some immobilization of the joint.

A strain is also called a pulled muscle. When too great a demand is placed on a muscle, it and the surrounding tendons can stretch and/or tear. The main symptom is pain; swelling and muscle spasm may also occur.

Muscle spasms and cramps are common. Sometimes they occur spontaneously, such as the calf muscle cramps that occur at night. Sometimes they are attributable to muscle strain (the charley horse that tightens thigh muscles in runners and other athletes). Muscles that are used often will go into spasm, such

as those in the thumb and fingers of writers (writers' cramp), as can muscles that have remained in one position for too long. Muscle spasms and cramps can also occur as direct consequences of dehydration; they are common in athletes who perspire excessively during hot weather.

Some injuries to muscles and joints occur so regularly that they are named for the activities associated with them. A good example is tennis elbow, a condition that results from repeated, vigorous movement of the arm, such as swinging a tennis racket, using a paintbrush, or pitching a baseball. Runners' knee can afflict joggers and other athletes. It is usually caused by sprains in the knee ligaments; there is pain and there may be partial or total immobilization of the knee. Achilles tendinitis, as the name suggests, is inflammation of the Achilles tendon in the heel. It is usually the result of excessive physical activity that causes small tears in the tendon. Pain and immobility are symptoms. Tendinitis can occur in other joints as well; elbows and shoulders are common sites. Tenosynovitis is inflammation of the synovial membrane that sheathes the tendons in the hand. It may be caused by bacterial infection or may be attributable to overexertion.

Tumors and cancerous growths in muscle tissue are rare. If a lump appears in muscle, it is usually a lipoma, a fatty deposit that is benign. One tumor, called rhabdomyosarcoma, however, is malignant and can be fatal.

TREATMENT AND THERAPY

The myopathies are a wide group of diseases, and treatment varies considerably among them. The muscular dystrophies also vary in their treatment methods. Physical therapy is recommended to prevent contractures, the permanent, disfiguring muscular contractions that are a feature of the disease. Orthopedic appliances and surgery are also used. Because these diseases are genetic, it is sometimes recommended that people with a familial history of muscular dystrophy be tested for certain genetic markers that would suggest the possibility of disease in their children.

Myasthenia gravis is treated with drugs that increase the number of neurotransmitters available where nerves and muscles come together. The drugs help improve the transmission of information from the brain to the muscle tissue. In some cases, a procedure called plasmapheresis is used to eliminate blood-borne substances that may contribute to the disease. Surgical removal of the thymus gland is helpful in alleviating symptoms in some patients.

In treating the many muscle disorders that are caused by athletic activity and excessive wear and tear on the muscle, the R-I-C-E formula is recommended. The acronym stands for rest-ice-compression-elevation: The patient must rest and not use or exercise the limb or muscle involved; an ice pack is applied to the injury; compression is supplied by wrapping a moist bandage snugly over the ice, reducing the flow of fluids to the injured area; and the injured limb is elevated. If there is a fracture involved, the limb must be properly splinted or otherwise immobilized before elevation. The ice pack is held in place for twenty minutes and removed, but the bandage is held in place. Ice therapy can be resumed every twenty minutes.

Heat is also part of the therapy for strains and sprains, but it is not applied until after the initial swelling has gone down, usually after forty-eight to seventy-two hours. Heat raises the metabolic rate in the affected tissue. This brings more blood to the area, carrying nutrients that are needed for tissue repair. Moist heat is preferred, and it can be supplied by an electrical heating pad, a chemical gel in a plastic bag, or hot baths and whirlpools. In using pads and chemical gels, there should be a layer of toweling or other material between the heat source and the body. The temperature for a whirlpool or hot bath should be about 106 degrees Fahrenheit. Only the injured part should be immersed, if possible. As in the ice treatments, heat should be applied for twenty minutes and can be repeated after twenty minutes of rest.

Analgesics are given for pain. Over-the-counter preparations such as aspirin, acetaminophen, or ibuprofen are used most often. Sometimes, when pain is severe, more potent medications are required. Steroids are sometimes prescribed to reduce inflammation, and nonsteroidal anti-inflammatory drugs (NSAIDs) can alleviate both pain and inflammation. If a strained muscle or tendon is seriously torn or otherwise damaged, surgery may be required. Similarly, if a sprain involves torn or detached ligaments, they may have to be surgically repaired.

Muscle spasms and cramps may require both manipulation and the application of heat or cold. The affected limb is gently extended to stretch the contracted muscle. Massage and immersion in a hot bath are useful, as are cold packs.

Tennis elbow, runners' knee, and tendinitis respond to R-I-C-E therapy. Ice is applied to the injured site, and the limb is elevated and allowed to rest. When tenosynovitis is caused by bacterial infection, prompt antibiotic therapy may be necessary to avoid permanent damage. When it is attributable to overexertion, analgesics may help relieve pain and inflammation. Rarely, a corticosteroid is used when other drugs fail.

Often, the injured site requires physical therapy for the full range of motion to be restored. The physical therapist analyzes the patient's capability and develops a regimen to restore strength and mobility to the affected muscles and joints. Physical therapy may involve massage, hot baths, whirlpools, weight training, and/or isometric exercise. Orthotic devices may be required to help the injured area heal.

An important aspect of sports medicine and the treatment of sports-related muscle disorders is prevention. Many painful, debilitating, and immobilizing episodes can be avoided by proper training and conditioning, intelligent exercise practice, and restriction of exertion. Before undertaking any sport or strenuous physical activity, the individual is advised to warm up by gentle stretching, jogging, jumping, and other mild muscular activities. Arms can be rotated in front of the body, over the head, and in circles perpendicular to the ground. Knees can be lifted and pulled up to the chest. Shoulders should be gently rotated to relax upper-back muscles. Neck muscles are toned by gently and slowly moving the head from side to side and in circles. Back muscles are loosened by bending forward and continuing around in slow circles.

If a joint has been injured, it is important to protect it from further damage. Physicians and physical therapists often recommend that athletes tape, brace, or wrap susceptible joints, such as knees, ankles, elbows, or wrists. Sometimes a simple commercial elastic bandage, available in various configurations specific to parts of the body, is all that is required. Neck braces and back braces are used to support these structures.

Benign muscle tumors require no treatment, or may be surgically removed. Malignant tumors may require surgery, radiation, and chemotherapy.

PERSPECTIVE AND PROSPECTS

With the increased interest in physical exercise in the United States has come increasing awareness of the dangers of muscular damage that can arise from improper exercise, as well as of the cardiovascular risks that lie in wait for weekend athletes. Warm-up procedures are universally recommended. Individual exercisers, those in gym classes, professional athletes, and schoolchildren, are routinely taken through procedures to stretch and loosen muscles before they start strenuous activity.

Greater attention is being paid to the special needs of young athletes, such as gymnasts. Over the years, new athletic toys and devices have constantly been developed for the young: Skateboards, skates, scooters, and bicycles expose children to a wide range of bumps, falls, bruises, strains, and sprains. Protective equipment and devices have been designed especially for them: Helmets, padding, and special uniforms give children more security in accidents. Similarly, adults should take the time and trouble to outfit themselves correctly for the sports and athletics in which they engage: Joggers should tape, wrap, and brace their joints; and cyclists should wear helmets.

Nevertheless, the incidence of sport- and athletic-related muscular damage is relatively high, pointing to the necessity for increased attention to prevention. The growth of sports medicine as a medical specialty helps considerably in this endeavor. Physicians and nurses in this area are trained to deal with the various problems that arise, and they are often expert commentators on the best means to prevent problems.

—*C. Richard Falcon*

See also Amyotrophic lateral sclerosis; Ataxia; Bell's palsy; Beriberi; Cerebral palsy; Chronic fatigue syndrome; Dystrophy; Exercise physiology; Guillain-Barré syndrome; Hemiplegia; Hypertrophy; Kinesiology; Motor neuron diseases; Multiple sclerosis; Muscles; Muscular dystrophy; Neurology; Neurology, pediatric; Numbness and tingling; Osteopathic medicine; Palsy; Paralysis; Paraplegia; Parkinson's disease; Physical rehabilitation; Poliomyelitis; Ptosis; Quadriplegia; Rabies; Rheumatoid arthritis; Sarcopenia; Seizures; Speech disorders; Sphincterectomy; Sports medicine; Tendon disorders; Tendon repair; Tetanus; Tics; Torticollis; Weight loss and gain.

FOR FURTHER INFORMATION:

Dragoo, Jason J. *Handbook of Sports Medicine.* Tempe, Ariz.: Renaissance, 1993. Dragoo covers the wide range of sports- and athletics-related disorders with clarity and precision. The text is intended for the general reader, and the illustrations are simple and clear.

Kirkaldy-Willis, W. H., and T. N. Bernard, Jr. *Managing Low Back Pain.* 4th ed. Philadelphia: Churchill Livingstone, 1999. This book covers the anatomy, biomechanics, pathophysiology, diagnosis, and management of low back pain from the perspective of a variety of disciplines. The aim of the book is to "help all those involved in the treatment of patients suffering from low back and leg pain."

Larson, David E., ed. *Mayo Clinic Family Health Book.* 2d ed. New York: William Morrow, 1996. Discusses both muscles and bones, underscoring the intimate relationship between disorders in the two systems. The text and illustrations are complete and easy to understand.

Ryan, Allan J., and Fred L. Allman, eds. *Sports Medicine.* 2d ed. San Diego, Calif.: Academic Press, 1989. Directed to the professional, but the text can be understood by the layperson. Particularly useful in outlining the contemporary status of sports medicine and how it relates to the training and care of the athlete.

MUSCLES

ANATOMY

ANATOMY OR SYSTEM AFFECTED: Arms, gastrointestinal system, legs, ligaments, musculoskeletal system

SPECIALTIES AND RELATED FIELDS: Cardiology, exercise physiology, orthopedics, osteopathic medicine, physical therapy, sports medicine

DEFINITION: Cardiac muscle, skeletal muscle, and smooth muscle—all of which have the ability to contract, making possible body movement, peristalsis (the movement of food through the gastrointestinal system), and the circulation of blood throughout the body.

KEY TERMS:

cardiac muscle: a type of muscle, found only in the heart, that makes up the major portion of the heart; involved in the movement of blood through the body

muscle contraction: the shortening of a muscle, which may result in the movement of a particular body part

muscle fibers: elongated muscle cells that make up skeletal, cardiac, and smooth muscles

musculature: the arrangement of skeletal muscles in the body

skeletal muscle: a type of muscle that attaches to bone and causes movement of body parts; the only type that is under conscious, voluntary control

smooth muscle: a type of muscle found in the walls of internal organs such as the stomach, intestines, and urinary bladder; involved in the movement of food through the digestive tract

STRUCTURE AND FUNCTIONS

More than half of the body weight of humans is made up of muscle. Three types of muscles are found in the body: skeletal muscle, cardiac muscle, and smooth muscle. These muscles are composed of different types of muscle cells and perform different functions within the body. The characteristics and functions of each of these three muscle types will be discussed separately, starting with skeletal muscle.

Skeletal muscles attach to and cover bones. This type of muscle is often referred to as voluntary muscle because it is the only muscle type that can be controlled or made to move by consciously thinking about it. Skeletal muscles perform four important functions: bringing about body movement, helping to maintain posture, helping to stabilize joints such as the knee, and generating body heat.

Nearly all body movement is dependent upon skeletal muscle. Skeletal muscle is needed not only to be able to run and jump but also to speak, to write, and to move and blink the eyes. These movements are brought about by the contraction or shortening of skeletal muscles. These muscles are attached to two bones or other structures by tough thin strips or cords of tissue known as tendons. When a muscle contracts or shortens, it pulls the tendons, which then pull on the bones or other structures to which they are connected. In this way, the desired movement is brought about.

Skeletal muscles also aid in the maintenance of posture. Posture is defined as the ability to maintain a position of the body or body parts: for example, the ability to stand or to sit erect. The constant force of gravity must be overcome in order to maintain a standing or seated posture. Small adjustments to the force of gravity are constantly being made through slight contractions of skeletal muscle.

Skeletal muscles—or, more appropriately, their tendons—help to maintain joint stability. Many of the tendons that connect muscles to bones cross movable joints such as the knee and the shoulder. These tendons are kept taut by the constant contraction of the muscles to which they are attached. As a result, they act as walls to prevent the joints from dislocating or shifting out of the normal positions.

More than 40 percent of the human body is composed of skeletal muscle. Skeletal muscles generate heat as they contract. As a result, skeletal muscles are of extreme importance in maintaining normal body temperature. When the body is exposed to cold temperatures, it begins to shiver. This shivering is the result of muscle contractions, which serve to generate body heat and maintain the body's normal temperature.

Skeletal muscles are made up of skeletal muscle cells. These cells are long and tubular-shaped and therefore are referred to as skeletal muscle fibers. In some instances, these muscle fibers may be a foot long. When individual skeletal muscle fibers are viewed under a microscope, they display bands that are referred to as striations. For this reason, skeletal muscle is often called striated muscle.

Each skeletal muscle, depending upon its size, is made up of hundreds or thousands of skeletal muscle fibers. These muscle fibers are surrounded by a tough connective tissue that holds the muscle fibers together. These muscle fibers and their surrounding connective tissue form a skeletal muscle. In the human body, there are more than six hundred skeletal muscles. It is the arrangement of these muscles in the body that is referred to as the musculature, or muscle system.

Smooth muscles are often referred to as involuntary muscles because they cannot be made to contract by conscious effort. Smooth muscles are typically found in the walls of internal organs such as the esophagus, stomach, intestines, and urinary bladder. The primary function of smooth muscles in these organs is to enable the passage of material through a tube or tract. For example, the contraction of smooth muscles in the intestines helps to move digested materials through the digestive system.

Smooth muscle is composed of smooth muscle cells. These cells differ from skeletal muscle fibers in that they are short and spindle-shaped. They also differ from skeletal muscle cells in that they are not striated. Furthermore, smooth muscle cells usually are not surrounded by a tough connective tissue to form a muscle; instead, they are arranged in layers.

Cardiac muscle is found only in the heart. Like smooth muscle, cardiac muscle cannot be made to contract by means of conscious effort. Like skeletal muscle, however, cardiac muscle is striated. The contraction of cardiac muscle results in the contraction of the heart. This, in turn, results in the pumping of blood throughout the body.

Although many differences exist among skeletal, smooth, and cardiac muscle, all have one thing in common—their ability to contract. The methods by which this contraction is brought about in skeletal muscle, however, are different from those used by smooth muscle and cardiac muscle.

In order for skeletal muscles to contract, they must first be electrically stimulated. This electrical stimulation is brought about by nerves that are closely associated with the muscle fibers. Each muscle fiber has a branch of a nerve, known as an axon terminal, that lies very close to it. This axon terminal does not touch the muscle fiber, but is separated from it by a tiny space known as the synaptic cleft (or gap). An electrical impulse from the nerve causes the release of a chemical called a neurotransmitter into the synaptic cleft. The specific type of neurotransmitter for skeletal muscle is known as acetylcholine. The neurotransmitter will then pass through the synaptic cleft to the muscle fiber membrane, where it will bind to a special site known as a receptor. When the neurotransmitter binds to the receptor, it causes an electrical impulse to travel down the muscle fiber. This, in turn, causes the contraction of the muscle fiber. When most or all of the muscle fibers contract, the result is the contraction of the entire muscle.

The muscle fibers and muscle will remain in a contracted state as long as the neurotransmitter is bound to the receptor on the muscle fiber membrane. In order for the muscle fiber to relax, the neurotransmitter must be released from the receptor to which it is bound. This is accomplished by the destruction of the neurotransmitter. Another chemical, known as an enzyme, is released into the synaptic cleft. This enzyme destroys the neurotransmitter; thus, the neurotransmitter is no longer bound to the receptor. In skeletal muscle, this enzyme is called acetylcholinesterase, because it destroys the neurotransmitter acetylcholine.

The contraction of cardiac muscle differs from that of skeletal muscle in that each cardiac muscle fiber does not have an axon terminal associated with it. Cardiac muscle is capable of making its own electrical impulse; it does not need a nerve to initiate the electrical impulse for every cardiac muscle fiber. An impulse is started in a particular place in the heart, called the atrioventricular (A-V) node. This impulse spreads from muscle fiber to muscle fiber. Thus, each cardiac muscle fiber stimulates those fibers next to it. The electrical impulse spreads so fast that nearly all

the cardiac muscle fibers contract at the same time. As a result, the single impulse that began in the A-V node causes the entire heart to contract.

DISORDERS AND DISEASES

Any type of muscle disorder has the ability to disrupt the normal functions performed by muscles. Skeletal muscle disorders can disrupt body movement and the ability to maintain posture. If these disorders affect the diaphragm, the principal breathing muscle, they can also be fatal.

Perhaps the most common and least detrimental muscle disorder is disuse atrophy. When muscles are not used, the muscle fibers will become smaller, a process called atrophy. As a result of the decrease in the diameter of the muscle fibers, the entire muscle also becomes smaller and therefore weaker.

Disuse atrophy occurs in such circumstances as when an individual is sick or injured and must remain in bed for prolonged periods of time. As a result, the muscles are not used and begin to atrophy. Disuse atrophy is also fairly common in astronauts. This occurs as a result of the lack of gravity against which the muscles must work. If a muscle does not work against a load or force, such as gravity, it will tend to decrease in size.

In general, disuse muscle atrophy is easily treated. The primary treatment is to exercise the unused muscle. Physical activity, particularly those activities in which the muscle must work to lift or pull a weight, will result in an enlargement in the diameter of the skeletal muscle fibers, and thus of the entire muscle. The increase in the diameter of the muscle fibers and muscle is referred to as hypertrophy.

Another common muscle disorder is a muscle cramp. A muscle cramp is a spasm in which the muscle undergoes strong involuntary contractions. These involuntary contractions, which may last for as short a time as a few seconds or as long as a few hours, are extremely painful. Muscle cramps appear to occur more frequently at night or after exercise, but their cause is unknown. Treatment for cramps involves rubbing and massaging the affected muscle.

Muscles are often overused or overstretched. When this is the case, it is possible for the muscle fibers to tear. When the muscle fibers are torn, the result is a muscle strain, more often referred to as a pulled muscle. Although pulled muscles may be painful, they are usually not serious. Treatment for pulled muscles most often involves the resting of the affected muscle. If the muscle fibers are torn completely apart, surgery may be required to reattach the muscle fibers.

Among the more serious skeletal muscle disorders is muscular dystrophy. The term "muscular dystrophy" is used to define those muscle disorders that are genetic or inherited. These diseases most often begin in childhood, but a few cases have been reported to begin during adult life. Muscular dystrophy results in progressive muscle weakness and muscle atrophy. The most common form of muscular dystrophy is known as Duchenne muscular dystrophy. This form of muscular dystrophy primarily affects males. In those affected with Duchenne muscular dystrophy, muscular weakness and atrophy begin to appear at three to five years of age. There is a progressive loss of muscle strength and muscle mass such that, by the age of twelve, those individuals afflicted with the disorder are confined to a wheelchair. Usually between the ages of fourteen and eighteen, the patients develop serious and sometimes fatal respiratory diseases as a result of the impairment of the diaphragm, the primary breathing muscle. The progressive deterioration of the muscles cannot be stopped, but may be slowed with exercise of the affected muscles.

Myasthenia gravis is also a severe muscle disorder. This disease results in excessive weakness of skeletal muscles, a condition known as muscle fatigue. Those with myasthenia gravis complain of fatigue even after performing normal everyday body movements. Although severe, myasthenia gravis is usually not fatal unless the diaphragm is affected.

Myasthenia results from a decrease in the availability of the receptors for acetylcholine. If fewer acetylcholine receptors are available on the muscle fibers, less acetylcholine binds to the muscle fiber receptors; this binding is needed for contraction to occur. As a result, fewer muscle fibers within the muscle contract. The fewer muscle fibers within the entire muscle that contract, the weaker the muscle.

Myasthenia gravis affects about one in every ten thousand individuals. Unlike Duchenne muscular dystrophy, myasthenia gravis may affect any group, and, overall, women are affected more frequently than men. Myasthenia gravis is usually first detected in the facial muscles, particularly those of the eyes and eyelids. Those afflicted have droopy eyelids and experience difficulty in keeping the eyes open. Other symptoms are weakness in those muscles involved in chewing and difficulty swallowing as a result of

weakening of the tongue muscles. In most patients, there is also some weakening of the muscles of the legs and arms.

The prognosis for the treatment of myasthenia gravis is very good. The most important treatment for the disorder is the use of anticholinesterase drugs. These drugs inhibit the breakdown of acetylcholine. As a result, there is a large amount of acetylcholine in the neuromuscular junction to bind with the limited number of acetylcholine receptors. This, in turn, increases the ability and number of the muscle fibers that are able to contract, resulting in an increase in muscle strength and the ability to use the muscles without fatigue.

Also of interest is the effect of pesticides and the way in which they affect muscle function. Some pesticides are classified as organic pesticides that inhibit the enzyme acetylcholinesterase. If acetylcholinesterase is inhibited, it will no longer break down the acetylcholine that is bound to the receptor on the skeletal muscle membrane. If the acetylcholine is not removed from the receptor, the muscle cannot relax and is therefore in a constant state of contraction. As a result, the respiratory muscles are unable to contract and relax, a process required for breathing. Thus, organic pesticides function to prevent the respiratory muscles from working, and an affected animal will die as a result of not being able to breathe.

Muscle fibers also require a blood supply in order to keep them alive. If the blood supply to the muscle fibers is inhibited, death of the muscle fibers can result. If enough muscle fibers are affected, death of the muscle can result. This most commonly occurs in cardiac muscle. If the blood supply to the cardiac muscle making up the heart is reduced or cut off, the result is a decrease in the ability of the cardiac muscle to contract. This, in turn, leads to heart failure.

PERSPECTIVE AND PROSPECTS

The study of muscles and musculature is as old as the study of anatomy itself. The first well-documented study of muscles was done by Galen of Pergamum in the first century. Galen made drawings of muscles and described their functions. In all, Galen described more than three hundred muscles in the human body, almost half of all the muscles now known.

The first refined drawings and descriptions of the skeletal muscles of the body were made in the late fifteenth century. Among those who stood out as muscle anatomists during this period was Leonardo da Vinci. Leonardo's drawings of the skeletal muscles of the body were magnificent. His chief interest in the muscles of the body, like Galen's, was their function. He accurately described, among many other muscles, the muscles involved in the movement of the lips and cheeks.

A major step to the understanding of muscle physiology did not occur until the late eighteenth century. Luigi Galvani in 1791 discovered the relationship between muscle contraction and electricity when he found that an electrical current could cause the contraction of a frog leg. The use of electrical stimulation to study muscle contraction and function was fully utilized in the mid-1800's by Duchenne de Boulogne. The actual measurement of the electrical activity in a muscle came about in 1929, with the invention by Edgar Douglas Adrian and Detlev Wulf Bronk of the needle electrode, which could be placed into the muscle to record the muscle's electrical activity. This recording of the electrical activity of the muscle is known as an electromyogram, or EMG. Electromyograms are important in the evaluation of the electrical activity of resting and contracting muscles. Since the discovery of EMGs, they have been used by anatomists, muscle physiologists, exercise physiologists, and orthopedic surgeons to study and diagnose muscle diseases. Furthermore, the knowledge gained from EMGs has led to the making of artificial limbs that can be controlled by the electrical impulses of the existing muscles.

Knowledge of muscle names, muscle anatomy, and movement, as well as muscle physiology, is needed for many medical fields. These fields include kinesiology, the study of movement; physical and occupational therapy; the treatment and rehabilitation of those who are disabled by injury; exercise physiology and sports medicine, in which the effects of exercise on muscle and the damage of muscle as a result of sports injuries are studied; and, finally, orthopedic surgery, which is the surgical repair of damaged bones, joints, and muscles.

—*David K. Saunders, Ph.D.*

See also Acupressure; Amyotrophic lateral sclerosis; Anesthesia; Anesthesiology; Ataxia; Bed-wetting; Bell's palsy; Breasts, female; Cells; Cerebral palsy; Chronic fatigue syndrome; Exercise physiology; Glycolysis; Guillain-Barré syndrome; Head and neck disorders; Hemiplegia; Kinesiology; Lower extremities; Mastectomy and lumpectomy; Motor neuron diseases; Multiple sclerosis; Muscle sprains, spasms, and disorders; Muscular dystrophy; Myomectomy; Orthopedic surgery; Orthopedics; Orthopedics, pediatric; Osteopathic medicine; Palsy; Paralysis; Paraplegia; Parkinson's disease; Physical rehabilitation; Poisoning; Poliomyelitis; Ptosis; Quadriplegia; Rabies; Respiration; Sarcopenia; Seizures; Speech disorders; Sphincterectomy; Sports medicine; Steroid abuse; Tendon disorders; Tendon repair; Tetanus; Tics; Torticollis; Trembling and shaking; Upper extremities; Weight loss and gain.

FOR FURTHER INFORMATION:

Guyton, Arthur C., and John E. Hall. *Textbook of Medical Physiology.* 10th ed. Philadelphia: W. B. Saunders, 2000. This textbook gives many examples of diseases and pathological conditions of skeletal and cardiac muscle. The text does an excellent job of describing how diseases and pathologies affect the normal functioning of the muscle. Although somewhat technical at times, the text is well written and understandable.

Hole, John W., Jr. *Essentials of Human Anatomy and Physiology.* 6th ed. Dubuque, Iowa: Wm. C. Brown, 1993. An introductory college anatomy and physiology book that is easy to read and understand. Provides a good general overview of skeletal, cardiac, and smooth muscle anatomy and function.

Marieb, Elaine N. *Essentials of Human Anatomy and Physiology.* 6th ed. San Francisco: Benjamin/Cummings, 2000. An excellent place to begin the study of muscles and musculature. This text uses little technical jargon and explains the jargon it does use. Provides good descriptions and drawings of the most important muscles.

_____. *Human Anatomy and Physiology.* 5th ed. Redwood City, Calif.: Benjamin/Cummings, 2000. Provides a detailed look at muscles and their functions. The explanations of muscle physiology are easily understood. Contains not only drawings of skeletal muscle but also pictures of dissected specimens.

Tortora, Gerard J., and Sandra R. Grabowski. *Principles of Anatomy and Physiology.* 9th ed. New York: John Wiley & Sons, 2000. This text clearly explains the functions of many individual muscles. Furthermore, it provides many examples of clinical applications involving muscles, including diseases and the use of medical tests for the diagnosis of muscle disease.

MUSCULAR DYSTROPHY

DISEASE/DISORDER

ANATOMY OR SYSTEM AFFECTED: Legs, muscles, musculoskeletal system

SPECIALTIES AND RELATED FIELDS: Genetics, pediatrics, physical therapy

DEFINITION: A group of related diseases that attack different muscle groups, are progressive and genetically determined, and have no known cure.

KEY TERMS:

disease: an interruption, cessation, or disorder of a body function or system, usually identifiable by a group of signs and symptoms and characterized by consistent anatomical alterations

distal: situated away from the center of the body; the farthest part from the midline of the body

DNA (deoxyribonucleic acid): a type of protein found in the nucleus of a cell comprising chromosomes that contain the genetic instructions of an organism

dystrophin: both the gene and the protein that are defective in Duchenne muscular dystrophy

dystrophy: an improper form of a tissue or group of cells (literally, "bad nourishment")

enzyme: a protein secreted by a cell that acts as a catalyst to induce chemical changes in other substances, remaining apparently unchanged itself in the process

fiber: a slender thread or filament; the elongated, threadlike cells that collectively constitute a muscle

genetic: imparted at conception and incorporated into every cell of an organism

muscle: a bundle of contractile cells that is responsible for the movement of organs and body parts

muscle group: a collection of muscles that work together to accomplish a particular movement

CAUSES AND SYMPTOMS

Muscles, attached to bones through tendons, are responsible for movement in the human body. In muscular dystrophy, muscles become progressively weaker. As individual muscle fibers become so weak that they die, they are replaced by connective tissue, which is fibrous and fatty rather than muscular. These replacement fibers are commonly found in skin and scar tissue and are not capable of movement, and the muscles become progressively weaker. There are several different recognized types of muscular dystrophy. These have in common degeneration of muscle fibers and their replacement with connective tissue. They are distinguished from one another on the basis of the muscle group or groups involved and the age at which individuals are affected.

The most common type is Duchenne muscular dystrophy. In this disease, the muscles involved are in the upper thigh and pelvis. The disease strikes in early childhood, usually between the ages of four and seven. It is known to be genetic and occurs only in boys. Two-thirds of affected individuals are born to mothers who are known to carry a defective gene; one-third are simply new cases whose mothers are genetically normal. Individuals afflicted with Duchenne muscular dystrophy suffer from weakness in their hips and upper thighs. Initially, they may experience difficulty in sitting up or standing. The disease progresses to involve muscle groups in the shoulder and trunk. Patients lose the ability to walk during their early teens. As the disease progresses, portions of the brain become affected, and intelligence is reduced. Muscle fibers in the heart are also affected, and most individuals die by the age of twenty.

The dystrophin gene normally produces a very large protein called dystrophin that is an integral part of the muscle cell membrane. In Duchenne muscular dystrophy, a defect in the dystrophin gene causes no dystrophin or defective dystrophin to be produced, and the protein will be absent from the cell membrane. As a result, the muscle fiber membrane breaks down and leaks, allowing fluid from outside of the cell to enter the muscle cell. In turn, the contents of affected cells are broken down by other chemicals called proteases that are normally stored in the muscle cell. The dead pieces of muscle fiber are removed by scavenging cells called macrophages. The result of this process is a virtually empty and greatly weakened muscle cell.

A second type is Becker's muscular dystrophy, which is similar to the Duchenne form of the disease. Approximately 3 in 200,000 people are affected, and it too is found only among males. The major clinical difference is the age of onset. Becker's muscular dystrophy typically first appears in the early teenage years. The muscles involved are similar to those of Duchenne muscular dystrophy, but the course of the disease is slower. Most individuals require the use of a wheelchair in their early thirties and eventually die in their forties.

Myotonic dystrophy is a form of muscular dystrophy that strikes approximately 5 out of 100,000 people in a population. Myotonia is the inability of a muscle group to relax after contracting. Individuals with myotonic dystrophy experience this difficulty in their hands and feet. On average, the disease first appears at the age of nineteen. The condition is benign, in that it does not shorten an affected person's life span. Rather, it causes inconveniences to the victim. Affected persons also experience a variety of other problems, including baldness at the front of the head and malfunction of the ovaries and testes. The muscles of the stomach and intestines can become involved, leading to a slowing down of intestinal functions and diarrhea.

Another type is limb girdle muscular dystrophy. The muscles of both upper and lower limbs—the shoulders and the pelvis—are involved. The onset of this dystrophy form is variable, from childhood to middle age. While the disorder is not usually fatal, it does progress, and victims experience severe disabil-

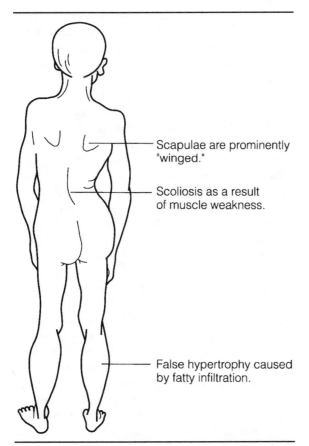

Scapulae are prominently "winged."

Scoliosis as a result of muscle weakness.

False hypertrophy caused by fatty infiltration.

Duchenne muscular dystrophy, the most common type, is characterized by prominently "winged" scapulae, scoliosis, false hypertrophy of the calves, and other less visible effects; children are the victims, usually not surviving beyond age twenty.

ity about twenty years after the disease first appears. While this variant is also genetically transmitted, men and women are about equally affected.

One type of muscular dystrophy found almost exclusively among individuals of Scandinavian descent is called distal dystrophy. It first appears relatively early in adult life, between the thirties and fifties. The muscles of the forearm and hand become progressively weaker and decrease in size. Eventually, the muscles of the lower leg and foot also become involved. This form of muscular dystrophy is not usually fatal.

Oculopharyngeal muscular dystrophy is a particularly serious form that involves the muscles of the eyes and throat. In this disease, victims are affected in their forties and fifties. There is progressive loss of control of the muscles that move the eyes and loss of the ability to swallow. Death usually results from starvation or from pneumonia acquired when the affected individual accidentally inhales food or drink.

A type of muscular dystrophy for which the location of the genetic abnormality is known is facioscapulohumeral muscular dystrophy; the defect is confined to the tip of the fourth chromosome. This disease initially involves the muscles of the face and later spreads to the muscles of the posterior or back of the shoulder. Eventually, muscles in the upper thigh are involved. The affected person loses the ability to make facial expressions and assumes a permanent pout as a result of loss of muscle function. As the condition advances, the shoulder blades protrude when the arms are raised. Weakness and difficulty walking are eventually experienced. As with other forms of muscular dystrophy, there is some variability in the degree to which individuals are affected. Occasionally, a variety of deafness occurs involving the nerves that connect the inner ear and the brain. Less commonly, victims become blind.

There are other variants of muscular dystrophy that have been recognized and described. These forms of the disease, however, are rare. The main problem facing physicians is differentiating accurately the variety of muscular dystrophy seen in a particular patient so as to arrive at a correct diagnosis.

TREATMENT AND THERAPY
The diagnosis of muscular dystrophy is initially made through observation. Typically, parents notice changes in their affected children and bring these concerns to the attention of a physician. The physician takes a

careful family history and then examines a suspected victim to make a tentative or working diagnosis. Frequently, knowledge of other family members with the condition and observations are sufficient to establish a firm diagnosis. Occasionally, a physician may elect to order physiological or genetic tests to confirm the tentative diagnosis. As Duchenne muscular dystrophy is the most common form of muscular dystrophy, it provides a convenient example of this process.

A diagnosis of Duchenne or any other form of muscular dystrophy is rarely made before the age of three. This form of the disease almost always occurs in boys. (Variants, rather than true Duchenne muscular dystrophy, are seen in girls, but this situation is extremely rare.) The reason for this finding is that the genetic defect occurs on the X chromosome that is found only in males. Approximately two-thirds of all victims inherit the defective chromosome from their mothers, who are asymptomatic carriers; thus, the condition is recessive and said to be X-linked. The disease occurs in the remaining one-third of victims as a result of a fresh mutation, in which there is no family history of the disease and the parents are not carriers.

Victims usually begin to sit, walk, and run at an older age than normally would be expected. Parents describe walking as waddling rather than the usual upright posture. Victims have difficulty climbing stairs. They also have apparently enlarged calf muscles, a finding called muscular hypertrophy. While the muscles are initially strong, they lose their strength when connective and fatty tissues replace muscle fibers. The weakness of muscles in the pelvis is responsible for difficulties in sitting and the unusual way of walking. Normal children are able to go directly from a sitting position to standing erect. Victims of Duchenne muscular dystrophy first roll onto their stomachs, then kneel and raise themselves up by pushing their hands against their shins, knees, and thighs; they literally climb up themselves in order to stand. These children also have a pronounced curvature of their lower backs, an attempt by the body to compensate for the weakness in the muscles of the hips and pelvis.

There is frequently some weakness in the muscles of the shoulder. This finding can be demonstrated by a physician, but it is not usually seen by parents and is not an early problem for the victim. A physician tests for this weakness by lifting the child under the armpits. Normal children will be able to support themselves using the muscles of the shoulder. Indi-

viduals with Duchenne muscular dystrophy are unable to hold themselves up and will slip through the physician's hands. Eventually, these children will be unable to lift their arms over their heads. Most victims of Duchenne muscular dystrophy are unable to walk by their teen years. The majority die before the age of twenty, although about one-quarter live for a few more years. Most victims also have an abnormality in the muscles of the heart that leads to decreased efficiency of the heart and decreased ability to be physically active; in some cases, it also causes sudden death. Most victims of Duchenne muscular dystrophy suffer mental impairment. As their muscles deteriorate, their measured intelligence quotient (IQ) drops approximately twenty points below the level that it was at the onset of the disease. Serious mental handicaps are experienced by about one-quarter of victims.

Other forms of muscular dystrophy are similar to Duchenne muscular dystrophy. Their clinical courses are also similar, as are the methods of diagnosis. The critical differences are the muscles involved and the age of onset.

Laboratory procedures used to confirm the diagnosis of muscular dystrophy include microscopic analysis of muscle tissue, measurement of enzymes found in the blood, and measurement of the speed and efficiency of nerve conduction, a process called electromyography. Some cases have been diagnosed at birth by measuring a particular enzyme called creatinine kinase. It is possible to diagnose some types of muscular dystrophy before birth with chorionic villus sampling or amniocentesis.

There is no specific treatment for any of the muscular dystrophies. Physical therapy is frequently ordered and used to prevent the remaining unaffected muscles from losing their tone and mass. In some stages of the disease, braces, appliances, and orthopedic surgery may be used. These measures do not reverse the underlying pathology, but they may improve the quality of life for a victim. The cardiac difficulties associated with myotonic dystrophy may require treatment with a pacemaker. For victims of myotonic dystrophy, some relief is obtained by using drugs; the most commonly used pharmaceuticals are phenytoin and quinine. The inability to relax muscles once they are contracted does not usually present a major problem for sufferers of myotonic dystrophy.

More useful and successful is prevention, which involves screening individuals in families or kinship groups who are potential carriers. Carriers are persons who have some genetic material for a disease or condition but lack sufficient genes to cause an apparent case of a disease or condition; in short, they appear normal. When an individual who is a carrier conceives a child, however, there is an increased risk of the offspring having the disease. Genetic counseling should be provided after screening, so that individuals who have the gene for a disease can make more informed decisions about having children.

Chemical tests are available for use in diagnosing some forms of muscular dystrophy. Carriers of the gene for Duchenne muscular dystrophy can be detected by staining a muscle sample for dystrophin; a cell that is positive for Duchenne muscular dystrophy will have no stained dystrophin molecules. The dystrophin stain test is also used to diagnose Becker's muscular dystrophy, but the results are not quite as consistent or reliable. Approximately two-thirds of carriers and fetuses at risk for both forms of muscular dystrophy can be identified by analyzing DNA. Among individuals at risk for myotonic dystrophy, nine out of ten who carry the gene can be identified with DNA analysis before they experience actual symptoms of the disease.

PERSPECTIVE AND PROSPECTS

Muscular dystrophy has been recognized as a medical entity for several centuries. Initially, it was considered to be a degenerative disease only of adults, and it was not until the nineteenth century that the disease was addressed in children with Guillaume-Benjamin-Amand Duchenne's description of progressive weakness of the hips and upper thighs. An accurate classification of the various forms of muscular dystrophy depended on accurate observation and on the collection of sets of cases. Correct diagnosis had to wait for the development of accurate laboratory methods for staining muscle fibers. The interpretation of laboratory findings depended on the development of biochemical knowledge. Thus, much of the integration of knowledge concerning muscular dystrophy is relatively recent.

Genes play an important role in the understanding of muscular dystrophy. All forms of muscular dystrophy are hereditary, although different chromosomes are involved in different forms of the disease. The development of techniques for routine testing and diagnosis has also occurred relatively recently. Specific chromosomes for all forms of muscular dystrophy

have not yet been developed. Considering initial successes of the Human Genome Project, an effort to identify all human genes, it seems likely that more precise genetic information related to muscular dystrophy will emerge.

There still are no cures for muscular dystrophies, and many forms are relentlessly fatal. Cures for many communicable diseases caused by bacteria or viruses have been discovered, and advances have been made in the treatment of cancer and other degenerative diseases by identifying chemicals that cause the conditions or by persuading people to change their lifestyles. Muscular dystrophy, however, is a group of purely genetic conditions. Many of the particular chromosomes involved are known, but no techniques are yet available to cure the disease once it is identified.

The availability of both a mouse model and a dog model of Duchenne muscular dystrophy, however, has facilitated the testing of gene therapy for this disease. Dystrophic mouse early embryos have been cured by injection of a functional copy of the dystrophin gene; however, this technique must be performed in embryos and is not useful for human therapy. Two avenues of research underway in these animal models are the introduction of normal muscle-precursor cells into dystrophic muscle cells and the direct delivery of a functional dystrophin gene into dystrophic muscle cells. It is hoped that these studies will lead to a cure for the disease.

In the meantime, muscular dystrophy continues to cause human suffering and to cost victims, their families, and society large sums of money. The disease is publicized on an annual basis via efforts to raise money for research and treatment, but there is little publicity on an ongoing basis. For these reasons, muscular dystrophy remains an important medical problem in contemporary society.

—*L. Fleming Fallon, Jr., M.D., Ph.D., M.P.H.;*
updated by Karen E. Kalumuck, Ph.D.

See also Dystrophy; Genetic counseling; Genetic diseases; Genetics and inheritance; Hypertrophy; Muscle sprains, spasms, and disorders; Muscles; Pediatrics; Physical rehabilitation; Screening.

FOR FURTHER INFORMATION:

Behrman, Richard E., ed. *Nelson Textbook of Pediatrics.* 16th ed. Philadelphia: W. B. Saunders, 2000. The forms of muscular dystrophy found in children are discussed in a logical and complete format.

Pictures clearly depict the difficulties in movement experienced by victims of Duchenne muscular dystrophy.

Bennett, J. Claude, et al., eds. *Cecil Textbook of Medicine*. 21st ed. Philadelphia: W. B. Saunders, 2000. The descriptions of muscular dystrophy are clear and detailed. The language used in the book is precise. Using multiple authors, each section is written by an internationally recognized expert.

Berkow, Robert, and Andrew J. Fletcher, eds. *The Merck Manual of Diagnosis and Therapy*. 17th ed. Rahway, N.J.: Merck Sharp & Dohme Research Laboratories, 1999. The more common forms of muscular dystrophy are discussed in clear, relatively nontechnical language. The entries are brief and succinct. This work is useful for an overview of muscular dystrophy; the more unusual and rarer forms of muscular dystrophy are not included.

Brown, Susan S., Jack A. Lucy, and Susan C. Brown, eds. *Dystrophin: Gene, Protein, and Cell Biology*. Cambridge, England: Cambridge University Press, 1997. This compilation of the latest research into the causes of muscular dystrophy at the molecular level is suitable for the nonspecialist with an introductory background in biology, as well as the specialist and clinician dealing with patients and their families affected by the disorder.

Robbins, Stanley L., Ramzi S. Cotran, and Vinay Kumar, eds. *Robbins' Pathologic Basis of Disease*. 6th ed. Philadelphia: W. B. Saunders, 1999. A complete discussion about the pathology of several forms of muscular dystrophy. Technical language is employed, but the book is well written. Photographs of microscopic sections of muscle are included, as well as descriptions of the clinical course of muscular dystrophy.

Tierney, Lawrence M., Jr., et al., eds. *Current Medical Diagnosis and Treatment: 2001*. 39th ed. New York: McGraw-Hill, 2000. In a brief and concise format, the diagnosis and management of muscular dystrophy are discussed. The section authors are recognized experts in their fields. Treatment protocols are included.

MUTATION

BIOLOGY

ANATOMY OR SYSTEM INVOLVED: Cells, immune system

SPECIALTIES AND RELATED FIELDS: Cytology, genetics, pathology

DEFINITION: An error in the process that copies genetic information for each new generation, resulting in an alteration in the organism that can be beneficial, harmful, or neutral.

KEY TERMS:

alleles: alternate forms of a gene; each person has two alleles of each gene, and these alleles may be the same or different; a person inherits one allele from each parent

chromosomes: the parts of a cell that contain genetic information, made of DNA covered with protein; each human cell has twenty-three pairs of chromosomes

deoxyribonucleic acid (DNA): a long, spiral-shaped molecule that makes up the bulk of chromosomes; the sequence of subunits contains the genetic information of the cell and organism

gene: the basic unit of inheritance; at the molecular level, a gene consists of a segment of DNA that codes for a particular protein

genotype: the genetic makeup of an individual; it is usually expressed as a list of alleles

heterozygous: having two different alleles for a particular gene

homozygous: having two identical alleles of a particular gene

meiosis: a special kind of cell division whereby four cells are produced; each cell has only half of the original number of chromosomes; meiosis produces the sex cells (eggs and sperm)

nucleotides: the subunits from which DNA is made

THE FUNCTION OF GENES

An individual is not a random assortment of characteristics. The way in which individuals look, their physiological makeup, their susceptibility to disease, and even how long they may live are determined by information received from their parents. The smallest unit of information for inherited characteristics is the gene. For each characteristic, an individual has two copies of the gene controlling that characteristic. The gene can have two forms, called alleles. For example, the alleles for eye color can be designated using the letters B and b, with the B allele carrying the information for brown eyes and the b allele specifying blue eyes. Thus the genotype, or genetic makeup, of an individual can be one of three types: BB, bb, or Bb. A BB individual will have brown eyes. A bb person will have blue eyes. A Bb individual will have brown eyes since the brown allele is dominant over the blue one. The dominant allele will always be expressed, whether present as two copies or only one. For a recessive allele to be expressed, an individual must have two recessive alleles (bb).

When a person reproduces, he or she passes on one allele for each gene to the child. Therefore, the child also has two alleles for each gene, one from each parent. A person with two identical alleles for a given gene is said to be homozygous for that trait and can pass on only one kind of allele. Someone with two different alleles for a particular gene is said to be heterozygous. A heterozygous person will pass on the dominant allele to 50 percent of his or her children, on average; the other 50 percent will receive the recessive allele. Alleles are passed on in the sex cells—the eggs and sperm. Eggs and sperm are produced by a special type of cell division, meiosis, that reduces by half the amount of genetic information carried by the cell. When an egg is fertilized by a sperm cell, the amount of genetic information is once again doubled. In "normal" cell division, called mitosis, the amount of genetic material in each cell is kept constant. After fertilization, the egg cell divides repeatedly by mitosis to produce the millions of cells that make up the embryo and later the adult organism.

If the genetic makeup of a couple for a given trait is known, the probable characteristics of their children for this trait can be predicted. For example, one can predict the eye color for children of a brown-eyed husband and blue-eyed wife. Assuming that the husband comes from a family of only brown-eyed people, one can be fairly certain that he is homozygous for this trait (BB). Since his wife has blue eyes, and blue is recessive, she must be homozygous for the other allele (bb). Their children will each have a brown allele from their father and a blue allele from their mother; they will all be heterozygous (Bb). Since brown is dominant, they will all have brown eyes.

One can take this example a step further and predict the outcome for the next generation. If one of this couple's brown-eyed sons marries a blue-eyed wife, one can predict the eye colors of their children using a simple diagram called a Punnett square. (Reginald Crundall Punnett contributed much to the early study of genetics.)

Using this simple tool, with the possible alleles in the sperm cells along the top and those from the eggs down the side, one can show all the possible combinations of inherited alleles (see figure 1). These

Figure 1. A Punnett Square Showing Alleles for Eye Color

		Father's Sperm Cells	
		B	b
Mother's Egg Cells	b	Bb	bb
	b	Bb	bb

boxes represent the genotypes of the fertilized eggs. In this case, one would expect about half of their children to have brown eyes (the Bb boxes) and half to have blue eyes (the bb boxes). Since chance determines exactly which sperm actually fertilizes the egg in every conception event, however, such a prediction is not always accurate. Nevertheless, the more children they have, the closer the actual percentage of brown-eyed or blue-eyed children will come to half.

Actually, the inheritance of eye color is somewhat more complicated than it is described above. Several genes contribute to eye color. Depending on the mix of dominant and recessive alleles for each gene involved, eye color can range from pale blue to dark brown. Other combinations produce green eyes.

In addition, many genes do not show complete dominance. For example, evidence shows that height is controlled by several genes that exhibit incomplete dominance. One homozygous individual (TT) will be tall, the other (tt) will be short, and the heterozygous individual (Tt) will be of medium height. The laws that determine how the alleles may be passed on from generation to generation, however, are exactly the same. One can use a simplified example of two people who are heterozygous for a hypothetical height gene (see figure 2, following page).

Since both parents are heterozygous, each will be able to produce two kinds of sex cells, those with "tall" alleles and those with "short" alleles. From all the possible outcomes shown in the boxes of the Punnett square, one would predict 25 percent tall (TT), 25 percent short (tt), and 50 percent medium-height (Tt) children.

If several genes are involved, a wide range of heights is possible. A person who is homozygous for the "tall" alleles in most of the height genes will be

Figure 2. A Punnett Square Showing Alleles for Height

		Father's Sperm Cells	
		T	t
Mother's Egg Cells	T	TT	Tt
	t	Tt	tt

very tall. Someone homozygous for most of the "short" alleles will be short. Someone who is heterozygous in most of these genes will be of medium height. Since even relatively short people will have some "tall" alleles, and since chance determines which sex cells are actually used, it is possible for two short people to have a tall child: By chance, the egg and sperm that united had more than the usual share of "tall" alleles.

The preceding examples have used genes that have only two alleles: brown or blue, tall or short. There are genes, however, for which more than two alleles are possible—although any one individual may have only two alleles in his or her genetic makeup. A good example of such a gene is the one that controls human blood type. There are three blood type alleles: A, B, and O. The A and B alleles are dominant, while the O allele is recessive. This allows for the various types of blood (see table).

This table allows one to see the mechanism of dominance. A person with an A allele produces a particular chemical in the blood. Similarly, the B allele causes the production of a different chemical. The O allele produces no chemical at all. If a chemical not already present in the blood is introduced, such as in a blood transfusion, the body will react against it, destroying the new blood. Since people with type O blood produce neither chemical, they are sometimes referred to as "universal donors." Their blood can be given safely to anyone. Similarly, people with AB blood can receive any other blood type because their bodies already contain both types of chemical.

One can also use a blood type example to show how parents can produce children that are genetically unlike both parents. The mother has type A blood and is heterozygous (AO), while the father has type B blood and is also heterozygous (BO). Their child could have any of the four blood types (see figure 3).

Although blood type is not an obvious visible feature, many genes that express themselves in an individual's appearance behave in a similar manner. Therefore, one should not be surprised to see two parents with a child who resembles neither of them.

The genes that control heredity actually consist of strands of deoxyribonucleic acid (DNA) that make up the chromosomes. Humans have twenty-three pairs of chromosomes in each cell. This explains how an individual can have two alleles for each gene, one on each chromosome of a pair. The exception is the sex chromosomes, which are different in males and females. Sex chromosomes come in two kinds, a relatively large X and a small Y. The X chromosomes can carry many more genes than the Y. Females have two X chromosomes and thus have two alleles for every gene found on the X chromosome. Males have only one X chromosome; therefore, they only have one allele for those genes carried on the X. The Y chromosome of the male has been shown to carry very little, although important, genetic information. Genes carried on the X chromosome are called sex-linked, since they typically are expressed in only one sex—the male. Females may be merely carriers of a sex-linked trait.

One sex-linked trait is the disorder called hemo-

The Relationship Between Genotype and Blood Type

Genotype	Blood Type	Comments
AA	A	These two genotypes produce identical blood types.
AO	A	
BB	B	These two genotypes produce identical blood types.
BO	B	
AB	AB	Both dominant alleles are expressed.
OO	O	With no dominant alleles, the recessive allele is expressed.

Figure 3. A Punnett Square Showing Alleles for Blood Type

		Father's Sperm Cells	
		B	O
Mother's Egg Cells	A	AB (AB blood)	AO (A blood)
	O	BO (B blood)	OO (O blood)

philia. A hemophiliac fails to produce a chemical which allows the blood to clot. This disorder is usually fatal if the hemophiliac is not constantly supplied with the clotting factor. Such an individual would simply bleed to death following even the slightest injury. Suppose that a woman who carries the trait for hemophilia marries a man who does not have the disorder. Hemophilia is a recessive condition; therefore, the woman has one normal X chromosome and one bearing the recessive allele (denoted by X_h). Since the normal allele directs the production of the clotting factor, her blood can clot and she is perfectly normal. Since her husband is not a hemophiliac, his one X chromosome must bear the normal allele. One can use a Punnett square to predict the likelihood of their children inheriting the disease (see figure 4). From this figure, one can see that their daughters should all be normal. About half of them will be carriers for the trait, but there is no way of knowing which ones they are. Of the sons, one half will be normal and the other half will suffer from hemophilia.

HOW MUTATIONS OCCUR

There is a variety of genetic information in the human population, leading to a diversity of internal and external features. The process of sexual reproduction randomly selects among that variety for each new individual who is born. Mutation is the process that created the variety originally, and it can continue to add to it today.

A human being begins as a single fertilized cell. That cell contains two copies of the genetic information in its twenty-three pairs of chromosomes. The

cell divides constantly during growth and development to produce the millions of cells that make up an adult. Each one of those cells, with very few exceptions, also has twenty-three pairs of chromosomes. In order for each cell to have its own double copy of information, the DNA that makes up the chromosomes must replicate, once for each cell division. This process of replication must ensure that the information contained in the DNA is copied exactly, and for the most part, it is.

To understand how a mistake can occur, one must look at the structure of DNA, the genetic blueprint. The DNA molecule resembles a spiral staircase. The outside rails are strings of sugar molecules hooked together by phosphate groups. The steps are made of bases that project from each sugar-phosphate backbone toward the middle. The information is contained in the sequence of base pairs that make up the steps of the staircase. The bases that can form such a pair are determined by their shape and bonding properties. Of the four bases, only two pairs are possible. Adenine (A) always pairs with thymine (T), leaving cytosine (C) and guanine (G) to form the other pair. This structure explains the accuracy with which DNA replicates. During replication, the original molecule unwinds from its spiral structure. The two strands separate, and a new complementary strand forms on each of the original strands. The order of bases on the new strand is determined by the original strand and the base-pairing rules. Where there is an A in the old strand, there must be a T in the new one. The other bases will not fit because they do not have the correct shape or bonding properties. Similarly, where the old

Figure 4. A Punnett Square Showing Alleles for Hemophilia

		Father's Sperm Cells	
		X	Y
Mother's Egg Cells	X	XX Normal Girl	XY Normal Boy
	X_h	XX_h Normal Girl (carrier)	X_hY Hemophiliac Boy

strand has a C, the new one must have a G. Each base is attached to a deoxyribose sugar and a phosphate group, all three forming a nucleotide. Once all proper nucleotides are linked together, the new strand is complete, the original DNA is rewound, and there are two molecules where there once was one.

The accuracy with which the DNA template is copied is impressive. It has been estimated that an error occurs only once for every 100,000 nucleotides copied. The replication of DNA is a chemical process which relies on random movements of molecules to put the correct ones together. There are enzymatic systems to make sure that only the correct nucleotides end up as part of the new DNA strand. There are also error detection and correction mechanisms that can remove an incorrect nucleotide and replace it with the correct one. This correction process reduces the error rate to one in 10 billion. Nevertheless, with the amount of DNA that has to be copied, mistakes do occur. If a mistake is made in a cell that produces an X or Y chromosome, the mistake will be passed on to future generations as a mutation.

The mistake will not be detected until the section of DNA that contains it is actually used by the cell to make a specific protein molecule. At the molecular level, a gene is a section of DNA that has the information necessary to make a particular protein molecule. Proteins are the working molecules of the body: They make up flesh and bone and the enzymes that speed up chemical reactions. The sequence of bases on a DNA molecule codes for the sequence of amino acids that makes up a protein molecule. Since there are twenty commonly used amino acids, and a protein can contain thousands of amino acids, there is an almost infinite number of different protein molecules. A mutation on a DNA molecule will usually mean that one amino acid in the protein for which it codes is changed.

Changing one unit in a thousand may not seem very significant, and usually it is not. Such a small change in a protein molecule generally has very little effect on the functioning of that molecule. Perhaps this mutation will make the molecule able to withstand a slightly higher temperature before breaking down. If the protein is an enzyme, the change may speed or slow its reaction time by a little bit. During human evolution, an individual may have been able to live slightly longer if the mutated protein was slightly improved in function. The longer that he or she lived, the greater was the chance that the individ-

ual could produce offspring—who would also have the mutated gene. In this way, positive, useful mutations became more common in the population. A change that made the protein less functional was less likely to be reproduced since the individual possessing the mutation may not have lived long enough to have children.

A slight change in a protein can make a very big difference. The hemoglobin (the oxygen-carrying protein in red blood cells) of a person with sickle-cell disease differs from normal hemoglobin by one amino acid. The amino acid, however, is in a critical position. With the changed amino acid, the hemoglobin clumps uselessly in the cell and does not carry oxygen. This is a lethal mutation, as a person afflicted with sickle-cell disease cannot live very long. One would assume that this mutation would not survive in the human population. Yet, in some parts of Africa, the mutant allele is carried by as much as 20 percent of the black population. To understand how this can be, one must consider the heterozygous individual. With one normal allele and one mutant one, such an individual makes both kinds of hemoglobin, including enough normal hemoglobin to be able to live comfortably under normal conditions. Moreover, the presence of the altered hemoglobin confers significant resistance to malaria. Because the heterozygous individual has a selective advantage over the other two genotypes, this mutant allele not only has been maintained but also has even increased in the black population in Africa.

PERSPECTIVE AND PROSPECTS

The modern study of genetics is conducted mostly at the molecular level. One project seeks to identify every human gene and its location on a specific chromosome. Dubbed the Human Genome Project, it is a cooperative venture among scientists worldwide. Such a map would tell researchers where each gene is located so that they could repair defective copies in people with genetic diseases. Genetic engineering techniques have already isolated many genes. For example, the gene for the production of insulin has been identified and extracted from human cells in culture. The gene has been inserted into the chromosomes of bacteria, and the bacteria are then grown in large quantities in commercial cultures. The insulin that they produce is harvested, purified, and made available to diabetics. This genuine human insulin is more potent than the insulin extracted from animals. In addition, such a process is essential for diabetics who suffer adverse reactions to the inevitable impurities that are found in insulin extracted from animals.

Ultimately, it should be possible to insert a functioning gene, like the one for insulin, directly into an afflicted person's chromosomes—thus curing the genetic disease. The cured individual, however, would still be able to pass the defective allele on to his or her children. The possibility of splicing genes into the chromosomes of sex cells does not seem likely in the near future.

More traditional genetics is also of value to prospective parents. A woman with a history of hemophilia in her family would want to know the chances that her children could inherit the disease. A genetic counselor would analyze the family tree of the woman and calculate a statistical probability. Some other genetic diseases can be detected in a fetus still in the womb. For example, a condition called phenylketonuria (PKU) can cause severe mental retardation and other medical problems. A genetic analysis of prospective parents with a family history of the condition could indicate the likelihood of PKU occurring in their children. If the chances are high, cells of the couple's child can be extracted and tested early in pregnancy. In the case of PKU, early detection can be used to prevent the effects of the disease. If the diet of the mother and then the newborn are carefully regulated, the toxic chemical that causes the disease will not accumulate in the fetus or newborn.

Genetic mutations have not stopped occurring in modern society. In fact, they are more likely. Many environmental factors have been shown to increase the mutation rate in animals. Several types of radiation and many chemicals can increase the mutation rate. This is why an X-ray technician will place a lead apron over the abdomen of a patient being X-rayed. Lead prevents the X rays from penetrating to the genital organs, where actively dividing DNA is particularly sensitive to the radiation. Such care should always be taken to protect the genetic makeup of future generations.

—James Waddell, Ph.D.

See also Bacteriology; Biostatistics; DNA and RNA; Embryology; Environmental diseases; Environmental health; Genetic counseling; Genetic diseases; Genetic engineering; Genetics and inheritance; Hemophilia; Human Genome Project; Microbiology; Oncology; Pathology; Phenylketonuria (PKU); Radiation sickness; Screening; Sickle-cell disease.

FOR FURTHER INFORMATION:
Campbell, Neil. *Biology: Concepts and Connections.* 5th ed. Redwood City, Calif.: Benjamin/Cummings, 1999. Chapters 13 ("Mendel and the Gene") and 16 ("From Gene to Protein") cover classical and molecular genetics, respectively. The text is accessible, and the many diagrams are useful.
Radman, Mirislav, and Robert Wagner. "The High Fidelity of DNA Duplication." *Scientific American* 259 (August, 1988): 40-46. Provides a readable account of the "proofreading" and error-correcting mechanisms that make mutations so rare. The author is careful to point out what is fact and what is speculation. The bibliography refers the reader to more technical articles on the subject.
Rusting, Ricki L. "Why Do We Age?" *Scientific American* 267 (December, 1992): 130-135. A review of contemporary research into the genetics of aging. Evidence is presented for the presence of genes that determine how long animals and humans may expect to live.
Stahl, Franklin W. "Genetic Recombination." *Scientific American* 256 (February, 1987): 90-101. This article describes how genes are constantly shuffled to make new genetic combinations for each generation. This process occurs when chromosomes exchange pieces during the cell divisions that produce the sex cells.

MYOCARDIAL INFARCTION. *See* **HEART ATTACK.**

MYOMECTOMY
PROCEDURE

ANATOMY OR SYSTEM AFFECTED: Reproductive system, uterus

SPECIALTIES AND RELATED FIELDS: General surgery, gynecology

DEFINITION: Myomectomy is the removal of benign smooth muscle tumors from the uterus. "Fibroids" and "myomas" are both terms for these common, benign growths. Frequently, they remain small and are asymptomatic. Others grow very large, distorting the normal size and shape of the uterus and causing severe pain and heavy bleeding during menstrual periods. Myomectomy is a method by which a surgeon removes only the fibroids and leaves the uterus intact. With the patient under local anesthesia, the surgeon passes the appropriate instrument through the dilated cervix into the uterus. Growths on the uterine wall can then be removed. Small fibroids can be viewed with a tiny camera inserted into the uterus and then detached with a laser, electric current, or scissors. After deeply embedded fibroids are surgically removed, the uterus may have to be reconstructed. Because of the complex and unpredictable arrangement of blood vessels to the fibroids, heavy bleeding may occur following myomectomy. Approximately 20 percent of patients will need additional surgery for recurrent fibroids. If the patient does not wish to have more children or any children, then hysterectomy (total removal of the uterus) is frequently recommended instead of myomectomy.

—*Karen E. Kalumuck, Ph.D.*

See also Dysmenorrhea; Genital disorders, female; Gynecology; Hysterectomy; Menorrhagia; Menstruation; Muscles; Reproductive system; Tumor removal; Tumors.

FOR FURTHER INFORMATION:

Altman, Roberta, and Michael Sarg. *The Cancer Dictionary.* New York: Facts on File, 1992.

Dollinger, Malin, Ernest H. Rosenbaum, and Greg Cable, et al. *Everyone's Guide to Cancer Therapy.* 3d ed. Kansas City, Mo.: Andrews and McMeel, 1997.

Hufnagel, Vicki. *No More Hysterectomies.* New York: New American Library, 1988.

Payer, Lynn. *How to Avoid a Hysterectomy.* New York: Pantheon Books, 1987.

MYOPIA

DISEASE/DISORDER

ALSO KNOWN AS: Nearsightedness

ANATOMY OR SYSTEM AFFECTED: Eyes

SPECIALTIES AND RELATED FIELDS: Ophthalmology, optometry

DEFINITION: A visual defect that impairs the perception of distant objects.

CAUSES AND SYMPTOMS

Nearsightedness (myopia) occurs when light from distant objects reaches a focal point in front of the retina, the photoreceptive tissue of the eye. Conse-

---

Myopia

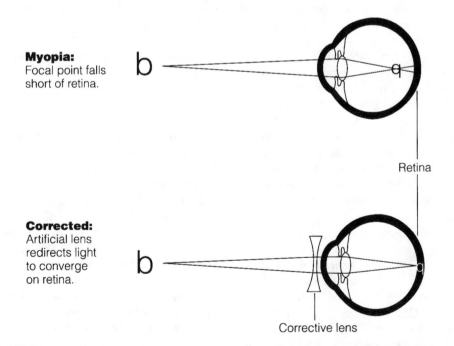

Myopia:
Focal point falls short of retina.

Corrected:
Artificial lens redirects light to converge on retina.

Retina

Corrective lens

Myopia is commonly termed "nearsightedness" because most light rays entering the eye will not resolve, or focus, on the retina unless they are coming from a very near distance; corrective lenses are required.

quently, vision of distant objects is blurred on the retina. The primary cause of myopia is an eyeball that is too long from front to back. Higher testosterone levels in the womb and a genetic predisposition have been advanced as possible causes of this condition. Research has also found that prolonged eyestrain, especially that which often accompanies long periods of reading, can distort the shape of the eye. This is one reason why well-educated people manifest higher rates of nearsightedness than less-educated individuals.

All children are born nearsighted; by the age of six months, however, vision begins to improve. Myopia is an uncommon problem in younger school-age children but begins to increase in prevalence as children move into their teenage years. From the twenties until the late sixties, the rate of visual deterioration tends to slow down. By the time people reach their seventies, however, the rate of visual decline accelerates again. People past the age of seventy are fourteen times as likely to experience myopia resulting in legal blindness as those in their twenties.

TREATMENT AND THERAPY

For several centuries, nearsightedness has been corrected by the use of a concave lens, which moves the focal point of light in myopic eyes closer to the retina. The first evidence for the use of concave lenses is found in a 1517 painting of Pope Leo X by Italian artist Raphael. As the twentieth century drew to a close, innovative surgical approaches were developed. Most of these procedures, such as laser surgery, move the focal point of light closer to the retina by changing the shape of the cornea.

—*Paul J. Chara, Jr., Ph.D.*

See also Aging; Blurred vision; Cataracts; Glaucoma; Eye surgery; Eyes; Laser use in surgery; Ophthalmology; Optometry; Optometry, pediatric; Sense organs; Visual disorders.

FOR FURTHER INFORMATION:

Anshel, Jeffrey. *Healthy Eyes, Better Vision: Everyday Eye Care for the Whole Family.* Los Angeles: Body Press, 1990.

Rubman, Robert H., and Howard Rothman. *Future Vision: Space-Age Techniques to Save Your Sight.* New York: Dodd, Mead, 1987.

Vaughan, Daniel, Taylor Asbury, and Paul Riordan-Eva, eds. *General Ophthalmology.* 15th ed. Norwalk, Conn.: Appleton and Lange, 1999.

MYRINGOTOMY

PROCEDURE

ANATOMY OR SYSTEM AFFECTED: Ears

SPECIALTIES AND RELATED FIELDS: Family practice, otorhinolaryngology

DEFINITION: The creation of an opening in the eardrum (tympanic membrane) to allow drainage of accumulated fluid in the middle ear.

INDICATIONS AND PROCEDURES

Fluid can collect in the middle ear as a result of infection or allergy; this fluid consists of blood, pus, water, and debris. An ear, nose, and throat specialist may surgically insert small tubes into the middle ear to facilitate drainage. Usually, local anesthesia is administered, particularly if the patient is a young child.

This procedure, called myringotomy, is used to relieve pain caused by pressure and to prevent temporary or permanent hearing loss. Physiologically, the problem involves blockage of the Eustachian tube, a narrow canal that connects the middle ear to the back of the nasal cavity. This tube regulates air pressure in the middle-ear cavity, allowing the hearing mechanism to function properly and helping to maintain a sense of balance.

Prior to performing a myringotomy, medical treatment may involve the prescription of antihistamines, decongestants, and perhaps steroids, which usually reduce the swelling of the Eustachian tube and sometimes preclude a myringotomy. After the procedure, improvement in hearing is usually immediate, and the middle-ear infection should heal. Antibiotic eardrops may be prescribed; three or four drops should be placed in each ear twice a day for five days. In approximately six to twelve months, the myringotomy tube will be expelled into the outer ear canal automatically and can be removed by a physician. Treatment may include follow-up visits every two months.

USES AND COMPLICATIONS

Postoperatively, it is not unusual for the patient to experience a certain amount of pulsation, popping, clicking, and other sounds in the ear. It is important during the postoperative period to make certain that the patient does not get water in his or her ear, especially when the tube is in place. When washing the hair or face, cotton covered with petroleum jelly may be placed in the outer part of the ear. For long-term protection, earplugs may be used during showering, bathing, and swimming. Diving, deep swimming, and any other activity that may place pressure on the eardrum are not recommended.

—John Alan Ross, Ph.D.

See also Ear infections and disorders; Ears; Hearing loss; Surgery, pediatric.

FOR FURTHER INFORMATION:
Davis, Hallowell, and S. Richard Silverman. *Hearing and Deafness*. 4th ed. New York: Holt, Rinehart & Winston, 1978.

Myringotomy. Eden Prairie, Minn.: Starkey Laboratories, 1983.

Pender, Daniel J. *Practical Otology*. Philadelphia: J. B. Lippincott, 1992.

Rosenthal, Richard. *The Hearing Loss Handbook*. New York: St. Martin's Press, 1975.

NAIL REMOVAL
PROCEDURE
ANATOMY OR SYSTEM AFFECTED: Feet, hands, nails

SPECIALTIES AND RELATED FIELDS: Dermatology, general surgery, podiatry

DEFINITION: The surgical removal of toenails and fingernails (onychectomy), which may be necessary if they become infected or undergo trauma.

INDICATIONS AND PROCEDURES
Ingrown toenails (onychocryptosis) is a common malady which may require nail removal. Poorly fitting shoes, improper nail cutting, and inborn defects can cause toenails to become ingrown. Infected and inflamed tissue around the nail (paronychia) can become a chronic condition requiring the removal of the nail. Fungal infections (onychomycosis) can cause nails to turn yellow, become brittle, and grow thick. While this condition can be treated by an antifungal agent, the treatment often fails; nail removal can be used to treat the problem more effectively. Nail removal is often used when nails are accidentally torn or injured. When nails are injured in a traumatic accident, X rays are often taken to check for fractures, shattered tendons, or unseen foreign bodies.

Adequate steps must be taken to numb the area prior to surgery. Chemical agents, such as lidocaine, are injected into the digit to achieve nerve blockage. In addition, it is often desirable to apply a tourniquet to the digit, using compression to drive blood away from the nail area. A few specialized medical instruments are often used when removing nails. The Freer septal elevator is used to pull nails away from the surrounding tissue. English nail splitters are used to cut through nails. Small skin or bone curettes are employed to remove tissue and debris from nail beds and folds.

USES AND COMPLICATIONS
Once the nail has been removed, the wound must be disinfected, dressed, and protected to prevent infection or trauma. These problems are the most serious complications that can result from the procedure.

—*Russell Williams, M.S.W.*

See also Feet; Fungal infections; Lower extremities; Nails; Upper extremities; Wounds.

FOR FURTHER INFORMATION:
Hilton, Lisette. "Nail Surgery Tips Include Need for More Biopsies." *Dermatology Times* 20, no. 9 (September, 1999): 28-29. While there are many practical points to keep in mind when considering nail surgery, one that stands out is the need for dermatologists to biopsy the nails more often.

Taylor, Robert B., et al., eds. *Family Medicine: Principles and Practice*. 5th ed. New York: Springer-Verlag, 1998. A comprehensive reference source providing clear guidelines for diagnosing and managing the common acute and chronic problems regularly encountered by the family practitioner.

NAILS
ANATOMY
ANATOMY OR SYSTEM AFFECTED: Hands, feet, skin

SPECIALTIES AND RELATED FIELDS: Dermatology, histology

DEFINITION: The thin, horny plates covering the dorsal ends of the fingers or toes.

KEY TERMS:

cuticle: cutaneous or skin tissue that surrounds the nail plate on its proximal sides and provides a protective barrier to the nail bed; it is attached to the proximal nail fold and to the nail plate

hyponychium: cutaneous tissue underlying the free nail at its point of separation from the nail bed; structurally similar to the cuticle

keratinocytes: matrix basal epithelial cells that differentiate, fill with keratin, and form the dead horny substance making up the nail plate

lunula: a whitish, crescent-shaped area at the end of the proximal nail fold that marks the end of the nail matrix and is the site of mitosis and nail growth

onychomycosis: common nail disorder in which fungal organisms invade the nail bed causing progressive changes in the color, texture, and structure of the nail

STRUCTURE AND FUNCTIONS
Nails function to protect fingers and toes against bumps and trauma. Fine touch is amplified and skillful manipulation of small objects with the fingers is enabled by the presence of nails. Nails also provide the ability to scratch, both as a temporary relief of an itch or in personal defense. Nails are important social communicators of beauty and sexuality and hence are the focus of a major cosmetic industry.

Biologically, nails are characterized as plates of tightly packed, hard epidermis cells filled with a protein called keratin. Nails are normally seen on the dorsal side (the side opposite the palm or sole) of all fingers and toes. The anatomy of the normal nail consists of a nail plate, proximal nail fold, nail bed, matrix, and hyponychium. These components are epithelial derived structures, like skin and hair, which emerge from the live germinative zone of the epidermis. These cells differentiate and form the horny layer, which is considered to be dead.

The nail plate is a relatively hard and flat, transparent, horny structure that is rectangular in shape. It rests on the underlying nail bed but typically extends beyond the bed as an unattached, free-growing edge reaching beyond the tip of the finger or toe. In the fingers, the thickness of the plate in adults increases from the proximal edge to the distal edge from about 0.7 millimeters to 1.6 millimeters. The terminal tip thickness varies considerably between persons.

Normally, a pinkish nail bed is seen through the transparent nail plate. Frequently in the thumb nail and sometimes in the other fingers, a whitish, semimoon-shaped structure called the lunula is seen that extends under the proximal nail fold. The borders of the nail plate are covered by skin structures: two lateral folds and a single proximal fold.

The proximal nail fold or the cuticle is the cutaneous or skin structure that is in continuity with the visible proximal border of the nail but overlies part of

The Anatomy of a Nail

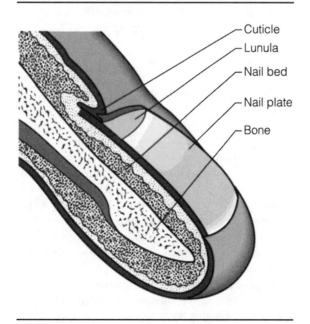

- Cuticle
- Lunula
- Nail bed
- Nail plate
- Bone

the nail root. The ventral side (underside) of the proximal nail fold provides physical protection to the germinative zone of the nail and aids in the physical attachment of the nail plate. About a fourth of the total surface area of the nail plate is located under the proximal fold. The cuticle is a layer of epidermis extending from the proximal nail fold and attached to the dorsal side of the nail. The cuticle functions to provide a physical seal against microbes and chemical irritants, which may otherwise enter the matrix and affect nail production.

The nail bed is the portion of the digit upon which the nail rests. The nail bed is highly vascular, with numerous capillaries, consists of epithelial tissue, and extends from the lunula to the point where the bed separates from the nail. A series of fine longitudinal folds in the nail bed corresponds to the undersurface structure of the nail. This arrangement enhances the adherence of the nail plate to the nail bed.

The nail matrix generally is considered the most proximal part of the nail bed and is bordered by the proximal nail fold. On the distal end it is bordered by the distal margin of the lunula. The nail matrix epithelium cells consist predominantly of keratinocytes in both a basal and spinous layer. Melanocytes and Langerhans' cells are intermingled with keratinocytes. It is within the matrix that the germinating center of nail growth is found. Basal epithelial cells increase in number through mitosis or division and then differentiate into keratinocytes, which are epithelial cells filled with keratin protein. These keratinocytes condense their cytoplasm, lose their nucleus, and form flat, horny-looking cells which are dead. As further cell division occurs in the nail matrix, the more distal keratinocytes are pushed out to form the nail plate.

The hyponychium consists of epidermis tissue that underlies the edge of the nail plate and extends from the nail bed to the distal groove. It functions to provide a defense against entry of bacteria under the free edge of the nail plate. Excessively vigorous cleaning may damage the hyponychium and allow for bacteria to enter more readily under the nail plate.

The turnover rate of matrix cells determines the growth rate of the nail. This rate varies with age, environmental conditions, nutritional status, and the specific digit. The growth rate proportionately increases with the length of the digit; thus the middle finger nail grows the fastest while the growth rate in the little finger is the slowest. Fingernails grow three times as rapidly as toenails. The growth rate is more rapid in the winter than in the summer. Furthermore, nails grow faster in young children than in older adults. It takes about six months for a fingernail to completely grow in. Male nails grow faster than female nails. Nails on the dominant hand grow faster than those on the other hand.

If nails are protected and untrimmed, they can grow to considerable lengths. Such long nails were prized by the wealthy classes in imperial Chinese culture as an indication of status. The practice of painting toenails red may have originated in the Ottoman seraglio, where it was a signal of menstrual status.

Nails continue to grow throughout life without a resting phase. Contrary to folk belief, nails cease growing when an individual dies. The matrix cells stop producing deoxyribonucleic acid (DNA) and dividing soon after death and thus the nail bed cannot grow longer. The appearance of nail growth after death is due to a retraction or shrinkage of nail matrix tissue, resulting in the apparent lengthening of the nail plate.

Professional grooming of the nails for both men and women is termed a manicure. Manicure procedures include cutting the nails according to fashion standards to improve their cosmetic appearance. A pedicure is the term applied to grooming the toenails. Typically, the nails are first soaked in a soapy solution to soften the nail plate and to remove dirt and debris. Currently it is fashionable to trim the nails to a delicate arc at the middle of the fingertip. The corners of the nail are typically filed. While this shape is attractive in creating the illusion of longer, slender fingers, it heightens the probability of nail plate fractures, hangnails, or ingrown nails. The cuticle, considered to be unattractive by manicurists, is typically minimized, partially removed, or traumatized. This may increase the incidence of fungal invasion and disease. Most of the problems associated with a manicure arise from excessive manipulation of the cuticle.

Nail polish typically consists of pigments suspended in a volatile solvent that also contains a film-forming agent. When the polish is applied to the finger, a covering film develops over the nail. The film is permeable to oxygen, which allows gas exchange to occur between the atmosphere and the nail plate. Resins and plasticizers are added to the polish to increase the flexibility of the film and to minimize chipping. The variety in nail polish color is due to the addition of coloring agents. Deep red nail polishes can cause a temporary yellowish staining of the nail plate.

Nail adornments are sometimes used. Frequently, small nail jewels or ribbons are applied to the fingernails immediately before the nail polish dries, allowing the decoration to adhere to the nail plate. Since some people frequently develop contact dermatitis to nickel, gold or nickel-free jewels should be selected. Artificial nail tips made of plastic also are glued to the nail tip to create the illusion of an elongated natural nail tip. The gluing may cause nail problems, since a portion of the natural nail is occluded by the glue. This occlusion inhibits oxygen transfer and stresses the nail plate. Frequently, the nail may thin and be unable to support its own weight after the plastic tip is removed. Removal of the plastic tip may result in nail pitting.

DISORDERS AND DISEASES

Nails are useful indicators of skin disease as well as of internal disorders. An abnormally pigmented band in the nail may indicate a malignant melanoma. A yellow nail may indicate psoriasis or a fungal infection. Pulmonary disease or smoking may also cause yellow or brownish nails. Antimalarial drugs may cause the nail to darken in appearance. Frequently, psoriasis causes pitting of nails and an acceleration in their growth rate. Chronic chest disease or a cyanotic congenital heart disorder is frequently associated with club-shaped deformity of the nail plate. Beau's lines, which are transverse depressions in the nail plates, are associated with illnesses such as coronary thrombosis, pneumonia, and severe injuries. Drug treatment may cause nail breakdown or destruction or complete shedding of the nail plate.

An unexplained aspect of nail physiology is its relationship to lung physiology. Hippocrates first described a connection between lung parenchymal disorders and an edema in the connective tissue beneath the lunula that results in clubbing. The relationship has long been recognized, but the causal link is still unexplained.

An ingrown nail results when a deformed nail grows improperly into the skin, or when the skin around the nails engulfs part of the nail. Wearing narrow, tight shoes can cause or worsen this pathology. Initially, symptoms may be slight or mild, but with time may come increasing pain. The affected area becomes reddish and, if not treated, may become infected. If infected, the area becomes swollen, inflamed, and painful. Blisters may develop. Treatment involves trimming away the nail from the infected area, allowing the inflammation to decline and the area to heal.

Clubbing is a disorder characterized by a bulblike enlargement of the nail with increased horizontal and longitudinal curvatures. Clubbing involves both fingers and toes and commonly begins at puberty. The disorder may be genetically inherited or acquired. Clubbed nails often have a spongy feel when pressure is placed on the proximal nail fold. This is due to the expanded soft tissue that underlies the nail. Acquired clubbing is often associated with another clinical pathology, most commonly pulmonary or cardiovascular disease. However, at times it is also associated with gastrointestinal inflammatory disease or cystic fibrosis.

A fungal infection is the cause of onychomycosis, which is the most common nail disorder. About half of all nail problems can be linked to this disease, which affects as many as 15 to 20 percent of people in North America. It is uncommon in children but more frequently seen in aged adults.

Several fungi may be the causal agents, although most belong to the group called dermatophytes. The fungi are present in soil, and indirect transmission to humans frequently occurs through public swimming pools and shower floors. Some yeasts and molds are also thought to cause this clinical condition. Alternatively, this infection is associated with athlete's foot infection. Typically this condition is found in toenails more frequently than fingernails. The presence of the fungus is furthered evidenced by scaling on the plantar surface of the foot, where it is often harbored.

In onychomycosis, the fungal organism invades the nail bed, causing a progressive change in the color, texture, and structure of the nail. The nail may turn white, thicken, and even detach from the nail bed. Debris from the infected nail often collects under its free edge. If untreated, the pathology may involve the entire nail plate, and rarely will the nail unit spontaneously heal itself.

Since several organisms may induce the pathology, effective treatment depends on matching the curative with the causal agent. Topically applied antifungals seldom are effective because most cannot penetrate the nail plate barrier to reach the causal organism. Systemically (orally) administered antifungal therapy frequently uses one of several drugs such as griseoful-vin, thiabendazole, or ketoconazole. These drugs are generally effective in halting further invasion of the fungus. While treatment continues the new growing nail is usually normal. Thus treatment typically continues until the old nail is replaced by new nail, and then the treatment is discontinued.

More than seventy tumors associated with parts of the nail have been found. Their origins may be from the epidermis, dermis, subcutaneous tissues, or the bone. The tumors may be found in the nail bed, nail matrix, hyponychium, or nail fold. The tumors may take various forms such as warts, erosion or ulceration of the nail bed, malignant neoplasms from underlying melanocytes, benign fibromas of the connective tissue, or squamous cell carcinomas. Diagnosis usually is made by taking a biopsy of the affected area. Treatment typically involves surgical removal of the tumor.

PERSPECTIVE AND PROSPECTS

The earliest cellular growth leading to nail formation can be seen histologically at eight weeks of human development, the end of the embryonic period. Microscopically, the cells forming the proximal edge of the nail field and the future matrix can be distinguished at this time. The earliest gross anatomical appearance of nails is seen on the finger digit surface at about nine weeks of development, the very early fetal stage. By eleven weeks of age, the nail field is seen clearly on the hand digits of the fetus. By twenty weeks of age, the fetus shows a nail plate and bed and a proximal cuticle. By thirty-two weeks, the third trimester of pregnancy, adult type nail structures are visible in the fetus, including a nail plate, matrix, and bed and a forming hyponychium.

Aging results in changes and disorders in nails. When people get older the color, contour, growth rate, surface texture, and thickness of the nail plate change. Some disorders are more prevalent with aging, such as brittle nails, splitting or fissuring of the nail plate, and increased infections. Aged nails appear dull and opaque, with a color varying from yellow to gray. Frequently in older persons, the lunula is decreased in size or is absent. The growth rate of nails decreases with aging. The most rapid period of growth is during the first thirty years; thereafter the rate steadily declines. With older persons, the nail plate thickness frequently increases, paralleled with discoloration and a loss of translucency of the nail plate.

For many years, blood and urine specimens have been used to detect and measure body concentrations of therapeutic drugs or drugs of abuse. During the past decade, alternative biological specimens, nails and hair, have been frequently used as the basis for drug detection. The basis for drug detection in nail clippings is that the dividing epidermal cells that form the nail plate also incorporate drugs from the systemic circulation. The subsequent cornification of these cells traps the drug within the forming nail plate. Drug detection methods involve taking a sample of nail clippings, and extracting and identifying drug molecules by using immunochemical or chromatographic techniques that are extremely sensitive and capable of detecting minute quantities of drug in the samples. As little as ten milligrams of nail clippings is required to detect the presence of drugs. Twenty-first century drug screening methods have detected amphetamines and cocaine in nail clippings. Using nail clippings for drug analysis and screening provides a long-term measure of drug exposure that potentially may represent months of drug use. Furthermore, nail clippings are relatively easy to collect and involve a noninvasive procedure; samples are easily stored, and once incorporated in the nail tissue most of the drugs are presumably stable.

Modern medicine at the beginning of the twenty-first century still lacks adequate descriptive science as well as understanding of the molecular mechanisms that control nail development and growth. To date, the specific genes or gene products that initiate nail growth have not been identified. The molecular basis for brittle nails, clubbing, and other nail pathologies is not known. Is onychomycosis affected by a systemic immune deficit? What causes yellow nail syndrome? Answers to these questions as well as additional information about the molecular control of nail physiology will greatly increase understanding and lead to better treatments for nail disorders.

—*Roman J. Miller, Ph.D.*

See also Fungal infections; Lower extremities; Nail removal; Pulmonary diseases; Skin; Skin disorders; Upper extremities.

FOR FURTHER INFORMATION:

Berkow, Robert, ed. *The Merck Manual of Medical Information, Home Edition.* Whitehouse Station, N.J.: Merck, 1997. This manual, written for home use, describes several common nail disorders. Symptoms, characteristics, and possible treatments are given.

De Berker, D. A. R., R. Baran, and R. P. R. Dawber. *Handbook of Diseases of the Nails and Their Management.* Cambridge, Mass.: Blackwell Science, 1995. Describes the normal physiology and pathology of nails. Superb color photographs vividly illustrate various nail diseases.

Hordinsky, Maria K., Marty E. Sawaya, and Richard K. Scher. *Atlas of Hair and Nails.* Philadephia: W. B. Saunders, 2000. This vividly illustrated atlas emphasizes nail disorders and special issues affecting nail physiology. Numerous colored photographs.

Williams, Peter. L., ed. *Gray's Anatomy: The Anatomical Basis of Medicine and Surgery.* 38th ed. New York: Churchill Livingstone, 1995. This classic anatomy text uses simple line drawings to illustrate the parts of a nail. The accompanying text accurately describes the parts of a nail and is well recognized as authoritative by health care professionals.

Zaias, Nardo. *The Nail in Health and Disease.* 2d ed. Norwalk, Conn.: Appleton & Lange, 1990. Describes in detail the anatomy and physiology of nails, specific disorders, and cosmetic care. Written for the health care professional, this well-illustrated text is also understandable for the average reader.

NARCOLEPSY

DISEASE/DISORDER

ANATOMY OR SYSTEM AFFECTED: Brain, nervous system, psychic-emotional system

SPECIALTIES AND RELATED FIELDS: Neurology

DEFINITION: An apparently inherited disorder of the nervous system characterized by brief, numerous, and overwhelming attacks of sleepiness throughout the day.

KEY TERMS:

cataplexy: brief periods of partial or total loss of skeletal muscle tone, usually triggered by emotional stimuli, which can cause the person to collapse

electroencephalogram (EEG): a recording of brain wave activity using electrodes attached to the scalp

excessive daytime sleepiness: a strong tendency to fall asleep, accompanied by reduced energy and lack of alertness during the entire day

hypnogogic hallucination: a bizarre, sometimes frightening, dreamlike occurrence just as one is falling asleep or just after waking

maintenance of wakefulness test: a polysomnographic technique to measure a person's ability to remain awake during repeated trials throughout the day

multiple sleep latency test: a polysomnographic technique to measure how quickly one falls asleep during repeated trials throughout the day

polysomnography: the continuous recording of brain waves, eye movements, skeletal muscle movements, and other body functions to determine bodily changes during the stages of sleep

REM sleep: a period of intense brain activity, often associated with dreams; named for the rapid eye movements that typically occur during this time

sleep paralysis: an inability to move voluntarily, occurring just at the beginning of sleep or upon awakening

CAUSES AND SYMPTOMS

Narcolepsy (*narco* meaning "numbness" and *lepsy* meaning "seizure") consists primarily of attacks of irresistible sleepiness in the daytime. The sleepiness is extreme; it has been described as the feeling that most people would experience if they tried to add columns of numbers in the middle of the night after forty-eight hours without sleep.

The narcoleptic's day is broken up by a series of brief and repetitive sleep attacks, perhaps even two hundred attacks in a single day. These transient, overpowering attacks of sleepiness may last from a few seconds to thirty minutes, with an average spell lasting two minutes. It is excruciatingly difficult, and frequently impossible, to ignore the urge to sleep, no matter how inconvenient or inappropriate. Narcoleptics typically fall asleep suddenly, on the job, in conversation, standing up, and even while eating, driving, or making love.

These sleep attacks result from an abrupt failure in resisting sleep, as opposed to a sudden surge in sleepiness, because narcoleptics are actually sleepy all day. The misconception that their daytime sleepiness is caused by insufficient nighttime sleep prompts undiagnosed patients to spend inordinately long hours in bed. Narcoleptics will be sleepy during the day regardless of how much sleep they get at night.

One of the most prominent and troubling features of narcolepsy is cataplexy, a sudden loss of muscle tone which causes the person to collapse. Cataplexy occurs during the daytime while the person is awake. It may involve all the muscles at once or only a select few, so the severity may range from total collapse to

the ground to partial collapse of a limb or the jaw. The cataplectic sometimes remains conscious, able to think, hear, and see, although vision may be blurred. At other times, there is a brief loss of consciousness, associated with an experience of dreaming. Although most attacks of cataplexy last less than a minute, occasionally they go on for as long as twenty minutes. Cataplexy is often triggered by enjoyable feelings, laughter, or excitement during which the person suddenly crumples into a heap. For other patients, a strong negative emotion, such as fear or anger, precipitates an attack.

Many narcoleptics notice the symptom of excessive daytime sleepiness for as much as a year before the onset of cataplexy. After many years of experiencing cataplexy, some patients find that less emotional stimulus is required to induce the muscle collapse and that increasingly more muscles are involved. Others find that this symptom diminishes, possibly because they have become adept at anticipating and avoiding the situations that trigger attacks. It has been noted that other hypersomnias—that is, other diseases of excessive sleepiness—do not include cataplexy; only narcoleptics suffer from this embarrassing and troubling symptom of muscle collapse.

Many narcoleptics also experience hypnogogic hallucinations, dreams that intrude into the waking state. In normal sleep, dreaming generally occurs approximately ninety minutes after falling asleep; narcoleptics begin their sleeping episodes with vivid dreams. These hallucinations are extremely realistic and often violent. The patient sees someone else in the room or hears someone calling his or her name, for the hallucinations are nearly always visual and are usually auditory. The vivid sights, sounds, and feelings characteristic of hypnogogic hallucinations are thought to occur while the person is awake, both during the day and just at the edges of nighttime sleep. Since narcoleptics typically fall asleep dozens if not hundreds of times a day, they can experience these disturbing hallucinations with great frequency. Somewhat more than 50 percent of daytime sleep attacks include hallucinations, while only about 7 percent are usually marked by cataplexy.

Approximately 40 to 60 percent of narcoleptics suffer another frightening symptom: sleep paralysis. This condition occurs at the beginning or end of sleep and renders immobile virtually every voluntary muscle, except those around the eyes. During sleep paral-

In the News: The Cause of Narcolepsy

Narcolepsy is a sleep disorder affecting humans as well as animals and is known to be a disease of the nervous system, but its biochemical and molecular basis has been a mystery. Recent studies in mice, dogs, and humans have now revealed a newly described neurotransmitter system that appears to be involved in narcolepsy and in the regulation of normal sleep patterns. The molecules implicated in narcolepsy are neuropeptides known as orexins (originally described as hypocretins). Changes in the hypocretin receptor 2 and prepro-hypocretin genes are able to produce narcolepsy in animals. In one study involving nine human subjects, hypocretin could not be detected in seven of the subjects. Other studies have produced hypocretin knockout mice, which have symptoms that are quite similar to those found in human narcoleptics. Hypocretins have been found to occur normally in the regions of the central nervous system that appear to be involved in the regulation of sleep. An autosomal recessive mutation has been discovered in narcoleptic dogs which alters the hypocretin receptor 2 gene. In humans, a similar disruption or deficiency in hypocretin is associated with most cases of narcolepsy, although it is still unclear as to what underlies the exact genetic predisposition to the disease.

—*Donald J. Nash, Ph.D.*

ysis, the mind is awake and one is aware of the external surroundings, but the muscles refuse to move. The paralysis usually lasts only a few seconds, but it may continue for as long as twenty minutes. Sleep researchers find that almost everyone has an episode of sleep paralysis that lasts a few seconds sometime during his or her lifetime. When the paralysis continues for more than a few seconds, however, it is usually a sign of narcolepsy. Although either sleep paralysis or hypnogogic hallucinations alone are distressing enough, they often happen simultaneously.

Because of their frequent, irresistible sleep attacks, narcoleptics often wobble back and forth between sleep and wakefulness in a state that has been likened to sleepwalking and is termed automatic behavior. When in this state, the person seems to behave normally but later does not remember extended periods of time. For example, narcoleptics might find themselves in a different building or several exits farther down a highway than they last remembered. Obviously, automatic behavior is very anxiety-producing; it is very troubling to narcoleptics to be unable to remember what they have done in the minutes or hours that have just passed.

In addition to these memory difficulties, some narcoleptics experience constant eye fatigue, difficulty focusing, and double vision. They also have a higher incidence of the heart abnormality called mitral valve prolapse, which affects blood flow to the left ventricle. The reason for this association is not clear.

Although narcolepsy is an illness of excessive daytime sleepiness, the nighttime sleep of those afflicted is far from normal as well. It is often troubled by restlessness and frequent awakenings, which are brief or may last for hours. Patients also experience many nightmares about murder and persecution. Many narcoleptics talk, cry out, or thrash about periodically during the night.

One narcoleptic in ten has the added complication of suffering from sleep apnea. This sleep disorder consists of recurrent interruptions in breathing during sleep. This further disturbance of nighttime sleep aggravates the narcoleptic's tendency to excessive daytime sleepiness.

Narcolepsy was once thought to be extremely rare. By 1989, however, the United States Department of Health estimated that 250,000 Americans suffer from this disease, which is more than the number afflicted by multiple sclerosis. The American Medical Association considers 250,000 to be a very conservative estimate and believes the number to be between 400,000 and 600,000.

Males and females are equally affected by narcolepsy. Although the disorder has been diagnosed in a five-year-old, its symptoms most frequently appear for the first time during adolescence. In about 75 percent of cases, the attacks begin between the ages of fifteen and twenty-five; only 5 percent of cases begin before the age of ten. Onset is rare after the age of forty; if narcolepsy seems to appear in an older person, it has probably existed undiagnosed for years.

Sleep researchers believe that the extra need for sleep characteristic of adolescence may make this stage of development particularly vulnerable for the onset of narcolepsy. Thus, this disorder may typically begin in adolescence because it is somehow triggered by the brain changes associated with sexual maturation.

Between two and five persons in one thousand in the general population of the United States have scattered episodes of excessive daytime sleepiness but are not considered narcoleptics. It is not until a person has one to several attacks each day that narcolepsy is suspected.

TREATMENT AND THERAPY

Narcolepsy is now known to be a disease of the nervous system. Although incurable, it can be successfully treated with various medications once it has been diagnosed. The diagnosis of narcolepsy, however, is often slow to occur. The average interval between the first appearance of symptoms and diagnosis is often as long as thirteen years. Because early symptoms are usually mild, narcoleptics typically spend years wondering whether they are sick or whether they merely lack initiative. They are often called lazy because they repeatedly nap during the day and are lethargic even when awake. Diagnosis is made more difficult by the wide range of severity of symptoms. For example, excessive daytime sleepiness may trouble a person for ten or twenty years before cataplexy appears. Patients may even occasionally experience a temporary or partial remission in their condition. Narcoleptics often fight off their sleep attacks by ingesting large amounts of caffeine and never realize that they have an actual disease until years later.

If narcolepsy is suspected, a polysomnographic study is done at a sleep disorders center to confirm the diagnosis. The most reliable confirmation of narcolepsy can be obtained by what is called the multiple sleep latency test (MSLT). The MSLT is easy, convenient, inexpensive, and very informative. The person is given four or five opportunities to lie down and fall asleep during the daytime. Normal individuals take fifteen to thirty minutes to fall asleep. In the MSLT, falling asleep in less than five minutes is considered abnormal. Those afflicted with narcolepsy always fall asleep in less than five minutes and often within a minute. The maintenance of wakefulness test (MOWT) is also used in the confirmation of narcolepsy. In the MOWT, the person is kept all day in a comfortable reclining position. Polysomnography is used to measure the patient's ability to stay awake and how many times he or she falls asleep.

Along with the MSLT and the MOWT, a thorough physical examination is needed to discover if the person has some other disorder that can mimic narcolepsy; an underactive thyroid gland, diabetes, chronic low blood sugar, anemia, and a malfunctioning liver can each cause excessive daytime sleepiness. Similarly, drug use, poor nutrition, emotional frustration, dissatisfaction, or poor motivation can also result in the type of sleepiness that a narcoleptic experiences.

When the diagnosis of narcolepsy is confirmed, treatment usually consists of stimulant medications such as dextroamphetamine, pemoline, or methylphenidate (Ritalin) during the daytime. These stimulant drugs can increase alertness and cut down the number of sleep attacks from perhaps several per day to several per month. Unfortunately, patients can quickly develop tolerance to these medications.

Even on low doses, some patients become irritable, aggressive, or nervous, or they may develop obesity and sexual problems. It is very important, therefore, to monitor a narcoleptic carefully, determining the lowest effective dose and the best times of day to take it. It may be months before the positive effects of drug therapy are fully experienced. The MSLT will often be given on a day that one takes the medication and on another when it is not taken, in order to evaluate the success of a given treatment.

Because specific drug and dosage schedules may have to be altered frequently, patients may repeatedly have to face drug withdrawal symptoms such as intensified sleepiness and disturbing dreams. To prevent adverse reactions, narcoleptics must often avoid certain foods and common medications. Their use of stimulant drugs may even be viewed as morally wrong, in these days of widespread drug abuse, by neighbors or coworkers who do not comprehend that narcolepsy is a disabling disease.

If cataplexy is present, medications other than amphetamines or Ritalin are required and useful. The class of drugs called tricyclic antidepressants, including protriptyline and imipramine, or the class of drugs called monoamine oxidase inhibitors may alleviate cataplexy. These medicines can often reduce attacks—for example, from three a day to three a month. In addition, effective treatment for cataplexy usually also relieves sleep paralysis and hypnogogic hallucinations.

Since the development of tolerance is common and these drugs can aggravate the symptom of sleepiness, determining the best timing and dose is critical. Another side effect of cataplexy drugs is impaired sexual function in males. Some men even discontinue these medications periodically for a day or two in order to sustain sexual relations. In addition, none of the drugs used for any symptoms of narcolepsy are safe to take during pregnancy.

In some cases, narcoleptics can be treated without medication if they carefully space naps during the day to relieve excessive sleepiness. Patients keep nap diaries to rate their alertness at regular intervals during the day. They then schedule short, strategically timed naps during those daytime periods when their sleep attacks are most likely to occur.

Naps are particularly valuable in treating children with narcolepsy because the consequences of a lifetime of medication on their development or on the course of their illness is unknown. Some children who show hyperactive behavior actually have narcolepsy; they are working frantically to overcome their persistent sleepiness and to keep themselves awake. Children with narcolepsy may also justifiably fear falling asleep, day or night, because of hallucinations and sleep paralysis.

It is evident that supportive counseling must be a strong component of treatment, whatever the patient's age. Sensitive medical monitoring can offer narcoleptics a measure of satisfactory daily living, but the use of stimulants to improve alertness may also make them more aware of their limitations and, therefore, more frustrated. Depression is not the cause of narcolepsy but may result primarily from the disruption in their lives and the feeling that they are denied the right to a "normal" life. Their constant sleepiness engenders feelings of inferiority and inadequacy. Narcoleptics usually refrain from mentioning their hallucinations and try to hide their automatic behavior for fear of being labeled insane. Loss of work, broken marriages, and social isolation are often witnesses to the crippling effects of narcolepsy.

Of all the people with narcolepsy seen at major sleep disorders centers, more than one-half have been completely disabled with respect to regular employment by the age of forty. With part-time, homebound, or self-employment, however, most narcoleptics can gain self-respect and help support themselves through work that is safe and tailored to their needs. They must be given tasks that can be divided into parts performed in relatively short time periods.

Drug and nap therapy can do little for narcoleptics without education of their families, friends, acquaintances, employers, and coworkers about the reality of this neurological disease. Most people find it hard to accept the notion that sleepiness cannot be controlled and insist that narcoleptics could be more alert if they tried harder. Narcoleptics are often stigmatized as slackers or incompetents, or assumed to be drug abusers or closet drinkers. It is most important that patients and all the people in their lives comprehend that excessive daytime sleepiness is not the patients' "fault."

Further help for narcoleptics seems to lie in animal studies, which may fill in many important pieces of the narcolepsy puzzle. The effects of the disease on behavior, the way in which it is inherited, and the benefits and risks of specific drugs continue to be evaluated in narcoleptic dogs.

PERSPECTIVE AND PROSPECTS

Once viewed as "all in the mind," narcolepsy is now recognized as a neurological disorder. Its origin is unknown, but research has already discovered evidence of possible causes. An understanding of narcolepsy both depended on and advanced the understanding of normal sleep and of other sleep disorders. Scientists define sleep as a reduction in awareness of and interaction with the environment, lowered movement and muscle activity, and partial or complete suspension of voluntary behavior and consciousness.

Although narcolepsy was named and described in 1880, it could not be genuinely studied until the 1930's, when the electroencephalograph (EEG) was developed to record brain activity during the various stages of sleep. By the 1940's, this advancement led to a description of the narcoleptic tetrad, the four usual symptoms of narcolepsy: excessive daytime sleepiness, cataplexy, sleep paralysis, and hypnogogic hallucinations.

In the 1950's, narcolepsy still only rated a paragraph in one neurology textbook, which mistakenly called it a rare variety of epilepsy. A major discovery occurred in 1960: Narcoleptics bypass the normal stages of light and deep sleep and fall directly into rapid eye movement (REM) sleep. Thus, sudden-onset REM period (or SOREMP) became the major distinguishing feature of this brain disorder.

It was soon noted that relatives of narcoleptics are sixty times more likely to have the disease than members of the general population. Clearly, there is a hereditary factor involved, and geneticists have joined the hunt for narcolepsy's cause. The hereditary aspects of the disease are particularly important to counselors because parents with narcolepsy may feel guilty if their child develops it. (Indeed, some patients abandon plans to have children.) Geneticists have found a gene which may be responsible for narcolepsy. Since the gene produces an antigen called DR2 on patients' white blood cells, which is not found in nonnarcoleptics, immunologists have also begun to search for the origins of narcolepsy.

The disease is thought to arise from a biochemical imbalance in the brain which disturbs the mechanism that activates the on/off cycle of sleep. Biochemists are studying the possible relationship of various brain chemicals called neurotransmitters to narcolepsy. A defect in the way in which the body produces or uses dopamine, acetylcholine, or some other neurotransmitter is suspected to precipitate narcolepsy, which never spontaneously disappears once it is developed.

Two interesting discoveries may help in the diagnosis of narcolepsy even before the classical clinical symptoms develop. There is some evidence that REM sleep is entered with abnormal rapidity years before the disorder develops. The drug physostigmine salicylate has no effect on normal dogs but elicits cataplexy in puppies with narcolepsy. Both these discoveries may be useful in screening the children of narcoleptics.

Because narcolepsy involves the fundamental processes of sleep, the combined efforts of neuroscientists, geneticists, biochemists, immunologists, and other scientists to unravel its mysteries will continue to yield important information about the basic mechanism of sleep—that state in which humans spend almost one-third of their lives.

—*Grace D. Matzen*

See also Apnea; Brain; Electroencephalography (EEG); Hallucinations; Memory loss; Nervous system; Neurology; Neurology, pediatric; Paralysis; Sleep disorders; Sleeping sickness; Unconsciousness.

FOR FURTHER INFORMATION:

Dement, William C. *The Sleepwatchers*. Stanford, Calif.: Stanford Alumni Association, 1992. A lively and often amusing book by the chair of the National Commission on Sleep Disorders Research. Traces the story of such research since the 1950's, when Dement first studied narcolepsy. Solid science that reads like a novel.

Dotto, Lydia. *Losing Sleep: How Your Sleeping Habits Affect Your Life*. New York: William Morrow, 1990. The intent of the author is to provide lay readers with basic scientific information to understand the impact of sleep problems on daily life. Dotto has a highly interesting style of writing. Includes a bibliography.

Hartmann, Ernest. *The Sleep Book*. Glenview, Ill.: Scott, Foresman, 1987. An easily understood discussion by a well-known pioneer in normal sleep and sleep disorders research. Contains a forty-page appendix of sleep disorders classification, centers, and specialists.

Hauri, Peter, and Shirley Linde. *No More Sleepless Nights*. Rev. ed. New York: John Wiley & Sons, 1996. Contains a brief description of narcolepsy, but there is an easy-to-understand chapter on basic sleep facts. Explains the need for and work of sleep disorders centers.

Poceta, J. Steven, and Merrill Mitler. *Sleep Disorders: Diagnosis and Treatment*. Totowa, N.J.: Humana Press, 1998. This volume fills an important need by making this field accessible to primary care physicians and giving them the tools and confidence to diagnose and treat those cases that do not need specialized help. It also makes clear which patients should be referred to a sleep disorder service and when.

Reite, Martin, John Ruddy, and Kim E. Nagel. *Concise Guide to Evaluation and Management of Sleep Disorders*. 2d ed. Washington, D.C.: American Psychiatric Press, 1997. Goals of this book are to provide a portable and practical approach to the diagnosis and treatment of sleep problems and a current summary of the classification of sleep disorders.

Sweeney, Donald R. *Overcoming Insomnia*. New York: G. P. Putnam's Sons, 1989. Although the major focus of this book is insomnia, its discussion of narcolepsy is quite adequate. Contains a bibliography and a useful list of the drugs used to treat sleep disorders.

Walsleben, Joyce A., and Rita Baron-Faust. *A Woman's Guide to Sleep: Guaranteed Solutions for a Good Night's Rest*. New York: Crown, 2000. Writing in an informal, easily comprehensible style, Walsleben, director of the Sleep Disorders Center at New York University School of Medicine, and freelancer Baron-Faust cover nearly every sleep disorder suffered by women.

NARCOTICS

TREAMENT

ANATOMY OR SYSTEM AFFECTED: Brain, nervous system, psychic-emotional system

SPECIALTIES AND RELATED FIELDS: Pharmacology

DEFINITION: The use of drugs from the opiate family, which mimic the action of the body's own painkilling substances, to treat pain, anxiety, coughing, diarrhea, and insomnia.

KEY TERMS:

agonist: a drug which acts in a fashion similar to that of a hormone or neurotransmitter normally found in the body

analgesia: the absence of pain; analgesics are compounds that stop the neurotransmission of pain messages

antagonist: a drug which acts to block the effects of a hormone or neurotransmitter normally found in the body

brain stem: the region between the brain and spinal cord that controls such functions as respiration and heart rate

central nervous system: the brain and spinal cord

dependence: a craving for a drug

endogenous: something naturally found in the body, such as neurotransmitters

exogenous: something originating outside the body and administered orally or by injection

neuron: a nerve cell which can conduct electrical impulses from one region of the body to another; it is capable of releasing neurotransmitters

neurotransmitter: a chemical substance released by one nerve cell to stimulate or inhibit the function of an adjacent nerve cell; a chemical message released from a neuron

opioids: drugs derived from opium; also known as narcotics or opiates

tolerance: the ability to endure ever-increasing amounts of a drug

THE EFFECTS OF NARCOTICS

Narcotics are drugs commonly used to treat pain (analgesics), suppress coughing, control diarrhea, and aid in anesthesia. These drugs are some of the oldest and most used agents. Most drugs are able to alter the effects of body functions by mimicking naturally occurring chemicals (as with agonists) or by blocking the physiological effects of these chemicals (as with antagonists).

Researchers have examined the many effects of the substances derived from the opium poppy, including morphine, codeine, and heroin. They have identified endogenous opioid-like chemicals called endorphins, dynorphins, and enkephalins that act as neurotransmitters; that is, some opioid compounds are normally found in the human nervous system as substances that allow nerve cells to communicate with one another. The synthetic opioid morphine mimics the actions of endorphins, dynorphins, and enkephalins by taking the place of these neurotransmitters. Scientists and physicians now know that morphine and related compounds produce their major effects by acting on the central nervous system, which includes the brain and spinal cord. In order to understand how opioids affect the body's response to pain, one must first understand the physiology of pain.

Any time tissues are damaged, they release chemical substances into the space outside the damaged cell, known as the extracellular space. Sensory neurons that have the ability to detect these chemicals are known as pain neurons. Once the chemicals bind to receptors on a pain neuron, the neuron is stimulated to send an electrical message to the spinal cord. Two actions occur once this message arrives. The first is an immediate initiation of a reflex which attempts to remove the tissue from the source of injury. For example, when one accidentally places an arm on a hot stove, a neural reflex causes the muscles of the limb to retract the arm from the burner. This is accomplished when the pain neuron releases a chemical message (neurotransmitter) in the spinal cord to stimulate neurons that control the muscles of the affected limb. This neurotransmitter is known as substance P. The second action of the sensory pain neuron is to inform the brain of the tissue damage, so that appropriate behavioral modification can take place. For example, one may become more cautious around the kitchen after burning one's arm on the stove. Notification of the brain is also accomplished by activating a second neuron using the neurotransmitter substance P, which will carry this electrical message toward the brain. Morphine and related opioids are very effective analgesics that seem to alter this pathway, thus dampening the transmission of pain messages.

Morphinelike drugs act at several sites in the nervous system. One of the most clinically important places is within the spinal cord at the region where the pain neurons release substance P. Opioids are known to reduce the amount of substance P that is released and thereby to decrease the stimulatory message in the neural pathway to the brain. If the pain impulses traveling to the brain are reduced, so is one's perception of pain. The second area of the nervous system known to be involved in regulating the perception of pain is a diffuse area of neurons located between the brain and spinal cord referred to as the brain stem. When researchers stimulate a region of the brain stem, the pain impulses traveling to the brain are reduced. Opioid peptides have been identified in this area which, as in the spinal cord, are probably responsible for reducing the pain message.

Because exogenous opioids must act to mimic endogenous opioids, one may wonder why there is a need for narcotic drugs if the body already produces the opioid-like endorphins and enkephalins. The reason is that every individual has a different degree of pain tolerance. How much pain one can endure also changes with certain circumstances. For example, one hardly notices the pain of a cut when participating in an exciting outdoor game. If the same wound occurs while one's attention is focused on it, however, the cut becomes noticeably painful. Perhaps the best explanation for the differing interpretation of pain during these activities and among different people is the endogenous opioid system. It is likely that the acupuncture pins used to block pain messages cause neurons to release increasing amounts of endorphins, enkephalins, and dynorphins. In the same way, with the administration of narcotics, one artificially increases the amount of opioids in the body in order to block pain impulses.

Opioids act on the brain stem to affect several systems other than the one associated with pain. They suppress coughing in a way that is similar to their effect on neural signals to decrease pain messages to the brain. Narcotics seem to inhibit release of the neurotransmitters responsible for the cough reflex. Unfortunately, opioids can activate another area in the brain stem to produce nausea and vomiting. This unwanted effect is related to the dose and type of drug used. Therefore, physicians can usually diminish the vomiting response with appropriate treatment selections. Perhaps the most dangerous problem with opioid usage is the effect that opioids have on the brain stem's regulation of respiration. When the brain stem senses that the level of carbon dioxide is too high, breathing is increased to rid the body of this excess waste gas. Narcotics decrease the responsiveness of the brain stem to carbon dioxide. Therefore, breathing rates tend to be inappropriately low, causing a buildup of carbon dioxide.

Constriction of the pupils of the eyes is a very common effect of opioids on the visual system. In fact, this constriction serves as an important diagnostic clue in examining a patient who has taken an overdose of a narcotic.

Opioids have a constipating effect, indirectly through the central nervous system and directly through their influence on the intestines. Opioids cause a decrease in peristalsis, the series of muscular contractions of the intestinal wall that would normally move food toward the anus.

Most opioid analgesics have no direct effect on the heart and blood vessels. Thus, they do not alter heart rate or rhythm or blood pressure to any significant degree. The only noticeable effect of narcotics on the cardiovascular system is a flushing and warming of the skin because of a slight increase in blood flow to the skin. Occasionally, this is accompanied by sweating. Kidney function tends to be depressed by opioids, which may be attributable to a decrease in the amount of blood that is filtered through the kidneys. There is also a decrease in the ability to urinate, as these drugs increase contraction of the muscle that prevents urine from leaving the bladder.

USES AND COMPLICATIONS

Medical personnel use this knowledge of how narcotics alter the body to the patient's advantage. Narcotics are used in the relief of pain and anxiety, as sedatives and anesthetics, to reduce coughing, and as a way to control diarrhea.

Opioid analgesics are among the most effective and valuable medications for the treatment of serious pain. Morphinelike drugs dampen the pain response but do not affect to a great extent other senses such as vision and hearing. They are often used to treat pain in the postoperative period, in which they effectively reduce or eliminate the short-term pain from tissue trauma that is caused by surgery. When pain is reduced, patients tend to eat, sleep, and recover much more rapidly. Physicians often prescribe narcotics such as meperidine (Demerol) or codeine on an as-needed basis. In this way, the patient, who knows firsthand the effectiveness of the drug, can control the frequency of analgesic administration. In fact, patients are usually advised to administer a small dose before the pain becomes too intense, thus decreasing the pain message before it reaches a high level and requires a relatively high dose to make the patient comfortable again.

A painful sensation consists of the neural response to the tissue damage and the patient's reaction to the stimulus. The analgesic properties of narcotics are related to their ability to diminish both pain perception and the reaction of the patient to pain. These drugs effectively raise the threshold for pain, perhaps because of the euphoria experienced by patients given opioids. For example, a patient in pain who is given morphine experiences a pleasant floating sensation with a great reduction in distress and anxiety. It is interesting to note, however, that subjects who are not in pain do not experience euphoria when given morphine. In fact, they tend to have an unpleasant response known as dysphoria, which often includes restlessness and a feeling of general discomfort.

Physicians and other health care workers must achieve a delicate balance between alleviating pain from known causes and masking pain as a warning signal from unexpected sources. For example, a patient having abdominal surgery would likely require relatively high doses of narcotic analgesics to reduce the postoperative pain. Yet the administration of an analgesic could mask the pain from an unexpected abdominal infection. Therefore, if used excessively, narcotics may prevent the early recognition of complications.

In addition to their analgesic effects, opioids tend to have a sedative effect and are often used as a pre-anesthesic drug or as an anesthetic. Potent opioids are used in relatively large doses to achieve general anesthesia, particularly in patients undergoing heart surgery. These narcotics are also commonly used during other surgeries in which it is important that heart function be affected only minimally. Examples of narcotic agents used in anesthesia include fentanyl (Sublimaze), sufentanil, and alfentanil.

Suppression of the cough reflex is a clinically useful effect of narcotics. The therapeutic doses of opioids needed to reduce coughing are much lower than the doses to achieve analgesia. The opioid derivatives most commonly used to suppress the cough reflex are codeine, dextromethorphan, and noscapine. How these agents work to reduce coughing is not known, but they are thought to act on the brain stem.

Diarrhea from almost any cause can be controlled with opioids. Diphenoxylate (Lomotil) and loperamide (Imodium), narcotics commonly used to treat diarrhea, do not possess analgesic properties. These drugs appear to act on the nerves within the intestinal tract to decrease muscular activity.

Like all drugs, narcotics have both beneficial and undesired effects. The toxic effects of an opioid depends on the dosage, the agent used, the clinical condition in which it is used, and an individual patient's response to the drug. Some of the more common unwanted effects include restlessness and hyperactivity instead of sedation, respiratory depression, nausea and vomiting, increased pressure within the brain, low blood pressure, constipation, urinary retention, and itching around the nose. Most of these conditions are of short duration and resolve themselves after the drug has been discontinued.

Patients, or more often narcotic drug abusers, may become tolerant and dependent upon these agents. These individuals, such as heroin abusers, have a strong craving for the drugs. These agents are abused for their euphoric effect at relatively high doses. The human body is very efficient in tolerating the effects of opioids. Their effects lessen somewhat with each succeeding dose, so that a higher dose must be taken to achieve the same effect. Physiological adaptation to the long-term use of opioids (two to three weeks) causes the development of tolerance for these drugs.

Exogenous opioids take the place of endogenous ones. Therefore, the nervous system and other physiological systems attempt to bring the levels of these neurotransmitters back to normal. First, the liver speeds up its metabolism of the drugs to eliminate them from the system more rapidly. Second, the regions of the nervous system that respond to opioids become desensitized by reducing the number of neural receptors that are available. Finally, after a few weeks of high levels of opioids, changes in other areas of the brain attempt to compensate for the rising opioid levels. Individuals who abruptly stop taking the drugs enter a period of withdrawal in which the symptoms are similar to a bad case of influenza. Morphine and heroine withdrawal symptoms usually start within twelve hours of the last dose. Peak symptoms of narcotic withdrawal occur after one to two days. Most symptoms gradually subside and are usually gone after one week. It should be emphasized that, under a physician's direction, the abuse potential of narcotics is very low.

There are certain clinical conditions in which opioid drugs should not be used or should be used with extreme caution. Because of the potential for respiratory depression with opioid treatment, these drugs should not be administered to patients with head injuries or impaired lung function. Most opioid drugs can cross the placenta and therefore should be avoided during pregnancy; with long-term use, the infant can be born addicted to narcotics.

Fortunately, some drugs can reverse the effects of narcotics. Three opioid antagonists are nalmefene, naloxone (Narcan), and naltrexone (Trexan). When these agents are given in the absence of an opioid agonist, they have no noticeable effect. When administered to a morphine-treated patient, however, they completely reverse the opioid effects almost immediately. These narcotic antagonists are particularly useful in treating patients who have taken an overdose of opioids. Such patients often arrive in the hospital emergency room not breathing and in a coma. These antagonists will normalize respiration, restore consciousness, and counteract other opioid effects. Interestingly, individuals who have become tolerant to and dependent upon opioids will immediately experience withdrawal symptoms when given naloxone or naltrexone.

PERSPECTIVE AND PROSPECTS

Narcotic drugs were originally found in the opium poppy five thousand years ago. Opium is obtained from the milky fluid of the unripe seed capsules of the poppy plant. The juice is dried in the air and forms a brown, sticky substance. With continued drying, the mass can be pulverized into powder. It is this powder that contains opioids. Morphine, codeine, and papaverine are the natural opioids that are used clinically. Most other narcotics are chemically derived.

The opium poppy, *Papaver somniferum*, was named after the Roman god of sleep, Somnis. Ancient Egyptian medical texts listed opium as a cure for illness and as a poison. Although opium was used extensively, the abuse potential was low because the poppy has a very bitter taste. Smoking opium became popular in eighteenth century China as a treatment for severe diarrhea and was also used as a socially acceptable drug mainly for its euphoric effects.

The opium poppy contains more than twenty distinct agents with a variety of potencies and unwanted effects. In 1806, a pharmacist refined opium into one active substance, morphine, which was found to be ten times as potent. Morphine was named after Morpheus, the Greek god of dreams, because the drug has powerful sedative effects. The discovery of other medically active agents quickly followed. Codeine and papaverine were identified next and found

to be slightly less potent than morphine. At this time, clinicians used these purified products rather than the crude opium juice.

Shortly after purified narcotics became available, so did the widespread use of hypodermic needles. This allowed physicians to administer narcotics directly into the bloodstream. The injected opioids would travel via the blood to the brain in as short a time as twenty seconds. In the United States, morphine found widespread use as an analgesic for wounded soldiers during the Civil War. It was one of the most powerful painkillers available to physicians, but its unrestricted availability created great potential for addiction with long-term use.

Opioids became so popular that hundreds of medications became available to the public. These tonics promised to cure everything from "tired blood" to common aches and pains. Their widespread, unregulated use produced a large number of addicts. At the beginning of the twentieth century, the U.S. government attempted to reduce the number of addicts by making it illegal to buy any opioid-containing compound without a prescription. Medical scientists tried to synthesize compounds with morphinelike characteristics but without the addictive effects.

Physicians now have available to them a wide range of narcotics with different pharmacological properties. For example, there are drugs without addictive, euphoric, or sedative properties that can treat coughing or diarrhea. Some of these are available without a prescription for the treatment of occasional coughing and diarrhea. Narcotic analgesics, however, are given only under the direction of a physician. For example, morphine is still used as a potent pain reliever; when it is used appropriately, there is little chance of addiction. It is likely that other clinical uses will be found for narcotic drugs as researchers learn more about the human body's own endogenous narcotics, the endorphins.

—*Matthew Berria, Ph.D.*

See also Addiction; Anesthesia; Anesthesiology; Coughing; Diarrhea and dysentery; Pain; Pain management; Pharmacology; Self-medication.

FOR FURTHER INFORMATION:

Camp, John F. "Patient-Controlled Analgesia." *American Family Physician* 44 (December, 1991): 2145-2150. This article describes the relatively new method of administering narcotics in which the patient controls the timing of drug administration.

Griffith, H. Winter. *Complete Guide to Prescription and Non-Prescription Drugs.* 7th ed. New York: Berkley, 1999. A complete guide to both prescription and nonprescription drugs, including major uses, unwanted effects, precautions, and interactions with other drugs. A highly organized, useful tool for the nonscientist.

Inaba, Darryl S., William E. Cohen, and Michael E. Holstein. *Uppers, Downers, All Arounders: Physical and Mental Effects of Psychoactive Drugs.* 4th ed. Ashland, Oreg.: CNS, 2000. Mainly covers drug abuse, but also contains brief descriptions of the history and medical uses for drugs with abuse potential. A reader-friendly book that offers numerous statements from drug addicts regarding their addiction and, in some cases, their recovery.

Ling, W., and D. R. Wesson. "Drugs of Abuse: Opiates." *Western Journal of Medicine* 152 (May, 1990): 565-572. This article reviews the ways that addiction can be treated. Also addresses the use of narcotic antagonists in the treatment of drug overdose.

Voth, Eric A., Robert L. Dupont, and Harold M. Voth. "Responsible Prescribing of Controlled Substances." *American Family Physician* 44 (November, 1991): 1673-1680. This article details some of the important problems in prescribing narcotics. Gives a description of characteristics that both health care workers and nonprofessionals can watch for in their attempts to identify drug abusers.

NASAL POLYP REMOVAL

PROCEDURE

ANATOMY OR SYSTEM AFFECTED: Head, nose

SPECIALTIES AND RELATED FIELDS: Family practice, general surgery, otorhinolaryngology

DEFINITION: The excision of benign growths that project from the mucous membrane lining the nasal cavity.

INDICATIONS AND PROCEDURES

Nasal polyps are swollen masses that project from the nasal wall. These benign structures are commonly found in patients with allergies. They may cause chronic nasal obstruction, which results in diminished air flow through the nasal cavity.

Once a polyp is detected, the physician may prescribe a nasal spray to reduce its size, such as the corticosteroids beclomethasone or flunisolide. This treatment is usually effective for small nasal polyps that cause only minor symptoms. When pharmacological management is not successful, however, the polyps should be removed surgically.

Surgical removal of nasal polyps (nasal polypectomy) is typically done as an outpatient procedure. It requires either general anesthesia or local anesthesia with sedation. After the patient is asleep or sedated, the lining of the nasal cavity is injected with a combination of local anesthesia and epinephrine to control pain and bleeding. The surgeon (usually an otorhinolaryngologist) visualizes the polyps with a headlight, and the polyps are removed with specialized, long surgical instruments inserted

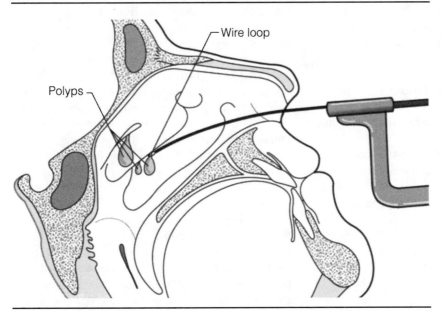

The Removal of Nasal Polyps

Wire loop

Polyps

Allergies or chronic sinus infections can lead to the development of nasal polyps, distended areas of the nasal lining. If they interfere with breathing or the sense of smell or if they cause frequent nosebleeds, the polyps may be removed with a wire loop.

into the nasal cavity. After the polyps are removed, the nasal passages are packed with ointment-coated gauze to help control bleeding and aid in the healing of the nasal mucosa. The gauze is removed in the physician's office a few days after the surgery. Once the packing is removed, the patient enjoys improved breathing through the nasal passages.

USES AND COMPLICATIONS

There are relatively few complications associated with nasal polyp removal. Some of the more common complications include bleeding from the surgical site, nasal and ear discomfort or anxiety as a result of the packing, and nausea from the anesthesia. The recurrence of nasal polyps after polypectomy is not unusual. Patients with cystic fibrosis have a high rate of occurrence of nasal polyps and often have recurrent problems.

—*Matthew Berria, Ph.D.,*
and Douglas Reinhart, M.D.
See also Allergies; Nasopharyngeal disorders; Otorhinolaryngology; Sense organs; Sinusitis; Smell.

FOR FURTHER INFORMATION:

Benjamin, Bruce, et al. *A Colour Atlas of Otorhinolaryngology.* Edited by Michael Hawke. Philadelphia: J. B. Lippincott, 1995.

Cody, D. Thane, et al. *Diseases of the Ears, Nose, and Throat.* Chicago: Year Book Medical, 1981.

Morelock, Michael. *Your Guide to Problems of the Ear, Nose, and Throat.* Philadelphia: G. F. Stickley, 1985.

NASOPHARYNGEAL DISORDERS
DISEASE/DISORDER

ANATOMY OR SYSTEM AFFECTED: Nose, respiratory system, throat

SPECIALTIES AND RELATED FIELDS: Family practice, occupational health, otorhinolaryngology

DEFINITION: Disorders of the nose, nasal passages (sinuses), and pharynx (mouth, throat, and esophagus).

KEY TERMS:

acute disease: a short and sharp disease process

chronic disease: a lingering illness

esophagus: the tube that leads from the pharynx to the stomach

larynx: the organ that produces the voice, which lies between the pharynx and the trachea; commonly called the voice box

nasopharyngeal: referring to the nose and pharynx (the upper part of the throat that leads from the mouth to the esophagus)

trachea: a tube that leads from the throat to the lungs; commonly called the windpipe

CAUSES AND SYMPTOMS

Nasopharyngeal disorders include all the diseases that can be present in the nasal cavity and the pharynx. These include the common cold, pharyngitis (sore throat), laryngitis (inflammation of the larynx), epiglottitis (inflammation of the lid over the larynx), tonsillitis (inflammation of the lymph nodes at the rear of the mouth), sinusitis (inflammation of the sinus cavities that surround the nose), otitis media (earache that is often associated with nasopharyngeal infection), nosebleed, nasal obstruction, halitosis (bad breath), and various other disorders.

The common cold is one of the most prevalent diseases that afflict humankind. Pharyngitis, or sore throat, often accompanies the common cold, or it may appear by itself. Acute infections can be caused by viruses or bacteria, often by certain streptococcus strains—hence the common term for the disorder, strep throat. Acute pharyngitis can also be caused by chemicals or radiation. As a chronic disorder, pharyngitis can be caused by lingering infection in other organs such as the lungs and sinuses, or it can be attributable to constant irritation from smoking, drinking alcohol, or breathing polluted air. The usual symptoms of pharyngitis include sore throat, difficulty in swallowing, and fever. The infected area appears red and swollen. Ordinarily, pharyngitis is not serious. If certain strains of streptococcus are the cause, however, then the infection may progress to rheumatic fever. This disease appears to be the result of an immune system reaction to some streptococcus bacteria. It can have painful effects in many parts of the body, such as in joints, and can do permanent damage to parts of the heart. In rare cases, rheumatic fever can be fatal.

Acute laryngitis is usually caused by a viral infection, but bacteria, outside irritants, or misuse of the voice are other causes. Ordinarily, the vocal cords produce sounds by vibrating in response to the air passing over them. When inflamed or irritated, they swell, causing distortion in the sounds produced. The voice becomes hoarse and raspy and may even diminish to a soft whisper. This distortion of sound is the main symptom of laryngitis, but there may also be a sore throat and congestion that causes constant coughing. The condition generally resolves itself and requires no treatment. Chronic laryngitis has the same symptoms but does not go away spontaneously. It may be caused by an infectious agent but more likely is attributable to some irritant activity, such as constantly misusing the voice, smoking, drinking alcohol, or breathing contaminated air.

The epiglottis is a waferlike tissue covered by a mucous membrane that sits on top of the larynx. It can become infected by such microorganisms as the bacteria *Haemophilus influenzae* type b in a condition called epiglottitis. Although the symptoms of epiglottitis can resemble those of pharyngitis, the infection can quickly progress to a very serious, life-threatening disorder. Epiglottitis usually afflicts children from two to four years of age, but adults can also be affected. The infection can begin rapidly, causing the epiglottis to swell and obstruct the airway to the lungs, creating a major medical emergency. Within twelve hours of the onset of symptoms, 50 percent of patients require hospitalization and intubation (insertion of a breathing tube into the trachea). The symptoms are high fever, severe sore throat, difficulty in breathing, difficulty in swallowing, and general malaise. As the airway becomes more and more occluded, the patient begins to gasp for air. The lack of oxygen may cause cyanosis (blue color in the lips, fingers, and skin), exhaustion, and shock.

Another disease associated with the larynx is croup, or laryngotracheobronchitis. As the medical name indicates, croup involves the larynx, the trachea, and the bronchi (the large branches of the lung). It is usually caused by a virus, but some cases are attributable to bacterial infection. Children from three to five years of age are the usual victims. This disease causes the airways to narrow because of inflammation of the inner mucosal surfaces. Inflammation causes coughing, but the narrowed airway causes the cough to be sharp and brassy, like the barking of a seal. Croup is usually relatively benign, but sometimes it progresses to a severe disease requiring hospitalization.

Various other disorders can afflict the larynx, such as damage to the vocal cords because of infection by bacteria, fungi, or other microorganisms. The vocal cords can also be damaged by misusing the voice, smoking, or breathing contaminated air. Polyps (masses of tissue growing on the surface), nodes (little knots of tissue), or "singers' nodules" may de-

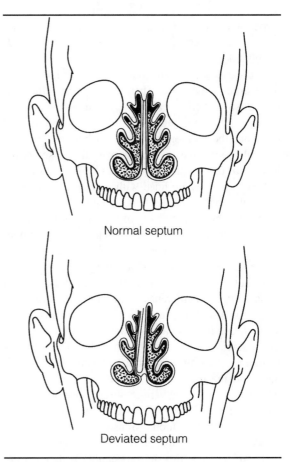

Normal septum

Deviated septum

A deviated septum is a malformation in the cartilage between the nostrils, either present at birth or caused by a blow to the nose.

velop. Sores called contact ulcers may form on the vocal cords.

Tonsillitis is an inflammation of two large lymph nodes located at the back of the throat, the tonsils. It may also involve the adenoids, lymph nodes located at the top of the throat. The function of these lymph nodes is to remove harmful pathogens (disease-causing organisms) from the nasopharyngeal cavity. At times, the load of microorganisms that they absorb becomes more than they can handle, and they become infected. The tonsils and adenoids may then become enlarged. A sore throat develops, along with a headache, fever, and chills. Glands of the neck and throat feel sore and may become enlarged. Young adults can also suffer from quinsy, or peritonsillar abscess. In this condition, one of the tonsils becomes infected and pus forms between the tonsil and the soft tissue surrounding it. Quinsy is characterized by pain in the throat and/or the soft palate, pain on swallowing, fever, and a tendency to lean the head toward the affected side.

The nasal sinuses are four pairs of cavities in the bone around the nose. There are two maxillary sinuses, so called because they are found in the maxilla, or upper jaw. Slightly above and behind them are the ethmoid sinuses, and behind them are the sphenoid sinuses. Sitting over the nose in the lower part of the forehead are the two frontal sinuses. All these sinuses are lined with a mucous membrane and have small openings that lead into the nasal passages. Air moves in and out of the sinuses and allows mucus to drain into the nose. In acute sinusitis, infection builds up in the mucous membrane of any or all of the sinuses. The membrane lining the sinus swells and shuts the opening into the nasal passages. At thesame time, membranes of the nose swell and become congested. Mucus and pus build up inside the sinuses, causing pain and pressure. Most often, sinusitis accompanies the common cold: The mucous membrane that lines the nose extends into the sinuses, so the infection of a cold can readily spread into the sinuses. The various viruses responsible for the common cold may be involved, as well as a wide group of bacteria. Chronic sinusitis can be caused by repeated infections that have allowed scar tissue to build up, closing the sinus openings and impeding mucus drainage, or may be the result of allergies.

Tissues in the nasopharyngeal cavity may be affected by conditions occurring in other parts of the body. For example, vocal cord paralysis may be caused by vascular accidents, certain cancers, tissue trauma, and other events.

Some infections in the nasopharyngeal cavity can spread to the ear through the Eustachian tubes that connect the two areas. Chief among the diseases of the ear that can be associated with nasopharyngeal disorders are the various forms of acute otitis media, an earache occurring in the central part of the ear. There are four basic types of otitis media. With the first type, serous otitis media, there is usually no infection, but fluid accumulates inside the middle ear because of the blockage of the Eustachian tube or the overproduction of fluid; the condition is usually mild, with some pain and temporary loss of hearing. The second type is otitis media with effusion; with this condition comes both infection and accumulation of fluid. The third form is acute purulent otitis media, the most serious type. Pus builds up inside the middle

ear, and its pressure may rupture the eardrum, allowing discharge of blood and pus. The fourth type is secretory otitis media, which usually occurs after several bouts of otitis media. Cells within the middle ear start producing a fluid that is thicker than normal and produced in greater amounts.

Chronic otitis media is bacterial in origin. It is characterized by a perforation of the eardrum and chronic pus discharge. The eardrum is a flat, pliable disk of tissue that vibrates to conduct sounds from the outside to the inner-ear structures. The perforation that occurs in chronic otitis media can be one of two types: a relatively benign perforation occurring in the central part of the eardrum or a potentially dangerous perforation occurring near the edges of the eardrum. The latter perforation can be associated with loss of hearing, increased discharge of pus and other fluids, facial paralysis, and the spread of infection to other tissues. When the perforation of chronic otitis media is near the edges of the eardrum, something called a cholesteatoma develops. This accumulation of matter grows in the inner ear and can be destructive to bone and other tissue.

The same organisms that cause otitis media can be responsible for a condition called mastoiditis. The mastoid process is a bone structure lined with a mucous membrane. Infection from otitis media can spread to this area and in severe cases can destroy the bone. Mastoiditis used to be a leading cause of death in children.

Nosebleeds are common and most often result from a blow to the nose, but they can also be caused by colds, sinusitis, and breathing dry air. The septum (the cartilaginous tissue that separates the nostrils) and the surrounding intranasal mucous membrane contain many tiny blood vessels that are easily ruptured. If an individual receives a blow to the nose, these vessels can break and bleed. They can also rupture because of irritation from a cold or other condition. Breathing very dry air sometimes causes the nasal mucous membrane to crust over, and bleeding can follow. Nosebleeds are not usually serious, but sometimes they are indicative of an underlying condition, such as hypertension (high blood pressure), a tumor, or another disease.

Nasal obstruction is common during colds and allergy attacks, but it can also be caused by a deviated septum, a malformation in the cartilage between the nostrils that can be congenital or caused by a blow to the nose. Also, nasal obstruction can be attributable to nasal polyps, nasal tumors, or swollen adenoids. A common source of nasal obstruction is overuse of nasal decongestants. These agents relieve nasal congestion by reducing intranasal inflammation and swelling. If used too often or too long, however, they can cause the very problem that they were intended to cure: Intranasal blood vessels dilate, the area swells, secretions increase, and the nose becomes blocked. This is known as rebound congestion, or in medical terminology, rhinitis medicamentosa (nasal inflammation that is caused by a medication).

Halitosis, or bad breath, can be considered a nasopharyngeal disorder in the sense that it can originate in the mouth. It can be caused by diseases of the teeth and/or gums, but the most common causes are smoking or eating aromatic foods such as onions and garlic. Bad breath may also be a sign of disease conditions in other parts of the body, such as certain lung disorders or cancer of the esophagus. Hepatic failure, a liver dysfunction, may be accompanied by a fishy odor on the breath. Azotemia, the retention of nitrogen in the blood, may give rise to an ammonia-like odor. A sweet, fruity odor on the breath of diabetic patients may accompany ketoacidosis, a condition that occurs when there are high levels of glucose in the blood. Sometimes, young children stick foreign objects or other materials into their noses; it has been reported that these materials can fester, causing severe halitosis. Bad breath is rarely apparent to the individual who has it, however offensive it may be to others. A good way to check one's breath is to lick the back of one's hand and smell the spot; malodor, if it exists, will usually be apparent.

TREATMENT AND THERAPY

Nasopharyngeal disorders are most often mild illnesses that can be treated at home. For example, acute pharyngitis or sore throat is easily managed most of the time. The patient is advised to rest, gargle with warm salt water several times a day, and soothe the pain with lozenges or anesthetic gargles. If the infection is caused by a virus, it usually will clear without further treatment. If the physician suspects, however, that the infection is bacterial in origin, throat smears may be taken so that the organism can be identified. If bacteria are discovered, antibiotic therapy will be undertaken to eradicate the pathogens. This is particularly important if the infection is caused by certain strains of streptococcus bacteria. In this case, it is vital to destroy the organism in

order to avoid the development of rheumatic fever.

In acute laryngitis caused by viral infection, the patient is advised to rest the voice, inhale steam, and drink warm liquids. If bacteria are the cause of the laryngitis, antibiotic therapy is undertaken. In treating chronic laryngitis, the physician must discover the cause and remove it. If allergy is the cause, antihistamine therapy could help. If the cause is bacterial, antibiotic therapy is used. If smoking or drinking alcohol is the problem, the patient should be counseled to stop. The simple palliative measures used for acute laryngitis—resting the voice, drinking warm liquids, and breathing steam—are also useful for chronic laryngitis.

Symptoms of epiglottitis are often similar to those of sore throat. If there is any evidence of difficulty in breathing, however, the patient should be seen by a physician quickly because an emergency situation may be developing. If epiglottitis is obstructing the airway, the patient should be treated in an intensive care setting. It is important to make an airway for the patient, and it may be necessary to insert a tube into the trachea to allow the patient to breathe.

Before the age of antibiotics, tonsillitis was often treated surgically, with both tonsils and adenoids removed. This procedure is now rare because the infection usually responds to antibiotic therapy. Similarly, in peritonsillar abscess or quinsy, antibiotics usually clear the condition satisfactorily. In some cases, accumulations of pus may be removed surgically. If the abscesses return, it may be advisable to remove the tonsils.

As a rule, the child with croup is treated at home. Because the disease is usually caused by viruses, antibiotics are not used unless bacteria are known to be involved. Steam is often used to help liquefy mucus deposits on the interior walls of the trachea, the larynx, and the bronchi. The patient is given warm liquids to drink and is closely watched so that any signs that the condition is getting worse will be detected. The following symptoms should alert the caregiver to the possibility that an emergency situation is developing and that medical help is needed quickly: drooling, difficulty in swallowing, difficulty in breathing, inability to bend the neck forward, blue or dark color in the lips, high-pitched sounds when inhaling, rapid heartbeat, and loss of consciousness.

The main goals of therapy for sinusitis are to control infection, relieve the blockage of the sinus openings to permit drainage, and relieve pain. When sinusitis is known to be of bacterial origin, an appropriate antibiotic will be used to eradicate the organism. Often, however, sinusitis is attributable to viral infection, and other procedures are used to treat it. Inhaling steam is useful for reducing swelling and promoting drainage, as are decongestant sprays and oral decongestants. Analgesics can be given for pain. In certain circumstances, the sinuses are drained surgically.

Acute otitis media is most often diagnosed with the aid of an otoscope, an instrument that the doctor uses to look at the eardrum and surrounding tissues. The eardrum will be a dull red color, bulging, and perhaps perforated. While a viral infection may precede otitis media, the causative microorganisms for this and related ear infections, such as mastoiditis, are usually bacteria. Antibiotics are used both to treat the infections and to prevent the spread of disease to other areas. The drugs are usually taken orally, although antibiotic ear drops are often given as well. Penicillin and its derivatives are used, as are erythromycin and sulfisoxazole. Antibiotic therapy for acute otitis media is usually continued for ten days to two weeks. Sometimes, pus and other fluids and solid matter build up in the inner ear. It may be necessary to pierce the eardrum in order to remove these deposits. To help relieve blockage of the Eustachian tubes, a topical vasoconstrictor may be used in the nose to reduce the swelling of blood vessels. Antihistamines could be helpful to patients with allergies, but otherwise they are not indicated.

For chronic otitis media, it is necessary to clean both the outer ear canal and the middle ear thoroughly. A mild acetic acid solution with a corticosteroid is used for a week to ten days. Meanwhile, aggressive oral antibiotic therapy is undertaken to eradicate the pathogen. The perforated eardrum associated with chronic otitis media can usually be repaired surgically with little or no loss of function, and the cholesteatoma must be surgically removed.

Simple nosebleed can be treated by pinching the nose with the fingers and breathing through the mouth for five or ten minutes, to allow the blood to clot. Also, a plug of absorbent paper or cloth can be inserted into the bleeding nostril. A nosebleed that does not stop easily should be seen by a physician.

Nasal obstruction resulting from colds or allergies is treated by appropriate medications, decongestants for colds, and antihistamines for allergies. A deviated septum may require surgery. The only therapy for rhinitis medicamentosa, or rebound congestion caused by overuse of nasal decongestants, is to stop the medication and endure the congestion for as long as it takes the condition to clear. Sometimes, it is necessary to consult a physician.

For simple halitosis caused by smoking or food, breath fresheners (with or without "odor-fighting" chemicals) are often used, even though they usually simply replace a "bad" odor with a "good" one. Some people firmly believe that chewing parsley or other leaves rich in chlorophyll will counteract the smell of garlic. When halitosis is attributable to tooth or gum disease, it will persist until the condition is cured. Halitosis may be of diagnostic value in certain situations where a characteristic odor could alert the physician to the possibility of a disease condition.

PERSPECTIVE AND PROSPECTS

Diseases and infections of the nasal cavity and throat have always been common among human populations, as have therapies to deal with them. Until the advent of antibiotics, some of these disorders were quite serious, especially in young children, but modern medications and surgeries, where appropriate, have greatly lessened the danger. Many over-the-counter drugs are now used to combat sore throats, sinus congestion, and other nasopharyngeal symptoms of the common cold, although colds themselves remain incurable because of the hundreds or thousands of different microorganisms that may be responsible. Despite the numerous medications that can be taken, however, more serious infections or diseases, such as chronic tonsillitis or laryngitis, require a doctor's care, with more potent, prescription drugs and surgery if needed. The treatments available to physicians and patients for the symptoms of nasopharyngeal disorders are many, but the search continues for better drugs and perhaps preventive measures such as vaccinations to address the causes of these conditions.

—*C. Richard Falcon*

See also Allergies; Choking; Common cold; Ear infections and disorders; Ears; Halitosis; Hearing loss; Laryngectomy; Laryngitis; Multiple chemical sensitivity syndrome; Nasal polyp removal; Otorhinolaryngology; Pharyngitis; Plastic surgery; Respiration; Rhinitis; Rhinoplasty and submucous resection; Sinusitis; Smell; Sore throat; Strep throat; Taste; Tonsillectomy and adenoid removal; Tonsillitis; Voice and vocal cord disorders.

FOR FURTHER INFORMATION:

Larson, David E., ed. *Mayo Clinic Family Health Book*. 2d ed. New York: William Morrow, 1996. A thorough and up-to-date medical text for the layperson. The section on nasopharyngeal diseases is quite complete and offers excellent anatomic illustrations.

Scott, Andrew. *Pirates of the Cell: The Story of Viruses from Molecule to Microbe*. New York: Basil Blackwell, 1987. Useful for understanding the virus families that are often responsible for nasopharyngeal disorders.

Smith, Lendon H. *The Encyclopedia of Baby and Child Care*. Rev. ed. Englewood Cliffs, N.J.: Prentice Hall, 1980. Nasopharyngeal diseases strike babies and children most often. This reference work lists all the familiar disorders with Smith's descriptions of their symptoms and his recommendations for treatment.

_____. *The New Complete Medical and Health Encyclopedia*. 4 vols. Chicago: J. G. Ferguson, 2000. The chapters on upper respiratory diseases in this work are thorough and clear, with good illustrations.

NATIONAL CANCER INSTITUTE (NCI)
ORGANIZATION

DEFINITION: A federal agency devoted to the study of cancer, as well as communication and education about this condition.

KEY TERMS:

carcinogenesis: the biological process of the initiation, promotion, and progression of cancer

epidemiology: the study of the relationships between a host, an agent, and an environment that lead to a condition or disease

OVERVIEW

The U.S. Department of Health and Human Services (DHHS) is the federal agency responsible for public health. The DHHS includes twelve divisions, one of which is the National Institutes of Health (NIH). The National Cancer Institute (NCI) is one of seventeen institutes within NIH. The NCI was established under the National Cancer Act of 1937 and is the principal federal agency for cancer research and training. Following special legislation in 1971, the scope of the NCI has continued to broaden through new initiatives and legislation.

The purpose of the NCI is to eliminate cancer as far as possible and to discover treatment for those cancers which cannot be eradicated. The NCI approaches these goals by supporting research, coordinating efforts in prevention and treatment, facilitating the movement of research findings into medicine, and providing education and resources for patients and their families, health educators, and scientists. The NCI conducts research in its own laboratories and clinics in Bethesda, Maryland, but also supports and coordinates research projects conducted by universities, hospitals, research foundations, and businesses throughout the United States and many other countries.

THE ORGANIZATION AND FOCUS OF THE NCI

The NCI is organized into the Office of the Director of NCI and eight divisions. Each division specializes in a different aspect of cancer research, although there is overlap among them. The divisions include the Division of Basic Sciences, the Division of Cancer Biology, the Division of Cancer Control and Population Sciences, the Division of Cancer Epidemiology and Genetics, the Division of Cancer Prevention, the Division of Cancer Treatment and Diagnosis, the Division of Clinical Sciences, and the Division of Extramural Activities.

The Division of Basic Sciences focuses on research relating to cellular, molecular, genetic, biochemical, and immunological mechanisms critical to the understanding, diagnosis, and treatment of cancer. Research in cancer cell biology, such as carcinogenesis and cancer immunology, falls within the realm of the Division of Cancer Biology. This division also examines the biological and health effects of exposures to ionizing and nonionizing radiation. The Division of Cancer Epidemiology and Genetics focuses on the special interests of genetic predisposition, lifestyle factors, environmental contaminants, occupational exposures, medications, radiation, and infectious agents, as well as epidemiological methods development. The efforts of the Division of Cancer Prevention center on early detection methods and the efficacy of nutritional or lifestyle changes on cancer prevention. The results of research in this area led to the 5 a Day for Better Health program. Initiated in 1991, this program is a collaborative effort between the food industry and the NCI, which encourages Americans to eat five or more servings of vegetables and fruits each day as part of a low-fat, high-fiber diet. The Division of Cancer Treatment and Diagnosis includes programs in biomedical imaging, cancer diagnosis, cancer therapy evaluation, developmental therapeutics, and radiation research.

The mission of the Division of Clinical Sciences is to take the scientific discoveries to the medical clinic. It has five major research areas: cancer genetics, cancer vaccines and immunotherapy, molecular therapeutics, experimental transplantation, and advanced technology. The clinical cancer genetics program integrates all aspects of clinical and laboratory medicine, particularly in studies of breast, colon, renal, and prostate cancer. Processes include molecular diagnostics, novel imaging techniques, and the molecular assessment of normal tissues in at-risk populations. The cancer vaccines and immunotherapy program investigates the clinical feasibility of using vaccines against known conditions associated with cancer, such as the human papillomavirus and human immunodeficiency virus (HIV), as well as with cancer-specific products, such as in melanoma and in lymphomas. The molecular therapeutics program is concerned with most clinical trial experiments. Important recent discoveries include the development of Taxol as an effective anticancer agent, the development of AZT as an important anti-HIV drug, and the use of adoptive immunotherapy in the treatment of malignant melanoma. The scientific thrust of the molecular therapeutics program is the belief that the analysis of the molecular profile of individual cancers will help determine the most effective chemotherapeutic approaches. The experimental transplantation program examines bone marrow biology in order to advance transplantation techniques and the effectiveness of this approach.

Integrating many programs and divisions is the advanced technology program. New technology is an essential key to identifying genetic elements involved in cancer initiation and progression, as well as in drug efficacy and drug resistance. Although many drugs have been discovered which inhibit the growth of cancer cells successfully, they also affect healthy cells. This causes side effects that have a negative impact on patients' health and quality of life. New therapeutics and technology are being investigated to minimize or eliminate these side effects and enhance the effectiveness of therapy.

The eighth division of the NCI is the Division of Extramural Activities, which is responsible for handling all applications for funding and for monitoring research which has received funding from the NCI. Extramural activities also include the oversight of scientific communications. To enhance communication, the NCI has a number of advisory boards and groups which provide the institute with input from the public, medical, and research communities.

In 1998, the Office of Cancer Complementary and Alternative Medicine was established to coordinate research and communication activities in the arena of complementary and alternative medicine, both within the NCI and with other agencies.

The NCI is strengthening the information base for cancer care decision making. Researchers, medical providers, and patients seek to understand better what constitutes quality cancer care. The NCI is concerned with both geographic and racial or ethnic disparities in who receives quality care. The Cancer Information Service, established in 1976, is the section of the NCI which is the link to the public, attempting to explain research findings in a clear, timely, and understandable manner. To this end, the Cancer Information Service helps develop education efforts targeting minority audiences and people with limited access to health care information or services.

Perspective and Prospects

To be successful in managing this range of responsibilities and breadth of mission, the NCI has a budget in the billions of dollars. Through the years, the work of the NCI has led to a decline in deaths due to cancer, even though advances in the treament of infectious deseases have made cancer the second leading cause of death in the United States. Creative and dedicated scientists at the NCI have goals to lower its numbers even further in the near future. The NCI will enhance collaborations among institutions and researchers so that priorities are targeted and goals are achieved. An important path to achieving these goals is a program to increase access to clinical trials. Achievement of research goals may also be expedited through a program of extraordinary opportunities for scientific areas of recent importance and promise.

—*Karen Chapman-Novakofski, R.D., L.D., Ph.D.*

See also Cancer; Chemotherapy; Clinical trials; Environmental diseases; Environmental health; Epidemiology; Genetics and inheritance; Nutrition; Oncology; Preventive medicine; Radiation therapy.

For Further Information:

National Cancer Institute. *The Cancer Information Service: A Fifteen-Year History of Service and Research.* Bethesda, Md.: Author, 1993.

_____. "CIS Research Consortium 1993-1997." *Preventive Medicine* 27, no. 5 (1998).

_____. *National Cancer Institute's Research Programs: Pursuing the Central Questions of Cancer Research.* Bethesda, Md.: Author, 1999.

_____. *NCI Fact Book.* Bethesda, Md.: Author, 1979- .

NATIONAL INSTITUTES OF HEALTH (NIH)

ORGANIZATION

DEFINITION: The National Institutes of Health (NIH), composed of more than twenty-five separate institutes, centers, and offices, is one of eight agencies constituting the United States Department of Health and Human Services.

KEY TERMS:

AIDSLINE: a database that is part of the National Library of Medicine (NLM) and is devoted to the topic of research on acquired immunodeficiency syndrome (AIDS)

CATLINE: the on-line catalog of books and manuscripts in the NLM

grant proposals: research plans that outline scientific methods to pursue new knowledge, the required budget, and the resulting products and significance of that work

institute: a specific subagency of the NIH that has the charge of advancing scientific discovery and clinical practice in a specific area of medical science

MEDLINE: a database that is available via the Internet featuring current and historical medical literature, research articles, monographs, presentations, and abstracts

HISTORY AND MISSION

The National Institutes of Health (NIH) is a U.S. federal agency that occupies a multibuilding campus in Bethesda, Maryland. It consists of a variety of offices, institutes focused on specific medical problems, research laboratories and centers, a center for scientific review, and a national medical library. Its main goal is to discover knowledge that will improve the state of public health for all persons, especially those in the United States. This goal extends to all medical conditions afflicting men, women, and children of all ethnic backgrounds. It also extends to seeking knowledge in areas of basic biological research, clinical research, and research on policy and practice in health care.

The National Institute of Health (precursor to the NIH) was formally established by the Ransdell Act of 1930, which bestowed the name on what was formerly called the Hygienic Laboratory (HL) of the Marine Hospital Service (MHS) in New York. The Ransdell Act also allowed for the establishment of fellowships for basic medical and biological research. The very beginnings of the NIH extend back to 1887, however, when basic laboratory work into medical problems was pursued by the MHS, the founding body of the United States Public Health Service (PHS). The MHS was formed in 1798 to provide hospital care for seamen, but by the 1880's it had shifted its focus to screening ship passengers for infectious diseases capable of starting epidemics.

New European research in the 1880's suggesting that microorganisms caused such diseases spurred American interest in medical research and helped form the original HL. Work by the HL continued, with the laboratory eventually moving from the MHS to its own Washington, D.C., campus. The study of microorganisms continued, extending from study of individual persons to studying the effects of bacteria on water and air pollution. Progress for such work was rewarded in 1901 with governmental money for the construction of a building (completed in 1904) to house the HL and further foster work focused on advancing the public health. Because the value of such work was not well-established, however, no permanent funding was provided, leaving the organization subject to ongoing evaluation and supplemental funding.

In 1902 the MHS was reorganized and renamed the Public Health and Marine Hospital Service (PHMHS); in 1912 it adopted the shortened name of the Public Health Service (PHS). During the intervening time, the HL continued its work and expanded to work in chemistry, pharmacology, zoology, immunology, and the regulation and production of vaccines and antitoxins. Additionally, new scientific staff were added to the staff of medical doctors already on board. Changes in the mission of the organization in 1912 also opened the door for the pursuit of research on noncontagious diseases and water pollution. This work continued during World War I in the form of examining sanitation, anthrax outbreaks, smallpox, tetanus, influenza, and other combat-related conditions. The success of the PHS's work in these areas caught the attention of legislators and resulted in the Ransdell Act of 1930, which established both the National Institute of Health and the practice of setting aside public monies for funding medical research. In 1937, the National Cancer Institute (NCI) was created. In 1944, the PHS formally designated the NCI as a component of the NIH, setting the pattern of a problem-focused structure within the NIH that continues to the present.

World War II led the NIH to focus almost exclusively on war-related problems. This involved examinations of fitness for military service and issues such as dental problems and syphilis. The effects of hazardous substances and conditions on workers in war industries; risks armed service professionals faced from lack of oxygen, cold temperatures, and blood clots while flying; burns, shock, bacterial infections, and fever; and the development of vaccines and therapies for tropical diseases such as malaria also composed much of its work during this time.

Successes established during the wars by such medical research led the PHS to take the 1944 Public Health Service Act to Congress. This act led to grant-funding mechanisms being extended from the NCI alone to the entire National Institute of Health. Additionally, an increasing public interest in health organizations caused Congress to create additional institutes for research on mental health, dental diseases, and heart disease between 1946 and 1949. In 1948, the National Heart Act allowed for the formal pluralization of the National Institutes of Health, rather than a singular institute with the NCI as a subinstitute. The Public Health Service Act of 1944 also provided funding for the Warren Grant Magnuson Clinical Center, which opened in 1953 to focus exclusively on clinical research on health.

From this point forward, each of the individual institutes now composing the NIH came into being. By 1960 there were ten institutes, by 1970 there were fifteen, and by 1998 there were twenty-four institutes and centers. As different health interests develop and advances in medical knowledge are needed, the NIH has responded by allocating its resources to pursue goals in those areas. This has been done both by developing institutes and also by creating specialized offices to pursue contemporary medical problems.

Illness and medicine know no boundaries, however, so the NIH has also maintained an interest in global public health issues. Such interest was formally shown in 1947, when grants were first awarded to investigators abroad. Similarly, in 1968, the John E. Fogarty International Center (FIC) was created to coordinate international research efforts, involving liaisons with the World Health Organization and a va-

riety of international research organizations. The FIC also supports language translation, documentation, and reviews of new health findings. It facilitates biomedical communications through its maintenance of the National Library of Medicine (NLM), MEDLINE, CATLINE, AIDSLINE, and numerous other databases for researchers, physicians, and the public at large. Similarly, focused consensus development conferences, where investigators and clinicians from around the world can meet to evaluate new and existing therapies, are another way that international interests are pursued. Since these conferences were initiated in 1977, more than one hundred such conferences have been held.

In keeping with its practical focus, the NIH has strived to seek out knowledge that yields new drugs, devices, and procedures that are useful not just for the government but for the public at large as well. In 1986, the Technology Transfer Act allowed for a partnership between NIH-funded research and the private sector. Encouraging researchers to examine possible commercial and practical applications of basic medical research to wide-reaching clinical or research use benefits overall scientific and health progress. Partnering with business allows private industries to take over the process of marketing and developing products in a manner more affordable to them than to the government, allowing the government to focus on development while benefiting through the use of the eventual marketed products.

ORGANIZATIONAL STRUCTURE AND METHOD

The NIH is organized to accomplish its goals by using its offices, institutes, and research centers. Research is conducted on the NIH campus in its own funded laboratories, as well as in the labs of scientists supported by NIH funding, who are stationed in institutes of higher education, teaching hospitals, and free-standing research institutions in the United States and other countries. In addition to supporting ongoing research, the NIH also supports research infrastructure by maintaining a library and a variety of printed and electronic resources to facilitate communication among its researchers, the larger scientific community, policymakers, and the public. Scientific research also is supported by developing one of the most valuable resources known to medicine: new researchers. The NIH sponsors a variety of training programs focusing on medical training and research in order to keep a large body of high quality scholars and investigators in development. Such programs extend from career development for postdoctoral researchers and predoctoral training, to high school level learning in the sponsoring of internships and other learning experiences for teenagers interested in medical science careers.

Funding for research and training programs outside of the NIH campus and research centers is facilitated through grant proposal programs that distribute federal tax monies devoted to such endeavors. Applicants to such programs are able to submit independent proposals for work, related to the goals of the NIH, that they believe is demanded by the state of science and knowledge. They are also able to submit proposals in response to program announcements and calls for proposals on specific topics as outlined by the institutes and offices of the NIH. Many different grant mechanisms exist for such proposals, from grants supporting the work of individual trainees, training programs for cohorts of researchers at different stages of career development, the ongoing work of career scientists, small grants for new or experimental work, focused projects, and even centers of research excellence where many researchers focus on the same topic of study. In addition, grant support is offered to sponsor conferences and academic meetings on special topics in health research and training.

In order to receive this funding, those wishing to be considered for receiving such grant monies need to submit proposals for confidential peer review through the Center for Scientific Review (CSR), which is part of the NIH structure. Proposals are reviewed by panels of experts who evaluate the research plans, goals, staff, environment, and overall innovation and merit of the work proposed. In addition, ethical considerations about the proposed research are reviewed and considered for both animal welfare and the welfare of human research participants. Emphasis on ethical issues has been a long-standing issue for medical research. It was, however, highlighted in the 1960's, when grantees receiving NIH grant monies were required to state the ethical principles guiding their research on humans, and in 1979, when written guidelines for research on human subjects were established. Once through peer review, proposals are reviewed again by a national advisory council to determine the priority of the work in addressing the goals of the NIH and its institutes and offices. After the proposals are approved by this council for advancement, the individual institutes (sometimes cooperating with specific NIH offices) work to fund them with the monies allotted. Unfortunately, not all proposals can be funded. It should be noted that even after funding, the work of the NIH Office for Protection from Research Risks continues so as to ensure that proper research ethics are followed through the life of the research.

Each year the CSR reviews more than thirty-eight thousand applications, while the NIH supports nearly thirty-five thousand grants nationally and internationally. Such work is facilitated by the various institutions and research offices that fall under the organizational umbrella of the NIH, each focusing on a discrete area of health interest. Some of the institutions involved include the NCI; the National Eye Institute; the National Heart, Lung, and Blood Institute; and the National Human Genome Research Institute. Also included are the National Institutes on Aging, Alcohol Abuse and Alcoholism, Allergy and Infectious Diseases, Arthritis and Musculoskeletal and Skin Diseases, Child Health and Human Development, Deafness and Other Communication Disorders, Dental and Craniofacial Research, Diabetes and Digestive and Kidney Diseases, Drug Abuse, Environmental Health Sciences, Mental Health, and Neurological Disorders and Stroke.

In addition to these institutes, the NIH has numerous offices focusing on specific issues or populations that need to be addressed in health research. These offices focus on contemporary issues of importance for research and include the Offices of Technology Transfer, AIDS Research, Research on Minority Health, Research on Women's Health, Behavioral and Social Sciences Research, Dietary Supplements, Medical Applications of Research, Rare Diseases, Science Policy, Biotechnology Activities, Science Education, and Information Technology. There are also offices that focus on the management of research, specific organizational issues at the NIH, or the communication of information from the NIH to members of the public. These include the Offices of Intramural Research, Extramural Research, Evaluation, Equal Opportunity, Human Resource Management, Financial Management, Procurement Management, Logistics Management, Contracts Management, Management Assessment, Communications and Public Liaison, and General Counsel, as well as the NIH Legal Advisor, and the Freedom of Information Act Office.

PERSPECTIVE AND PROSPECTS

The NIH has been responsible for supporting some very influential research for more than one hundred years, garnering more than eighty Nobel Prizes for NIH-supported work. More vaccines against infectious diseases are available than ever before. The successful mapping of the human genome has set the stage for enhanced genetic testing and the development of gene therapies. Substantial decreases in mortality rates have been achieved for heart disease and strokes. Survival rates for individuals afflicted by cancer have increased, as have survival rates for infants with respiratory distress syndrome. Recovery from spinal cord injuries has been enhanced so as to lessen the probability of long-term disability. Advances in the pharmacological and behavioral treatment of mental health problems such as depression, anxiety, bipolar disorder, and schizophrenia have been achieved. Preventive approaches in dentistry have been highly successful in stopping and slowing dental problems.

Given such successes, billions of dollars of federal tax monies continue to be devoted to the NIH budget to foster continued scientific advances. New work focused on improving prevention, screening, assessment, diagnosis, and treatment for conditions such as AIDS, alcoholism and drug dependence, Alzheimer's disease, arthritis, blindness, communication disorders, diabetes, heart disease, kidney disease, lung cancer, lupus, mental illnesses, Parkinson's disease, stroke, and other persisting conditions continues on a daily basis. While great successes have been achieved to date with the majority of the population, new research is needed that will focus on specialized approaches that may enhance health for women, minorities, youth, and the elderly. The combination of these needs, past successes, and governmental commitment to improving the state of the public health ensures that the NIH will continue onward with its mission for the foreseeable future.

—*Nancy A. Piotrowski, Ph.D.*

See also Childhood infectious diseases; Disease; Environmental diseases; Environmental health; Epidemiology; Immunization and vaccination; Occupational health; World Health Organization.

FOR FURTHER INFORMATION:

Eberhart-Philips, Jason. *Outbreak Alert: Responding to the Increasing Threat of Infectious Diseases*. Oakland, Calif.: New Harbinger, 2000. Emphasizes the importance of public health to national health; defines and identifies infectious diseases posing a public health threat and how the current way that society functions relates to this threat.

Garrett, Laurie. *Betrayal of Trust: The Collapse of Global Public Health*. New York: Hyperion, 2000. Discusses global public health, putting the status of health in the United States in perspective on some very basic matters related to public health.

Institute of Medicine. *Scientific Opportunities and Public Needs: Improving Priority Setting and Public Input at the National Institutes of Health*. Washington, D.C.: National Academy Press, 1998. Provides an overview of scientific and popular perceptions of the needed long-term health interests of the United States, as well as other global health concerns.

Lappé, Marc. *Breakout: The Evolving Threat of Drug-Resistant Disease*. San Francisco: Sierra Club Books, 1995. Discusses perspectives on and causes of diseases, the long-term impact of the use of antibiotics, and how disease and disruption of the global ecosystem are related.

Tulchinsky, Theodore H., and Elena A. Varavikova. *The New Public Health: An Introduction for the Twenty-first Century*. San Diego, Calif.: Academic Press, 2000. Discusses global perspectives on how organizational structures of health care and other public activities affect the state of public health and health care service delivery.

NAUSEA AND VOMITING

DISEASE/DISORDER

ANATOMY OR SYSTEM AFFECTED: Brain, gastrointestinal system, nervous system, stomach

SPECIALTIES AND RELATED FIELDS: Gastroenterology, otorhinolaryngology

DEFINITION: Nausea is an unpleasant subjective sensation, accompanied by epigastric and duodenal discomfort, which often culminates in vomiting, the regurgitation of the contents of the stomach.

KEY TERMS:

affect: the emotional reactions associated with experience

antiemetics: drugs that prevent or relieve the symptoms of nausea and/or vomiting

chemoreceptor trigger zone: a sensory nerve ending in the brain which is stimulated by and reacts to certain chemical stimulation localized outside the central nervous system

emesis: the act of vomiting

psychogenic: of mental origin

psychotropics: drugs that affect psychic function, behavior, or experience

CAUSES AND SYMPTOMS

Nausea is defined as a subjectively unpleasant sensation associated with awareness of the urge to vomit. It is usually felt in the back of the throat and epigastrium and is accompanied by the loss of gastric tone, duodenal contractions, and reflux of the intestinal contents into the stomach. Retching is defined as labored, spasmodic, rhythmic contractions of the respiratory muscles (including the diaphragm, chest wall, and abdominal wall muscles) without the expulsion of gastric contents. Vomiting, or emesis, is the forceful expulsion of gastric contents from the mouth and is brought about by the powerful sustained contraction of the abdominal muscles, the descent of the diaphragm, and the opening of the gastric cardia (the cardiac orifice of the stomach).

Nausea and vomiting are important defense mechanisms against the ingestion of toxins. The act of emesis involves a sequence of events that can be divided into three phases: preejection, ejection, and postejection. The preejection phase includes the symptoms of nausea, along with salivation, swallowing, pallor, and tachycardia (an abnormally fast heartbeat). The ejection phase comprises retching and vomiting. Retching is characterized by rhythmic, synchronous, inspiratory movements of the diaphragm, abdominal, and external intercostal muscles, while the mouth and the glottis are kept closed. As the antral (cavity) portion of the stomach contracts, the proximal (nearest the center) portion relaxes and the gastric contents oscillate between the stomach and the esophagus. During retching, the hiatal portion of the diaphragm does not relax, and intraabdominal pressure increases are associated with a decrease in intrathoracic pressure.

In contrast, relaxation of the hiatal portion of the diaphragm (near the esophagus) permits a transfer of intraabdominal pressure to the thorax during the act of vomiting. Contraction of the muscles of the anterior abdominal wall, relaxation of the esophageal sphincter, an increase in intrathoracic and intragastric pressure, reverse peristalsis (movement of the contents of the alimentary canal), and an open glottis and mouth result in the expulsion of gastric contents. The postejection phase consists of autonomic and visceral responses that return the body to a quiescent phase, with or without residual nausea.

The complex act of vomiting, involving coordination of the respiratory, gastrointestinal, and abdominal musculature, is controlled by what researchers label the emetic center. This center in the brain stem has access to the motor pathways responsible for the visceral and somatic output involved in vomiting, and stimuli from several areas within the central nervous system can affect this center. These include afferent (inward-directed) nerves from the pharynx and gastrointestinal tract, as well as afferents from the higher cortical centers (including the visual center) and the chemoreceptor trigger zone (CTZ) in the area postrema (a highly vascularized area of the brain stem). The CTZ can be activated by chemical stimuli received through the blood or the cerebrospinal fluid. Direct electrical stimulation of the CTZ, however, does not result in emesis.

Clinical assessment of nausea and vomiting usually focus on the occurrence of vomiting, that is, the frequency and number of episodes. Nausea, however, is a subjective phenomenon unobservable by another. Few data collection instruments that measure separately the patient's experience of nausea and vomiting and his or her symptom distress have been reported in the literature. In fact, the Rhodes Index of Nausea and Vomiting (INV) Form 2 is the only available tool that measures the individual components of nausea, vomiting, and retching. This index measures the patient's perception of the duration, frequency, and distress from nausea; the frequency, amount, and distress from vomiting; and the frequency, amount, and distress from retching (dry heaves). The INV score provides a measurement of the total symptom experience of the patient.

While the causes of nausea and vomiting are numerous—they include gastrointestinal diseases, infections, intracranial disease, toxins, radiation sickness, psychological trauma, migraines, and circulatory syncope—three of the most common causes are motion sickness (air, sea, land, or space), pregnancy, and anesthesia administered during operative procedures.

The sequence of symptoms and signs that constitute motion sickness is fairly characteristic. Premonitory symptoms often include yawning or sighing, lethargy, somnolence, and a loss of enthusiasm and concern for the task at hand. Increasing malaise is directed toward the epigastrium, a sensation best described as "stomach awareness," which progresses to nausea. Diversion of the blood flow from the skin toward the muscles results in pallor. A feeling of warmth and a desire for cool air is often accompanied by sweating. Frontal headache and a sensation of disorientation, dizziness, or light-headedness may also occur. As symptoms progress, vomiting occurs early in the sequence of symptoms for some; in others, malaise is severe and prolonged and vomiting is delayed. After vomiting, there is often a temporary improvement in well-being; however, with continued provocative motion, symptoms build again and vomiting recurs. The symptoms may last for minutes, hours, or even days.

The most coherent explanation for the development of motion sickness is provided by sensory conflict theory. Motion sickness is generally thought to occur as the result of a "sensory conflict" between information arising from the semicircular canals and organs of the vestibular system, visual and other sensory input, and the input that is expected on the basis of past experience or exposure history. It is argued that conflicts between current sensory inputs are by themselves insufficient to produce motion sickness since adaptation occurs even though the conflicting inputs continue to be present. Visual input alone, however, can produce symptoms of motion sickness, such as watching motion pictures shot from a moving vehicle or looking out of the side window (as opposed to the front window) of a moving vehicle.

Nausea and/or vomiting in the early morning during pregnancy, so-called morning sickness, is so common that it is accepted as a symptom of normal pregnancy. Occurring soon after waking, it is often retching rather than actual vomiting and usually does not disturb the woman's health or her pregnancy. The symptoms nearly always cease before the fourteenth week of pregnancy. In a much smaller proportion of cases, approximately 1 in 1,000 births, the vomiting becomes more serious and persistent, occurring throughout the day and even during the night. The term "hyperemesis gravidarum" is given to this serious form of vomiting. Theories on the etiology of morning sickness have tended to be grouped under four main areas: endocrine (caused by estrogen and progesterone levels), psychosomatic (a conscious or unconscious wish not to be pregnant), allergic (a histamine reaction), and metabolic (a lack of potassium).

Nausea and vomiting occur frequently as unpleasant side effects of the administration of anesthesia in many clinical procedures. Most postoperative vomiting is mild, and only in a few cases will the problem persist so as to cause electrolyte disturbances and dehydration. The factors affecting postoperative nausea and vomiting may be divided into two categories: by the type of patient and surgery, and by the anesthetic and preoperative and postoperative medication uses.

Patients with a history of motion sickness have a predisposition to postoperative vomiting. Nearly 43 percent of patients who vomited following previous surgery vomited again, whereas slightly more than 14 percent of those who did not vomit previously had an emetic episode at their next operation. Patients undergoing their first anesthetic procedure had an incidence of vomiting of approximately 30 percent.

No direct association between vomiting and age has been found. That vomiting may be hormonally related, however, is suggested by the higher incidence of nausea and vomiting in the latter half of the menstrual cycle. Other factors that may affect nausea and vomiting associated with anesthesia include patient weight (female obese patients being particularly more vulnerable), amount of hydration, metabolic status, and psychological state.

With regard to the type of surgery performed, the highest incidence of nausea and vomiting appears to be associated with abdominal surgery, as well as ear, nose, and throat surgery, with middle-ear surgery being the major category. The length of surgery, and therefore the duration of anesthesia, also has a direct effect on nausea and vomiting. Short (thirty-minute to sixty-minute) operations using cyclopropane had an emetic incidence of 17.5 percent, while operations lasting one and a half to three and a half hours had an incidence of 46.4 percent.

Most of the causes of vomiting associated with general anesthesia are expected to be eliminated with regional or spinal anesthesia. The type of anesthesia used also has an effect on nausea and vomiting. Research indicates that cyclopropane, ether, and nitrous oxide are potent emetics.

TREATMENT AND THERAPY

Since the generation of sensory conflict underlies all motion environments that give rise to motion sickness, practical measures that reduce conflict are likely to reduce motion sickness incidence. Motion sickness can be minimized if the subject has the widest possible view of a visual reference in which the earth is stable. Passengers aboard ships are less likely to be seasick if they remain on deck at midship, where vertical motion is minimized, and view the horizon. In a car or bus, individuals should be in a position to see the road directly ahead, since the movement of this visual scene will correlate with the changes in the direction of the vehicle. While head movements in a rotating environment are known to precipitate motion sickness, there is no clear experimental evidence that they elicit nausea in mild linear oscillation. Thus, some nonpharmacologic remedies for motion sickness are restricting head movements, lying in a supine position, or closing the eyes. In addition, the use of acupressure wrist bands has proven effective in combating motion sickness.

Pharmacologically, the drug hyoscine hydrobromide (also called hyoscine or scopolamine) emerged as a valuable prophylactic drug following extensive research during World War II into the problems of motion sickness in troops transported in aircraft, ships, and landing craft. It remains one of the most effective drugs for short-duration exposures to provocative motion. Doses in excess of 0.6 milligram, however, are very likely to lead to drowsiness, and there is much experimental evidence that hyoscine impairs short-term memory. Hyoscine can be absorbed transdermally, and in order to extend the duration of action, a controlled-release patch was developed to deliver 1.2 milligrams on application and 0.01 milligram hourly thereafter. There is substantial evidence of its sustained effectiveness, but, perhaps as a result of variable absorption rates, there is an increased risk of blurred vision after more than twenty-four hours of use.

Amphetamines, ephedrine, and a number of antihistamines (such as dimenhydrinate) have been found to be clinically useful in motion sickness. Following oral administration, these drugs are generally slower than hyoscine in reaching their peak efficacy, but they have a longer duration of action.

For most susceptible subjects, whose exposure to motion sickness-inducing stimuli is infrequent, prophylactic drugs offer the only useful treatment. When exposure to provocative stimuli is more frequent, as for example in professional aircraft pilots, spontaneous adaption occurs during training and an initially high incidence of motion sickness decreases with time.

In medical conditions in which the cause is relatively unknown, it is usual to find a wide variety of suggested therapies; nausea and vomiting during pregnancy and hyperemesis gravidarum (the serious, persistent form of vomiting in pregnancy) are no exception. Prior to 1968, treatments numbered approximately thirty. In subsequent years, however, suggested therapy has been mainly drugs of the antiemetic variety. Yet since the thalidomide tragedy (in which severe deformities occurred in the children of women who took this drug), there has been a reluctance to use drugs of any kind during early pregnancy. Probably the only value of drug therapy is at the stage of morning sickness, when antiemetics or mild sedatives may counter the feeling of nausea and prevent women from experiencing excessive vomiting and entering the vicious cycle of dehydration, starvation, and electrolyte imbalance. Once the patient has reached the stage of hyperemesis gravidarum, much more basic therapy is required, and the regimen calls for correction of dehydration, carbohydrate deficiency, and ionic deficiencies. This program is best managed by intravenous therapy, with or without the addition of vitamin supplements and sedative agents.

Nonpharmacologic self-care actions for morning sickness fall into the three broad categories of manipulating diet, adjusting behavior, and seeking emotional support. Some of the most effective self-care actions are getting rest, eating several small meals rather than three large ones, avoiding bad smells, avoiding greasy or fried foods, avoiding cooking, and receiving extra attention and support.

In terms of postoperative nausea and vomiting caused by anesthesia, it has been found that routine antiemetic prophylaxis of patients undergoing elective surgical procedures is not indicated, since fewer than 30 percent of patients experience postoperative nausea and vomiting. Of those who develop these symptoms, many have transient nausea or only one or two bouts of emesis and do not require antiemetic therapy. In addition, commonly used antiemetic drugs can produce significant side effects, such as sedation. Nevertheless, antiemetic prophylaxis may be justified in those patients who are at greater risk for developing postoperative nausea and/or vomiting. Such therapy is often given to patients with a history of motion sickness or to those undergoing gynecologic procedures, inner-ear procedures, oral surgery (in which the jaws are occluded by wires, causing a high risk of breathing in vomitus), and operations on the ear or eye and plastic surgery operations (in order to avoid disruption of delicate surgical work).

Many different antiemetic drugs are available for the treatment of postoperative nausea and vomiting. Researchers have found it difficult to interpret the results of antiemetic drug studies because the severity of postoperative vomiting and the response to therapeutic agents can be influenced by many variables in addition to the antiemetic drug being studied. Even with the use of the same drugs in a homogeneous population undergoing the same procedure, the severity of emesis varies from individual to individual.

Because antiemetic drugs have differing sites of action, better results can be obtained by using a multi-drug approach. If a combination of drugs with a similar site of action is used, however, the incidence of side effects may be increased. There are few data regarding combination antiemetic prophylaxis or therapy for postoperative nausea and emesis. Drug combinations have been avoided in postsurgical patients because of concerns about additive central nervous system toxicity. An exception is the combination of low-dose droperidol and metoclopramide, which appears to be more effective than droperidol alone for outpatient gynecologic procedures.

Although a full stomach is best avoided before any operative procedure, with situations such as emergencies, in which danger from vomiting is acute, a rapid sequence of administering anesthesia (induction) and clearing the air passage (intubation) remains the method of choice to avoid nausea and vomiting in patients with a full stomach. After the procedure, it is recommended that the patient minimize movement in order to avoid nausea and vomiting. Also, it has been found that avoiding eating solid food for at least eight hours after a surgical procedure is helpful in preventing postoperative nausea and vomiting.

Perspective and Prospects

Though it has existed for as long as there have been human beings, the symptom of nausea has never received much attention in health care practice or research. In fact, until the early 1970's the sensation of nausea was frequently dismissed as merely a passing phenomenon. The rationale for this dismissal was most likely the understanding that nausea is self-limiting (it always passes with time), is never life-threatening in itself, is probably psychogenic in nature (at least to some degree), and, being subjective, is very difficult to measure. In addition, in the past the most predictable nausea was related to pregnancy, which may also explain the lack of attention given to it.

Until the late 1980's, there was still little research being conducted on the nausea associated with pregnancy, although it is a common symptom. The historical lack of interest in nausea and vomiting during pregnancy may be traced to the fact that, since the symptoms generally persist only through the first trimester, health care professionals have viewed the problem as relatively insignificant. As more pregnant women work outside the home in demanding positions, however, these women have exhibited less tolerance for illness. Demands upon the health care industry and upon personal physicians for more research and effective treatment have become more widespread.

While it is surprising that nausea has received scant attention in the history of clinical research, it is even more astonishing that vomiting, an observable behavior, has received so little attention as well. Although vomiting is a primitive neurologic process that has remained almost unchanged in the evolution of animals, the mechanisms that regulate the behavior remain virtually unknown.

One reason for the paucity of information on the subject of nausea in particular stems from the lack of a reliable animal model. This fact has hampered research aimed at establishing the etiological basis for nausea and its relationship to vomiting. While some species of lower animals, for example rats, cannot vomit, it is not known whether rats experience the phenomenon of nausea. Thus no effective means of measuring nausea in lower animals has been devised.

Since the early 1970's, there has been a noticeable increase in research on nausea as a drug side effect because it was so frequently seen in cancer chemotherapy clinical trials sponsored by the National Cancer Institute and the American Cancer Society. As more powerful chemotherapy agents and aggressive combinations were clinically investigated, patients began to experience severe, potentially life-threatening nausea and vomiting. Yet it was still the symptom of vomiting that began to receive attention; nausea was either coupled with the investigation of vomiting, with the two treated as a unit, or it was ignored. Nevertheless, efforts continued to improve antiemetic drugs until nausea began to be seen as a separate but related symptom.

Aside from the pharmacological investigations of new drugs and drug combinations in the treatment of nausea and vomiting, an interesting branch of scientific investigation has begun the process of exploring alternative ways of managing these symptoms. Behavioral interventions, such as progressive muscle relaxation, biofeedback, imagery, or music therapy, have been used to alleviate postchemotherapy anxiety. These methods may also be used to treat other patients suffering from the symptoms of nausea and vomiting, such as pregnant women.

Another noninvasive, nonpharmacologic measure that has been considered in the relief of nausea and vomiting is transcutaneous electrical nerve stimulation

(TENS). Several research studies indicate that TENS may be useful in alleviating chemotherapy-related nausea and vomiting, including delayed nausea and vomiting. Side effects from using TENS units are negligible, and with further study they may prove to be an acceptable, helpful relief measure.

—Genevieve Slomski, Ph.D.

See also Anesthesia; Botulism; Bulimia; Colitis; Crohn's disease; Digestion; Eating disorders; Food biochemistry; Food poisoning; Gastroenterology; Gastroenterology, pediatric; Gastrointestinal disorders; Gastrointestinal system; Heartburn; Indigestion; Influenza; Lactose intolerance; Motion sickness; Multiple chemical sensitivity syndrome; Poisoning; Poisonous plants; Pregnancy and gestation; Radiation sickness; Salmonella infection; Stomach, intestinal, and pancreatic cancers; Ulcer surgery; Ulcers; Vagotomy.

FOR FURTHER INFORMATION:

Blum, Richard H., W. LeRoy Heinrichs, and Andrew Herxheimer. *Nausea and Vomiting: Overview, Challenges, Practical Treatments and New Perspectives for Primary Care Professionals, Multidisciplinary Students, and All Persons Thoughtful and Curious.* Philadelphia: Whurr, 2000. Discusses such topics as drugs to prevent and control nausea and vomiting, pregnancy nausea and vomiting, allergy and immunology, anesthesiology, and gastroenterology.

Funk, Sandra G., ed. *Key Aspects of Comfort.* New York: Springer, 1989. This work, which discusses the management of pain, fatigue, and nausea, functions both as an introduction to these topics and as a sourcebook for treatment.

Kucharczyk, John, et al. *Nausea and Vomiting.* Boca Raton, Fla.: CRC Press, 1991. After an introductory chapter on pioneers in emesis research, discusses the mechanisms of emesis, including respiratory muscle control, digestive tract activity, and neural mechanisms; the clinical characteristics and consequences of vomiting; and antiemetic therapies.

Preboth, Monica. "Drug for Radiation-Induced Nausea and Vomiting." *American Family Physician* 60, no. 8 (November 15, 1999): 2436. Granisetron has been approved by the FDA for the prevention of nausea and vomiting associated with radiation, including total body irradiation and fractionated abdominal radiation.

Simini, Bruno. "More Oxygen May Equal Less Postoperative Nausea." *The Lancet* 354, no. 9190 (No-

vember 6, 1999): 1618. A new report indicates that high oxygen concentrations during and after surgery can decrease postoperative nausea. Earlier studies had shown oxygen to have antiemetic properties.

Sleisenger, Marvin H., ed. *The Handbook of Nausea and Vomiting.* New York: Caduceus Medical/Parthenon, 1993. A short manual for dealing with the symptoms and causes of nausea and vomiting. Includes a bibliography and an index.

NECK INJURIES AND DISORDERS. *See* HEAD AND NECK DISORDERS.

NECROSES. *See* FROSTBITE; GANGRENE.

NECROTIZING FASCIITIS
DISEASE/DISORDER

ANATOMY OR SYSTEM AFFECTED: Blood vessels, muscles, skin

SPECIALTIES AND RELATED FIELDS: Bacteriology, critical care, dermatology, emergency medicine, epidemiology, histology, plastic surgery, vascular medicine

DEFINITION: An invasive bacterial infection that occurs in the connective tissue between the skin and muscle known as the fascia, cutting off blood flow; it must be urgently treated surgically and, even in the best circumstances, has a high mortality rate.

CAUSES AND SYMPTOMS

Although it had been identified in the past, in 1994 there were numerous headline newspaper reports describing a new "flesh-eating bacteria." These articles detailed the devastating effect of seemingly minor wounds infected with streptococcal bacteria. Patients quickly become very sick, with a rapidly progressive downward course, even from trauma resulting in a deep muscle bruise or muscle strain or in "minor" cuts and scrapes.

In the former nonpenetrating injuries, it is likely that the bacteria were already present in the blood and then seeded the site of damage. Most of these patients, however, did not recall any prior recent infection that may have made them susceptible. Penetrating injuries, where the normally protective barrier of the skin has been broken, were often minor and not originally treated as contaminated or infected. Other cases of necrotizing fasciitis are caused by surgical infections and bowel contamination. These cases are more rare and often found to have a mixture of bacteria, such as staphylococci or *Escherichia coli* (*E. coli*).

Patients with necrotizing fasciitis have fever, inflammation, severe pain, and blistering at the site of infection. If this cellulitis is not recognized and urgently treated, the infection will quickly spread in the layers of connective tissue just under the skin known as the fascia. As the bacteria multiply, they cause blood vessels supplying the skin to form clots and thus cut off blood flow to the skin. Without nutrients, oxygen, and the ability to remove waste products, the skin dies. Once this occurs, the nerves are destroyed and the patient no longer has the excruciating pain. The skin at this point appears to be "eaten away." The possibility exists that the underlying muscle adjacent to the fascia will become infected. Thus, the potential for muscle death as well as skin death is of great concern, particularly if the infection begins in the arms, legs, abdomen, or back, as these areas have large muscle groups directly underlying the skin. In necrotizing fasciitis, the extremities and the area around the genitals and anus (perineum) are most commonly and extensively involved. Multiplication and movement of these streptococcal bacteria and their toxins into the bloodstream produces a shocklike state.

TREATMENT AND THERAPY

The patient with necrotizing fasciitis must be stabilized quickly in an intensive care unit, where fluids can be administered and heart and lung condition can be closely monitored. The only lifesaving treatment available is extensive surgical debridement to remove the necrotic (dead) tissue and slow the spread of the bacteria. Antibiotics including penicillins, clindamycin, and gentamicin are given to help eradicate the pathogen. Because the infection spreads so rapidly, death often results even with heroic surgical and drug therapy unless the condition is diagnosed and treated early. Fortunately, these infections remain relatively rare.

—*Matthew Berria, Ph.D.*

See also Antibiotics; Bacterial infections; Bacteriology; Dermatology; Epidemiology; Shock; Skin; Skin disorders; Streptococcal infections; Wounds.

FOR FURTHER INFORMATION:

Finegold, Sydney M., and William J. Martin. *Bailey and Scott's Diagnostic Microbiology.* 6th ed. St. Louis: C. V. Mosby, 1998.

Roemmele, Jacqueline A., and Donna Batdorff. *Surviving the Flesh-Eating Bacteria: Understanding, Preventing, Treating, and Living with the Effects of Necrotizing Fasciitis.* Garden City Park, N.Y.: Avery, 2000.

Shaw, Michael, ed. *Everything You Need to Know About Diseases.* Springhouse, Pa.: Springhouse Press, 1996.

NEONATOLOGY

SPECIALTY

ANATOMY OR SYSTEM AFFECTED: All

SPECIALTIES AND RELATED FIELDS: Cardiology, critical care, embryology, genetics, obstetrics, pediatrics, perinatology

DEFINITION: A subspecialty of pediatrics that involves the care of newborn infants from birth through the first month of life, especially those infants with life-threatening conditions such as prematurity, genetic defects, and serious illnesses.

KEY TERMS:

congenital disorders: abnormalities present at birth that occurred during fetal development as a result of genetic errors, exposure to toxins and microorganisms, or maternal illness

incubator: in the nursery, a plexiglass unit that encloses the premature or sick infant to allow strict temperature regulation

intrauterine growth retardation: the condition of infants who are born significantly smaller than the standard for the number of weeks that they have spent in the uterus

neonatal intensive care unit: a hospital nursery with advanced equipment and specially trained staff to maintain the vital functions of sick newborns and to monitor their progress closely

neonatal period: the first month of life; derived from the Greek *neo* (meaning "new") and the Latin *natum* (meaning "birth")

prematurity: strictly defined, birth before a full-term pregnancy (thirty-eight weeks); more commonly associated with birth before thirty-five weeks

respirator: a machine which inflates and deflates the lungs, imitating normal breathing; connected to the patient through a tube placed into the windpipe (endotracheal tube)

respiratory distress syndrome: a life-threatening illness primarily of premature infants; immature lungs lack a vital substance that keeps the tiny air sacs (alveoli) from collapsing upon exhalation

SCIENCE AND PROFESSION

Neonatology has grown dramatically since its beginnings in the late 1960's, and neonatologists have become an integral part of the obstetric-pediatric team at major medical centers throughout the world. In large part because of an ever-expanding technological base and marked advances in scientific research, these health care professionals have greatly changed the outlook for premature and sick newborns. The last decades of the twentieth century saw a dramatic reduction in infant mortality in industrialized nations, where better prenatal care and advanced neonatal care significantly improved the chances of survival for millions of infants.

As a subspecialty of pediatrics, neonatology is concerned with the most critical time of transition and adjustment—the first four weeks of life, or the neonatal period—whether the infant is healthy (a normal birth) or sick (as a result of genetic problems, obstetric complications, or medical illness). By the early 1970's, it became increasingly clear to health administrators that hospitals throughout the United States had varying abilities to care for medical and pediatric cases requiring the most sophisticated staff and equipment. Consequently, they developed a system that designated hospitals as either level I (small, community hospitals), level II (larger hospitals), or level III (major regional medical centers also called tertiary care centers). It was in the last group that the most advanced neonatal care could be delivered. In these major centers, there are two types of nurseries, separating the normal healthy infant from the sick or high-risk infant: the routine nursery and the neonatal intensive care unit (NICU).

Routine nurseries are the temporary home of the vast majority of newborns. The services of the neonatologist are rarely needed here, and the general pediatrician or family practitioner observes and examines the infant for twenty-four to forty-eight hours to be sure that it has made a smooth transition from intrauterine to extrauterine life. These babies soon leave the hospital for their homes. Those neonates with minor problems arising from multiple births, difficult deliveries, mild prematurity, and minor illness are easily managed by their primary care physician in consultation with a neonatologist, perhaps at another hospital. It is in the neonatal intensive care unit, however, that the most difficult situations present themselves. Here several teams of pediatric subspecialists—surgeons, cardiologists, anesthesiolo-

gists, and highly trained nurses, along with many other health professionals—are led by a neonatologist, who coordinates the team's efforts. These newborns have life-threatening conditions, often as a result of extreme prematurity (more than six weeks earlier than the expected date of delivery), major birth defects (genetic or developmental), severe illness (such as overwhelming infections), or being born to drug- or alcohol-addicted mothers. They require the most advanced technological and medical interventions, often to sustain life artificially until the underlying problem is corrected. It is in this setting that the most dramatic successes of neonatology are found.

After hours of being inside a forcefully contracting uterus and sustaining the stress of passing through a narrow birth canal, the newborn emerges into a dry, cold, and hostile environment. The umbilical cord, which has provided oxygen and nutrients, is clamped and cut; the fluid-filled lungs must now exchange air instead, and the respiratory center of the infant's brain begins a lifetime of spontaneous breathing, usually heralded by crying. The vast majority of neonates make this extraordinary adjustment to extrauterine life without difficulty. At one minute and again at five minutes, the newborn is evaluated and scored on five physical signs: heart rate, breathing, muscle tone, reflexes, and skin tone. The healthy infant is vigorously moving, crying, and pink regardless of race. These Apgar scores, named for founder Virginia Apgar, evaluate the need for immediate resuscitation. A brief physical examination follows, which can identify other life-threatening abnormalities.

It is essential to remember that the medical history of a neonate is in fact the medical and obstetric history of its mother, and seemingly normal infants may develop problems shortly after birth. Risk factors include middle-aged or very young mothers; difficult deliveries; babies with Rh-negative blood types; mothers with diabetes mellitus, kidney disease, or heart disease; and concurrent infections in either the mother or the baby. Anticipating these problems of the healthy newborn by using the Apgar scores and the results of the physical examination allows the proper assignment of the infant to the nursery or NICU.

The NICU is a daunting place containing high-tech equipment, a tangle of wires and tubes, the sounds of beeps and alarms, and tiny, fragile infants. All this technology serves two simple purposes: to monitor vital functions and to sustain malfunctioning or nonfunctioning organ systems. Looked at individually,

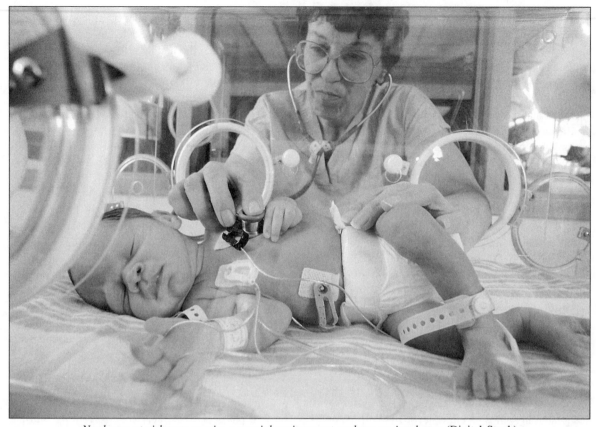

Newborns at risk may require a special environment such as an incubator. (Digital Stock)

however, the machines and attachments become much more understandable. The incubator, perhaps the most common device, maintains a warm, moist environment of constant temperature at 37 degrees Celsius. Small portholes with rubber gloves allow people to stroke the child safely. Generally, the infants will have small electrodes taped on their chests, connected to video monitors that record the heart and breathing rates and that will sound alarms if significant deviations occur. These monitors will also record blood pressure through an arm or thigh cuff. In order to ensure immediate access to the blood, for delivering medications and taking blood for testing, catheters (plastic tubes) are placed into larger arteries or veins near the umbilicus, neck, or thigh (in adults, intravenous access is found in the arms).

The remaining equipment is used for the very serious business of life support, in particular the support of the respiratory system. Maintaining adequate oxygenation is critical and can be accomplished in several ways, depending on the baby's needs. The least stressful are tubes placed in the nostrils or a face

mask, but these methods require that breathing be spontaneous although inadequate. More often, unfortunately, neonates with the types of problems that bring them to an intensive care unit cannot breathe on their own. In these cases, a tube must be connected from the artificial respirator into the windpipe (the endotracheal tube). Warm, moistened, oxygen-rich air is delivered under pressure and removed from the lungs rhythmically to simulate breathing. Tranquilizers and paralytic agents are used to calm and immobilize the infant. Sick or premature infants are also generally unable to feed or nurse naturally, by mouth. Again, several methods of feeding can be employed, depending on the problems and the length of time that such feedings will be needed. For the first few days, simple solutions of water, sugar, and protein can be given through the intravenous catheters. These lines, because of the very small, fragile blood vessels of the newborn, are rarely able to carry more complex solutions. A second method, known as gavage feeding, employs tubing that is inserted through the nose directly into the stomach. Through that tube, infant formula (water, sugar, protein, fat, vitamins, and minerals) and, if available, breast milk can be given.

As the underlying problems are resolved, the infant is slowly weaned, first feeding orally and then breathing naturally. Next, the infant will be placed in an open crib, and gradually the tangled web of tubes and wires will clear. With approval from the neonatologist, the baby is transferred to the routine nursery, a transitional home until discharge from the hospital is advisable.

DIAGNOSTIC AND TREATMENT TECHNIQUES

Neonatology has amassed an enormous body of knowledge about normal neonatal anatomy and physiology, disease processes, and, most important, how to manage the wide variety of complications that can occur. Specific treatment protocols have been developed that are practiced uniformly in all neonatal intensive care units. Approximately 12 percent of all neonates in the United States require admission to the NICU. Short-term stays (twenty-four to forty-eight hours) are meant to observe and monitor the infant with respiratory distress at birth that required immediate intervention. Long-term stays, lasting from several weeks to months, are the case for the sickest newborns, most commonly those with severe prematurity and low birth weight (less than 1,500 grams), respiratory distress syndrome (also known as hyaline membrane disease), congenital defects, and drug or alcohol addictions.

Infants born prematurely make up the major proportion of all infants at high risk for disability and death, and each passing decade has seen younger and younger babies being kept alive. While many maternal factors can lead to preterm delivery, often no explanation can be found. The main problem of prematurity lies in the functional and structural immaturity of vital organs. Weak sucking, swallowing, and coughing reflexes lead to an inability to feed and the danger of choking. Lungs that lack surfactant, a substance that coats the millions of tiny air sacs (alveoli) in each lung to keep them from collapsing and sticking together after air is exhaled, cause severe breathing difficulty as the infant struggles to reinflate them. An immature immune system cannot protect the newborn from the many viruses, bacteria, and other microorganisms that exist. Inadequate metabolism causes low body temperature and inadequate use of food or medications. Neurological immaturity can lead to mental retardation, blindness, and deafness.

Aggressive management of the preterm baby begins in the delivery room, with close cooperation between the obstetrician and the neonatologist. Severely preterm infants, some born after only twenty weeks of pregnancy, require immediate respiratory and cardiac support. Placement of the endotracheal tube, assisted ventilation with a handheld bag, and delicate chest compressions similar to the cardiopulmonary resuscitation (CPR) done on adults to stimulate the heartbeat are each accomplished quickly. Once the respiratory and circulatory systems have been stabilized, excess fluid will be suctioned, while a brief physical examination is performed to note any abnormalities that require immediate attention. As soon as transport is considered safe, the newborn is sent to the NICU. If the infant has been delivered at a small, community hospital, this may involve ambulance or even helicopter transport to the nearest tertiary care center.

Once in the unit, the neonate will be placed in an incubator and attached to video monitors that record heart rate, breathing, and blood pressure. The endotracheal tube can now be attached to the respirator machine, and intravenous or intra-arterial catheters will be placed to allow the fluid and medication infusions and the blood drawing for the battery of tests that the neonatologist requires. Feeding methods can be set up as soon as the infant has stabilized. Within a short time after delivery, the premature newborn has had a flurry of activity about it and is surrounded by the most sophisticated equipment and staff available. Supporting the immature organs becomes the first priority, although the ethical issues of saving very sick infants must soon be addressed as complications begin to occur. Nearly 15 percent of surviving preterm infants whose birth weights were less than 2,000 grams have serious physical and mental disabilities after discharge. The majority, however, grow to lead normal, healthy lives.

Congenital defects are common, with nearly 7 percent of the American population having some physical or cosmetic deformity, although most are not serious. Unfortunately, nearly 2 percent of all newborns have life-threatening abnormalities that require immediate attention and admission to the NICU. It is estimated that the majority of miscarriages are a direct result of congenital defects that are incompatible with life. Many infants that do survive development and delivery die shortly after birth despite the most sophisticated and heroic attempts to intervene. The causes of such defects are arbitrarily assigned to two broad categories, although a combination of these factors is the most likely explanation: genetic errors (such as breaks, doubling, and mutations) and environmental insults (such as chemicals, drugs, viruses, radiation, and malnutrition). In the United States, among the most common birth defects that require immediate intervention are heart problems, spina bifida (an open spine), and tracheoesophageal fistulas and esophageal atresias (wrongly connected or incomplete wind and food pipes).

The birth of a malformed infant is rarely expected, and the neonatologist's team plays a key role in its survival. Congenital heart disease is the most prevalent life-threatening defect. During development in utero, the umbilical cord supplies the necessary oxygen; it is not until birth, when that lifeline is cut, that the neonate's circulatory and respiratory systems acquire full responsibility. At delivery, all may appear normal, and the one-minute Apgar score may be high.

Several minutes later, however, the pink skin color may begin to darken to a purplish blue (cyanosis), indicating that insufficient oxygen is being extracted from the air. Immediately, the infant receives rescue breathing from the bag mask. Upon admission to the neonatal unit, the source of the cyanosis must be determined. A chest X ray may provide significant information about the anatomy of the heart and lungs, but special tests are usually needed to pinpoint the problem. Catheters that are threaded from neck or leg vessels into the heart can reveal the pressure and oxygen content of each chamber in the heart and across its four valves. Echocardiograms, video pictures similar to sonograms generated by sound waves passing through the chest, enhance the data provided by the X rays and catheterizations, and a diagnosis is made. Based on the physical signs and symptoms of the newborn, a treatment plan is devised.

Because of the nature of congenital defects and structural abnormalities, their correction generally re-

Number of Infant Deaths in the United States			
Cause of Death	*1980*	*1990*	*1994*
Congenital anomalies	9,220	8,239	6,854
Disorders relating to short gestation and low birth weight	3,648	4,013	4,254
Sudden infant death syndrome (SIDS)	5,510	5,417	4,073
Respiratory distress syndrome	4,989	2,850	1,567
Newborn affected by maternal complications of pregnancy	1,572	1,655	1,296
Newborn affected by complications of placenta, cord, and membranes	985	975	948
Accidents and adverse effects	1,166	930	889
Infections specific to the perinatal period	971	875	828
Pneumonia and influenza	1,012	634	559
Intrauterine hypoxia and birth asphyxia	1,497	762	537
All other causes	14,956	12,001	9,905
Total	**45,526**	**38,351**	**31,710**

Source: Statistical Abstract of the United States 1997. Washington, D.C.: GPO, 1997.

quires surgery. Openings between the heart's chambers (septal defects), valves that are too narrow or do not close properly, and blood vessels that leave or enter the heart incorrectly are all common defects treated by the pediatric heart surgeon. Because of the delicacy of the operation and the vulnerability of the newborn, surgery may be postponed until the baby is larger and stronger while it is provided with supplemental oxygen and nutrients. The risk of such operations is high, and depending on the degree of abnormality, several operations may be required.

Another group of infants who have benefited from advances in neonatology are those born to drug-addicted women. The lives of these infants are often complicated by congenital defects and life-threatening withdrawal symptoms. For example, heroin-addicted babies are quite small, are extremely irritable and hyperactive, and develop tremors, vomiting, diarrhea, and seizures. The newborn must be carefully monitored in the unit, and sedatives and antiseizure medications are given, sometimes for as long as six weeks. Cocaine and its derivatives frequently cause premature labor, fetal death, and maternal hemorrhaging during delivery. Infants that do survive often have serious congenital defects and suffer withdrawal symptoms. The risk of acquired immunodeficiency syndrome (AIDS) adds another dimension to an already complicated picture.

PERSPECTIVE AND PROSPECTS

Throughout human history, maternal and neonatal deaths have been staggering in number. Ignorance and unsanitary conditions frequently resulted in uterine hemorrhaging and overwhelming infection, killing both mother and baby. Highly inaccurate records at the beginning of the twentieth century in New York City show maternal death averaging 2 percent; in fact, the rate was probably greater, since most births occurred at home. Neonatal deaths from respiratory failure, congenital defects, prematurity, and infection loom large in these medical records. The expansion of medical, obstetric, and pediatric knowledge and technology that began after World War II has dramatically lowered maternal and infant mortality. It should not be forgotten, however, that nonindustrialized nations, the majority in the world, remain devastated by the neonatal problems that have plagued civilization for thousands of years.

Ironically, the problems associated with neonatology in Western nations are now at the other end of the spectrum: saving and prolonging life beyond what is natural or "reasonable." As neonatology advanced scientifically and technically, saving life took precedence over ethical issues. The famous and poignant story of "Baby Doe" in the early 1980's illustrates the dilemmas that occur daily in neonatal intensive care units. Baby Doe was a six-pound, full-term male born with Down syndrome and three severe congenital defects of the heart, trachea, and esophagus. These malformations were deemed surgically correctable, although the underlying problem of Down syndrome, a disease characterized by mental retardation and particular facial and body features, would remain. The parents would not agree to any operations and requested that all treatment be withheld. He was given only medication for sedation and died within a few days. The case was related by the attending physician in a letter to *The New England Journal of Medicine*. Enormous controversy was sparked. On July 5, 1983, a law was passed in effect stating that all handicapped newborns, no matter how seriously afflicted, should receive all possible life-sustaining treatment, unless it is unequivocally clear that imminent death is inevitable or that the risks of treatment cannot be justified by its benefit. The legislators believed that Baby Doe had been allowed to die because of his underlying condition (Down syndrome).

Since then, attorneys, ethicists, juries, and the courts have used the example of Baby Doe, and the law that grew from it, to interpret many cases that have come to light. Life-and-death decisions are made on a daily basis in the neonatal care unit. They are always difficult, but they usually remain a private matter between the parents and the neonatologist. These cases become public matters, however, when the family disagrees with the medical staff. Then the question of what is in the best interest of the child is compounded by who will pay for the treatments and who will care for the baby after it is discharged.

Such ethical dilemmas will continue as expertise and technology grow. A multitude of questions, previously relegated to philosophy and religion, will arise, and the benefits of saving a life will have to be weighed against its quality and the resources necessary to maintain it.

—Connie Rizzo, M.D.

See also Apgar score; Birth defects; Blue baby syndrome; Bonding; Cardiology, pediatric; Cesarean section; Childbirth; Childbirth complications; Chlamydia; Circumcision, male; Cleft lip and palate; Cleft lip and palate repair; Cognitive development; Colic; Congenital heart disease; Craniosynostosis; Critical care, pediatric; Cystic fibrosis; Developmental stages; Down syndrome; Embryology; Endocrinology, pediatric; Failure to thrive; Fetal alcohol syndrome; Gastroenterology, pediatric; Genetic diseases; Genetics and inheritance; Hematology, pediatric; Hemolytic disease of the newborn; Hydrocephalus; Jaundice, neonatal; Motor skill development; Multiple births; Nephrology, pediatric; Neurology, pediatric; Obstetrics; Orthopedics, pediatric; Pediatrics; Perinatology; Phenylketonuria (PKU); Premature birth; Pulmonary medicine, pediatric; Rh factor; Shunts; Sudden infant death syndrome (SIDS); Surgery, pediatric; Tay-Sachs disease; Toxoplasmosis; Urology, pediatric; Well-baby examinations.

FOR FURTHER INFORMATION:

Avery, Gordon B., Mary A. Fletcher, and Mhairi G. MacDonald, eds. *Neonatology: The Pathophysiology and Management of the Newborn*. 5th ed. Philadelphia: J. B. Lippincott, 1999. This excellent text, used as a main reference for neonatologists, provides a thorough scientific background, including the anatomy, physiology, and biochemistry of all known abnormal conditions. As one of the most respected sources in the field, it can be technical and involved at times, but it is well worth the effort.

Behrman, Richard E., ed. *Nelson Textbook of Pediatrics*. 16th ed. Philadelphia: W. B. Saunders, 2000. This bible of pediatrics is notable not only for its breadth and scope but also for its clarity and accessibility. The several chapters devoted to neonatology, intensive care, prematurity, and congenital defects provide a good overview in the context of pediatrics as a whole.

Cunningham, Nicholas, ed. *Columbia University College of Physicians and Surgeons: Complete Guide to Early Child Care*. New York: Crown, 1990. A very well written and organized book meant for health professionals as well as parents; the finest of this type. Its material is thorough but not too technical, so it is accessible to a wider audience. A good place to start for an overview before turning to more difficult texts.

Levin, Daniel, et al., eds. *Essentials of Pediatric Intensive Care*. 2d ed. St. Louis: Quality Medical, 1997. This superb paperback focuses on the daily routine of the neonatal intensive care unit. Good photographs and diagrams explain the technology

and the procedures used. Often used as a supplement to hardcover neonatology texts, but it can be used alone.

NEPHRECTOMY

PROCEDURE

ANATOMY OR SYSTEM AFFECTED: Abdomen, kidneys, urinary system

SPECIALTIES AND RELATED FIELDS: General surgery, nephrology, oncology, urology

DEFINITION: The removal of the kidney, which may be performed to treat disorders and disease or for the purpose of transplantation.

KEY TERMS:

adrenal gland: a small hormone-producing gland which is adjacent to the upper pole of the kidney

donor nephrectomy: a procedure in which a kidney is removed for transplantation into another patient; the kidney can be removed from a person who is brain-dead but whose heart is still beating (cadaveric donor nephrectomy) or from a relative of the recipient (a living related donor)

nephroureterectomy: a procedure similar to a radical nephrectomy, with the additional removal of the ureter and a cuff of the bladder; performed to treat transitional cell carcinomas of the ureters and the pelvis of the kidneys

radical nephrectomy: a procedure in which a kidney is removed along with the covering layers of tissue and the adjacent adrenal gland; performed with cancerous conditions

renal cell carcinoma (RCC): cancer of the small tubules of the kidney; generally known as kidney cancer

simple nephrectomy: a procedure in which a kidney is removed but the covering layers of tissue and the adjacent adrenal gland are left intact; usually performed to treat benign (noncancerous) conditions

transitional cell carcinoma (TCC): cancer arising from the lining of the urine-collecting system of the kidneys, ureters, and bladder

ureters: the tubes that drain urine from the kidneys to the bladder

INDICATIONS AND PROCEDURES

A kidney may be removed for several reasons, including congenital defects, trauma, cancer, inflammation, and transplantation. Congenital problems, or birth defects, associated with the kidneys include abnormal development, nonfunctional cysts, blockage, tumors, and cysts that are functional but which cause difficulty in breathing because of their large size. A kidney may be removed if the organ or its main blood vessels have been damaged beyond repair by trauma, such as a gunshot wound. Cancer is one of the most common reasons for nephrectomy; kidney cancers include renal cell carcinomas, transitional cell carcinomas, and tumors in the capsules of the kidneys or in surrounding layers of tissue. Infections or abscesses in the kidney that are beyond medical treatment and that become life-threatening also necessitate a nephrectomy. Finally, a kidney may be removed from a donor for transplantation.

Depending on the underlying disease and the surgeon's preference and experience, the kidney can be approached from the front, side, or back. In certain situations, the chest is also opened. The incisions used to reach the kidney are similar for simple, radical, and donor nephrectomies, but the steps that follow differ once the abdomen has been entered. For nephroureterectomy, in which the kidney, the connecting ureter, and a part of the bladder are removed, the surgeon makes either one long, S-shaped incision starting in the flank and ending near the bladder, or two separate incisions.

In the frontal approach to nephrectomy, the patient lies on his or her back and the abdomen and peritoneal cavity are opened. The intestines near the kidney are pushed to the side, and the kidney is approached from the front. The advantage of this approach includes better evaluation of the liver and the structures surrounding the kidney, better control of the blood vessels, and easy removal of clots from veins if necessary. The disadvantages of this approach are the possibility of adhesions developing in the intestines and lung complications after the surgery.

In the side approach, the patient is placed on his or her side and the incision is made through the eleventh or twelfth ribs. The kidney is approached from behind. This type of incision involves cutting into muscle and results in significant postoperative pain. The main advantage is that the peritoneal cavity is not entered.

In the back approach, known as dorsal lumbotomy, the patient is placed facedown and a muscle-splitting incision is used. The kidney is approached from behind. This method is usually used for simple nephrectomy. Its primary advantages are less postoperative pain and avoidance of the peritoneal cavity. Its main disadvantage is a limited view of the surgery site.

In simple nephrectomy, after the kidney has been exposed, Gerota's fascia (the covering envelope of the kidney) is opened, and the fat around the kidney is dissected. The adjacent blood vessels and the connecting ureter are tied and cut, and the kidney is removed. In radical nephrectomy, the adjacent adrenal gland and surrounding lymph glands are also removed in the one block. For nephroureterectomy, the ureter is not cut close to the kidney but is dissected all the way down to the bladder. A 2-centimeter cuff of bladder is cut off, the entire specimen is removed, and the hole in the bladder is closed.

The techniques used with kidney transplantation differ for cadaveric donor nephrectomy and living related donor (LRD) nephrectomy. For cadaveric donor nephrectomy, the abdominal aorta (the main artery bringing blood to the kidney) and the inferior vena cava (the main vein taking blood away from the kid-

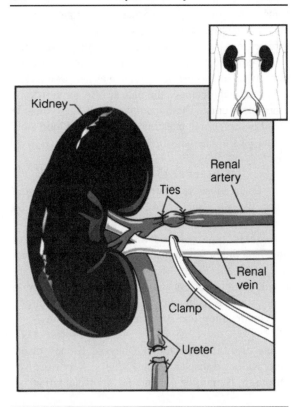

Nephrectomy

The removal of a kidney may be necessary because of disease or because the kidney is intended for transplantation into another patient; the inset shows the location of the kidneys.

ney) are isolated above and below the kidneys and cannulated with pipes to irrigate both kidneys with cold preservation fluid. Both kidneys and ureters, along with their related blood vessels, are removed. For LRD nephrectomy, the kidney is dissected along with its blood vessels and ureter. Great care is taken to obtain the maximum length of ureter and blood vessels without causing damage to the donor.

USES AND COMPLICATIONS

The major complications of nephrectomy during surgery are bleeding, damage to surrounding structures, and problems related to anesthesia. Therefore, there is significant evaluation of the patient before surgery. A battery of tests may be performed, including blood testing, urinalysis, electrocardiography, and X rays. A thorough medical examination is done to determine whether the patient can be placed under anesthesia safely. The patient's blood is also typed and cross-matched in the event that a transfusion is required. Good surgical skills, the availability of blood for transfusion, and proper anesthesia techniques usually ensure that any complications which occur are not life-threatening. Nevertheless, the patient may also experience complications during the procedure that are not directly related to the surgery, such as a heart attack.

After a nephrectomy, the patient is at some risk for other problems. These complications may include bleeding, infection, intestinal obstruction, blood clots in the legs or lungs, or a heart attack.

PERSPECTIVE AND PROSPECTS

Significant advances have been made in nephrectomy since the first such procedure was performed by Gustav Simmons in 1869. Thorough preoperative evaluation; improved anesthesia techniques; a greater understanding of anatomy, physiology, and pathology (including the nature of infections and microorganisms); and the discovery of antibiotics have all led to better surgical techniques. As a result, the death rate for nephrectomy operations is only 1 percent.

—*Saeed Akhter, M.D.*

See also Adrenalectomy; Dialysis; Kidney disorders; Kidney transplantation; Kidneys; Nephritis; Nephrology; Nephrology, pediatric; Transplantation.

FOR FURTHER INFORMATION:

Hinman, Frank. *Atlas of Urologic Surgery.* 2d ed. Philadelphia: W. B. Saunders, 1998. This is an excellent book with very useful diagrammatic and graphic details of operations and good descriptions of both old and new procedures.

Marshall, Fray F., ed. *Textbook of Operative Urology.* Philadelphia: W. B. Saunders, 1996. This book presents the most current information on indications for operation, preoperative management, operative technique, postoperative management, and complications specific to each procedure.

Novick, Andrew C., and Stevan B. Streem. "Surgery of the Kidney." In *Campbell's Urology,* edited by Patrick Walsh et al. 7th ed. Philadelphia: W. B. Saunders, 1998. A chapter in a classic urology text, which maintains its encyclopedic approach while following a new organ systems orientation. Halftone illustrations and contributions by multiple authors.

NEPHRITIS
DISEASE/DISORDER

ANATOMY OR SYSTEM AFFECTED: Abdomen, kidneys, urinary system

SPECIALTIES AND RELATED FIELDS: Internal medicine, nephrology

DEFINITION: Nephritis refers to an inflammation of the kidneys. Pyelonephritis is caused by a bacterial infection and may be acute or chronic; it is generally the result of bladder infection that has spread to the kidneys or from the reflux of urine to the kidneys because of a congenital defect. Nephritis can also be caused by glomerulonephritis, an inflammation of the glomeruli (the functioning units of the kidneys) that may result from an improper response of the immune system to bacteria. Metabolic disorders, such as kidney stones and gout, may also be responsible for kidney infection. Renal failure can result from many of these conditions.

—*Jason Georges and Tracy Irons-Georges*

See also Glomerulonephritis; Gout; Kidney disorders; Kidneys; Nephrectomy; Nephrology; Nephrology, pediatric; Renal failure; Stone removal; Stones.

FOR FURTHER INFORMATION:

Cameron, Stewart. *Kidney Disease: The Facts.* 2d ed. New York: Oxford University Press, 1986.

Legrain, Marcel, and Jean-Michel Suc Legrain, et al. *Nephrology.* Translated by M. Cavaille-Coll. New York: Masson, 1987.

Whitworth, Judith A., and J. R. Lawrence. *Textbook of Renal Disease.* 2d ed. New York: Churchill Livingstone, 1994.

NEPHROLOGY

SPECIALTY

ANATOMY OR SYSTEM AFFECTED: Abdomen, blood, kidneys, urinary system

SPECIALTIES AND RELATED FIELDS: Biochemistry, biotechnology, endocrinology, genetics, hematology, internal medicine, urology

DEFINITION: The field of medicine that deals with the anatomy and physiology of the kidneys.

KEY TERMS:

analyte: any chemical substance undergoing measurement; includes charged electrolytes found in the blood, such as sodium or potassium

creatinine: a nitrogen-containing by-product of metabolism; levels of creatinine may be indicative of kidney function

endocrine: referring to a process in which cells from an organ or gland secrete substances into the blood; these substances in turn act on cells elsewhere in the body

glomerulonephritis: inflammation of the glomeruli, the clusters of blood vessels and nerves found throughout the kidney

nephritis: any disease or pathology of the kidney that results in inflammation

nephron: the structural and functional unit of the kidney; composed of the renal corpuscle, the loop of Henle, and renal tubules

nephrotic syndrome: an abnormal condition of the kidneys characterized by a variety of conditions, including edema and proteinuria; often accompanies glomerular dysfunction and diabetes

renal: pertaining to the kidney

urea: a waste product of protein metabolism which represents the form in which nitrogen is eliminated from the body

SCIENCE AND PROFESSION

Nephrology is the branch of medicine that deals with the function of the kidneys. As a consequence, a nephrologist frequently deals with problems related to homeostasis, that is, the maintenance of the internal environment of the body. The most obvious function of the kidneys is their ability to regulate the excretion of water and minerals from the body, at the same time serving to eliminate nitrogenous wastes in the form of urea. While such waste material, produced as by-products of cell metabolism, is removed from the circulation, essential nutrients from body fluids are retained within the renal apparatus. These nutrients include proteins, carbohydrates, and electrolytes, some of which help maintain the proper acid-base balance within the blood. In addition, cells in the kidneys regulate red blood cell production through the release of the hormone erythropoietin.

The human excretory system includes two kidneys, which lie in the rear of the abdominal cavity on opposite sides of the spinal column. Urine is produced by the kidneys through a filtration network composed of 2 million nephrons, the actual functional units within each kidney. Two ureters, one for each kidney, serve to remove the collected urine and transport this liquid to the urinary bladder. The urethra drains urine from the bladder, voiding the liquid from the body.

Each adult human kidney is approximately 11 centimeters in length, with a shape resembling a bean. When the kidney is sectioned, three anatomical regions are visible: a light-colored outer cortex; a darker inner region, called the medulla; and the renal pelvis, the lowest portion of the kidney. The cortex consists primarily of a network of nephrons and associated blood capillaries. Tubules extending from each nephron pass into the medulla. The medulla, in turn, is visibly divided into about a dozen conical masses, or pyramids, with the base of the pyramid at the junction between the cortex and medulla and the apex of the pyramid extending into the renal pelvis. The loops (such as the loop of Henle) and tubules within the medulla carry out the reabsorption of nutrients and fluids that have passed through the capsular network of the nephron. The tubules extend through the medulla and return to the corticol region.

There are approximately 1 million nephrons in each kidney. Within each nephron, the actual filtration of blood is carried out within a bulb-shaped region, Bowman's capsule, which surrounds a capillary network, the glomerulus. In most individuals, a single renal artery brings the blood supply to the kidney. Since the renal artery originates from a branch of the aorta, the body's largest artery, the blood pressure within this region of the kidney is high. Consequently, hypotension, a significant lowering of blood pressure, may also result in kidney failure.

The renal artery enters the kidney through the renal pelvis, branching into progressively smaller arterioles and capillaries. The capillary network serves both to supply nutrition to the cells that make up the kidney and to collect nutrients or fluids reabsorbed from the loops and tubules of the nephrons. Renal capillaries also enter the Bowman's capsules in the form of balls or coils, the glomeruli. Since blood pressure remains high, the force filtration in a nephron pushes about 20 percent of the fluid volume of the glomerulus into the cavity portion of the capsule. Most small materials dissolved in the blood, including proteins, sugars, electrolytes, and the nitrogenous waste product urea, pass along within the fluid into the capsule. As the filtrate passes through the series of convoluted tubules extending from the Bowman's capsule, most nutrients and salts are reabsorbed and reenter the capillary network. Approximately 99 percent of the water that has passed through the capsule is also reabsorbed. The material which remains, much of it waste such as urea, is excreted from the body.

Nephrology is the branch of medicine that deals with these functions of the kidney. Loss of kidney function can quickly result in a buildup of waste material in the blood; hence kidney failure, if untreated, can result in serious illness or death. Within the purview of nephrology, however, is more than the function of the kidneys as filters for the excretion of wastes. The kidneys are also endocrine organs, structures that secrete hormones into the bloodstream to act on other, distal organs. The major endocrine functions of the kidneys involve the secretion of the hormones renin and erythropoietin.

Renin functions within the renin-angiotensin system in the regulation of blood pressure. It is produced within the juxtaglomerular complex, the region around Bowman's capsule in which the arteriole enters the structure. Cells within the tubules of the nephron closely monitor the blood pressure within the incoming arterioles. When blood pressure drops, these cells stimulate the release of renin directly into the blood circulation.

Renin does not act directly on the nephrons. Rather, it serves as a proteolytic enzyme which activates another protein, angiotensin, the precursor of which is found in the blood. The activated angiotensin, called angiotensin II, has several effects on kidney function that involve the regulation of blood pressure. First, by decreasing the glomerular filtration rate, it allows more water to be retained. Second, angiotensin II stimulates the release of the steroid hormone aldosterone from the adrenal glands, located in close association with the kidneys. Aldosterone acts to increase sodium retention and transport by cells within the tubules of the nephron, resulting in increased water reabsorption. The result of this complex series of hormone interactions within the kidney is a close monitoring of both salt retention and blood pressure and volume. In this manner, nephrology also relates to the pathophysiology of hypertension—high blood pressure.

The kidneys also regulate the production of erythrocytes, red blood cells, through the production of the hormone erythropoietin. Erythropoietin is secreted by the peritubular cells associated with regions outside the nephrons in response to lowered oxygen levels in the blood, also monitored by cells within the kidney. The hormone serves to stimulate red cell production within the bone marrow. Approximately 85 percent of the erythropoietin in blood fluids is synthesized within the kidneys, the remainder by the liver.

Since proper kidney function is related to a wide variety of body processes, from the regulation of nitrogenous waste disposal to the monitoring and control of blood pressure, nephrology may deal with a number of disparate syndromes. The kidney may represent the primary site of a disease or pathology, an example being the autoimmune phenomenon of glomerulonephritis. Renal failure may also result from the indirect action of a more general systemic syndrome, as is the case with diabetes mellitus. In many cases, the decrease in kidney function may result from any number of disorders, which poses many problems for the nephrologist.

Proper function of the kidney is central to numerous homeostatic processes within the body. Thus nephrology by necessity deals with a variety of pathophysiological disorders. Renal dysfunction may involve disorders of the organ itself or pathology associated with individual structures within the kidneys, the glomeruli or tubules. Likewise, the disorder within the body may be of a more general type, with the kidney being a secondary site of damage. This is particularly true of immune disorders such as lupus (systemic lupus erythematosus) or diabetes. Conditions that affect proper kidney function may result from infection or inflammation, the obstruction of tubules or the vascular system, or neoplastic disorders (cancers).

Immune disorders are among the more common processes that result in kidney disease. They may be of two types: glomerulonephritis or the more general nephrotic syndrome. Glomerulonephritis can result either from a direct attack on basement membrane tissue by host antibodies, such as with Goodpasture's syndrome, or indirectly through deposits of immune (antigen-antibody) complexes, such as with lupus. Nephritis may also be secondary to high blood pressure. In any of these situations, inflammation resulting from the infiltration of immune complexes and/or from the activation of the complement system may result in a decreased ability of the glomeruli to function. Treatment of such disorders often involves the use of corticosteroids or other immunosuppressive drugs to dampen the immune response. Continued recurrence of the disease may result in renal failure, requiring dialysis treatment or even kidney transplantation.

Activation of the complement system as a result of immune complex deposition along the glomeruli is a frequent source of inflammation. Complement consists of a series of some dozen serum proteins, many of which are pharmacologically active. Intermediates in the complement pathway include enzymes that activate subsequent components in a cascade fashion. The terminal proteins in the pathway form a "membrane attack complex," capable of significantly damaging a target (such as the basement membrane of a Bowman's capsule). Activation of the initial steps in the pathway begins with either the deposition of immune complexes along basement membranes or the direct binding of antibodies on glomerular surfaces. The end result can be extensive nephrotic destruction.

Nephrotic syndrome, which can also result in extensive damage to the glomeruli, is often secondary to other disease. Diabetes is a frequent primary disorder in its development; approximately one-third of insulin-dependent diabetics are at risk for significant renal failure. Other causes of nephrotic syndrome may include cancer or infectious agents and toxins.

DIAGNOSTIC AND TREATMENT TECHNIQUES

Nephrologists can measure glomerular function using a variety of tests. These tests are based on the ability of the basement membranes associated with the glomeruli to act as filters. Blood cells and large materials such as proteins dissolved in the blood are unable to pass through these filters. Plasma, the liquid portion of the blood containing dissolved factors involved in blood-clotting mechanisms, is able to pass through the basement membrane, the driving force for filtration being the hydrostatic pressure of the blood (blood pressure).

The glomerular filtration rate (GFR) is defined as the rate by which the glomeruli filter the plasma during a fixed period of time. Generally, the rate is determined by measuring either the time of clearance of the carbohydrate inulin from the blood or the rate of clearance of creatinine, a nitrogenous by-product of

metabolism. Though the rate may vary with age, it generally is about 125 to 130 milliliters of plasma filtered per minute.

Any significant decrease in the GFR is indicative of renal failure and can result in significant disruptions of acid-base or electrolyte balance in the blood. A decrease in the GFR can sometimes be observed through measurements of urine output. Healthy individuals usually excrete from one to two liters of urine per day. If the urine output drops to less than 500 milliliters (0.5 liter) per day, a condition known as oliguria, the body suffers a diminished capacity to remove metabolic waste products (urea, creatinine, or acids). Taken to an extreme, in which the filtering capacity is completely shut down and urine formation drops below 100 milliliters per day (anuria), the resulting uremia may cause death in a matter of days.

Anuria may have a variety of causes: kidney failure; hypotension, in which blood pressure is insufficient to maintain glomerular filtration; or a blockage in the urinary tract. As waste products, fluids, and electrolytes (especially sodium and potassium) build up, the person may appear puffy, be feverish, and exhibit muscle weakness. Heart arrhythmia or failure may also occur. Mediation of the problem, in addition to attempts to alleviate the reasons for kidney dysfunction, include regulation of fluid, protein, and electrolyte uptake. Medications are also used to increase the excretion of potassium and tissue fluids, assuming that the cause is not a urinary blockage.

The nephrologist or other physician may also monitor kidney function through measurements of serum analytes or through observation of certain chemicals within the urine. The levels of blood, urea, and nitrogen (BUN), nitrogenous substances in the blood, present a rough measure of kidney function. Generally, BUN levels change significantly only after glomerular filtration has been significantly disrupted. The levels are also dependent on the amount of protein intake in the diet. When changes occur as a result of renal dysfunction, BUN levels can be a useful marker for the progression of the disease. A more specific indicator of renal function can be the creatinine concentration within the blood. Serum creatinine, unlike BUN levels, is not related to the diet. In the event of renal failure, however, changes in BUN levels usually can be detected earlier than those of creatinine.

As the glomeruli lose their ability to distinguish large from small molecules during filtration, protein can begin to appear in the urine, the condition known as proteinuria. Usually, the level of protein in the urine is negligible (less than 250 milligrams per day). A transient proteinuria can result from heavy exercise or minor illness, but persistent levels of more than 1 gram per day may be indicative of renal dysfunction or even complications of hypertension. Generally, if the problem resides in the loss of tubular reabsorption, levels of protein generally are below 1 to 2 grams per day, with that amount usually consisting of small proteins. If the problem is a result of increased glomerular permeability caused by inflammation, levels may reach greater than 2 grams per day. In cases of nephrotic syndrome, excretion of protein in the urine may exceed 5 grams per day.

Measurement of urine protein is a relatively easy process. A urine sample is placed on a plastic stick with an indicator pad capable of turning colors, depending on the protein concentration. Analogous strips may be used for detection of other materials in urine, including acid, blood, or sugars. The presence of either red or white blood cells in urine can be indicative of infection or glomerulonephritis.

In addition to the filtration of blood fluids through the nephrons, the reabsorption of materials within the tubules results in increased urine concentration. A normal GFR within a healthy kidney produces a urine concentration three or four times as great as that found within serum. As kidney failure progresses, the concentration of urine begins to decrease, with the urine becoming more dilute. The kidneys compensate for the decreased concentration by increasing the amount of urine output: The frequency of urination may increase, as well as the volume excreted (polyuria). In time, if renal failure continues, the GFR will decrease, resulting in the retention of both analytes and water.

Determination of urine concentration is carried out following a brief period of dehydration: deprivation of fluids for about fifteen hours prior to the test. This dehydration will result in increased production by the hypothalamus of antidiuretic hormone (ADH), or vasopressin, a chemical which decreases the production of urine through increased renal tubule reabsorption of water. The result is a more concentrated urine. Following the dehydration period, the patient's urine is collected over a period of three hours and assessed for concentration. Significantly low values may be indicative of kidney disease.

A battery of tests in addition to those already described may be utilized in the diagnosis of kidney disease. These may include intravenous pyelography (in which a contrast medium is injected into the blood and followed as it passes through the kidneys), kidney biopsy, and ultrasound examinations. Diagnosis and course of treatment depend on an evaluation of these tests.

PERSPECTIVE AND PROSPECTS

The roots of modern nephrology date from the seventeenth century. In the early decades of that century, the English physician William Harvey demonstrated the principles of blood circulation and the role of the heart in that process. Harvey's theories opened the door for more extensive analysis of organ systems, both in humans and in other animals. As a result, in 1666, Italian anatomist Marcello Malpighi, while exploring organ structure with the newly developed microscope, discovered the presence of glomeruli (what he called Malpighian corpuscles) within the kidneys. Malpighi thought that these structures were in some way connected with collecting ducts in the kidneys that had recently been found by Lorenzo Bellini. Malpighi also suspected that these structures played a role in urine formation.

Sir William Bowman, in 1832, was the first to describe the true relationship of the corpuscles discovered by Malpighi to urine secretion through the tubules. Bowman's capsule, as it is now called, is a filter which allows only the liquid of the blood, as well as dissolved salts and urea within the blood, into the tubules, from which the urine is secreted. It remained for Carl Ludwig, in 1842, to complete the story. Ludwig suggested that the corpuscles function in a passive manner, in that the filtrate is filtered by means of hydrostatic pressure through the capsule into the tubules and from there concentrated as water and solutes are reabsorbed.

The first definitive work on urine formation, *The Secretion of the Urine*, was published by Arthur Robertson Cushny in 1917. In the monograph, Cushny offered a thorough analysis of the data published on kidney function. Though Cushny was incorrect in some of his conclusions, the work catalyzed intensive research activity on the functions of the kidney. A colleague of Cushny, E. Brice Mayrs, made the first attempt to determine the glomerular filtration rate, measuring the clearance of sulfate in rabbits. In 1926, the Danish physiologist Poul Brandt Rehberg demonstrated the superiority of creatinine as a marker for glomerular filtration; the "guinea pig" for the experiment was Rehberg himself.

A pioneer in renal physiology, Homer William Smith, began his research while serving in the United States Army during World War I. Until he retired in 1961, Smith was involved in much of the research related to renal excretion. It was Smith who developed inulin clearance as a measure of the GFR; his later years dealt with studies on mechanisms of solute excretion.

With the newer technology of the 1970's and 1980's, more accurate methods for analysis became available. These have included ultrasound scanning, intravenous pyelography, and angiography. In addition, better understanding of immediate causes of many kidney problems has served to control or prevent some forms of renal failure.

—Richard Adler, Ph.D.

See also Abdomen; Abdominal disorders; Adrenalectomy; Blood and blood disorders; Cysts; Diabetes mellitus; Dialysis; Edema; Glomerulonephritis; Internal medicine; Kidney disorders; Kidney transplantation; Kidneys; Lithotripsy; Nephrectomy; Nephritis; Nephrology, pediatric; Renal failure; Stone removal; Stones; Terminally ill: Extended care; Transplantation; Urinalysis; Urinary system; Urology; Urology, pediatric; Transplantation.

FOR FURTHER INFORMATION:

Cameron, Stewart. *Kidney Disease: The Facts*. 2d ed. New York: Oxford University Press, 1986. A brief but thorough discussion of types of kidney disease. Written in a style which falls between detailed analysis and cursory treatment. Some knowledge of biology is helpful.

Legrain, Marcel, and Jean-Michel Suc Legrain, et al. *Nephrology*. Translated by M. Cavaille-Coll. New York: Masson, 1987. A basic text on the function of the kidney. The book provides an overview of kidney structure, diseases of the kidney, and their treatment. Also included is a chapter dealing with appropriate diets for the prevention or alleviation of kidney disease.

Tanagho, Emil A., and Jack W. McAninch, eds. *Smith's General Urology*. 15th ed. Norwalk, Conn.: Appleton and Lange, 2000. A text within the Appleton and Lange series of medical publications. An outstanding overview of kidney structure and function. Written at a level appropriate for readers with a basic knowledge of biology, but contains enough detail that it can also serve as a reference work.

Wallace, Robert A., Gerald P. Sanders, and Robert J. Ferl. *Biology: The Science of Life*. 4th ed. New York: HarperCollins, 1996. Included in the chapter on excretion is a fine description of the human excretory system. Written on a basic level, the section includes useful diagrams and a concise discussion of kidney function written for those with only rudimentary knowledge of the field.

Whitworth, Judith A., and J. R. Lawrence. *Textbook of Renal Disease*. 2d ed. New York: Churchill Livingstone, 1994. A detailed analysis of kidney anatomy and function, with an emphasis on types of disease. The book provides a fine description of the effects of systemic problems on renal dysfunction. Also included are sections on imaging and diagnosis.

NEPHROLOGY, PEDIATRIC

SPECIALTY

ANATOMY OR SYSTEM AFFECTED: Abdomen, blood, kidneys, urinary system

SPECIALTIES AND RELATED FIELDS: Biochemistry, biotechnology, endocrinology, genetics, hematology, internal medicine, neonatology, pediatrics, urology

DEFINITION: The specialty involving the diagnosis and treatment of kidney disorders and diseases in children and adolescents.

KEY TERMS:

dialysis: the process of separating crystalloid molecules in solution by diffusion through a semipermeable membrane (essentially, a machine performing the function of the nephrons in the kidney)

glomerulus: one of the very small units in the kidney, where blood is filtered through a membrane

immunology: the science concerned with various phenomena of immunity, increased sensitivity, and allergy

nephrology: the medical science of the kidneys and their function

nephron: the basic functioning unit of the kidney, consisting of the glomerulus plus a series of collecting and transport tubules; there are approximately one million nephrons in each kidney

renal: referring to the kidneys

urea: a nitrogenous molecule found in the blood and urine; the largest component of urine besides water

SCIENCE AND PROFESSION

Pediatric nephrology is a major subspecialty limited to children and adolescents that involves the study of normal and abnormal kidney (renal) function. This discipline not only relates to kidney diseases and renal dysfunction but also places heavy emphasis on the kidneys' adaptive role in many diseases and disorders of nonrenal origin. Pediatric nephrologists are doctors of medicine or osteopathy who have completed three years of pediatric residency training, followed by two or three years in a pediatric nephrology fellowship.

The kidneys are among the most interesting and complex organs in the human body. Kidney diseases often involve the fields of immunology, oncology, genetics, chemistry, physiology, biotechnology, and both gross anatomy and microanatomy (histology). While the cognitive aspects of nephrology dominate the day-to-day work of its specialists, hands-on procedures such as renal biopsies and renal dialysis add variety and interest. Pediatric nephrologists spend approximately 60 percent of their time dealing with primary renal disease, while 40 percent of their time is spent with diseases and conditions of nonrenal origin, especially in critically ill children.

While the kidneys have many functions, their main role is filtering metabolic wastes from the blood and eliminating them via the urinary tract. The process of filtering blood, concentrating its wastes, and reabsorbing water and useful metabolic components (such as protein, sodium, and potassium salts) is accomplished with an elaborate system of passive and active mechanisms in the nephrons in each kidney. The kidneys respond to many factors, including blood volume, blood pressure, the salt and acid content of the blood, nitrogenous wastes (urea), and even hormonal and neural (nerve) stimuli. The kidneys deliver feedback to other vital organs with chemical messengers via the bloodstream and also through the nervous system.

Several key areas in pediatric nephrology make it unique from adult nephrology: immature renal function in infancy, growth retardation in chronic renal disease, and the role of genetics.

DIAGNOSTIC AND TREATMENT TECHNIQUES

The patient's history, a physical examination, and routine urinalysis are the cornerstones of diagnosis in nephrology. Urinalysis is one of the most available, fastest, and least expensive tests in clinical medicine. Frequently, diagnosis is made or suspected from a routine urinalysis done in screening or as part of a routine physical. The test can reveal evidence of in-fection; microscopic traces of blood, protein, or sugar; and many other abnormalities. Often, early diagnosis of silent renal disease will aid in early intervention, treatment, and the prevention of advanced disease and morbidity. In addition to blood chemistry tests—such as for sodium, potassium, glucose (sugar), and blood, urea, and nitrogen (BUN)—many quantitative tests are available to measure other aspects of renal function.

Dramatic advances in imaging techniques have been made. X rays, ultrasound, computed tomography (CT) scans, magnetic resonance imaging (MRI), and nuclear scans are making detailed anatomical diagnosis possible in noninvasive ways. Very small tumors and structural abnormalities can be identified. Some scans can provide useful information on renal function.

Renal biopsy with a percutaneous (through-the-skin) technique, using a large-bore needle, was developed in the 1960's. The samples allow detailed examination at microscopic and submicroscopic (electron microscopy) levels. Since many renal diseases reveal a characteristic thickening from immunoglobulin deposits and inflammation of membranes in the glomerulus, exact diagnoses are often made by biopsy alone or in conjunction with immunological tests.

In the early part of the twentieth century, the treatment of renal diseases was limited to symptomatic and supportive measures. By the 1940's and 1950's, the advent of antibiotics allowed definitive treatment of kidney and urinary tract infections. Since that era, chemotherapy and immunotherapy have developed rapidly, and many primary renal diseases are now being treated successfully by such methods. Immunotherapy also plays a major role in renal transplantation.

In chronic renal disease, in which the total renal function becomes inadequate to sustain life, children can be treated successfully with renal dialysis. Evolving from pioneer efforts in the 1960's and early 1970's, dialysis is now done routinely for such children, including infants. The effectiveness, safety, and efficiency of the procedure have improved dramatically. Now infants and toddlers usually have peritoneal (abdominal cavity) dialysis conducted at home. Older children usually have hemodialysis about three times a week at a dialysis center. The dialysis machine is connected to a cannula (tubing) that is placed in the patient's arm.

Severe growth retardation is a major problem associated with chronic renal disease in children, often compounded by psychological problems such as severe depression. A combination of improved aggressive nutritional and metabolic support plus treatment with growth hormone has improved the health and mental well-being of these children.

By the early 1970's, kidney transplantation was being done on children. This operation is performed by urologists and pediatric surgeons. Originally, rejection rates and other complications were very high. Results have improved dramatically, and in the United States a national collaborative database reported in 1993 that five years after live donor grafts, 75 percent of the kidneys had not been rejected. This procedure allows thousands of children to lead healthy, normal lives.

The study of renal function in newborns, especially premature ones, has led to sophisticated intensive care for critically ill infants. Pediatric nephrologists may also act as consultants for older children with critical illnesses, injuries, poisonings, and even trauma. Such cases often involve sophisticated intravenous (IV) fluid therapy. Because of temporary renal failure, some of these cases require dialysis.

PERSPECTIVE AND PROSPECTS

The progress in renal dialysis and transplantation has been remarkable. Continued advances in effectiveness, success rates, safety, and convenience are certain. The gene that causes familial polycystic kidney disease has been identified. Such discoveries, coupled with advances in genetics, may revolutionize therapy and even prevent some renal diseases through genetic engineering.

—*C. Mervyn Rasmussen, M.D.*

See also Abdomen; Abdominal disorders; Adrenalectomy; Blood and blood disorders; Diabetes mellitus; Dialysis; Edema; Glomerulonephritis; Internal medicine; Kidney disorders; Kidney transplantation; Kidneys; Nephrectomy; Nephritis; Nephrology; Pediatrics; Renal failure; Systems and organs; Transplantation; Urinalysis; Urinary system; Urology; Urology, pediatric.

FOR FURTHER INFORMATION:

Bock, Glenn H., Edward J. Ruley, and Michael P. Moore. *A Parent's Guide to Kidney Disorders*. Minneapolis: University of Minnesota Press, 1993. A good overview. Nicely organized, with a glossary.

Faris, Mickie Hall. *When Your Kidneys Fail: A Handbook for Patients and Their Families*. Rev. 2d ed. Los Angeles: National Kidney Foundation of South-

ern California, 1991. A handbook for patients and their families. Easy to read, and contains an excellent glossary.

Orsini, Jenoveva. "Comprehensive Care for Children with Renal Disease." *The Exceptional Parent* 29, no. 9 (September, 1999): 36, 38. With commitment, patience, and the support of an outstanding pediatric nephrology team, parents of children with kidney disease and renal failure can provide the care and attention that will enhance the health of their children. Topics such as nutrition, medication, dialysis, and transplantation are addressed.

Postlethwaite, R. J. *Clinical Paediatric Nephrology*. 2d ed. Boston: Butterworth-Heinemann, 1994. Discusses kidney diseases in infants and children. Includes a bibliography and an index.

NERVOUS SYSTEM
ANATOMY

ANATOMY OR SYSTEM AFFECTED: Ears, nerves, spine
SPECIALTIES AND RELATED FIELDS: Neurology
DEFINITION: The major control system of the body, which synchronizes physiologic activity by interpreting incoming stimuli and which is responsible for memory and reasoning; it is composed of the central nervous system (the brain and spinal cord) and the peripheral nervous system (nerve processes, sensory receptors, and ganglia).

KEY TERMS:
cerebrospinal fluid (CSF): the extracellular fluid of the central nervous system; it flows through the ventricles of the brain and the central canal of the spinal cord, circulating nutrients and providing a cushion for the brain
effector: a general term referring to skeletal, smooth, and cardiac muscles or glands that respond to impulses produced by the nervous system
glial cells: nonexcitable cells of the nervous system; they include astrocytes, microglial cells, oligodendrocytes, and Schwann cells
receptors: membrane-bound proteins with specific binding sites for neurotransmitters
synapse: a juncture between neurons or between neurons and muscle

STRUCTURE AND FUNCTIONS

The nervous system serves as the major control system of the human body. It is responsible for the synchronization of body parts, the integration of physiologic activity, the interpretation of incoming stimuli, and all intellectual activity, including memory and abstract reasoning. The nervous system regulates these activities by communication between various nerve cells; by controlling the actions of skeletal, smooth, and cardiac muscle; and by stimulating the secretion of products from various glands of the body.

Anatomically, the nervous system is divided into the central nervous system, which is composed of the brain and the spinal cord, and the peripheral nervous system, which includes all nervous structures outside the central nervous system—primarily, nerve processes, sensory receptors, and a limited number of cells of the nervous system that are located in special structures known as ganglia. Ganglia are found at various locations throughout the body. They are the only locations of neurons outside the central nervous system. Information from incoming cells can be transmitted to the ganglion cells, which in turn can transmit that information to other locations.

Although the brain and the spinal cord contain several different types of cells that are morphologically unique, there is only one functional cell present, which by convention is always referred to as the neuron. The neuron is one of the few cells in the body that cannot reproduce; a fixed number of these cells develop in infancy, and the number never increases. The number of neurons can, however, decrease in the event of injury or disease.

The neuron consists of a cell body that is similar to that of the typical animal cell familiar to most people. In addition, the neuron has extensions called processes. In the typical neuron, there are two types of processes: dendrites and axons.

Usually a neuron has many dendrites. Dendrites are very short, receive information from nearby cells, and relay that information to the cell body. Each cell has only a single axon, which may be very long, extending up and down the spinal cord or from the spinal cord to the ends of the fingers or toes. The axons conduct information from the cell bodies to the effectors—that is, the muscles and glands—or to other neurons.

Functionally, the nervous system is divided into two areas: the somatic nervous system and the autonomic nervous system. The somatic system controls posture and locomotion by stimulating the skeletal muscles. It is responsible for knowing where the body is in space and for ensuring that there is sufficient muscle contraction (tone) to maintain posture. Responses of the somatic system occur through the motor neurons.

The Nervous System

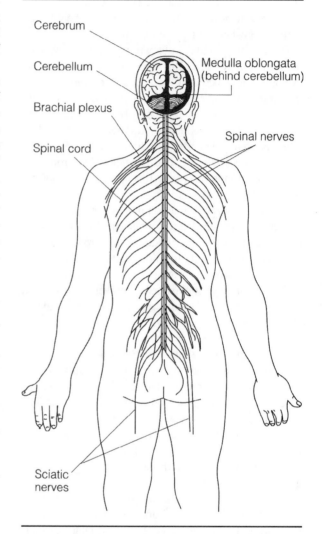

The autonomic nervous system regulates the internal activities through the innervation, or nerve stimulation, of the smooth muscles or the glands. It is anatomically different from the somatic nervous system in that the stimulation of body parts always involves two neurons. The cell body of the second neuron in the sequence is located in a ganglion outside the central nervous system.

The autonomic nervous system is broken down further into two divisions: the sympathetic and the parasympathetic. The sympathetic system is also known as the "fight or flight" reaction, since it evolved from the mechanism in lower animals by which an animal would prepare to fight a predator or run from it. More commonly, it is referred to in humans as the adrenaline response, which is active during stressful situations, strenuous physical activity, public performance, or competition.

The parasympathetic system, which is responsible for the digestive functions of the body, controls stimulation of salivary gland secretions, increased blood flow to digestive organs, and movement of materials through the digestive system. The sympathetic and parasympathetic systems usually function in balance; the parasympathetic system predominates after meals, and the sympathetic system predominates during periods of stress or physical activity.

Neurons communicate with other neurons or effectors through the release of chemical messengers known as neurotransmitters. At the termination of the axon, there is a widened area known as the synaptic knob. It produces and/or stores neurotransmitters. The effects of neurotransmitters are always localized and of short duration. There are many types of neurotransmitters, some of which are well known, such as acetylcholine and norepinephrine.

Neurotransmitters are released in response to an electrical impulse that is conducted along the axon. Once released, a neurotransmitter binds to cells that have appropriate receptors on their dendrites. Neurotransmitters may either stimulate or inhibit the activity of the second cell. If there is significant stimulation of the second cell, it will conduct the information along its axon and release a neurotransmitter from the axon terminal, which will in turn stimulate or inhibit the next neuron or effector. There must be a mechanism for the immediate removal of neurotransmitters from the synaptic cleft if the stimulation of the second neuron is to cease and if other impulses are to be conducted.

Neurotransmitters can influence only those cells that have the appropriate receptors on their surfaces. It is through the neurotransmitter-receptor complex that neurotransmitters are able to influence cells, and any alteration of the number of receptors or type of receptors on a cell membrane will lead to an alteration of cellular functioning.

The axons of some neurons are covered with multiple layers of a cell membrane known as myelin. The myelin is produced by specialized cells in the brain known as oligodendrocytes and by cells in the peripheral axons known as Schwann cells. Myelin serves as an insulator for axons and is effective in speeding up the conduction of nerve impulses. It is essen-tial for the normal functioning of the nervous system.

The brain and spinal cord are enclosed by three membranes of dense connective tissue called the meninges. The meninges separate the nervous system from other tissue and from the skull and spinal cord. The meninges are, from the outside inward, the dura mater, the arachnoid mater, and the pia mater. Many of the blood vessels of the brain travel through the meninges; therefore, the surface of the brain is very vascular and is subject to bleeding or clotting after trauma.

DISORDERS AND DISEASES

Diseases of the nervous system can be arranged into several general categories: infections, congenital diseases, seizure disorders, circulatory diseases, traumatic injury, demyelinating diseases, degenerative diseases, mental diseases, and neoplasms.

Infections of the nervous system are described according to the tissues infected. If the meninges are infected, the disease is known as meningitis; if the brain tissue is infected, the disease is referred to as encephalitis. The development of abscesses in the nervous tissue can also occur. The conditions described can be caused by viruses, bacteria, protozoa, or other parasites.

In most cases, the organism that causes meningitis is spread via the bloodstream. It is also possible, however, for infections to be spread from an infected middle ear or paranasal sinus, a skull fracture, brain surgery, or a lumbar puncture. The infectious agent can usually be determined by analyzing the spinal fluid. Bacterial infections are treated with antibiotics, while viral infections receive only supportive treatment.

An abscess of nervous tissue is usually a complication resulting from an infection at some other anatomical site, particularly from middle-ear infections or sinus infections. Abscesses may also occur following penetrating injuries. The abscess can create pressure inside the skull, and, if left untreated, it may rupture and lead to death.

Viral encephalitis is an acute disease that is often spread to humans by arthropods from animal hosts. After a carrier insect bites a human, the virus is spread to the brain of the human via the bloodstream. The specific causative agent often goes undiagnosed. Some well-known forms of encephalitis are herpes simplex encephalitis, poliomyelitis, rabies, and cytomegalovirus encephalitis. In addition, some forms of encephalitis fall into the category of slow virus infections, which have latent periods as long as several years between the time of infection and the development of encephalitis.

Other serious infections include neurosyphilis, which occurs in the late stages of untreated syphilis infections; toxoplasmosis, a protozoan infection that is extremely dangerous to fetuses but rarely causes serious problems in adults; cerebral malaria; and African trypanosomiasis, which is also known as sleeping sickness.

Congenital diseases of the brain vary in the degree of malfunction they produce. Spina bifida is a general term for a group of disorders in which the vertebrae do not develop as they should. As a result, the spinal cord may protrude from the lower back. In some cases, the effects may be so minimal as to produce no symptoms; in other cases, however, these malformations may lead to major neurologic impairment.

Hydrocephalus is another congenital malformation. It may lead to an increase in the size of the ventricles of the brain. It may be caused by blockage of the flow of spinal fluid, which in the fetus may lead to expanded brain size. In some cases, the spinal fluid produced by the nervous system fills the ventricles and limits the space available for the growing brain and nervous tissue. The result under these conditions is the presence of larger-than-normal ventricles and a smaller-than-normal amount of nervous tissue.

A seizure disorder is any sudden burst of excess electrical activity in the neurons of the brain. Epilepsy is a general term for seizure disorders. The condition may be mild and have only minimal effects, or it may be severe, leading to convulsions. The cause is often unknown, but epilepsy may result from infection, trauma, or neoplasms.

Cerebrovascular accident (CVA) is the term used to describe a variety of malfunctions of the blood circulation in the nervous system that are not a result of trauma. More commonly, the term "stroke" is used to describe the condition. Strokes have many causes that generally fall into two categories: ischemic and hemorrhagic.

Ischemic strokes are those in which the nervous tissue is deprived of oxygen as a result of an impairment of blood flow to the area. An ischemic stroke is often the result of a blood clot that blocks the blood vessels leading to the brain or the blood vessels in the brain itself. Although there are other causes, these are the most common. Since the cells can live for only a few minutes without oxygen, the consequence of an ischemic stroke can be neurological impairment or even death.

In hemorrhagic strokes, there is bleeding in the brain itself. It may be caused by hypertension or by the rupture of a weakened blood vessel, which is known as an aneurysm. Both ischemic and hemorrhagic strokes lead to the death of neurons in the affected area. The degree of damage to the brain is determined by the number of cells destroyed by the oxygen deprivation.

Traumatic injury to the brain can generally be classified as penetrating or nonpenetrating. Penetrating injuries produce a risk of infection as well as bleeding at the site of the wound. Since many large blood vessels are located in the meninges, even injuries that penetrate only into the meninges may be sufficient to cause serious injury. Nonpenetrating injuries may also cause bleeding of the meninges, which can limit blood flow to the nervous tissue or put excessive pressure on the tissue.

Injury to the spinal cord may result in severing the spinal cord from the brain. If this should occur, communications between the brain and any structures below the area of the injury are lost, as is all sensory and motor function in those areas. Since neurons are unable to regenerate and axon repair is limited, there is little hope for reversal of this condition, although extensive research is being conducted in this area.

Demyelinating diseases are those that result in changes in the myelin sheaths of neurons. The most common example is multiple sclerosis, which affects myelin in the central nervous system but not in the peripheral nervous system. Although there are varying degrees of severity, the condition causes limb weakness, impaired perception, and optic neuritis, among other things. Some cases present only mild symptoms, while others are degenerative and can lead to death—in some patients, within months. Many patients, however, survive for more than twenty years. The cause of the disease is not yet clear, although viral infections have been associated with some demyelinating diseases.

Degenerative diseases are those in which there is a gradual decline in nervous function. The disease may be hereditary, as in the case of Huntington's disease, or may occur without any apparent genetic basis, as in the case of Parkinson's disease. Parkinson's disease involves the death of certain neurons in the brain and a decreased concentration of neurotransmitters.

As the disease progresses, there is a gradual loss of motor ability and, ultimately, a complete loss of motor function. Not much is known about neurotransmitter replacement or mechanisms to stop degenerative diseases.

Little is known about mental diseases such as schizophrenia and manic depression. They appear to involve abnormal levels of neurotransmitters or errors in the membrane receptors associated with those neurotransmitters. Success in localizing the causes of these diseases has been slow in coming; there has been much more success in the development of medications to treat them.

Cancer of the brain can be primary or metastatic. Metastatic tumors, the more common variety, can arise from any source. Of the primary neoplasms, the most common are those derived from glial cells, which are responsible for more than 65 percent of all primary neoplasms. The second most common are neoplasms resulting from transformation of cells of the meninges. Since neurons cannot divide, neuron tumors are almost nonexistent except in children.

PERSPECTIVE AND PROSPECTS

When the control system of the body experiences a malfunction, the effects are wide ranging. Since the nervous system has the responsibility of regulating so many diverse activities, nervous system injury or disease must be treated immediately if the patient is to survive. This problem is further complicated by the fact that the brain is a difficult organ to study, because of its location within the skull and because its cells are vital and can be studied only after they have died.

Disease or injury of the cells of the nervous system—especially the brain—creates problems that are unique to that organ for several reasons, including the facts that those cells cannot repair themselves and cannot divide. In addition, the cells of the brain are restricted to a limited area. The cells of the nervous system are unique in that they are so highly specialized that they are not capable of cell division. As a result, humans have the greatest number of neurons during early childhood. Any neural injury or disease that kills cells results in a decreased number of neurons. In addition, neurons are not very good at repairing themselves. Furthermore, the space in the skull is tightly packed with cells and cerebrospinal fluid. There is no room for the blood that might appear as the result of an injury or the fluid accumulation that might be caused by tissue infection or tumors. Any of these conditions will increase the pressure within the skull and will also increase the extent of the injury to the nervous tissue.

Although there is no mechanism for replacing cells that have died, the prognosis is not totally bleak. There are cells in the brain that can, in the event of disease or injury, assume the responsibilities of the dead cells. For example, a person who has lost the capacity to speak following a stroke may be retaught to speak using cells that previously did not perform that function.

Among the problems with which the nervous system must cope, there are many things that can go wrong at the synapse of a neuron. The cell may produce too little or too much neurotransmitter. It is possible that the neurotransmitter may not be released on cue or that, if it is released, the postsynaptic cells will not have the appropriate receptors. There also may be no mechanism for removal of the neurotransmitter from the synaptic cleft. These are only a few of the problems that can interfere with communication between neurons and between neurons and other effectors. As science learns more about the communication system of neurons, efforts to correct these problems will intensify. Already there are many drugs available that can alter activity at the synapse. Correcting these errors can lead to methods for the treatment of mental diseases.

Someday it may be possible to transplant healthy neurons from one person to another. This procedure may permit physicians to prevent total paralysis in a person who has suffered a broken neck or total loss of motor function in an individual who suffers from Parkinson's disease. In 1990, normal neurons were grown in tissue culture for the first time. Such scientific breakthroughs will lead to more and better treatments for individuals who suffer from diseases of the nervous system.

—Annette O'Connor, Ph.D.

See also Acupressure; Acupuncture; Alzheimer's disease; Amnesia; Amputation; Anesthesia; Anesthesiology; Aneurysmectomy; Aneurysms; Anxiety; Aphasia and dysphasia; Apnea; Aromatherapy; Ataxia; Autism; Balance disorders; Bell's palsy; Biofeedback; Brain; Brain disorders; Carpal tunnel syndrome; Cells; Cerebral palsy; Cluster headaches; Coma; Computed tomography (CT) scanning; Concussion; Craniotomy; Cysts; Dementias; Disk removal; Dizziness and fainting; Dyslexia; Ear infections and disorders; Ear surgery; Ears; Electrical shock; Electroencephalography (EEG); Encephalitis; Epilepsy; Fetal alcohol syndrome; Fetal tissue transplantation; Ganglion removal; Guillain-Barré syndrome; Hallucinations; Head and neck disorders; Headaches; Hearing loss; Hemiplegia; Hydrocephalus; Laminectomy and spinal fusion; Lead poisoning; Learning disabilities; Leprosy; Lower extremities; Lumbar puncture; Memory loss; Meningitis; Mental retardation; Migraine headaches; Motor neuron diseases; Motor skill development; Multiple sclerosis; Narcolepsy; Neuralgia, neuritis, and neuropathy; Neurofibromatosis; Neurology; Neurology, pediatric; Neurosurgery; Numbness and tingling; Paget's disease; Palsy; Paralysis; Paraplegia; Parkinson's disease; Physical rehabilitation; Poisoning; Poliomyelitis; Porphyria; Premenstrual syndrome (PMS); Quadriplegia; Rabies; Reflexes, primitive; Sciatica; Seizures; Sense organs; Shingles; Shock therapy; Skin; Sleep disorders; Snakebites; Spina bifida; Spinal cord disorders; Spine, vertebrae, and disks; Strokes; Sympathectomy; Systems and organs; Tetanus; Tics; Touch; Toxicology; Trembling and shaking; Unconsciousness; Upper extremities; Vagotomy.

FOR FURTHER INFORMATION:

Affifi, A. K., and R. A. Bergman. *Functional Neuroanatomy: Text and Atlas*. New York: McGraw-Hill, 1998. Written by a physician and an anatomist, this book is designed to be an integrated neuroscience textbook and atlas covering the regions of the central nervous system. The peripheral nervous system, however, is not covered.

Barondes, S. H. *Molecules and Mental Illness*. New York: W. H. Freeman, 1992. A well-written book that describes the chemistry and physiology of mental illness. Provides a good background for understanding the pathology of mental illness.

Bigner, Darell D., Roger W. McLendon, and Janet M. Bruner, eds. *Russell and Rubinstein's Pathology of Tumours of the Nervous System*. 6th ed. 2 vols. London: Arnold, 1998. This classic work of neuroscience has been completely redesigned from its previous edition. Collected together are the writings of thirty different authors, who approach neurooncology from a number of different perspectives.

Hanaway, J. *The Brain Atlas: A Visual Guide to the Human Central Nervous System*. Bethesda, Md.: Fitzgerald Science Press, 1998. This book provides an overview of modern neuroimaging. Particularly helpful is the display of magnetic resonance images and photographs of sections of fixed brain on facing pages.

McCance, Kathryn L., and Sue E. Huether. *Pathophysiology: The Biologic Basis for Disease in Adults and Children*. 2d ed. St. Louis: C. V. Mosby, 1994. This book, which was written for nurses, describes the physiologic basis of diseases. There is an extensive section on diseases of the nervous system.

Underwood, J. C. E., ed. *General and Systematic Pathology*. 2d ed. Edinburgh, Scotland: Churchill Livingstone, 1996. A well-developed pathology book written for students that contains illustrations and tables. Although some terms will be unfamiliar to the layperson, most of the material is presented in a straightforward manner.

NEURALGIA, NEURITIS, AND NEUROPATHY

DISEASE/DISORDER

ANATOMY OR SYSTEM AFFECTED: Nerves, nervous system, spine

SPECIALTIES AND RELATED FIELDS: Neurology

DEFINITION: Pathological conditions affecting the peripheral nerves of the body and interfering with the proper functioning of those nerves.

KEY TERMS:

autonomic neuropathy: a disorder involving the nerves that work independently of conscious control, and including those nerves that go to small blood vessels, sweat glands, the urinary bladder, the gastrointestinal tract, and the genital organs

axon: the portion of a neuron that carries electrical impulses away from the nerve cell body

mononeuropathy: a neuropathy involving only one peripheral nerve

nerve: a bundle of sensory and motor neurons held together by layers of connective tissue

neuralgia: pain associated with a nerve, often caused by inflammation or injury

neuritis: inflammation of a nerve

neuron: a nerve cell that is capable of conducting electrical impulses; several different types of neurons exist, including motor neurons, sensory neurons, and interneurons

neuropathy: a disorder that causes a functional disturbance of a peripheral nerve, brought about by any cause

peripheral nervous system: the portion of the nervous system found outside the brain and spinal cord

polyneuropathy: a disease that involves a disturbance in the function of several peripheral nerves

CAUSES AND SYMPTOMS

Peripheral nerves, those nerves found outside the brain and spinal cord, function to carry information between the central nervous system and the other portions of the body. These peripheral nerves consist of a bundle of nerve cells, also called neurons, which are wrapped in a protective sheath of connective tissue. A nerve consisting of neurons that only carry impulses toward the central nervous system is termed a sensory nerve. Nerves that contain only neurons that carry information from the central nervous system to the periphery of the body are called motor nerves, because they usually carry information telling a particular body part to move. Most nerves, however, consist of both sensory and motor neurons and are thus called mixed nerves.

The nerves of the peripheral nervous system can be divided into two different categories, cranial nerves and spinal nerves. Cranial nerves come directly out of the brain and supply information to and about the head and neck. There are twelve pairs of cranial nerves. Spinal nerves come directly out of the spinal cord and provide information to and from the arms, legs, chest, gut, and all other parts of the body not supplied by cranial nerves. In humans, there are usually thirty-one pairs of spinal nerves. Both cranial and spinal nerves can be affected by neuropathies.

Neurons (nerve cells) are highly specialized structures designed to convey information from one part of the body to another. This information is passed along in the form of electrical impulses. Neurons consist of three main parts: a cell body, which contains the nucleus and is the control center of the entire neuron; dendrites, which are slender, fingerlike extensions that convey electrical impulses toward the cell body; and an axon, which is a slender extension that carries electrical impulses away from the cell body.

Most of the dendrites and axons of peripheral nerves are covered with a white, fatty substance called myelin. Myelin acts to protect and insulate axons and dendrites. By insulating the axons and dendrites, myelin actually speeds up the rate at which an electrical impulse can be carried along these two structures. Damage to the myelin sheath surrounding axons and dendrites can greatly impair the function of a nerve.

Often, when a nerve becomes pinched, damaged, or inflamed, the result is excessive electrical stimulation of the nerve, which will be registered as pain. The pain associated with the damaged nerve is referred to as neuralgia. One of the most common forms of neuralgia occurs upon the striking of the "funny bone." This area around the elbow is the spot where the ulnar nerve is easily accessible. The ulnar nerve runs from just under the shoulder to the little finger, and when the ulnar nerve is struck near the elbow it is compressed or pinched, leading to pain or a tingling sensation from the elbow down to the little finger.

Compression of nerves for prolonged periods can also lead to neuralgia. The most common example of compression neuralgia is carpal tunnel syndrome. In this syndrome, the median nerve becomes compressed at the wrist, usually as a result of an inflammation of the tendon sheaths of the tendons located on either side of the median nerve. The swelling of these tendon sheaths causes the compression of the median nerve, which may initially lead to neuralgia. As this condition progresses, it can lead to a loss of feeling along the palm side of the thumb and the index and middle fingers. This condition is most common in people who use their fingers for rigorous work over prolonged periods of time, such as operators of computer terminals.

Sciatica is another common form of neuralgia, in which pain is associated with the sciatic nerve. The sciatic nerve is the longest nerve in the human body, running from the pelvis down the back of the thigh to the lower leg and then down to the soles of the feet. The symptoms of sciatica include sharp pains along the sciatic nerve. The pain may involve the buttocks, hip, back, posterior thigh, leg, ankle, and foot. Sciatica can result from many different causes, but the most common cause is from a ruptured intervertebral disk which puts pressure on, or causes a pinching of, the sciatic nerve.

Neuritis is defined as the inflammation of a nerve or of the connective tissue that surrounds the nerve. Many diseases can lead to the inflammation of peripheral nerves. Perhaps the most common disease leading to neuritis is shingles. Shingles are caused by the occurrence of herpes zoster, a virus that attacks the dorsal root ganglion, a place near the spinal cord that houses the cell bodies of neurons. A rash, swelling, and pain progress from the dorsal root ganglion along one or more spinal nerves. The rash along the course of the spinal nerves usually disappears within two or three days, but the pain along this path can persist for months.

Leprosy is another disease that leads to the inflammation of nerves. Leprosy is a bacterial disease caused by *Mycobacterium leprae*. These bacteria invade the cells that make up the myelin sheath that surrounds the nerve. The result is a noticeable swelling of the nerves affected, primarily those that are close to the skin. Many times, this swelling will lead to neuralgia and, if left untreated, to muscle wasting.

"Neuropathy" is a general term used to describe a decrease in the function of peripheral nerves which may be caused by many factors. The first signs of a neuropathy are usually a tingling, prickling, or burning sensation in some part of the body. This is followed by a sensory loss; the inability to perceive touch, heat, cold, or pressure; and a weakness in the muscles in the area affected. This weakness may eventually lead to a loss of muscle termed muscular atrophy. Neuropathies may affect sensory neurons, motor neurons, or both and can occur in both spinal and cranial nerves. A neuropathy may develop over a few days or many years. Neuropathies can be caused by a number of factors, including toxic exposure to solvents, pesticides, or heavy metals; viral illness; certain medications; metabolic disturbances such as diabetes mellitus; excessive use of alcohol; vitamin deficiency; loss of blood to the nerve; or cold exposure.

Neuropathies can be categorized based on the number of nerves that they affect, whether it is the myelin sheath surrounding the axon that is affected or the axon itself is destroyed, and the amount of time before symptoms of the neuropathy occur and progress. Thus, neuropathies are usually broken down into four different types: polyneuropathy, in which more than one nerve is affected; mononeuropathy, in which only one nerve is affected; axonal neuropathy, in which the axon is affected and degenerates; and demyelinating neuropathy, in which the myelin sheath surrounding the nerve is destroyed. Each of the four categories can be further subdivided based on the time frame in which the symptoms occur. Those neuropathies that appear over days are termed acute, those that appear over weeks are termed subacute, and those neuropathies whose symptoms slowly appear over months or years are termed chronic.

Another type of neuropathy is autonomic neuropathy, a condition which affects the nerves of the autonomic nervous system. These are the peripheral nerves that go to the sweat glands, small blood vessels, gastrointestinal tract, urinary bladder, and genital organs. These nerves are referred to as autonomic since they automatically provide information between these organs and the central nervous system without the individual's conscious effort. The symptoms associated with this form of neuropathy include loss of control over urination, difficulty swallowing food, occasional stomach upset, diarrhea, impotence, and excessive sweating.

The most common cause of neuropathies in the Western world is diabetes mellitus, while leprosy is the more common cause of neuropathies elsewhere. It is estimated that at least 70 percent of all diabetics have some degree of peripheral neuropathy. In most of these cases, the neuropathy is very slight and causes the patient no noticeable symptoms. In about 10 percent of those diabetics with a neuropathy, however, the symptoms will be serious.

Treatment and Therapy

Often, the first notable feature of a neuropathy that prompts a patient to seek medical attention is a tingling, prickling, or burning sensation in a particular area of the body. The occurrence of these sensations without any external stimuli is termed paresthesias. Since diabetes is the most common cause of neuropathy in the Western world, the sensations experienced by a diabetic patient can serve as an example of the symptoms that are associated with common neuropathies. These patients may first notice the above-mentioned symptoms in the balls of the feet or tips of the toes. As the neuropathy progresses, patients may lose feeling in their feet and experience a weakness in the muscles of the feet, leading to a difficulty in flexing the toes upward. This makes walking difficult, and many patients remark that they feel as if they are walking on stumps. This condition may lead to difficulties in maintaining balance. The neuropathy will begin to affect the legs above the ankles and then travel up the legs, eventually leading to atrophy of the leg muscles.

As the neuropathy worsens, it is critical that patients seek help because they can no longer feel pain. This situation is dangerous, as the patient may no longer sense the pain that can be caused by injuries from sharp objects or even a pebble in the shoe. If unnoticed, these injuries lead to ulcers that can easily become infected.

The first step in treating a neuropathy is to diagnose the type of neuropathy affecting the patient. A patient's medical history is taken to identify any recent viral or bacterial illness, any exposure to toxic substances such as pesticides or heavy metals, the patient's habits concerning alcohol use, or any other illness or injury that might have brought about a possible neuropathy. Next, a physical exam will be performed to determine if the patient's sensations regarding touch, pain, pressure, or temperature have been affected, as well as the ability of the patient to react to these stimuli. The physician may also feel the affected area to determine if the nerve or nerves are inflamed and enlarged.

If the patient's history and the physical examination point toward a neuropathy, further testing using electrodiagnostic tests will be performed. These tests measure the speed at which an electrical impulse travels down a nerve, which is called the nerve conduction velocity. Motor nerve conduction velocity is measured by stimulating the nerve with electrodes placed on the skin above the nerve. Stimulation of the nerve is typically done at two different sites. Using the arm as an example, one electrode would be placed on the inside of the arm at the elbow. The time that it takes for the impulse to reach a recording electrode on the thumb would be measured. A second site at the wrist would be tested to determine the time that it takes for the electrical impulse to reach the recording electrode on the thumb. The time that it took for the impulse to travel from the wrist to thumb would be subtracted from the amount of time that it took for the impulse to go from the inside of the arm at the elbow to the thumb. The resulting value would then be divided by the distance between the site at the wrist and the site at the elbow, giving a nerve conduction velocity value measured in meters per second.

The typical nerve conduction velocity for the motor and sensory peripheral nerves of adults is approximately 40 to 80 meters per second. If a neuropathy is the result of demyelination, the affected nerve will have a much slower nerve conduction velocity. If the neuropathy is a result of axonal damage, then the nerve conduction velocity is usually not altered from normal. Thus, electrodiagnostic testing helps to determine if the neuropathy is a demyelination neuropathy or an axonal neuropathy. Such a determination is important because the different neuropathies are caused by different diseases and are thus treated differently. Electrodiagnostic tests can also provide useful information regarding the site of the neuropathy and whether the neuropathy is affecting sensory neurons, motor neurons, or both.

The last diagnostic test to be performed, if other methods are inconclusive, is a biopsy of the affected nerve. This procedure involves the surgical removal of a portion of the afflicted nerve. The small sample of nerve will be placed under a microscope and examined for specific changes in the nerve. The nerve sample may also be subjected to various biochemical studies to determine if metabolic disturbances have occurred. Nerve biopsies are rarely performed, however, and are usually not recommended.

Once the type of neuropathy afflicting the patient has been determined, treatment can begin. Unlike axons in the central nervous system, axons in the peripheral nervous system are capable of regenerating under certain conditions. If the neuropathy is the result of exposure to toxic substances such as pesticides or heavy metals, removal of the patient from the exposure to such substances is the simple cure. If the neuropathy is the result of viral or bacterial infections, the treatment and recovery from these infections will also usually correct the neuropathy. The same principle applies to neuropathies caused by metabolic diseases and vitamin deficiencies: Corrections of these problems will lead to the correction of the neuropathy.

Should the neuropathy be of the mononeuropathy type and caused by trauma, anti-inflammatory drugs such as corticosteroids may be used or surgery may be performed to repair the nerve. If the mononeuropathy is caused by compression, as in carpal tunnel syndrome, surgery may also be needed to increase the space around the nerve and thus relieve the compression. Surgery is also used to remove tumors on the nerve that might be causing a neuropathy.

The time required to recover from a neuropathy is dependent on the severity and type of neuropathy. Recovery from demyelination is typically quicker than recovery from axonal neuropathies. If only the myelin surrounding the axon is damaged, and not the axon itself, the axon can quickly replace the damaged myelin. Demyelinating neuropathies usually require three to four weeks for recovery. In contrast, recovery from axonal neuropathies may take from two months to more than a year, depending on the severity of the neuropathy.

Perspective and Prospects

Perhaps the earliest documentation of peripheral neuropathies occurred during biblical times, when the term "leprosy" was coined. It is likely, however, that this term was employed rather loosely, as it was used to describe not only the disease leprosy but also a number of skin diseases not involving neuropathies, such as psoriasis.

The actual diagnosis of neuropathies and their subsequent categorization did not occur until the advent of electrical diagnostic testing. The earliest use of electricity to study nerve function occurred in 1876 when German neurologist Wilhelm Erb noted that the electrical stimulation of a damaged peripheral nerve below the site of injury resulted in muscular contraction. In contrast, electrical stimulation at a site above the injured nerve brought about no activity in the muscle. Erb concluded that the injury blocked the flow of electrical impulses down the nerve.

The actual use of electrical diagnostic testing did not take place until the late 1940's, when electrodes and an oscilloscope, an instrument that measures electrical activity, were used to measure the rate at which an electrical impulse could travel down a nerve. This discovery allowed the testing of nerve function and would become useful in the discrimination between axonal and demyelinating neuropathies. During this period, the invention of the electron microscope and the discovery of better nerve-staining techniques enhanced the ability of scientists to study the physiological and anatomical changes that occur in nerves with the onset of neuropathies.

Neuropathies received considerable attention in 1976 when approximately five hundred cases of the neuropathy called Guillain-Barré syndrome occurred in the United States following a national vaccination program for swine flu. The reason that the swine flu vaccine caused this neuropathy has never been discovered, but this syndrome often occurs after an upper-respiratory tract or gastrointestinal infection.

Those suffering from neuropathies that result from exposure to toxic substances, viral or bacterial infections, or metabolic diseases have a good prognosis of recovery if the underlying cause of the neuropathy is treated. The prognosis of recovery is not as good for those who suffer neuropathies as a result of hereditary diseases. Advances made in genetic research and continued research in gene therapy may someday greatly increase the prognosis of recovery for those suffering from hereditary neuropathies.

—*David K. Saunders, Ph.D.*

See also Brain disorders; Carpal tunnel syndrome; Cerebral palsy; Cluster headaches; Diabetes mellitus; Encephalitis; Epilepsy; Guillain-Barré syndrome; Hallucinations; Headaches; Hemiplegia; Lead poisoning; Leprosy; Meningitis; Migraine headaches; Motor neuron diseases; Multiple sclerosis; Nervous system; Neurology; Neurology, pediatric; Neurosurgery; Numbness and tingling; Pain; Palsy; Paralysis; Paraplegia; Parkinson's disease; Quadriplegia; Sciatica; Seizures; Shingles; Sympathectomy; Tics; Vagotomy.

FOR FURTHER INFORMATION:
Kandel, Eric R., James H. Schwartz, and Thomas M. Jessell. *Principles of Neural Science.* 4th ed. New York: Elsevier, 2000. Although this book is used in many college graduate courses, the discussion involving peripheral neuropathies should be understandable to the general reader. Provides examples of neuropathies, their syndromes, causes, diagnosis, and history.

Margolis, Simeon, and Hamilton Mosses III, eds. *The Johns Hopkins Medical Handbook: The One Hundred Major Medical Disorders of People over the Age of Fifty.* Rev. ed. Garden City, N.Y.: Random House, 1999. This book deals primarily with neuropathies associated with diabetes mellitus, discussing the symptoms and dangers of neuropathies in diabetic patients.

Marieb, Elaine N. *Essentials of Human Anatomy and Physiology.* 6th ed. Redwood City, Calif.: Benjamin/Cummings, 2000. An excellent book to begin the study of the peripheral nervous system. This text is easy to understand, as it uses little technical jargon and explains the jargon that it does use. Provides good descriptions and drawings of most parts of the peripheral nervous system.

NEUROFIBROMATOSIS
DISEASE/DISORDER

ANATOMY OR SYSTEM AFFECTED: Bones, nervous system, skin

SPECIALTIES AND RELATED FIELDS: Dermatology, genetics, neurology, orthopedics, plastic surgery

DEFINITION: A genetic disease affecting the nervous system, skin, and bones that produces multiple nerve tumors (neurofibromas), deeply pigmented areas of skin (café-au-lait spots), and bone deformities.

CAUSES AND SYMPTOMS

Most infants born with neurofibromatosis, which is also known as Von Recklinghausen disease, have few symptoms until puberty. Disease progression and signs and symptoms vary from mild (in about one-third of affected children) to moderate and severe disfigurement and organ failure. The disease causes abnormal growths of nerve tissue along the peripheral nerve tracts of the head, neck, trunk, and extremities, usually involving the brain and spinal cord (the central nervous system) later. These so-called neurofibromas appear as multiple, visible growths lying beneath the skin. Also typical are the many areas of deeply pigmented skin, known as café-au-lait (coffee-and-milk) spots. In addition, severely disfiguring bone defects of the skull and spine can be caused by neurofibromas.

Some patients lead nearly normal lives, with only cosmetic problems from the café-au-lait spots and visible neurofibromas. Most patients, however, experience serious consequences from deep growths and skeletal deformities. Depending on the size and location of these tumors, they can cause blindness, deafness, mental retardation, seizures, pain, and paralysis. Other organs, especially the kidneys and glands, are frequently damaged as well. The most feared complication is the transformation of these benign tumors into cancerous ones.

TREATMENT AND THERAPY

No cure exists for neurofibromatosis. Supportive therapy includes surgical removal of the neurofibromas and reconstructive plastic surgery for the sometimes severe disfigurement that can result from deep tumors and bone deformities. The skull, spine, and eye sockets are particularly affected. Social isolation and embarrassment are serious problems with neurofibromatosis, and counseling is essential. The prognosis is variable depending on the size and location of the tumors. Both cancer and organ failure can shorten the patient's life.

Because neurofibromatosis is genetic, occurring in one in three thousand births, genetic analysis of the parents is essential if there is a family history of the disease. Prenatal testing can determine if the fetus has inherited the defect. Research is now focusing on correcting the genetic error in the developing fetus.

—*Connie Rizzo, M.D.*

See also Bone disorders; Bones and the skeleton; Dermatology; Dermatopathology; Genetic diseases; Genetics and inheritance; Nervous system; Neuralgia, neuritis, and neuropathy; Neurology; Neurology, pediatric; Skin; Skin cancer; Skin disorders; Skin lesion removal; Tumor removal; Tumors.

FOR FURTHER INFORMATION:

Adams, Raymond D., Maurice Victor, and Allan H. Ropper. *Adams and Victor's Principles of Neurology.* 7th ed. New York: McGraw-Hill, 2000.

Gaudin, Anthony J., and Kenneth C. Jones. *Human Anatomy and Physiology.* New York: Harcourt Brace Jovanovich, 1989.

Nicholls, John G., A. Robert Martin, and Bruce G. Wallace. *From Neuron to Brain.* 4th ed. Sunderland, Mass.: Sinauer Associates, 2000.

NEUROLOGY

SPECIALTY

ANATOMY OR SYSTEM AFFECTED: Brain, ears, hands, head, muscles, musculoskeletal system, nerves, nervous system, psychic-emotional system, spine

SPECIALTIES AND RELATED FIELDS: Audiology, endocrinology, genetics, physical therapy

DEFINITION: The study of the structure and function of the nervous system.

KEY TERMS:

axon: the cellular extension of the neuron that conducts electrical information, transmitting it to the dendrite of the next neuron through the synaptic gap between them

cellular automaton: a self-reproducing entity and mathematical model for complex systems, including animal nervous systems

dendrite: the extension of the neuron that receives electrical information from neurotransmitters moving across the synaptic gap from the axon of a preceding neuron

neuroglial cell: a supportive cell for neurons within the central nervous system of animals

neuron: the principal nervous system cell that conducts electrical information from its dendritic extensions, through its cell body, to its axonic extensions, and on to other cells

neurotransmitter: a chemical messenger or hormone which relays electrical information across a synapse from the axon of one neuron to the dendrite of another neuron

plasticity: a phenomenon of many animal nervous systems, particularly those in higher vertebrates, in which central nervous system neurons grow in patterns based upon input information

Schwann cell: a supportive cell for neurons in the peripheral nervous systems of vertebrate animals that wraps around and insulates axons using the protein myelin

synapse: the gap between the transmitting axon of one neuron and the receiving dendrite of another neuron

von Neumann machine: a cellular automaton or machine which can think and self-replicate; based on the attempts of the physicist John von Neumann to duplicate the human nervous system in computers

THE PHYSIOLOGY OF THE NERVOUS SYSTEM

Neurology is the study of the nervous system, an intricate arrangement of electrically conducting nerve cells that permeate the entire animal body. Nervous tissue, which represents a principal means of cell-to-cell communication within animals, is one of four principal adult tissues found within the organs of most animals. The remaining three adult tissues—epithelia, connective tissue, and muscle—rely heavily on nervous tissue for their proper functioning, particularly muscle tissue.

Nervous tissue is a primary characteristic of most animal species, the exceptions including thousands of species of the animal phyla Porifera (sponges) and Coelenterata (consisting of hydra, sea anemones, and jellyfish). Nervous tissue is a prominent tissue in every other major animal phylum, including the primitive platyhelminths (flatworms) and nematodes (roundworms).

Evolutionarily, nerve tissue arose from cells that primarily were endocrine in origin. Endocrine cells are hormone producers that secrete hormones for distribution through the organism via the organism's bodily fluids and circulatory systems. Hormones and closely related chemical messengers called neurotransmitters are molecules that are produced in one part of the organism (such as by an endocrine cell or gland), travel through the organism, and target cells in another part of the organism. Hormones or neurotransmitters usually are composed of proteins (long chains of amino acids, or polypeptides) or of fats such as steroids. These chemical messengers affect gene expression within their target cells. Hormones and neurotransmitters determine whether genes are active or inactive. In active genes, the deoxyribonucleic acid (DNA) of the gene encodes messenger ribonucleic acid (mRNA), which encodes protein. An inactive gene does not encode protein. All events within the target cell are influenced by the presence or absence of gene-encoded proteins.

Hormones are effective cell-to-cell communicative and control molecules within all organisms, including animals. In animals, however, hormones and neurotransmitters have become elaborated as parts of extensive nervous systems. The nervous systems of animals have developed according to the evolution of a specialized nervous cell type called a neuron.

The neuron, a specialized, electrically conducting cell, is the basic unit of the nervous system. A neuron is unlike many other cells because it can assume diverse shapes and can assume (relatively) great lengths, sometimes spanning many centimeters. A neuron consists of a cell body containing a nucleus, where the genetic information resides, and numerous organelles, including the energy-producing mitochondria and protein-synthesizing ribosomes. There may be a few or many cellular extensions of its cytoplasm and membrane that twist the neuron into a very distorted appearance. The two principal types of extensions are axons and dendrites.

A dendrite is an electrically receiving extension of a neuron; it receives electrical information from another neuron. An axon is an electrically transmitting extension of a neuron; it transmits electrical information to another neuron. An axon of one neuron transmits electrical information to the dendrite of another neuron. Yet the two neurons are not in direct contact; the axon does not touch the dendrite. A gap called a synapse separates the axon from the receiving dendrite.

Electrical information crosses the synapse via a special type of hormone called a neurotransmitter, a protein encoded by the genes and synthesized by the ribosomes of the neuron. Electrical information traveling along the axon of a neuron triggers the release of a specified quantity of neurotransmitter proteins at the synapse. The neurotransmitters diffuse across the synapse where, upon making contact with the dendritic membrane of the next neuron, they depolarize the dendrite and allow the electrical information transmission to continue unabated.

Actual electrical conduction in a neuron involves membrane depolarization and the influx of sodium ions and the efflux of potassium ions. Electrical conduction along a neuronal segment involves the depolarization of the membrane with the movement of sodium cations into the neuron. Electrical conduction for a particular neuronal segment ends with repolarization of the neuronal membrane as potassium cations move across the neuronal membrane and out of the neuron. The passing electrical action potential, which is measured in millivolts, involves simultaneous depolarization and repolarization in successive regions of the neuron. The initial depolarization is triggered by neurotransmitters contacting the dendritic membrane. Sodium and potassium ion pumps continue the successive stages of depolarization and repolarization along the dendrites, cell body, and axons of the neuron until neurotransmitters are released from a terminal axon across a synaptic gap to depolarize the membrane of the next neuron.

Within animal nervous systems, neurons are very plastic: They grow in specified patterns, much like crystals, in response to stimuli and contacts with other neurons. A neuron may have one or many axonic and dendritic extensions. A neuron with one dendrite and one axon is termed bipolar. A neuron with many dendrites and many axons is termed multipolar; such a neuron makes many contacts with other neurons for the transmission of electrical information along many different neural pathways.

Animal nervous systems usually consist of centralized, concentrated neurons that form the center of nervous control, called the central nervous system. In vertebrate animals, the central nervous system consists of the billions of neurons composing the brain and spinal cord. Additionally, peripheral neurons extend throughout the animal body, permeating virtually every cell and tissue region and thus forming the peripheral nervous system, composed of billions of dispersed neurons.

Functionally, neurons are of three principal types: sensory, motor, and internuncial neurons. Sensory neurons detect stimuli and transmit the electrical information from the stimulus toward the central nervous system. The sensory neurons are arranged one after another, transmitting the electrical action potential from axon to neurotransmitter to dendrite, and so on. The central nervous system processes this information, usually utilizing an intricate array of connected internuncial neurons and specialized neuronal regions devoted to specific bodily functions. Once the central nervous system has processed a response to the stimulus, the response is effected by motor neurons, which transmit electrical information back to the body. Motor neurons will transmit electrical information between each other in the same fashion as sensory neurons. The motor neurons, however, often will terminate at some effector tissue, usually a muscle. Neurotransmitters released from the last motor neuron will depolarize the muscle membranes and trigger the biochemical and physical contraction of muscle. The muscle responds to the stimulus.

The primary purpose of nervous systems in ani-

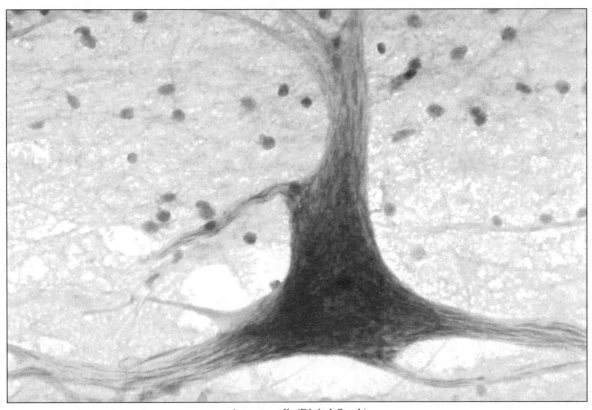

A nerve cell. (Digital Stock)

mals is to respond to stimuli, both internal and external. Sensory neurons detect stimuli and direct this information to the central nervous system, where internuncial neurons process the information to appropriate decision centers, which direct a response along a chain of motor neurons to a muscle or muscles that physically respond to the initial stimulus. This chain of nervous communication is called a reflex arc. Virtually every activity in the body requires reflex arcs involving central and peripheral nervous system sensory, internuncial, and motor neurons.

The neurons of vertebrate animal nervous systems are very plastic and make trillions of neuron-to-neuron interconnections for the accurate processing of information, the reception of stimuli information, and the direction of response information along reflex arcs. Within the central and peripheral nervous systems of the human body, millions of information transfer processes occur by reflex arcs every second along trillions of neuronal interconnections. The number of such electrical information transfers that must occur accurately every moment within the body is staggering, yet the human nervous system accomplishes these amazingly intricate tasks with ease. No supercomputer yet devised even comes close to the complexity and efficiency of the vertebrate animal nervous system.

SCIENCE AND PROFESSION

Neurologists attempt to understand the structure of the nervous system, including the functioning of the neuron, neuronal plasticity, supporting nerve cells (neuroglia and Schwann cells), neurotransmitters, neuronal patterning in learning, how vision and hearing occur, nerve disorders, and the embryological development of the nervous system.

Neurons are among the most flexibly specialized cells in animal tissues. Animal nerve tissue is derived from embryonic ectodermal tissue. The ectoderm is a tissue layer of cells formed very early in animal development. Very early in development following conception, all animals undergo a blastula stage, in which the embryo is a hollow sphere of roughly five hundred cells. A region of the blastula called the blastopore folds to form a channel of cells through the blastula, thus initiating the gastrula stage.

The gastrula has three embryonic tissues: ectoderm, mesoderm, and endoderm. The ectoderm and endoderm continue to divide and differentiate into epithelial cells. Mesodermal cells multiply and differentiate

into muscle and connective tissue cells. Dorsal ectodermal cells (cells that will become the back side of the organism) fold inward to form a nerve cord. The neurons of this nerve cord multiply and differentiate into central and peripheral nervous tissue.

In humans, the dorsal nerve cord becomes the billions of centralized neurons composing the spinal cord. The neurons in the anterior region of the spinal cord will fold, multiply, and differentiate into the various brain regions. The complete, fully functional human brain has approximately one hundred billion neurons that grow plastically and form trillions of interconnections for the accurate processing of electrical information.

The embryonic brain consists of three principal enfolded regions: the prosencephalon (forebrain), the mesencephalon (midbrain), and the rhombencephalon (hindbrain). Each of these three embryonic regions folds and differentiates further. The prosencephalon neurons multiply and differentiate to become the cerebrum, thalamus, and hypothalamus. The mesencephalon region becomes the corpora quadrigemina and cerebral peduncles, areas that connect other brain regions and coordinate sensory and motor impulses for basic reflexes. The rhombencephalon becomes the cerebellum, pons, and medulla oblongata; these are brain regions that control basic bodily processes such as coordination, prediction of movements, and maintenance of heart rate and respiration.

Furthermore, special regions of brain tissue develop into external sensory apparatuses: eyes for vision, ears for hearing and balance, nasal and tongue chemoreceptors for smell and taste. Millions of sensory neurons flow from these special sense organs to highly complicated brain regions that analyze, interpret, learn from, and react to these sensory stimuli. Neurophysiologists attempt to decipher the mechanisms by which the brain processes information. For example, the hundreds of thousands of retinal neurons in the eye collect light images reflected from objects, convert these diverse stimuli into thousands of bits of electrical information, and combine this information along an optic nerve. The optic nerve then transmits the electrical information of vision to the posterior occipital region of the cerebrum within the brain, where millions of visual processing neurons position the inverted, reversed visual image and interpret it.

How the brain neurons process such information is poorly understood and is the subject of intense study. While neurophysiologists have a fairly good understanding of nervous system structure, nervous system function represents a tremendous challenge to investigating scientists.

Structurally, neurons are supported by nerve cells called neuroglia in the central nervous system and Schwann cells in the peripheral nervous system. Neuroglia include four cell types: astrocytes, ependyma, microglia, and oligodendrocytes. Astrocytes stabilize neurons, ependyma allow cerebrospinal fluid exchange between brain ventricles and neurons, microglia clean up dead and foreign tissue, and oligodendrocytes insulate neurons by wrapping around them and secreting an electrically insulating protein called myelin. In the peripheral nervous system, Schwann cells behave much like oligodendrocytes; they wrap around axons and electrically insulate the axons with myelin for the efficient conduction of electrical information.

Specific neurological research is focused on neuronal plasticity in learning, the effects of various neurotransmitters upon neural activity, and diseases of the central nervous system. Various models of neuronal plasticity have been proposed to explain how learning occurs in higher vertebrates, including humans and other mammals. Most of these neuronal processing models involve the spatial patterning of neural bundles, which orient information in space and time. The plastic growth of these neurons in specified directions and locking patterns contributes to memory, learning, and intelligence in higher mammals such as primates (which include humans and chimpanzees) and cetaceans (dolphins and whales).

Neurotransmission can be affected by a variety of physical states and chemical influences. The extensive use and misuse of pharmaceuticals and drugs can have serious effects upon the nervous system. Furthermore, developmental errors of the nervous system and aging can contribute to various diseases and disorders.

PERSPECTIVE AND PROSPECTS

The nervous system of humans and higher vertebrate animals presents a tremendous variety of exciting research possibilities. The brain, the seat of human consciousness, represents a mystery to scientists even with the intense scientific scrutiny devoted to this organ. The brain is studied to understand how humans learn and how they might accelerate this exceptional ability. The intricate connections between billions of very plastic cerebral cortical neurons enable millions of electrical information impulses to direct millions of simultaneous activities every second. Brain structure, neural pathways, and techniques of learning and cognition are studied indirectly in human subjects and more directly in other intelligent mammals such as chimpanzees, gorillas, dolphins, and whales. These studies include analyses of the senses as well as poorly understood extrasensory perceptions that no doubt are linked to exceptional nervous system activity.

Researchers in the field of artificial intelligence attempt to generate cellular automatons, machines that can think and self-replicate. Artificial intelligence research began with the work of the brilliant physicist and computer pioneer John von Neumann, who attempted to mimic the human nervous system within computer systems—systems that have been called von Neumann machines. Yet no true thinking machines have been developed. The best supercomputers yet devised by humans may process data far more rapidly than the human brain, but they are no match for the human brain's capacity to process millions of data items simultaneously.

While the basic physical and chemical mechanisms of neuronal function have been deciphered by neurological scientists, research into neurotransmission across synaptic gaps continues. One principal neurotransmitter at muscular junctions is acetylcholine, which triggers muscle contractions following a motor neural impulse. When acetylcholine is not needed, it is destroyed by a molecule called acetylcholinesterase. Two types of molecular poisons can affect neuromuscular activity: acetylcholine inhibitors, which compete with acetylcholine; and antiacetylcholinesterases, which inhibit acetylcholinesterase and, therefore, accelerate acetylcholine activity. Acetylcholine competitors (such as atropine, nicotine, caffeine, morphine, cocaine, and valium) block acetylcholine at neuromuscular junctions, thereby stopping muscular contractions and producing flaccid paralysis; death can result if the heart or respiratory muscles are affected. Antiacetylcholinesterases, such as the pesticides sevin and malathion, leave acetylcholine free to contract muscles endlessly, thereby causing convulsions.

Neurology also is devoted to understanding the biochemical and genetic basis for various neurological disorders, including Alzheimer's disease, parkinsonism, seizures, abnormal brain wave patterns, paralysis, and coma. Neurological research also is concerned with the nature of pain, the sense organs, and viral diseases of the nervous system, such as meningitis, encephalitis, herpes simplex virus 2, and shingles. The complexity of the human nervous system has inspired an enormous variety and quantity of research.

—*David Wason Hollar, Jr., Ph.D.*

See also Alzheimer's disease; Amnesia; Anesthesia; Anesthesiology; Aneurysmectomy; Aneurysms; Aphasia and dysphasia; Apnea; Ataxia; Attention-deficit disorder (ADD); Audiology; Balance disorders; Bell's palsy; Biofeedback; Biophysics; Brain; Brain disorders; Carpal tunnel syndrome; Cerebral palsy; Cluster headaches; Concussion; Craniotomy; Creutzfeldt-Jakob disease and mad cow disease; Critical care; Critical care, pediatric; Cysts; Dementias; Disk removal; Dizziness and fainting; Dyslexia; Ear infections and disorders; Ear surgery; Ears; Electrical shock; Electroencephalography (EEG); Emergency medicine; Encephalitis; Epilepsy; Fetal tissue transplantation; Ganglion removal; Grafts and grafting; Guillain-Barré syndrome; Hallucinations; Head and neck disorders; Headaches; Hearing loss; Hemiplegia; Laminectomy and spinal fusion; Learning disabilities; Lower extremities; Lumbar puncture; Memory loss; Ménière's disease; Meningitis; Migraine headaches; Motor neuron diseases; Motor skill development; Multiple sclerosis; Narcolepsy; Nervous system; Neuralgia, neuritis, and neuropathy; Neurofibromatosis; Neurology, pediatric; Neurosurgery; Numbness and tingling; Otorhinolaryngology; Palsy; Paralysis; Paraplegia; Parkinson's disease; Physical examination; Poliomyelitis; Porphyria; Prion diseases; Psychiatry; Psychiatry, child and adolescent; Psychiatry, geriatric; Quadriplegia; Rabies; Reflexes, primitive; Sciatica; Seizures; Sense organs; Shock therapy; Skin; Sleep disorders; Smell; Snakebites; Spina bifida; Spinal cord disorders; Spine, vertebrae, and disks; Strokes; Sympathectomy; Taste; Tay-Sachs disease; Tetanus; Tics; Touch; Trembling and shaking; Unconsciousness; Upper extremities; Vagotomy.

For Further Information:

Alberts, Bruce, et al. *Molecular Biology of the Cell.* 3d ed. New York: Garland, 1994. Leading molecular biologists have collaborated to produce this valuable textbook describing the genetics, biochemistry, and developmental biology of eukaryotic cells. Chapter 18, "The Nervous System," is extensively detailed.

Chiras, Daniel D. *Biology: The Web of Life.* St. Paul, Minn.: West, 1993. Chiras's outstanding biology textbook is an excellent introduction to the subject. Chapter 17, "The Nervous System: Integration, Co-ordination, and Control," is an excellent presentation of neurons, the brain, and the senses for the beginning biology student.

Lilly, John C. *Programming and Metaprogramming in the Human Biocomputer.* Rev. 4th ed. New York: Julian Press, 2000. Lilly, a controversial and pioneering neurophysiologist, presents the results of a five-year study of the effects of LSD on cognitive abilities in humans and dolphins in this work.

Nicholls, John G., A. Robert Martin, and Bruce G. Wallace. *From Neuron to Brain.* 4th ed. Sunderland, Mass.: Sinauer Associates, 2000. In this comprehensive work, three leading neurophysiologists describe contemporary knowledge of the neuron: its structure, its function, and its roles in the central and peripheral nervous systems.

Rich, Elaine, and Kevin Knight. *Artificial Intelligence.* 2d ed. New York: McGraw-Hill, 1991. Rich and Knight have assembled a fascinating textbook in which the major ideas of artificial intelligence are presented. They discuss major models for intelligent automata, parallel reasoning, knowledge representation techniques, and neural networks.

Snyder, Solomon H. "The Molecular Basis of Communication Between Cells." *Scientific American* 253, no. 4 (October, 1985): 132-141. In this scientific survey article, Snyder describes the structures and functions of neurotransmitters and related hormones. This article is one of several in a *Scientific American* edition devoted to "The Molecules of Life."

Neurology, pediatric
Specialty

Anatomy or system affected: Brain, ears, hands, head, muscles, musculoskeletal system, nerves, nervous system, psychic-emotional system, spine

Specialties and related fields: Audiology, endocrinology, genetics, neonatology, pediatrics, perinatology, physical therapy

Definition: The treatment of nervous system disorders in infants and children.

Key terms:

autonomic nervous system: the body system that regulates involuntary vital functions and is divided into sympathetic and parasympathetic divisions

brain stem: the medulla oblongata, pons, and mesencephalon portions of the brain, which perform motor, sensory, and reflex functions and contain the corticospinal and reticulospinal tracts

cerebrum: the largest and uppermost section of the brain that integrates memory, speech, writing, and emotional response

lesion: a visible local tissue abnormality such as a wound, sore, rash, or boil, which can be benign, cancerous, gross, occult, or primary

neurologic: dealing with the nervous system and its disorders

paralysis: the loss of muscle function or sensation as a result of trauma or disease

pediatric: pertaining to neonates, infants, and children up to the age of twelve

SCIENCE AND PROFESSION

Neurologic illness and injury are principal causes of chronic disability when they occur in children because they result in the development of abnormal motor and mental behaviors and/or in the loss of previously existing capabilities, with a common problem in children being musculoskeletal dysfunction. Pediatric neurology involves the ongoing assessment of an infant's or child's neurologic function, which requires the pediatric neurologist to identify problems; set goals; use appropriate interventions, including physical therapy, teaching, and counseling; and evaluate the outcome of treatment.

The pediatric neurologist looks for certain positive or negative signs of dysfunction in the nervous system. Positive signs of neurologic dysfunction include the presence of sensory deficits; pain; involuntary motor events such as tremor, chorea, or convulsions; the display of bizarre behavior or mental confusion; and muscle weakness and difficulty controlling movement. Negative signs are those which represent the loss of function, such as paralysis, imperception of external stimuli, lack of speaking ability, and/or loss of consciousness.

The major manifestations of neurologic disease include disorders of motility, such as motor paralysis, abnormalities of movement and posture caused by extrapyramidal motor system dysfunction, cerebellum dysfunction, tremor, myoclonus, spasms, tics, and disorders of stance and gait; pain and other disorders of somatic sensation, headache, and backache, such as general pain and localized pain in the craniofacial area, back, neck, and extremities; disorders of the special senses, such as smell, taste, hearing, vision, ocular movement, and pupillary function, as well as dizziness and equilibrium disorders; epilepsy and disorders of consciousness, such as seizures and related

disorders, coma and related disorders, syncope, and sleep abnormalities; derangements of intellect, behavior, and language as a result of diffuse and focal cerebral disease (such as delirium and other confusional states, dementia, and Korsakoff's syndrome), lesions in the cerebrum, and disorders of speech and language; and anxiety and disorders of energy, mood, emotion, and autonomic and endocrine functions, such as lassitude and fatigue, nervousness, irritability, anxiety, depression, disorders of the limbic lobes and autonomic nervous system, and hypothalamus and neuroendocrine dysfunction.

DIAGNOSTIC AND TREATMENT TECHNIQUES

The pediatric neurologist begins with a medical history of the infant or child to determine if the problem is congenital or acquired, chronic or episodic, and static or progressive. The focus of the pediatric neurologist in taking the patient's history is on genetic disorders, the medical history of family members, and perinatal events, with an emphasis on the mother's health, nutrition, medications, and tobacco, alcohol, or drug use during pregnancy. Considerable information about a child's or infant's behavior or neuromuscular function can be obtained by observation of the child's alertness and curiosity, trust or apprehension, facial and eye movements, limb function, and body posture and balance during simple motor activities. If possible, the pediatric neurologist will ask the child about instances of weakness, numbness, headaches, pain, tremors, nervousness, irritability, drowsiness, loss of memory, confusion, hallucinations, and loss of consciousness. Headaches, abdominal pain, or reluctance to attend school are often associated with neurologic disturbances, with contributing factors including subtle mental retardation, specific learning disabilities, and depression. Disorders of movement include tics, developmental clumsiness, ataxia, chorea, myoclonus, or dystonia.

A complete neurologic examination includes an evaluation of mental status, craniospinal inspection, cranial nerve testing, sensory testing, musculature evaluation, an assessment of coordination, and autonomic function testing. Mental status evaluation involves the assessment of orientation, memory, intellect, judgment, and affect. Craniospinal inspection includes the palpation, percussion, and auscultation of the cranium and spine. Cranial nerve testing assesses the motor and sensory function of the head and neck. Sensory testing measures peripheral sensations, including responses to pinprick, light touch, vibration, and fine movement of the joints. In musculature evaluation, weakness is associated with altered tendon reflexes, indicating lower motor neuron lesions, whereas exaggerated tendon reflexes are associated with an extensor response of the big toe following plantar stimulation (Babinski's sign). In coordination assessment, smooth fine and gross motor movements demand integrated function of the pyramidal and extrapyramidal systems, whereas hyperreflexia, increased muscle stiffness, and problems with muscle coordination reflect spasticity. The evaluation of autonomic function involves bowel and bladder function, emotional state, and symmetry of reflex activity, particularly resting muscle tone and positioning of the head. Additional diagnostic aids include lumbar puncture (spinal tap), complete blood count (CBC), myelography, electroencephalography (EEG), and computed tomography (CT) scanning.

PERSPECTIVE AND PROSPECTS

Pediatric neurologists have been greatly assisted in their recognition of neurologic disease in infants and children by recently developed brain-imaging techniques, such as CT scanning and magnetic resonance imaging (MRI). Event-mediated evoked potentials are also used to assess the conduction and processing of information within specific sensory pathways. These advances have enabled an accurate evaluation of the integrity of the visual, auditory, and somatosensory pathways and the uncovering of single and multiple lesions within the brain stem and cerebrum. Particularly noteworthy are CT scanning and sonographic detection of clinically silent intracranial hemorrhages in premature infants.

Recent success in assisting premature infants has produced a population of patients at risk for developing cerebral palsy, mental retardation, epilepsy, and various learning disorders. The recent higher incidence of neurologic disease in the pediatric age group probably results from the increased ability of medical science to detect nervous system disturbances and from the increased survival rate of premature infants. Neurologic patients are compromised in nearly every aspect of living and have a high incidence of psychiatric problems, and their recovery is often slow and unpredictable. Because medical advances have resulted in an increased survival rate following serious neurological insult, more individuals are in need of long-term rehabilitation. The financial cost associated with this care presents an ongoing challenge to health care systems and to researchers examining effective means to restore function.

—Daniel G. Graetzer, Ph.D.,
and Charles T. Leonard, Ph.D., P.T.

See also Amnesia; Anesthesia; Anesthesiology; Aphasia and dysphasia; Apnea; Ataxia; Attention-deficit disorder (ADD); Audiology; Biofeedback; Biophysics; Brain; Brain disorders; Carpal tunnel syndrome; Cerebral palsy; Cluster headaches; Concussion; Craniotomy; Creutzfeldt-Jakob disease and mad cow disease; Critical care, pediatric; Dizziness and fainting; Dyslexia; Ear infections and disorders; Ear surgery; Ears; Electrical shock; Electroencephalography (EEG); Emergency medicine; Encephalitis; Epilepsy; Ganglion removal; Grafts and grafting; Guillain-Barré syndrome; Hallucinations; Head and neck disorders; Headaches; Hearing loss; Laminectomy and spinal fusion; Learning disabilities; Lower extremities; Lumbar puncture; Memory loss; Ménière's disease; Meningitis; Migraine headaches; Motor neuron diseases; Motor skill development; Multiple sclerosis; Narcolepsy; Nervous system; Neuralgia, neuritis, and neuropathy; Neurofibromatosis; Neurology; Neurosurgery; Numbness and tingling; Otorhinolaryngology; Palsy; Paralysis; Paraplegia; Pediatrics; Physical examination; Poliomyelitis; Porphyria; Prion diseases; Psychiatry, child and adolescent; Quadriplegia; Rabies; Reflexes, primitive; Seizures; Sense organs; Skin; Sleep disorders; Smell; Snakebites; Spina bifida; Spinal cord disorders; Spine, vertebrae, and disks; Sympathectomy; Taste; Tay-Sachs disease; Tetanus; Tics; Touch; Trembling and shaking; Unconsciousness; Upper extremities.

FOR FURTHER INFORMATION:

Adams, Raymond D., Maurice Victor, and Allan H. Ropper. *Adams and Victor's Principles of Neurology.* 7th ed. New York: McGraw-Hill, 2000. This classic "teaching text" in neurology is completely revised and features a new art program and the latest advances in diagnosis and treatment. Includes new coverage of papillary function, sleep, syncope, inherited metabolic disease, degenerative disease, epilepsy, and cerebellar disease.

Behrman, Richard E., ed. *Nelson Textbook of Pediatrics.* 16th ed. Philadelphia: W. B. Saunders, 2000. This standard pediatric textbook has been around for years and deservedly so. Minimal medical jargon makes it readable by laypersons.

Fenichel, G. M. *Clinical Pediatric Neurology.* 4th ed. Philadelphia: W. B. Saunders, 2001. Thoroughly revised and updated. The main neurological disorders of childhood are uniquely organized by presenting signs, which offers a practical approach to diagnosis and management.

Kempe, C. H., et al., eds. *Current Pediatric Diagnosis and Treatment.* 9th ed. Los Altos, Calif.: Appleton & Lange, 1987. This softcover textbook is one in a series of publications, each covering a different medical science. All are well respected for clear, well-organized reviews. The chapters cover the gamut of pediatrics; three chapters are devoted to the newborn and to genetic and congenital diseases.

Volpe, J. J. *Neurology of the Newborn.* 4th ed. Philadelphia: W. B. Saunders, 2000. New edition of a scholarly, thorough, single-author reference for pediatricians, obstetricians, or neurologists on diagnosis and treatment of neurological disorders in the newborn. Well-referenced and illustrated.

NEUROSIS

DISEASE/DISORDER

ANATOMY OR SYSTEM AFFECTED: Psychic-emotional system

SPECIALTIES AND RELATED FIELDS: Psychiatry, psychology

DEFINITION: A chronic mental disorder characterized by distressing and unacceptable anxiety.

CAUSES AND SYMPTOMS

A neurosis is experienced at a level of severity that is less than psychotic but significant enough to impair a person's functioning. The term "neurosis" includes nine psychological states: hysteria, obsessions and compulsions, phobias, some depressions, some traumatic reactions, addictions, psychosomatic disorders, some sexual disorders, and anxiety. A person tends to continue suffering from one of the recurrent and continuing reactions noted above, if not treated for the neurosis.

Hysteria features somatic symptoms resembling those of a physical disease without actual physical illness (for example, a headache without organic cause). Phobias are abnormal fears that arise because an inner fear is displaced onto an object or situation outside the individual (for example, impotence to deal with fear of intimacy). Obsessions (recurrent thoughts) and compulsions (repetitively performed behaviors) bear little relation to the person's needs and are expe-

rienced by the person as foreign or intrusive (for example, repeated hand washing). Depression is a mood of sadness, unhappiness, hopelessness, loss of interest, difficulty concentrating, and lack of a sense of self-worth. Addictions are the use of substances or self-defeating behaviors to fulfill one's need for love instead of loving self or another person (for example, addiction to gambling). Psychosomatic disorders are organic illnesses caused by psychological distress (for example, peptic ulcer). Sexual disorders are the avoidance of developing adult sexual competency by immature sexual behavior (for example, exhibitionism). Traumatic reactions in the past delay or impair normal development in the present (for example, childhood sexual abuse leads to difficulty with intimacy as an adult). Anxiety is experienced as a generalized anxious affect which is pervasive and without a known cause (for example, a person chronically worrying that "something bad will happen").

TREATMENT AND THERAPY

All the forms of neuroses listed above need treatment to be resolved. All have the potential to become borderline or overtly psychotic disorders under stress. Treatment involves entering psychotherapy to understand better and therefore manage neurotic symptoms. It often can require the use of psychoactive medications for the treatment of anxieties, depressions, obsessions, and addictions. Treatment can be received from family physicians and general internists at the first level of intervention. Patients refer to psychiatrists, psychologists, social workers, and substance counselors for more advanced interventions.

PERSPECTIVE AND PROSPECTS

Sigmund Freud (1856-1939), Alfred Adler (1870-1937), Carl Jung (1875-1961), and Karen Horney (1885-1952) all made major contributions toward understanding neuroses. All four were Austrian-born physicians who helped invent modern psychology, eventually leaving Austria to work in either Great Britain or America.

Freud founded psychoanalysis with his work on the causes and treatment of neurotic and psychopathic states. The methods that he developed form the root of all "talking therapies." Freud proposed that psychological conflicts produce neuroses according to the following pattern. Inner conflicts are produced by fears or guilt around one's emerging sexual drives. The conflicts, if not resolved on a conscious level, are repressed on the unconscious level, where they drive a person to act according to one or more of the various neurotic symptoms.

Adler was one of the four original members of Freud's psychoanalytic school. With his emphasis on the person as a whole being and on the importance of willpower, he created an individual psychology for the twentieth century. Adler said that neurotic persons form a rigid way of thinking about themselves and others. They then project that rigid thought process onto the world. They proceed to operate as though the world accepted their rigid thinking as real. This tendency is at the basis of the neurotic thought processes of sadism, hatred, intolerance, envy, and irresponsibility.

Jung was the only member of Freud's inner circle who was formally trained as a psychiatrist. He founded analytic psychology, which studies mental behavior as complexes of behavior, emotion, thought, and imagery. He opened up psychology to religious and mystical experiences. Jung wrote that neuroses are a dissociation of the personality caused by splitting. A person has a conscious set of values or beliefs which conflict with an opposite set of feelings. The person, rather than resolving the problem, maintains the rational-emotive split as one or more of the forms of neuroses.

Horney developed a psychoanalytic theory of humans who evolve within their culture, family, and environment. She was sensitive to the negative effects of a male-dominated psychology, attempting to explain women's experiences. Horney believed that neuroses are disturbances in the relationship of self-to-self and self-to-other. If one's development in childhood is disturbed from its normal pattern, the adult will use one of three neurotic coping styles: compliance, aggressiveness, or detachment.

These four psychologists agreed that neuroses are a childhood developmental defect which impairs the adult's rational-emotional integration, appearing as one or more of the indirect symptoms of anxiety.

—*Gerald T. Terlep, Ph.D.*

See also Addiction; Anxiety; Bipolar disorder; Delusions; Depression; Hypochondriasis; Midlife crisis; Obsessive-compulsive disorder; Panic attacks; Paranoia; Phobias; Postpartum depression; Post-traumatic stress disorder; Psychiatric disorders; Psychiatry; Psychiatry, child and adolescent; Psychiatry, geriatric; Psychoanalysis; Psychosis; Psychosomatic disorders; Schizophrenia; Stress.

FOR FURTHER INFORMATION:

Cleve, Jay. *Out of the Blues*. Reprint. Minneapolis: CompCare, 1996. Presents methods of coping with neurotic depression, stemming from Alfred Adler's belief that neurosis comes from overly rigid thinking.

Leibenluft, Ellen, ed. *Gender Differences in Mood and Anxiety Disorders: From Bench to Bedside*. Washington, D.C.: American Psychiatric Press, 1999. Mood and anxiety disorders are the most common psychiatric illnesses psychiatrists and other physicians treat. Moreover, most anxiety disorders, as well as depressive disorders, are at least twice as common in women (except for obsessive-compulsive disorder).

Lindesay, James, ed. *Neurotic Disorders in the Elderly*. Oxford, England: Oxford University Press, 1995. Addresses neuroses in old age, including possible complications. Provides a bibliography and an index.

March, J., and K. Mulle. *OCD in Children and Adolescents: A Cognitive-Behavioral Treatment Manual*. New York: Guilford Press, 1998. The primary purpose of this book is to describe a cognitive-behavioral treatment program which eliminates or alleviates obsessive-compulsive disorder symptoms in children and adolescents.

Rapoport, Judith. *The Boy Who Couldn't Stop Washing*. New York: Penguin Group, 1989. A classic description of the neurosis of obsessive-compulsive behaviors. Based upon Sigmund Freud's understanding of neurosis as an illness.

Roth, Geneen. *When Food Is Love*. New York: Plume, 1991. Reviews the neurotic abuse of foods as an addiction. Roth's work reflects Carl Jung's understanding of the importance of love and spirit for each person.

NEUROSURGERY

PROCEDURE

ANATOMY OR SYSTEM AFFECTED: Bones, brain, glands, head, nerves, nervous system, psychic-emotional system, spine

SPECIALTIES AND RELATED FIELDS: General surgery, neurology, psychiatry

DEFINITION: Surgery involving the brain, spinal cord, or peripheral nerves, including craniotomy, lobotomy, laminectomy, and sympathectomy.

KEY TERMS:

aneurysm: the swelling of a blood vessel, which occurs with the stretching of a weak place in the vessel wall

cannula: a tube or hypodermic needle implanted in the body to introduce or extract substances

commissurotomy: the severing of the corpus callosum, the fiber tract joining the two cerebral hemispheres

hematoma: a localized collection of clotted blood in an organ or tissue as a result of internal bleeding

lesion: a wound or tumor of the brain or spinal cord

lobectomy: the removal of a lobe of the brain, or a major part of a lobe

lobotomy: the separation of either an entire lobe or a major part of a lobe from the rest of the brain

trephination: the opening of a hole in the skull with an instrument called a trephine

INDICATIONS AND PROCEDURES

Neurosurgery refers to any surgery performed on a part of the nervous system. Brain surgery may be used to remove a tumor or foreign body, relieve the pressure caused by an intracranial hemorrhage, excise an abscess, treat parkinsonism, or relieve pain. In cases of severe mental depression or untreatable epilepsy, psychosurgery (such as lobotomy) may alleviate the worst symptoms. Surgery may be performed on the spine to correct a defect, remove a tumor, repair a ruptured intervertebral disk, or relieve pain. Surgery may be performed on nerves to remove a tumor, relieve pain, or reconnect a severed nerve.

Most brain operations share some common procedures. Bleeding from the numerous tiny blood vessels in the brain is controlled by use of an electric needle, a finely pointed instrument that shoots a minute electric current into the vessel and seals it. (This same instrument can be used as an electric knife for bloodless cutting.) Brain tissue is kept moist by continued washing with a dilute salt solution. The brain tissue itself is handled with damp cotton pads attached to the end of forceps.

If the brain is swollen, it may be treated by intravenous injections of urea. The resulting increase in the salt concentration of the blood draws the water away from the brain. In addition to drawing off excess water, the brain's size is temporarily reduced, giving the surgeon extra room to maneuver. To help reduce bleeding within the brain, the patient's blood pressure can be lowered by half temporarily through an injection of a drug into the blood. The patient's temperature is also reduced, which lowers the brain's need

for oxygen and ensures that the reduced blood flow will not be deleterious.

An operation in which a hole is cut into the skull is called a craniotomy. The instrument used is called a trephine (trepan); it resembles a corkscrew with a short, nail-like tip and a threaded cutting disk. The size of the opening that is made ranges from 1.5 centimeters (0.6 inches) to 3.8 centimeters (1.5 inches) in diameter and, if necessary, may be enlarged with an instrument called a rongeur. This type of surgery is performed to insert needles or cannulas and to remove subdural hematomas. If too much of the bony skull has to be removed (or is fractured by accidental means), a substitute for the bone is inserted. The substitute is usually made of plastic, such as acrylic.

A depressed fracture of the skull, especially if it is a compound fracture (involving an open laceration), is surgically treated as soon as possible. Because an open wound is an easy way for bacteria to enter the body and cause infection, disinfection and closure are done quickly. The patient is often conscious and requires local anesthesia, so that consciousness is maintained. The surgeon drills burr holes at the edges of the depression, lifts the bone fragments, and places them in their original positions. Some pieces of bone may be too damaged to be used, and they are discarded. If the hole is large, a later surgery may close the hole with a metal or plastic plate or with a graft from a rib. Another method of filling large holes is the use of metal or fabric mesh; these materials suffice because scalp tissue and heavy muscle are protective as well.

Surgery for parkinsonism will not cure the disease but will help alleviate some of its symptoms. The major symptoms are tremor, stiffness, weakness, and slowed movements. Neurosurgery can be used to reduce or stop the shaking. Surgery to the directly affected areas, however, is all but prohibited by their unavailability: The sites are so deep in the brain that the knife would damage or destroy other vital brain tissue.

When pain becomes unbearable, such as the pain associated with cancer, the nerves carrying these pain messages can be interrupted anywhere between the brain and the cancerous region. The nerve to the affected organ can be severed, the nerve roots of the spinal cord can be cut, or the cut can be made within the spinal cord.

Hypophysectomy is the surgical removal of the pituitary gland. It is usually performed to slow the growth and spread of endocrine-dependent malignant

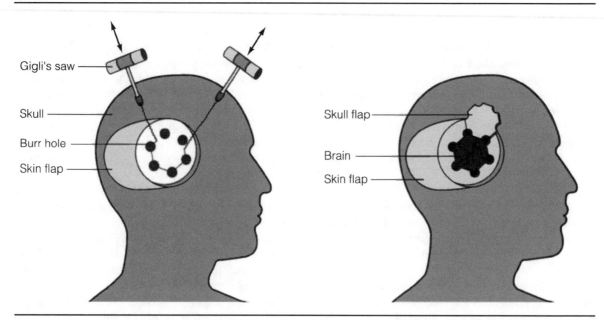

Craniotomy, the opening of the skull, is the first step taken to perform neurosurgery on the brain.

tumors of the breast, ovary, or prostate gland. It may also be used to stop the deterioration of the retina that may come with diabetes mellitus or to remove a pituitary tumor. Hypophysectomy is considered only as a last resort when cryosurgery or radioactive implants fail to destroy the pituitary tissue. There are two ways to reach a diseased pituitary gland by surgery. One way is to go through the nose. The skull is entered through the sphenoid sinus, and the floor of the bony saddle of the middle of the skull is cut to reach the gland. The second means is by craniotomy. The skull is opened through an incision in the hairline above the forehead. A flap of bone, hinged at eyebrow level, is brought forward so that the surgeon can see the entire affected area clearly. The gland is completely excised.

Psychosurgery is now considered only as a last resort, when nothing else can possibly work. It is rarely undertaken because of the availability of so many drugs to control mental illnesses. In the cases when a lobotomy is performed, it can be done under local anesthesia through tiny holes drilled in the roof of the eyes' orbits. An instrument is then inserted to separate the lobes of the brain.

A laminectomy is performed to relieve compression of the spinal cord caused by injury (the displacement of a bone) or by the degeneration of a disk; it may also be used to find and remove a displaced intervertebral disk. A laminectomy is performed under general anesthesia. The surgeon makes an incision in the back, vertically over the tips of the vertebral bones. The large, thick muscles that lie on either side are peeled back from the surface of the bones. The lamina itself is the part of a vertebral bone that forms the back wall of the spinal canal. When the laminae are cut away, the spinal canal is opened so that the spinal cord covering can be cut. Once the cord is exposed, a particular condition can be treated. It may then be necessary to fuse the vertebrae. The removal of the laminae causes little interference with support or motion of the spine, although recovery from the surgery requires that the patient remain prone for several days to keep the spine in alignment.

Fusion of the vertebrae is the surgical joining of two or more spinal vertebrae to stabilize a segment of the spinal column following severe trauma, a herniated (ruptured) disk, or a degenerative disease. The surgery is performed under general anesthesia. The cartilage pads are removed from between the posterior portions of the affected vertebrae. Bone chips are cut from the vertebral ridges and inserted as a replacement for the removed cartilage. Postoperative motion must be limited until the articulating bones heal.

Severe pain that cannot be controlled by analgesics (painkillers) may be treated by surgery. One procedure, a cordotomy, removes a section of the spinal cord so that most of the nerve fibers that transmit pain messages to the brain are destroyed. At first, the patient does experience less pain, but after a few months, the pain recurs and is worse than before. The recurrence of pain is likely attributable to the reconstruction of some axons that carry ascending messages. Other painful conditions can be treated with surgery. Trigeminal neuralgia (or tic douloureux) is one such condition. These severe attacks of stabbing pain in the face may last a minute or more. The trigeminal nerve can be injected with a concentrated alcohol solution, which will prevent it from working for a year or two. This condition is usually treated surgically by drilling a burr hole in the temple and cutting across the lower two-thirds of the nerve trunk at the site.

A sympathectomy surgically interrupts a part of the sympathetic nerve pathways. It is used to relieve the pain of vascular disease. The surgery involves removing the sheath from around an artery. This sheath carries the sympathetic nerve fibers that control vasoconstriction. Once the sheath is removed, the vessel relaxes and expands so that more blood travels through it.

USES AND COMPLICATIONS

While neurosurgery offers the hope of recovery to sufferers of tumors, aneurysms, and brain injuries, it may result in complications that can bring disability, coma, or even death. Therefore, three considerations must be taken into account before neurosurgery is performed. First, these surgeries involve more high-risk procedures than most other types. Second, diseases that necessitate neurosurgical treatment often render patients wholly or partially incompetent to understand the implications of their surgery. Third, sometimes matching the appropriate surgery to the patient's condition is an uncertain process. Even standard neurosurgical procedures have not been proven in every event.

Because the diagnosis of a brain tumor is often seen as fatal, many believe that surgery has little value as therapy, especially for malignant tumors. Others suggest, however, that the more radical the surgery, the greater the chance of survival for the patient. The problem arises when a tumor is found within the center area of the brain, where the primary sensory and motor cortices are situated. Surgical methods of the past tended to exacerbate the problems of the patient.

The use of lasers and microscopy, however, may increase the chance of successful treatment. Using these tools, incisions of no longer than 2 centimeters can be made. Using the microscope, the surgeon can guide the laser to the tumor, which is gently melted and vaporized—all without disturbing the brain. This method is especially useful for reaching deep-seated tumors.

Stereotaxic surgery is a means by which monitoring devices are inserted into the brain cortex. These devices can detect lesions, stimulate or record areas within the cortex, or in some other way study the brain. The two things necessary to perform this surgery are a stereotaxic atlas (or map) of the brain and the instrumentation for the procedure. The atlas is a series of individual maps, each representing a slice of the brain. The stereotaxic instrument consists of two parts: a head holder, which maintains the patient's head in a particular position and orientation, and an electrode holder, which holds the device that is to be inserted.

The purpose of the lesion method of stereotaxic surgery is to remove, damage, or destroy a part of the brain in such a way that the behavior of the patient can be monitored to determine the functions of the affected area, or lesion. Surgery to produce lesions is an extremely precise, and therefore dangerous, surgery. Structures within the brain are tiny, convoluted, and tightly packed; it is likely that any surgery performed on an area will damage adjacent areas. There are four different methods of producing lesions.

Aspiration lesions are performed when the lesion is in a more accessible area of the brain, where the surgeon can see it clearly and can use the proper instruments. The cortical tissue is aspirated by a handheld pipette, and then the tougher white matter layers are peeled away. Deeper lesions are cut away with high-frequency (radiofrequency) currents passed through carefully placed electrodes. The heat of the current destroys the tissue. The amount of tissue to be removed is regulated through control of the current's duration and intensity. In the third method, a nerve or tract to be removed can be cut with a scalpel. A tiny incision severing the nerve does not have to do damage to surrounding tissues, so the lesion is small.

The fourth method is cryogenic blockade. Blockade is a preferable alternative because virtually no structural damage results and a return to normal temperature causes neural activity to resume. In this method, a coolant is pumped through the tip of an implanted cryoprobe to cool the area. When the tissue is cooled, the neurons do not fire. The temperature must remain above freezing, however, to prevent destruction of the tissue. Although the result is not a true lesion, since function returns, this cooled area acts as a lesion because the behavior that it governs is interrupted. Consequently, cryogenic blockade is said to produce a reversible lesion.

A commissurotomy, or cutting apart of the two cerebral hemispheres, may be performed in cases of severe epilepsy if no other treatment is successful. After the two halves are separated (the brain stem is left intact), each hemisphere maintains all the centers that mediate its functions, except that each cortex sees only half the world. For example, visual messages are crossed so that the opposite hemisphere is stimulated by only one eye's input. If both eyes and both hemispheres are working, however, vision should be unaffected. In fact, no real deficits should occur in these patients' behavior. They retain the same verbal intelligence, reasoning, perception, motor coordination, and personality because of the brain's extraordinary ability to preserve unity, or oneness.

Commissurotomies were first performed in the hope of reducing the severity of convulsions and seizures associated with epilepsy. The rationale was that the severity of the convulsions would be reduced if discharges could be limited to the hemisphere from which they originated. The benefits far surpassed expectations; many patients never experience another convulsion.

Studies of lobotomized patients, especially those who have undergone a frontal lobotomy, have provided insight into the importance of these lobes. Frontal lobotomies are generally performed to lessen psychoses that cannot be treated successfully by any other means or to relieve unbearable pain, such as that induced in the latter stages of cancer.

Lobotomies are somewhat controversial. It has been shown that the surgery results in diminished anxiety and concern in the patient, but in some patients this reaction is extreme, causing them to lose their ethical standards. Their judgment and planning ability are decreased. Actions and behavior are not necessarily matched to stimuli; they may be inappropriate or badly timed: For example, crying may be a response to a comic situation. One patient may plan a meal but forget how to cook, and another may urinate in public while dressed for a formal occasion. Thus, although a lobotomy does not diminish intellect,

memory, or consciousness to the extent that injury to other parts of the brain does, it is debasing. Perseverance or the ability to continue some activity is decreased, and patients often cannot deal with or overcome challenges.

PERSPECTIVE AND PROSPECTS

People living in the Stone Age often performed trephination. This operation consisted of boring or making holes in the skull and removing pieces or disks of bone. Trephination was likely performed to release evil spirits or demons: There is little evidence of fractures of the skulls that have been found, and the pieces of skulls that were excised were preserved and worn as talismans. Today, surgeons in some tribal cultures perform the same surgery; in some cases, some are done for ritual purposes, while others are performed for head injuries as well as headache, dizziness, and epilepsy. Trephination provided the groundwork for brain surgery as it is still practiced.

Perhaps the most intriguing possibility for future research is transplanting brains or brain tissue. Brain transplants have come a long way from their portrayal in science fiction. In 1971, the first real evidence that transplanted tissue could survive was found. These successful attempts were made in rats. Further studies have shown that transplants have a higher survival rate in tissue richly vascularized with sufficient room to grow. It is hoped that neurotransplant surgery can be used to treat brain damage. One approach would be to develop procedures of implantation that would stimulate the regeneration of the patient's own tissue. A second approach would be to replace damaged tissue with healthy tissue of the same type.

The major question that will have to be answered before successful regeneration is accomplished is why neurons of the peripheral nervous system (PNS) regenerate but the neurons of the central nervous system (CNS) do not. One hypothesis would be that they are too structurally different. This theory is disputed by studies that show CNS neuron regeneration in the peripheral nervous system, while PNS neurons do not regenerate in the central nervous system. Other evidence to refute the hypothesis is that peripheral sensory neurons regenerate until they reach the spinal cord, then regeneration ceases. Therefore, perhaps there is an environmental factor within the central nervous system that prohibits regeneration, such as scar tissue that forms only in the area of CNS damage. Experiments to prove or disprove this theory are inconclusive. The other possibility is that the insulating cells wrapped around CNS neurons are different enough from the Schwann cells of PNS neurons that regeneration is discouraged.

Attempts to replace damaged tissue with healthy tissue have been most useful in treating Parkinson's disease (with its rigidity, tremors, and lack of spontaneous movement). One type of tissue used for replacement is fetal neural tissue. It not only survives but also innervates adjacent tissue, releases neurotransmitters (in this case dopamine), and alleviates the symptoms of parkinsonism. Even though this procedure is highly successful, it is unlikely that fetal tissue transplantation will become common. The use of fetal tissue raises serious ethical questions regarding the harvesting of donor tissue from human fetuses. A possible substitute for neural tissue is autotransplantation with some of the patient's own adrenal medulla. This tissue could be used because it too releases dopamine. Investigations thus far have been controversial, but the operation is being performed worldwide.

—Iona C. Baldridge

See also Aneurysmectomy; Brain; Brain disorders; Craniotomy; Cysts; Electroencephalography (EEG); Fetal tissue transplantation; Ganglion removal; Laminectomy and spinal fusion; Laser use in surgery; Lumbar puncture; Nervous system; Neurology; Neurology, pediatric; Pain; Pain management; Parkinson's disease; Positron emission tomography (PET) scanning; Psychiatric disorders; Psychiatry; Spina bifida; Spinal cord disorders; Spine, vertebrae, and disks; Stem cell research; Tics; Tumor removal; Tumors.

FOR FURTHER INFORMATION:
Cotman, Carl W., and James L. McGaugh. *Behavioral Neuroscience*. New York: Academic Press, 1980. Describes all the facets of the nervous system and the mechanisms that determine behavior. Each chapter concludes with key word definitions and references. This textbook is best read by those with some experience in biology or psychology.

Pinel, John P. J. *Biopsychology*. 4th ed. Boston: Allyn & Bacon, 2000. A textbook for introductory courses in biopsychology, which studies a combination of neurology and behavior. The chapters are rich in case studies and illustrations, and they conclude with key word definitions and references.

Post, Kalman, et al., eds. *Acute, Chronic, and Terminal Care in Neurosurgery*. Springfield, Ill.: Charles C Thomas, 1987. An interesting compilation of chapters written by various health care workers on the various aspects of neurosurgery. The procedures themselves are not the focus of the pieces, but medical care, ethics, and facing death are addressed.

NIGHTMARES
DISEASE/DISORDER

ANATOMY OR SYSTEM AFFECTED: Psychic-emotional system

SPECIALTIES AND RELATED FIELDS: Family practice, pediatrics, psychiatry, psychology

DEFINITION: Anxiety-provoking, scary, unpleasant, and frightening dreams that disturb sleep, causing children to cry in their sleep or awake in an emotionally upset, typically anxious state.

KEY TERMS:

dream sleep: sleep during which dreaming occurs and rapid eye movements are produced

night terrors: episodes characterized by screaming and rapid awakening from deep sleep; sometimes confused with nightmares

rapid eye movement (REM) sleep: the stage of sleep in which dreaming occurs; in addition to rapid eye movements, which are easily visible through closed eyelids, characterized by facial and body movements, changes in heart and breathing rates, inhibition of certain (deep) reflexes, and increased blood flow to the brain

CAUSES AND SYMPTOMS

Nightmares have intrigued people for centuries, inspiring a range of explanations about what causes them. It is now known that they occur in all children shortly after the developmental stage of the "terrible two's," which overlaps but is not the same as the chronological age of two.

Two concurrent developments mark this period of growth. The first is intellectual and cognitive. Children develop the ability to conceptualize, process, and recall information in ways that they could not before and begin reporting that they had dreams the previous night. These dreams usually involve things they wish for, playful fantasies, and daytime activities. The second development is emotional. At this stage, children are growing beyond the autonomy and individuation issues that characterize the infamous "terrible two's." They start involuntarily to experience strong aggressive feelings and desires to control, and they direct these emotions toward those with whom they have the most trouble in establishing their autonomy: parents and siblings. At the same time, children also experience anxiety from speculating about what would happen if their feelings were ever directly expressed. This intellectual and emotional combination gives rise to vividly intense nightmares, what children commonly refer to as "bad dreams."

In addition to aggressive impulses, nightmares may involve big dogs, snakes, insects, or other dangerous animals; monsters; giants; a "bad man"; or harm coming to them or someone in their family. During nightmares, children sense their own helplessness and vulnerability, which adds to the awful feelings experienced afterward. Children who dream that they are victorious over the threat—for example, they beat up the monster—usually report that they have had "good dreams" and are not frightened.

Nightmares affect boys and girls equally, although individually children experience, or recall the experience, with wide-ranging frequency. Some will have few nightmares throughout this preschool period; others will have many. Regardless of the baseline, all children will experience an increase in frequency during times of worsening stress. Both a marked increase in the frequency of nightmares and the experience of having a single frequently recurring nightmare have psychological significance and causes. Rapid awakening after any dream is associated with good recall, which is also true with nightmares.

Night terrors also begin around this time, although, unlike nightmares, not all children experience them. They occur with regularity only between the ages of two and six. Night terrors are characterized by screaming and rapid awakening from deep sleep during the first third of the night, with vague or no recollection of the scary dream or image that presumably caused them. The child is terrified, hard to comfort, and difficult to awaken fully. Episodes last from ten to twenty minutes. It is often more upsetting for parents to witness a child thrashing and screaming than it is for the children who experience night terrors, as there is usually no recollection of the episodes the next morning.

Electroencephalogram (EEG) testing during night terrors shows the electrical activity in the brain as similar to that which occurs during small seizures, although night terrors are neither seizures nor caused by seizures and should not be treated as such. Usually, when night terrors occur, either the preceding day or the period right before bedtime has been particularly challenging or difficult. Night terrors may be a way in which children work off the psychological steam that they have built up as a result.

Treatment and Therapy

Nightmares are often problematic because parents are uncertain about what to do. Do they look under the bed or in the closet for the "bogeyman"? Do they keep the lights on all night? Do they let the child sleep with them after having a nightmare? Parents can help a child who has had a bad dream and who is afraid of monsters by looking under the bed or opening the closet together, while reassuring the child that they both know nothing is there.

All children experience imagined fears like monsters or spiders. These fears need to be taken seriously because they are real to the children having them. It is important that parents not scold or embarrass already frightened children or tell them that they should not feel the way they do. Parents should not discount or dismiss fears of imaginary and fantasized threats. Children need to feel that when their fantasies and worries get out of control, as in nightmares, someone can take charge and provide safety, security, and reassurance. Children must know that their worries and fears are important to their parents and caregivers.

When nightmare frequency begins to signal an underlying adjustment problem, nightmares should be thought of as an expression of intense anxiety caused by something or someone. In such cases, professional help in the form of a child therapist should be sought.

Night terrors, as disturbing as they can be, usually do not require professional intervention. In most cases, a calm, reassuring parent is all that a child needs to be comforted, to settle down, and to resume the sleep cycle. When the frequency of night terrors becomes problematic, parents should consult a sleep disorder specialist, whose professional discipline is usually medicine or psychology. In both disciplines, treating sleep disorders is a specialized area of clinical practice, and most physicians and psychologists are not trained to treat them.

—Paul Moglia, Ph.D.

See also Anxiety; Cognitive development; Developmental stages; Emotions: Biomedical causes and effects; Phobias; Psychiatry, child and adolescent; Sleep disorders; Sleepwalking.

FOR FURTHER INFORMATION:

Brazelton, T. Berry. *Touchpoints: Your Child's Emotional and Behavioral Development.* New York: Addison-Wesley, 1992. Brazelton is a knowledgeable physician with years of experience with thousands of children, and he brings that experience to bear on virtually every issue faced by families with kids, from birth through age six.

_____. *What Every Baby Knows.* New York: Ballantine, 1987. This guide offers helpful hints for rearing your child and a discussion of child psychology. Includes an index.

Ferber, Richard. *Solve Your Child's Sleep Problems.* New York: Simon & Schuster, 1985. Based on Ferber's research as the director of Boston's Center for Pediatric Sleep Disorders at Children's Hospital, this book is a practical, easy-to-understand guide to common sleeping problems for children ages one to six. Detailed case histories on night waking, difficulty sleeping, and more serious disorders such as sleep apnea and sleepwalking help illustrate a wide variety of problems and their solutions.

Spurr, Pam. *Understanding Your Child's Dreams.* New York: Sterling, 1999. Illuminating real-life case histories show just how much youthful dreams reveal, and a dictionary of common images will help the reader with interpretation. Includes extraordinary color drawings to help children visualize and focus on their dreams.

NONINVASIVE TESTS

PROCEDURES

ANATOMY OR SYSTEM AFFECTED: All

SPECIALTIES AND RELATED FIELDS: Cardiology, emergency medicine, nuclear medicine, obstetrics, pathology, preventive medicine, radiology

DEFINITION: Diagnostic techniques that do not involve the collection of tissue or fluid samples or the introduction of any instrument into the body; most noninvasive tests involve imaging or the measurement of electrical activity.

KEY TERMS:

computed tomography (CT) scanning: a method of producing images of cross sections of the body

diagnosis: recognition of diseases based on physical examination, the microscopic and chemical results of laboratory findings, and an analysis of imaging results

Doppler shift: the increase in frequency of sound waves as the source of the waves approaches the observer or instrument; Doppler techniques are often used to assess blood flow in body channels such as veins

echocardiogram (EC): a graph of cardiac motion and heart valve closure produced by sending sound waves to the heart and recording their deflections

electrocardiogram (EKG or ECG): a diagnostic tool used to detect disturbances in the electrical activity of the heart

magnetic resonance imaging (MRI): a procedure using magnetic fields to determine blood vessel condition, fluid flow, and tissue contours and to detect abnormal masses

signal-averaged electrocardiogram (SAECG): a sophisticated EKG which detects subtle and potentially lethal cardiac conduction defects

sonography: the use of sound waves deflected from internal body organs to find growing masses (including fetuses) and abnormal lesions; also called ultrasound

X radiology: the use of ionizing radiation of short wavelength to detect abnormalities in primarily dense portions of the body

INDICATIONS AND PROCEDURES

Noninvasive tests are used in the initial diagnosis of a disease or abnormality and for the monitoring of certain conditions and body processes. Most such tests involve imaging techniques. Primary among them are X radiology, computed tomography (CT) scanning, magnetic resonance imaging (MRI), electrocardiography (EKG or ECG), and ultrasound.

Diagnostic X-ray examinations are often the first step in complex technological solutions to medical diagnoses and health problems. New uses for diagnostic X rays are constantly being devised. It is common practice for hospitals to require chest X rays for all outpatients visiting X-ray departments; and hospital inpatients are usually given chest X rays before admission or surgery.

Computed tomography (CT) scanning, also known as computed axial tomography (CAT) scanning, uses a computer to interpret multiple X-ray images in order to reconstruct a cross-sectional image of any area of the body. The inventors of the procedure for CT scanning were awarded a Nobel Prize in 1979.

After the patient is placed in the CT scanner, an X-ray source rapidly rotates around it, taking hundreds of pictures. The pictures are electronically recorded and stored by a computer. The computer then integrates the data into cross-sectional "slices." The CT scanner can assess the composition of internal structures, which it is able to discriminate from fat, fluid, and gas. The scanner can show the shape and size of various organs and lesions and has the capability of detecting abnormal lesions as small as 1 or 2 millimeters in diameter.

Magnetic resonance imaging (MRI), unlike CT scanning (which uses X rays), uses magnetic fields passing through the body to detect details of anatomy and physiology.

MRI equipment consists of a tunnel-like magnet that creates a magnetic field around the patient. This magnetic field causes the hydrogen atoms found in the body—water has two hydrogen and one oxygen atom in the molecule—to line up. At the same time, a radio frequency signal is quickly transmitted to upset the uniformity of the formation. When the radiofrequency signal is turned off, the hydrogen atoms return to their proper lineup, and a small current is generated. By detecting the speed and volume with which the atoms return, the computer can display a diagnostic image on a monitor.

MRI is noninvasive, and no pain or radiation is involved. The procedure takes from fifteen to forty-five minutes, depending on the number of views needed. Diagnostic X rays rely on variations of density on film, and areas of soft tissue, for example, produce little or no shadow and are difficult to distinguish in any detail. MRI images, on the other hand, allow tumors, muscles, arteries, and vertebrae to be seen with great clarity.

Monitoring and providing electrical support to the heart constitute other useful noninvasive techniques. A healthy heart generates electrical impulses rhythmically and spontaneously; this activity is controlled by the sinoatrial (S-A) node, the heart's natural pacemaker. From there, the impulses pass through specialized conduction tissues in the atria and into the atrioventricular (A-V) node. Then the electrical impulses enter the ventricular conduction system, the bundle of His, and the right and left bundle branches. From the bundle branches, the impulses spread into the ventricles through the network of Purkinje fibers. The spread of electrical stimulation through the atria and the ventricles is known as depolarization. The standard electrocardiogram (ECG or EKG) records this activity from twelve different angles. The EKG records the heart's electrical activity and provides vital information concerning its rate, rhythm, and con-

duction system status. Detecting changes in the EKG can help to diagnose ventricular conduction problems and ventricular hypertrophy.

The signal-averaged electrocardiogram (SAECG) is another noninvasive procedure that is a promising diagnostic tool for many cardiac patients. Unlike the standard twelve-lead EKG, the SAECG can detect conduction abnormalities that often precede sustained ventricular tachycardia—which is second only to myocardial infarction (heart attack) as the leading cause of sudden death. The SAECG records the heart's electrical activity via six electrodes applied to the frontal and posterior chest walls. The SAECG can often pick up repolarization delays that occur when ischemic (damaged) tissue impedes the passage of electrical impulses through a portion of the myocardium, a condition which can lead to ventricular tachycardia.

A valuable weapon in the battle against sudden cardiac death is the temporary pacemaker, which provides support for the heart's electrical conduction system. Four types of temporary devices are available to manage cardiac arrhythmias. One of these is a noninvasive temporary pacemaker, known as Zoll NTP, a transcutaneous pacemaker which can provide vital support when there is no time to prepare for an invasive procedure. Such pacemakers are also used when invasive procedures are contraindicated.

Another method for diagnosing heart problems is echocardiography, a technique for recording echoes of ultrasonic waves when these waves are directed at areas of the heart. The principle is similar to that used in the sonar detection of submarines and other underwater objects. In this very simple and painless procedure, the patient lies on a table while a small, high-frequency generator (transducer) is moved across the chest. The instrument projects ultrasonic waves and receives the returning echoes. As the waves pass through the heart, their behavior differs, depending on whether there is any calcification present, whether there is a blood clot or any other mass in the cavity of the heart, whether certain heart chambers are enlarged, whether the valves within the heart open and close in the proper fashion, and whether any part of the heart is thicker than it should be.

Sonography, or ultrasound, imaging and the images produced are unique: Patients can hear their blood flowing through the carotid arteries of the neck, and physicians can see a brain tumor or watch a human fetus suck its thumb. Some physicians believe that this simple and inexpensive imaging technique will be the basis for the development of fetal medicine as a subspecialty. Sonography uses sound waves to look within the body by using a piezoelectric crystal to convert electric pulses into vibrations that penetrate the body. These sound waves are reflected back to the crystal, which reconverts them into electric signals. Many doctors foresee much growth in the use of ultrasound as a noninvasive procedure.

USES AND COMPLICATIONS

Historically, diagnostic X rays have been used for the detection of metal objects, cavities in teeth, and broken bones. Films of various parts of the body, such as the abdomen, skull, and chest, have been taken ever since X rays were first discovered in the late 1800's. Dentists and orthodontists use X rays to check for jaw fractures, tooth misalignment, gum disease, tartar deposits, impacted teeth, and bone cancer. Chronic illnesses that can be detected by X rays include arthritis, tuberculosis, osteoporosis, emphysema, ulcers, pneumonia, and urinary tract infections.

The CT scanner uses a series of narrow, pencil-like X-ray beams to scan the section of the body under investigation. CT scans allow the rapid diagnosis of brain abnormalities, cysts, tumors, and blood clots. Newly developed body scanners assist in the early detection of cancers and other diseases of the internal organs.

Magnetic resonance imaging has undergone an explosive growth in applications. In 1982, there were only six machines in operation. Hospitals often used a portable MRI device, which can be driven from place to place with a tractor-trailer truck. As the cost for MRI machines decreases, however, more hospitals are purchasing this equipment instead of sharing it.

The MRI machine is able to differentiate the brain's gray matter (nerve cells) from the brain's white matter (nerve fibers). Gray matter contains 87 percent water, and white matter contains 72 percent water. Thus, since MRI detects the protons in the hydrogen in water, a great difference in contrast between the two types of brain material is seen on the resulting scan. MRI is also useful in detecting and monitoring the progression of multiple sclerosis because the fatty tissue that normally exists around nerve fibers deteriorates and these abnormal, fat-free areas can be clearly imaged.

MRI research seeks ways of analyzing the numerous chemical elements found in the body and aids in the study, diagnosis, treatment, and cure of a host of human diseases.

EKGs are useful in the detection of irregularities in the heart's electrical conduction system. This technology can also help in the diagnosis of ventricular hypertrophy, pulmonary emboli, and intraventricular conduction problems.

Echocardiograms, based on sound waves, are used to detect infarcts (areas of necrosis, or tissue death), valve closure between heart chambers, and abnormal thickening of myocardial muscle. Sonography is perhaps best known for its contribution to diagnostic medicine in the study of human fetal development. Determining the age of a developing embryo is now standard procedure, and clear images can be obtained at five weeks of gestation, when the embryo is only 5 millimeters long. Fetal weight can be determined by volume, and fetal anatomy can also be studied. Congenital heart defects can be spotted very early, and neural brain defects can be discovered as well.

The great advantage of ultrasound is that it emits no ionizing radiation and thus can be used on pregnant women without danger to the fetus. Ultrasound can detect gallstones, kidney stones, and tumors and can monitor blood flow. Its applications have grown exponentially since its discovery.

The American Cancer Society estimates that one in every four people in the United States will develop cancer at some point in his or her life. These statistics suggest the enormous problem that cancer presents to American society. Cancer detection, as early as possible, is of primary importance because aggressive treatment can be initiated to deter further progression of the disease. The roles of X rays, MRI, and CT scanning in determining the source and extent of the malignancy are vital in the treatment of cancer.

Mammography is a subset of X-ray imaging which is useful in detecting breast cancer. The equipment used in mammography is designed to image breast tissue, which is usually soft and of uniform density. Very small changes in density can be identified in fine detail, including small areas of calcification. Radiation doses must also be kept to a minimum. The film interpretation of mammograms is difficult, but early detection of breast cancer is often possible.

In the United States, the Public Health Service, in a memo dated June 1, 1993, delegated authority for implementing the Mammography Quality Standards Act (MQSA) of 1992 to the Food and Drug Administration (FDA). MQSA is intended to ensure that mammography is reliable and safe. The act makes it unlawful for any facility to provide services unless it is accredited by an approved private nonprofit or state body and it has received federal certification indicating that it meets standard for quality. Each facility must also pass an annual inspection conducted by approved federal personnel. The law was enacted in response to the need for safe, early detection of breast cancer. Mammography is the most effective technique for early detection of this type of cancer.

Given a choice, most persons would prefer a non-invasive diagnostic tool. The earliest used diagnostic tool was the X ray. X rays were discovered in 1895 by a German professor named Wilhelm Conrad Röntgen. The first X rays were produced in a Crookes tube, a pear-shaped, glass tube in which two electrodes, the cathode (negative electrode) and anode (positive electrode), were placed at right angles to each other. The tube was then evacuated of gas. In Röntgen's first experiment, the cathode was "excited" with an electrical current, producing a beam of cathode rays, or electrons. These electrons were directed across the tube from the cathode and struck the glass, causing it to glow and, at the same time, producing X rays, which excited a fluorescent screen. In a modern X-ray tube, the cathode ray strikes a target in the anode rather than the glass. Modern equipment also uses high-energy electricity in order to energize the tube at the high voltages necessary for producing X rays.

Radiology has come far. From a medical discipline with a limited but vital function (that of aiding diagnosis), it has become interventional. It is a field that has moved into therapy—repairing a growing variety of abnormalities, averting surgery, and sometimes achieving results beyond the reach of surgery.

In addition to the simple X ray, physicians now have more powerful diagnostic devices: MRI, CT scanning, and sonography. Cardiac conditions and abnormalities are quite easily analyzed via the ECG or echocardiogram. Where once the diagnosis of gallstones required a two-day X-ray test and 12 grams of diarrhea-causing pills, now ultrasound allows a diagnosis to be made painlessly and noninvasively, in ten to fifteen minutes.

The computer has been the core in the revolution in imaging. As more information becomes available and the density of information grows exponentially, larger and faster computers have been developed to assimilate this information. Computer visualization both interprets data and generates images from data in order to provide new insight into disease states through visual methods. Visualization and computation promise to play a key role in diagnostic medicine.

—*Jane A. Slezak, Ph.D.*

See also Computed tomography (CT) scanning; Electrocardiography (ECG or EKG); Electroencephalography (EEG); Imaging and radiology; Magnetic resonance imaging (MRI); Mammography; Physical examination; Radiation therapy; Screening; Ultrasonography; Urinalysis.

FOR FURTHER INFORMATION:
Galton, Lawrence. *Med Tech*. New York: Harper & Row, 1985. A book for laypeople which explains, in simple terms, advanced therapies and techniques used in medicine. Elucidates the controversies, dangers, and costs of treatment and answers specific questions regarding medical research.

Merva, Jean. "SAECG: A Closer Look at the Heart." *RN* 56 (May, 1993): 51-53. Describes the use of signal-averaged EKGs.

Sochurek, Howard. *Medicine's New Vision*. Easton, Pa.: Mack, 1988. The many forms of radiology are described, with illustrative images of several diagnostic modalities including MRI, CT scanning, ultrasound, and radiation therapy.

Solomon, Jacqueline. "Take the EKG One Step Further." *RN* 55 (May, 1992): 56-60. Discusses the diagnostic use of EKGs.

Wolbarst, Anthony Brinton. *Looking Within: How X-Ray, CT, MRI, Ultrasound, and Other Medical Images Are Created*. Berkeley: University of California Press, 1999. Modern medical imaging has changed perceptions of the overall workings of the human body. The author explains how imaging tools work and what noninvasive imaging procedures do to and for the patient.

NOSEBLEEDS
DISEASE/DISORDER

ALSO KNOWN AS: Epistaxis

ANATOMY OR SYSTEM AFFECTED: Blood, blood vessels, circulatory system, nose, throat

SPECIALTIES AND RELATED FIELDS: Emergency medicine, family practice, general surgery, hematology, internal medicine, otorhinolaryngology, pediatrics

DEFINITION: Bleeding from the nose.

KEY TERMS:

mucosa: the moist membrane covering the internal nose, mouth, sinuses, respiratory tract, gastrointestinal tract, and other sites in the body

nasal polyp: a small growth, usually benign, on the nasal mucosa

nasal septum: the midline wall inside the front of the nose that separates the nostrils

CAUSES AND SYMPTOMS

The nose is a highly vascular area and is therefore a common site of bleeding. Most nosebleeds are benign. They may result from local causes that affect the mucosa of the nose directly. They can also result from systemic causes, which affect the body as a whole.

The major cause of nosebleeds is irritation of the nasal mucosa. Simple trauma from nose picking is the most common in children. Chronic irritation can be associated with allergies, a dry environment or changes in the weather, smoking or the inhalation of smoke, or the inhalation of caustic substances, such as cocaine. Sneezing as a result of recurrent colds or infections of the nose and throat can be associated with nosebleeds. The use of medications such as decongestants, antihistamines, and allergy/cold nasal sprays may also result in nosebleeds because of local irritation.

Trauma to the nose may result from blunt injury, such as those associated with sports or other accidents. Occasionally, children may place small objects high in the nose; these objects may go undetected for periods of time before eventually causing infection and bleeding. Rarely, bleeding may be caused by structural problems, such as nasal polyps, malignant growths, or deviation of the midline nasal septum.

Systemic causes of nosebleeds include underlying bleeding disorders, fevers, bacterial or viral infections, high blood pressure, cancer, and liver or kidney problems. Bleeding disorders should be considered in cases where the bleeding is recurrent and/or prolonged or if there is a significant family history of bleeding problems. Medications such as aspirin, ibuprofen (or other anti-inflammatory agents), anticoagulants, or steroids may produce a transient or short-lived coagulation defect that may cause nosebleeds.

TREATMENT AND THERAPY

Most nosebleeds can be stopped sitting upright (or by holding a young child on one's lap) and gently squeezing the front or anterior of the nose closed for five to ten minutes. It is important to seek medical attention if the bleeding does not stop or if there is continued bleeding or oozing of blood. Occasionally, nasal packing (placement of gauze inside the nose) or other procedures may be required to control severe bleeding. People with coagulation problems need special consideration and require specific medical treatment.

Efforts to keep the nasal mucosa from becoming too dry may be helpful in preventing recurrent nosebleeds. Applying petroleum jelly or other moisturizing agents inside the nose or using a humidifier in the home to keep the air moist may also be helpful.

Most nosebleeds are not life-threatening, but they can be very frightening for patients, especially children and their parents or caregivers. When caring for a child who is bleeding, it is important to remain calm to help decrease the child's anxiety and to assess and begin to treat the bleeding.

—*Frank E. Shafer, M.D.*

See also Allergies; Bleeding; Blood and blood disorders; Common cold; Otorhinolaryngology; Respiration; Sneezing.

FOR FURTHER INFORMATION:

Owen, Charles A., E. J. Walter, and John H. Thompson. *The Diagnosis of Bleeding Disorders.* 2d ed. Boston: Little, Brown, 1975.

Ratnoff, Oscar D., and Charles D. Forbes, eds. *Disorders of Hemostasis.* 3d ed. Philadelphia: W. B. Saunders, 1996.

Thompson, Arthur R., and Laurence A. Harker. *Manual of Hemostasis and Thrombosis.* 3d ed. Philadelphia: F. A. Davis, 1983.

NUCLEAR MEDICINE
SPECIALTY

ANATOMY OR SYSTEM AFFECTED: Bones, gallbladder, glands, kidneys, musculoskeletal system

SPECIALTIES AND RELATED FIELDS: Cardiology, endocrinology, internal medicine, radiology

DEFINITION: The field of medicine that employs radioactivity for both diagnostic and therapeutic purposes; the former involves imaging techniques, while the latter uses large amounts of radioactive material to destroy cells.

KEY TERMS:

cathode-ray tube: a display device used for the presentation of nuclear medicine data; it displays images in real time

collimator: a device used for restricting and directing gamma rays by passing them through a grid made of metal, which absorbs the rays

gamma radiation: electromagnetic radiation of a short wavelength that is emitted by the nucleus of a radionuclide during radioactive decay

half-life: a unique characteristic of a radionuclide defined by the time during which its initial activity is reduced to one half; this period varies among radionucleotides from less than one-millionth of a second to millions of years

pharmacological stress testing: a procedure wherein a pharmacological agent is administered to a patient in order to increase blood flow to the heart, thereby enabling coronary artery disease, if present, to manifest itself

radionuclide: a species of atom (of natural or artificial origin) having a specified number of protons and neutrons in its nucleus which exhibits radioactivity

radiopharmaceutical: a sterile, radioactively tagged compound that is administered to a patient for diagnostic or therapeutic purposes

scintillation: the production of flashes emitted by luminescent substances when excited by high-energy radiation

tomography: the term that describes all types of body-section imaging techniques; that is, a visual representation restricted to a specified section or "cut" of tissue within an organ

tracer: a radioactive substance introduced into the body, the progress of which may be followed by means of an external radioactivity detector; it must not affect the process that it is used to measure

SCIENCE AND PROFESSION

Nuclear medicine is the branch of medicine that uses radioactive substances in the diagnosis and treatment of diseases. A discussion of such technology requires an understanding of the nature of radioactivity and the tools employed by specialists in this medical field.

Radioactivity is the spontaneous emission of particles from the nucleus of an atom. Several kinds of emissions are possible. Gamma-ray emission is the type with which nuclear medicine imaging is concerned. The activity of radionuclides is measured in terms of the number of atoms disintegrating per unit time. The basic unit of measurement is the curie. Radiopharmaceuticals that are administered are in the microcurie or millicurie range of activity. Most radionuclides used in nuclear medicine are produced from accelerators, reactors, or generators. Accelerators are devices that accelerate charged particles (ions) to bombard a target. Cyclotron-produced radionuclides that are used frequently in nuclear medicine include gallium 67, thallium 201, and indium 111. The core of a nuclear reactor consists of material undergoing nuclear fission. Nuclides of interest in nuclear medicine that are formed from reactors include molybdenum 99, iodine 131, and xenon 133.

In generator systems, a "parent" isotope decays spontaneously to a "daughter" isotope in which the half-life of the parent is longer than that of the daughter. The parent is used to generate a continuous supply of the relatively short-lived daughter radionuclides and is therefore called a generator. The most commonly used generator system is molybdenum 99 (with a half-life of sixty-seven hours) and technetium 99m (with a half-life of six hours). The daughter, technetium 99m, is the most widely used radioisotope in nuclear medicine. It is obtained from the generator in a physiologic sodium chloride solution as the pertechnetate ion. It can be used alone to image the thyroid, salivary glands, or gastric mucosa, or it can be labeled to a wide variety of complexes that are picked up physiologically by various organ systems.

The scintillation camera, or Anger camera (named for its inventor, Hal O. Anger), is the most commonly used static imaging device in nuclear medicine. The scintillation camera produces a picture on a cathode-ray tube of the distribution of an administered radio nuclide within the target organ of a patient. It uses the gamma rays emitted by the nuclide and collimator to create the image as a series of light flashes on a disk-shaped sodium iodide crystal. The system determines the location of each scintillation and then produces a finely focused dot of light on the face of the cathode-ray tube in a corresponding position. The complete picture is then produced on photographic film. The camera normally contains two parts, the head and the computer console. The head serves as the gamma-ray detector. It absorbs incoming gamma rays and generates electrical signals that correspond to the positions where the absorptions took place. These signals are sent to a computer to be processed and to produce a picture that can be displayed on film or stored on disk for video display.

The collimator normally consists of a large piece of lead with many small holes in it. There are many types of collimators. The most commonly used are parallel-hole types. The holes are of equal, constant cross section, and their axes form a set of closely spaced, vertical, parallel lines. The material between the holes are called septa.

Putting this all together, the radioisotope, once injected or ingested, travels to the target organ. Gamma rays from the target organ are emitted in all directions. The collimator allows only those gamma rays traveling in a direction essentially parallel to the axis of its holes to pass through to the crystal. The crystal is made of sodium iodide, with a small amount of thallium impurity. The thallium is transparent and emits light photons whenever it absorbs a gamma ray. This action by the collimator causes the light flashes in the crystal to form an image of the nuclide distribution located below it. This image will preserve gray-scale information, since the number of gamma rays received by any given region of the crystal will be directly proportional to the amount of nuclide located directly below that region.

Single photon emission computed tomography (SPECT) is a tomographic imaging technique employing scintillation cameras to display the information at a given depth in sharp focus, while blurring information above and below that depth. There are two distinct methods of SPECT, each based on the type of images produced. The first, longitudinal section tomography, provides images of planes parallel to the long axis of the body. The second method, transverse section tomography, is perpendicular to the long axis of the body. Transverse section tomography with a rotating gamma camera has received wide clinical acceptance, partly because of the information that it provides and its multiple-use capability, since these systems can perform routine planar imaging as well as SPECT imaging. In this system, the gamma camera is a device mounted to a gantry and capable of rotating 360 degrees around the patient. These systems must be interfaced with a computer. The orbit around the patient is circular, and from 32 to 180 equiangular images are acquired over a 360-degree arc. Image acquisition is by computer. The images are stored digitally, and image reconstruction is achieved by filtering each projection, with geometric correction for photon attenuation. Noise reduction is generally accomplished by the application of filters. The efficiency of rotating systems can be improved by incorporating additional detectors (most often two or three), which rotate around the patient. Virtually any organ in the body for which an appropriate radiopharmaceutical exists can be studied with SPECT techniques.

No overview of nuclear medicine would be complete without a brief description of positron emission tomography (PET) scanning. Positron-emitting radionuclides, such as carbon 11, nitrogen 13, oxygen 15, and fluorine 8 (a bioioteric substitution for hydrogen), are isotopes of elements that occur naturally in organic compounds. These tracers enter into the biochemical processes in the body so that blood flow; oxygen, glucose, and free fatty acid metabolism; amino acid transport; pH; and neuroreceptor densities can be measured. A positron is an antimatter electron. This positron-emitting radiopharmaceutical is distributed in a patient's system. As a positron is emitted, it travels several millimeters in tissue until it meets a free electron and annihilation occurs. Two gamma rays appear and are emitted 180 degrees apart from each other. A scintillation camera could be used to detect these gamma rays, but a collimator is not needed. Instead, the patient is surrounded by a ring of detectors. By electronically coupling opposing detectors to identify the pair of gamma rays simultaneously, the location where the annihilation event must have occurred (the coincidence) can be determined. The raw PET scan consists of a number of coincidence lines. Reconstruction could simply be the drawing of these lines as they would cross and superimpose wherever there is activity in the patient. In practice, the data set is reorganized into projections.

DIAGNOSTIC AND TREATMENT TECHNIQUES

Nuclear medicine is widely used in the diagnosis and prognosis of coronary artery disease, especially in conjunction with either physical stress testing (treadmill or bicycle exercise) or pharmacological stress testing. The patient is instructed to exercise on the treadmill until his or her heart rate has significantly increased. At peak exercise, a radioisotope, usually thallium 201 or technetium 99m, is injected into a vein. Stress images are obtained. Because the injected tracer corresponds to the blood flow through the arteries that supply oxygen to the heart muscle, those vessels that have a blockage exhibit decreased flow, or decreased tracer delivered to that area of the heart. Rest images are also obtained. Rest and stress images are compared, and differences in the intensity of the tracer, analyzed by a computer, help to identify blocked arteries and the extent of the blockage. This technique is also used in follow-up of patients who have undergone bypass surgery or angioplasty to determine if blockage has recurred.

Nuclear cardiology is also used to measure the ejection fraction (the amount of blood ejected by the left ventricle to all parts of the body) and motion of the heart. Patients with cardiomyopathy, coronary artery disease, or congenital heart disease often have decreased function of the heart. Certain medications used in cancer therapy can also damage the heart muscle. These patients are followed closely to determine if they are developing toxicity from their drug therapy. In these studies, commonly called MUGA scans, a small portion of the patient's blood is extracted. A radioactive tracer is tagged to this blood, which is then reinjected. The gamma camera takes motion pictures of the beating heart and, through the aid of computers, calculates the ejection fraction.

Nuclear medicine can be very helpful in locating primary or metastatic tumors throughout the body, and it is unique in its ability to assess the viability of a known lesion and its response to radiation or chemotherapy. Breast cancer, lymphomas (especially low-grade), differentiated thyroid cancer, and most sarcomas (both bone and soft tissue) are tumors that will metabolize the appropriate injected radiopharmaceutical. The resulting images will show increased localization in an active tumor but none in those masses that have been destroyed by treatment.

By injecting a radioisotope that has been tagged by bone-seeking agents, doctors can view images of an entire skeleton. Multiple fractures, metastatic disease, osteomyelitis, osteoporosis, and Paget's disease are but a few diseases that can be identified quickly and with minimal exposure of the patient to radiation.

Functional as well as anatomical information can be obtained by using nuclear medicine techniques to image the genitourinary tract, especially the kidneys. A perfusion study may be performed as the first phase of structural imaging. This study is done primarily to evaluate the vascularity (amount of blood vessels) of renal (kidney) masses. Cystic lesions and abscesses are usually avascular (having few or no blood vessels), and tumors are usually moderately or highly vascular. Uncommonly occurring arteriovenous (A-V) malformations show high vascularity. An evaluation of blood flow may also be important in patients who have received a kidney transplant. Anatomical renal imaging is performed to evaluate the position, size, and shape of the kidneys. Renal function studies have proven to be very sensitive in the diagnosis of both bilateral and unilateral kidney disease. By following specific tracers through the kidneys, doctors are able to evaluate the filtration by the glomeruli (capillary tufts) and the function of the tubules. Radionuclide cystography (imaging of the bladder), although not performed routinely, is extremely useful in diagnosing vesicoureteral reflux (urine reflux from the bladder back to the ureters), a relatively common problem in children.

Radionuclide imaging plays a significant role in the diagnosis of disease involving the gastrointestinal tract. Swallowing function, esophageal transit, gastroesophageal reflux, gastric emptying, gallbladder function, pulmonary aspiration of liver disease, and gastrointestinal bleeding can all be evaluated with nuclear medicine. The application of radioactive materials in the endocrine system provides historical benchmarks in the field of nuclear medicine with the use of radioiodine to assess the dynamic function of the thyroid gland. Radioiodine uptake testing is important and useful in the diagnosis of thyroid disease, specifically hyperthyroidism and hypothyroidism, thyroiditis, and goiters. Thyroid imaging is employed for the detection and functional evaluation of solitary or multiple thyroid nodules and the evaluation of aberrant thyroid tissue, metastases of thyroid cancer, and other tumors containing thyroid tissue.

The therapeutic value of nuclear medicine is best demonstrated in its role in the treatment of Graves' disease, toxic adenoma, toxic multinodular goiter, and metastatic thyroid carcinoma. The purpose of the therapeutic application of radioiodine to hyperthyroidism (an overactive thyroid) is to control the disease and return the patient to a normal state. The accumulation and retention of radioiodine, with the subsequent radiation effects upon the thyroid cells, underlie the basic principle behind radionuclide therapy. The treatment of thyroid carcinoma with radioiodine is directed toward the control of metastatic foci and palliation of patients with thyroid carcinoma. Not all thyroid tumors localize radioiodine. Therefore, care must be taken for proper patient selection by assuring a tumor's response to iodine.

Monoclonal antibody imaging has become important not only diagnostically but therapeutically as well. Antibodies with perfect specificity for antigens of interest—in this case, malignancies—are produced. These antibodies are labeled with a large dose of radioactivity and injected into the patient. This "magic bullet" is then directed only to the antigen-producing areas. As in thyroid treatment, the radiation effect destroys only those cells to which the radioactivity is attached, leaving the noncancerous cells undamaged. Although this treatment is primarily a research protocol, the future role of radioactive monoclonal antibodies in the treatment of malignant disorders could be significant.

Clinical applications of PET scanning have focused on three areas: cardiology, oncology, and neurology/psychiatry. The principal clinical utility of PET in cardiology lies primarily in accurately differentiating infarcted, scarred tissue from myocardium, which is viable but not contracting because of a reduced blood supply. PET offers a noninvasive procedure to distinguish tissue viability, which allows more accurate patient selection for surgery and angioplasty than conventional approaches. In cancer cases, PET can determine cellular viability and the growth of tumor tissue. It can directly measure the effectiveness of a given radiation or chemotherapy regimen on the metabolic process within the tumor. PET can differentiate tumor regrowth from radiation necrosis.

Because of the unique ability of PET scanning to assess metabolic function, it can aid in the diagnosis of dementia and other psychoses as well as offer possible effective treatment of these disorders. PET is also helpful in detecting the origin of seizures in patients with complex epilepsy and can be used to locate the lesion prior to surgical intervention. Strokes are the third most common cause of death in the United States. A total of 1.6 million people are affected, 40 percent of whom are in need of special services. PET can determine the viability of brain tissue, permitting the clinician to select the most effective (and least invasive and expensive) form of treatment.

Nuclear imaging techniques are quite safe. Allergic reactions to isotopes are essentially nonexistent. In fact, the few that have been reported can be traced back to a contaminant in the injected dose. The radiation burden is far less than that of fluoroscopic radiographic examination and is equal to that of one chest X ray, regardless of the picture produced.

PERSPECTIVE AND PROSPECTS

Natural radioactivity was discovered in the late 1800's. The first medical success with a radioisotope was Robert Abbe's treatment of an exophthalmic goiter with radon in 1904. In 1934, the Joliot-Curies produced artificial radioisotopes, specifically phospho-

rus 32. In 1938, Glenn T. Seaborg synthesized iodine 131. Phosphorus 32 was used to treat chronic leukemia and iodine 131 to treat thyroid cancer. Both treatments fell victim to radiation hysteria fueled by the aftermath of World War II and the dropping of the atomic bomb on Hiroshima. For a decade, nuclear medicine was equated with the "atomic cocktail" and was used only sporadically as a therapeutic modality. In 1949, the first gamma camera was introduced by Benjamin Cassen. It was called a "tap scanner" because as it measured radioactivity, it would tap ink on a piece of paper. The intensity of the ink mark was directly proportional to the radioactivity that was being scanned. The first nuclear medicine image was that of a thyroid gland.

Although discovered in the late 1930's, the imaging properties of the short-lived technetium 99m were not understood until the early 1960's. The six-hour half-life and its chemical properties were ideally suited to imaging with the newly introduced scintillation camera in 1965. From that time on, nuclear medicine grew in its role as a diagnostic tool, with technetium agents becoming the primary radiopharmaceuticals employed in the detection of disease.

With the addition of computers and array processors to the technology, tomographic imaging is becoming increasingly useful in the localization and quantification of disease states. Improved body attenuation correction and computerized three-dimensional imaging enable physicians to quantify the size and extent of abnormalities quite accurately. When one examines the relative role and costs of a transmission computed tomography (CT) scanning versus SPECT, a number of factors must be kept in mind. On the side of advantage of SPECT are the low costs compared to CT scanning. Additionally, no contrast is required in the SPECT study, which lessens the chance of adverse patient reaction. CT scanning is still primarily an anatomic diagnostic tool, while SPECT, by employing physiological radiopharmaceuticals, demonstrates the functional features of organs. By repeated imaging during the course of treatment, minute changes in the physiologic biochemical process can be detected and appropriately addressed.

Because of the physiologic nature of nuclear medicine, the development of radiopharmaceuticals to detect other disease states is essential for further growth in this field. It is interesting that much activity in this area is now centered on the treatment of diseases, primarily malignant ones. It seems as if radiation phobia has run its course and researchers will be permitted to develop the "magic bullet" that will target only those cells that it has been programmed to destroy. As PET scanning becomes more frequently used, new positron radiopharmaceuticals will be introduced. Theoretically, all biochemical reactions in the body can be imaged, if the proper radiopharmaceutical is produced.

Much of the human body can now be visualized employing anatomic, physiologic, or biochemical modalities. Nuclear medicine minimized its original emphasis on therapy and developed a new form of physician diagnosis, a physiological radiology now called imaging. This all goes back to an offhand remark made by Hippocrates to a student: "You really ought to look at a patient before making a diagnosis."

—Lynne T. Roy

See also Biophysics; Imaging and radiology; Invasive tests; Magnetic resonance imaging (MRI); Noninvasive tests; Nuclear radiology; Positron emission tomography (PET) scanning; Radiation therapy; Radiopharmaceuticals.

FOR FURTHER INFORMATION:

Bernier, D. R., P. E. Christian, J. K. Langan, and J. D. Wells, eds. *Nuclear Medicine Technology and Techniques*. St. Louis: C. V. Mosby, 1989. A comprehensive text which encompasses the spectrum of nuclear medicine technology from basic and applied mathematics, physics, chemistry, and biology to the details of performance and principles of interpretation of individual nuclear medicine procedures, regulations, and patient care.

Brucer, Marshall. *A Chronology of Nuclear Medicine*. St. Louis: Heritage, 1990. In an immensely enjoyable book, the author traces the history of nuclear medicine from the 1600's, when Robert Boyle defined a new intellectual discipline that would eventually be called "science," through the April 28, 1986, Chernobyl nuclear accident in the Soviet Union.

Iskandrian, Abdulmassih S. *Nuclear Cardiac Imaging: Principles and Applications*. Philadelphia: F. A. Davis, 1987. Many strides have occurred in the field of nuclear cardiology since the 1970's. These developments have had considerable impact on reshaping the entire field of cardiovascular medicine. This book provides an in-depth analysis of relevant pathophysiologic concepts and the results of the most commonly available cardiac imaging modalities.

Iturralde, Mario P. *Dictionary and Handbook of Nuclear Medicine and Clinical Imaging*. Boca Raton, Fla.: CRC Press, 1990. This medical dictionary provides overview information to those readers unfamiliar with the field of nuclear medicine science and clinical imaging. Clear definitions of terms are provided in an easy-to-use reference.

Taylor, Andrew, David M. Schuster, and Naomi P. Alazraki. *A Clinician's Guide to Nuclear Medicine*. Reston, Va: Society of Nuclear Medicine, 2000. Aimed at the medical professional, this handy guide covers many aspects of nuclear medicine. Includes bibliographical references and an index.

NUCLEAR RADIOLOGY
PROCEDURE

ANATOMY OR SYSTEM AFFECTED: Bones, brain, glands, kidneys, musculoskeletal system, nervous system

SPECIALTIES AND RELATED FIELDS: Nuclear medicine, radiology

DEFINITION: The use of radiopharmaceuticals for the diagnosis of disease and the assessment of organ function.

KEY TERMS:

collimator: a device that directs photons into a crystal for their detection

gamma camera: a system composed of a cesium-iodide crystal, collimator, and computer which is used to detect radioactivity and create an image of its distribution

radioisotope: a radioactive atom

radiopharmaceutical: the combined form of a pharmaceutical labeled with a radioisotope

INDICATIONS AND PROCEDURES

Nuclear radiology, also known as nuclear medicine, is similar to conventional radiology in that radiation is used to look inside the patient's body. Unlike conventional radiology, however, nuclear radiology looks not only at the anatomy of the patient but also at the functioning of the organ of interest. In conventional radiology (X rays), the radiation or X-ray photon is produced by accelerating electrons, elemental negative charges, up to 50,000 to 125,000 volts and then ramming them into a metal anode. The physical act of stopping the electrons causes about 0.2 percent of the electrons to give off the accelerating energy as packets of energy called photons. This radiation is then directed by the lead housing of the X-ray tube toward the patient. The radiation transmitted through the patient is then recorded on either film or an image-intensifying tube. Nuclear radiology differs from conventional radiology because there is no X-ray tube generating the radiation. The radiation comes from the pharmaceuticals injected into the patient. The source of the radiation is from a radioactive atom attached to a pharmaceutical (therapeutic drug). The physiological action and distribution of the pharmaceutical determines the diagnostic ability of the radiation given to the patient. The radiation can be emitted in any direction from the atom. The radiation, which travels in the direction of a piece of cesium-iodine crystal and through a collimator or set of lead holes, is detected. The cesium-iodine crystal with the accompanying computer is known as a gamma camera.

The radioactive atom currently used in most nuclear radiology departments is an isotope of technetium. The isotope is in a semistable state known as a metastable state. When it becomes unstable and decays, it emits a single photon with the energy equivalent of that of an electron accelerated in a 140,000 volt potential (140 keV). After the emission of this single photon, the technetium atom is nonradioactive. The number of photons given off is dependent on the number of technetium atoms present in the metastable state. The time required for half of those present to emit the photons is called its half-life. The half-life of technetium is 6.02 hours. Because of its ease of production and reasonable half-life, technetium is used in many pharmaceuticals.

Specialty isotopes are also used. Gaseous isotope of xenon 133 is used for some lung studies. Xenon has a more complicated decay than does technetium. Xenon decays by release of an energetic electron to unstable states of cesium 133. Cesium 133 gives off six gamma rays, with the predominate one being 80.9 keV. The half-life of xenon is 5.31 days. Xenon, being a noble gas, is chemically inert.

An isotope that can be used without being attached to a pharmaceutical is thallium 201. Thallium can be used in cardiac studies since it is readily taken up in the cardiac tissue. When thallium 201 decays, it becomes mercury 201. As mercury 201 becomes stable, it gives off high-energy X rays and gamma rays with the predominant energy being between 68.8 and 80 keV. Iodine is another isotope that does not necessarily need to be attached to a pharmaceutical. The three isotopes of iodine used are iodine 123, 125, or 131. All give off gamma rays that can be detected, pre-

dominant being 159.1, 35.4, and 364.4 keV, respectively. Iodine 131 also gives off energetic electrons when it decays and as such is used when energetic electrons are desired for therapy purposes. The emission of energetic electrons can damage surrounding tissues. Iodine 123 and iodine 125 decay by absorbing an electron from the atom and only emit gamma rays. The use of one over the other depends on the cost, with iodine 123 more costly because of its 13-hour half-life. Iodine 125 has a half-life of 60.2 days. Iodine 131 has a half-life of 8.06 days. Other isotopes are used for specialty purposes, such as chromium 51, which can be used to attach to red blood cells. Chromium has a half-life of 27.7 days, with a predominant gamma emission of 320 keV.

A collimator is employed to force only the radiation from the front of the crystal through a known path to be detected. A collimator can consist of a piece of metal, usually lead, with one or multiple holes. The size and length of the hole determine the number of photons that will reach the crystal. The collimator works because it absorbs the photons that are not directed along the axis of the hole. The higher the energy of the photon being directed, the thicker the sides of the holes, known as septa, must be. The smaller the hole, the better the spatial resolution and ease of detecting small concentrations of the isotope of interest. The longer the hole, the better defined the path will be from the crystal face out through the hole to the patient. The limitations of the size and length are dictated by the need to detect sufficient number of photons to give a diagnostic result. Unlike conventional radiology, in which the films are acquired in a short time (usually a fraction of a second), nuclear radiology can require fifteen to thirty minutes or more to acquire enough photons for a clinician to make a diagnostic determination.

PERSPECTIVE AND PROSPECTS

The main organs that nuclear medicine studies are blood, brain, heart, thyroid gland, parathyroid glands, liver, kidneys, lungs, and bones. Blood studies use several different pharmaceuticals and radioisotopes depending on what is being measured. These studies involve the measurement of the blood volume or blood filtration. Brain studies use technetium with several different pharmaceuticals. Some pharmaceuticals will not pass the blood-brain barrier and can be used to detect bleeding in the cranial compartment. Others pass easily through the blood-brain barrier and can be used to detect sections of the brain that are either hyperactive or hypoactive. Heart studies are involved in determining the health of the cardiac muscles. By the use of thallium and new, additional technetium-labeled pharmaceuticals, the viability of heart tissue after a heart attack can be assessed, along with the thickness of cardiac structures such as the septa between the right and left ventricles. Other properties such as the filling and ejection fractions can be determined in this study. Thyroid studies look at the size and location and are easiest to use with iodine isotopes. A different thallium-labeled radiopharmaceutical can be used to look at the same properties of the parathyroid glands. Liver studies involve the determination of areas that are not functioning and that are revealed as voids on a scan. These pharmaceuticals use technetium as the labeled isotope. Kidney studies, which determine whether the kidneys are filtering the blood properly and in sufficient quantities, use technetium as the labeled isotope. Lund studies determine if all the lobes of the lungs are filling properly by using inhalation isotope of xenon or aerosol compounds labeled with technetium. The health of the alveoli can be determined by introduction of a radiopharmaceutical that congregates in the alveolar space. Bone studies are involved in determining whether new bone is being formed.

—*Anthony J. Wagner, Ph.D.*

See also Biophysics; Imaging and radiology; Invasive tests; Magnetic resonance imaging (MRI); Nuclear medicine; Positron emission tomography (PET) scanning; Radiation therapy; Radiopharmaceuticals.

FOR FURTHER INFORMATION:

Saha, Gopal B. *Physics and Radiobiology of Nuclear Medicine.* New York: Springer, 2000. A textbook and study guide for medical residents preparing to take the American Board of Radiology examination, especially those specializing in nuclear radiology. Reviews the fundamental physics of radiology, the instrumentation, radiobiology, dosimetry, and safety regulations.

Sorenson, James A., and Michael E. Phelps. *Physics in Nuclear Medicine.* 2d ed. Orlando, Fla.: Grune & Stratton, 1987. This excellent book covers the necessary physical principles in detail for an understanding of radionuclide properties and the nuclear medicine instrumentation techniques for imaging. The authors have considerable experience in this field.

NUMBNESS AND TINGLING
DISEASE/DISORDER

ANATOMY OR SYSTEM AFFECTED: Legs, muscles, musculoskeletal system, nerves, nervous system, skin

SPECIALTIES AND RELATED FIELDS: Neurology, physical therapy

DEFINITION: Abnormalities of sensation that are attributable to nerve damage or disorders.

Symptoms. Patients commonly report various sensory aberrations that are often described as "pins and needles," tingling, prickling, burning of varying severity, or sensations resembling electric shock. The accepted term for these symptoms is "paresthesias" or "dysesthesias." When severe enough to be painful, they can be referred to as painful paresthesias.

The other major sensory symptom is a reduction or loss of feeling in an area of skin. Most patients use the relatively unambiguous term "numbness"; however, the more formal medical term is "hypesthesia." Paresthesias and hypesthesias are usually restricted to a part rather than all of the cutaneous territory of a damaged root or nerve.

The distribution of nonparesthetic pain is seldom as anatomically specific as the paresthesias themselves. Patients with carpal tunnel syndrome, for example, often have arm and shoulder pain that suggests compression of a cervical root rather than of the distal median nerve (a combined motor and sensory nerve). The paresthesias, by contrast, are usually localized to the tips of the fingers innervated by the median nerve. Similarly, in patients with cervical or lumbosacral radiculopathies (any diseased condition of the roots of spinal nerves), the distribution of pain in the upper or lower limbs often correlates poorly with the root involved. The paresthesias, however, are felt usually either along the entire area or, more commonly, in the distal part of the skin area innervated by the damaged root (the dermatome).

Examination. In attempting to localize the site of a lesion, the physician innervates major muscles from the spinal nerve roots (myotomes) through the plexuses, the individual peripheral nerves and their branches, and also the cutaneous areas supplied by each of these components of the peripheral nervous system. Traditionally, the site of the lesion can be deduced from which muscles and nerves are involved and from where the various branches of the peripheral nerves arise.

In motor examination, the muscles and tendon reflexes are examined first because weakness and reflex changes are often easier to elicit than are sensory signs. The muscles are first examined for atrophy. Since muscles become atrophic when denervated, the focal atrophy can sometimes identify accurately a nerve lesion. The lack of atrophy in a weak muscle either indicates an upper motor neuron lesion or raises the suspicion of spurious weakness. A systematic examination of individual muscles is then performed.

In sensory examination, the patient describes the area of sensory abnormality, which often tells as much as a formal examination. Testing light touch with the examiner's finger is frequently all that is required for confirmation. If this reveals no abnormality, retesting with a pin may disclose an area of sensory deficit. Pinpricks in normal and abnormal areas are compared.

It is important to examine the entire course of an affected nerve for bone, joint, or other abnormalities that may be causing the nerve damage. Local tenderness of the nerve and/or a positive Tinel's sign (paresthesias produced in the area of the nerve when the nerve is tapped or palpated) may also help to identify the site. Many normal persons experience mild tingling when nerves such as the ulnar at the elbow or the median at the wrist are tapped lightly, so this finding is significant only when the nerve is very sensitive to light percussion. Conversely, a badly damaged nerve may be totally insensitive to percussion or palpation.

Nerve conduction studies and the electromyographic examination of muscles evaluate the function of large-diameter, rapidly conducting motor and sensory nerve fibers. These two complementary techniques are valuable tools in the accurate assessment of focal peripheral neuropathies, helping in the localization of the nerve lesion and the assessment of its severity.

Diagnosis. Peripheral nerves causing sensory symptoms may be damaged anywhere along their course from the spinal cord to the muscles and skin that they innervate. The site of a focal neuropathy (the focus of neurologic disease) may therefore be in the nerve roots, the spinal nerves, the ventral or dorsal rami (branches), the plexuses (network of nerves), the major nerve trunks, or their individual branches. The character, site, mode of onset, spread, and temporal profile of sensory symptoms must be established and precipitating or relieving factors identified. These features—

and the presence of any associated symptoms—help identify the origin of sensory disturbances, as do the physical signs. Sensory symptoms or signs may conform to the territory of individual peripheral nerves or nerve roots. Involvement of one side of the body, or of one limb in its entirety, suggests a central lesion. Distal involvement of all four extremities suggests polyneuropathy (several neurologic disorders), a cervical cord or brain-stem lesion, or, when symptoms are transient, a metabolic disturbance such as hyperventilation syndrome. Short-lived sensory complaints may be indicative of sensory seizures or cerebral ischemic phenomena (local and temporal deficiency of blood supply caused by obstruction of the circulation to a part) as well as metabolic disturbances. In patients with cord lesions, there may be a transverse sensory level. Dissociated sensory loss is characterized by the loss of some sensory modalities and the preservation of others. Such findings may be encountered in patients with either peripheral or central disease and must therefore be interpreted in the clinical context in which they are found.

The absence of sensory signs in patients with sensory symptoms does not mean that symptoms have a nonorganic basis. Symptoms are often troublesome before signs of sensory dysfunction have had time to develop.

—*Genevieve Slomski, Ph.D.*

See also Carpal tunnel syndrome; Nervous system; Neuralgia, neuritis, and neuropathy; Neurology; Neurology, pediatric; Pain; Sense organs; Spinal cord disorders; Spine, vertebrae, and disks.

FOR FURTHER INFORMATION:

Bellenir, Karen, ed. *Back and Neck Disorders Sourcebook.* Detroit: Omnigraphics, 1997. A reference for lay readers on the causes and consequences of spinal cord disorders, recognizing symptoms, current treatment options, prevention strategies, and sources of help.

Mathers, Lawrence H. *The Peripheral Nervous System: Structure, Function, and Clinical Correlations.* Menlo Park, Calif.: Addison-Wesley, 1985. Discusses diseases of the peripheral nervous system. Includes bibliographical references and an index.

Rothman, Richard H., and Frederick Simeone. *The Spine.* 3d ed. Philadelphia: W. B. Saunders, 1992. Discusses diseases and abnormalities of the spine and evaluates surgical remedies. Includes bibliographical references and an index.

NURSING

SPECIALTY

ANATOMY OR SYSTEM AFFECTED: All

SPECIALTIES AND RELATED FIELDS: Critical care, emergency medicine, geriatrics and gerontology, neonatology, nutrition, pediatrics, perinatology, preventive medicine, public health

DEFINITION: A helping profession which focuses on the care of the sick and disabled and on the maintenance of the health and well-being of all individuals.

KEY TERMS:

assessment: the systematic process of collecting, validating, and communicating patient data; these data will include information gathered from the patient's history and from physical examination and laboratory test results

healing: the restoration to a normal physical, mental, or spiritual condition

health: a condition in which all functions of the body, mind, and spirit are normally active

holistic: the philosophy that individuals function as complete units or integrated systems and are not understood merely through their parts

illness: the condition of being sick or diseased

nurture: the act or process of raising or promoting development and well-being

service: work done or duty performed for another or others

treatment: any specific procedure used for the cure or improvement of a disease or pathological condition

THE ROLE OF NURSING

It is difficult at times to distinguish nursing from medicine, since there are so many ways in which they interrelate. Whereas some people think that nursing began with Florence Nightingale (1820-1910), nursing is as old as medicine itself. Throughout history, there have been periods when the two fields functioned interdependently and times when they were practiced separately from each other. It seems likely that the role of the mother-nurse would have preceded the magician-priest or medicine man. Even the seeds of medical knowledge were sown by the natural remedies used by the mother.

Over the course of human history, the words "nurse" and "nursing" have had many meanings, and the connotations have changed as tribes became highly developed and sophisticated nations. The word "nurse" comes from the Latin *nutrix*, which means "nursing mother." The word "nursing" originated from the Latin *nutrire*, meaning "to nourish." The word "nurse" as a noun was first used in the English language in the thirteenth century, being spelled "norrice," then evolving to "nurice" or "nourice," and finally to the present "nurse." The word "nurse" as a verb meant to suckle and to nourish. The meaning of both the noun and the verb have expanded to include more and more functions related to the care of all human beings. In the sixteenth century, the meaning of the noun included "a person, but usually a woman, who waits upon or tends the sick." By the nineteenth century, the meaning of the verb included "the training of those who tend the sick and the carrying out of such duties under the supervision of a physician."

With the origin of nursing as mother care came the idea that nursing was a woman's role. Suckling and nurturing were associated with maternal instincts. Ill or helpless children were also cared for by their mothers. The image of the nurse as a loving and caring mother remains popular. The true spirit of nursing, however, has no gender barriers. History has seen both men and women respond to the needs of the sick.

The role of the nurse has certainly expanded from that of the mother in the home, nourishing infants and caring for young children. Care of the sick, infirm, helpless, elderly, and handicapped and the promotion of health have become vital aspects of nursing as a whole. In history, the role of nursing developed with the culture and society of a given age. Tribal women practiced nursing as they cared for the members of their own tribes. As tribes developed into civilizations, nursing began to be practiced outside the home. As cultures developed, nursing care became more complex, and qualities other than a nurturing instinct were needed to do the work of a nurse. Members of religious orders, primarily those composed of women, responded by devoting their lives to study, service, and self-sacrifice in caring for the needs of the sick. These individuals were among the educated people of their time, and they helped set the stage for nursing to become an art and a science.

It was not until the nineteenth century that the basis of nursing as a profession was established. The beliefs and examples of Florence Nightingale laid that foundation. Nightingale was born in Italy in 1820, but she grew up in England. Unlike many of the children of her time, she was educated by governesses and by her father. Against the wishes of her family, she trained to be a nurse at the age of thirty-one. Amid enormous difficulties and prejudices, she organized and managed the nursing care for a military hospital in Turkey during the Crimean War. She returned to England after the war, where she established a school to train nurses. Again, she encountered great opposition, as nurses were considered little more than housemaids by the physicians of the time. Because of her efforts, the status of nurses was raised to a respected occupation, and the basis for professional nursing in general was established.

Nightingale's contributions are noteworthy. She recognized that nutrition is an important part of nursing care. She instituted occupational and recreational therapy for the sick and identified the personal needs of the patient and the role of the nurse in meeting those needs. Nightingale established standards for hospital management and a system of nursing education, making nursing a respected occupation for women. She recognized the two components of nursing: promoting health and treating illness. Nightingale believed that nursing is separate and distinct from medicine as a profession.

Nightingale's methods and the response of nursing to the Civil War casualties in the 1860's pointed out the need for nursing education in the United States. Schools of nursing were established, based on the values of Nightingale, but they operated more like an apprenticeship than an educational program. The schools were also controlled by hospital administrators and physicians.

Types of Nursing

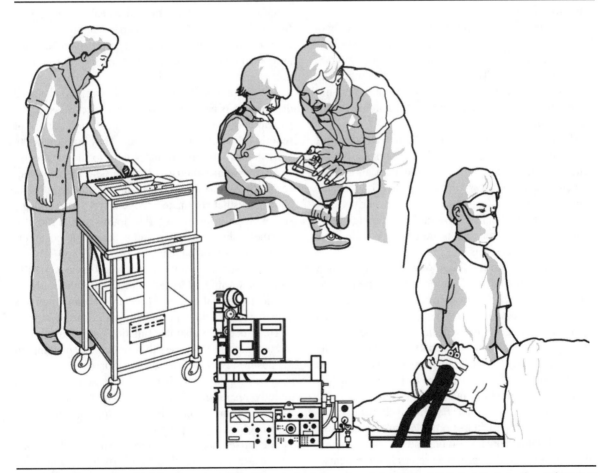

Nurses may become involved in many areas of health care, including the administration of diagnostic tests, the performance of physical examinations, and assistance during surgical procedures.

In 1896, nurses in the United States banded together to seek standardization of educational programs, to establish laws to ensure the competency of nurses, and to promote the general welfare of nurses. The outcome of their efforts was the American Nurses Association. In 1900, the first nursing journal publication, *The American Journal of Nursing*, was founded.

The impact of World War II also pointed out the need to base schools of nursing on educational objectives. Many women had responded to the need for nurses during the war. A great expansion in medical knowledge and technology had taken place, and the roles of nurses were expanding as well. Nursing programs developed in colleges and universities and offered degrees in nursing to both women and men.

While there were impressive changes in the expectations and styles with which nursing care has been delivered from ancient times to the twentieth century, the role and function of the nurse have been and continue to be diverse.

The nurse is a caregiver, providing care to patients based on knowledge and skill. Consideration is given to physical, emotional, psychological, socioeconomic, and spiritual needs. The role of the nurse-caregiver is holistic and integrated into all other roles that the nurse fulfills, thus maintaining and promoting health and well-being.

The nurse is a communicator. Using effective and therapeutic communication skills, the nurse strives to establish relationships to assist patients of all ages to manage and become responsible for their own health needs. In this way, the nurse is also a teacher who assists patients and families to meet their learning needs. Individualized teaching plans are developed and used to accomplish set goals.

The nurse is a leader. Based on the self-confidence gained from a nursing education and experience, the nurse is able to be assertive in meeting the needs of patients. The nurse facilitates change to improve care for patients, whether individually or in general. The nurse is also an advocate. Based on the belief that patients have a right to make their own decisions about health and life, the nurse strives to protect their human and legal rights in making those choices.

The nurse is a counselor. By effectively using communication skills, the nurse provides information, listens, facilitates problem-solving and decision-making abilities, and makes appropriate referrals for patients.

Finally, the nurse is a planner, a task that will call forth qualities far beyond nurturing and caring. In an age confronted with controversial topics such as abortion, organ transplants, the allocation of limited resources, and medical research, the role of nurses will continue to expand to meet these challenges in the spirit that allowed nursing to evolve and become a respected profession.

SCIENCE AND PROFESSION

While the nurse-mother of ancient times functioned within a very limited framework, the modern nurse has the choice of many careers within the nursing role. The knowledge explosion of the twentieth century has created many job specialties from which nurses can choose a career. The clinical nurse specialist is a nurse with experience, education, or an advanced degree in a specialized area of nursing. Some examples are enterostomal therapy, geriatrics, infection control, oncology, orthopedics, emergency room care, operating room care, intensive and coronary care, quality assurance, and community health. Nurses who function in such specialties carry out direct patient care; teach patients, families, and staff members; act as consultants; and sometimes conduct research to improve methods of care.

The nurse practitioner is a nurse with an advanced degree who is certified to work in a specific aspect of patient care. Nurse practitioners work in a variety of settings or in independent practice. They perform health assessments and give primary care to their patients.

The nurse anesthetist is a nurse who has also successfully completed a course of study in anesthesia. Nurse anesthetists make preoperative visits and assess patients prior to surgery, administer and monitor anesthesia during surgery, and evaluate the postoperative condition of patients.

The nurse midwife is a nurse who has successfully completed a midwifery program. The nurse midwife provides prenatal care to expectant mothers, delivers babies, and provides postnatal care after the birth.

The nurse administrator functions at various levels of management in the health care field. Depending on the position held, advanced education may be in business or hospital administration. The administrator is directly responsible for the operation and management of resources and is indirectly responsible for the personnel who give patient care.

The nurse educator is a nurse, usually with a master's degree, who teaches or instructs in clinical or educational settings. This nurse can teach both theory and clinical skills.

The nurse researcher usually has an advanced degree and conducts special studies that involve the collection and evaluation of data in order to report on and promote the improvement of nursing care and education.

DUTIES AND PROCEDURES

Creativity and education are the keys to keeping pace with continued changes and progress in the nursing profession. Nurses are expected to play many roles, function in a variety of settings, and strive for excellence in the performance of their duties. A service must be provided that contributes to the health and well-being of people. The following examples of nursing—an operating room nurse and a home health nurse—provide a limited portrait of how nurses function and what roles they play in medical care.

Operating room nurses function both directly and indirectly in patient care and render services in a number of ways. Operating room nurses, usually known as circulating nurses, briefly interview patients upon their arrival to the operating room. They accompany patients to specific surgery rooms and assist in preparing them for surgical procedures. They are responsible for seeing that surgeons correctly identify patients prior to anesthesia. They are also directly attentive to patients when anesthesia is first administered.

Circulating nurses perform the presurgical scrub, which is a cleansing of the skin with a specified solution for a given number of minutes. It is their overall responsibility to monitor aseptic (sterile) techniques in certain areas of the operating room and to deal with the situation immediately if aseptic techniques are broken. They count the surgical sponges with surgical technologists before the first incision is made, throughout the procedure as necessary, and again before the incision is closed. They secure needed items requested by surgical technologists, surgeons, or anesthesia personnel: medications, blood, additional sterile instruments, or more sponges. At times, they prepare and assist with the operation of equipment used for surgeries, such as lasers, insufflators (used for laparoscopic surgery), and blood saver and reinfuser machines. They arrange for the transportation of specimens to the laboratory. They may also be instrumental in sending communications to waiting family members when the surgery takes longer than anticipated. When the surgery is completed, they accompany patients to the recovery room with the anesthesia personnel.

Home health nurses, on the other hand, function in a very different manner. This type of nurse usually works for a private home health services agency, or as part of an outreach program for home services through a hospital. Referrals come to the agency or program via the physician, through the physician's office, by way of the social services department in a hospital, or by an individual requesting skilled services through the physician.

The following scenario is an example of a patient whom a home health nurse may be requested to see: a seventy-six-year-old man who was hospitalized with a recent diagnosis of diabetes mellitus, for which he is now insulin-dependent. He also has an open wound on his right ankle. The number of days allowed for hospitalization for his diagnosis has expired, but he still needs help using a glucometer to take his blood sugar readings and assistance with drawing up his insulin. He still has questions about how to manage his diabetes, especially the dietary parameters. He is unable to manage the wound care on his right ankle. His wife is willing to assist him, but she has no knowledge about diabetes or wound care.

The home health nurse performs the following assessments on the initial visit: general physical condition, the patient's level of knowledge and understanding and his ability to manage his diabetic condition, all medications used, and the patient's understanding of the actions, side effects, and interactions of these medications. An assessment is made of the home setting in general: the patient's safety, the support system, and any special needs, such as assistive devices. If services such as physical therapy, occupational therapy, or speech therapy are needed, the nurse makes these referrals. If the patient requires additional in-home services, a referral to a medical social worker is made. Wound care is performed, and the nurse will then set up a plan of care, with the patient's input, for follow-up visits. Guidelines requested by the physician, as well as approval needed by health insurance companies covering the cost for home health services, will be taken into consideration when planning ongoing visits. If the home health agency has a nurse who is a diabetic specialist, the nurse can either consult with that specialist about the care of this patient or have the diabetic specialist make a home visit.

PERSPECTIVE AND PROSPECTS

From the beginning of time, nursing and the role of the nurse have been defined by the people and the society of a particular age. Nursing as it is known today is still influenced by what occurred over the centuries.

In primitive times, people believed that illness was supernatural, caused by evil gods. The roles of the physician and the nurse were separate and unrelated. The physician was a medicine man, sometimes called a shaman or a witch doctor, who treated disease by ritualistic chants, by fear or shock techniques, or by boring holes into a person's skull with a sharp stone to allow the evil spirit or demon an escape. The nurse, on the other hand, was usually the mother who tended to family members and provided for their physical needs, using herbal remedies when they were ill.

As tribes evolved, the centers for medical care were temples. Some tribes believed that illness was caused by sin and the displeasure of gods. The physician of this age was a priest and was held in high regard. The nurse was a woman, seen as a slave, who performed menial tasks ordered by the priest-physician. There was no respect for either women or human life.

Living in the same era were Hebrew tribes who used the Ten Commandments and the Mosaic Health Code to develop standards for ethical human relationships, mental health treatment, and disease control. Nurses visited the sick in their homes, practiced as midwives, and provided for the physical and spiritual needs of family members who cared for the ill. These nurses provided a family-centered approach to care.

With the advent of Christianity, the value of the individual was emphasized, and the responsibility for recognizing the needs of each individual emerged. Nursing gained an elevated position in society. A spiritual foundation for nursing was established as well. The first organized visiting of the sick was done by deaconesses and Christian Roman matrons of the time. Members of male religious orders also cared for the sick and buried the dead.

During the time of the Crusades, there were both male and female nursing orders, and nursing at this time was a respected vocation. Men usually belonged to military nursing orders, who cared for the sick, on one hand, and defended the building when under attack, on the other. In medieval times, hospitals became a place to keep, not cure, patients. There were no methods of infection control. Nursing care was largely custodial, and the practice of accepting individuals of low character to supplement inadequate nursing staffs became common.

The worst era in nursing history was probably from 1500 to 1860. Nursing at this time was not a respected profession. Women who had committed a crime were sent into nursing as an alternative to serving a jail term. Nurses received poor wages and worked long hours under deplorable conditions. Changes in the Reformation and the Renaissance did little or nothing to improve the care of the sick. The attitude prevailed that nursing was a religious and not an intellectual occupation. Charles Dickens quite aptly portrayed the nurse and nursing conditions of the time through his immortal caricatures of Sairey Gamp and Betsey Prig in *Martin Chuzzlewit* (1843-1844).

It was not until the middle of the nineteenth century, when the works of Florence Nightingale revolutionized nursing care in a military hospital in Turkey, that this situation began to change. She later became instrumental as an authority for nursing care and nursing management in England, Australia, the United States, and Canada. Nightingale also developed the first organized nurse training program, in spite of vehement physician opposition. The school, known as the Nightingale Training School for Nurses, opened in 1860 in England. Through her efforts, nursing became a respected occupation once more, the quality of nursing care improved tremendously, and the foundation was laid for modern nursing education.

As innovations in health care have an impact on nursing, nurses' roles will continue to expand in the future. Nursing can also be a background from which both men and women begin to bridge gaps of service where other affiliations are needed: computer science, medical-legal issues, health insurance agencies, and bioethics, to name a few. The words of Florence Nightingale still echo as a challenge to the nursing profession:

> May the methods by which every infant, every human being will have the best chance of health, the methods by which every sick person will have the best chance of recovery, be learned and practiced! Hospitals are only an intermediate state of civilization never intended, at all events, to take in the whole sick population.

Nursing will continue to meet this challenge to improve the quality of health care around the world.

—*Karen A. Mattern*

See also Aging: Extended care; Allied health; Anesthesiology; Cardiac rehabilitation; Critical care; Critical care, pediatric; Emergency medicine; Geriatrics and gerontology; Holistic medicine; Hospitals;

Immunization and vaccination; Neonatology; Nursing; Nutrition; Pediatrics; Physical examination; Physician assistants; Preventive medicine; Surgical procedures; Surgical technologists; Terminally ill: Extended care.

FOR FURTHER INFORMATION:

Dolan, Josephine A., M. Louise Fitzpatrick, and Eleanor K. Herrmann. *Nursing in Society: A Historical Perspective.* 15th ed. Philadelphia: W. B. Saunders, 1983. A concise yet systematic history of nursing for those who wish to orient themselves in this field without having to explore extensive and detailed documents.

Donahue, M. Patricia. *Nursing: The Finest Art.* 2d ed. St. Louis: C. V. Mosby, 1996. A presentation of the proud heritage of nursing. Describes the emergence of nursing using a global approach. The text is accompanied by reprints of paintings, photographs, and other illustrations pertinent to nursing, making it a breathtaking photojournalistic work.

Taylor, Carol, Carol Lillis, and Priscilla LeMone, eds. *Fundamentals of Nursing.* Philadelphia: J. B. Lippincott, 1989. A textbook that intends to capture the unique essence of both the art and the science of nursing. Distills what the person beginning the study of nursing needs to know and presents this information in a straightforward manner.

NUTRITION

SPECIALTY

ANATOMY OR SYSTEM AFFECTED: Gastrointestinal system, glands, hair, intestines, mouth, nails, stomach, teeth

SPECIALTIES AND RELATED FIELDS: Alternative medicine, biochemistry, exercise physiology, family practice, gastroenterology, geriatrics and gerontology, gynecology, internal medicine, pediatrics, preventive medicine, psychology, public health

DEFINITION: The study of those substances found in foods that are needed by the body for maintenance, growth, and repair, as well as those substances that increase the risk of disease.

KEY TERMS:

essential nutrient: a substance that must be included in the diet because it cannot be synthesized by the body

kilocalorie: the unit of measurement of food energy; a kilocalorie is the amount of heat needed to raise the temperature of one kilogram of water one degree Celsius; also known as a Calorie

nutrients: substances needed by the body for maintenance, growth, and repair; the six classes of nutrients are carbohydrates, fats, proteins, vitamins, minerals, and water

recommended daily (or dietary) allowance (RDA): the amount of nutrients needed daily by a healthy person to maintain health; age and gender affect the listed RDAs

SCIENCE AND PROFESSION

The science of nutrition studies the intake, digestion, absorption, and utilization of foods in the body. The goal of this research is to identify disorders caused by dietary deficiencies or imbalances and to devise strategies to prevent or correct these conditions.

Nutritional research may involve several different methods of inquiry. Epidemiological studies allow researchers to investigate relationships between disorders in populations and dietary habits. The results are of value but must be interpreted carefully. For example, there is a correlation between the amount of meat consumed by a population and the incidence of colon cancer in members of that population. Diets that are high in meat are, however, often high in fat and low in vegetables, fruits, and fiber. If these factors are not considered, false conclusions may be drawn.

Data from human populations may suggest hypotheses that can be tested in animals. Such experiments provide researchers with an opportunity to control dietary factors in a way that would not be possible in human studies. In a typical study of this type, the control group of laboratory animals receives a complete diet. During the same time period, the experimental group receives an identical diet, with a single substance removed or added. Researchers then record any differences between the health of the experimental group and the health of the control group.

Conclusions drawn from animal testing may not always apply to human dietary needs. The species used in an experiment can influence the results. Some early vitamin C experiments used rabbits as test animals until it was discovered that rabbits can synthesize vitamin C. Guinea pigs, like humans, cannot synthesize vitamin C and therefore are more suitable for such experiments. Some animal research may conflict with human epidemiological data. Saccharin was nearly banned in the United States because experiments linked its use to bladder tumors in rats. After 100 years, however, little evidence linking its use to human cancer has been found, and it has been allowed to remain on the market as long as warnings are displayed on products containing it.

Another type of research analyzes the chemical and physical characteristics of nutrients and determines their amounts in various foods. Nutrients are divided into six classes based on their chemical composition: carbohydrates, lipids, proteins, vitamins, minerals, and water. Carbohydrates, lipids, and proteins provide energy that is used by the body, while vitamins, minerals, and water do not. An intake of 3,500 kilocalories more than the amount of energy used in metabolism and physical activity will result in a weight gain of one pound. Conversely, a deficit of kilocalories will result in a comparable weight loss.

The carbohydrate class is composed of sugars, starches, and fiber. Sugars and starches are digested and converted to glucose, the primary fuel used by cells for metabolic processes. Sugars, which are simple carbohydrates, are the quickest source of energy. A cup of sucrose (table sugar) provides about 770 kilocalories of energy but otherwise has little nutritional value. Other examples of sugars include maltose, dextrose, and fructose. Starches are complex carbohydrates and, if eaten in more natural form, have nutritional value in addition to their energy content. A cup of whole wheat flour provides 400 kilocalories of energy and is a source of vitamins and minerals. Fibers are substances taken primarily from plant cell walls that are too complex to be broken down by human digestive enzymes. Although not a source of energy, fiber is considered necessary for intestinal health.

Lipids include such compounds as fats, oils, and cholesterol. Saturated fats, which are solid at room temperature, generally are associated with meat and other animal products. Polyunsaturated fats, commonly called oils because they are liquid at room temperature, are generally derived from plant sources. Fats, a more concentrated source of energy than carbohydrates, contain 9 kilocalories per gram. A cup of oil, for example, would contain approximately 1,800 kilocalories. The human body can make most of the fats and oils it needs from carbohydrates and proteins. A small amount of dietary fat is necessary to supply essential fatty acids, which cannot be synthesized by the body. Although cholesterol is used by the body to make steroid hormones and other compounds, it is also manufactured by the body and therefore does not have to be supplied in the diet. Cholesterol is found in animal cell membranes; therefore, unlike fat, it cannot be trimmed from meat.

Proteins contain 4 kilocalories of energy per gram. Proteins are made up of many smaller molecules called amino acids. There are twenty amino acids that are used in different combinations and quantities to make up the proteins found in living organisms. Of these twenty, eight cannot be manufactured by the human body. Therefore, the right kind of protein, in sufficient amounts, must be included in the diet to provide these essential amino acids. While meat contains these, the proper combinations of foods from plants can also supply them.

Vitamins, which are less complex than carbohydrates, lipids, and proteins, are needed in very small amounts. Although not a source of energy, they are required in order to extract energy from glucose. The water-soluble vitamins (B complex and C) are absorbed and, after being dissolved in plasma, are carried to the tissues. Because they are excreted if not used within a matter of hours, sufficient amounts of water-soluble vitamins must be eaten daily. Excess amounts of fat-soluble vitamins (A, D, E, and K) settle out in fatty tissues of the body, so reserves of these vitamins can be maintained.

Minerals are elements or simple inorganic compounds. They perform a wide variety of functions in the body. Calcium, for example, is an important structural component of bones and teeth, and calcium ions are necessary to the processes of blood clotting and muscle contraction. Minerals are also needed to maintain the acid-base balance and support electrical activities in the body.

Water makes up approximately 60 percent of the weight of the body. Water, the primary component of plasma and tissue fluid, is needed to transport many materials throughout the body. The watery fluid surrounding the brain and spinal cord, and found in joint cavities, acts as a shock absorber. In molecular form, water is used in the chemical reactions of synthesis and digestion. A human can live without food for several weeks but may die in a matter of days without water.

DIAGNOSTIC AND TREATMENT TECHNIQUES

Nutritionists apply the information gathered by researchers when they design diets appropriate for individuals. Healthy individuals should follow diets that maintain the body and prevent nutritional deficiencies and other diseases. Individuals who are ill need to follow diets that will aid the healing process or that are directly related to the treatment of their diseases.

A deficiency disease is one in which the person has the pattern of symptoms associated with a lack of a specific nutrient. Diets containing inadequate amounts of a nutrient may result in subclinical deficiencies with minor changes in a person's health. For example, vitamin C is used by the immune system and is also needed to make collagen, a protein found in skin, bones, tendons, and other tissues. An individual with scurvy will not be able to maintain and repair these tissues. Thus, broken bones and wounds will not heal properly, and life-threatening infections can occur. A person with a subclinical deficiency may not be ill enough to seek medical help but will have wounds that heal slowly and have less resistance to infectious diseases. Adding foods, such as citrus fruits, or vitamin C supplements to the diet will cure scurvy and prevent its return.

Often, other dietary factors, illness, or medications will complicate a nutritional condition. The high amounts of folic acid found in vegetarian diets can mask a deficiency of vitamin B_{12}, which is found in meat. Vitamin B_{12} is needed both for the production of red blood cells and for the maintenance of the nervous system. Folic acid can maintain red blood cell production, resulting in normal blood tests, but nerve damage may occur because of the B_{12} deficiency. Some individuals have pernicious anemia, a disorder resulting from an inability to transfer vitamin B_{12} from the intestine into the bloodstream. In this case, ingesting the right food or vitamin supplement is ineffective; only vitamin B_{12} injections will adequately treat the disease.

The presence of an illness may change dietary needs and practices. A person with an infectious disease requires a nutrient-dense diet to strengthen his or her resistance to the disease; additional water intake helps to reduce fever and remove toxins from the body. Medications may also complicate dietary needs.

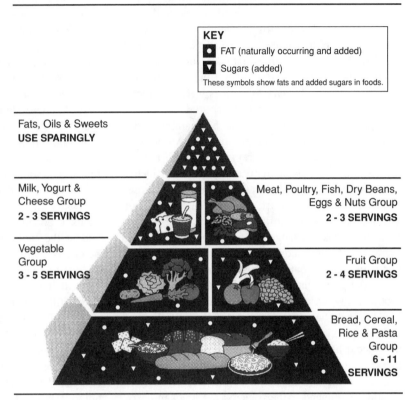

The Food Guide Pyramid

KEY
- FAT (naturally occurring and added)
- Sugars (added)

These symbols show fats and added sugars in foods.

Fats, Oils & Sweets
USE SPARINGLY

Milk, Yogurt & Cheese Group
2 - 3 SERVINGS

Meat, Poultry, Fish, Dry Beans, Eggs & Nuts Group
2 - 3 SERVINGS

Vegetable Group
3 - 5 SERVINGS

Fruit Group
2 - 4 SERVINGS

Bread, Cereal, Rice & Pasta Group
6 - 11 SERVINGS

For example, dairy products may block the action of antibiotics such as tetracycline.

Some diseases require a special diet as part of their treatment. Individuals with diabetes lack sufficient amounts of insulin to process sugar, and their blood glucose levels can rise to dangerous levels if dietary carbohydrates, especially sugars, are not limited. Phenylketonuria (PKU) is a genetic disorder resulting in an inability to process the amino acid phenylalanine. A diet low in phenylalanine must be followed to prevent the buildup of toxins in the body. Food allergies are controlled by removing the allergy-causing foods from the diet; however, care must be taken to replace lost nutrients. For example, a person who is allergic to milk and dairy products must ingest calcium from another source.

In developing countries, lack of food and nutritional deficiencies are serious health problems. In developed countries, the problem of nutritionally related diseases is based on food choice rather than on food availability. In 1989, *The Surgeon General's Report on Nutrition and Health* identified diet as a contributing factor in five of the ten leading causes of death in the United States: heart disease, cancer, stroke, diabetes, and atherosclerosis. Other conditions with dietary causes include osteoporosis, dental diseases, high blood pressure, and intestinal disorders. The typical Western diet is high in meat, fat, salt, sugars, and refined carbohydrates, and low in fruits, vegetables, and whole grains. Dietary guidelines were developed based on epidemiological and other studies.

First, a normal weight should be maintained by balancing energy intake and expenditure. An individual whose weight is 20 percent higher than normal for his or her sex, age, height, and build is considered obese. Obesity is a risk factor in arthritis, hypertension, diabetes, and heart disease. The source of kilocalories may also influence weight gain; dietary fat is more easily changed to fat in the human body. Increased physical activity is an important nondietary factor in weight control. An individual who is more than 10 percent underweight may also have health problems. When energy intake and fat stores are too low, the body begins to use protein from muscles and organs as an energy source. Dangerous weight loss may occur as a result of infectious diseases, chemotherapy, starvation diets, and eating disorders.

Second, the amount of dietary fat and cholesterol should be reduced. Atherosclerosis, a thickening of the arterial cell walls triggered by cholesterol, impedes blood flow throughout the body. As arterial diameters decrease, the blood pressure is raised. Heart disease results when the coronary arteries are affected, and strokes may occur if the arteries leading to the brain are blocked. The reduction of dietary cholesterol is important. Because the liver manufactures cholesterol in response to fat, however, the total dietary fat should make up less than 30 percent of the daily Calorie intake. An individual with other risk factors, such as a family history of heart disease or a sedentary lifestyle, must be especially careful of the amount of fat in the diet. High-fat diets are also associated with cancers of the breast and colon.

Third, there should be a dietary emphasis on foods containing complex carbohydrates and fibers, such as whole grains, fruits, and vegetables. Starches provide a steady source of energy and are less likely to cause blood glucose problems than are sugars. Fiber retains water in the intestine, which helps to move intestinal contents. Low-fiber diets increase pressure on the intestinal wall, contributing to constipation, hiatal hernias, and diverticulosis.

Fourth, a healthy diet includes little sugar in any form. Dental caries (cavities) and gum diseases are more likely to occur in people who have diets that are high in sugar. A high intake of sugar may result in an overproduction of insulin, causing an abrupt drop in blood sugar, a condition called reactive hypoglycemia. Excess dietary sugar also has been linked to some behavioral problems.

Fifth, there should be a reduction of dietary sodium. Sodium chloride (table salt), soy sauce, and monosodium glutamate (MSG), a flavor enhancer, are the most common sources of sodium. In ancient times, salt was a precious commodity because of its scarcity, but modern diets contain more salt than is necessary. Salt, which is found naturally in some foods, is added to food during processing, in cooking, and at the table. Certain high-risk groups, such as people of African ancestry and those with a family history of hypertension, should take special care to limit their sodium consumption.

Sixth, alcoholic beverages should be used in moderation, if at all. Alcohol is a toxin that must be neutralized by the liver. Niacin and thiamine are used in this process, and a person whose alcohol consumption interferes with nutrition may have the symptoms associated with deficiencies of these vitamins. Alcohol interferes with the processing of lipids, resulting in an accumulation of fat in the liver. If too much alcohol is ingested, the excess is released from the liver and transported in the bloodstream to the brain and other parts of the body. Although alcohol is not a nutrient, it contains 7 kilocalories of energy per gram and can contribute to obesity.

In summary, a healthy diet will include a wide variety of foods to achieve an appropriate balance, incorporating increased amounts of fruits, vegetables, and whole grains and maintaining adequate, but lower, amounts of high-fat animal and dairy products. This variety will ensure ingestion of the essential nutrients and decrease the risk of many chronic diseases.

Perspective and Prospects

In the sixteenth century, when explorers began to take longer trips at sea, scurvy became an occupational hazard. It was not unusual for a crew to lose more than half its number to scurvy and its complications. In the 1700's, a British physician discovered that citrus fruits or their juices could prevent and cure scurvy. By the end of that century, British ships were supplied with adequate citrus fruits to supply their crews during a long voyage. At that time, the mechanism by which the fruit acted to counteract scurvy was not known.

In 1876, stimulated by acceptance of the germ theory of disease, researchers focused their attention on microbiology. Because they were successful in finding microbial causes for many disorders, they were puzzled when some diseases did not fit this pattern. One of these, beriberi, was prevalent in countries where rice was "polished" by removing the hulls. A physician in Indonesia noticed that chickens that were fed polished rice developed beriberi, but those that were fed the hulls did not. He correctly deduced that it was not the presence of a microorganism but the absence of a component contained in rice hulls that caused the disorder. Changing the diet of the men in his care confirmed his conclusion. His findings led researchers to look for nutritional causes for other diseases.

While beriberi was being studied in Asia, public health authorities in the United States were concerned with the problem of pellagra. The symptoms of this disease included peeling skin, diarrhea, and mental illness. In the early 1900's, more than 10,000 people with pellagra died each year. The highest incidence occurred among people in the Southern states who depended on corn as their major source of food. Researchers thought that pellagra was caused by bacteria or molds in the corn. In the 1930's, researchers determined that corn was low in niacin; they found that pellagra was caused by a niacin deficiency and could be cured by administering niacin supplements.

Agencies of the United States government became involved in nutritional issues as part of public health concerns. Efforts have included both education and legislation. In 1917, the United States Department of Agriculture (USDA) published its first set of nutritional guidelines, *What the Body Needs*, which listed five food groups. As nutritional research continued, the guidelines were revised and an emphasis was placed on preventing nutritional deficiencies by including a variety of foods in the diet. In 1977, the U.S. Senate published *Dietary Goals for the U.S.*, which recommended weight control and the consumption of less fat, salt, cholesterol, and sugar. Subsequent publications have also emphasized the prevention of diseases associated with dietary excess and imbalance.

Legislation may also be enacted to alleviate nutritional problems. A 1936 survey determined that people who depended on white bread and pasta in their diets had a high incidence of several nutrient deficiencies. Chemical analysis determined that white flour, which has had the hull and bran removed, contains starch but few other nutrients. Based on these studies, Congress passed the Enrichment Act in 1942. This requires processors to add iron, thiamine, riboflavin, and niacin to refined flour products.

As consumers became more knowledgeable about healthy nutritional practices, they expressed concern about the misinformation or lack of information provided by food labels. In 1992, regulations were adopted that required more nutritional information on food labels. Now, consumers can compare the nutrients in a packaged food with their daily nutritional needs. The goal of such efforts is to educate the public regarding healthy dietary practices, to aid consumers in making wise choices, and to reduce the incidence of nutrition-based diseases.

—Edith K. Wallace, Ph.D.

See also Aging: Extended care; Anorexia nervosa; Antioxidants; Beriberi; Breast-feeding; Bulimia; Cardiac rehabilitation; Cholesterol; Digestion; Eating disorders; Enzyme therapy; Exercise physiology; Failure to thrive; Food biochemistry; Gastroenterology; Gastroenterology, pediatric; Gastrointestinal system; Gastrostomy; Geriatrics and gerontology; Hirschsprung's disease; Holistic medicine; Hypercholesterolemia; Jaw wiring; Kwashiorkor; Lactose intolerance; Lipids; Malabsorption; Malnutrition; Metabolism; Nursing; Obesity; Pinworm; Roundworm; Scurvy; Sports medicine; Supplements; Tapeworm; Taste; Tropical medicine; Ulcer surgery; Ulcers; Vagotomy; Veterinary medicine; Vitamins and minerals; Weaning; Weight loss and gain; Weight loss medications; Worms.

FOR FURTHER INFORMATION:

Foods That Harm, Foods That Heal: The A-Z Guide to Safe and Healthy Eating. Pleasantville, N.Y.: Reader's Digest, 1997. This source provides a practical listing of how to use nutritional choices to benefit one's health, as well as how to avoid common mistakes that can lead to illness.

Sizer, Frances Sienkiewicz, and Eleanor Noss Whitney. *Hamilton/Whitney's Nutrition: Concepts and Controversies.* Rev. 6th ed. St. Paul, Minn.: West, 1994. This widely used introductory college textbook is well written and enjoyable to read. The "concepts" sections provide information on nutrients and the nutritional needs of different age groups. The "controversy" essays focus on specific issues and present different viewpoints.

Spallholz, Julian E., L. Mallory Boylan, and Judy A. Driskell. *Nutrition: Chemistry and Biology.* Boca Raton, Fla.: CRC Press, 1999. This book is composed of seventeen chapters that are subdivided into seven sections, including macronutrients, micronutrients, bioavailability of nutrients, cellular metabolism, energy utilization, and metabolic aspects.

U.S. National Institutes of Health. *Diet, Nutrition, and Cancer Prevention.* Bethesda, Md.: National Institutes of Health, 1988. This brochure begins with a list of general guidelines for a healthy diet, then focuses on the relationship of diet to cancer. The inclusion of dietary fiber, cruciferous vegetables, and vitamins A and C is linked to lowered risk; high fat consumption is linked to increased risk.

U.S. Public Health Service. Office of the Surgeon General. *The Surgeon General's Report on Nutrition and Health.* Washington, D.C.: Government Printing Office, 1988. This book summarizes a 712-page government report for the general public. Conclusions and recommendations are based on a four-year examination of more than 2,500 scientific studies. Emphasizes the shift from the prevention of deficiencies to the prevention of chronic illnesses.

Vaughn, Lewis, Sharon Faelten, and William Gottlieb, eds. *The Complete Book of Vitamins and Minerals for Health.* Emmaus, Pa.: Rodale Press, 1988. Compiled by the editors of *Prevention* magazine, this book for the general reader includes not only vitamins and minerals but also detailed information on other nutrients, supplementation, special health problems, disease-prevention strategies, and recipes.

OBESITY

DISEASE/DISORDER

ANATOMY OR SYSTEM AFFECTED: Endocrine system, gastrointestinal system, glands, intestines, psychic-emotional system, skin, stomach

SPECIALTIES AND RELATED FIELDS: Endocrinology, family practice, internal medicine, nutrition, psychiatry, psychology

DEFINITION: A condition in which the body carries abnormal or unhealthy amounts of fat tissue, leading the individual to weigh in excess of 20 percent more than his or her ideal weight.

KEY TERMS:

adipose tissue: fat; a soft tissue of the body composed of cells (adipocytes) that contain triglyceride, a compound consisting of glycerol and fatty acids; in obesity, there may be increased numbers of adipocytes, and the cells may contain an increased amount of triglyceride

basal metabolic rate (BMR): the minimal energy expended for maintenance of the vegetative functions of the body (respiration, heat production, and so on), expressed as calories per hour per square meter of body surface

body mass index (BMI): weight in kilograms divided by height in meters, squared (kg/m^2); since this value is relatively independent of height and sex, the same standard values can be used for all adults, both men and women

Calorie: 1 kilocalorie, which is the amount of heat (energy) needed to raise the temperature of 1 kilogram of water by 1 degree Celsius

metabolism: the sum of the physical and chemical processes by which living matter is produced, maintained, and transformed

resting metabolic rate (RMR): similar to the BMR, but more easily measured (the subject is resting rather than in a truly basal state)

CAUSES AND SYMPTOMS

Obesity is a condition in which the body accumulates an abnormally large amount of adipose tissue. Fat normally makes up about 15 to 18 percent of body weight in young men, 20 to 25 percent in young women, and 30 to 40 percent in older adults. Because it is not practical to measure body fat content directly but it is easy to measure weight and height, the body mass index (BMI), which correlates closely with body fat, is often used to identify and quantify obesity.

To set a dividing line between the normal and the obese, medical professionals use the concept of ideal body weight. Statistics compiled by life insurance companies have revealed the body weight (depending on a given individual's height, sex, and frame size) that is associated with the lowest mortality rate; this figure is assumed to be the individual's ideal weight. Because health problems associated with obesity have been observed to increase significantly when body weight is more than 20 percent higher than ideal weight, or when the BMI exceeds 27, obesity is often defined by these limits. If these criteria are used, it is estimated that about 23 percent of men and 30 percent of women in the United States are obese.

An important function of adipose tissue is to store energy. If the intake of energy, in the form of food calories (usually measured in kilocalories, or Calories), is greater than the expenditure of energy, then the excess calories are stored, mainly in the adipose tissue, with a resulting gain in weight. Expenditure of energy depends largely on the resting metabolic rate or resting energy expenditure, defined as the calories used each day to maintain normal body metabolism. Additional calories are expended by exercise or other activity, by the digestion and metabolism of food, and by other metabolic processes. Because of this simple relationship between energy intake, energy utilization, and energy storage, weight gain can occur only when there is increased caloric intake, decreased caloric expenditure, or both.

Genetic factors appear to be very important in determining the presence or absence of obesity. Body weight tends to be similar in close relatives, especially in identical twins, who share the same genetic makeup. The extent to which genetic factors affect food intake, activity level, or metabolic processes is not known.

One theory holds that each individual has a "setpoint" that determines body weight. When food intake is decreased, experiments have shown less weight loss than predicted by the caloric deficit, suggesting that the body has slowed its metabolic rate, thus minimizing the deviation from the original weight. Many believe that physiologic regulation of body weight, which tends to maintain a preferred weight for each individual, explains some of the difficulty in treating obesity. The discovery and role of leptin in regulating weight helps to explain this apparent setpoint of weight for each individual (see the article on leptin).

There are other causes of obesity as well. Producing lesions in the hypothalamus, a part of the brain, can make animals eat excessively and become obese, and rare cases of obesity in humans are attributable to disease of the hypothalamus. In hypothyroidism, a condition in which the thyroid gland produces too little thyroid hormone, the metabolic rate is slowed, which may cause a mild gain in weight. In Cushing's syndrome, which is caused by excessive amounts of the adrenal hormone cortisol or by drugs that act like cortisol, there is an accumulation of excessive fat in the face and trunk, which disappears when the disease is cured or the drug is stopped. Weight gain has also occurred with the use of other drugs, including some antidepressants and tranquilizers.

While most physicians and the public assume that the main factor causing obesity is excessive food intake in relation to physical activity, it has not been possible to prove that overweight people eat more than slender people. This may be the case because it is very difficult to measure food intake under normal conditions, or perhaps because obese individuals tend are taken. Some experts believe, however, that differences in metabolic efficiency and the physiologic set point for body weight are the principal causes of obesity in some people, rather than excessive food intake. The basal metabolic rate (BMR) varies fairly widely among persons of the same age, sex, and body size, and studies have shown large differences in the daily caloric intake needed to maintain a constant body weight in normal people; these observations support the possibility that metabolic differences could contribute to obesity.

Many health problems are associated with obesity. The majority of people who develop non-insulin-dependent diabetes mellitus are overweight, and manifestations of the disease commonly improve or disappear if the individual succeeds in losing weight. Hypertension (high blood pressure) is more common with obesity, and weight loss may lower the blood pressure enough to lessen or avoid the need for medication. Arteriosclerosis, or "hardening of the arteries," is more prevalent in obese persons and causes an increased risk for heart attacks and strokes. Certain forms of cancer are more prevalent with obesity: cancer of the colon, rectum, and prostate in men and cancer of the uterus, gallbladder, ovary, and breast in women. Severe obesity can cause difficulties in breathing, with sleepiness resulting from inadequate oxygen delivery to the tissues and sometimes from interruption of sleep at night. In addition, conditions such as arthritis may be worsened by the additional strain that obesity places on weight-bearing parts of the body.

The distribution of excess adipose tissue differs among individuals. Two main patterns have been described: android obesity (more commonly affecting men), in which fat accumulates mainly in the abdomen and upper body; and gynoid obesity (more common in women), in which fat accumulates mainly in the hips, thighs, and lower body. This distinction has received much attention because persons with android obesity are more likely to suffer from diabetes, hypertension, and cardiovascular disease. The closest association with these diseases is seen when sensitive measurements of abdominal visceral fat mass are made with computed tomography (CT) scanning, a special X-ray technique. A simple measurement of the waist circumference compared with the hip circumference—the waist-to-hip ratio—can also be used to identify those obese individuals at greater risk for diabetes and cardiovascular disease.

TREATMENT AND THERAPY

Many obese people are highly motivated to lose weight because of the common perception that a slim body build is more attractive than an obese one. Many other overweight individuals desire to lose weight because of health problems related to obesity. As a result, the human and financial resources devoted to weight loss efforts are extensive. Unfortunately, the long-term results of the treatment of obesity are successful in only a minority of cases.

The only measures useful in the treatment of obesity are those that decrease the intake or absorption of calories or those that increase the expenditure of calories. The basis for any long-term weight reduction program is a low-calorie diet. The average daily calorie intake in the United States is approximately 1,600 Calories for women and 2,300 Calories for men; decreasing an individual's intake, usually to between 800 and 1,500 Calories, will result in weight loss, provided that energy expenditure does not decrease. A balanced diet, with 20 percent to 30 percent of the calories derived from fat (considerably less fat than is found in the typical American diet) is usually recommended. Many unbalanced diets, or "fad diets," have enjoyed periods of popularity. Rice diets, low carbohydrate diets, vegetable diets, and other special diets may produce rapid weight loss, but long-term persistence with an unbalanced diet is rare and the lost weight is often regained.

Many patients fail to lose weight with low-calorie diets. More severe calorie restriction can be achieved with very-low-calorie diets that provide only 400 to 800 Calories daily. This level of caloric restriction is unsafe unless a very high proportion of the diet consists of high-quality protein, with correct amounts of other nutrients such as vitamins and minerals. These requirements can be met with special formula diets under careful medical supervision. Such a program is recommended for severely obese patients who are otherwise healthy enough to tolerate this degree of caloric restriction.

Because most people find it difficult to lower their calorie intake, behavioral management programs may be combined with dietary restrictions. Dieters can be taught techniques for self-monitoring of food intake, such as keeping a daily log of meals and exercise, which will increase the awareness of eating behavior as well as point out ways in which that behavior can be modified. There are techniques for reducing exposure to food and the stimuli associated with eating, such as keeping food out of sight, keeping food handling and preparation to a minimum, and eliminating the occasions when food is eaten out of habit or as part of a social routine. Ways can be sought to increase the social support of friends and family for weight-losing behavior and for reinforcement of compliance with dietary restrictions. Interestingly, the "diet merry-go-round" which many mildly obese individuals experience—restricting their caloric intake until a weight goal is achieved, ending the diet only to resume over-eating and regain the weight lost—often results in higher weight. Over time, such a pattern can "cycle" the individual to a dangerously high weight. Such individuals tend to experience more success if they can adjust their long-range eating behavior to moderate, rather than restrictive, intake of food. Many physicians would prefer to see their obese patients remain relatively stable in weight, reducing slowly over time, to avoid physical stress and ensure success.

Because obesity is caused by an excess of calorie intake over calorie expenditure, another approach to weight loss is to increase energy utilization by increasing physical activity. Some studies have shown that overweight individuals are less active than their nonobese counterparts. This fact could contribute to their obesity, since less energy utilization results in more energy available for storage as fat. Decreased

activity could also be a result of obesity, since a heavier person must do more work, by carrying more pounds, than a nonobese person who walks or climbs the same distance.

Each pound of fat contains energy equal to about 4,000 Calories. If an obese person expends 400 extra Calories each day by walking briskly for one hour, it will take ten days for this activity to result in the loss of one pound. In a year, this increased calorie expenditure would result in a thirty-six-pound weight loss. More vigorous exercise, such as running, swimming, or calisthenics, would lead to more rapid weight loss, but might not be advisable for every person because of the increased prevalence of certain health problems in obese individuals, such as heart disease, hypertension, and musculoskeletal disorders. For this reason, any exercise program that involves vigorous physical activity should be undertaken with medical supervision.

Exercise as part of a weight-loss program has additional benefits. The function of the cardiovascular system may be improved, and muscles may be strengthened. Exercise will lead to loss of adipose tissue and gain in lean body mass as weight is lost, a change in body composition that is beneficial to overall health. Although some fear that physical activity will lead to an increase in appetite, studies show that any increase in food intake that occurs after exercise is usually not great enough to match the calories expended by the exercise.

Drugs that decrease appetite are occasionally used to help people comply with a low-calorie diet. Some appetite suppressants act like adrenaline and may cause such side effects as nervousness, irritability, and increased heart rate and blood pressure. Other drugs may stimulate serotonin, a chemical transmitter in the central nervous system that decreases appetite, and may cause drowsiness as a side effect. The use of these drugs is controversial because of their side effects and their limited effectiveness in promoting weight loss.

Several surgical procedures have been used to treat severe obesity that has impaired the patient's health and has resisted other treatment. Operations that decrease the absorption of food by bypassing a section of the small bowel have largely been abandoned because of long-term complications of diarrhea and liver disease. The operation now most commonly performed is gastroplasty, which creates a small pouch in the stomach with a narrow outlet through which all food must pass. This procedure decreases the effective volume of the stomach, causing fullness and nausea if more than small amounts of solid food are eaten. Patients have lost about half of their excess weight after one and one-half to two years, but some weight may be regained after this period. Gastroplasty has produced fewer serious complications than intestinal bypass operations. Care must be taken to avoid certain foods that might cause blockage of the narrowed opening from the surgically created stomach pouch, and the benefit of the operation can be overcome by eating soft or liquid foods, which can be consumed in large quantities. The long-term benefit of this procedure is being evaluated.

PERSPECTIVE AND PROSPECTS

Fat has several important functions in the human body. It serves as a cushion for the body frame and internal organs, it provides insulation against heat loss, and it is a storage site for energy. Fat stores energy very efficiently since it contains approximately 9 Calories per gram, compared with approximately 4 Calories per gram in protein and carbohydrate. The presence of reserve stores of energy in the form of fat is particularly important when regular food intake is interrupted and the body becomes dependent on its fat deposits to maintain a source of fuel for daily metabolism and physical activity.

In affluent, culturally advanced societies, however, where food is abundant and modern conveniences greatly reduce the need for physical exertion, many people tend to accumulate excessive amounts of fat, since energy that is taken in but not utilized is stored in the adipose tissue. In the United States, as many as one person in four may become obese. This is an important public health problem because obesity increases the risk of diabetes, hypertension, cardiovascular disease, and other illnesses. Also, many overweight men and women are distressed by the effects of their weight on their social interactions and self-image. Therefore, many obese individuals desire to lose weight.

Unfortunately, the results of weight-loss programs and countless individual efforts at dieting to achieve this goal have often been disappointing. Short-term weight loss can often be achieved; programs utilizing low-calorie diets, behavior modification, exercise, and sometimes appetite-suppressing drugs usually lead to a weight loss of ten to thirty pounds or more over a period of several weeks or months. The problem is

that after a year or more, the great majority of these dieters have regained the lost weight. It appears that the maintenance of a low-calorie diet and an increase in physical activity require a degree of commitment and willingness to endure inconvenience, self-deprivation, and sometimes even physical discomfort that most people can accept for short periods of time but not indefinitely. There are exceptions—some people do succeed in maintaining long-term weight loss—but more commonly dieters return to or surpass their original weight. It is as if the body's set point can be overcome temporarily by intense effort, but not permanently.

Because of the poor prognosis for long-term weight loss, some experts now question the extent to which efforts should be devoted to the treatment of obesity. Nevertheless, because one cannot predict which obese individuals will succeed in achieving long-term weight reduction and because of the important health benefits of maintaining a normal body weight, most physicians agree that serious efforts should be made to treat obesity. Overweight individuals should identify the modifications in their diet and lifestyle that would be most beneficial and should attempt, with medical supervision, to initiate and maintain the behavior needed to bring about permanent weight loss.

—E. Victor Adlin, M.D.;
updated by Karen E. Kalumuck, Ph.D.

See also Arteriosclerosis; Cholesterol; Cushing's syndrome; Diabetes mellitus; Eating disorders; Endocrine disorders; Endocrinology; Exercise physiology; Glands; Heart disease; Hormones; Hyperadiposis; Hypercholesterolemia; Hyperlipidemia; Hypertension; Insulin resistance syndrome; Leptin; Malnutrition; Metabolism; Nutrition; Thyroid disorders; Weight loss and gain; Weight loss medications.

FOR FURTHER INFORMATION:

Barinaga, Marcia. "Obesity: Leptin Receptor Weighs In." *Science* 271 (January 5, 1996): 29. This article presents a summary of leptin receptor research accessible to the nonspecialist, as well as prospects for obesity drug research.

Bennett, J. Claude, et al., eds. *Cecil Textbook of Medicine.* 21st ed. Philadelphia: W. B. Saunders, 2000. This textbook offers a brief review of all aspects of the problem of obesity by a recognized authority in the field.

Bjorntorp, Per, and Bernard N. Brodoff, eds. *Obesity.* Philadelphia: J. B. Lippincott, 1992. A very comprehensive, multiauthor book on all aspects of obesity, from basic considerations of metabolism, body composition, and etiology, to practical questions of the psychological and medical consequences and the various methods of treatment.

Bray, G. A., ed. "Obesity: Basic Considerations and Clinical Approaches." *Disease-a-Month* 35 (July, 1989): 449-537. This volume contains a series of review articles by leading experts in many areas of obesity, including the causes and basic physiology, diagnosis and prevalence, complications, and treatment with diet, behavioral management, drugs, and surgery. An authoritative review of the entire topic.

Consensus Development Conference Panel. "Gastrointestinal Surgery for Severe Obesity: Consensus Development Conference Statement." *Annals of Internal Medicine* 115, no. 12 (1991): 956-961. Describes a consensus reached by leading surgeons, gastroenterologists, endocrinologists, psychiatrists, and nutritionists on the status of surgical procedures for the treatment of severe and intractable obesity.

Hirsch, J., and R. L. Leibel. "Clinical Review 28: Biological Basis for Human Obesity." *The Journal of Clinical Endocrinology and Metabolism* 73 (December 1, 1991): 1153-1157. Reviews the long-term results of the treatment of obesity by all available methods, and emphasizes the fact that effective treatment for most patients is not yet available.

Rink, Timothy J. "In Search of a Satiety Factor." *Nature* 372 (December 1, 1994): 372-373. A history of the research into weight regulation and a description of how leptin supports prior theories are presented in a general news format. References are provided for further reading.

OBSESSIVE-COMPULSIVE DISORDER
DISEASE/DISORDER

ANATOMY OR SYSTEM AFFECTED: Psychic-emotional system

SPECIALTIES AND RELATED FIELDS: Psychiatry, psychology

DEFINITION: An anxiety disorder characterized by intrusive and unwanted but uncontrollable thoughts, by the need to perform ritualized behavior patterns, or both; the obsessions and/or compulsions cause severe stress, consume an excessive amount of time, and greatly interfere with a person's normal routine, activities, or relationships.

KEY TERMS:

anal stage: the stage of psychosexual development in which a child derives pleasure from activities associated with elimination

anxiety: an unpleasant feeling of fear and apprehension

biogenic model: the theory that every mental disorder is based on a physical or physiological problem

major affective disorder: a personality disorder characterized by mood disturbances

monoamine oxidase inhibitors: antidepressant compounds used to restore the balance of normal neurotransmitters in the brain

phobia: a strong, persistent, and unwarranted fear of a specific object or situation

Tourette's syndrome: a childhood disorder characterized by several motor and verbal tics that may develop into the compulsion to shout obscenities

tricyclics: medications used to relieve the symptoms of depression

CAUSES AND SYMPTOMS

Obsessive-compulsive disorder (OCD) is an anxiety disorder that is characterized by intrusive and uncontrollable thoughts and/or by the need to perform specific acts repeatedly. Obsessive-compulsive behavior is highly distressing because one's behavior or thoughts are no longer voluntarily controlled. The more frequently these uncontrolled alien and perhaps unacceptable thoughts or actions are performed, the more distress is induced. A disturbed individual may have either obsessions (which are thought-related) or compulsions (which are action-related), or both. At various stages of the disorder, one of the symptoms may replace the other.

OCD affects 1 to 2 percent of the population; most of those afflicted begin suffering from the disorder in early adulthood, and it is often preceded by a particularly stressful event such as pregnancy, childbirth, or family conflict. It may be closely associated with depression, with the disorder developing soon after a bout of depression or the depression developing as a result of the disorder. OCD is more likely to occur among intelligent, upper-income individuals, and men and women are equally affected. A fairly high proportion (as much as 50 percent) do not marry.

Obsessions generally fall into one of five recognized categories. Obsessive doubts are persistent doubts that a task has been completed; the individual is unwilling to accept and believe that the work is done satisfactorily. Obsessive thinking is an almost infinite chain of thought, targeting future events. Obsessive impulses are very strong urges to perform certain actions, whether they be trivial or serious, that would likely be harmful to the obsessive person or someone else and that are socially unacceptable. Obsessive fears are thoughts that the person has lost control and will act in some way that will cause public embarrassment. Obsessive images are continued visual pictures of either a real or an imagined event.

Four factors are commonly associated with obsessive characteristics, not only in people with OCD but in the general population as well. First, obsessives are unable to control mental processes. Practically, this means the loss of control over thinking processes, such as thoughts of a loved one dying or worries about hurting someone unintentionally. Second, there may be thoughts and worries over the potential loss of motor control, perhaps causing impulses such as shouting obscenities in church or school, or performing inappropriate sexual acts. Third, many obsessives are afraid of contamination and suffer irrational fear and worry over exposure to germs, dirt, or diseases. The last factor is checking behavior, or backtracking previous actions to ensure that the behavior was done properly, such as checking that doors and windows are shut, faucets are turned off, and so on. Some common obsessions are fear of having decaying teeth or food particles between the teeth, fear of seeing fetuses lying in the street or of killing babies, worry about whether the sufferer has touched vomit, and fear of contracting a sexually transmitted disease.

Compulsions may be either mild or severe and debilitating. Mild compulsions might be superstitions, such as refusing to walk under a ladder or throwing salt over one's shoulder. Severe compulsions become fixed, unvaried ritualized behaviors; if they are not practiced precisely in a particular manner or a prescribed number of times, then intense anxiety may result. Even these strange behaviors may be rooted in superstition; many of those suffering from the disorder believe that performing the behavior may ward off danger. Compulsive acts are not ends in themselves but are "necessary" to produce or prevent a future event from occurring. Although the enactment of the ritual may assuage tension, the act does not give the compulsive pleasure.

Several kinds of rituals are typically enacted. A common ritual is repeating; these sufferers must do everything by numbers. Checking is another compul-

sive act; a compulsive checker believes that it is necessary to check and recheck that everything is in order. Cleaning is a behavior in which many compulsives must engage; they may wash and scrub repeatedly, especially if the individual thinks that he or she has touched something dirty. A fourth common compulsive action is avoiding; for certain superstitious or magical reasons, certain objects must be avoided. Some compulsives experience a compelling urge for perfection in even the most trivial of tasks; often the task is repeated to ensure that it has been done correctly. Some determine that objects must be in a particular arrangement; these individuals are considered "meticulous." A few sufferers are hoarders; they are unable to throw away trash or rubbish. All these individuals have a constant need for reassurance; for example, they want to be told repeatedly that they have not been contaminated.

No cause for OCD has been isolated. Therapists even disagree over whether the obsessions increase or decrease anxiety. Three theories exist that attempt to explain the basis of OCD psychologically: guilt, anxiety, and superstition. Sigmund Freud first proposed that obsessive thoughts are a replacement for more disturbing thoughts or actions that induce guilt in the sufferer. These thoughts or behaviors, according to Freud, are usually sexual in nature. Freud based his ideas on the cases of some of his young patients. In the case of a teenage girl, for example, he determined that she exchanged obsessive thoughts of stealing for the act of masturbation. The thoughts of stealing produced far fewer guilt feelings than masturbation did. Replacing guilt feelings with less threatening thoughts prevents one's personal defenses from being overwhelmed. Other defense mechanisms may be parlayed into OCD. Undoing, one of these behaviors, is obliterating guilt-producing urges by undergoing repetitive rituals, such as handwashing. Since the forbidden urges continue to recur, the behavior to replace those urges must continue. Another mechanism is reaction formation. When an unacceptable thought or urge is present, the sufferer replaces it with an exactly opposite behavior. Many theorists believe that both obsessive and compulsive behaviors arise as a consequence of overly harsh toilet training. Thus the person is fixated at the anal stage and, by reaction formation, resists the urge to soil by becoming overly neat and clean. A third mechanism is isolation, the separation of a thought or action from its effect. Detachment or aloofness may isolate an individual from aggressive or sexual thoughts.

Although there is disagreement among therapists regarding the role of the anxiety associated with OCD, some theorize that OCD behaviors develop to reduce anxiety. Many thought or action patterns emerge as a way of escape from stress, such as daydreaming during an exam or cleaning one's room rather than studying for a test. If the stress is long-lasting, then a compulsive behavior may ensue. This theory may not answer the problem of behaviors such as hand-washing. If this theory is always viable, then washers should feel increased anxiety at touching a "contaminated" object and washing should relieve and reduce those feelings. While this does occur in some instances, it does not explain the origin of the disorder.

The superstition hypothesis proposes a connection between a chance association and a reinforcer that induces a continuation of the behavior. Many theorists believe that the same sequence is involved in the formation of many superstitions. A particular obsessive-compulsive ritual may be reinforced when a positive outcome follows the behavior; anxiety results when the ritual is interrupted. An example would be a student who only uses one special pencil or pen to take exams, based on a previous good grade. In actuality, there is seldom a real relationship between the behavior and the outcome. This hypothesis, too, fails to explain the development of obsessions.

A fourth theory is accepted by those who believe that mental disorders are the result of something physically or physiologically amiss in the sufferer, employing data from brain structure studies, genetics, and biochemistry. Indeed, brain activity is altered in those suffering from OCD, and they experience increased metabolic activity. Whether the activity is a cause or an effect, however, is unclear. Studies of genetics in families, at least in twins, reinforce the idea that genetics may play a small role in OCD because there appears to be a higher incidence of the disorder in identical twins than in other siblings. Yet these results may be misleading: Because all the studies were carried out on twins who were reared together, environment must be considered. Relatives of OCD sufferers are twice as likely as unrelated individuals to develop the same disorder, indicating that the tendency for the behavior could be heritable.

TREATMENT AND THERAPY

While obsessional symptoms are not uncommon in the general population, a diagnosis of OCD is rare.

Perhaps between five thousand and ten thousand Americans are affected by this mental disorder, although many sufferers are too horrified to admit to their symptoms.

Diagnostic techniques evaluating OCD have not changed much since the nineteenth century. There may be confusion about whether the patient is actually suffering from schizophrenia or a major affective disorder. When depression is also noted, it is important to determine whether the OCD is a result of the depression or the depression is a result of the OCD. If such a determination is not possible, both disorders must be treated.

In cases where differentiation between OCD and schizophrenia is necessary, the distinction can be made by determining the motive behind the ritualized behavior. Stereotyped behaviors are symptomatic of both disorders. In the schizophrenic, however, the behavior is triggered by delusions rather than by true compulsions. People suffering from true delusions cannot be shaken from them; they do not resist the ideas inundating the psyche and even rituals may not decrease the feelings associated with these ideas. On the other hand, obsessive people may be absolutely certain of the need to perform their ritual while other aspects of their thinking and logic are perfectly clear. They generally resist the ideas that enter their minds and realize the absurdity of the thoughts. As thoughts and images intrude into the obsessive person's mind, the person may appear to be schizophrenic.

Other disorders having symptoms in common with OCD are Tourette's syndrome and amphetamine abuse. What seems to separate the symptoms of these disorders from those experienced with OCD is that the former are organically induced. Thus, the actions of a sufferer from Tourette's syndrome may be mechanical since they are not intellectually dictated or purposely enacted. In the case of the addict, the acts may bring pleasure and are not resisted.

"Normal" people also have obsessive thoughts; in fact, the obsessions of normal individuals are not significantly different from the obsessions of those with OCD. The major difference is that those with the disorder have longer-lasting, more intense, and less easily dismissed obsessive thoughts. The importance of this overlap is that mere symptoms are not a reliable tool to diagnose OCD, since some of the same symptoms are experienced by the general population.

Assessment of OCD separates the obsessive from the compulsive components so that each can be examined. Obsessional assessment should determine the triggering fears of the disorder, both internal and external, including thoughts of unpleasant consequences. The amount of anxiety that these obsessions produce should also be monitored. The compulsive behaviors then should be examined in the same light.

The greatest chance for successful treatment occurs with patients who experience mild symptoms that are usually obsessive but not compulsive in nature, with patients who seek help soon after the onset of symptoms, and with patients who had few problems before the disorder began. Nevertheless, OCD is one of the most difficult disorders to treat. Types of treatment fall into four categories: psychotherapy, behavioral therapy, drug therapy, and psychosurgery.

When psychotherapy is attempted, it usually begins with psychoanalysis. Whether psychoanalysis will be successful is often determined by the stressor or inducer of the thought or action and the personality of the patient. The major goal of this psychoanalytical approach is to find and then remove an assumed repression so that the patient can deal honestly and openly with whatever is actually feared. Some analysts believe that focusing on the present is most beneficial, since delving into the past may strengthen the defensive mechanism (the compulsive behavior). If the patient attempts to "return" to the mitigating event, the analyst should intervene directly and actively and bring the patient back to the present by encouraging, pressuring, and guiding him or her.

The most effective treatment for controlling OCD is the behavioral approach, in which the therapist aids the patient in replacing the symptoms of the obsession or compulsion with preventive or replacement actions. Aversive methods may include a nonvocal, internal shout of "stop!" when the obsessive thoughts enter the mind, the action of snapping a rubber band on the wrist, or physically restraining oneself if the compulsive action begins. This latter approach may be so uncomfortable and disconcerting to the patient that it may work only under the supervision supplied by a hospital.

Behavioral therapy may also help by breaking the connection between the stimulus (what induces the compulsion or obsession) and anxiety. Response prevention involves two stages. First, the patient is subjected to flooding, the act of exposing the patient to the real and/or imagined stimuli that cause anxiety. This process begins with brief exposure to the stressors while the therapist assesses the patient's thoughts,

feelings, and behaviors during the stimulus period. In the second stage, the patient is flooded with the stimuli but restrained from acting on those stressors. Although flooding may produce intense discomfort at first, the patient is gradually desensitized to the stimuli, causing the resulting anxiety to decrease. The therapist must expend considerable time preventing the response, discussing the anxiety as it appears, and supporting the patient as the anxiety abates. To be effective, treatment must also occur in the home with the guidance and support of family members who have been informed about how best to interact with the patient. While behavioral treatment can help to control OCD, it does not generally "cure" the disorder. If the patient is also depressed, successful treatment with behavioral therapy is even less likely.

Drugs commonly used to treat OCD that have met with some success include antidepressants, tricyclics, monoamine oxidase inhibitors, LSD, and tryptophan. Although a psychiatrist may prescribe tranquilizers to reduce the patient's anxiety, these drugs are usually not adequate to depress the frequent obsessive thoughts or compulsive actions. Antidepressants may occasionally benefit those who are suffering from depression as well as OCD; as depression is lifted, some of the compulsive behavior is also decreased. Monoamine oxidase inhibitors (MAOIs) are used most effectively in treating OCD associated with panic attacks, phobias, and severe anxiety. When medication is halted, however, the patient often relapses into the previous obsessive-compulsive state.

Some psychosurgeons may resort to psychosurgery to relieve a patient's symptoms. The improvement noted after surgery may simply be attributable to the loss of emotion and dulling of behavioral patterns found in any patient who has undergone a lobotomy. Because such surgery may result in a change in the patient's intellect and emotional response, it should be considered only in extreme, debilitating cases. Newer surgical techniques do not destroy as much of the cerebral cortex. These procedures separate the frontal cortex from lower brain areas in only an 8-centimeter square area.

Perspective and Prospects

Descriptions of OCD behavior go back to medieval times; a young man who could not control his urge to stick out his tongue or blurt out obscenities during prayer was reported in the fifteenth century. Medical accounts of the disorder and the term "obsessive-compulsive" originated in the mid-1800's. At this time obsessions were believed to occur when mental energy ran low. Later, Freud stated that OCD was accompanied by stubbornness, stinginess, and tidiness. He attributed the characteristics to a regression to early childhood, when there are perhaps strong urges to violence or to dirty and mess one's surroundings. To avoid acting on these tendencies, he theorized, an avoidance mechanism is employed, and the symptoms of obsession and/or compulsion appear. Other features related to this regression are ambivalence, magical thinking, and a harsh, punitive conscience.

An unpleasant consequence of OCD behavior is the effect that the behavior has on the people who interact with the sufferer. The relationships with an obsessive person's family, school mates, or coworkers all suffer when a person with OCD takes up time with uncontrollable and lengthy rituals. These people may feel not only a justifiable concern but also resentment. Some may feel guilt over the resentful feelings because they know the obsessive-compulsive cannot control these actions. An obsessive-compulsive observing these conflicting feelings in others may respond by developing depression or other anxious feelings, which may cause further alienation.

Although not totally disabling, OCD behaviors can be strongly incapacitating. A famous figure who suffered from OCD was millionaire and aviator Howard Hughes (1905-1976). A recluse after 1950, he became so withdrawn from the public that he only communicated via telephone and intermediaries. His obsession-compulsion was the irrational fear of germs and contamination. It began with his refusal to shake hands with people. If he had to hold a glass or open a door, he covered his hand with a tissue. He would not abide any of his aides eating foods that gave them bad breath. He disallowed air conditioners, believing that they collected germs. Because Hughes acted on his obsessions, they became compulsions.

Most parents will agree that children commonly have rituals to which they must adhere or compulsive actions they carry out. A particular bedtime story may be read every night for months on end, and children's games involve counting or checking rituals. It is also not atypical for adults without psychiatric disorders to experience some mild obsessive thoughts or compulsive actions, as seen in an overly tidy person or in group rituals performed in some religious sects. Excessively stressful events may trigger obsessional thoughts as well. Some behaviors commonly called

compulsions are not truly compulsive in nature. For example, gambling, drug addiction, or exhibitionism are not clinically compulsive because these addictive behaviors bring some pleasure to the person. The anxiety ensuing from these addictive behaviors is appropriate by society's standards; compulsive behavior produces anxiety that is considered inappropriate to the situation.

—Iona C. Baldridge

See also Addiction; Anorexia nervosa; Anxiety; Bipolar disorder; Bulimia; Depression; Eating disorders; Grief and guilt; Neurosis; Panic attacks; Paranoia; Phobias; Post-traumatic stress disorder; Psychiatric disorders; Psychiatry; Psychiatry, child and adolescent; Psychiatry, geriatric; Psychoanalysis; Schizophrenia; Stress; Tics.

FOR FURTHER INFORMATION:

American Psychiatric Association. *Diagnostic and Statistical Manual of Mental Disorders: DSM-IV-TR*. Rev. 4th ed. Washington, D.C.: Author, 2000. The bible of the psychiatric community, this is a compendium of descriptions of disorders and diagnostic criteria widely embraced by clinicians. Included is an extensive glossary of technical terms, making this volume easy to understand.

Barlow, David H., ed. *Clinical Handbook of Psychological Disorders*. 2d ed. New York: Guilford Press, 1993. This collection defines and describes psychological disorders and uses case histories as illustrations for treatment. The chapter on OCD provides a series of tests that can be given to determine the presence and severity of this disorder.

Davison, Gerald C., and John M. Neale. *Abnormal Psychology*. 8th ed. New York: John Wiley & Sons, 2001. This college text addresses the causes of psychopathology and treatments commonly used to treat various disorders. The book is well organized, readable, and interesting. An extensive reference list and a glossary are included.

Frances, Allen, John P. Docherty, and David A. Kahn. "Treatment of Obsessive-Compulsive Disorder." *Journal of Clinical Psychiatry* 58 (1997): 5-72. This article gives the most up-to-date recommendations for treating obsessive-compulsive disorder. It may be particularly useful to individuals or family members of individuals seeking treatment.

Oltmans, Thomas F., John M. Neale, and Gerald C. Davison. *Case Studies in Abnormal Psychology*. 5th ed. New York: John Wiley & Sons, 1999. A sample of twenty clinical case histories of abnormal psychology. Included are descriptions of a given disorder, ways to view and treat the disease, and the origin and causes of the disease.

Sue, David, Derald Sue, and Stanly Sue. *Understanding Abnormal Behavior.* 6th ed. Boston: Houghton Mifflin, 2000. Recognized disorders of the mind and common successful treatments of these disorders are discussed in this college text. Well organized and understandable.

OBSTETRICS

SPECIALTY

ANATOMY OR SYSTEM AFFECTED: Reproductive system, uterus

SPECIALTIES AND RELATED FIELDS: Embryology, genetics, gynecology, neonatology, perinatology

DEFINITION: The medical science dealing with pregnancy and childbirth, including the health of both mother and unborn infant and the successful delivery of the child and the placenta at the time of birth.

KEY TERMS:

amniocentesis: a technique by which a very fine needle is inserted through a pregnant woman's abdomen to collect fetal amniotic fluid cells for genetic analysis

birth defect: a genetic abnormality in the tissue development of a certain body part of the fetus; in some cases the defect is minor, but in others it may be medically dangerous to the fetus and/or mother

gestation: the period from conception to birth, in which the fetus reaches full development in order to survive outside the mother's body

gynecology: the scientific study of the female anatomy and physiology and the diseases that afflict women

obstetrics: the scientific study of pregnancy and childbirth, which concerns the health of the mother and the fetus during the course of a pregnancy

Pap smear: a simple diagnostic test for the presence of cervical cancer, involving the removal of cervical tissue cells and the subsequent biopsy of these cells

placenta: a blood barrier between the mother's circulatory system and the fetal circulatory system, across which essential oxygen and nutrients pass to the fetus

Rh₀(D) immune globulin (human): a type of gamma globulin protein injected into Rh-negative mothers who may have an Rh-positive fetus in order to protect the fetus from an immune reaction

trimester: an arbitrary division of a human pregnancy into three-month divisions based on developmental changes in the fetus over time

ultrasonography: a specialized technique by which high-intensity sound waves penetrate bodily tissues and, via computer imaging, generate an image of the fetus inside the mother's uterus

SCIENCE AND PROFESSION

Obstetrics is the scientific study of pregnancy and childbirth in women. Once conception has occurred and a woman is pregnant, major physiological changes occur within her body as well as within the body of the developing embryo or fetus. Obstetrics deals with these changes leading up to and including childbirth. As such, obstetrics is a critical branch of medicine, for it involves the complex physiological events by which every person comes into existence.

The professional obstetrician is a licensed medical doctor whose area of expertise is pregnancy and childbirth. Often, the obstetrician is also a specialist in the closely related science of gynecology, the study of diseases and conditions that specifically affect women. The obstetrician is knowledgeable concerning the detailed female anatomy and physiology, major bodily changes that occur during and following pregnancies, necessary medical diagnostic procedures for monitoring fetal and maternal health, and the latest technologies for facilitating a successful pregnancy and childbirth with minimal complications.

In in vivo fertilization, pregnancy begins with the fertilization of a woman's egg by a man's sperm following sexual intercourse, the chances of which are highest if intercourse takes place during a two-day period following ovulation. Ovulation is the release of an unfertilized egg from the woman's ovarian follicle, which occurs roughly halfway between successive periods during her menstrual cycle. Fertilization usually occurs in the upper one-third of one of the woman's Fallopian tubes connecting the ovary to the uterus; upon entering the woman's vagina, sperm must travel through her cervix to the uterus and up the Fallopian tubes, only one of which contains a released egg following ovulation.

Once fertilization has occurred, the first cell of the new individual, called a zygote, is slowly pushed by cilia down the Fallopian tube and into the uterus. Along the way, the zygote undergoes several mitotic cellular divisions to begin the newly formed embryo, which at this point is merely a bundle of undifferentiated cells.

Upon reaching the uterus, the multicellular embryo implants itself into the endometrium, the nerve- and blood-rich epithelial lining of the uterus, and the pregnancy has started. The woman's body will elevate production of the female steroid hormone progesterone, which maintains the endometrium and ensures the continuation of the pregnancy. Failure of the embryo to be implanted in the endometrium and subsequent lack of progesterone production will cause release of the endometrium as a bloody discharge; the woman will menstruate, and there will be no pregnancy.

Therefore, menstrual cycles do not occur during a pregnancy, although there may be periodic yellowish discharges from a woman's vagina during her pregnancy at times that coincide with her usual menstrual periods. The embryo will grow and develop over the next nine months of gestation. Early events in embryonic development will be numerous mitotic cellular divisions, converting the one-celled zygote into the trillion-celled complete human organism; cellular specialization through the hormonal control of gene regulation; and the grouping of cells into tissues and tissues into organs.

Early during the pregnancy, the embryo releases human chorionic gonadotropin, a protein which penetrates the mother's bloodstream and eventually makes its way to her urine. A home pregnancy test of her urine will be positive if human chorionic gonadotropin is present.

The developing new human is considered an embryo for the first eight weeks of the pregnancy. During this time, billions of cells have formed from repeated cellular divisions, and the cells have specialized by gene regulation into four principal tissue types: epithelial tissue, covering body surfaces inside and out; connective tissue, eventually forming cartilage, bone, fat, and blood; nervous tissue, conducting electrical impulses as an information pathway; and muscle tissue, for contractility and the movement of body parts both large and small. These four tissue types combine in various ways to form all organ types, and the organs are linked by function to form the major organ systems, including the nervous, endocrine, circulatory, skeletal, digestive, excretory, and integumentary systems.

The embryo's heart forms and begins beating at

roughly five and one-half weeks following conception. During the first eight weeks, the embryo successively develops three pairs of kidneys, of which the last pair will become the fully functional kidneys; the preceding two vestigial pairs degenerate or are modified for use in other organ systems. Based on the presence or absence of a Y chromosome in every cell of the embryo, hormonally induced genetic changes will occur within the embryo to cause the individual to be male (if the Y chromosome is present) or female (if the Y chromosome is absent).

By the end of the first three months of the pregnancy, the developing human is considered to be a fetus. All the major organ systems have formed, although not all systems can function yet. The fetus is surrounded by a watery amniotic fluid within an amniotic sac. The umbilical cord connects the fetal navel to the placenta and the mother's blood supply. The placenta is a blood barrier separating the maternal and fetal circulatory systems. Across the placenta, oxygen and nutrients from the mother's blood can diffuse to the fetal blood vessels in the umbilical cord, to the fetal abdomen, and to the fetal stomach and liver. Waste products from the fetus cross the placenta from the umbilical cord to the mother's blood for removal from her body via the kidneys.

The first three months of the pregnancy constitute the first trimester. The second and third trimesters, covering the middle three months and final three months, respectively, of the pregnancy, involve full organ system development; massive cell divisions of certain tissues such as nervous, circulatory, and skeletal tissue; and preparation of the fetus for survival as an independent organism. The fetus cannot survive outside the mother's body, however, until the third trimester. Up to birth, the fetal lungs are deflated, and the fetal circulatory system is modified so that the pulmonary artery connects to the aorta and the two heart atria are connected; both of these configurations are unlike those of babies and adults.

Changes also occur in the mother. Increased levels of the female steroid hormone estrogen create increased skin vascularization (that is, there are more blood vessels near the skin) and the deposition of fat throughout her body, especially in the breasts and the buttocks. The growing fetus and stretching uterus press on surrounding abdominal muscles, often creating abdominal and back pain. Reasonable exercise is important for the mother to stay healthy and to deliver the baby with relative ease. A proper diet also is important for the nourishment of her body and that of the fetus.

Late in the pregnancy, the protein hormones prolactin and oxytocin will be produced by the woman's pituitary gland. Prolactin activates milk production in the breasts, which will continue to enlarge. Oxytocin causes muscular contractions, particularly in the breasts and in the uterus during labor. Near the time of birth, drastically elevated levels of the hormones estrogen and oxytocin will cause progressively stronger contractions (labor pains) until the baby is forced through the vagina and out of the woman's body to begin its independent physical existence. The placenta, or afterbirth, is discharged shortly thereafter.

DIAGNOSTIC AND TREATMENT TECHNIQUES

The role of the obstetrician is to monitor the health of the mother and unborn fetus during the course of the pregnancy and to deliver the baby successfully at the time of birth. Once the fact of the pregnancy is established, the obstetrician is trained to identify specific developmental changes in the fetus over time in order to ensure that the pregnancy is proceeding smoothly.

The mother often is placed on a diet which is high in protein and essential vitamins and minerals but low in fats and sugars. She is prescribed a complex vitamin supplement, including folic acid, to replenish her body's nutrient supplies that are being depleted by the developing fetus. The use of caffeine (including soft drinks), tobacco, alcohol, and most medications (including aspirin) is strongly discouraged because of possible ill effects on the fetus, and sometimes on the mother, during the pregnancy.

During an examination, which may occur monthly early in the pregnancy but weekly during the late months of the pregnancy, the obstetrician will perform a physical examination of the mother. Her abdomen will be measured, and the vaginal/cervical region may be checked. Early in the pregnancy, a Pap smear of cervical tissue will be conducted to identify the presence of any cancerous tissue that would endanger the mother.

Periodic tests monitor the mother's blood glucose levels, especially if she is diabetic or has a family history of diabetes, as well as the levels of maternal and fetal hormones. Blood tests also can monitor the existence of certain fetal birth defects, such as spina bifida.

If the mother has an Rh-negative blood type, as a result of the inherited absence of the Rh factor on her red blood cells, and the father has an Rh-positive blood type, the fetus probably will have an Rh-positive blood type. When this is the case, the mother will be given a shot of $Rh_0(D)$ immune globulin (human), also known under the brand name of RhoGAM, at roughly the twenty-sixth week of her pregnancy and again several weeks following childbirth. If she does not receive RhoGAM and the fetus is Rh-positive, then some fetal red blood cells may cross the placenta into her bloodstream and activate her immune system to attack the fetal blood; the first child will be anemic, but further pregnancies will miscarry because of the mother's immunization against Rh-positive fetuses. RhoGAM clears the mother's blood of any Rh-positive fetal blood, thereby preventing her immune system from being activated and enabling her to have a healthy child and more healthy children later.

The correct development of the fetus and the presence of any birth defects can be assessed by two powerful techniques known as amniocentesis and ultrasonography. Amniocentesis involves the injection of a very fine needle through the pregnant woman's abdomen and into her uterus to reach the amniotic fluid surrounding the fetus. The amniotic fluid contains excess cells sloughed off from the fetus. These cells can be collected, and fetal cell chromosomes can be ordered into a karyotype by which any chromosomal abnormalities can be identified. The presence of extra chromosomes beyond the normal two copies of every chromosome, such as trisomy 21 leading to Down syndrome, can be determined. Other chromosomal abnormalities, such as chromosome translocations and inversions, also can be identified. The presence of serious chromosome abnormalities identified early in the pregnancy may lead the pregnant woman to choose an abortion. The sex of the fetus can be determined by amniocentesis as well.

Ultrasonography involves the beaming of high-intensity sound waves into the uterus; the reflected sound waves are recorded into a computer, which generates an image of the uterine contents. With proper positioning, the fetus can be located and physically assessed by the obstetrician. Measurements can be made of body proportions, including the skull cephalic index, body length, and spinal curvature and development. Body organs can be identified and an assessment can be made of their functioning. If the fetal position allows it, external reproductive organs can be identified to determine the sex of the fetus. Most obstetricians allow their patients to make a videocassette recording of the ultrasound. Both amniocentesis and ultrasonography are optional; however, many obstetricians choose to perform at least one ultrasound no earlier than the end of the first trimester.

During a typical pregnancy examination, the physician can listen for the fetal heartbeat and thereby assess proper cardiac functioning. Advances in acoustic technology enable amplification of the heartbeat so that it can be heard by both doctor and patient.

Near the time of childbirth, the obstetrician will determine the position of the fetus; most babies exit the mother's vagina headfirst. Certain conditions involving the mother and/or fetus require a cesarean section, in which the baby is surgically removed from the uterus. A cesarean section may be performed when the baby would otherwise be born feetfirst, in what is called a breech presentation, or when serious complications arise, such as the baby becoming entangled in the umbilical cord.

At the time of childbirth, the obstetrician and the delivery staff support the mother through the final stages of labor and the birth of the child. Upon delivery, the umbilical cord is clamped and cut, and the baby is assisted in its first breaths of life. The placenta is collected for biopsy to ensure the absence of cancerous tissue.

PERSPECTIVE AND PROSPECTS

Obstetrics is central to medicine because it deals with the very process by which all humans come to exist. The health of the fetus and its mother in pregnancy is of primary concern to the doctor. The field of obstetrics has blossomed as a sophisticated specialty from the days when general practitioners delivered babies. Advances in medical technology have enabled more precise analysis and monitoring of the fetus inside the mother's uterus, and obstetrics has therefore become a complicated specialty in its own right.

The obstetrician assesses the state of the mother and the proper development of the unborn fetus throughout the pregnancy with a variety of general techniques and specialized apparatuses. The mother is advised about the proper diet and the proper care of her body during rapid physiological changes. She must eat certain foods and vitamins while abstaining from foods and chemicals that might damage the fetus. Many substances, including caffeine and drugs, have been demonstrated to affect the gene regulation of fetal cells, thereby causing mutations and abnor-

mal tissue development. The obstetrician is scientist, medical practitioner, and adviser to the mother so that she and her child proceed through the pregnancy with minimal discomfort.

Technology such as computer imaging, ultrasonography, and amniocentesis, among other techniques, allows the obstetrician to collect a much larger supply of fetal data than was available to the general practitioner of the 1960's. Increased data availability enables the obstetrician to monitor the pregnancy closely, identifying early problems. Drugs such as RhoGAM make it possible for some couples to have more children. Improvements in genetic screening promise to identify lethal genes such as those producing cystic fibrosis and Tay-Sachs disease early in the pregnancy, so that abortion can be an option. Such a decision might save individuals and their loved ones the misery of a painful, eventual death early in life.

The medical science of obstetrics continues to advance. The field has increased the number of live births and healthy children while decreasing infant mortality rates in most parts of North America and Europe. As with most fields, however, it is not without controversies, such as abortion. Nevertheless, obstetrics is an essential component of medical science.

—*David Wason Hollar, Jr., Ph.D.*

See also Amniocentesis; Birth defects; Breastfeeding; Breasts, female; Cesarean section; Childbirth; Childbirth complications; Chorionic villus sampling; Conception; Critical care; Down syndrome; Eclampsia; Ectopic pregnancy; Embryology; Emergency medicine; Episiotomy; Family practice; Fetal alcohol syndrome; Genetic counseling; Genetic diseases; Genital disorders, female; Gonorrhea; Growth; Gynecology; In vitro fertilization; Incontinence; Miscarriage; Multiple births; Neonatology; Obstetrics; Perinatology; Postpartum depression; Pregnancy and gestation; Premature birth; Reproductive system; Rh factor; Rubella; Spina bifida; Stillbirth; Toxoplasmosis; Ultrasonography; Urology.

FOR FURTHER INFORMATION:

Gabbe, Steven G., Jennifer R. Niebyl, and Joe Leigh Simpson, eds. *Obstetrics: Normal and Problem Pregnancies.* 4th ed. New York: Churchill Livingstone, 2001. This mammoth work surveys the entirety of pregnancy, from conception to following childbirth, including sections on female anatomy and physiology. Numerous authorities have contributed to this work, including obstetricians from such prestigious medical schools as Yale University, The Johns Hopkins University, and the University of California at Los Angeles.

Gaudin, Anthony J., and Kenneth C. Jones. *Human Anatomy and Physiology*. New York: Harcourt Brace Jovanovich, 1989. Gaudin and Jones's introductory textbook in human anatomy and physiology is geared toward health science majors, both premedical and prenursing. They describe the subject matter in appropriate detail, with excellent illustrations and supporting material. Chapter 28, "Development and Inheritance," is a thorough discussion of the issues confronting obstetricians in their practices.

Grant, Harvey D., et al. *Brady Emergency Care*. Rev. 7th ed. Englewood Cliffs, N.J.: Brady Prentice Hall Education, Career & Technology, 1995. A detailed survey of patient care for the training of emergency medical technicians (EMTs) and paramedics. Chapter 16, "Childbirth," deals with the basics of the birthing process, obstetrics, and problems that may arise during a pregnancy or during birth. An excellent source of basic medical information.

Hood, Gail Harkness, and Judith R. Dincher. *Total Patient Care: Foundations and Practice of Adult Health Nursing*. 8th ed. St. Louis: Mosby Year Book, 1992. A comprehensive introduction to nursing care for various types of patients, ranging from the aged to pregnant women. Chapter 20, "Problems Affecting Sexuality," concerns human reproductive anatomy, diagnostic procedures, ultrasonography, and other important aspects of reproduction and obstetrics.

Memmler, Ruth L., Barbara J. Cohen, and Dena L. Wood. *Memmler's Structure and Function of the Human Body*. 7th ed. Philadelphia: J. B. Lippincott, 2000. This short but thorough work is an excellent introduction to human anatomy and physiology for the layperson. Chapter 20, "Reproduction," is a concise survey of human reproductive anatomy and processes and of the major events of pregnancy and childbirth.

Wallace, Robert A., Gerald P. Sanders, and Robert J. Ferl. *Biology: The Science of Life*. 4th ed. New York: HarperCollins, 1996. Chapter 11, "Going Beyond Mendel," discusses the genetics of Rh incompatibility and RhoGAM. Chapter 43, "Animal Development," describes fetal development in mammals, with an emphasis on human development during the three trimesters.

OBSTRUCTION
DISEASE/DISORDER

ANATOMY OR SYSTEM AFFECTED: Abdomen, gastrointestinal system, intestines

SPECIALTIES AND RELATED FIELDS: Gastroenterology

DEFINITION: Partial or complete closure of the channels through which food normally passes; it may be silent, or it may cause either acute and life-threatening or chronic and debilitating illness.

KEY TERMS:

biliary tract: the series of ducts that drain bile from the liver and gallbladder into the intestine

colon: the large intestine except for the cecum and rectum; includes the ascending colon, transverse colon, descending colon, and sigmoid colon

distal: away from the point of origin; for example, the stomach is distal to the esophagus

endoscopic retrograde cholangiopancreatography: an endoscopic procedure in which dye is injected into the common bile duct and pancreatic ducts for visualization with X rays

endoscopy: the process of passing a fiber-optic instrument into the gastrointestinal tract for visualization; upper endoscopy is also called esophagogastroduodenoscopy, whereas lower endoscopy is called sigmoidoscopy or colonoscopy, depending on how far the scope is inserted

esophagus: the tube that extends from the pharynx to the stomach

gut: the gastrointestinal tract; includes the esophagus, stomach, and small and large intestines

peristalsis: the series of involuntary muscular contractions that propel material along the gastrointestinal tract

proximal: toward the point of origin; for example, the small intestine is proximal to the large intestine

small intestine: the organ that extends from the stomach to the large intestine; its three regions are the duodenum, jejunum, and ileum

CAUSES AND SYMPTOMS

The gastrointestinal (GI) tract runs from the mouth to the anus and includes the throat, esophagus, stomach, small intestine, large intestine, and rectum. Accessory glands whose secretions drain into the GI tract include the liver, gallbladder, and pancreas. Because the GI tract is essentially a hollow tube, its inner channel being called its lumen, it is susceptible to being closed off. The same holds true for the biliary tree, which is a series of ducts draining bile from the liver and gallbladder into the duodenum, and the pancreatic duct, which drains secretions from the pancreas into the duodenum.

Obstruction of the gastrointestinal tract is a blockage severe enough to impair the transit of materials through the lumen. Although often caused by narrowing, that term differs from obstruction in that a narrowing may be without consequences. A partial obstruction is one in which there is still some flow through the narrowing; in complete obstruction, there is no flow.

Obstruction of these organs or ducts may be mechanical or functional. Mechanical obstructions result when a problem arises from within the bowel lumen (intraluminal), from within the wall of the organ (mural), or from something outside the organ causing its lumen to be narrowed (extrinsic). Functional obstructions are caused by some motor abnormality, such as spasm or lack of peristalsis, causing impaired transit of materials.

An example of an intraluminal obstruction is a gallstone occluding the cystic duct. The liver produces bile, a fluid that has various functions including excretion of bilirubin, which is a breakdown product of hemoglobin, the protein inside red blood cells that carries oxygen. Bile also contains bile salts and cholesterol, substances that help break down large fat globules in the duodenum into smaller droplets, initiating fat digestion. Bile from the liver flows through tiny ducts that eventually unite to form the common hepatic duct. The gallbladder, a hollow sac that stores bile, joins the common hepatic duct via the cystic duct; these two ducts unite to form the common bile duct, which drains bile into the duodenum.

If there is excess cholesterol in bile, it tends to form gallstones. These stones most often form in the gallbladder, but they may form in other areas of the biliary tree such as in the common bile duct. If the stones are formed in the gallbladder but do not occlude the cystic duct, bile may still flow in and out of the organ. If the stones become impacted in the cystic duct, however, they cause obstruction to the flow of bile, leading to inflammation of the gallbladder, called acute cholecystitis.

With cystic duct obstruction, the impacted stone and some of the components of bile cause the gallbladder to become inflamed. The inflamed lining secretes fluid into the gallbladder; this fluid cannot escape because the cystic duct is occluded by the

gallstone. The accumulating fluid causes the gallbladder to become distended.

This inflamed gallbladder causes abdominal pain that often lasts several hours. It is also associated with nausea, vomiting, and a fever. The fever may be attributable to a bacterial infection of the bile: When not flowing well, bile tends to be a good place for bacteria to multiply. The stones may pass through the cystic duct and occlude the common bile duct. In this situation, there is no route for bile to flow into the duodenum. Therefore it backs up, dilating the common bile duct, and is reabsorbed into the bloodstream. This causes jaundice, or a yellowish pigmentation of the skin; it may be associated with dark-colored urine.

There are ways to distinguish between acute cholecystitis caused by cystic duct obstruction and biliary tract infection (cholangitis) caused by obstruction of the common bile duct. Ultrasonography is excellent for detecting stones in the gallbladder and dilated bile ducts, but it is not as good at detecting stones in the common duct. In order to detect such stones, endoscopic retrograde cholangiopancreatography (ERCP) may be performed. In this study, an endoscope is passed through the mouth, esophagus, and stomach and into the duodenum. A catheter is inserted into the opening of the common bile duct, and dye is injected. The dye outlines stones in the common bile duct.

An example of a mechanical obstruction caused by a mural process is an esophageal obstruction caused by a cancer which grows from the walls of the esophagus into its lumen. The most common symptom of esophageal obstruction is dysphagia, or a sensation of food sticking in the throat after being swallowed. If food becomes impacted in the narrowed region, it may cause an aching sensation in the chest wall.

The obstruction is evaluated with a barium esophagram, in which barium is swallowed and an X ray of the esophagus is taken. It may show findings such as severe narrowing of the lumen of the esophagus. Endoscopy is then performed, which can be used to visualize the area, looking for evidence of cancer, and to take a piece of the lining of the esophagus for evaluation under the microscope.

An example of an extrinsic mechanical obstruction is one caused by scar tissue, or adhesions, compressing a portion of the small intestine. Adhesions may be caused by previous abdominal surgery. If they cause obstruction, the bowel proximal to the obstruction dilates to a diameter that is larger than normal. Its function changes: Normally the small intestine absorbs fluid, whereas in obstruction it secretes fluid. Since intestinal contents cannot pass through the narrowing, vomiting occurs.

Normally, the bacterial content of the small intestinal lumen is kept low because of the continuous flow of contents through it. During small bowel obstruction, this flow is partially or completely diminished, enabling bacteria to overgrow in the small intestine. These bacteria may pass through the wall of the small intestine into the bloodstream, causing a systemic infection or even death.

An example of a functional obstruction is a disorder called chronic intestinal pseudo-obstruction (CIP). The prefix "pseudo" means "false": A pseudo-obstruction is a disorder in gastrointestinal motility that results in diminished peristalsis through the diseased segment of gut, creating an illness similar to a mechanical obstruction but without any occlusion of the lumen. There are a variety of causes of CIP, which can involve the different regions of the gastrointestinal tract. It may occur as part of the spectrum of some systemic diseases, or it may be of unknown cause (idiopathic).

If the esophagus is involved, dysphagia and heartburn are predominant symptoms, resulting from decreased esophageal peristalsis. Everyone experiences occasional reflux, or the backward flow of stomach acid into the esophagus. Normal esophageal peristalsis keeps this acid in the stomach; if peristalsis is diminished, then the acid may cause heartburn. If the stomach and small intestine are involved, symptoms include nausea, vomiting, bloating, and abdominal discomfort. The abdomen may become extremely distended. Since the flow of small intestinal contents is slowed, overgrowth of bacteria that are normally present only in the colon occurs. These bacteria may take up so much vitamin B_{12} in the gut that a deficiency results. Bacterial overgrowth may also cause diarrhea. If the colon is extensively involved and exhibits markedly diminished peristalsis, abdominal distension and constipation result. An abdominal X ray may show that the colon has become very dilated, a condition called megacolon.

TREATMENT AND THERAPY

Obstructions caused by gallstones can be treated in several ways. If the stones are in the gallbladder and are obstructing the cystic duct, surgery is often performed within a day or two. One technique for removing the gallbladder is laparoscopic cholecystectomy, which involves making a small incision in the

abdominal wall and inserting an instrument called a laparoscope. The structures of the biliary tree are identified, and dye is injected into the cystic duct to obtain a cholangiogram, an X ray that helps identify where the stones are located. After cholangiography, clips are placed along the cystic duct, and the duct is cut between the clips (similar to cutting the umbilical cord between the ties). Bile and stones are evacuated from the gallbladder, which is then removed. The advantages of laparoscopic cholecystectomy over other surgical approaches are that the laparoscopic approach is less invasive, causes less scarring and less pain, and allows a more rapid recovery.

If the stones are in the common bile duct, one way to remove them is endoscopically. The endoscope is advanced into the duodenum, and the opening of the common bile duct is visualized. An instrument is passed through the endoscope into the opening of the common bile duct. Electrical current is applied, creating a small incision in the opening of the common bile duct. This enlarges the opening, and sometimes bile and stones come gushing out into the duodenum. If the stone is still in the common duct, a balloon-tipped catheter is passed into the common bile duct and advanced up above the stone. The balloon is inflated, and the catheter is pulled out of the common duct, bringing the stone with it. If this procedure fails, other options include surgery or extracorporeal shock-wave lithotripsy. This involves generating shock waves and focusing them onto the stone, causing it to break into tiny fragments.

Despite progress made in the care of esophageal cancer patients, the overall five-year cure rate did not change from the 1950's to the 1990's. A main treatment goal is to relieve the symptom of dysphagia. This can be done by passing dilators down through the narrowed area, stretching it so that food, saliva, and liquids can pass. Because the tumor is undoubtedly growing, repeated dilations are necessary. This treatment obviously does nothing to reduce the mass of the tumor, but it helps relieve the symptom of dysphagia.

Two treatments aimed at reducing the tumor mass are surgical removal of the tumor and radiation therapy. Before deciding that surgery is a viable option, several factors need to be taken into consideration, including the potential risks of surgery. For example, surgery performed on patients with advanced heart or lung disease has a very high mortality risk. If the tumor involves the lower esophagus, that area can be removed and the stomach can be sewn to the remaining end of the esophagus. This surgery can be dangerous: Mortality rates from the operation range from 2.8 to 17 percent.

Another treatment, which is effective if the tumor is of a specific cell type called a squamous cell carcinoma, is to irradiate the tumor, attempting to kill tumor cells by focusing beams of radiation onto the mass. This procedure produces survival rates that are roughly equal to surgical survival rates and avoids the risk of surgery. The most common way to apply radiation is to focus it onto the chest wall using an external source. The radiation energy penetrates into the area on which it is focused—the esophageal tumor. One complication of radiation therapy is that the radiation, which kills rapidly dividing cells, cannot distinguish between cancer cells and those lining the wall of the esophagus. Therefore the lining of the esophagus may become very inflamed, a condition called radiation esophagitis. Another approach for applying radiation is with a delivery system such as a specialized radioactive device which fits inside the lumen of the esophagus and delivers radiation locally.

Small bowel obstructions can be fatal. Their treatment first consists of generalized care, such as correcting fluid deficits. All oral intake is stopped, and a nasogastric tube, which is a tube inserted into the nose and passed into the stomach, is hooked up to suction to try to decompress the dilated loops of bowel. Since surgery may be imminent, it is important to optimize the functions of various organ systems so that the mortality risk of surgery is minimized. The likelihood of needing surgery depends on whether the obstruction is partial or complete: About 81 percent of partial small bowel obstructions and about 16 percent of complete obstructions resolve without surgery. This likelihood also depends on the cause of obstruction. For example, many partial obstructions resulting from adhesions resolve with conservative treatment, whereas obstructions caused by a loop of intestine twisting at its base, called a volvulus, carry a high probability of needing surgery.

The treatment of CIP is difficult: Nothing is curative, and nothing slows the progression of the diseases causing pseudo-obstruction. The most effective drug for increasing intestinal motility is probably cisapride. Some studies show that it improves symptoms and hastens the transit of material through the gut. Antibiotics to treat bacterial overgrowth in the small intestine are sometimes used in CIP, especially in cases where diarrhea is present. Dietary measures may be somewhat helpful, including lowering fat, lactose, and fiber. Vitamin supplementation may be necessary, especially with injectable vitamin B_{12}.

Occasionally, surgery is helpful in CIP, especially for a localized problem. Because the disease often causes widespread gut involvement, however, surgery will not cure the problem. Nevertheless, when the problem is caused by the lower esophageal sphincter (LES) failing to open properly, creating a distal esophageal obstruction, a myotomy (or cutting of the circular smooth muscle in the LES) may improve dysphagia symptoms. If the stomach or colon is massively dilated, it may need to be removed. Sometimes removal of portions of the small intestine may be helpful. Once abdominal surgery has been performed, it may be difficult to distinguish future attacks of CIP from mechanical bowel obstruction caused by adhesions.

Alternative forms of nutrition may need to be considered. For example, if the disease mainly affects the esophagus and stomach, a feeding tube could be placed into the small intestine. If the gut has such widespread involvement that jejunal feeding would be fruitless, parenteral nutrition, which is the administration of nutrition intravenously, may be necessary.

PERSPECTIVE AND PROSPECTS
Since obstructions of various areas in the gastrointestinal tract can be life-threatening, they served as the sources of some of the most exciting diagnostic and therapeutic advances in medicine during the twentieth century.

The earliest way to diagnose mechanical obstruction, such as small bowel obstruction, was by exploratory surgery. Then came X-ray studies, which were initially able to outline the gastrointestinal tract first by plain-film studies that showed various findings such as loops of small intestine dilated with air that suggested obstruction. Later, the addition of contrast dyes, given either by mouth or by rectum, increased the ability to outline the anatomy of the GI tract and to diagnose obstructions.

Endoscopy has revolutionized the ability to diagnose mechanical obstructions that are attributable to various causes. Developed initially using a rigid endoscope, which was difficult to position and required that the patient be put under general anesthesia, endoscopes now are flexible, only about one centimeter in diameter, and easily passed well into the duodenum.

The instruments passed through the endoscope have also been greatly improved. There are instruments for removing coins lodged in the esophagus, inserting feeding tubes through the stomach wall, injecting drugs to stop the bleeding in ulcers, burning tumors with ulcers, and cutting the opening of the common bile duct for removing stones impacted in it.

Surgical techniques have improved. Crohn's disease can cause inflammation and segments of narrowing of the intestine called strictures; these strictures can cause problems such as mechanical small bowel obstructions. Surgeons used to remove the strictured areas, plus a significant margin of small intestine on either side of the stricture, in the belief that such removal would eliminate the diseased segments of the small intestine. The disease tends to recur, however, and a patient needing repeated operations to remove strictures might end up with a small intestine so short that it would be unable to absorb fluids and nutrients. Therefore, the individual could have massive diarrhea and malabsorption of nutrients and need to be fed intravenously. By the 1990's, surgical treatment for Crohn's disease sought to relieve the stricture but preserve as much small intestine as possible.

In the 1970's, therapy for biliary stones began to move away from traditional surgery and toward the use of stone-dissolving medications, endoscopic techniques, lithotripsy, and laparoscopy.

Manometry, which involves the measurement of pressure inside the GI tract, has been especially useful in helping scientists understand the physiology of functional obstruction and its relationship to emotions. For example, in 1987, L. D. Young and coworkers published an article describing how exposing research subjects to experimental noise and complicated thinking problems would increase the pressure inside the esophagus, in effect concluding that it increased the strength and speed of esophageal muscle contractions.

—*Marc H. Walters, M.D.*

See also Abdomen; Abdominal disorders; Cancer; Cholecystectomy; Cholecystitis; Cholesterol; Colon and rectal polyp removal; Colon and rectal surgery; Colon cancer; Colon therapy; Colonoscopy; Constipation; Crohn's disease; Diarrhea and dysentery; Endoscopy; Gallbladder diseases; Gastroenterology; Gastroenterology, pediatric; Gastrointestinal disorders; Gastrointestinal system; Heartburn; Intestinal disorders; Intestines; Laparoscopy; Lithotripsy; Nausea and vomiting; Peristalsis; Pyloric stenosis; Radiation therapy; Stone removal; Stones; Tumor removal; Tumors.

FOR FURTHER INFORMATION:

Ganong, William F. *Review of Medical Physiology.* 19th ed. Stamford, Conn.: Appleton and Lange, 1999. This classic text has a nice section emphasizing normal gastrointestinal physiology, which would provide a solid background for understanding obstruction.

Robbins, Stanley L., Ramzi S. Cotran, and Vinay Kumar, eds. *Basic Pathology.* 6th ed. Philadelphia: W. B. Saunders, 1997. An introductory pathology textbook that is less detailed than that used by physicians, but it still contains a wealth of information on the various disorders that can cause obstruction of the GI tract.

Sleisenger, Marvin H., and John S. Fordtran, eds. *Sleisenger and Fordtran's Gastrointestinal and Liver Disease: Pathophysiology, Diagnosis, Management.* 6th ed. 2 vols. Philadelphia: W. B. Saunders, 1998. The best comprehensive textbook of gastrointestinal diseases and physiology. Contains excellent chapters on all disorders mentioned in the text, as well as some beautiful endoscopic photographs.

Tortora, Gerard J., and Sandra R. Grabowski. *Principles of Anatomy and Physiology.* 9th ed. New York: John Wiley & Sons, 2000. An outstanding textbook of human anatomy and physiology. A good place to start before reading more advanced gastroenterology and journal articles.

OCCUPATIONAL HEALTH

SPECIALTY

ANATOMY OR SYSTEM AFFECTED: All

SPECIALTIES AND RELATED FIELDS: Environmental health, epidemiology, internal medicine, preventive medicine, psychology, public health, pulmonary medicine, toxicology

DEFINITION: The diagnosis, treatment, and prevention of diseases and injuries that can occur in the workplace or that result from a person's employment.

SCIENCE AND PROFESSION

The discovery that eighteenth century chimney sweeps were prone to developing testicular cancer is often cited as the first example of an acknowledged occupational illness. In fact, physicians and other health care professionals had been aware for many centuries that certain jobs were linked to particular medical disorders: Millers developed coughs, and hatmakers

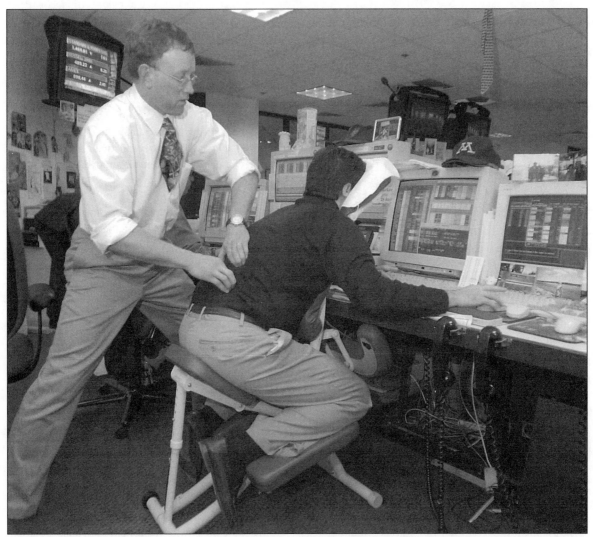

A massage therapist helps an employee relieve stress in the workplace. Some businesses are finding that such preventive measures as stress reduction, ergonomic design, and exercise sessions help keep medical costs down and increase productivity. (AP/Wide World Photos)

became mentally unbalanced. Textbooks urged physicians to consider a patient's occupation both in diagnosing and in treating illness. The emergence of occupational health as a distinct specialty within the medical professions is, however, a relatively recent phenomenon.

The Industrial Revolution brought with it not only the separation of one's home life from one's work life but also an increased risk of injury from factory machinery. Spinning jennies, power looms, mill wheels and belts, and early assembly line processes all carried the risk of accidental amputations, mangled limbs, and other permanently crippling injuries. Not surpris-

ingly, much of the early emphasis of occupational health focused on safety. While company doctors treated the injured workers, engineers sought ways to reduce the job hazards.

By the twentieth century, several different but related specialties had evolved that focused on different aspects of occupational health. Industrial hygienists combine training in engineering and public health and attempt to improve safety in the workplace by providing education and training for workers and by redesigning the work area to eliminate hazards. Doctors of occupational medicine are employed by both government and industry to diagnose and to treat occupational illnesses and work-related disabilities. Public awareness of occupational health issues has led to the passage of legislation creating such agencies as the United States Occupational Safety and Health Administration (OSHA). All occupational health specialists in the United States must work within guidelines established by OSHA. There is a high cost to society from such disabilities as the black lung disease suffered by coal miners and the toxic or radioactive exposure experienced by workers ranging from hospital laboratory technicians to pipefitters and welders. As a result, occupational health has become an ever-expanding, complex, and important medical specialty.

Diagnostic and Treatment Techniques

Because occupational health problems can affect any part of the human anatomy, their diagnostic and treatment techniques are drawn from all areas of medical science. If a worker is injured on the job or suffers from an easily recognizable problem, such as a repetitive motion disorder, diagnosis and treatment can be quite straightforward. In the case of repetitive motion, problems such as carpal tunnel syndrome, which is sometimes experienced by word processing operators, might be treated by advising patients to change their work posture, providing them with splints to align the wrists and hands properly, employing corrective surgery to alleviate pain, and redesigning the work site to prevent future problems. The treatment for many on-the-job injuries will also include an extensive course of physical and rehabilitative therapy to allow the worker to return to work eventually, either at the old job or at a new one.

Many occupational health problems, however, are not as readily diagnosed as carpal tunnel syndrome. The industrial hygienist and the doctor of occupational medicine often must rely on the expertise of epidemiologists and toxicologists to determine the substances to which occupational exposure may be responsible for a worker's ill health. In cases where workers complain of vague symptoms such as chronic fatigue, nausea, or neuropathy (loss of nerve function), an accurate diagnosis can prove elusive. The medical literature contains numerous examples of occupational illnesses that mimicked other common disorders. For example, doctors misdiagnosed a cosmetologist as suffering from multiple sclerosis (a degenerative disease of the central nervous system) when she was actually experiencing nerve damage caused

by many years of exposure to the chemical solvents used to apply and remove artificial fingernails. Because many occupational illnesses can take years or even decades to appear, in some cases an accurate diagnosis may never be achieved. Once a diagnosis is made, treatment for an occupational illness caused by exposure to chemicals, for example, can be as simple as assigning the worker to tasks that eliminate exposure or as technologically sophisticated as using dialysis or chemical chelation to remove toxins from a patient's blood.

Perspective and Prospects

Occupational health is one of the most challenging specialties in modern medicine. Practitioners must combine skills and knowledge gleaned from a wide spectrum of related skills. The proliferation of technologically complex methods and materials in the workplace has resulted in occupational exposures and illnesses that were unknown until the twentieth century. At the time that occupational health first emerged as a distinct concern in the medical community, industrial hygiene focused almost exclusively on safety in the workplace. If the factory could be designed so that workers did not risk losing a limb whenever they operated machinery, the hygienist could feel a sense of accomplishment.

Workplace safety remains a concern in occupational health, but obvious hazards such as poorly lit work areas or exposed moving parts on machines have been joined by a host of subtler threats to workers' well-being. Epidemiologists and toxicologists have linked on-the-job exposure to dust, heavy metals, radiation, solvents and other chemicals, and even blood-borne pathogens to a host of cancers, disabling diseases, reproductive problems, and other concerns. Yet, not only must the industrial hygienist and doctor of occupational medicine worry about protecting workers from these physical hazards but the modern occupational health specialist must also be concerned with the long-term effects of repetitive motions, noise exposures, and even emotional stress. As the influence of workers' jobs on those workers' health and on the health of their families is recognized as a major factor in a family's overall well-being, the importance of the occupational health specialist becomes increasingly obvious within modern society. Occupational health specialists employed in government, industry, and private practice, each approaching the question of worker wellness from a slightly different perspective, all fill a vital and expanding niche in modern medical practice.

—*Nancy Farm Mannikko, Ph.D.*

See also Allied health; Altitude sickness; Asphyxiation; Biofeedback; Cardiac rehabilitation; Carpal tunnel syndrome; Environmental diseases; Environmental health; Hearing loss; Interstitial pulmonary fibrosis (IPF); Law and medicine; Lead poisoning; Lung cancer; Lungs; Multiple chemical sensitivity syndrome; Nasopharyngeal disorders; Occupational health; Preventive medicine; Pulmonary diseases; Pulmonary medicine; Pulmonary medicine, pediatric; Radiation sickness; Skin disorders; Stress; Stress reduction; Tendon disorders; Tendon repair; Toxicology.

FOR FURTHER INFORMATION:

Caplan, Robert D., et al. *Job Demands and Worker Health: Main Effects and Occupational Differences.* Ann Arbor: University of Michigan, 1980. Discusses such topics as job stress, occupational diseases, psychological occupational medicine, and industrial hygiene. Includes bibliographical references.

Cralley, Lester V., Lewis J. Cralley, George D. Clayton, and John Jurgiel, eds. *Industrial Environmental Health: The Worker and the Community.* New York: Academic Press, 1972. A detailed catalog of known workplace hazards, including toxic materials, radiation, and noise. The emphasis is on monitoring techniques and a thorough survey of the literature.

Durbin, Paul T., ed. *A Guide to the Culture of Science, Technology, and Medicine.* New York: Free Press, 1980. Discusses the social aspects of science and technology. Includes bibliographical references and an index.

Koren, Herman. *Illustrated Dictionary of Environmental Health and Occupational Safety.* Boca Raton, Fla.: Lewis, 1996. Detailed illustrations enhance the definitions and provide visual tools for understanding. Definitions are supplemented with synonyms, acronyms, and abbreviations, all of which are cross-referenced.

Sadhra, Steven, and Krishna Rampal, eds. *Occupational Health Risk Assessment and Management.* Malden, Mass.: Blackwell Science, 1999. This book is divided into four sections with three appendices. Intended as a textbook, each of the twenty-eight chapters written by recognized specialists in the field, contains a list of references to original material.

ONCOLOGY

SPECIALTY

ANATOMY OR SYSTEM AFFECTED: All

SPECIALTIES AND RELATED FIELDS: Critical care, cytology, general surgery, genetics, immunology, pathology, pharmacology, radiology

DEFINITION: The study of cancer—its causes, its possible spread throughout and destruction of the body, and its medical treatment.

KEY TERMS:

cancer: a tumorous growth of abnormal cells that invade other tissues, choke off available resources, and eventually destroy major organs and the organism

carcinogen: a chemical or radiation mutagen that causes changes in genes, leading to the cancerous state in a cell

cellular transformation: the process in which a cell becomes cancerous, which begins with abnormal changes in gene expression and cell differentiation

hormone: a chemical messenger, usually composed of protein or steroid, that controls the gene expression within target cells and thereby affects cellular development

mutagen: a chemical or an ionizing radiation that causes a change in the nucleotide sequence of the DNA of a gene, possibly affecting the gene's normal expression

mutation: a change in the nucleotide sequence of the DNA (that is, the genetic information) of a gene

oncogene: a gene within the chromosomes of all the cells of an individual organism that triggers cancerous cellular transformation when it is expressed incorrectly

protein kinase: an enzyme type that often is encoded by oncogenes; this enzyme attaches phosphate molecules to certain amino acids on specifically targeted proteins

tumor: an uncontrollable growth of cells within a tissue region that may be benign (noninvasive) or malignant (invasive cancer)

virus: an obligate intracellular parasite, composed of nucleic acid protected by a protein capsid, which reproduces inside cells

SCIENCE AND PROFESSION

Oncology is the scientific study and treatment of cancers, tumors, and other abnormal tissue growths. This field is an important part of medical science because of the prevalence of cancer within the human population, particularly in the progressively older populations of Western societies, in which people enjoy life-prolonging medical advances. Cancer ranks second only to heart disease as a killer of people in Western nations. Its victims number in the hundreds of thousands each year.

The study of cancer and its various physiological manifestations involves an understanding of several diverse biological disciplines, including genetics, developmental biology, embryology, neurology, endocrinology, and general physiology. The oncologist must synthesize information from these scientific fields in diagnosing, monitoring, and treating the disease. The oncologist works closely with the cancer patient's physician, surgeons, laboratory technicians, radiation therapists and chemotherapists, and pharmacists in treating cancerous tumors.

A tumor is an abnormal growth of cells within a specific tissue or organ beyond that tissue or organ's normal developmental pattern. Tumors may be either benign or malignant. Benign tumors are noninvasive; benign tumor cells multiply more rapidly than normal cells within a single, localized region that grows larger and larger. A benign tumor does not spread to other body regions. A malignant tumor, however, is invasive; it grows rapidly and uncontrollably. A malignant tumor is a cancer that consists of grotesquely aberrant cells that break off and are carried through the affected individual's bloodstream to other body regions, where they lodge and overcrowd or outcompete normal body cells.

Cells function normally as a result of the hormonal control of thousands of protein-encoding genes located on twenty-three pairs of chromosomes. The order of nucleotide nitrogen bases on a gene's deoxyribonucleic acid (DNA) polynucleotide chain serves as the genetic code. A change in the nucleotide sequence of DNA is called a mutation. A substance causing a mutation, which is called a mutagen, may be ionizing radiation (for example, ultraviolet light, X rays, gamma radiation) or a chemical. The DNA of a gene encodes ribonucleic acid (RNA), which encodes protein. Thus, an alteration in the nucleotide sequence of DNA, such as the replacement of a cytosine by an adenine nitrogen base, affects the messenger RNA nucleotide information sequence and, subsequently, the protein amino acid sequence. Proteins serve important structural, enzymatic, and hormonal roles within and between cells. A mutation within the DNA nucleotide sequence of a particular cellular gene affects the resulting protein encoded by that gene. Consequently, a variety of cellular functions are affected in sequence. In some cases, the cell is transformed into a cancerous state.

Mutagens that alter certain genes and then trigger cellular transformation into a cancerous state are called carcinogens. Only certain mutagens are carcinogens. An altered gene encodes a protein that has an incorrect amino acid sequence, thereby altering the normal functioning of the protein. An aberrant protein enzymatically or hormonally alters the functioning of other molecules within the cell, thereby directing the cell into the cancerous state.

The precise genes and proteins that are affected in transformed cells have not been identified completely. It appears that certain cancer-causing genes called oncogenes are involved, as well as certain oncogene-encoded enzymes called protein kinases. Protein kinases attach phosphate molecules to certain amino acids on certain cellular proteins, thereby altering the functioning of the proteins and triggering developmental changes within the cell. Certain viruses can also trigger these changes by activating oncogenes and protein kinases. The cell becomes cancerous as a result of these influences.

DIAGNOSTIC AND TREATMENT TECHNIQUES

Oncologists must confront a variety of cancers that affect many different tissues. The six most common cancers affecting American women are breast, colon, lung, uterine, ovarian, and lymphatic cancers, whereas the five most prevalent cancers affecting American men are prostate, lung, colon, bladder, and lymphatic cancers, according to the American Cancer Society. Oncologists must identify and treat these tumors as rapidly and as efficiently as possible.

The successful treatment of cancer begins with its early detection. The classic seven warning signs of cancer are a sore that does not heal, a lump on the body, a persistent cough, difficulty in swallowing, unusual bleeding, a change in a wart or mole, and a change in bladder or bowel movements. The presence of cancer in a patient can be identified by an oncologist by means of several techniques, including cytological (cellular) analysis, biopsy, and direct observation. Cytological techniques employ the microscopic examination of discarded cells from the suspected cancerous region. Biopsy involves the surgical removal of suspected cancerous tissue from an individual and the subsequent chemical and microscopic analysis of the removed tissue cells. Cancer cells are morphologically and chemically distinct from normal body cells.

Cancerous cell masses can be directly observed within the body by means of probing tubes that contain fiber-optic imaging devices and that can be inserted into body cavities. Such medical technology can visualize directly the trachea, bronchi, and larger bronchioles of the lungs; the esophagus and stomach; the colon and rectum; and the reproductive organ passageways, such as the vagina and cervix. Cancerous tumors also can be located via more elaborate techniques, such as computed tomography, magnetic resonance imaging, mammography, radioactive isotopes, X rays, and ultrasound.

Computed tomography (CT) scanning is an enhanced X-ray survey of selected regions of the patient's body. The patient lies within the device, which rotates and X-rays around the patient, thereby generating a three-dimensional, computer-enhanced image of the tumor. Conventional X rays can identify many tumors; however, computed tomography can penetrate deeper tissues with greater sensitivity. Mammography is an example of a regular X-ray treatment that utilizes low-energy X rays beamed at a woman's breasts. Mammography is recommended yearly for women of age fifty or older.

Similarly, the ingestion of certain radioactive isotopes such as iodine can be used to localize tumors. Certain elemental isotopes concentrate in specific body tissues and organs. The radioactive isotope concentrates in a particular tissue, the tissue is imaged, and any abnormal growths can be detected. Magnetic resonance imaging and ultrasound utilize magnetic fields and sound waves, respectively, to image interior tissues and abnormalities in tissue growth.

Once the presence of cancer and the type of cancer have been established, prompt treatment must ensue. The oncologist must determine the appropriate course of treatment. Surgical removal of the tumor may be possible. Radiotherapy and chemotherapy can be used in conjunction with, or instead of, surgery. Radiotherapy, or radiation therapy, involves the killing of the cancerous tumor by using a concentrated beam of ionizing radiation such as X rays or gamma rays, or by using an ingested radioactive isotope (such as cobalt 60) that will concentrate in the target cancerous tissue. Chemotherapy involves the internal administration of cytotoxic (cell-killing) chemicals to the patient; cancer cells are particularly susceptible to these chemicals.

Treatment for all forms of cancer involves combinations of chemotherapy and radiation therapy. Cancer cells are more sensitive to these treatments than are normal body cells, and they are killed more easily as a result. Early detection of cancer is critical to the success of such treatments. Accessible cancers, such as skin cancers, can be removed surgically or frozen.

Common chemicals used in cancer chemotherapy include alkylating agents, antimetabolites, antibiotics, plant alkaloids, human and synthetic hormones, and enzymes. All these chemicals kill cells, especially cancer cells. Examples of alkylating agents are cisplatin for the treatment of testicular and ovarian cancers, cyclophosphamide for the treatment of breast and lymphatic cancers, and mechlorethamine for the treatment of Hodgkin's disease. A typical antimetabolite is 5-fluorouracil, which is used for the treatment of breast and colon cancer. Examples of antibiotics are mitomycin-C and actinomycin-D. Vincristine is a plant alkaloid that is used to treat leukemia. The human male hormone testosterone and the female hormone progesterone are both used to treat breast cancer, while the female hormone estrogen is used to treat prostate cancer.

Radiation therapies include concentrated beams of X rays or gamma rays aimed at target cancerous tissues or the ingestion of specific radioactive isotopes that concentrate in target cancerous tissues. Both radiation and chemical therapies for cancer have numerous side effects, because normal cells are damaged as well as cancerous cells in both treatments. Such side effects include nausea, weakness, vomiting, diarrhea, loss of hair, and anemia.

In cases of certain tissue tumors and cancers, such as leukemia and bone cancer, tissue transplants from carefully matched individuals have been very effective in saving the lives of these cancer patients. The advent of molecular cloning and the use of tissue-specific viral gene vectors provide another avenue by which the oncologist will treat cancer in the future.

The oncologist's goals are to remove and/or kill the cancerous growth and to arrest its spread (metastasis) to other body tissues. The prevention of metastatic spreading is of critical importance, because the establishment of tumors in multiple body regions makes treatment much more difficult and patient death much more likely. Also, the oncologist must help the patient to cope psychologically with the disease and the possibility of dying.

Oncological research and the treatment of neoplastic (cancerous) tissues represent formidable tasks for medical science. Cancer is the number-two killer of Americans, and tumors are responsible for countless other ailments and millions of dollars of medical expenses. The use of surgery, cytotoxic chemical agents, and radiation to destroy or remove cancers has proven to be effective in saving thousands of lives. The incidence of cancer is increasing, however, and hundreds of thousands of people die from cancer each year.

Perspective and Prospects

Cancer is an increasing problem in Western societies, where medical science is increasing longevity and where industry and business place extraordinary levels of stress upon individuals. Most theories of aging maintain that accumulated genetic mutations in somatic cells during organismal development contribute to the breakdown of body systems, particularly the immune system. Aging is contained for much of an individual's life. Aging accelerates, however, following the end of an individual's period of reproduction. Although cancer can occur at any age, its probability of occurrence accelerates with aging.

Cancer cells are present in the bodies of all humans. Out of approximately 1,000 trillion cells within the human body, it is inevitable that mistakes will occur frequently within the gene regulation mechanisms of certain cells. Humans and other life-forms are exposed continuously to radiation and carcinogenic chemicals of varying types. A critical gene within a critical cell eventually will mutate so that the cell follows a cancerous pathway.

A healthy person with a strong immune system, however, quickly will destroy these mutated, transformed cancers. Individuals having weakened immune systems as a result of stress, aging, illness, and so forth are more susceptible to cancer because the mutated cells have the opportunity to multiply and spread rapidly throughout the body before the person's immune system can respond. Many scientists are beginning to identify aging and stress as diseases, and cancer as a symptom of these diseases.

As the body ages, more and more mutations accumulate, thereby increasing the probability that cancer cells will develop, survive, and multiply. At the same time, the aging immune system cannot respond to abnormal cells and infections as rapidly. Consequently, cancer cells elude the victim's immune system and spread to other body regions.

Evidence is implicating stress as a contributor to incidences of disease, illness, cancer, aging, and premature death in the human population. Stress causes abnormal elevations in nerve and endocrine (hormonal) systems that affect a tremendous variety of cellular and tissue-specific processes within the human body. Elevated levels of hormones for prolonged periods of time can permanently alter the gene expression of certain body tissues, causing these tissues to develop abnormally. Stress is a major problem in fast-paced, technological societies, and it is probably no coincidence that heart disease and cancer are the two principal killers of people in such societies.

Additionally, certain cancers may be infectious. In 1910, Peyton Rous determined that the Rous sarcoma virus, which infects chickens, can trigger cancerous tumors. Subsequent investigators corroborated Rous's findings, and nearly two dozen viruses have been identified that are capable of initiating cellular transformation in animals. Such oncogenic viruses either carry an oncogene or activate oncogenes in their host cells when they infect cells. All viruses must infect cells in order to reproduce. Some viruses can insert their genetic material into the host cell's DNA, thereby affecting the expression of host-cell genes at the viral insertion point; this may be one method of oncogenic viral cellular transformation into cancer. Among the oncogenic viruses that infect humans are hepatitis B; the papillomavirus, which also causes warts; and the Epstein-Barr virus. The Epstein-Barr virus usually causes infectious mononucleosis. In a region of western central Africa, however, humans develop a deadly lymph node cancer called Burkitt's lymphoma when exposed to the virus—a phenomenon that has baffled oncologists.

Genetic damage caused by chemicals and radiation to which humans are exposed has a substantial effect upon the incidences of tumors and cancer. The link between ionizing radiation (for example, ultraviolet light, X radiation, gamma radiation) and cancer has been established. The links between various chemicals and cancer are more difficult to sustain, however, often leading to controversies over the banning of certain substances and the health risks associated with contact with such substances (for example, saccharin or motor oil). The Ames test for chemical mutagens is a very effective assessment of whether a chemical is mutagenic; it was developed by biochemist Bruce Ames and his colleagues at the University of California at Berkeley in the 1970's.

The problems posed by cancer are immense and will require decades of intense medical research. Advances in oncological research are saving many lives each year. Understanding gene regulation within living cells and developing more effective diagnostic techniques and cancer-inhibiting treatments are important steps in conquering this dreaded disease.

—*David Wason Hollar, Jr., Ph.D.*

See also Amputation; Biopsy; Blood testing; Bone cancer; Bone grafting; Bone marrow transplantation; Breast biopsy; Breast cancer; Breasts, female; Cancer; Carcinoma; Cells; Cervical, ovarian, and uterine cancers; Chemotherapy; Colon and rectal polyp removal; Colon cancer; Cystectomy; Cytology; Cytopathology; Dermatology; Dermatopathology; Endometrial biopsy; Gene therapy; Genital disorders, female; Genital disorders, male; Gynecology; Hematology; Histology; Hodgkin's disease; Hysterectomy; Imaging and radiology; Immunology; Immunopathology; Kaposi's sarcoma; Laboratory tests; Laryngectomy; Liver cancer; Lung cancer; Lymphadenopathy and lymphoma; Malignancy and metastasis; Malignant melanoma removal; Mammography; Mastectomy and lumpectomy; National Cancer Institute (NCI); Nephrectomy; Parathyroidectomy; Pathology; Plastic surgery; Proctology; Prostate cancer; Prostate gland removal; Radiation therapy; Sarcoma; Screening; Serology; Skin cancer; Skin lesion removal; Stomach, intestinal, and pancreatic cancers; Stress; Terminally ill: Extended care; Thyroidectomy; Tumor removal; Tumors.

FOR FURTHER INFORMATION:

Alberts, Bruce, et al. *Molecular Biology of the Cell.* 3d ed. New York: Garland, 1994. Leading molecular biologists collaborated to produce this valuable textbook describing the genetics, biochemistry, and developmental biology of eukaryotic cells. Chapter 11, "Cell Growth and Division," discusses tumorigenesis, cancer cells, and viral-induced cancers. Numerous other chapters are devoted to gene regulation and hormones.

Gaudin, Anthony J., and Kenneth C. Jones. *Human Anatomy and Physiology.* New York: Harcourt Brace Jovanovich, 1989. Gaudin and Jones's introductory anatomy and physiology textbook is a valuable reference. Chapter 3, "Cell Structure and Organization," provides a thorough, clear discussion of gene regulation and cancer formation.

Glass, Leon, and Michael C. Mackey. *From Clocks to Chaos: The Rhythms of Life.* Princeton, N.J.: Princeton University Press, 1988. Glass and Mackey's book is a scientific discussion of how chaos applies to the normal physiological functioning of the human body and its various tissues and organs. They cite numerous research studies to support their arguments.

Harnett, Paul, John Cartmill, and Paul Glare, eds. *Oncology: A Case-Based Manual.* Oxford: Oxford University Press, 1999. More than eighty cases are used to illustrate and discuss management of patients with cancer. The editors introduce this slim text with an emphasis on data that the practicing physician should know but might have difficulty finding elsewhere in a digestible form.

Hood, Gail Harkness, and Judith R. Dincher. *Total Patient Care: Foundations and Practice of Adult Health Nursing.* 8th ed. St. Louis: Mosby Year Book, 1992. Hood and Dincher's comprehensive textbook provides a strong introduction to health care for the nursing or premedical student. Chapter 9, "The Patient with Cancer," includes valuable data describing the types of cancer, American Cancer Society information, diagnostic techniques, and cancer treatments.

Joesten, Melvin D., David O. Johnson, John Netterville, and James L. Wood. *World of Chemistry.* 2d ed. Philadelphia: W. B. Saunders College, 1991. This textbook is both a valuable reference and an excellent introduction to environmental chemistry for anyone who has had no prior exposure to the subject. Chapter 16, "Toxic Substances," describes mutagens, carcinogens, and teratogens in detail.

OPHTHALMOLOGY

SPECIALTY

ANATOMY OR SYSTEM AFFECTED: Eyes

SPECIALTIES AND RELATED FIELDS: General surgery, optometry

DEFINITION: The study of the anatomy and physiology of the eye, as well as treatment of vision problems or diseases, ranging from corrective lenses to delicate surgery.

KEY TERMS:

ciliary body: a ring of tissue that surrounds the eye; the uveal portion of this tissue contains the ciliary muscle that adjusts the degree of curvature of the lens

cornea: the transparent portion of the first layer of the eye *keratitis:* a state of inflammation of the cornea that may cause partial or total opacity, leading to loss of vision

retina: the key sensory element located in the eye's inner layer

sclera: the opaque portion of the outer layer of the eye; commonly referred to as the "white of the eye"

SCIENCE AND PROFESSION

Among the sense organs and functions in the body, probably the most complex are the eye and the process of vision that it supports. Ophthalmologists study both the anatomy and the physiology of the eye in order to understand and treat common and rare eye diseases.

The principal anatomical element of vision is the eyeball, or eye globe, located in the right and left orbital openings of the skull. It is embedded in a complex system of tissues surrounded by ocular muscles that control its movement. Adjacent to the eye and also within the bony orbit is the lacrimal gland, which is responsible for keeping the eye moist. Only the front one-third of the globe is exposed. This exposed area is made up of the central transparent portion, the cornea, and a surrounding white portion, which is only part of the sclera, the main component mass of the globe itself. The sclera is a very dense collagenous (protein-rich) structure which has two large openings (the anterior and posterior scleral foramina) and a number of smaller apertures that allow for the passage of nerves and blood vessels into the eye. It is through the posterior scleral foramen that three main components sustaining the eye's functions pass: the optic nerve, the central retinal vein, and the central retinal artery.

The eye has three main layers, within which are further specialized divisions. The outer layer consists essentially of the transparent cornea and opaque sclera. The middle layer, called the uvea, is made up of the choroid, which is the outer coating of the layer; the ciliary body, which contains key eye muscles that affect the degree of curvature in the lens; and the iris, which, with the lens located immediately behind it, separates the anterior from the posterior chambers of the eye. This iris itself has two layers, the stroma and the epithelium. The latter is immediately recognizable to the layperson, since its cells are markedly pigmented, giving to each individual a characteristic eye color.

It is the opening in the iris, called the pupil, that allows the passage of light into the inner layer of the eye, which contains the key sensory portion of the organ, the retina. Before light reaches the inner layer and the retina, it passes through the lens of the eye, located immediately behind the iris (which it supports), and through the largest area of open space within the eye, the vitreous cavity. This posterior cavity, like the smaller forward cavity of the eye, is filled with a transparent hydrogel called aqueous humor, made up mainly of water (about 95 percent of its total mass) in a collagenous framework within which the main component is hyaluronic acid. The aqueous humor is very similar to plasma but lacks its protein concentration. The pupil of the eye serves a purpose similar to the diaphragm (or f-stop) on a camera; it opens wider (dilates) or closes (contracts) according to the intensity of light striking the eye. (This reaction explains why, after a few minutes in an apparently totally dark room, the eye adjusts at least in part to the lower intensity of light.) For purposes of examining the internal structures of the eye, ophthalmologists sometimes place special drops in the eye to cause the pupil to dilate.

The lens of the eye, which is held in place behind the pupil by zonular fibers, consists of onionlike lens fibers. These are the product of epithelial cells that "migrate" from their place of origin in a germinative zone next to the edges of the lens to the anterior portion of the concentric structure of the lens. The central or internal layers of lens fibers, called the embryonic nucleus, represent the earliest cell specialization processes before birth. By contrast, the anterior and posterior lens fibers are constantly renewed at the surface.

As light passes through the transparent lens fibers, the phenomenon of refraction results, in the simplest possible explanation, both from the concentric shape of the lens itself and from a differential in the index of refraction occurring in the "younger" outside layers of lens fibers and that of the "older" central layers; the latter have a greater index of refraction than the former. Another phenomenon that increases the refractive power of the lens occurs when the zonular fibers that hold it in place relax under the influence of the ciliary muscle, making the lens more spherical in shape. The resultant increase in refractive power is called accommodation.

It is the retina, located in the last layer of the eye, that receives the light images passing through the lens and transmits them to the brain via the optic nerve. Physiologists consider the nerve-related function of the retina to be comparable in many details with all other sensory phenomena in the body, including touch and smell. The retina itself consists of a very thin outer layer, called the retinal pigment epithelium, and an inner layer, the sensory retina. On the surface of the retina, one finds a layer of photoreceptor cells. Once affected by the absorption of light rays reaching them from the lens, these cells form synapses with an intermediate layer of modulator cells. A synaptic relationship may be defined as an excitatory functional contact between two nerve cells, causing either a chemical or an electrical response. The modulator cells—referred to as neurones when their function is to receive synaptic transmissions from receptor cells—in turn pass the "message" of light to ganglion cells forming the innermost cellular layer of the retina. These cells transmit electrical discharges through the optic nerve to the brain, where they are registered as images.

DIAGNOSTIC AND TREATMENT TECHNIQUES

Ophthalmologists must deal with a wide variety of problems affecting the eyes, ranging from injuries to the diagnosis of vision problems that can be corrected with eyeglasses or contact lenses. Perhaps the most important area of applied ophthalmology, however, involves treating the diseases that may occur in several areas of the eye.

An entire category of diseases can appear in the conjunctiva, the thin mucous membrane that lines the inner portion of the eyelid and covers the exterior of the sclera. Conjunctivitis refers to inflammatory conditions that may attack this membrane. Some conditions cause mere irritation, while others may lead to serious infections. In acute catarrhal, or mucopurulent, conjunctivitis, the conjunctival blood vessels become congested with mucus and then with pus, which accumulates on the margins of the eyelids. If untreated, this form of contagious, easily transmitted infection begins to affect the cornea, by causing prismatic distortions and eventually abrasions that may infect the cornea itself. A more serious form of conjunctivitis is referred to as purulent conjunctivitis; it is sometimes associated with complications of the sexually transmitted disease gonorrhea.

Inflammation of the cornea, or keratitis, usually comes from the passage of virulent organisms from the conjunctival sac, which, although exposed to the external environment, may not itself react to the presence of bacteria. There are many different types of keratitis. Individuals may be vulnerable to infections in the cornea as a result of abrasions (one of the main reasons that all ophthalmologists recommend against rubbing the eye to remove irritating particles) or because of abnormal conditions affecting the surface of the cornea. Among the latter, opthamologists list excessive dryness in the eye and the side effects of malnutrition leading to a condition called keratomalacia, which is common in underdeveloped countries.

Bacteria such as pneumococci (the primary contributor to pneumonia in the lungs) may cause infections that result in corneal ulceration, the most common form of keratitis. In such cases, the area affected by the ulceration may increase considerably as epithelial tissue in the cornea attaches itself to the ulcer. Corneal ulcers may be removed by surgery, although the effect of remaining scar tissue may reduce the level of vision. The prospect of success in corneal transplant operations has not eliminated the need for ulcer removal surgery, since transplants depend on the availability of "fresh" cornea donors.

Another form of corneal infection, herpes zoster (a form of skin rash also called shingles), is caused by the virus that causes chickenpox; it tends to be common among aged patients whose cellular immunity systems suffer from decreased efficiency. In herpes zoster ophthalmicus, an infection that begins in the eye spreads via the nasociliary branch of the ophthalmic nerves and appears as red blotches on the surface of the skin (usually near the eye orbits on the side of the infection only). Zoster attacks are accompanied by rather severe pain. Ophthalmologists use several key drugs to treat this condition, including Distalgesic, Fortral, or Pethidine. Resultant depression in the patient may be relieved by prescribing amitriptyline.

Inflammation and possible infection of other regions of the eye also occur. Some zones, such as the sclera, tend to be more resistant to invasion because of the density of their fibrous tissues. Superficial inflammation of the sclera, called episcleritis, may be transitory but recurrent. Ophthalmologists will prescribe the anti-inflammatory drug Tandearil in the form of drops. More serious but much less common is the condition called scleritis, which extends much deeper into the tissue of the sclera and may affect the cornea and the uveal tract in the middle layer of the eye. Treatment of scleritis involves the use of steroid therapy, such as the corticosteroid drug prednisolone, often supplemented with Tandearil.

Uveitis is a term that applies to inflammations that occur in the uveal tract. The name suggests that such complications are not limited to one or another of the parts of the uveal zone (the iris or the ciliary body): All are affected and must be treated simultaneously.

The most common vision problem is myopia (nearsightedness). While most people still choose to correct nearsightedness with contact lenses or glasses, laser techniques such as photorefractive keratectomy (PRK) and laser in situ keratomileusis (LASIK) have shown some promise in treating myopia. Early enthusiasm for radial keratotomy has waned because of erratic results.

The most widely known eye disorders are probably glaucoma and cataracts. Glaucoma occurs when pressure caused by an excessive amount of aqueous humor increases inside the eyeball, specifically in the area of the retina. Impairment of vision may be slight, occurring at first in the peripheral area of sight. Further deterioration, however, may lead to blindness in the eye. Regular treatment with drugs that reduce the production of aqueous humor is necessary in patients suffering from chronic glaucoma. Acute glaucoma, which is very sudden, represents only about one-tenth of recorded cases. It must be treated within less than a week to avert permanent blindness.

Cataracts occur when there is a loss of full transparency in the lens of the eye. Cataracts occurring among children are congenital or hereditary in origin. Cataract-like damage to the lens of the eye may also result from exposure to the sun's rays (which is especially dangerous when one views the sun without protection during eclipses), extreme heat, X rays, or nuclear radiation. Most characteristically, however, cataracts (from slight to advanced stages) are associated with the aging process. Formerly, cataract surgery was difficult and the recovery period slow, so patients were advised to wait as long as possible to have cataracts removed. Improvements in surgical techniques and materials mean that patients no longer need to wait until their vision is severely impaired to have this surgery. Most cataract extractions are combined with implantation of an intraocular lens, so that patients do not need to wear specially prescribed contact lenses or thick glasses following surgery.

Ophthalmologists make use of laser surgery for an increasing number of eye disorders. Lasers are used to treat eye problems caused by diabetes and hyper-

tension, to treat or prevent some types of glaucoma, and to treat other, rarer eye conditions. Macular degeneration, an important cause of decreased central vision, may be arrested by laser therapy, but the technique does not repair existing damage.

Microsurgical techniques have further revolutionized eye care and have led to more effective management of conditions (such as retinal detachment) that formerly caused blindness.

PERSPECTIVE AND PROSPECTS

Knowledge of the anatomy and physiology of the eye evolved gradually through history and then spectacularly in the latter half of the twentieth century. The most extraordinary advances in the later period were made in the field of eye surgery. For an understanding of how vision itself worked, it took centuries for surprisingly unscientific views to cede to the first modern theories and then, with the advance of anatomical dissection, the practical possibility of examining both normal and abnormal conditions of the organ in the laboratory.

An early but not widespread theory of how the eye sees, held into the Middle Ages, depended on what now seems to be the fantastic conception of *eidola*, or "skins." Those who believed this theory held (in part correctly) that something must be leaving the objects that one perceives through the eyes. This "something" was thought to be a skinlike picture that, once detached from the object in question, actually entered the eye (after an unexplainable physical contraction) through the pupil, the aperture in the eye that is visible in many different animals. Another widespread theory was a prescientific version not of light rays but of "visual rays" that were thought to leave the interior of the eye, returning to record the colors and shapes of objects encountered.

Historians generally agree that the twelfth century Arab scientist Ibn al-Haitham, known in the West as Alhazen, was the first to suggest that rays of light entered the eye to stimulate what he called the "sensorium." Although Alhazen's theory predated a scientific explanation of the nature of light itself, he based his views on the phenomenon of the lingering image on the eye's "sensorium" of strong light, particularly that of the sun, even after the eyelids closed out the object emitting light. He went as far as to propose a basic theory of refraction of light inside the eye. According to his theory, the sensorium recorded images according to an exact formula that reconstituted both the "shape" and the "order" in which rays are received by the eye, depending on the angle at which they strike the spherical surface of the cornea. Alhazen even warned that, although the eye's sensorium always duplicated this formula exactly, the observer (actually, the observer's brain) could be "tricked" by the reproduction of certain ray patterns that might resemble something that was not "real"—the optical illusion.

Alhazen's views would be examined and extended during the late sixteenth and mid-seventeenth centuries in the West by the scientific pioneers of optics, specifically the Italian Francesco Maurolico (died 1575) and the famous German astronomer Johannes Kepler (1571-1630). Kepler's best-known work complemented that of his Italian contemporary Galileo Galilei (1564-1642), marking a breakthrough in the science of optics and the use of lenses to make telescopes in order to explore the skies. Only in later generations, however, did the ophthalmological relevance of some of his findings concerning the measurement of light reflected off the objects "seen" by a lens become clear.

As specialized interest in the eye progressed along with the constant advance of science in the eighteenth and nineteenth centuries, exact observation of the internal features of the organ of vision hinged on both the historical progress of anatomical dissection and the development of instruments to look into the living eye. One of the principal figures who contributed to the latter field was the Swedish ophthalmologist Allvar Gullstrand (1862-1930). Gullstrand received the Nobel Prize in Physiology or Medicine in 1911 for his application of physical mathematics to the study of refraction of light in the eye. He gained additional worldwide attention for his research on astigmatism (the failure of rays to be focused by the lens accurately on a single central point) and for devising the so-called slit lamp for viewing the interior of the eye through the use of an intense beam of light.

In the area of eye surgery, a major landmark was achieved in the 1960's when the Spanish ophthalmologist Ramón Castroviejo began to develop a method for surgical transplant of fully transparent corneas from deceased donors to replace damaged corneas in eye patients.

—Byron D. Cannon, Ph.D.;
updated by Rebecca Lovell Scott, Ph.D.
See also Aging: Extended care; Albinos; Astigmatism; Biophysics; Blindness; Blurred vision; Cataract

surgery; Cataracts; Color blindness; Conjunctivitis; Corneal transplantation; Eye surgery; Eyes; Geriatrics and gerontology; Glaucoma; Laser use in surgery; Macular degeneration; Microscopy, slitlamp; Myopia; Optometry; Sense organs; Trachoma; Visual disorders.

For Further Information:

Davson, Hugh. *Physiology of the Eye.* 5th ed. New York: Academic Press, 1990. The eleven-chapter section called "The Mechanism of Vision" provides a technical but generally readable treatment of the photochemical and electrophysiological aspects of vision. Another section deals in detail with the muscular mechanisms that aid the eye in its work.

Miller, Stephen J. H. *Parsons' Diseases of the Eye.* 18th ed. New York: Churchill Livingstone, 1990. This study of the basic ophthalmological disorders and diseases was first published in 1907. Miller's updating in this edition supplements, on the basis of research at the beginning of the 1980's, common diagnoses and prognoses for each vital area of the eye.

Newell, Frank W. *Ophthalmology.* 8th ed. St. Louis: C. V. Mosby, 1996. Although clearly technical in its treatment of the subject, this textbook, revised over a twenty-year period, is widely cited.

Palay, David A., and Jay H. Krachmer. *Ophthalmology for the Primary Care Physician.* St. Louis: C. V. Mosby, 1997. While this text is aimed at physicians, it is well illustrated, and much of the material is in an outline format. The sixteen chapters cover the diagnosis and treatment of the eye problems seen in the primary care setting.

Ronchi, Vasco. *Optics: The Science of Vision.* Translated by Edward Rosen. Rev. ed. New York: Dover, 1991. Originally published in Italian in 1955, this textbook deals in quite readable detail with the principles of optics as they relate to the eye itself.

Yanoff, Myron, and Jay S. Duker. *Ophthalmology.* London: Mosby, 1999. Discusses such topics as the anatomy and histology of the eye and ocular physiology and physiopathology. Includes bibliographical references and an index.

Optometry

Specialty

Anatomy or system affected: Eyes
Specialties and related fields: Ophthalmology
Definition: A field involving the provision of eye exams, the prescription of corrective lenses, and

the diagnosis and treatment of eye disease, but not eye surgery.

KEY TERMS:

clinical refraction: the determination of appropriate optical powers and related parameters to promote optimal visual acuity

contact lens: a small, shell-like glass or plastic lens that rests directly on the external surface of the eye to serve as a new anterior surface and thus correct refractive error as an alternative to spectacles, to protect the eye, or to serve as a prosthetic device promoting a more normal appearance of a disfigured eye

ophthalmologist: a physician who specializes in the comprehensive care of the eyes and the visual system; ophthalmologists provide visual, medical, and surgical eye care and diagnose general diseases of the body

prism: an optical element or component that, by virtue of two nonparallel plane faces, deviates the path of a beam of light

spectacles: a pair of ophthalmic lenses held together with a frame or mounting; also called glasses

SCIENCE AND PROFESSION

Optometry has been defined as "the art and science of vision care" by Monroe J. Hirsch and Ralph E. Wick in *The Optometric Profession* (1968). The American Optometric Association has stated that "Doctors of Optometry are independent primary health care providers who specialize in the examination, diagnosis, treatment and management of diseases and disorders of the visual system." Optometrists examine eyes and the visual system. They prescribe spectacles and contact lenses, optimize binocularity (the manner in which the two eyes work together), and improve visual function. Optometrists are trained to detect, treat, and manage disorders and diseases of the eyes and related structures.

Optometry is one of the youngest of the learned professions, which were originally restricted to law, medicine, and theology. Following the earlier lead of organized medicine, optometrists successfully organized and passed the first optometry practice law in 1901. Optometrists today complete a university education and then spend four additional years in a specialized school or college of optometry to receive the O.D. (doctor of optometry) degree. Many optometrists spend an additional year training in special-interest residency programs after graduation. Optometrists

practice independently in private offices, although increasing numbers of optometrists also work in groups, the military, public health agencies, and university and hospital environments.

Distinctions are made between optometrists, ophthalmologists, and opticians. Ophthalmologists are physicians who diagnose and treat eye diseases and who perform eye surgery. They complete a premedical university education, four years of medical school, one year of internship, and three or more years of specialized training in ophthalmology. Many ophthalmologists also complete one or more years of fellowship subspecialty training. Opticians are technicians trained in the manufacture and dispensing of optical aids.

DIAGNOSTIC AND TREATMENT TECHNIQUES

A portion of the eye examination performed by optometrists is called clinical refraction. To the physicist, refraction is the bending of light as it passes through an interface separating two differing media (such as water and air). Refraction, however, has also come to mean the clinical evaluation of the human visual system. Clinical refraction generally results in a spectacle prescription; such a prescription will contain the spherical optical power, and the astigmatic optical power and its axis when appropriate, that are necessary to provide optimally focused light on the retina for each eye.

A clinical refraction also includes an assessment of binocularity, which is the way in which both eyes are used simultaneously such that each retinal image contributes to the final visual percept. (The retina is the inner nerve layer of the eye upon which the optics of the eye focuses the image of the outside world.) Much effort is made, during a refraction, to attain maximum visual comfort by optimizing binocularity. Occasionally, it is necessary to utilize a prismatic element in the spectacle prescription as well as optical powers to this end. In other cases, the clinician may suggest a course of eye exercises to assist the patient in achieving improved binocularity without, or in supplement to, spectacles. Some patients may be found to suffer from severe binocular dysfunction and are referred for surgical consideration.

Near vision is tested during a refraction, especially for those people more than forty years of age who might require optical assistance for near work. The cornea is the clear, circular "window" in the front of the eye through which the colored iris is seen. Behind the iris is a crystalline lens. The cornea and the lens act together to focus light on the retina. The cornea provides most of the refractive power of the eye, and the lens serves to fine-tune the image in a process called accommodation. As one ages, however, the ability to accommodate deteriorates. Some form of near correction, either with two pairs of spectacles or with some form of bifocal, is then necessary. Only minimal optical power is needed at first, but as the aging process continues, the need for stronger near correction increases.

For a given patient, an analysis of binocularity, the determination of near vision requirements, and a consideration of additional occupational or avocational tasks (such as sports) make up his or her "functional vision." For some patients, the data gleaned in a standard refraction will provide the optometrist with all the information necessary to recommend comfortable visual correction for all tasks. For other patients, some additional thought and consideration may be required. For example, a very tall, fifty-year-old patient may not require as strong a reading correction as another shorter individual of the same age because the former has longer arms and is more used to holding reading material at a greater distance than the latter. In addition, providing visual care to patients using computers and video display terminals has become a rapidly growing subarea in functional vision.

No clinical refraction would be complete without an assessment of ocular health. This examination consists of observation of the eyes and related structures, as well as a testing of function. Good visual acuity, in and of itself, is fairly good evidence that the function of the eye is normal. Some ocular diseases, however, may occur and—at least initially—leave central vision intact. The structures of the eye are inspected with the assistance of instruments such as a clinical biomicroscope, or slitlamp microscope, to examine the outer ocular structures, and an ophthalmoscope, which allows inspection of the structures of the inner eye. Pupillary dilation with pharmaceutical agents in the form of drops allows inspection of the peripheral retina. The pressure in the eye should be tested, a process called tonometry, and the field of vision evaluated. Many optometrists also bear the responsibility for the treatment of certain ocular diseases.

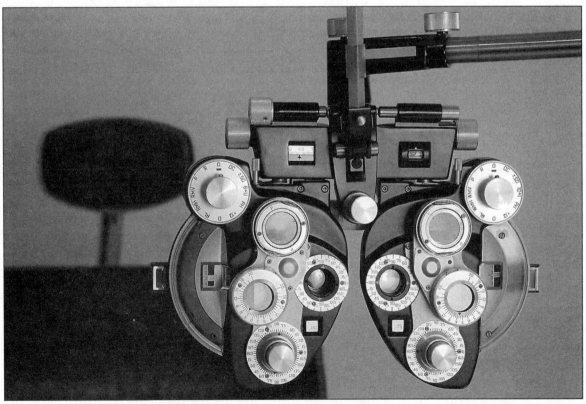

A device called a phoropter, which is used to evaluate a patient's vision. (Digital Stock)

As is true for all professionals, when the management of a specific problem is beyond one doctor's training, interest, or licensure, referral is made to another more appropriate doctor. For example, a patient with an age-related cataract (clouding of the crystalline lens) may be referred to an ophthalmologist for surgery, and an optometrist who suspects multiple sclerosis will refer the patient to a neurologist.

There are subspecialty areas in optometry, such as the prescription of appropriate visual aids for patients with particularly poor vision, known as low vision rehabilitation. Other subspecialty areas include industrial vision, developmental vision and vision therapy, and ocular disease. Contact lens care has become a large subspecialty in optometry. In fitting contact lenses, the curvature of the cornea, the quality of the patient's tears, and the health of the ocular surface and associated structures (such as eyelids) are all important considerations. Contact lenses are usually intended as devices to provide vision as an alternative to spectacles (although there are occasions when contact lenses may be used as prosthetics, to cover a damaged eye, or as therapy for a specific disease). The clinician must modify the original refractive findings to adjust for the placement of the lens because it will rest directly on the ocular surface instead of being attached to a frame half an inch from the eye. The contact lens must be designed so that the surface of the eye is not compromised by its presence. The proper contact lens care system is vitally important for the initial and continued success of a contact lens fitting. Continuing professional supervision is essential in maintaining optimal vision and safe contact lens wear.

Perspective and Prospects

Evidence suggests that spectacles were first used to assist human vision in Europe at about the end of the thirteenth century. Organizations of spectacle makers

Focal Disorders

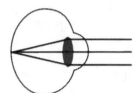

Normal sight:
Rays focus on retina.

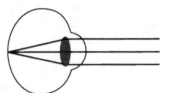

No correction necessary.

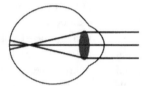

Myopia (nearsightedness):
Rays focus in front of retina.

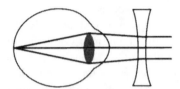

Bi-concave lens corrects nearsightedness. Light rays passing through lens are altered.

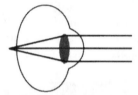

Hyperopia (farsightedness):
Rays focus behind retina.

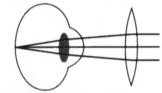

Bi-convex lens corrects farsightedness. Light rays passing through lens are altered.

were formed in Europe in the fourteenth and fifteenth centuries. These guilds policed the quality of spectacles and the working conditions under which their manufacture occurred. Spectacles were sold to the public in stores and by peddlers. Individuals self-selected the lens or lenses that seemed most appropriate to them for their visual tasks. Retailers selling spectacles eventually began to assist their clientele in making an informed selection. Over time, spectacle vendors evolved into opticians. Some "refracting" opticians tested vision to provide what they believed to be the most appropriate correcting lenses for a particular person. Physicians at that time did not recommend or examine the eyes for spectacles, preferring the use of medication for eye difficulties.

The impetus for optometry's modern development and legal recognition in the United States began with a confrontation between optometry and ophthalmology. A New York refracting optician named Charles Prentice referred a patient to Henry D. Noyes, an ophthalmologist, in 1892. Noyes wrote Prentice a thank-you note for the referral, but suggested that Prentice should not have charged a fee (of three dollars) for his services—such being the right reserved to professionals such as physicians. Prentice responded, defending his practice of charging for his services. Noyes sent Prentice's letters to another ophthalmologist named D. B. St. John Roosa, who expressed his opinion that Prentice was in violation of the law by charging a fee for his services. By 1895, Roosa had announced that he would seek legislation to prevent opticians from practicing, and Prentice responded by organizing the Optical Society of the State of New York. This society eventually introduced a bill to the New York legislature to regulate the "practice of optometry." Optometry was defined as refraction, dispensing (that is, selling) spectacles, and related services.

This bill was quite controversial and never came to a vote. Later, however, another New York optometrist, Andrew J. Cross, while visiting Minnesota to teach a program in optics, scoffed at the notion that Minnesota could pass an optometry practice act before New York. Thus inspired, the Minnesotans passed their law, which included a regulatory board, in 1901. Arguing that optometry was separate and distinct from medicine, optometrists proceeded to obtain practice acts in all the states over the next twenty-three years.

Optometrists sought to be professionals rather than businesspeople and developed an agenda which included the formation of organizations: Both the American Optometric Association (AOA) and the American Academy of Optometry were established early in the twentieth century. Efforts were made both to reduce the commercial aspects of practice and to improve educational standards. A code of ethics and stringent rules of conduct were adopted by the AOA.

The first American optometric schools were extensions of apprenticeships and offered short courses (one to two weeks) in refraction. Eventually, private schools were established to train both physicians and non-physicians. Academic programs developed from these independent schools, such as the Southern California College of Optometry and the Illinois College of Optometry. A milestone two-year optometry course began at Columbia University in New York in 1910; Cross and Prentice were instrumental in preparing the curriculum. Ohio State University began a four-year program in 1915, and the University of California, Berkeley, established an optometry course in 1923.

By 1992, seventeen schools and colleges of optometry trained optometrists in the United States; many of the university programs also provided academic postgraduate studies. Similar programs were created in England, Australia, Canada, Europe, Asia, Africa, and South America.

Optometrist and lawyer John G. Classe credits the major change in the way optometry developed in the latter half of the twentieth century to contact lenses and modern tonometry. Prior to technical improvements in contact lenses and tonometry, the practice of optometry was limited and nonmedical. The commercial success of contact lenses brought about research in physiology, which in turn expanded biological knowledge and improved contact lenses. The ability to use a tonometer without drops to test for increased intraocular pressure (a condition called glaucoma) gave optometrists additional responsibility in ocular disease management. Unfortunately, the subsequent changes in practice placed optometry in even greater direct conflict with ophthalmology.

In a meeting held in January, 1968, many of the leaders of the schools and colleges of optometry, the chair of the AOA's Council on Optometric Education, and the editor of the *Journal of the American Optometric Association* unofficially discussed the future of the profession. Court decisions had ruled that optometrists had the legal responsibility to detect, diagnose, and refer ocular disease, and many optometrists were frustrated by the limited scope of their practice. This group believed that optometry should discard its original concept of being a drugless profession dedicated solely to ocular function. They argued that optometric education should be expanded in the fields of ocular pharmacology, anatomy, physiology, and pathology so that optometrists would become primary entry points into the health care system for patients. Finally, it was concluded that the state laws which govern the practice of optometry should be updated to allow the optometrist to practice what he or she was taught, including the appropriate use of pharmaceutical agents.

In 1971, Rhode Island became the first state to amend its optometry law to permit the use of diagnostic pharmaceutical drugs. Despite continued opposition from ophthalmology, all fifty states followed over the next twenty years. In 1976, West Virginia became the first state to permit the use of therapeutic drugs, and thirty-two states had enacted similar laws by 1993.

It should be noted, however, that ophthalmologists continue to oppose the expansion of optometry's scope of practice, believing that a physician—medically trained to appreciate both the local and the systemic natures of ocular disease and treatment—is best qualified to treat ocular disease. Optometry is a health care profession providing eye care to a large segment of the public. It remains a field in transition, however, and it is not clear how the dual professions of optometry and ophthalmology, as they become more similar clinically and legally, will work out their future relationship.

—Barry A. Weissman, O.D., Ph.D.

See also Aging: Extended care; Astigmatism; Biophysics; Blurred vision; Cataracts; Eyes; Geriatrics and gerontology; Glaucoma; Myopia; Ophthalmology; Optometry, pediatric; Sense organs; Strabismus; Trachoma; Visual disorders.

FOR FURTHER INFORMATION:

Classe, John G. "Optometry: A Legal History." *Journal of the American Optometric Association* 59, no. 8 (1988): 641-650. This outstanding paper provides a summary of the history of the profession from a legal standpoint, including much of the more recent history not available elsewhere.

Cline, David, Henry W. Hofstetter, and John R. Griffin. *The Dictionary of Visual Science*, 4th ed. Radnor, Pa.: Chilton, 1989. A comprehensive dictionary of visual science, which is very complete and well organized.

Eger, Milton J. "Now It Can and Should Be Told." *Journal of the American Optometric Association* 60, no. 4 (1989): 323-326. This paper, written by a former editor of the *Journal of the American Optometric Association*, provides insight into the deliberations and conclusions of a very important, although unofficial, meeting which helped to redirect the course of the profession of optometry in the United States.

Gregg, James R. *History of the American Academy of Optometry*. Washington, D.C.: American Academy of Optometry, 1987. This text covers the history of the academic arm of the profession of optometry. It is quite well written and focuses on many of the early proponents of academics and professionalism in the field.

Millodot, Michel. *Dictionary of Optometry and Visual Science*. Oxford, England: Butterworth-Heinemann, 1998. Millodot, of Hong Kong Polytechnic University, defines forty-two hundred of the most commonly used terms in optometry and visual science, often with clinical advice.

OPTOMETRY, PEDIATRIC

SPECIALTY

ANATOMY OR SYSTEM AFFECTED: Eyes

SPECIALTIES AND RELATED FIELDS: Neurology, ophthalmology

DEFINITION: The diagnosis and treatment of vision problems and of diseases and injuries to the eye in infants and children.

KEY TERMS:

amblyopia: a problem, related to strabismus but not as severe, in which one eye does not function in conjunction with its partner; also called lazy eye

astigmatism: a visual disorder in which the eyeball is misshapen, causing the resulting image to be distorted

esotropia: a condition in which the eye is turned inward

exotropia: a condition in which the eye is turned outward

hyperopia: a visual disorder, commonly called farsightedness, in which the vocal point of the image falls behind the retina; farsighted people are able to see objects better from a distance than from a short range

myopia: a visual disorder, commonly called nearsightedness, in which the focal point of the image falls in front of the retina; nearsighted people are able to see objects better from a short range than from a distance

nystagmus: jerky eye movements

strabismus: a disorder of vision in which one or both eyes are turned inward or outward

vision: the process by which the brain gives meaning to the images that it receives from the eye through the optic nerve

SCIENCE AND PROFESSION

The pediatric optometrist has received special training in the diagnosis and treatment of visual disorders in children beyond the four years of optometry college that is required for the doctor of optometry (O.D.) degree. Those who choose pediatric optometry as a specialty must, during a one-year residency, develop competency in the diagnosis and treatment of childhood visual disorders as well as develop knowledge about the various aspects of child development. They must learn to prescribe and carry out vision therapy that can help children overcome problems of eye movement, eye coordination, and perception.

The optometrist is concerned with the health and functioning of all parts of the eye: the eyelids, which act as a filter; the cornea, which covers the outer part of the eye, bends light for focusing, allows the light to pass to the retina, and protects the eye from infection; the conjunctiva, which covers the underside of the lid and allows for the proper wetting of the cornea; the lachrymal system, a glandular system that produces and eliminates tears; the orbit, the bony structure that holds the eyeball; the extraocular muscles, which control eye movement; the lens, which provides focus; and the pupil, which regulates the amount of light that enters the eye. Optometry is also concerned with the visual pathway, the route that light takes from an image through the pupil, through the lens, to the optic nerve, and to the brain for interpretation. Optometry also considers problems related to the visual field, which describes the area that can be seen to the left, to the right, up, down, and in front.

In general, children suffer the same range of visual problems that adults suffer, even cataracts and glaucoma. While the vast majority of cataracts are not congenital and occur beyond the age of fifty, a cataract can be present at birth or develop at any time. One of every 10,000 births produces a baby with congenital glaucoma.

Conditions such as amblyopia or strabismus, in which one eye does not function properly with the other eye, are treated by pediatric optometrists. These conditions are characterized by eye turns that may be esotropic (inward) or exotropic (outward). Esotropic turning usually occurs at birth, while exotropic turning generally occurs after six months of age. Whether the eye turns are inward or outward, the pediatric optometrist must work with the patient to establish or restore binocularity, the process of two eyes working together to send an image to the brain; individuals who do not have binocularity have problems with depth perception and distance judgment.

Like adults, children have problems with farsightedness, nearsightedness, and astigmatism, as well as with eye injuries and diseases of the eye such as conjunctivitis, a highly contagious infection of the conjunctiva. Various diseases occurring in childhood, such as rubella and juvenile-onset diabetes, might affect eye functioning and create visual disorders.

Even though children have many of the same eye and vision problems as adults, childhood is a special developmental period. Eye or vision problems can significantly affect the quality of a child's early years as well as the quality of the child's future. A child's ability to read well, to do well in school, to play sports, and to interact effectively with peers may all be hampered by poor eye health or by vision problems. Pediatric optometrists must have knowledge of all aspects of human development and must understand how vision problems can impact development.

DIAGNOSTIC AND TREATMENT TECHNIQUES

Upon the initial examination of a child, the pediatric optometrist first takes the child's health history. A health history is important because many types of diseases, such as diabetes, and many kinds of physical conditions, such as high blood pressure, can create vision problems. The optometrist also obtains a family medical history, since certain visual problems are genetically based.

Next, the pediatric optometrist examines the patient's eyes for disease and injury. Certain tests are performed to determine visual acuity, perception, and reaction. An optometrist may prescribe visual therapy to improve or correct problems related to binocularity, perception, or reaction. Corrective lenses are prescribed to correct problems of acuity. When glasses are needed, the optometrist may work with an optician to make sure that the child receives eyewear that is flattering, as eyewear can affect the child's social life.

In cases of amblyopia and strabismus, surgery may be indicated. If so, the pediatric optometrist refers the patient to a pediatric ophthalmologist. Modern practice generally involves the use of vision therapy to train the eyes to work together. Sometimes, surgery is performed for strabismus, but often such surgery is only cosmetic; vision therapy is still required. Pediatric cases involving glaucoma, cataracts, or tumors also require the optometrist to work closely with an ophthalmologist.

PERSPECTIVE AND PROSPECTS

Research indicates that cultures that rely heavily on work requiring close visual examination, such as reading, have much higher incidences of vision problems than do other cultures. Thus, in the modern world, where there is a high dependence on literacy skills and computer use for recreational purposes, for communication, and for job functions, it is likely that all aspects of pediatric optometry will grow in the fore-seeable future.

—*Annita Marie Ward, Ed.D.*

See also Blindness; Blurred vision; Conjunctivitis; Diabetes mellitus; Eye surgery; Eyes; Myopia; Optometry; Sense organs; Strabismus; Styes; Visual disorders.

FOR FURTHER INFORMATION:

D'Alonzo, Thomas L. *Your Eyes: A Comprehensive Look at the Understanding and Treatment of Vision Problems.* Clifton Heights, Pa.: Avanti, 1991.

Rosner, Jerome. *Pediatric Optometry.* Stamford, Conn.: Appleton & Lange, 1996.

Seiderman, Arthur S., and Steven E. Marcus. *20/20 Is Not Enough: The New World of Vision.* New York: Alfred A. Knopf, 1989.

ORCHITIS

DISEASE/DISORDER

ANATOMY OR SYSTEM AFFECTED: Genitals, reproductive system

SPECIALTIES AND RELATED FIELDS: Family practice

DEFINITION: Orchitis is an inflammation of the testes, or testicles, usually caused by a generalized infection such as mumps, scarlet fever, or typhoid. It typically involves only one testicle. The patient can experience vomiting, fever, tenderness, and great swelling of the affected testicle. Orchitis caused by bacterial infection is treated with antibiotics, while orchitis resulting from viral infections can only be treated with rest, support for the testicles, and pain-relieving drugs. Chronic cases can be caused by syphilis, tuberculosis, and parasitic infections.

—*Alvin K. Benson, Ph.D.*

See also Antibiotics; Bacterial infections; Mumps; Parasitic diseases; Reproductive system; Scarlet fever; Sexually transmitted diseases; Testicles, undescended; Testicular surgery; Testicular torsion; Tuberculosis; Typhoid fever and typhus; Viral infections.

FOR FURTHER INFORMATION:

Coe, R. P. K. "Primary Mumps Orchitis with Meningitis." *The Lancet* 1, no. 6333 (January 13, 1945): 49-50.

Gilbaugh, James H. *A Doctor's Guide to Men's Private Parts.* New York: Crown, 1989.

Glenn, James F. *Glenn's Urologic Surgery.* 5th ed. Philadelphia: J. B. Lippincott, 1998.

ORGANS. *See* SYSTEMS AND ORGANS.

ORTHODONTICS

SPECIALTY

ANATOMY OR SYSTEM AFFECTED: Gums, mouth, teeth

SPECIALTIES AND RELATED FIELDS: Dentistry

DEFINITION: A dental specialty in which the teeth are straightened and moved into positions in the jaws that yield a correct and attractive arrangement.

KEY TERMS:

analgesic: a medication (such as aspirin) that reduces or eliminates pain

dental arch: the arched bony part of the upper and lower jaws, in which the teeth are found

lingual: related to the tongue; in orthodontics, the inner sides or faces of the teeth

malocclusion: an incorrect fit of the upper and lower teeth when they are brought together

mastication: the act of chewing food

occlusion: the fit of the upper and lower teeth when they are brought together

SCIENCE AND PROFESSION

The term "orthodontics" comes from the Greek words meaning "straight teeth." It is practiced by the dental specialist called an orthodontist. Orthodontists graduate from dental school and then specialize in orthodontics. To explore orthodontics as a field, one must first consider teeth and the mouth. Ideally, thirty-two human teeth are arranged in appropriate orientations in the dental arches of each jaw. Four incisors are located in the center of each arch; on either side of them are a cuspid or canine tooth, followed by two bicuspids (premolars) and three molars.

The first molar on the side of each jaw is viewed as particularly important to orthodontics. Appropriate tooth development within the jaw and correct tooth eruption enable proper dental health, which keeps teeth in the mouth for most of an individual's life. They also ensure appropriate mastication of food and good digestive health, as well as self-confidence with an attractive smile.

Teeth are rarely optimally placed in the jaws. One important reason for this is heredity. This facet of orthodontics relates to the teeth and to jaws. The genes that control the size and shape of human teeth and jaws vary considerably. In addition, the genes for teeth and jaws are highly individualized and often poorly related to one another. Hence, it is likely that orthodontic problems caused by tooth-jaw mismatch will occur.

Other aspects of the development of irregular tooth positioning arise from living. In some cases, teeth are damaged by decay, oral diseases, or injury. In others, poor oral habits such as thumb sucking move them out of appropriate positions. In many cases, minor problems may be handled by restorative dentistry, such as filling dental caries or placing crowns. Most treatment of poorly positioned teeth, however, is carried out by orthodontists on nearly 5 million Americans per year. The majority of these patients are children, but many adults are presently undergoing orthodontic treatment.

There are several main goals of orthodontic treatment involving the bones of the jaws and the teeth. First, occlusion is improved so that all teeth engage one another properly for chewing and swallowing. Speech patterns are also improved, because almost twenty letter sounds involve interactions between tooth, tongue, and jaw movements. Another goal is increased resistance to decay and periodontal disease, which cause havoc in mouths where teeth are too close together or misaligned in other ways. The final orthodontic goal is improved appearance, which is for many individuals the primary reason for undergoing treatment.

Most orthodontic problems are termed malocclusions and are caused by defects of teeth and/or the jaws. Malocclusions are often classified according to the system developed by Edward H. Angle, the origi-

nator of orthodontics. Three occlusion classes exist, defined by relationships between the upper and lower first molars.

In normal occlusion (class I), the lower first molars are seen slightly farther forward than their upper counterparts when the mouth is closed. This relationship positions the rest of the teeth for optimum chewing. When the arch length of either jaw is too small for all the teeth to be in appropriate positions, they become crowded. Also, in some individuals bimaxillary protrusion occurs, in which the front teeth of the jaws flare outward. These occurrences are unattractive and lead both to tooth decay and to periodontal disease.

Classes II and III are malocclusions that can be considered together. They are caused by improper positioning in the closed mouth of the lower first molars, either very far back or very far forward. In the first case (class II), the position of the first molars produces buck teeth because of the protrusion of the upper jaw in the closed mouth. The resulting problems are uncosmetic appearance and the ease with which buck teeth can be knocked out. Class II malocclusion is most often attributable to a hereditary size mismatch of the jawbones. Class III malocclusion is often termed crossbite. It causes the lower jaw to be positioned so that the lower front incisors are in front of the upper ones. In some cases, this problem is treated by orthodontics; in others, surgery is required.

The Angle classification system does not include faulty vertical relationships of the jaws, which produce other problems. Examples are overbite, which hides the lower teeth entirely in the closed jaw, and open bite, which leaves a gap between the upper and lower front teeth in the closed mouth. These situations may be asymmetric and make closures lopsided.

Functional malocclusions are also caused by thumb sucking, chewing of the lower lip, or tongue thrusting. With thumb sucking, class II malocclusion may result or be enhanced, or open bite may occur. Chewing the lower lip will cause the upper front teeth to flare outward, and tongue thrusting (often a consequence of mouth breathing because of asthma) may cause open bite, crossbite, or class II malocclusion.

Defects of the teeth themselves occur as well. They are caused by overretention or underretention of the baby teeth and missing or lost permanent teeth. These conditions cause the remaining teeth to drift in the mouth and should be corrected as soon as possible in order to preclude occlusion problems.

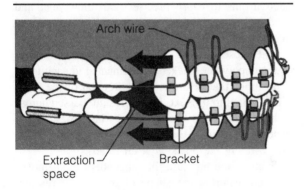

The most common orthodontic appliances are braces, which can be used to realign crooked teeth or correct malocclusion (such as underbite or overbite). In cases of tooth overcrowding, some teeth may be extracted, and the remaining teeth may be repositioned to fill the extraction space (shown here).

DIAGNOSTIC AND TREATMENT TECHNIQUES

The first stage of orthodontic treatment is an extensive diagnostic procedure that requires several office visits. First, the orthodontist compiles a complete dental and medical history. Then, the patient's mouth and teeth are examined thoroughly. This effort, accomplished in one visit, leads to a preliminary treatment plan. During the next visit, complete X rays of the jaws are taken to show their relationship to each other, dental impressions of the teeth and jaws are made, and color photographs of the face and mouth are taken.

On the third visit, the patient is given a comprehensive diagnosis, and a treatment plan is described. At this point, the patient is informed about the problems to be treated, the probable consequences if they are left untreated, the steps to be used and their duration, the results that are expected, and any possible treatment complications. The overall cost of the treatment is also discussed. After agreement is reached, treatment begins and may require up to several years of visits at varied intervals. The process begins with the use of orthodontic appliances worn to move the teeth to new positions. After this, a simpler appliance called a retainer is worn until the bone of the tooth sockets, remodeled by the earlier treatment, is able to maintain the new dental arrangement.

Patient compliance with treatment instructions is crucial. Short-term noncompliance can lengthen the treatment period greatly; extreme noncompliance may completely destroy the endeavor. Most aspects of modern orthodontic treatment are relatively painless. If soreness occurs, it may usually be relieved quickly by combining salt water gargles, temporary soft diets, and mild analgesics. Soreness caused by the rubbing of metal appliance parts against the inside of the cheeks or lips may be prevented by application of a wax supplied by the orthodontist. Pain that lasts for more than several days should be reported; it can usually be alleviated by an office visit where the orthodontist adjusts the offending portion of the appliance.

Throughout the course of orthodontic treatment, it is recommended that patients keep careful written records of orthodontic instructions and a complete daily record of use of the orthodontic appliance prescribed. The orthodontic appliances also need to be kept clean, stored carefully if removable, and guarded carefully during sports or other physical activities. The teeth must also be kept clean to prevent tooth decay. In addition, hard or sticky foods must be avoided.

The mechanical devices used by orthodontists vary widely. Their purposes are to direct jaw growth, to move selected teeth, to alter the behavior of the jaw muscles, and to maintain the position of the teeth once they have been moved. These appliances operate on two main principles. First, bone growth slows when pressure is applied against it and accelerates when the bone is kept in traction. This is how desired facial bone growth is attained. Second, when pressure is applied to the bone in tooth sockets, bone growth slows on the side to which the pressure is applied. Conversely, the growth of bone is stimulated on the other side of the tooth. This is the principle that generates tooth movement in the mouth. Applied properly, the combination of jaw and tooth treatment achieves results that can be fine-tuned over the treatment period. A lengthy treatment period ensures the minimum amount of pain while this movement occurs.

There are two main categories among the many orthodontic appliances used: fixed and removable appliances. Each category has numerous subcategories, and there are variants within each subcategory. Fixed appliances are firmly affixed in the mouth for the duration of treatment. They are made of metal cylinders shaped to fit snugly around individual teeth and cemented in position. The main fixed appliance types are bracketed appliances, lingual arch wires, habit control appliances, and space retainers.

Bracketed appliances, usually called braces, move teeth and direct growth of bone in the dental arches. Although braces are often disliked by patients on aesthetic grounds, orthodontists view them as an unrivaled means to cause precise tooth movement and directed bone growth. They are made up of several components. First, bands (metal cylinders) are applied around chosen anchor teeth. Then, metal or sturdy synthetic polymer brackets are cemented to each tooth in positions that determine the direction of the force to be applied to it. Next, arch wires are passed across each bracket to the anchor teeth, where they are attached to the bands. Elastic or wire ligatures keep the arch wires in the brackets at all times.

Much of the pressure that engenders tooth movement comes from the shape of the arch wires and their composition. Elastic bands are also used to provide special treatment to a given tooth or tooth group. These bands must be removed before eating and replaced daily. When necessary, external headgear is used to apply pressure to teeth and/or jaws, either pulling them forward or pushing them backward.

Lingual bracketed appliances, a newer device often called "invisible braces," are fixed appliances attached to the teeth on the inside of the dental arch. They are not externally visible except for the bands on the anchor teeth. Thus, they are advantageous aesthetically. They do not function as well as standard braces, however, and often interfere with normal speech. Other fixed appliances include lingual arch wires, habit control devices, and space retainers. They are not discussed here.

A wide variety of removable appliances is also used. They are either entirely or partly removable by wearers. Removable appliances are most effective when worn constantly, but they can be removed at meals and on special occasions. Their use gives much less precise results than fixed appliances, however, and requires the continuous, unflagging cooperation of patients. Active, partly removable appliances put pressure on teeth and jaws. Functional appliances, which are completely removable, alter the pressure created by the muscles of the mouth and so act on the teeth and bones (for example, lip bumpers, which keep lips away from teeth).

Removable habit control appliances and space retainers are used, respectively, to prevent activities such as thumb sucking and to maintain desired spaces between teeth until the new dental arrangements have stabilized. They are specially designed bands, acrylic plates, and/or combinations. Space retainers exert enough pressure on teeth to keep them in place but not to move them. Special headgear may also be used as an auxiliary to in-the-mouth appliances. In some cases, diseased or extra teeth must be extracted as part of the treatment regimen.

PERSPECTIVE AND PROSPECTS

Orthodontics has changed markedly since its inception. The changes include efforts at making braces more appealing and a changing clientele, evolving from one in which most patients were children to a population having many adult customers. The new direction in producing more cosmetic bracketed appliances arises from several factors.

First is the development of stronger and better synthetic polymer and ceramic replacements for metals, allowing the creation of materials that are less visible and that still produce the unrivaled therapeutic capabilities of bracketed appliances. A second factor is the interest of adults in orthodontic treatment. This discriminating population wishes to appear as attractive as possible, even in braces, and has both the independence of judgment and the monetary power to drive trends toward the use of such materials.

The adult move toward orthodontics in the United States is founded partly on the funding of orthodontic work by entities as diverse as Medicaid for welfare recipients and third-party group dental insurance plans. In addition, the adult public is being made more aware that it is not necessary to live out life with an uncosmetic smile simply because orthodontic treatment was not attempted in childhood or adolescence.

Considerable research has been carried out in the treatment of problems associated with orthodontics, including the root tip resorption that often halts such treatment. It is hoped that a combination of these endeavors and factors will continue to improve orthodontics.

—Sanford S. Singer, Ph.D.

See also Bones and the skeleton; Dentistry; Jaw wiring; Orthodontics; Periodontal surgery; Teeth; Tooth extraction.

FOR FURTHER INFORMATION:

Holt, Robert Lawrence. *Straight Teeth: Orthodontics and Dental Care for Everyone.* New York: William Morrow, 1980. Provides excellent information on teeth; orthodontic principles, procedures, and appliances; and dental health procedures that can help maintain good dentition and cut dental and orthodontic costs. A handy glossary is included.

Houston, W. J. B., C. D. Stephens, and W. J. Tulley. *A Textbook of Orthodontics.* 2d ed. Boston: Butterworth-Heinemann, 1992. This dental handbook covers all aspects of the field of orthodontics. Includes a bibliography and an index.

Klatell, Jack, Andrew Kaplan, and Gray Williams, Jr., eds. *The Mount Sinai Medical Center Family Guide to Dental Health.* New York: Macmillan, 1991. This excellent family reference work has a fine, well-illustrated chapter on orthodontics. Procedures, appliances, and patient "dos and don'ts" are included. A wide variety of related dental options is also described.

Mitchell, Laura, Nigel E. Carter, and Bridget Doubleday. *An Introduction to Orthodontics.* New York: Oxford University Press, 2001. This book provides a concise but comprehensive introduction to clinical orthodontics. It is designed to appeal to both undergraduate dental students and the practicing dentist. It is both easy to read and fully illustrated.

ORTHOPEDIC SURGERY

PROCEDURE

ANATOMY OR SYSTEM AFFECTED: Bones, feet, hands, hips, joints, knees, legs, ligaments, muscles, musculoskeletal system, nervous system, spine, tendons

SPECIALTIES AND RELATED FIELDS: General surgery, orthopedics, physical therapy, podiatry, rheumatology, sports medicine

DEFINITION: Surgical procedures involving the bones or joints.

KEY TERMS:

polymethylmethacrylate: a material used in the fixation of bones

valgus: a musculoskeletal deformity in which a limb is twisted outward from the body

varus: a musculoskeletal deformity in which a limb is twisted toward the body

INDICATIONS AND PROCEDURES

Orthopedic surgery encompasses a number of different procedures carried out to repair injuries affecting the skeletal system and joints or to repair tissues associated with these structures. Such surgery may also attempt to correct associated neurological injury. In addition, orthopedic surgery is used to correct musculoskeletal problems that may be congenital in origin.

Among the congenital conditions for which orthopedic surgery may be warranted are bowlegs (valgus knees) and knock-knees (varus knees). In the case of bowlegs caused by a congenital malformation, one or both legs are twisted outward at the knee. In knock-knees caused by congenital conditions, the knees are curved inward, causing the lower legs to twist away from the body.

Treatment begins with a thorough evaluation of the problem. Based on X-ray analysis, an orthopedic surgeon may make a decision as to whether surgery can be used in the correction of the problem. During the surgical procedure itself, the affected limbs are properly aligned; they are splinted upon completion of the surgery. The chances of success are greatest in younger children. In an analogous situation, if a limb is twisted during fetal development, the child may exhibit misalignment of the structure following birth. Since bone at this stage of life is only beginning its growth, maintaining the limb in a splint may correct the problem. If necessary, the surgeon may decide to realign the limb at the joint through orthopedic surgery.

Tumors that originate in bone are uncommon. If they occur, such growths must be removed as quickly as possible because of the speed with which they spread to adjacent and distant structures in the body if the tumor is cancerous. The first signs of bone cancer include pain and swelling in the affected region. Spontaneous fractures may occur. X-ray and biopsy analyses are necessary to confirm the diagnosis of cancer. If the tumor is benign, it may be removed through surgery. Osteomas, which are tumors that arise from connective tissue within the bone, may require radiation or chemotherapy in addition to surgical removal.

Commonly, orthopedic surgery is used to correct fractures or dislocations. As with any procedure, a thorough evaluation is necessary prior to a final decision. This evaluation often includes X-ray and computed tomography (CT) analyses. If the injury involves the spine, treatment must both correct the problem and prevent secondary injury to the spinal cord. Fractures to the vertebral column may produce fragments that pose a threat to the spinal cord. Under these conditions, orthopedic surgery is used to immobilize or straighten the spinal column; this may involve external braces or an internal brace such as a Harrington distraction rod. The patient may be immobilized for weeks to months, depending on the extent of the injury and the course of treatment.

USES AND COMPLICATIONS

One of the most common applications of orthopedic surgery is the repair of trauma or fractures to bones. For example, a blow to the face, either intentional or accidental, may result in fractures to the nose or facial bones. Injuries to other skeletal structures, including the spine, may also result from the incident. This is particularly true if the source of the injury was an automobile accident. Upon clinical examination by a physician, it may be apparent that facial bones have been fractured. X-ray analysis may be used to confirm the initial diagnosis. Proper repair and restoration of features will be the primary concern of the orthopedic surgeon, assuming that the injuries are not life-threatening. In the event of facial injuries, damage to teeth and other periodontal regions will also be a consideration. In many cases, wire fixation may be a sufficient course of treatment. If more severe, the fracture may require screw-plate fixation, particularly in complicated fractures.

If uneventful or uncomplicated, the healing of such

injuries usually requires about six weeks of immobilization. The procedure and immobilization, however, are inherently uncomfortable. If a muscle tear is severe or significant, resulting in a pull to the bone or joint, an associated fracture may heal improperly because of the dislocation of tissue. Proper evaluation of surgical options, including the use of metallic plates, can limit any such complications.

Although cancers originating in bone tissue are uncommon, they nevertheless present problems for the orthopedic surgeon. Fractures related to tumor development are generally treated in much the same way as uncomplicated breaks. If damage to the bone, either through the tumor itself or as a result of therapy, is severe, even surgical repair may not be sufficient to heal the structure and allow mobility or normal function. If the fracture is near the joint, the bone may require realignment or resection, resulting in a shortening of the structure. In some cases, internal fixation with polymethylmethacrylate bone cement may be used to augment repair.

PERSPECTIVE AND PROSPECTS

The introduction of CT scanning technology in the 1970's allowed for much more detailed evaluation of bone and joint injuries. Much of the technology is best applicable in a post-traumatic situation, evaluating the result of injury rather than its cause. Magnetic resonance imaging (MRI) is based on different technology but produces results that are similar to CT scans.

The destruction of bone as a function of aging or of disease is not well understood. Degenerative bone disease as a result of arthritis is among the most common of arthritic conditions, affecting nearly half of middle-aged adults in some manner. Such conditions, particularly among the elderly, remain to be fully addressed.

The ability to carry out bone transplants, developed extensively in the latter half of the twentieth century, allowed for at least partial replacement of damaged bone. Replacement structures may come from the patient's own body or from a cadaver. In addition, orthopedic technology has resulted in artificial prostheses for the replacement of most joints in the body.

Joint replacements are dramatic. Individuals with crippling deformities can have nearly normal function restored through replaced joints. The most commonly replaced joints include hips and knees. Other joints can also be replaced. Individuals who have their hips and knees replaced usually start walking on the replaced joint in the first or second postoperative day. Complete rehabilitation requires several months.

—Richard Adler, Ph.D.;
updated by L. Fleming Fallon, Jr.,
M.D., Ph.D., M.P.H.

See also Amputation; Arthroplasty; Arthroscopy; Bone grafting; Bunions; Disk removal; Fracture repair; Hammertoe correction; Hammertoes; Heel spur removal; Hip fracture repair; Hip replacement; Jaw wiring; Kneecap removal; Laminectomy and spinal fusion; Orthopedics; Orthopedics, pediatric; Physical rehabilitation.

FOR FURTHER INFORMATION:

Bentley, George, and Robert B. Greer, eds. *Orthopaedics*. 4th ed. Oxford, England: Linacre House, 1993. A standard textbook of orthopedic surgery. Although the text is quite technical, a nonphysician can easily understand the diagrams.

McCallaghan, John, and Aaron Rosenberg, eds. *The Adult Hip*. Philadelphia: Lippincott-Raven, 1997. A standard reference text on surgery of the hip. Complementing the text are more than 1,300 full-color and black-and-white illustrations, including drawings by a noted medical illustrator.

Tapley, Donald F., et al., eds. *The Columbia University College of Physicians and Surgeons Complete Home Medical Guide*. Rev. 3d ed. New York: Crown, 1995. This book is easy for nonmedical readers to understand. It is most likely to be found in a library.

Tierney, Lawrence M., Jr., et al., eds. *Current Medical Diagnosis and Treatment: 2001*. 39th ed. New York: McGraw-Hill, 2000. This book is revised annually and provides information relating to medical conditions that are associated with orthopedic surgery. It is an excellent and concise text but is written for professionals.

Way, Lawrence W., ed. *Current Surgical Diagnosis and Treatment*. 11th ed. Norwalk, Conn.: Appleton & Lange, 1998. This book is intended for professionals and provides up-to-date information concerning orthopedic surgical procedures.

ORTHOPEDICS

SPECIALTY

ANATOMY OR SYSTEM AFFECTED: Bones, feet, hands, hips, joints, knees, legs, ligaments, muscles, musculoskeletal system, nervous system, spine, tendons

SPECIALTIES AND RELATED FIELDS: Physical therapy, podiatry, rheumatology, sports medicine

DEFINITION: The field of medicine concerned with the prevention and treatment of disorders, either developmental or caused by injury or disease, that are associated with the skeleton, joints, muscles, and connective tissues.

KEY TERMS:

articulation: a joint between two bones of the skeleton; also called an arthrosis

bursa: a connective tissue sac filled with fluid that reduces friction at joints

collagen: a fibrous protein found in skin, bone, ligaments, tendons, and cartilage

inflammation: the reaction of tissue to injury, with its corresponding redness, heat, swelling, and pain

ligament: a structure of tough connective tissue that attaches one bone to another bone

synovial: referring to the lubricating fluid in the joints or the membrane surrounding the joints

tendon: a structure of tough connective tissue that attaches a muscle to a bone

SCIENCE AND PROFESSION

Orthopedics is the branch of medicine primarily concerned with the movement of the human body and its parts, as well as disorders that affect its function. Such activities as maintaining posture, walking, doing manual work, and exercising involve a complex relationship between the nervous system, muscular system, and skeletal system. While orthopedists must be familiar with the nervous system, they focus primarily on the prevention and treatment of disorders of the skeleton and muscles. They also have expertise in the proper development of these systems in childhood and the changes that occur as a result of aging.

When a person decides to make a movement, the brain sends signals to the muscles. The muscles contract and, by pulling on the bones to which they are attached, cause that part of the body to move. The anchor point for the muscle is the origin, and the attachment point to the bone that is being moved is the insertion. Muscles work in groups to perform a movement. The principal muscle involved is the prime mover, or agonist. The muscles that help the prime mover are called synergists. When a prime mover contracts, the muscle on the opposite side of the bone, termed the antagonist, must relax. An illustration of this would be the muscle and bone interaction involved in the flexing of the arm. The biceps muscle, anchored to bone in the shoulder, contracts, pulling on the bone in the lower arm to which it is attached by a tendon. Its synergist, the brachialis, also contracts. On the back of the upper arm, its antagonist, the triceps muscle, relaxes to allow the arm to bend. When the arm is extended, the triceps becomes the prime mover for that action, and the biceps is the antagonist.

The skeletal system is made of bone and cartilage. Bone cells, called osteocytes, take in nutrients from the blood and constantly renew the bony matrix. The chemical composition of bone includes calcium and phosphorus salts, which provide stiffness. The fibrous protein collagen gives bones some flexibility. Cartilage cells, called chondrocytes, manufacture cartilage, which is a mass of collagen and elastic fibers imbedded in a gelatin-like substance. The nature of this structure gives cartilage more flexibility than bone, which makes it an ideal substitute for bone in certain areas. The ribs, for example, are attached by cartilage to the sternum or breastbone. This arrangement allows for the expansion of the chest during breathing.

Tendons, ligaments, and bursas are also part of the skeletal and muscular systems. Tendons attach muscles to bones. They are made of fibrous tissue so strong that, under stress, the muscle will tear or the bone will break before the tendon will be damaged. Ligaments, which are also made of fibrous tissue, attach bones to other bones and provide stability at the joints. Bursas are fluid-filled connective tissue sacs that lie between muscle and bone, tendon and bone, or other areas around joints. They reduce the damage that occurs to the softer tissue as it rubs against bone with each movement. Because of their close interdependence, the skeleton, attached muscles, and other associated structures are often referred to as the musculoskeletal system.

The health of the musculoskeletal system during childhood is of primary importance to an individual in attaining full growth and function as an adult. In the early developmental stages of the embryo and fetus, a skeleton of cartilage is formed. This structure is replaced with bone in a process called ossification that continues for years after birth. Good nutrition is vital to this process. In particular, the body requires adequate amounts of protein, calcium, and vitamin D. The ends of a long bone are separated from the shaft of the bone by cartilage until the child reaches full growth. Care should be taken when participating in sports, since damage to these areas could affect the growth of that limb. Hormonal production influences the development of the skeleton. Adequate amounts of growth hormone are needed to ensure that proper growth is attained. At puberty, sex hormones, especially testosterone, stimulate the final growth spurts and completion of the adult skeleton.

Young adults have attained their full growth, but the skeleton must renew itself continuously to remain strong and maintain its ability to repair injury. A woman of childbearing age must eat a healthy diet since she may need to nourish a fetus that, in turn, is developing its own skeleton. Both men and women must take care to exercise, since the stress of activity not only builds muscle but also sends messages to the bone to maintain its strength. Calcium and vitamin D intake must continue, or the bones may begin to dissolve some of their calcium matrix. Automobile accidents, work injuries, and sports injuries are more likely to occur at this stage of life.

As adults age, metabolic and other cellular processes become less efficient, and care must be taken to maintain functions and prevent further losses. At one time, disorders such as osteoarthritis and osteoporosis were considered an inevitable part of the aging process. While heredity is certainly a risk factor in these conditions, a substantial body of evidence has been accumulated showing that some degenerative processes can be traced to lifestyle and diet. Osteoarthritis is the type of joint tissue degeneration that is associated with wear and tear on the joints. A person who is obese puts excessive pressure on the skeletal system, especially the hips, knees, and ankles. This pressure increases the damage to the joints. A person who fails to exercise begins to lose flexibility in the joints, and muscles become weaker.

Osteoporosis occurs as bones become porous and brittle. As osteocytes age, they become less efficient at calcium absorption and renewal of the bony matrix. At a time in life when more calcium is needed to make up for this inefficiency, most people consume fewer dairy products, either because of lactose intolerance or because of the ingestion of other beverages. Older women are at particular risk because their bones are lighter than are those of men. After the menopause, women lose some of the protection that estrogen provided by stimulating the absorption of calcium and thus bone renewal. If older people lose the ability to move as surely as before and their reflexes slow down, injuries are likely to occur as a re-

sult of falls. These injuries are much more serious if the bones are brittle. Even if osteoporosis is not a factor, fractures and other injuries in an older individual do not heal as quickly as they would in a younger person.

Because of their knowledge of developmental processes, orthopedists, as well as pediatricians, are able to advise parents concerned about their growing children and the appropriate precautions for sports activities. Recommendations are made by orthopedists with regard to the design and utilization of safety equipment to prevent or reduce injury. Advice on nutrition and exercise for adults may also be given by physicians in an effort to reduce the incidence of problems as a person ages, allowing continuation of an active, independent life.

DIAGNOSTIC AND TREATMENT TECHNIQUES

In nonemergency situations, patients with some pain or disorder of the muscles, bones, or joints are usually referred to an orthopedic surgeon. The first office visit begins with a review of the condition, during which the physician will take a general medical history and obtain a history of the current complaint. This history will include the time frame from onset, any action that may have initiated the condition, and

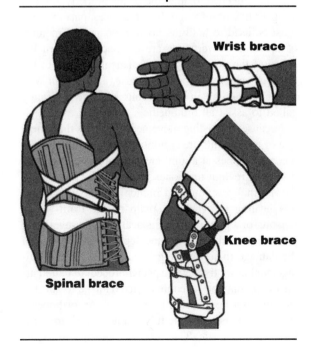

Common Orthopedic Braces

Wrist brace

Knee brace

Spinal brace

a description of any difficulty in movement that the patient is having. A physician will then perform a physical examination to determine the specific areas affected and observe range-of-motion exercises to determine if function has been lost.

X rays or other imaging methods are ordered to see whether any structural defect can be seen. Blood tests may be ordered if a disease process is expected. Once a diagnosis has been made, a physician may prescribe medication, order physical therapy or home exercises, schedule surgery, or take other therapeutic measures to correct the condition. The types of abnormalities treated by orthopedists generally fall into one of three categories: injuries caused by accidents, repetitive motion disorders, and diseases affecting the skeleton, skeletal muscles, or joints.

The most common situation in which a patient sees an orthopedist is after an accidental injury. If the injury is severe, the patient may be transported to a hospital emergency room, with care taken to keep the injury site immobilized until a physician can see the patient. The type of treatment needed will be determined by the type and severity of the injury. In a closed or simple fracture, the skin is unbroken; the bones are manipulated back in line and then immobilized with a plaster cast or brace. An open or compound fracture occurs when the ends or fragments of the bone protrude through the skin. In this case, or if surgery is needed to align the bones properly, there is a higher risk of infection. In some cases, pins or wires must be used to hold the bone in position. Fractures of the skull or vertebrae are of special concern because of the possibility of permanent damage to the brain or spinal cord; a neurologist (a physician with specialty training in the nervous system) is usually called to assist an orthopedic surgeon.

Because of twisting movements, injuries that affect one or more joints are common. A dislocation occurs when the bones at a joint are separated. An orthopedist must realign the bones as closely as possible to the original positions and immobilize the joint to allow healing to occur. A sprain results from severe twisting of a joint without dislocation. The severity of joint injury and recovery time depend on the extent of the damage to surrounding ligaments, tendons, cartilage, and other tissues. A special procedure called arthroscopy may be scheduled since damage to soft tissue may not be revealed in an X ray. An orthopedic surgeon inserts a flexible tube, called an arthroscope, into the injury site. This tube, combined with lights

and a camera, allows the surgeon to view the joint cavity, to see if any abnormality is present, and, if possible, to repair it.

Some damage to the musculoskeletal system is not the result of a single accident but of actions that are repeated over a long period of time as a part of work duties or recreational activities. These are termed repetitive motion disorders. For example, bursitis, or inflammation of the bursas, may arise in a baseball pitcher's shoulder or a tennis player's elbow. Because the same motion is repeated over and over, the rub of the bursa and other soft tissue over bone causes irritation and inflammation, resulting in pain each time the movement is attempted. Treatment consists of reducing the inflammation by using cortisone or other similar drugs, usually by injection at the affected site, coupled with rest. Resumption of the activity may occur following recommendations from an orthopedist or therapist on a change in technique aimed at reducing the trauma. In some cases, the condition becomes chronic, and the patient may have to discontinue the activity altogether.

Many occupations arising in the mid-twentieth century involved relatively small movements of the hands and wrists. A worker on an assembly line who installs a specific part and an employee who uses a computer keyboard all day are examples of people at high risk for repetitive motion disorders. An understanding of the structure of the wrist leads to better understanding of the problem involved. The median nerve leads from the spinal cord through a tunnel in the carpal bones of the wrist and then branches out to the fingers. It is encircled, together with tendons leading to the fingers, by the transverse carpal ligament. When constant friction causes swelling of the tendons and tissues adjacent to the nerve, the nerve is pinched, resulting in pain, tingling, and weakness in the hand and fingers. This condition is termed carpal tunnel syndrome. Therapy may include changing work positions, wearing a splint to hold the wrist straight, using medications to reduce inflammation, and injecting cortisone at the injury site. If the problem continues, surgery may be needed. In this procedure, the orthopedic surgeon makes an incision in the wrist and cuts the transverse carpal ligament, thus releasing the pressure on the nerve and tendons. If the motion or activity that initially caused carpal tunnel syndrome is not stopped, the condition is likely to recur.

Diseases can affect the bones and joints. Congenital defects and inheritance may result in deformities that can be treated by orthopedic devices or surgery. Hormone therapy may be used by a physician to help a child attain full growth. Nutritional disorders, such as rickets, may cause the softening of the bones, with the corresponding bowed-leg deformity. Caused by a vitamin D deficiency, rickets must be treated not only with vitamin therapy but also with braces to keep the legs straight while the bones harden. Multiple myeloma is a form of cancer that invades the bone and bone marrow and must be treated with chemotherapy as well as surgery to remove the tumor. Infections such as gangrene affect the limbs and, if not treated in time, may necessitate amputation by the orthopedic surgeon.

Of all the diseases of the musculoskeletal system, arthritis and related disorders affect the most people. "Arthritis" is a general term referring to inflammation of a joint. Osteoarthritis is a degenerative disease that results to some extent from the aging process, although it can be exacerbated by obesity, lifestyle, or injury. Arthritis can also be caused by infection or by deposits of uric acid crystals, a condition called gout. The most serious form of joint disease is rheumatoid arthritis, a term that is sometimes used to encompass a group of related disorders. These diseases are classified as autoimmune conditions because the body is making antibodies against itself—in this case, against the tissues associated with the joints. The disease process itself is often treated by a specialist called a rheumatologist, who tries various medications to alleviate the condition. An orthopedic surgeon may be called upon to help correct the deformities resulting from the disease or to replace defective joints with artificial ones. Special care must be taken in cases of juvenile rheumatoid arthritis, since the growth process may also be affected. Lupus erythematosus, ankylosing spondylitis, and scleroderma are some of the other autoimmune diseases that affect the musculoskeletal system.

PERSPECTIVE AND PROSPECTS

In the study of prehistoric humans, a major source of information is their skeletal remains. Archaeologists have found evidence of broken bones that were set and healed, indicating some rudimentary attempts at the treatment of injuries. Examination of hieroglyphs shows that ancient Egyptians set bones and used wooden splints held in place by the same gum and bandages that were used to wrap mummies. There were no medical specialties, and the treatment of

wounds and fractures was part of the duties of any medical practitioner.

The branch of medicine known as orthopedics had its start in the eighteenth century. A physician named Jean André Venel opened an institute in Switzerland with the purpose of correcting skeletal deformities in children. The term "orthopedics" is actually a combination of two Greek words: *orthos*, meaning "straight" or "correct," and *pais*, meaning "child." Treatment of congenital deformities such as clubfoot and defects caused by rickets or injury was the primary function of this type of clinic.

In the nineteenth century, the development of quick-setting plaster for casts aided physicians in the immobilization of broken bones after they were set. The development of anesthesia and antiseptic techniques to prevent infection allowed the practice of orthopedic surgery to expand. Research using the microscope added to the understanding of the structure and function of bone as a living tissue.

In 1895, Wilhelm Conrad Röntgen discovered that radiation from a cathode-ray tube would produce a photographic image of the bones of his hand. By the early twentieth century, the medical X ray came into widespread use, providing an invaluable diagnostic tool for orthopedists. In the 1940's and 1950's, better understanding of radioactive phenomena allowed the development of safer X-ray equipment and techniques. In the 1970's and 1980's, other imaging techniques, such as computed tomography (CT) scanning and magnetic resonance imaging (MRI), increased the ability of orthopedic surgeons to diagnose and treat musculoskeletal disorders.

One of the greatest orthopedic surgical advances has been in the ability to treat badly damaged limbs. At one time, the best the orthopedic surgeon could do for some patients was to amputate the limb to prevent the spread of infection and the development of gangrene, then help them cope with the amputations by use of artificial limbs. More sophisticated techniques, incorporating the use of the microscope with computer-directed surgical instruments, allow the reattachment of limbs in many cases by enabling the surgeon to connect even the smallest blood vessels and nerves.

If amputation is necessary, artificial limbs, or prostheses, have also become more sophisticated. Artificial hands have become functional as a result of computer technology that enables the patient to direct the movement of the fingers by contracting and relaxing arm muscles. New plastics and other materials are being developed and used for synthetic joint replacements which increase the mobility of, and decrease the pain for, arthritic patients.

Joints are now routinely replaced. The most common replacements are hip and knee joints, although techniques have been developed to replace other joints in the body. The surgery is performed in a hospital. Recipients are encouraged to begin to use their replaced joints within twenty-four to forty-eight hours after surgery. Complete rehabilitation requires several months of increasingly intense physical activity and exercise. Contemporary materials have an expected useful life of twenty or more years.

A better understanding of the natural healing process at the cellular level has also allowed advances in the treatment of fractures. It has been found that attaching a device that generates a weak electric current can increase the rate of healing in some patients. This current stimulates the multiplication of osteocytes and the growth of new bone in the area.

As the understanding of disease and of degenerative processes increases, better treatments can also be devised. Osteoporosis, for example, is known to be a preventable condition when a correct diet and sufficient physical exercise are obtained throughout life. After the menopause in women, treatment with estrogen replacement therapy gives further protection against osteoporosis. New imaging devices allow osteoporosis to be detected at an earlier stage and more aggressive treatment measures to be applied. The genetic factor in diseases and conditions that trigger autoimmune disorders are other areas of research that are being pursued. While accidents will always occur, orthopedic research into the injury process can help devise methods of prevention, as well as new treatments for the orthopedic problems that do arise.

—Edith K. Wallace, Ph.D.;
updated by L. Fleming Fallon, Jr.,
M.D., Ph.D., M.P.H.

See also Amputation; Arthritis; Arthroplasty; Arthroscopy; Bone cancer; Bone disorders; Bone grafting; Bones and the skeleton; Bowlegs; Bunions; Bursitis; Cancer; Chiropractic; Craniosynostosis; Disk removal; Dwarfism; Ewing's sarcoma; Feet; Flat feet; Foot disorders; Fracture and dislocation; Fracture repair; Geriatrics and gerontology; Growth; Hammertoe correction; Hammertoes; Heel spur removal; Hip fracture repair; Hip replacement; Jaw wiring; Kinesiology; Kneecap removal; Knock-knees; Laminectomy and spinal fusion; Lower extremities; Muscle sprains, spasms, and disorders; Muscles; Neurofibromatosis; Orthopedic surgery; Orthopedics, pediatric; Osgood-Schlatter disease; Osteoarthritis; Osteochondritis juvenilis; Osteogenesis imperfecta; Osteomyelitis; Osteopathic medicine; Osteoporosis; Paget's disease; Physical examination; Physical rehabilitation; Pigeon toes; Podiatry; Rheumatoid arthritis; Rheumatology; Rickets; Scoliosis; Slipped disk; Spina bifida; Spinal cord disorders; Spine, vertebrae, and disks; Sports medicine; Tendon disorders; Tendon repair; Upper extremities.

FOR FURTHER INFORMATION:

Brewer, Earl J., and Kathy C. Angel. *Parenting a Child with Arthritis*. Los Angeles: Lowell House, 1992. Written for parents and others concerned with juvenile arthritis. The nature of the disease process, available medications, and surgical treatments are discussed.

McIlwain, Harris. *Winning with Osteoporosis*. 2d ed. New York: John Wiley & Sons, 1993. This book is informative and written in an easy-to-read style. It is intended for general readers.

Marcus, Robert, David Feldman, and Jennifer Kelsey, eds. *Osteoporosis*. Philadelphia: Current Medicine, 2000. This book offers a comprehensive, authoritative reference on osteoporosis, covering all aspects of the disease, from basic biology, anatomy, physiology, and pathophysiology to preclinical issues, experimental medicine, management, and therapeutics.

Tennenhaus, Norra. *Relief from Carpal Tunnel Syndrome and Other Repetitive Motion Disorders*. New York: Dell Books, 1991. This book for the general reader provides an overview of the problem of repetitive motion disorders. The author explains the development of these conditions and discusses various treatment options.

Tortora, Gerard J., and Sandra R. Grabowski. *Principles of Anatomy and Physiology*. 9th ed. New York: John Wiley & Sons, 1996. This introductory college textbook offers an excellent survey of human anatomy and physiology. Six chapters are devoted to the musculoskeletal system. In addition to normal structure and function, each chapter includes sections on abnormalities (including both injuries and diseases) and their treatment.

Trien, Susan F., and David Pisetsky. *The Duke University Medical Center Book of Arthritis*. New York:

Fawcett Columbine, 1992. This book, directed to the general reader, describes the normal functioning of the musculoskeletal system and the autoimmune disorders that affect it. In addition to rheumatoid arthritis and osteoarthritis, other inflammatory diseases such as lupus erythematosus, tendinitis, and bursitis are discussed.

ORTHOPEDICS, PEDIATRIC
SPECIALTY

ANATOMY OR SYSTEM AFFECTED: Bones, feet, hands, joints, knees, legs, ligaments, muscles, musculoskeletal system, nerves, nervous system, tendons

SPECIALTIES AND RELATED FIELDS: Exercise physiology, neonatology, orthopedics, pediatrics, physical therapy, rheumatology, sports medicine

DEFINITION: The evaluation and treatment of diseases and injuries of the musculoskeletal system and related nerves in infants and children.

KEY TERMS:

cerebral palsy: a group of nonprogressive disorders of the upper neurologic system resulting in abnormal muscle tone and lack of muscular control

computed tomography (CT) scanning: a computer-assisted method of taking X rays that allows the detailed examination of cross sections of the body

congenital defect: an anatomic deformity present at birth; it is not necessarily hereditary

SCIENCE AND PROFESSION

The pediatric orthopedic surgeon has received additional training in the management of the orthopedic problems of infants and children. Four years of medical school are followed by one year of internship, in either general surgery or primary care. Next come four years of orthopedic residency, then an additional year of fellowship in pediatric orthopedics. After completing training, this specialist usually works in a community with a large referral hospital or in a children's hospital.

The word "orthopedics" comes from two Greek root words, *orthos* ("correct" or "straight") and *pais* ("child"). Childhood musculoskeletal diseases were the original reason for which orthopedic surgery was developed early in the twentieth century. As polio, tuberculosis, and dietary deficiencies came under control, however, the practice of orthopedics grew to encompass adult bone and joint diseases and injuries as well. Nevertheless, a number of orthopedic surgeons continued to work primarily with children.

Infants and children may suffer from a number of congenital musculoskeletal deformities such as clubfoot, hand deformities, congenital dislocation of the hip, and deformities of the spine. Treatment for these disorders may include splints, braces, casts, and surgery. The goal of therapy is to achieve function that is as near normal as possible in the affected part of the skeletal system. Normal appearance, while secondary to function in importance, is also a goal. Some defects require a combination of therapies or repeated operations over a number of years. As the child's musculoskeletal system grows and develops, the mechanics of normal movement change. The pediatric orthopedic surgeon must be aware of these dynamic changes in order to adjust the therapy.

Cerebral palsy, a neuromuscular disorder of infancy and childhood, requires considerable orthopedic evaluation and therapy. As a result of damage to the nerves in the brain that control muscle use, the affected muscles develop abnormal tone (spasticity) and weakness (paralysis). The child cannot control these muscles normally. The asymmetric pull of muscles leads to deformities of the bones and joints and to increasing difficulty in movement as the child grows. Using a combination of splints, braces, and physical and occupational therapy, the pediatric orthopedic surgeon works to keep function as normal as possible in the affected extremities. At times, surgery is necessary to release especially tight muscles. Unfortunately, very little can be done to correct the underlying neurologic defect.

The pediatric orthopedic surgeon also deals with spinal deformities. These conditions may be congenital or may be the result of illness or of some types of surgery, such as removal of a portion of a lung. Scoliosis, the lateral curvature of the spine, may be attributable to factors outside the spine, such as cerebral palsy, or to intrinsic factors in the spine itself. Spinal deformity requires regular observation and the initiation of therapy if the curvature becomes too great. Treatment may involve different types of back braces or, in severe cases, back surgery.

A worry to parents, although often not a significant problem, is the in-toeing and out-toeing that may often be noticed in infants and young children. The pediatric orthopedic surgeon can usually reassure the family that there is no serious problem. Severe toeing problems, however, may require special shoes, splints, or casts.

Childhood fractures must be treated differently from those of adulthood. Children's bones grow at their ends, and growth continues into young adulthood. A fracture at or near the end of a bone may damage the growth area, leading to the loss of normal growth after the injury. Pediatric fractures may be difficult to diagnose, since the growing parts of the bones are cartilage and are not visible on X rays. The pediatric orthopedic surgeon looks for subtle signs of fracture when the growth areas may be involved and follows the patient closely.

DIAGNOSTIC AND TREATMENT TECHNIQUES

The pediatric orthopedic surgeon's practice is divided between the operating room and the clinic. The pediatric specialist spends relatively more time in the clinic than his or her adult practice counterpart because the large percentage of pediatric practice in orthopedics involves chronic deformities.

While taking the patient's history is important, the pediatric orthopedic surgeon relies heavily on a careful and thorough examination of the child's bones, joints, and nervous system. Radiographic studies, especially routine X rays and computed tomography (CT) scans, are often helpful in the evaluation.

Pediatric orthopedic operations must often be carefully planned. It is important for the parents to be involved, so that they can be educated about the child's disorder and can help make appropriate decisions regarding therapy.

PERSPECTIVE AND PROSPECTS

Childhood illnesses and deformities were the original impetus for the development of orthopedic surgery as a specialty early in the twentieth century. Despite the conquest of polio and tuberculosis in the mid-twentieth century, the need for pediatric orthopedic surgeons continued into the 1990's. Improved techniques and innovative procedures, such as bone transplantation and metal implants, allow the correction of more musculoskeletal deformities and suggest a bright future for the specialty.

—*Thomas C. Jefferson, M.D.*

See also Amputation; Arthritis, juvenile rheumatoid; Arthroplasty; Arthroscopy; Bone cancer; Bone disorders; Bone grafting; Bones and the skeleton; Bowlegs; Cancer; Chiropractic; Craniosynostosis; Dwarfism; Ewing's sarcoma; Feet; Flat feet; Foot disorders; Fracture and dislocation; Fracture repair; Growth; Kinesiology; Knock-knees; Lower extremities; Neurofibromatosis; Orthopedic surgery; Orthopedics; Osgood-Schlatter disease; Osteochondritis juvenilis; Osteogenesis imperfecta; Osteomyelitis; Osteopathic medicine; Paget's disease; Pediatrics; Physical examination; Physical rehabilitation; Pigeon toes; Podiatry; Rickets; Scoliosis; Spina bifida; Spinal cord disorders; Spine, vertebrae, and disks; Sports medicine; Tendon disorders; Tendon repair; Upper extremities.

FOR FURTHER INFORMATION:

Kaplan, Deborah. "How to Avoid Orthopedic Pitfalls in Children." *Patient Care* 33, no. 4 (February 28, 1999): 95-116. Missing an orthopedic diagnosis can be hazardous to patients' health. A list of the most common pitfalls in pediatric orthopedic disorders is presented.

Leet, Arabella I., and David L. Skaggs. "Evaluation of the Acutely Limping Child." *American Family Physician* 61, no. 4 (February 15, 2000): 1011-1018. The differential diagnosis of the acutely limping child is explored. The challenge to the family physician is to identify the cause of the limp and determine whether further observation or immediate diagnosis work-up is indicated.

Patel, Hema, and Victor Bialik. "Hip Dysplasia in Infants." *Pediatrics* 104, no. 6 (December, 1999): 1418. Since the 1960's, it has been recognized that up to 90 percent of infants with developmental dysplasia of the hip, identified at birth by any diagnostic method, require absolutely no intervention.

Rose, Rene, Andy Fuentes, Brenda J. Hamel, and Cynthia J. Dzialo. "Pediatric Leg Length Discrepancy: Causes and Treatments." *Orthopedic Nursing* 18, no. 2 (March/April, 1999): 21-31. Leg length discrepancies have multiple causes with a number of treatment options available to accomplish a goal of equal or near equal leg lengths at skeletal maturity.

Thompson, George H., "Common Orthopedic Problems of Children." In *Nelson Essentials of Pediatrics*, edited by Richard E. Behrman and Robert M. Kliegman. 3d ed. Philadelphia: W. B. Saunders, 1998. A chapter in a great text for medical students rotating through pediatrics. It has thorough explanations of diseases and treatments.

Wenger, Dennis R., and Mercer Rang. *The Art and Practice of Children's Orthopaedics*. New York: Raven Press, 1993. A thorough look at pediatric orthopedics, which includes bibliographical references and an index.

OSGOOD-SCHLATTER DISEASE
DISEASE/DISORDER

ANATOMY OR SYSTEM AFFECTED: Bones, knees, legs, tendons

SPECIALTIES AND RELATED FIELDS: Family practice, orthopedics, pediatrics

DEFINITION: Osgood-Schlatter disease, or osteochondrosis, is the partial separation of the epiphysis (growing end) of the tibia, or shin, from the rest of the bone shaft. Severe disease can cause enlargement of the epiphysis and persistent pain. It generally results from either a single violent trauma or repetitive stress on the tendon surrounding the kneecap through flexing of the quadriceps muscle. Osgood-Schlatter disease usually affects adolescent boys. The condition often resolves itself; immobilization may speed up this process.

—*Tracy Irons-Georges*

See also Bone disorders; Bones and the skeleton; Orthopedic surgery; Orthopedics; Orthopedics, pediatric.

FOR FURTHER INFORMATION:
Goldberg, Kathy E. *The Skeleton: Fantastic Framework*. Washington, D.C.: U.S. News Books, 1982.

Thompson, George H. "Common Orthopedic Problems of Children." In *Nelson Essentials of Pediatrics*, edited by Richard E. Behrman and Robert M. Kliegman. 3d ed. Philadelphia: W. B. Saunders, 1998.

Tortora, Gerard A., and Sandra R. Grabowski. *Principles of Anatomy and Physiology*. 9th ed. New York: John Wiley & Sons, 2000.

OSTEOARTHRITIS
DISEASE/DISORDER

ANATOMY OR SYSTEM AFFECTED: Feet, hands, hips, joints, knees, legs, spine

SPECIALTIES AND RELATED FIELDS: Rheumatology

DEFINITION: Osteoarthritis is a degenerative disease of the cartilage in the joints that may also cause inflammation in the surrounding tissues. Although it can be found in all joints, osteoarthritis commonly affects the fingers, feet, knees, hips, and spine. Often, sufferers of osteoarthritis experience joint stiffness and pain, especially during cold, damp weather and when the weather changes. It is thought to be caused by stress on the joints over time or by injury to the joint lining. Symptoms can usually be relieved, but the degeneration in the joints is permanent. Osteoarthritis can be avoided by maintaining a normal weight and engaging in regular physical activity throughout life.

—*Jason Georges and Tracy Irons-Georges*

See also Arthritis; Bursitis; Gout; Obesity; Rheumatoid arthritis; Rheumatology.

FOR FURTHER INFORMATION:
Dong, Collin, and Jane Banks. *New Hope for the Arthritic*. New York: Ballantine Books, 1990.

Eades, Mary Dan. *Arthritis: Reducing Your Risk*. New York: Bantam Books, 1992.

Pisetsky, David S., and Susan Trien Flamholtz. *The Duke University Medical Center Book of Arthritis*. New York: Fawcett Columbine Press, 1992.

OSTEOCHONDRITIS JUVENILIS
DISEASE/DISORDER

ALSO KNOWN AS: Legg-Calvé-Perthes disease, coxa plana, pseudocoxalgia

ANATOMY OR SYSTEM AFFECTED: Bones, circulatory system, hips, joints

SPECIALTIES AND RELATED FIELDS: Orthopedics, vascular medicine

DEFINITION: The disturbance of the blood supply to the tops of the thigh bones, resulting in their destruction.

CAUSES AND SYMPTOMS
Osteochondritis juvenilis is believed to be the result of trauma and damage to the blood vessels that serve the thigh bone. The patient, who in 80 percent of cases is male, usually experiences tenderness in the hip joint area during the early stages of the disease, accompanied by limping, pain in the thigh or knee, and limited movement of the leg. Usually it is difficult to rotate the leg or move it sideways. In 90 percent of cases, only one leg is affected. In such cases, one leg is shorter than the other, and the child favors the affected leg. If the disease is not treated, atrophy of the thigh results.

TREATMENT AND THERAPY
Most cases of osteochondritis juvenilis do not require treatment beyond observation, particularly with children under the age of six who have a small amount of damage. For children over six with most of the joint affected, a more aggressive therapy is needed.

Physical therapy, coupled with braces and crutches or bed rest with traction, is used only in the most severe cases. For most children, a Scottish Rite brace is used. Such a brace is belted around the waist and wrapped around the thighs, with a bar holding the knees apart so that the legs are held at a slight angle away from the body. The child wears the brace until the bone begins to form again, usually in six months.

If the child is more than eight years old, if the brace is too restrictive for an active child, or if the brace must be worn more than six months, surgical correction is recommended. In these cases, the affected bone is cut away and the tip of the thigh bone placed back into its socket. Occasionally, the hip bone must be cut away instead.

—*Rose Secrest*

See also Bone disorders; Bones and the skeleton; Circulation; Lower extremities; Orthopedics; Orthopedics, pediatric; Vascular system.

FOR FURTHER INFORMATION:

Goldberg, Kathy E. *The Skeleton: Fantastic Framework*. Washington, D.C.: U.S. News Books, 1982.

Thompson, George H. "Common Orthopedic Problems of Children." In *Nelson Essentials of Pediatrics*, edited by Richard E. Behrman and Robert M. Kliegman. 3d ed. Philadelphia: W. B. Saunders, 1998.

Wenger, Dennis R., and Mercer Rang. *The Art and Practice of Children's Orthopaedics*. New York: Raven Press, 1993.

OSTEOGENESIS IMPERFECTA

DISEASE/DISORDER

ANATOMY OR SYSTEM AFFECTED: Bones, ears, ligaments, musculoskeletal system, spine, teeth

SPECIALTIES AND RELATED FIELDS: Biochemistry, dentistry, genetics, orthopedics, pediatrics

DEFINITION: A genetic disorder of variable severity that results in frequent bone breaks.

KEY TERMS:

chondrocytes: cartilage cells

collagen: organic material that provides a matrix for bone formation

osteoblasts: bone-forming cells

osteogenesis: new bone formation and repair during development and after trauma

osteogenesis imperfecta congenita: a genetic disorder of collagen formation that begins to show signs during gestation

osteogenesis imperfecta tarda: a genetic disorder of collagen formation that begins to show signs after infancy

CAUSES AND SYMPTOMS

Osteogenesis imperfecta, a rare genetic disorder occurring in 1 in 20,000 people, affects the formation of collagen, which in turn alters bone formation, as collagen provides the foundation for mineralization of developing and healing bone. As the name implies, patients with this disorder have imperfect bone formation, resulting in multiple, recurrent fractures.

Bones are composed of a complex matrix including strands of cross-linked collagen. Collagen is produced by chondrocytes in newly forming bone. Osteoblasts then add the mineral matrix (calcium salts), which forms a complex with collagen to create bone. Children with osteogenesis imperfecta do not produce collagen molecules that allow for a well-organized, strong, stable structure. Fractures can take place without outside stresses such as those occurring in a fall. Normal muscle contractions can produce enough force in some children to induce a bone break.

The long-term outcome of the disease is variable. Most severely affected infants die from complications of lung disease. Patients with less severe disease usually survive but have fractures of their long bones. Most breaks occur between the ages of two and three and again during puberty, between ten and fifteen. From late adolescence through the adult years, the fracture incidence drops unless the patient becomes pregnant, is nursing, or becomes inactive.

There are two main types of osteogenesis imperfecta. The more severe form, osteogenesis imperfecta congenita, affects bone development during gestation and results in bone fractures before birth. These children continue to have fractures without adequate bone repair. Because of the malformation of bony tissues and frequent fractures, they do not grow normally and have numerous bone deformities.

Other tissues with abundant collagen are also affected in osteogenesis imperfecta congenita. Because these tissues include tendons and ligaments, joints become more mobile and less stable. The small bones in the middle ear are similarly affected, resulting in otosclerosis, in which the ossicles stiffen and do not allow the normal transition of sound from the eardrum to the inner ear. Thus, patients have hearing difficulties and subsequent language delays. Because the white parts of the eyes (the sclera) are composed of mainly collagen, these patients tend to have bluish sclera. They also have thinner skin that bleeds easily. Epistaxis (nosebleeding) is likewise common and difficult to control. Patients have deformed teeth, as tooth development is also affected. They tend to have elevated body temperatures, causing them to sweat excessively; because this can become dangerous during surgery under general anesthesia, the anesthesiologist should be made aware of such a possibility. It is important to note that the nervous system, and thus the intelligence, of children with osteogenesis imperfecta congenita is not affected.

The second type of osteogenesis imperfecta is known as osteogenesis imperfecta tarda. Patients with this type have a slower onset and milder course of disease. Fractures begin after birth, do not occur as frequently, and tend to heal better, causing less deformity.

Treatment and Therapy

Unfortunately, there is no effective way to control osteogenesis imperfecta with medication. Drug therapies include the hormones calcitonin, estrogen, and testosterone and supplements of fluoride, calcium, and magnesium. Hormonal therapy seems to stabilize the bone matrix by stimulating bone-forming cells (osteoblasts) and inhibiting the cells which break down bone tissue (osteoclasts). This is likely why patients tend to improve during and after puberty, since levels of these hormones naturally rise.

Activity is encouraged, as exercise strengthens bones. Activities with a high potential for fractures, however, should be avoided. If fractures occur, pediatric orthopedic specialists often place metal rods in the long bones when repairing a fracture to help prevent deformities.

Perspective and Prospects

Unfortunately, the prognosis for some children with osteogenesis imperfecta is poor, and most are confined to wheelchairs as adults. Others are more fortunate and have relatively few fractures after adolescence.

Some advancements in the understanding of osteogenesis imperfecta have occurred using molecular biology techniques to help identify the errors in collagen formation. It is hoped that these data will result in future gene therapy techniques.

—*Matthew Berria, Ph.D.*

See also Bone disorders; Bones and the skeleton; Ear infections and disorders; Ears; Fracture and dis-

location; Genetic diseases; Hearing loss; Hip fracture repair; Orthopedics; Orthopedics, pediatric.

For Further Information:

Behrman, Richard E., ed. *Nelson Textbook of Pediatrics*. 16th ed. Philadelphia: W. B. Saunders, 2000. Offers detailed information intended mainly for pediatricians.

Green, Morris. *Pediatric Diagnosis: Interpretation of Symptoms and Signs in Infants, Children, and Adolescents*. 6th ed. Philadelphia: W. B. Saunders, 1998. An excellent text providing information on physical diagnosis.

Hay, William W., and Jessie R. Groothuis, eds. *Current Pediatric Diagnosis and Treatment*. 15th ed. Norwalk, Conn.: Appleton and Lange, 2000. A basic pediatric text detailing general pediatric diseases.

Jones, Kenneth L. *Smith's Recognizable Patterns of Human Malformation*. 5th ed. Philadelphia: W. B. Saunders, 1997. This classic text discusses pediatric malformations.

Schwartz, M. William, ed. *The Five-Minute Pediatric Consult*. Baltimore: Williams & Wilkins, 1997. Summarizes information on pediatric diseases in a concise format.

Tierney, Lawrence M., Jr., et al., eds. *Current Medical Diagnosis and Treatment: 2001*. 39th ed. New York: McGraw-Hill, 2000. A general medical text with information appropriate for older children and adults.

Van De Graaff, Kent M., and Stuart I. Fox. *Concepts of Human Anatomy and Physiology*. 5th ed. Dubuque, Iowa: Wm. C. Brown, 2000. A basic anatomy and physiology textbook. See especially chapters 8, 9, and 10.

Osteomyelitis

Disease/disorder

Anatomy or system affected: Bones, joints

Specialties and related fields: Bacteriology, orthopedics

Definition: A secondary bacterial infection of the bone and bone marrow.

Causes and Symptoms

After a cut, open bone fracture, or puncture wound to the heel becomes infected, a secondary infection, caused 80 percent of the time by the bacterium *Staphylococcus aureus*, can take place. In children, the bacterium usually enters the body via an infection of the mucous membranes in the throat or an infected sore on the body. In the case of a heel puncture, a bacterium that breeds in old athletic shoes, called *Pseudomonas aeruginosa*, can be the culprit. In children, osteomyelitis tends to be located at the growing ends of the long bones.

Osteomyelitis is generally accompanied by fever, drowsiness, dehydration, bone pain, and swelling and redness in the affected region. When a joint near the infected area is flexed, severe pain and tenderness can result. With a heel puncture, the heel tends to hurt and swell, but there is often no fever. Over time, the bacteria form pus.

TREATMENT AND THERAPY

If osteomyelitis is discovered within seven to ten days from the onset of the infection, large doses of antibiotics can be administered with success. In children, oral antibiotics are not recommended because compliance is hard to achieve. Patients must ingest two to four times the recommended daily dose of the antibiotic over four to six weeks, which can cause severe side effects. Usually, children are hospitalized and given intravenous antibiotics. During this time, the affected bones should not be exposed to undue stress until easy, pain-free movement is achieved. Risks during the time of treatment include broken bones and the onset of severe osteoporosis.

In severe cases or in cases in which the infection was not discovered early, surgery that removes the infected bone or bone marrow is necessary. If the osteomyelitis is not treated, the infection enters the bloodstream and the disease becomes chronic. Extensive bone damage, arthritis, and extrusion of pus will follow. Treatment may involve occasional removal of pus and pieces of dead bone or, in extreme cases, amputation.

—Rose Secrest

See also Antibiotics; Arthritis; Bacterial infections; Bone disorders; Bone marrow transplantation; Bones and the skeleton; Orthopedics; Orthopedics, pediatric.

FOR FURTHER INFORMATION:

Esterhai, John L. *Adult Posttraumatic Osteomyelitis of the Tibia*. Philadelphia: Lippincott, Williams & Wilkins, 1999.

Norden, Carl W., ed. *Osteomyelitis*. Philadelphia: W. B. Saunders, 1990.

Pankey, George A. *Osteomyelitis*. Research Triangle Park, N.C.: Glaxo, 1992.

OSTEOPATHIC MEDICINE
SPECIALTY

ANATOMY OR SYSTEM AFFECTED: Bones, muscles, musculoskeletal system

SPECIALTIES AND RELATED FIELDS: Critical care, emergency medicine, family practice, geriatrics and gerontology, internal medicine, physical therapy, preventive medicine, public health

DEFINITION: The practice of medicine as dictated by the philosophy of treating the individual instead of merely the disease, by the belief that the musculoskeletal system is crucial to the health of the entire body, and by an emphasis on the interrelatedness of all bodily systems.

KEY TERMS:

allopathic medicine: the traditional course of study leading to a doctorate in medicine; most practicing physicians are allopathic physicians

family medicine: the practice of medicine in which the physician cares for the basic needs of the family and emphasizes preventive health care, as well as the importance of the patient's environment

immune system: the system of the body that is responsible for the maintenance of health; includes the spleen, thymus, bone marrow, and the lymphatic system

Medical College Admission Test (MCAT): a test of problem-solving skills taken by all candidates to medical school in the United States; used to predict which students will be successful

musculoskeletal system: the system of the body consisting of the muscles and skeleton particularly in relation to their role in the maintenance of health

obstetrics/gynecology: the practice of medicine which deals with the health of the female reproductive system; includes care of the pregnant woman and delivery of her baby, as well as care for infertile couples who need assistance in becoming pregnant

osteopathy: philosophy of medicine which emphasizes the treatment of the whole person, rather than only the disease; from the Greek *osteo*, meaning bone, and *pathos*, meaning to suffer or be in sympathy with

THE HISTORY OF OSTEOPATHY

Osteopathy is a medical philosophy which treats disease in the context of the whole person, taking into consideration the functions and interrelationships of all body systems as well as such factors as nutrition, environment, and psychology. The first college of osteopathic medicine was founded in Kirksville, Missouri, in 1892, by Andrew Taylor Still, a frontier physician and Civil War surgeon. A hundred years later, there were fifteen colleges of osteopathic medicine located in various parts of the United States.

Still was the son of the Reverend Abraham Still, a doctor as well as a minister. As a youth, Andrew often accompanied his father on house calls, where he helped with basic medical procedures. His study of medicine led to a doctorate of medicine (M.D.), and he was licensed in the state of Missouri.

During the Civil War and in his practice as a frontier doctor, Still became frustrated by his inability to cure patients using the available techniques. The suffering of his patients was difficult for him to tolerate. The lack of knowledge about diseases and their treatment drove him to reconsider ways to improve the lot of the ill and injured. He also suffered a great personal loss when an epidemic of spinal meningitis spread through Kansas. Three of his children died of the disease, and three others died shortly after they were born. These tragedies nearly caused Still to abandon his career, but, in spite of the fact that the practice of modern medicine was in its infancy, he was determined to find the answers that would help him conquer disease and improve the health of his patients.

After the war ended, Still spent his life studying, observing, comparing, and experimenting in the treatment of disease. His observations closely paralleled the theories that the Greek physician Hippocrates proposed two thousand years earlier, primarily in the belief held by Hippocrates that the nature of human beings is the physician of the disease. Both Still and Hippocrates encouraged the physician to concentrate on the patient, not the disease.

Still wanted to establish the first school of osteopathy at Baker University in Baldwin, Kansas. He was refused permission to do so, however, because his philosophy of medicine did not conform to the accepted medical practice of the day. He was ostracized in Kansas, and in 1874, he moved to Missouri, where he was still licensed as a doctor and was legally able to practice medicine. As an itinerant doctor, he gained fame throughout the area and was affectionately known as the "bonesetter." It was during this time that he perfected his practice of osteopathy. Still's reputation and popularity spread, and he soon required assistance in treating the patients who sought him out. He established the first school of osteopathic med-

icine in Kirksville, Missouri, as the American School of Osteopathy under the law governing scientific institutions in 1892.

In 1894, he received a new charter from the state of Missouri for an educational institution. By the authority of the charter, the school could have awarded an M.D. degree, but Still wanted his degree to be different and chose to award a doctor of osteopathy (D.O.) degree instead. During the next few years, osteopathic colleges became a fad, and at one time, thirty-seven of them existed, many of which were correspondence or diploma schools.

The American School of Osteopathy taught the art of manipulative therapy. Still and his followers believed that if they could regulate and correct malfunctions of musculoskeletal function, they could return the body to a healthful state. When possible, they also eliminated the use of drugs to treat disease. Although this approach now sounds extreme, at that time few, if any, drugs were on the market, and most had severe side effects.

At the time that Still was establishing the roots of osteopathy, many significant advances were made in medical knowledge and techniques, including germ theory, the development of antiseptic surgery, the development of anesthesia, and the reorganization of medical education. The emphasis of Still on the treatment of the entire person has taken on more importance in modern times with the development of the fields of holistic medicine and preventive care.

SCIENCE AND PROFESSION

The philosophy of osteopathic medicine suggests that a human being is an ecologically and biologically unified whole. Among its tenets are that the various body systems are joined through the nervous, endocrine, and circulatory systems and that if one region of the body is diseased, the entire body is diseased.

There are five basic premises of osteopathy. First, the unity of all body parts is a benefit which assists in the maintenance of health and the resistance to disease. Second, when the body is properly nourished and structural relationships are normal, the body is able to adapt to physiologic changes that might otherwise put the body out of balance. Third, a healthy body depends on a healthy circulatory system and a nervous system that is able to conduct information to all areas of the body. Fourth, the musculoskeletal system does more than simply provide a framework for the body, and its normal function is critical to a healthy body. Fifth, it is not in the patient's best interest for the physician to treat only one aspect of the disease; the physician must treat the entire body and mind if the patient is to be cured. In modern times, the osteopathic physician uses manipulative therapy—in which rhythmic stretching and thrusting movements are used to realign joints and muscles properly—as one of many tools to cure the patient.

Osteopathic physicians and allopathic physicians have much in common. Both are members of the health care community who are fully trained physicians, who have taken a prescribed amount of undergraduate work, and who received four years of training in a medical school. After completing medical school, osteopathic physicians take a one-year rotating internship in hospitals with approved intern training programs. They may then enter a medical specialty program which may require a three- to four-year residency program.

Both allopathic and osteopathic medical programs use scientifically accepted methods of diagnosis and treatment. In the United States, the graduates of these programs are licensed by the same state medical boards and can practice in all phases of medicine in all states.

Admission to a college of osteopathic medicine in the United States requires a minimum of three years of preprofessional education in an accredited college or university. Virtually all students in osteopathic school, however, have been awarded undergraduate degrees. Many osteopathic students were science majors in undergraduate school, but all areas of study are represented. Most schools require a minimum of two semesters of study in biology, physics, and inorganic and organic chemistry. Students are also required to take the Medical College Admission Test (MCAT), submit letters of recommendation, and demonstrate an understanding of osteopathic medicine.

During the first two years in a college of osteopathic medicine, students receive basic science and preclinical instruction in a classroom or laboratory environment. Students are required to take courses in anatomy, biochemistry, physiology, pharmacology, pathology, and microbiology.

Schools are organized along one of two lines. They teach either by discipline or by system. In a discipline curriculum, the student concentrates on one subject at a time, such as biochemistry or physiology. In those programs with a curriculum that is organized by system, the student will study one organ system from the perspective of various basic science disciplines. For example, when studying the circulatory system, the student would concentrate on the anatomy, biochemistry, physiology, and pathology of the blood vessels and heart before moving on to another system.

Most students of osteopathy are required to take the first part of an examination prepared by the National Board of Examiners in Osteopathic Medicine and Surgery near the end of their second year. At the end of the second year or in the third year, the student concentrates on clinical instruction. Students of osteopathy may do clinical rotations in teaching hospitals, community hospitals, or physicians' offices in both urban and rural areas. Clinical instruction is designed to give the student experience in the diagnosis and treatment of a patient's symptoms. Students also attend seminars and conferences which are more specialized and which emphasize the disease process and the healing process.

The second part of the national boards is taken during the last year, and the third part is taken after the student has received the D.O. degree. After completion of the degree, the student participates in a one-year rotating internship in an approved hospital prior to selection of a residency program. Sixty-nine percent of all doctors of osteopathy enter one of the primary care specialties, including general practice, general internal medicine, obstetrics/gynecology, and pediatrics.

DIAGNOSTIC AND TREATMENT TECHNIQUES

Osteopathic medicine stresses the interdependence of structure and function. The application of manipulative therapy, and in particular joint mobilization, has been a hallmark of osteopathic medicine since its inception. Osteopathic physicians recognize human beings as complex biomechanical, biophysical, and biochemical organisms. They believe that structural disturbances can have wide-ranging effects that may spread to interconnecting systems. The biologic foundations of osteopathic medicine are based in the concepts of holism, homeostasis, unity of the body, environmental influences, and health-versus-disease.

Holism suggests that humans are whole beings that are not resolvable into component parts and that each "whole" is more than the sum of its parts. This premise can also be extended to mean that people are not isolated units—they are a part of their surroundings and thus are a part of their environment and the universe. The increased tendency toward specialization in health care would seem to be in conflict with this principle. Osteopathic medicine suggests a need to increase the number of generalists or primary care physicians to ensure adequate care of the whole person. It further requires time to know and understand the patient as a person in his or her own environment.

The concept of body unity suggests that the normal healthy body contains all the elements necessary to maintain optimum function. Osteopathic physicians would argue that when disease alters body function, there is adequate flexibility within the system to compensate for change and to return the body to a state of wellness. This concept is similar to the principle of general physiology known as homeostasis.

Homeostasis recognizes the fact that essential body functions such as acidity of the blood, body temperature, and blood pressure are maintained within relatively narrow limits. It is not unusual for these parameters to drift slightly from the norm, but they must be quickly and efficiently returned to normal if the body is to survive. Deviations that cannot be readjusted quickly lead to poor body function and even death. Therefore, the body expends much time and energy in maintaining homeostasis, which prevents changes in the environment from having a significant effect on body function.

The philosophy of osteopathic medicine presents the position that musculoskeletal function is important in the maintenance of homeostasis. If this system is "out of line" or in any way unhealthy, the body will have a more difficult time maintaining homeostasis. It further argues that a healthy musculoskeletal system is necessary for a healthy immune system and that an unhealthy immune system can interfere with homeostasis.

The role of the environment in health is emphasized by the osteopathic physician. There is general agreement that a healthy environment contributes to a healthy body. A healthy environment here refers not only to the working and living environment of the patient but also to all associates and family members who are directly involved with the patient.

The concept of health-versus-disease is central to the philosophy of osteopathic medicine. The osteopathic physician is not as concerned with the treatment of the disease as with the cause of the disease and the methods that can be used to prevent its continuation or recurrence. The concept of health implies that all components of the body are functioning as a unit and that all are contributing to the maintenance of homeostasis. Consequently, properly functioning circulatory, nervous, and endocrine systems are required. Disease, on the other hand, is present when cells do not receive appropriate circulation and/or nervous or endocrine regulation, causing a breakdown in the immune system or impairment of the adaptative mechanisms.

Although there are many similarities between allopathic and osteopathic physicians, some distinctions can be made. While the allopathic physician's philosophy emphasizes the value of the type of intervention used, the osteopathic physician stresses the importance of the body's ability to heal itself. Osteopathic medicine recognizes the musculoskeletal system as an important factor in the body's efforts to resist and overcome illness and disease. The major factor that separates osteopathic medicine from allopathic medicine is manipulative treatment, which is often called biomechanics. Osteopathic manipulative treatment is used in conjunction with other practices to provide the body with the means to cure itself.

PERSPECTIVE AND PROSPECTS

In 1894, when Andrew Taylor Still opened the first osteopathic medical school in Kirksville, Missouri, the medical community was skeptical of the methods of the osteopathic physician. Although Missouri was the first state to recognize an osteopathic medical school, there was resistance to licensing the graduates. In 1896, Vermont was the first state to enact legislation legalizing the licensing of osteopathy. Licensing in Missouri followed in 1897. By 1924, thirty-eight states had legally recognized osteopathy. In 1897, the American Osteopathic Association was formed to establish professional standards of practice. Its objectives were to promote the public health and to maintain high standards of medical education in osteopathic colleges.

Members of the American Medical Association (AMA) were not as accepting of osteopathic physicians as was the general public. When World War I broke out, some allopathic physicians claimed that the osteopaths were insufficiently trained for military service. Although there was widespread disagreement across the country, these allopathic physicians were successful, and the osteopathic physicians were kept at home. This situation ultimately proved to be to the benefit of osteopathy: While allopaths were serving in foreign countries, health care in the United States was left to osteopaths.

In 1923, the AMA continued its efforts to limit the practice of osteopathic physicians by declaring that it was unethical for M.D.'s to consult with D.O.'s. In 1938, M.D.'s were forbidden to engage in any professional relationship with D.O.'s.

Acceptance of osteopathic physicians finally came in 1967, when the AMA voted to negotiate for the merger of the two professions. The American Osteopathic Association was not interested in such a merger, but allopaths and osteopaths were allowed to work side by side in hospitals, community health clinics, and offices throughout the United States.

In the United States in 1993, there were 32,000 osteopathic physicians across the nation, constituting 10 percent of practicing physicians and delivering 15 percent of American health care. The education of osteopathic physicians is expected to have an increasingly important role in the United States as people continue to emphasize preventive and family medicine. In efforts to cut costs and to improve the availability of health care, the United States government and health care insurance providers have stressed the need for primary care—an area that has always been important to the osteopathic physician.

Two monthly journals are available in libraries throughout the United States: *The Journal of the American Osteopathic Association* and *The D.O.* These journals contain research studies from osteopathic physicians, as well as articles regarding the profession and the education of its students.

—*Annette O'Connor, Ph.D.*

See also Alternative medicine; Bones and the skeleton; Exercise physiology; Family practice; Holistic medicine; Massage; Muscle sprains, spasms, and disorders; Muscles; Nutrition; Physical rehabilitation; Preventive medicine.

FOR FURTHER INFORMATION:

American Association of Colleges of Osteopathic Medicine. *The Education of the Osteopathic Physician*. Rev. ed. Rockville, Md.: Author, 1990. In addition to a thorough discussion of the educational requirements for entrance into an osteopathic medical school, this book outlines the courses required for the osteopathic physician.

Lederman, Eyal. *Fundamentals of Manual Therapy: Physiology, Neurology, and Psychology*. New York: Churchill Livingstone, 1997. This text discusses orthopedic manipulation as a means of therapy. Includes a bibliography and an index.

Siegel, Irwin M. *All About Bone: An Owner's Manual*. New York: Demos Medical, 1998. Includes chapters on osteoporosis, arthritis, fractures, scoliosis, and low back pain.

OSTEOPOROSIS
DISEASE/DISORDER

ANATOMY OR SYSTEM AFFECTED: Back, bones, hips, legs, spine

SPECIALTIES AND RELATED FIELDS: Geriatrics and gerontology, nutrition, orthopedics, physical therapy

DEFINITION: A condition resulting from reduced bone mass; fractures are the major complications and are associated with significantly increased risks of morbidity and mortality, especially in older women.

KEY TERMS:

biochemical diagnostic procedures: a series of blood tests to evaluate the presence or absence of diseases, such as those aggravating osteoporosis

bone densitometry: a technique of bone scanning to measure mineral content, calcium content, and density

bone mineral density: the amount of mineralized bone, reported in grams per square centimeter of bone tissue, as measured by densitometry

cancellous bone: also called spongy or trabecular bone; bone that makes up 20 percent of the bone mass, is present in the ends of the long bones and throughout the vertebrae, provides the microstructure that gives bone its strength, and is the site for osteoporotic fractures

dual energy X-ray absorptiometry (DEXA): a method used to evaluate the regional and total bone mineral content considered the standard or criterion measure for bone mineral density

fracture risk: an estimate of the likelihood that a fracture will occur in an individual

hormone replacement therapy: treatment protocols using estrogens, with or without progesterone, to reduce the rate of bone mineral loss which occurs after the menopause

CAUSES AND SYMPTOMS

Bone is constantly being remodeled by cells: Old bone is reabsorbed by the osteoclasts, and new bone is formed by the osteoblasts. Several factors control these processes of bone formation and resorption, which are about equal in adults. In children, formation exceeds resorption, and the bone mass increases. In old age, however, bone resorption exceeds bone formation and bone mass is lost. When bone mass is reduced, the bone becomes mechanically weak and vulnerable to fractures. This condition of reduced bone mass is known as osteoporosis and is part of the aging process. At this time, there is no known cure for osteoporosis, which emphasizes that prevention is the only strategy for combating bone mineral loss and the development of osteoporosis.

Type I osteoporosis is related to aging alone. It has two forms: postmenopausal (occurring in women between the ages of fifty-one and sixty-five, with fractures of the vertebrae and wrist) and senile (occurring in both men and women past the age of seventy, with fractures of the hip and vertebrae). Type II osteoporosis is associated with an underlying disease such as hyperparathyroidism or multiple myeloma and may occur in younger as well as older individuals. A third type has been found in young women who are amenorrheic (having no menstrual cycles) in association with eating disorders. Osteoporotic fractures are occurring in women in their twenties and thirties who have been amenorrheic for several years. Because it was found in athletic women, the link between eating disorders, amenorrhea, and osteoporosis was named the Female Athlete Triad. No matter the type of osteoporosis, it remains a clinically silent disease until a fracture occurs. In the United States, one to three million fractures related to osteoporosis occur yearly. The frequency of osteoporosis and related fractures is expected to increase in parallel with the increase in the older population. Women are more vulnerable to this condition, especially after the menopause. As the life span for men increases, however, so will their risk for osteoporosis.

In the early postmenopausal period, the distal end of the radius and ulna are particularly susceptible to fractures; a few years later, the patient is likely to sustain vertebral fractures. The most common presentation of such a fracture is a sudden onset of very severe, localized back pain, often occurring spontaneously. The pain is so severe that it incapacitates the patient and may require the administration of narcotics for relief. Unlike the pain caused by a disk rupture, this pain does not radiate to the legs, although some radiation anteriorly may be present. The pain usually lasts about four weeks and is then spontaneously relieved unless nerve compression or secondary arthritic changes complicate the condition.

When multiple vertebrae have collapsed, the body height is reduced and the patient's arms appear to be disproportionately long. Normally, both measurements—body height and arm span—are equal. In osteoporosis complicated by several vertebral fractures, body height is reduced, but the arm span is unchanged. When multiple thoracic vertebrae collapse, kyphosis (an increased spinal curvature) develops, a condition sometimes referred to as dowager's hump. The space between the ribs and the pelvic cavity is also reduced. When lumbar vertebrae are collapsed, the lower end of the ribs may lie over the pelvic cavity. At this stage, the patient's lung functions may be compromised because the chest move-

Osteoporosis

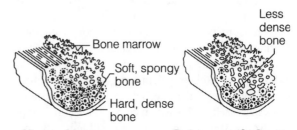

Normal bone **Osteoporotic bone**

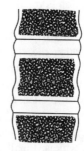

Normal vertebral body

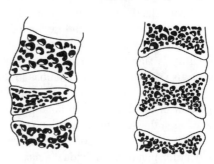

Osteoporotic vertebral bodies

Osteoporosis leads to bone that is less dense, more brittle, more easily broken, and degenerative.

ments are limited. Pneumonia is a common, fatal complication.

Progressive and long-standing osteoporosis may be complicated by fractures of the femoral neck. Although most of these fractures are preceded by a fall, it is probable that in some cases the bones are so weakened and fragile that they fracture spontaneously and cause the patient to fall. Fractures of the femoral neck are associated with significant mortality and morbidity risks, with 12 to 20 percent of the patients dying within six months of the fracture and about half losing the ability to live independently.

A number of factors predisposing an individual to osteoporosis have been identified. Some of these factors cannot be changed. For example, the older patients are, the more likely they are to develop osteoporosis. Furthermore, although both sexes are affected by osteoporosis, women tend to be more vulnerable because, in addition to the accelerated rate of bone loss which occurs at the menopause, women tend to have smaller skeletons than men do and, therefore, are likely to reach the threshold at which bone fragility is increased well before men do. Whites in Europe and North America are more susceptible to osteoporosis than are African Americans or Chicano/Latinos, in whom this condition is relatively rare. The reasons for these racial differences are not well known. It is possible, however, that African Americans have larger skeletons than the other races, and weight may be a factor in both African Americans and Chicano/Latinos. Asians have about the same bone densities as whites. Because a difference in stature means that their hip axis length is shorter and therefore less likely to fracture, however, they have about half the number of hip fractures as whites. Finally, people with large body frames are less likely to develop osteoporosis than those with small body frames, probably because their bone reserve allows them to lose bone for a longer period before reaching the threshold at which the bone fragility is significantly increased. Genetic research has also determined that variations in the gene for the vitamin D receptor (VDR) may contribute to 7 to 10 percent of the difference in bone mass density because of its influence on calcium intake. For those with a family history of osteoporosis, this factor could lead to identification of an individual's risk factor and enable early intervention.

A number of risk factors that can be reversed have also been identified. A low dietary calcium intake is associated with a reduced bone mass and an increased fracture rate. Conversely, an elevated calcium intake, particularly before puberty, is associated with an increased mass. In 1994, the National Institutes of Health consensus statement recommended an increase in daily calcium, and in 1997 the National Academy of Sciences' Dietary Reference Intake (DRI), formerly the Recommended Dietary Allowance (RDA), increased from 800 milligrams per day to 1,300 milligrams at age nine up to age eighteen. Some researchers are recommending a daily intake of 1,300 to 1,500 milligrams for all young people during puberty and up to at least age thirty to obtain optimal peak bone mass. Women during pregnancy and lactation also need a higher amount, up to 1,300 milligrams. Men from age thirty to sixty-four should take in 1,000 milligrams, increasing to 1,200 milligrams at age sixty-five. Women from age nineteen to the menopause should take in 1,000 milligrams, increasing to 1,200 milligrams when they are no longer producing estrogen. Women on hormone replacement therapy (HRT) may only need 1,000 milligrams. Amenorrheic women should be taking in 1,300 to 1,500 milligrams. The maximum allowable intake has been increased from 2,000 to 2,500 milligrams. Higher doses may be detrimental, as they may cause the formation of kidney stones, so the benefit must be weighed against the risk in each case. Getting the greatest percent of the calcium from the diet is preferred, but, if it is to be taken as a supplement, no more than 500 milligrams should be taken at one time and always with meals. Calcium is not absorbed well, so having stomach acid present, as well as vitamin D and protein, enhances the absorption.

Physical inactivity is associated with a reduced bone mass and therefore an increased predisposition to developing osteoporosis. There is also evidence that people who have a sedentary lifestyle are more susceptible to osteoporosis than those who are physically active. During the formative years, exercise is imperative to develop the highest bone density possible. Then throughout the rest of life, exercise is essential to slow the rate of bone loss. Research on amenorrheic and eumenorrheic young female athletes has contributed much to the body of knowledge of the relationship of exercise to bone density. It is not only the exercise that is important but also the presence of estrogen (or testosterone in males) that enhances the process of bone formation. Several factors modulate the response of the skeleton to exercise. These include the subject's age and gender; the intensity, frequency, and type of exercise; and the subject's endocrinal status. The current recommendation for exercise in relationship to osteoporosis is preventive: a variety of exercise, both weight-bearing and vigorous, to be done regularly (thirty to sixty minutes per day, three to five days per week) throughout life. Variety is essential because no single exercise stresses all bones equally. The stimulus to build bone comes from the muscle that is attached to the bone pulling on the attachment site, which makes the bone remodel itself to resist the stress.

In the elderly, exercise may have a secondary benefit. Often, a fracture is precipitated by a fall, and the cause of the fall may be a loss of balance or coordination. Maintaining an active lifestyle helps with balance and coordination as well as confidence, all of which may help in the prevention of a fall. Studies in the elderly have demonstrated that a general exercise such as walking is not enough to maintain gains in bone density for very long. Exercise studies of one or two years' duration show a decline begins after about one year. To combat that loss, a regular strength training regimen, targeting the most common fracture sites, done two or three times a week for twenty minutes to stimulate specific bones, should be added to any other activities that are done.

Cigarette smoking is associated with osteoporosis; however, the underlying mechanism is not clearly understood. It is possible that cigarette smokers are more likely to lead a sedentary life and have a reduced dietary calcium intake than nonsmokers. Cigarette smoking may have a direct effect on the bone cells, or it may have an indirect effect by modulating the release of substances which may affect the activity of these cells, such as the parathyroid hormone or calcitonin secretion.

At one time, caffeine ingestion was thought to have a significantly adverse effect on calcium absorption. The craze of drinking lattes (espresso coffee mixed with hot milk) stimulated more research, and the findings suggested that the advantage of drinking about 14 ounces of milk in a latte resulted in an increased calcium intake of about 400 milligrams. The amount of calcium lost as a result of the caffeine amounted to only about one teaspoon of milk, which is insignificant. Since many American women surveyed have been drinking little or no milk, the popularity of lattes may have a beneficial effect on the members of the thirty- to fifty-year-old population, who seem to be drinking them the most.

A number of drugs may induce osteoporosis. Among them, cortisone preparations are particularly notorious. Therefore, the long-term administration of these drugs should be avoided. If cortisone must be administered, then the lowest effective dose should be chosen. Studies are underway on a drug, etidronate (Didronel), which, when given along with corticosteroid drugs, may act as a bone-sparing therapy and lower the chance of fractures in people who must take the corticosteroids. The long-term administration of potent diuretics also should be avoided, as they induce a negative calcium balance by increasing renal urinary calcium excretion. Milder diuretics, on the other hand, may actually induce a positive calcium balance by reducing renal calcium excretion. Other drugs that have been added to the list include anticonvulsive drugs, antacids that contain aluminum, some forms of cancer chemotherapy, and heparin, which is used to prevent blood clots. For a person at risk for osteoporosis, anytime that medications are prescribed, calcium interaction should be considered.

TREATMENT AND THERAPY

Several tests are available to confirm the diagnosis of osteoporosis, quantify its degree, and identify underlying diseases that might cause or aggravate the osteoporosis.

Plain X rays used to be the only way to evaluate patients with osteoporosis. Although they are helpful in assessing bone involvement from other diseases, they are not useful for the detection of early osteoporosis because the characteristic appearances are only seen when at least 40 percent of the bone mass has been lost. In the 1990's, a new analysis technique was developed using a simple X ray of the hand and then computer analysis. It is able to reveal as little as 1 percent bone loss.

The most accurate technique now available to measure bone density uses a technique called dual energy X-ray absorptiometry (DEXA). DEXA is based on the principle that if a beam of radiation is directed at a bone, the amount of radiation trapped by the bone is proportional to the amount of mineral and calcium inside. By knowing the amount of radiation aimed at the bone and the amount reaching a detector crystal across the bone, the amount of mineral can be calculated. In order to differentiate the radiation trapped by the surrounding muscles and fat from the radiation trapped by the bone itself, radiation with two different peaks (which are absorbed to a different extent by bone and soft tissue) is used. The exposure to radiation is minimal, one-fiftieth the radiation as in a chest X ray. The same densitometry machine can do whole-body or single-site readings, making it even more useful for diagnosis. The only problem is that the number of DEXA machines available for diagnosis does not allow everyone to be assessed. Therefore, the criteria for who should be screened is determined by perceived risk. The physician must assess a patient's known risks to determine when and how often densitometry should be done.

Bone density determination is useful in deciding whether HRT should be recommended in women at risk for osteoporosis. If the patient's bone density is at or below the low percentile of a normal population, then such therapy is indicated. If it is above the upper percentile, HRT may not be necessary, at least as far as bone mass is concerned. If the patient is in the midrange, then another densitometry measurement a year later may be indicated. The information obtained from bone densitometry is also useful in monitoring the bone mass of patients requiring long-term cortisone therapy in order to determine whether bone loss is occurring and therefore whether some other medication needs to be prescribed.

Osteoporosis therapy includes several options. Several drugs are currently being used or investigated for use; the most commonly prescribed is HRT. HRT is effective in arresting the bone loss that occurs after the menopause, and even increasing the bone mass, particularly if started within the first five years and combined with calcium and exercise. The main drawback of this therapy is that estrogens alone increase the risk of uterine cancer, but if they are combined with progesterone, the risk is eliminated, as the latter hormone exerts a protective effect on the uterus. Such therapy also reduces the risk of developing cardiovascular diseases.

The effect of HRT on the incidence of breast cancer is controversial, and it is recommended that a mammogram be done beforehand and at yearly intervals thereafter. Estrogen therapy often induces breast enlargement and some tenderness, both of which are usually self-limited (running a definite, limited course). Complications such as strokes have been overemphasized in the past, occurring at a time when large doses of estrogen were used for contraception. Furthermore, many patients were at an increased risk of developing these complications because of coexistent hypertension and/or cigarette smoking.

If HRT is administered on a cyclical pattern, then menstrual periods are likely to resume. These can be avoided if the hormones are administered continuously, in the form of either tablets or patches placed over the skin, which must be replaced twice a week. Subcutaneous implants, which can be left in the skin for much longer periods, are being evaluated.

Calcitonin, a hormone produced by the thyroid gland, specifically inhibits the osteoclasts, which are the bone resorbing cells. As a result, there is a relative increase in the rate of bone formation, and the bone mass increases. After the initial increase, however, the bone mass tends to stabilize, and the continued administration of calcitonin beyond this point may be associated with an actual decline in bone mass. Many physicians, therefore, administer calcitonin in cycles of six to twelve months. One of the main advantages of calcitonin is that, unlike HRT, it is effective in both sexes and in patients of all ages, including the very old. Calcitonin also appears to have an analgesic effect, which may be quite useful following a vertebral collapse. The main disadvantages of calcitonin are cost and form of administration. A synthetic form that is administered as a nasal spray has received Food and Drug Administration (FDA) approval. This is a relief to patients who have had to give themselves a daily injection. The only disadvantage of this drug is that it does not appear to be as effective in thickening bones as other drugs being studied.

Another drug that has recently received FDA approval for use in women is alendronate. It is the first nonhormonal osteoporosis drug. In very large studies, dramatic increases in bone density have been seen, along with less fractures. The cost is about the same as calcitonin, but considerably more than HRT. The cost, coupled with the lack of long-term use studies to determine side effects, suggests that alendronate should be the drug of choice for the elderly with severe bone loss rather than a preventive measure for a newly postmenopausal woman, unless her risk is very high.

Several other drugs are showing promise in controlled studies, including slow-release sodium fluoride, calcitriol, and raloxifene. Sodium fluoride causes significant increases in bone densities, as much as 5 percent a year for four years. The side effects, however, include peptic ulcers, and, unfortunately, the bone that is built is sometimes brittle. Also, fluoride can be toxic, so the levels must be monitored carefully. The slow-release form seems to avoid some of the side effects, but larger studies need to be completed before the drug can be approved. Calcitriol is used in many countries as a treatment for osteoporosis. Currently, it is only used in the United States to treat a bone disorder that can result from kidney dialysis. Calcitriol helps in the absorption of calcium and stimulates osteoblasts. Raloxifene is a compound that attaches to estrogen receptors in the body. It is thought that the drug might mimic the estrogen effect on the bones, but it will take several more years of testing before raloxifene could be available.

Calcium supplements are useful if the patient's dietary calcium intake is less than required. There is no evidence to support any beneficial effect of supplements if the daily dietary intake of calcium exceeds the DRI. Unfortunately, only 14 percent of girls and 35 percent of boys aged twelve to nineteen are achieving the DRI. According to the FDA, either supplementation or education needs to occur in this population in order to avoid an epidemic of osteoporosis in the future. Similarly, if the daily vitamin D intake is below the recommended level of 400 milligrams in the elderly population, supplementation is recommended. Vitamin D supplements may also be necessary in patients who are taking a medication that interferes with vitamin D metabolism, such as anticonvulsant drugs which increase the rate of vitamin D breakdown in the liver. The determination of proper dosage is based on some vitamin D formation from sunlight. If a person is not exposed to a minimum of twenty minutes of sunlight a day, the requirement increases by 200 milligrams. An excessive vitamin D and calcium intake, however, may lead to the development of kidney stones. Furthermore, excessive vitamin D (greater than 1,000 milligrams a day) may increase the rate of bone resorption and, because vitamin D is lipid soluble and it is stored in the body-fat tissue, its toxicity may last for months.

Although fluorides are sometimes used in the treatment of osteoporosis, they are associated with a high incidence of adverse effects, such as gastritis, kidney damage, and joint pain. In addition, investigators are trying to identify the optimum fluoride dose that will encourage the deposition of calcium in the bone and yet keep the side effects to a minimum.

Considerable research has been conducted on the use of different preparations, such as growth hormone, testosterone, and anabolic steroids, in the treatment of osteoporosis, particularly in men. Some experts are recommending that in men with low testosterone,

a biweekly injection or the daily application of a testosterone patch may be needed. More research is needed on men with the new drugs that have been approved for use for women. Also, studies of heart disease risk or prostate problems in men using testosterone need to be conducted.

PERSPECTIVE AND PROSPECTS

Osteoporosis is a major public health problem, affecting at least 25 million Americans, with about 1.5 million fractures occurring each year. It is often silent until a fracture occurs. Up to one of every five older patients sustaining a hip fracture dies within six months of the fracture. One-half of the survivors need some help with their daily living activities, and as many as 25 percent of these patients need care in a nursing home. The 1995 estimated cost for treating osteoporotic fractures was nearly $14 billion.

The early diagnosis of osteoporosis and the ability to quantify its degree have represented major strides in the diagnosis, management, and prevention of this disease. It is now recommended that all women approaching the menopause be checked to determine a base-line density reading and to help with prevention and possible treatment options. Indeed, physicians can now identify patients with early osteoporosis and assess their response to treatment accurately. Additionally, modifiable risk factors increasing the likelihood of developing osteoporosis have been identified; these include a low dietary calcium intake, cigarette smoking, excessive alcohol use, amenorrhea, anorexia nervosa or bulimia nervosa, and a sedentary lifestyle. Education of the public, therefore, has an important part to play in the prevention and management of osteoporosis. Working with young people may be the best way to combat osteoporosis. For many people, making the right choices early in life may have great influence in preventing this debilitating disease later in life. For the older adult, attempts are being made to develop "risk profiles" which can be used to estimate the individual patient's fracture risk. This in turn will allow physicians to identify those in the population who are particularly likely to benefit from specific therapy. Moreover, the increased understanding of bone formation, bone resorption, and bone metabolism has led to a considerable amount of research work on the development of effective treatment programs. Drugs that can build strong bones, or ones that can prevent further bone loss, will need to be continually studied in both men and women, and ev-

erything that can be done to reduce side effects from these or other drugs that affect calcium stores in the bones must be a top priority of research dollars spent.
—*Ronald C. Hamdy, M.D., Larry Hudgins, M.D., and Sharon Moore, M.D.; updated by Wendy E. S. Repovich, Ph.D.*

See also Aging; Aging: Extended care; Amenorrhea; Anorexia nervosa; Bone disorders; Bones and the skeleton; Eating disorders; Estrogen replacement therapy; Exercise physiology; Fracture and dislocation; Fracture repair; Hip fracture repair; Hormone replacement therapy; Hormones; Malnutrition; Menopause; Nutrition; Orthopedic surgery; Orthopedics; Preventive medicine; Spinal cord disorders; Spine, vertebrae, and disks; Sports medicine; Supplements; Vitamins and minerals.

FOR FURTHER INFORMATION:
Bilger, Burkhard. "Bone Medicine." *Health* 10, no. 3 (1996). This article summarizes the new drugs approved by the FDA for the treatment of osteoporosis in women, as well as other drugs that are being researched for approval.
Byyny, Richard, and Leonard Speroff. *A Clinical Guide for the Care of Older Women.* Baltimore: Williams & Wilkins, 1990. Outlines specific treatment protocol for hormone replacement therapy and nonhormonal therapy for osteoporosis treatment.
Heaney, Robert P. "Osteoporosis." In *Nutrition in Women's Health,* edited by Debra A. Krummel and Penny M. Kris-Etherton. Gaithersburg, Md.: Aspen, 1996. This chapter highlights the role of nutrition in the prevention and treatment of osteoporosis in the postmenopausal woman.
Isselbacher, Kurt J., et al., eds. *Harrison's Principles of Internal Medicine.* 14th ed. New York: McGraw-Hill, 1998. This text contains a chapter outlining the physiology, pathophysiology, diagnosis, and treatment of bone metabolism.
Meredith, C. M. "Exercise in the Prevention of Osteoporosis." In *Nutrition of the Elderly,* edited by Hamish Munro and Gunter Schlierf. Nestle's Nutrition Workshop Series 29. New York: Raven Press, 1992. This report emphasizes the positive effect of sustained exercise programs on bone mineral stabilization.
Petersen, Marilyn D., and Diana L. White, eds. *Health Care of the Elderly: An Information Sourcebook.* Newbury Park, Calif.: Sage, 1989. D. W. Belcher's article "Prevention of Osteoporosis in the Elderly" discusses accepted treatment modulations to reduce the acceleration of osteoporosis in patients at risk.
Rosen, Clifford J., Julie Glowacki, and John P. Bilezikian, eds. *The Aging Skeleton.* San Diego, Calif.: Academic Press, 1999. This book is a substantial addition to the texts available in the area of osteoporosis. Its large-format pages are divided into forty-nine chapters that range widely across such topics as the biology of aging, determinants of peak bone mass, the biology of age-related bone loss, assessment of bone loss, the epidemiology of osteoporotic fractures, and the therapeutics of osteoporosis.
Snow-Harter, Christine, and Robert Marcus. "Exercise, Bone Mineral Density, and Osteoporosis." In *Exercise and Sport Sciences Reviews.* Vol. 19. Baltimore: Williams & Wilkins, 1991. A review of the role exercise plays in the development and retention of bone density and osteoporosis.
Van Horn, Linda, and Annie O. Wong. "Preventive Nutrition in Adolescent Girls." In *Nutrition in Women's Health,* edited by Debra A. Krummel and Penny M. Kris-Etherton. Gaithersburg, Md.: Aspen, 1996. Discusses the role that nutrition in the adolescent may play in the prevention of osteoporosis later in life.

OTOPLASTY
PROCEDURE

ANATOMY OR SYSTEM AFFECTED: Ears, skin

SPECIALTIES AND RELATED FIELDS: Audiology, family practice, general surgery, pediatrics, plastic surgery

DEFINITION: Cosmetic or reconstructive surgery performed on the outer ear.

INDICATIONS AND PROCEDURES

Otoplasty is performed to improve the appearance of the outer ear, typically to flatten protruding ears or to repair or reconstruct a missing or badly damaged ear. Since the ears have reached 90 percent of their adult size by the time a child reaches age five, the surgery can be performed either at this early age or later.

The first step in flattening protruding ears is to remove a flap of skin from the back of each ear. The underlying cartilage is then remolded, and the two edges of the wound are stitched together, bringing the ear closer to the head. Dressings are applied to the ears and left for a few days, when they are replaced by a headband that is worn for several weeks. The stitches are removed approximately one week after the surgery.

The reconstruction of a missing or badly damaged ear is a complex procedure that typically involves more than one operation, and long healing intervals are necessary between operations. The first step is to remove a piece of cartilage from a rib and sculpture it to resemble a normal ear. The cartilage is then transferred to a fold of skin where the ear will be located. A skin graft may be necessary. Dressings are applied to the ear for up to two weeks, and the stitches are then removed. In many cases, hearing in the reconstructed ear may not be normal. As long as hearing is normal in the other ear, however, no attempt is usually made to improve hearing in the reconstructed ear.

USES AND COMPLICATIONS

Possible complications associated with otoplasty operations include sensitivity of the ear to cold weather, especially during the first year after surgery, and skin graft failure. On rare occasions, excessive bleeding or infection of the surgical wounds may arise. For minor pain, the patient can take acetaminophen or ibuprofen. As the ear heals, a hard ridge usually forms along the incision, but it will gradually recede. The scar will be hidden in the crease between the scalp and the ear.

—*Alvin K. Benson, Ph.D.*

See also Ear infections and disorders; Ears; Hearing loss; Plastic surgery; Surgery, pediatric.

FOR FURTHER INFORMATION:

Converse, J. M. *Reconstructive Plastic Surgery.* 2d ed. Philadelphia: W. B. Saunders, 1977.

Sabiston, David C., Jr., ed. *Textbook of Surgery.* 16th ed. Philadelphia: W. B. Saunders, 2001.

Suddarth, Doris S., ed. *The Lippincott Manual of Nursing Practice.* 7th ed. Philadelphia: J. B. Lippincott, 2000.

Zuckerman, Barry S., and Pamela A. M. Zuckerman. *Child Health: A Pediatrician's Guide for Parents.* New York: Hearst Books, 1986.

OTORHINOLARYNGOLOGY

SPECIALTY

ANATOMY OR SYSTEM AFFECTED: Ears, nose, respiratory system, throat

SPECIALTIES AND RELATED FIELDS: Audiology, neurology, pediatrics, plastic surgery

DEFINITION: The study of the diseases and disorders of the ears, nose, and throat.

KEY TERMS:

audiometer: an electronic device, often used in combination with a computer, that measures a patient's range of hearing

fenestration: the surgical opening of a passage in a closed or narrowing ear canal through which sound can pass

mastoidectomy: the surgical removal of the temporal or mastoid bone, which is located behind the ear

maxillofacial surgery: surgery of the face and neck, a form of cosmetic and reconstructive surgery

otologist: a medical doctor who specializes in diseases and disorders of the ear

stapedectomy: the surgical removal of all or part of the stapes or innermost ossicle of the ear

tomography: an X ray used in combination with sophisticated computers to create an image of a specific organ, blotting out everything in front or behind

SCIENCE AND PROFESSION

Otorhinolaryngology—whose practitioners are often referred to simply as otolaryngologists or ear, nose, and throat (ENT) doctors—is a medical specialty that requires a doctor of medicine degree followed by a hospital or medical center residency ranging from four to five years, depending on the institution in which it is served. Many physicians in this field develop subspecialties, for which additional training is requisite. Among the most common subspecialties are oncology of the head and neck, ear surgery, pediatric otolaryngology, and maxillofacial surgery.

The scope of the otorhinolaryngologist's job is broad and overlaps several other medical specialties, notably general surgery, neurosurgery, plastic surgery, pediatrics, ophthalmology, and oncology. The otorhinolaryngologist treats all diseases and lesions that occur above the clavicle or collarbone except for those belonging to two categories: diseases and disorders of the eyes, which fall into the province of ophthalmology, and brain lesions, which are usually treated by neurosurgeons.

Otorhinolaryngology has existed as a specialty since the late nineteenth century. The need for it was great because ear, nose, and throat problems had, through the centuries, been among the most persistent killers of human beings. The areas affected have much to do with the ability to take in food and air. They also are directly connected with speech, smell, taste, hearing, and balance. Dysfunction of the ears, nose, or throat can profoundly affect a person's well-being physically, emotionally, and socially.

Among the medical conditions and diseases that most frequently come under the purview of otorhinolaryngology are the following: cleft lip and palate deformities (which are often treated as well by plastic surgeons); thyroid tumors (which are also treated by oncological surgeons); skin cancers (which also fall within the practices of plastic surgeons and oncological surgeons); face lifts, the treatment of facial lacerations, and other reconstructive surgery (which plastic surgeons also handle); lumps on the salivary glands (which are sometimes treated by oncological surgeons); and jaw injuries, including fractures (which are treated by maxillofacial surgeons, many of them board-certified in otorhinolaryngology).

Some of the surgery once done by otorhinolaryngologists is now virtually unnecessary because of the development of antibiotics. For example, drugs can combat effectively the kinds of infections that used to result in mastoiditis (inflammation of the mastoid bone), which frequently required a mastoidectomy. The flexible fiber-optic endoscope permits doctors to look into areas that previously could be exposed only through surgery. Advances in research have revealed that nasal polyps, which had a high rate of recurrence and were removed on a continuous basis, can usually be treated effectively with antibiotics, making such surgery unnecessary.

Until the mid-twentieth century, the most serious operation performed by otorhinolaryngologists was the laryngectomy (removal of the larynx, or voice box). By the end of the century, however, many practitioners in this specialty were routinely performing surgeries on tongue cancers and thyroid tumors because otorhinolaryngologists are often the ones who initially dis-

The Anatomy of the Nose and Throat

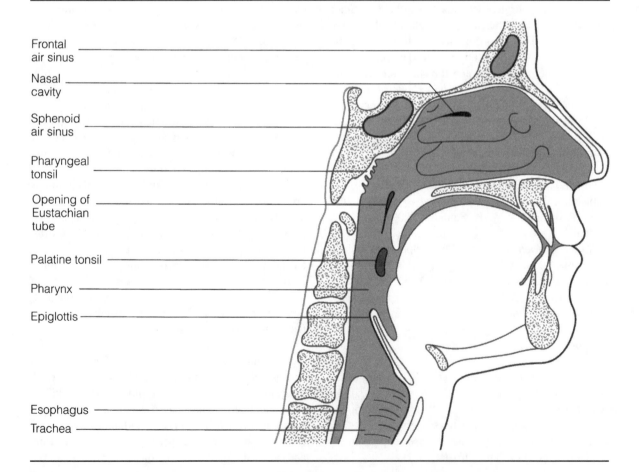

Frontal air sinus

Nasal cavity

Sphenoid air sinus

Pharyngeal tonsil

Opening of Eustachian tube

Palatine tonsil

Pharynx

Epiglottis

Esophagus

Trachea

cover these conditions during head and neck examinations.

Because otorhinolaryngologists have long dealt with the grafting of bone and skin and the surgical management of skin flaps, much reconstructive and cosmetic surgery now falls into their specialty. Removal of tumors from the base of the skull, the interior ear canal, or the posterior cranial depression by means of modified craniotomies can be done by otorhinolaryngologists, who sometimes work in tandem with neurosurgeons in such cases.

DIAGNOSTIC AND TREATMENT TECHNIQUES

The illnesses treated by otorhinolaryngologists have plagued the human race throughout history but could not be treated effectively until technology was developed that enabled physicians to look into the crowded crevices deep inside the body that were the source of many illnesses. In 1854, Manuel Garcia invented a concave mirror with a hole in its center through which doctors, attaching the implement to their heads, could peer as light from the mirror illuminated a patient's ears, nose, and throat. Doctors discovered that, using the reflecting head mirror in combination with an angled mirror held as far back as possible in the throat, they could illuminate the laryngeal area and the pharynx as well as the area behind the nose, all previously unavailable for visual inspection. Eventually, rather than examining affected areas with the bare eye, physicians had available to them, imbedded in the eyepiece of a hollow instrument with a light at the end, a magnifying telescope through which they could examine remote cavities with considerable ease and in great detail.

Modern otorhinolaryngologists can also examine patients under mild local anesthetic with sophisticated endoscopes, flexible devices that can easily be inserted into the nose, mouth, or ear of the patient. Such procedures are usually carried out in the doctor's office or in a hospital on an outpatient basis. These endoscopes, originally lighted with bulbs that heated up and burned out quickly, now carry light through light-bearing fiberoptic strands. In combination with small magnifying devices and cameras designed for this purpose, physicians can examine almost any area of the ears, nose, and throat and create color images, which can be invaluable in determining the presence of disease and in making an accurate diagnosis.

Modern technology has also made available to otorhinolaryngologists laser scalpels that permit extremely intricate surgery and accurate electronic audiometers. Audiometers eliminate the subjectivity of past tests of hearing acuity: In the nineteenth century, doctors either whispered into patients' ears, increasing the volume until their whispers could be heard, or used tuning forks to determine how much their patients could hear.

Treatment of disorders and diseases of the ear, nose, and throat have changed rapidly with the introduction of increasingly sophisticated surgical equipment and with the development of new drugs to control many conditions that once could be managed only by surgery. Computers have also been a valuable tool in diagnosing many of the problems that fall within this specialty.

All the anatomical areas with which otorhinolaryngologists must deal are interconnected; therefore a disease that begins in the ears can affect the nose and the throat, and vice versa. The most common diseases of the ears include deafness and Ménière's disease, an illness caused by an accumulation of fluid in the ear's labyrinth that results in loss of balance. Both of these disorders are most common among people over fifty, although they can afflict people at any age. One out of every ten thousand babies born in the United States has some hearing deficit, and many—particularly those whose mothers contracted rubella (German measles) during pregnancy—are almost totally deaf.

Otologists (physicians who treat diseases and disorders of the ear) have made considerable headway in treating some forms of deafness, particularly conductive deafness, which results from a narrowing of the ear canal to the point of closure. Shortly before 1920, it was discovered that considerable hearing can be restored through fenestration—that is, through making a small surgical opening in the eardrum through which sound can pass. The complications associated with this procedure have been largely overcome with stapedectomy (the removal of all or part of the stapes, one of the bones of the middle ear) and the insertion of a prosthetic device, which is made of wire or Teflon and used in combination with a gelatin sponge or the patient's own veins, connective tissue, and fat. Although fenestration is highly successful in cases in which deafness is conductive, it does not alleviate deafness whose cause is sensorineural, so-called nerve deafness, which is often treated palliatively with hearing aids. These devices are constantly improving, however, as they are decreasing in size and increasing in effectiveness.

Tumors of the inner ear can now be successfully removed through a translabyrinthine approach. The ear canal is entered with tiny, well-illuminated laser instruments to which magnifying devices are attached. Such surgery is often performed by otologists, although many undertake it collaboratively with a neurologist. Pituitary tumors, once the responsibility almost solely of neurosurgeons who performed craniotomies to reach the diseased area of the brain, are often treated by otorhinolaryngologists, who approach the tumor through the nose. Thus the tumor can be removed without the need for debilitating surgery.

From the earliest beginnings of otorhinolaryngology, the larynx has been among the parts of the anatomy most often treated by its practitioners. The laryngectomy, with its radical side effect of rendering the patient unable to speak, was once the treatment of choice for malignant laryngeal tumors. Such tumors can now be treated successfully with radiation, obviating the need for more drastic treatment. Teflon injections have been used to treat patients whose vocal cords have been compromised by surgery or by radiation. Because the larynx is in the area of the thyroid glands, otorhinolaryngologists also possess expert knowledge of thyroid disorders and may perform a thyroidectomy (removal of the thyroid), a procedure that is now emphasized in their residencies.

Two of the most frequent surgical procedures of the field in the mid-twentieth century were the removal of the tonsils (tonsillectomy) and of the adenoids, the masses of lymphoid tissue in the lining at the back of the tongue that produce white blood cells, which fight disease. Tonsils and adenoids were once removed routinely if children suffered from frequent colds. Now this surgery is discouraged because it has been discovered that the tonsils and adenoids help children develop a resistance to infection. When these tissues become inflamed, they can be treated conservatively and successfully through medication.

Otorhinolaryngologists regularly work in concert with physicians in other specialties, particularly neurosurgery. An internist treating a patient who suffers from loss of balance usually refers that patient to an otologist, who orders diagnostic tests to check for fluid in the inner ear, which would suggest Ménière's disease. If such tests fail to reveal a buildup of fluid in the inner ear, the otologist usually refers the patient to a neurologist or neurosurgeon to check for other causes, including a tumor or a disorder in the central nervous system.

Otologists sometimes perform plastic surgery on ears that are abnormally protrusive. This reduction is a form of cosmetic surgery. By the end of the twentieth century in the United States, it was common for otorhinolaryngologists to perform most cosmetic and reconstructive surgeries related to these areas of the body. Consequently, residencies in this specialty offer considerable training in plastic surgery, especially in the procedures that otorhinolaryngologists have come to perform routinely in connection with thyroid, nasal, and other surgeries. They are often the physicians of choice in cases of cleft lip and cleft palate, the treatment of which normally falls largely within the province of reconstructive surgery. Because much cosmetic and reconstructive surgery involves the face, maxillofacial surgeons are often otorhinolaryngologists.

The common cold, although usually treated by an internist or family doctor if it is referred to a physician at all, sometimes involves complications such as bronchitis, pneumonia, or ancillary infections of the ears and sinuses. In such cases, an otorhinolaryngologist may be consulted for treatment. Dealing with the common cold is merely a waiting game: Colds generally go away after a week or ten days. Colds afflict the average adult about four times a year and the average child twice that often (because young children have not yet built up the immunity that prevents infection).

Perspective and Prospects

Many of the illnesses that fall within the purview of otorhinolaryngology became more threatening and more frequent when the Industrial Revolution of the eighteenth century caused the relocation of large numbers of people from rural to urban settings. Cities grew as factories opened. Living conditions were often deplorable and, at best, overcrowded. Added to this situation was the pollution of the air by the waste products expelled by smokestack industries. Wherever pollution is prevalent, diseases of the upper-respiratory tract are endemic.

The eighteenth century spawned conditions that compromised the environment and severely affected humans, but until physicians had a way of examining the body's more remote crevices, the diagnosis and treatment of ear, nose, and throat problems were difficult. Such treatments as bleeding frequently killed rather than cured patients. Surgery was a treatment of last resort because the major anesthetic was whiskey. Patients sometimes died of shock from the unbearable pain that they suffered during surgical procedures.

Once physicians had reliable means of seeing into the body by using such equipment as reflective mirrors, endoscopes, X rays, tomography, and ultrasonography, they could treat many illnesses nonsurgically. It is hoped that in the future even less invasive surgery will be done in all fields of medicine, including otorhinolaryngology.

Even when surgery is indicated, in the field of otorhinolaryngology it can often be performed without an incision by entering the body through the ear canal, nose, or throat. Advanced technology has produced surgical instruments that, in combination with computer imaging, work precisely and with less trauma. In cases where incisions are necessary, the opening is often so small that it is almost undetectable a year after the procedure.

—*R. Baird Shuman, Ph.D.*

See also Aromatherapy; Audiology; Cleft lip and palate; Cleft lip and palate repair; Common cold; Ear infections and disorders; Ear surgery; Ears; Epiglottitis; Halitosis; Hearing loss; Hearing tests; Laryngectomy; Laryngitis; Ménière's disease; Motion sickness; Myringotomy; Nasal polyp removal; Nasopharyngeal disorders; Nosebleeds; Otoplasty; Pharyngitis; Plastic surgery; Quinsy; Rhinitis; Rhinoplasty and submucous resection; Sense organs; Sinusitis; Smell; Sneezing; Sore throat; Strep throat; Taste; Tonsillectomy and adenoid removal; Tonsillitis; Voice and vocal cord disorders.

FOR FURTHER INFORMATION:

Benjamin, Bruce, et al. *A Colour Atlas of Otorhinolaryngology*. Edited by Michael Hawke. Philadelphia: J. B. Lippincott, 1995. This atlas explores the diseases that can affect the ears, nose, and throat. Includes a bibliography.

Chasnoff, Ira J., Jeffrey W. Ellis, and Zachary S. Fainman, eds. Rev. ed. *The New Illustrated Family Medical and Health Guide*. Lincolnwood, Ill.: Publications International, 1994. The fourteen-page chapter on disorders of the ear, nose, and throat is distinctly directed toward a nonspecialized audience. The text is enhanced by useful illustrations.

Crumley, Roger L. "Otolaryngology—Head and Neck Surgery." In *Planning Your Medical Career: Traditional and Alternative Opportunities*, edited by T. Donald Rucker and Martin D. Keller et al. Garrett Park, Md.: Garrett Park Press, 1986. Presents a comprehensive overview of the field in language that, although occasionally specialized, is, on the whole, not difficult for readers who lack a medical background.

Gulya, Aina J., and William R. Wilson. *An Atlas of Ear, Nose, and Throat Diagnosis and Treatment*. New York: Parthenon, 1999. Authoritative, up-to-date color atlas and textbook on diagnosing and treating ear, nose, and throat disorders. Published expressly for otorhinolaryngology physicians, it contains more than ninety distinctive color photographs along with many other figures and tables.

Woodson, Gayle E. *Ear, Nose, and Throat Disorders in Primary Care*. Philadelphia: W. B. Saunders, 2001. Discusses such topics as the examination of the head and neck; hearing loss, tinnitus, and otalgia; dizziness and vertigo; facial paralysis; the nose and sinus disease; and the oral cavity and throat.

OVARIAN CANCER. *See* CERVICAL, OVARIAN, AND UTERINE CANCERS.

OVARIAN CYSTS
DISEASE/DISORDER

ANATOMY OR SYSTEM AFFECTED: Reproductive system

SPECIALTIES AND RELATED FIELDS: Gynecology

DEFINITION: Benign growths that develop in the ovaries.

CAUSES AND SYMPTOMS

Ovarian cysts may occur at any age, individually or in numbers, on one or both ovaries. The cyst consists of a thin, transparent outer wall enclosing one or more chambers filled with clear fluids or jellylike material. Such cysts range in size from that of a raisin to that of a large orange. The normal ovary measures 3 centimeters by 2 centimeters; the cystic ovary requiring investigation is one which is enlarged to more than twice its normal size. Large cysts may cause a feeling of fullness in the abdominal area or pain on vaginal intercourse. Often, however, there are no apparent symptoms, and the cyst is discovered only during a routine gynecologic examination when the physician, on manual examination, discovers that one ovary is considerably enlarged. At that point, it is important to rule out malignancy, since ovarian cancers in their early stages also have no warning symptoms and can occur at any age.

Polycystic ovaries (ovaries containing multiple cysts) causing significant enlargement occur in a va-

Dermoid Cysts

Dermoid cysts are a relatively common form of ovarian cyst, often found in younger women.

riety of conditions. For example, polycystic ovaries can result from an enzyme deficiency in the ovaries which interferes with the normal biosynthesis of hormones, resulting in the release of an abnormal amount of androgen (a substance producing or stimulating the development of male characteristics).

Many ovarian cysts—some authorities say more than half—are functional; that is, they arise out of the normal functions of the ovary during the menstrual cycle. These cysts are relatively common. A cyst can form when a follicle (a small, spherical, secretory structure in the ovary) has grown in preparation for ovulation but fails to rupture and release an egg; this type is called a follicular cyst. Sometimes the structure formed from the follicle after ovulation, the corpus luteum, fails to shrink and forms a cyst; this is called a corpus luteum cyst.

Another type of ovarian cyst most often found in younger women is the dermoid cyst, which contains particles of teeth, hair, or calcium-containing tissue that are thought to be an embryologic (developmental) remnant; such cysts usually do not cause menstrual irregularity and are very common. Dermoids are bilateral in 25 percent of cases, making careful examination of both ovaries mandatory. The cyst has

a thickened, white, opaque wall and is more buoyant than other types of cysts.

Ovarian cysts cause problems when they become very large, when they rupture and cause severe internal bleeding, or when a cyst's pedicle (a tail-like appendage) suddenly twists and cuts off its blood supply, creating severe pain and possibly gangrene. Rupture of a cyst is followed by the acute onset of severe lower abdominal pain radiating to the vagina and lower back. The most severe symptoms of pain and collapse are associated with rupture of a dermoid cyst, as the cyst contents are extremely irritating to the peritoneum, the serous membrane reflected over the viscera and lining the abdominal cavity.

Torsion (twisting) of a cyst may occur at any age but most often in the twenties; it may be associated with pregnancy. A twisted dermoid cyst is the most common, probably because of its increased weight. The onset of pain often occurs in the umbilical region and radiates to one or the other side of the pelvis. Pain on the right is frequently confused with appendicitis. Hemorrhage may sometimes occur from a vessel in the wall of the cyst or within the capsule.

TREATMENT AND THERAPY

The diagnosis of an ovarian cyst is determined by the patient's age, medical and family history, and symptoms and by the size of the enlarged ovary. In women under thirty, after a manual examination, physicians will usually wait to see if the ovary will return to its normal size. If it does not and pregnancy has been ruled out, a pelvic X ray and/or sonogram (the use of sound to produce an image or photograph of an organ or tissue) can determine the exact size of the ovaries and distinguish between a cyst and a solid tumor. In older women (over forty), X rays and sonograms may be done sooner. If uncertainty still exists, the physician may recommend laparoscopy, the visual examination of the abdominal cavity using a device consisting of a tube and optical system inserted through a small incision. The physician may also suggest the option of a larger incision and a biopsy.

In the case of the functional ovarian cyst, if no severe pain or swelling is present, the physician may choose to wait for one or two more menstrual cycles to be completed, during the course of which this type of cyst frequently disappears of its own accord. Sometimes this process is hastened by administering oral contraceptives for several months, which establishes a very regular menstrual cycle. Women already taking oral contraceptives rarely develop ovarian cysts.

In the case of torsion or rupture, surgical treatment is indicated, preferably the removal of the cyst only and preservation of as much of the normal ovarian tissue as possible. Sometimes, with a very large cyst, the ovary cannot be saved and must be removed, a procedure called oophorectomy or ovariectomy.

—Genevieve Slomski, Ph.D.

See also Biopsy; Cyst removal; Cysts; Genital disorders, female; Infertility in females; Laparoscopy.

FOR FURTHER INFORMATION:

Adashi, Eli Y., and Peter C. K. Leung, eds. *The Ovary (Comprehensive Endocrinology)*. New York: Raven Press, 1993. Contributed by leading investigators, the material presented in this volume links molecular and cellular physiology with traditional physiology. Moving from follicular and oocyte maturation to ovulation and corpus luteum formation, it addresses all phases of the ovarian life cycle.

Kovacs, Gabor. *Polycystic Ovary Syndrome*. New York: Cambridge University Press, 2000. This publication provides an essential guide to the diagnosis of polycystic ovary syndrome and its etiology, pathology, and effective medical management. This comprehensive account summarizes the most recent advances in the molecular basis of the syndrome, its genetic basis, and long-term health effects.

Mahajan, Damodar K., ed. *Polycystic Ovarian Disease*. Philadelphia: W. B. Saunders, 1988. In addition to polycystic ovary syndrome, this text discusses Stein-Leventhal syndrome. Includes bibliographical references and an index.

Peters, Hannah. *The Ovary: A Correlation of Structure and Function in Mammals*. Berkeley: University of California Press, 1980. Discusses the growth and development of the ovaries as well as their physiology. Includes bibliographical references and an index.

Zuckerman, Solly. *The Ovary*. 2d ed. 3 vols. New York: Academic Press, 1977. Volume 1 discusses the general aspects of the ovary. Volumes 2 and 3 cover the physiology and the regulation of oogenesis and steroidogenesis, respectively.

OXYGEN THERAPY
PROCEDURE

ANATOMY OR SYSTEM AFFECTED: Lungs, respiratory system

SPECIALTIES AND RELATED FIELDS: Alternative medicine, emergency medicine, exercise physiology, immunology, pulmonary medicine, sports medicine

DEFINITION: Oxygen therapy, also known as oxygen inhalation therapy, is the use of concentrated oxygen to treat disease or to enhance physical performance. It can be administered either through a hyperbaric oxygen chamber or by the inhalation of pure oxygen. In the hyperbaric oxygen chamber, the patient sits or lies in a stainless steel chamber filled with pure oxygen at high pressure. Medically approved uses of the hyperbaric oxygen chamber include the treatment of burns, carbon monoxide poisoning, and decompression sickness (the "bends"). Other uses that are not approved by the medical community include the treatment of arthritis, cancer, multiple sclerosis, and acquired immunodeficiency syndrome (AIDS), among other conditions. The inhalation of pure oxygen is practiced by some athletes, especially football players, who may occasionally be seen on the sidelines breathing oxygen through a mask attached to an oxygen tank. They believe that the increase in oxygen consumption will enhance their performance under aerobically challenging circumstances, such as running. From a scientific standpoint, this belief is strictly a psychological illusion: The use of oxygen in this manner provides no actual physical benefit. Viruses and bacteria may be spread through the sharing of an inhalation apparatus.

—Karen E. Kalumuck, Ph.D.

See also Alternative medicine; Burns and scalds; Exercise physiology; Poisoning; Respiration; Sports medicine.

FOR FURTHER INFORMATION:

Goldberg, Burton, comp. *Alternative Medicine: The Definitive Guide*. Puyallup, Wash.: Future Medicine, 1993.

Jacobs, Jennifer, ed. *The Encyclopedia of Alternative Medicine: A Complete Family Guide to Complementary Therapies*. Rev. ed. Boston: Journey Editions, 1997.

Kastner, Mark, and Hugh Burroughs. *Alternative Healing: The Complete A-Z Guide to over 160 Different Alternative Therapies*. New York: Henry Holt, 1996.

PACEMAKER IMPLANTATION

PROCEDURE

ANATOMY OR SYSTEM AFFECTED: Chest, circulatory system, heart

SPECIALTIES AND RELATED FIELDS: Biotechnology, cardiology

DEFINITION: The introduction into the heart of a permanent instrument that uses electrical pulses to regulate its rhythm.

KEY TERMS:

atrium: one of the two upper chambers of the heart; the right atrium receives blood returning through the veins; the left atrium receives oxygenated blood from the lungs

catheter: a thin tube that can be inserted into blood vessels, such as a vein leading into the heart, to carry electrical wires or optical fibers

circus movement: electrical impulses in the heart that continue firing instead of reaching a normal resting phase, causing heart flutter and fibrillation

electrocardiogram (ECG or EKG): a recording of electrical signals generated by the heart that are detected by electrodes placed on the chest, arms, and legs; used to diagnose heart abnormalities

fibrillations: rapid and chaotic contractions of the heart muscle that are usually fatal when they occur in the ventricles because of insufficient blood flow

heart block: a delay or blockage of the electrical signal traveling through the heart muscle, which upsets the synchronization between contractions of the upper and lower chambers

sinoatrial (S-A) node: a cluster of cells above the right atrium that emit electrical signals that initiate contractions of the heart; also called natural pacemaker cells

ventricles: the two lower chambers of the heart; the right ventricle pumps blood to the lungs, and the left ventricle pumps oxygenated blood to the body

INDICATIONS AND PROCEDURES

The first human-made pacemaker, which used electronic pulses to stimulate a regular heart rhythm, was built in the 1950's. Since then, the device has evolved into a sophisticated and reliable instrument. It was miniaturized so that it could be implanted under the skin of the patient. Tiny batteries that would last from five to fifteen years were developed. A microprocessor that can sense the need for different heart rates during sleep or strenuous exercise has become a standard component. Most recently, a small automatic defibrillator was incorporated into the pacemaker to supply several large jolts of electrical energy in case of heart stoppage or other emergencies.

The normal rhythm of a healthy heart is regulated by natural pacemaker cells. These unique cells are located at the sinoatrial (S-A) node near the top interior of the heart, where blood empties from the veins into the right atrium. Electrical impulses originating at the S-A node travel to the atrioventricular (A-V) node, which is located where the four chambers of the heart come together. From there, the signal is relayed to the ventricles, causing the muscle fibers to contract. This pumping action forces blood to flow from the two ventricles to the lungs and the body arteries.

If the natural pacemaker cells or the nerve pathways do not function properly, the heart may beat too rapidly, too slowly, irregularly, or not at all. For example, the condition called heart block interrupts or delays the electrical signal at the A-V node. It can happen that only every second or third pacemaker signal triggers a contraction. Sometimes, the ventricles will start a contraction on their own, but it will not be synchronized with the blood flow from the atrium. An artificial electronic pacemaker can be used to overcome heart block.

The electrical activity of the heart is observed in an electrocardiogram (ECG or EKG). Metal electrodes are placed in contact with a patient's left arm, right arm, left leg, and sometimes the chest. After suitable amplification, the signal can be displayed on a video screen or recorded by an ink pen on moving paper.

For a healthy heart, the normal ECG pattern starts with a small pulse (the P wave), which is followed by a group of three closely spaced pulses (the QRS complex) and a final small pulse (the T wave). This pattern is repeated approximately seventy-two times per minute for a person sitting at rest.

In brief, the P wave indicates contraction of the atrium, the QRS complex shows contraction of the ventricles, and the T wave represents the muscles' return to the resting state. If the heart "skips a beat" because of a heart block at the A-V node, the ECG will show a missing or delayed pulsation in the otherwise regular pattern. This is where electronic stimulation is needed.

Two other serious malfunctions of the heart's electrical system are flutter and fibrillation. Flutter is a very rapid but still constant rhythm that may produce 200 to 300 beats per minute. Fibrillations are much

Locations of Internal Pacemakers

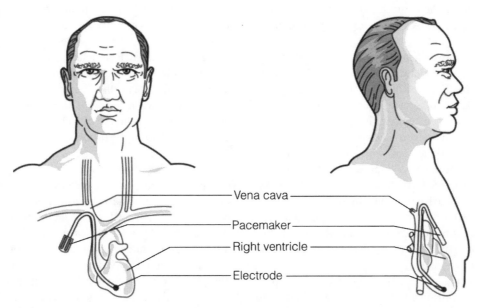

Vena cava

Pacemaker

Right ventricle

Electrode

Transvenous Implantation

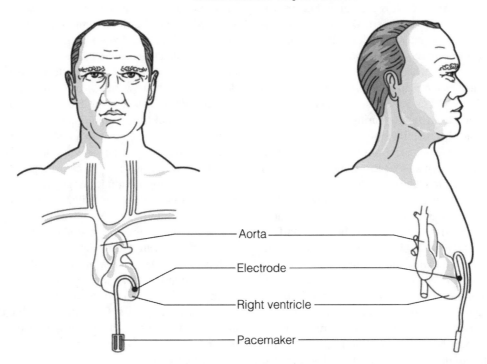

Aorta

Electrode

Right ventricle

Pacemaker

Epicardial Implantation

more serious, causing chaotic, random contractions that can occur as often as 500 times per minute. There is insufficient time between contractions for blood to fill the ventricles. Pumping action becomes very inefficient, and death is likely to occur if the fibrillations continue.

To restore normal heart rhythm, a defibrillator is used to send a strong electric shock through the ventricular muscle fibers, which inactivates the heart's electrical system for several seconds. An electronic pacemaker may then replace the natural pacemaker cells to prevent the recurrence of fibrillations.

The cause of flutter and fibrillation is a process called "circus movement." Suppose the electrical impulses are diverted from their normal pathway by thickened or dead heart tissue. In such a case, the timing may be thrown off so that the ventricles are restimulated to contract again without waiting for the pacemaker's signal. Therefore, the heart is unable to reach its resting state.

In the ECG pattern, flutter shows up as a rapid pulsation with an indistinct QRS complex. Fibrillation is indicated by irregularly spaced pulses of random size that have no pattern at all. It is something like electrical noise coming from the heart, with no synchronization. Heart cells at many locations fire at random, producing ripples similar to those made by a handful of pebbles thrown into a lake.

The first artificial pacemaker was developed by Paul Zoll in 1952. When a patient suffering from heart block went into heart failure during surgery, Zoll inserted a needle electrode into the man's chest and applied regular voltage pulses from an external circuit. After two days, the man's heart resumed beating on its own, and the circuit was disconnected.

A portable artificial pacemaker was developed in 1957 by C. W. Lillehei and Earl Bakken. The electrode was inserted directly against the outer surface of the heart, and a battery pack and timer circuit were worn around the patient's waist. Three years later, the pacemaker was miniaturized sufficiently to be implanted under the skin of the patient's chest. This has the advantage of reducing the risk of infection.

The next major improvement was to redesign the fixed-rate pacemaker so that it could respond to variable demand during exercise or sleep. The demand pacemaker has a built-in sensor that monitors the heart's electrical system. An electronic microprocessor is programmed to recognize abnormal ECG pulses. Generally, the demand pacemaker is set to deliver a trigger pulse only when the heart rate falls below a certain point.

For people with a potential for unpredictable heart stoppage or fibrillation, an automatic implantable defibrillator has been developed. The unit, which is comparable to the external defibrillators used by emergency medical technicians, can deliver several large jolts directly to the heart. Since implanted batteries are quite small, the circuit requires some time to recharge between shocks. The circuit is quite similar to the flash attachment of a camera, with its "slow charge, fast discharge" process.

USES AND COMPLICATIONS

The implantation of a pacemaker may become necessary as a result of a coronary artery disease, in which a buildup of plaque leads to irregularities in the heart's rhythm. Coronary artery disease is the leading cause of death in the United States. It claims more than half a million American lives per year and disables another 2 million. It is primarily a disease of modern, industrial society, and is less frequently found in more rural, underdeveloped countries. In the United States, the death rate from heart attacks increased sharply after 1920, reached a peak in the mid-1960's, and has declined substantially since then.

A heart attack is usually caused by an oxygen deficiency in the heart muscle. The attack may come suddenly and without warning, but most often there is previous tissue damage that has weakened the heart over a period of time. A buildup of plaque in the coronary artery, called atherosclerosis, can reduce the flow rate to a dangerously low level. The heart muscle tries to compensate for its reduced pumping power and may develop rhythmic irregularities. Eventually, heart block or ventricular fibrillations can ensue, leading to heart failure and death.

The famous Framingham study, initiated in 1948, has been following the medical histories of approximately 5,000 men and women in order to identify the most important risk factors for heart disease. For example, the rate of heart disease among male smokers in this study was three times as high as that among nonsmokers. (This result is in addition to the much higher rate of lung cancer among smokers.) Other risk factors are excessive alcohol consumption, lack of exercise, high blood cholesterol, emotional or physical stress, and excess weight. Some unalterable risk factors are age, sex, and a family history of heart disease. The decline in heart attack deaths in recent years has been attributed to widespread changes of lifestyle to reduce the risk factors, as well as to improvements in medical diagnosis and treatment.

Modern pacemakers are remarkably reliable and safe. One of the few precautions for pacemaker wearers is to avoid standing near a microwave oven or an airport radar transmitter. The problem is that the metal wire going into the heart acts like an antenna; it can pick up stray microwave radiation, which can disrupt the electronics in the sensitive pacemaker circuit. Also, the battery in a pacemaker must be changed at five- to ten-year intervals to ensure proper operation.

Thousands of people receive implanted pacemakers each year. The procedure has become so routine that even small community hospitals are equipped to handle it. Many patients with heart block and irregular rhythm, especially elderly patients, have benefited greatly from this technological development.

The creation of effective electronic pacemakers depends on an understanding of the structure and function of the human heart. Also, instruments such as X-ray machines and electrocardiographs are indispensable for monitoring an individual patient's response. This section will review the progress of the medical ideas and the instruments that were the essential prerequisites for modern pacemakers. A good starting point is the pioneering studies of human anatomy made by Leonardo da Vinci (1452-1519) and Andreas Vesalius (1514-1564).

Leonardo dissected and studied the human body and made anatomical sketches in his notebooks. He recognized that the heart had four chambers and drew the heart valves in detail. His interest in anatomy was that of an artist rather than that of a physician.

Vesalius was a professor of medicine at the University of Padua, in Italy. He taught anatomy and wrote a famous seven-volume treatise on the structure of the human body that had many excellent illustrations. His knowledge of anatomy came from the dissection of animals and of human cadavers obtained at night from pauper's graves. Some of his anatomical investigations contradicted traditional medical doctrine and brought him into conflict with the Church. Like Galileo, he believed that experimental information was superior to ancient textbooks.

William Harvey, a British physician, received his medical degree from the University of Padua in 1602. He is known for formulating the first accurate description of the circulation of the blood through the body. He showed that the volume of blood is fairly constant, so the function of the heart is to act as a recirculating pump. He had a clear understanding of the way in which the right ventricle pushes blood through the lungs and the left one circulates it to the rest of the body. There was, however, one missing link in Harvey's theory: How did the blood get from the arteries to the veins for its return flow? The invention of the microscope in the 1670's made it possible to see the tiny, previously invisible capillaries, thus providing final confirmation of the circulation process.

The scientific investigation of electricity began in the 1700's. Benjamin Franklin studied lightning rods, and scientists learned how to build a friction machine that produced electricity in the laboratory. Taking an electric shock became an amusing, although somewhat dangerous, entertainment at parties.

About 1790, the Italian anatomist Luigi Galvani made an important, though accidental, discovery. A metal scalpel lying near an electrostatic machine came into contact with the leg of a recently dissected frog, causing a sudden twitching of the muscle. Evidently, there was a connection between the electric shock and the muscle contraction.

The modern pacemaker that stimulates the heart muscle works in the same way that Galvani's scalpel worked; however, a major evolution in physiological knowledge and medical practice had to take place before the pacemaker could be developed.

Mary Wollstonecraft Shelley picked up the idea of animal electricity and popularized it in her famous science-fiction story *Frankenstein*, which was published in 1809. If electricity could make a dead muscle twitch, perhaps enough electricity could make a dead body come to life. Shelley's story was a frightening exaggeration. Nevertheless, present-day emergency medical technicians use electric shocks to revive a stopped heart—an accepted procedure for a person at the borderline between life and death.

The nineteenth century was a fertile period for new inventions and discoveries in electrical technology. Among these were the telephone, the electric light bulb, and radio waves. The most basic diagnostic tool for checking the heart is the stethoscope. Its invention is attributed to a French physician in the early 1800's who first used a kind of ear trumpet with a flexible hollow tube. Measuring blood pressure is done routinely today to indicate possible heart problems. The method of using a tourniquet on the arm together with a mercury column pressure gauge was not invented until 1896.

Wilhelm Conrad Röntgen was experimenting with high voltages in his laboratory in 1896 when he observed a mysterious new type of radiation, which he called X rays. Unlike light, X rays were able to pass through black paper, wood, and even thin metal sheets. They could cause certain paints to glow in the dark and could expose photographic film that was still in its light-tight box. For the medical profession, the discovery of X rays was a major breakthrough.

The immediate usefulness of X rays was to show broken bones, objects that had been swallowed, bullets or shrapnel embedded in tissue, and large tumors. The heart and lungs, however, showed up only as faint outlines. Physicians learned to inject opaque dye into the blood vessels to increase the contrast. A new technique of inserting a catheter through a vein directly into the heart chambers was developed after experimentation was performed with animals. Combining catheters and X rays, doctors could obtain diagnostic information about the interior of the heart.

X-ray technology has been improved in recent years. Electronic image intensifiers were developed in the 1950's in order to brighten the dim pictures on a fluorescent screen. A major breakthrough in the 1970's was the invention of computed tomography (CT) scanning. Instead of using film or a fluoroscope, a computer generates images of the heart and other internal organs on a video screen. For the pacemaker, X-ray apparatus is indispensable to observe the electrode's precise placement into the interior of the heart.

The heart is a mechanical pump, but its rhythm is controlled by electrical impulses. The instrument that provides essential electrical information about the heart to the physician is the electrocardiograph. It was invented in 1903 by the Dutch physician Willem Einthoven. The voltage fluctuations produced by the heart are typically only one-thousandth of a volt at the peak, so a very sensitive meter is necessary to observe them.

A typical electric meter has a coil of wire mounted between the poles of a magnet. When current flows through the coil, the coil rotates. A pointer is attached to the coil, indicating the amount of current by its deflection. Einthoven's ingenious adaptation was to hang the coil from a very thin fiber that allowed it to rotate with almost no resistance. Attached to the fiber was a small mirror. A beam of light shining on the mirror would be deflected to different angles as the mirror

rotated. This so-called "string galvanometer" worked very well and won for Einthoven the 1924 Nobel Prize in Physiology or Medicine.

The interpretation of normal and abnormal electrocardiogram patterns requires training and experience on the part of the physician. (Some correlations between abnormal ECGs and malfunctions of the heart will be discussed in the following section on pacemaker applications.)

The electrodes of most pacemakers are installed with a catheter that is inserted through a vein, through the right atrium, through the valve, and finally touches the inside of the right ventricle. The first human heart catheterization is credited to Werner Forssmann in 1929, when he was a young intern at a hospital in Berlin, Germany. He requested permission to try the procedure on a patient, but his supervisor refused. Forssmann then decided to try it on himself. He anesthetized his left elbow, opened a vein, and inserted the catheter tube. As he pushed it up the arm, he watched its progress on an X-ray fluoroscope, which he had to view by reflection in a mirror held by a nurse. When the catheter had gone in 65 centimeters, Forssmann asked an X-ray technician to record it on film to prove that it had entered his heart. During the next two years, he repeated the procedure several times, but criticism by his medical colleagues forced him to discontinue it. He became a small-town doctor and was amazed to learn in 1956 that he had been awarded the Nobel Prize for Medicine.

Accumulated knowledge about the structure of the heart, improvements in surgery, the development of new drugs, and the availability of modern instrumentation have all contributed to a substantial improvement in the medical treatment of heart ailments in modern times.

The development of artificial heart valves, the heart-lung machine, the success of heart bypass surgery, the use of laser beams for surgery, and the use of drugs to control high blood pressure are recent developments.

An important contribution from the field of electronics was the development of the transistor in the early 1950's. It made possible the whole technology of miniaturized electronics, replacing the bulky vacuum tubes that were used in old radio circuits. Implantable pacemakers and microprocessor sensors would not have been possible without transistors.

Human ingenuity no doubt will continue to develop new instruments for cardiac diagnosis and rehabilitation, building on the accomplishments of the innovators of the past.

—Hans G. Graetzer, Ph.D.

See also Arrhythmias; Cardiac rehabilitation; Cardiology; Cardiology, pediatric; Circulation; Electrocardiography (ECG or EKG); Exercise physiology; Heart; Heart attack; Heart disease; Heart valve replacement; Vascular medicine; Vascular system.

FOR FURTHER INFORMATION:

Cameron, John R., James G. Skofronick, and Roderick M. Grant. *Medical Physics: Physics of the Body.* Madison, Wis.: Medical Physics, 1992. A well-written, college-level textbook applying the laws of physics to the human body. A section dealing with the cardiovascular system discusses blood pressure, fluid flow, electrical (ECG) impulses, mechanical forces, and instruments such as the defibrillator and the pacemaker.

Corona, Gyl Garren. "Pacemakers: Keeping the Beat Today." *RN* 62, no. 12 (December, 1999): 50-52. Today's permanent pacemakers not only send electrical impulses to the right atrium and ventricle, they can be programmed to respond to a variety of metabolic cues, bringing medicine ever closer to duplicating the heart's own pacing system.

Davis, Goode P., and Edwards Park. *The Heart: The Living Pump.* Washington, D.C.: U.S. News Books, 1981. An excellent book about the structure and functioning of the heart, with many full-color photographs and diagrams, intended for a general audience of nonspecialists. Good explanations of the electrocardiogram, rheumatic fever, coronary bypass surgery, and new diagnostic technology. Highly recommended.

Jensen, J. Trygve. *Physics for the Health Professions.* 3d ed. New York: John Wiley & Sons, 1982. An elementary textbook for future medical practitioners, with helpful diagrams and informative explanations. The chapter "Electricity" contains a good selection of topics, including bioelectricity, modern instruments such as ECGs and pacemakers, and electrical safety hazards in the hospital.

Sonnenberg, David, Michael Birnbaum, and Emil A. Naclerio. *Understanding Pacemakers.* New York: Michael Kesend, 1982. The authors discuss the way in which the normal heart works, rhythm disorders that may occur, the way in which a pacemaker is surgically implanted, and new developments in pacemaker technology and technique.

Urone, Paul Peter. *Physics with Health Science Applications.* New York: Harper & Row, 1986. An introductory work describing how the principles of physics apply to human physiology. A chapter on basic electric circuits is followed by a discussion of the electrical hazards of medical instruments. Contains a thorough description of bioelectricity, including electrocardiograms and the artificial pacemaker.

PAGET'S DISEASE
DISEASE/DISORDER

ANATOMY OR SYSTEM AFFECTED: Bones, musculoskeletal system, nervous system, spine

SPECIALTIES AND RELATED FIELDS: Internal medicine, orthopedics

DEFINITION: Paget's disease is characterized by a progressive thickening and weakening of the bones. As the disease progresses, movement becomes impaired, resulting in fractures that heal slowly and cause deformities. In the head, neck, and spine, enlarged bones may compress sensory nerves and curve the spine abnormally, inducing forms of nerve paralysis. Complications include high blood pressure, kidney stones, gout, bone cancer, and congestive heart failure. Drugs can halt the process and control the pain; however, there is no cure for Paget's disease.

—Jason Georges and Tracy Irons-Georges

See also Bone disorders; Bones and the skeleton; Fracture and dislocation.

FOR FURTHER INFORMATION:

Goldberg, Kathy E. *The Skeleton: Fantastic Framework.* Washington, D.C.: U.S. News Books, 1982.

Larson, David E., ed. *Mayo Clinic Family Health Book.* 2d ed. New York: William Morrow, 1996.

Marieb, Elaine N. *Human Anatomy and Physiology.* 5th ed. Redwood City, Calif.: Benjamin/Cummings, 2000.

Seeley, Rod R., Trent D. Stephens, and Philip Tate. *Anatomy and Physiology.* 5th ed. St. Louis: Mosby Year Book, 2000.

PAIN
DISEASE/DISORDER

ANATOMY OR SYSTEM AFFECTED: All

SPECIALTIES AND RELATED FIELDS: Family practice, internal medicine, neurology, psychiatry

DEFINITION: Physical distress often associated with a disorder or injury.

Causes and Symptoms

Pain has been described by Harold Merskey as "an unpleasant experience which is primarily associated with tissue damage or described in terms of such damage, or both." It is a highly personal sensation which may be acute to one person and have only a moderate effect on another. Pain is unique from all other sensations because it also involves suffering, which may lead to consequences in the psychological and sociological behavior of the patient.

The sensory mechanism of pain occurs via the nerves, which transfer pain signals to the brain in the form of electric impulses to which the brain responds in various ways. The transfer of the information to the central nervous system (nociception) occurs through the sense organs (nociceptors), which convert physical, thermal, or chemical stimulations along the peripheral nerves to the spinal cord and from there to the higher brain centers. The nociceptors lie on the skin, blood vessels, muscles, and bones of the indi-

vidual. They are of two general types: A-delta fibers and the C-fibers. The A-delta fibers provide fast and short-lasting pain (such as that associated with sudden impact to a toe). The C-fibers are responsible for the slow, unpleasant feeling that follows. As the injury takes place, spinal reflexes, which are stimulating circuits between the nociceptors and the spinal cord, are produced. Spasms follow, which are responsible for the sensation of pain, and the circulation around the injured muscle is temporarily disturbed. Certain chemicals, called prostaglandins, are released and create pain when they come in contact with the nociceptors. The spinal cord is responsible for the transmission of pain and at the same time modulates the impulses.

The sensory nerves that transmit injury signals connect with spinal cord pathways at junctions called synapses. Injury signals are transferred to the spinal cord through two kinds of pathways. The first one has long nerve fibers that connect directly with the

Referred Pain

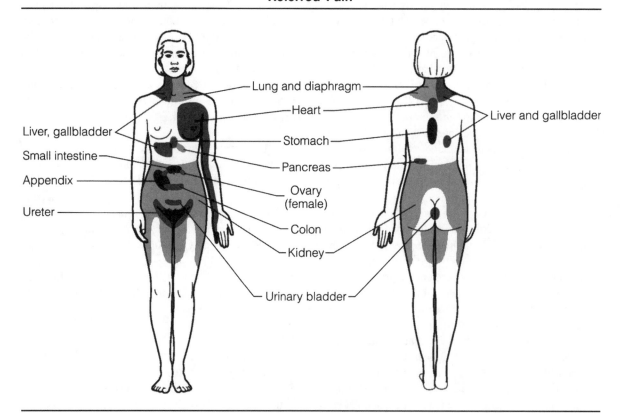

Internal organs do not have the same type of neural sensors found in surface tissues; as a result, damage to internal organs may manifest itself in areas of the body away from the organ's location.

thalamus, from which point other neurons reach to the cerebral cortex. Via this path, the site and intensity of the damaging stimulation is rapidly transmitted as a sharp feeling which is accurately localized by the patient and is often referred to as first pain. The second pathway has long and short fibers with a large number of synapses and is responsible for the slow transfer of the unpleasant, confusing pain feeling and the physiological reactions that accompany it. This type of pain, also known as second pain, may increase in intensity with continuous tissue irritation.

The feeling of pain is a reflection of a tissue-damaging stimulus, which in some cases may be defective: The pain sensation may be erroneously recorded. This is particularly evident in patients whose limb, such as the foot, was recently amputated but who can still feel a crushing pain in the area where the foot once was.

When the pain of an injury or disease never completely disappears with all healing treatments or when pains (such as headache, and lower back, abdominal, and joint pains) appear, disappear, and recur for no apparent reason, the condition is termed chronic pain. Pains such as arthritis, which is prevalent among older people, and various forms of cancer are attributed to physical conditions. Such conditions require medical therapy, which often involves surgery. Surgery may lead to a worse condition, however. If the pain persists, the patient tends to become increasingly anxious, discouraged, helpless, and hypochondriacal and may lose sleep. Occasionally, chronic pain may arise because of psychological depression and disappear only when the patient's depression is lessened. If this does not occur, the patient may tend to become alcoholic or addicted to drugs or may suffer a mental breakdown. Multidisciplinary pain clinics have been established in many Western countries to help patients cope with chronic pain, but generally finding a cure is a difficult process.

Scientific studies suggest that chronic pain may be caused by the depletion of the critical neurotransmitter serotonin, which creates hypersensitivity to tissue irritation. The pain-controlling system of the body needs serotonin to transmit the impulses across the gaps (synapses) between connecting neurons. Preliminary results suggest that low levels of serotonin are observed in depressed people.

The human body also possesses a pain-inhibition system which is controlled by chemicals called enkephalins and endorphins. The timing effect of the enkephalins is rather short. Their function is to act as neurotransmitters in the spinal cord, where they block the transmission of pain signals. Endorphins exist in the brain and are believed to control pain in the brain stem. They bind to the receptors and are responsible for some cases of injury in which pain appears to be nonexistent, at least at the time of incidence.

TREATMENT AND THERAPY

The subject of many years of clinical and laboratory research, pain relief may be achieved several different ways. In the mid-1800's, anesthetics such as ether and chloroform were first introduced in surgery, replacing the traditional wine. Others such as procaine are currently being used in dentistry. Controversial methods of pain relief include acupuncture and hypnosis, as well as the use of marijuana in a clinical setting. Common pain relievers that are used in cases of inflammation are aspirin, acetaminophen, and ibuprofen. Opium and such related drugs as morphine mimic the naturally produced substances that activate pain-inhibiting systems in the brain stem and spinal cord. Morphine is administered extensively to terminally ill patients because it triggers the activation of pain-inhibiting neurons. Opioids, however, display side effects such as nausea and are highly addictive when used over a prolonged period of time. The side effects are reduced dramatically when the opioid is directly injected to the area adjacent to spinal receptors. Other methods include massage and electrically stimulated treatments that reduce the pain gates at the spinal cord, while at the same time increasing the blood circulation to the pain-affected area.

—*Soraya Ghayourmanesh, Ph.D.*

See also Acupressure; Acupuncture; Amputation; Arthritis; Brain disorders; Cancer; Depression; Hypochondriasis; Narcotics; Nervous system; Neuralgia, neuritis, and neuropathy; Pain management; Self-medication.

FOR FURTHER INFORMATION:

Shipton, Edward A. *Pain: Acute and Chronic*. New York: Oxford University Press, 1999.

Swanson, David W., ed. *Mayo Clinic on Chronic Pain*. Rochester, Minn.: Mayo Clinic, 1999.

Vertosick, Frank T., Jr. *Why We Hurt: The Natural History of Pain*. New York: Harcourt Brace, 2000.

Wall, Patrick D. *Pain: The Science of Suffering*. Edited by Steven Rose. New York: Columbia University Press, 2000.

PAIN MANAGEMENT

PROCEDURE

ANATOMY OR SYSTEM AFFECTED: All

SPECIALTIES AND RELATED FIELDS: Alternative medicine, anesthesiology, critical care, emergency medicine, geriatrics and gerontology, oncology, pharmacology, physical therapy, psychiatry, psychology

DEFINITION: Any treatment or management technique to lessen, eliminate, or make pain more tolerable.

INDICATIONS AND PROCEDURES

Pain is described by most people by its intensity. When treating pain, doctors look at several other properties. Recent onset of pain is termed acute pain. Long-standing pain or pain that returns periodically is termed chronic pain.

Pain is not easily treated because doctors cannot measure pain directly. The patient must be able to communicate the pain's intensity, location, pattern (such as throbbing, steady, or comes-and-goes), and type (such as crushing, burning, sharp, or dull). In addition, factors that make the pain better or worse must be known.

Generally, the best way to treat pain is to prevent its occurrence. Failing that, a number of different interventions should be used together. Whatever treatment is used, the therapy must be tailored both to the patient and to the nature and severity of the pain. When medications are used, review of some important principles is essential, such as the pharmacology, duration of effectiveness, and optimal dose of a certain medication. Even the route of administration must be considered in every case.

Treatment may include combinations of simple analgesics, narcotics, and other treatments. Combinations take advantage of the additive pain relief while sparing the patient potential side effects. When choosing pain medications, a step-wise approach is often used. It starts with the simple analgesics: aspirin, acetaminophen, and nonsteroidal anti-inflammatory drugs (NSAIDs). These medications are generally well tolerated, although aspirin and NSAIDs can produce gastrointestinal distress ranging from mild heartburn to bleeding ulcers.

For more severe pain, the second step often includes a narcotic analgesic with or without the simple analgesics. Narcotics are very potent and have a potential for addiction. Furthermore, they may produce problems such as confusion, nausea and vomiting, constipation, and drowsiness.

The third step in pain control involves alternative methods of pain control. Treatments here include physical therapy, nerve-blocking injections, transcutaneous electrical nerve stimulation (TENS), or behavioral approaches. The later method seeks to identify the causes of preventable pain (physical or mental) and takes steps to minimize pain.

—*Charles C. Marsh, Pharm.D.*

See also Acupressure; Acupuncture; Alternative medicine; Anesthesia; Anesthesiology; Biofeedback; Chiropractic; Hypnosis; Meditation; Narcotics; Pain; Pharmacology; Self-medication.

FOR FURTHER INFORMATION:

Cousins, Michael J., and P. O. Bridenbaugh, eds. *Neural Blockade in Clinical Anesthesia and Management of Pain*. 3d ed. Philadelphia: J. B. Lippincott, 1998.

Ferrari, Lynne R., ed. *Anesthesia and Pain Management for the Pediatrician*. Baltimore: The Johns Hopkins University Press, 1999.

Ferrer-Brechner, Theresa. *Common Problems in Pain Management*. Chicago: Year Book Medical, 1990.

Loeser, John D., ed. *Bonica's Management of Pain*. 3d ed. Philadelphia: Lippincott, Williams & Wilkins, 2001.

PALPITATIONS

DISEASE/DISORDER

ANATOMY OR SYSTEM AFFECTED: Circulatory system, heart, psychic-emotional system

SPECIALTIES AND RELATED FIELDS: Cardiology, internal medicine

DEFINITION: Palpitation is the sensation of being aware of the heartbeat, generally because it is beating rapidly or more forcefully than normal. Such a sensation is common after strenuous exercise and in times of stress or fear. Palpitation may also be attributable to heart disorders such as arrhythmia, tachycardia, and atrial fibrillation, which are characterized by rapid and/or irregular heartbeats. Ectopic heartbeats are moments of palpitation in which an individual at rest experiences a sequence of rapid beating followed by a pause; the most common causes for such a sensation are alcohol or caffeine consumption and heavy smoking, not heart disease.

—*Jason Georges and Tracy Irons-Georges*

See also Addiction; Alcoholism; Anxiety; Arrhythmias; Cardiology; Cardiology, pediatric; Exercise physiology; Heart; Heart disease; Panic attacks; Stress; Stress reduction.

FOR FURTHER INFORMATION:

Burch, George E., and Travis Winsor. *A Primer of Electrocardiography*. 6th ed. Philadelphia: Lea & Febiger, 1972.

McGoon, M. *The Mayo Clinic Heart Book*. New York: William Morrow, 1993.

Wallwork, John, and Rob Stepney. *Heart Disease*. Oxford, England: Basil Blackwell, 1987.

Zaret, Barry L., Marvin Moser, and Lawrence S. Cohen, eds. *Yale University School of Medicine Heart Book*. New York: William Morrow, 1992.

PALSY

DISEASE/DISORDER

ANATOMY OR SYSTEM AFFECTED: Muscles, musculoskeletal system, nerves, nervous system

SPECIALTIES AND RELATED FIELDS: Neurology, physical therapy

DEFINITION: A paralysis or partial paralysis that is usually accompanied or followed by muscle weakness and muscle wasting over the affected area; in some cases, there may be residual electrical activity present, but the amount is usually small and the activity cannot be controlled.

KEY TERMS:

Bell's palsy: paralysis of the seventh cranial nerve (facial nerve)

cerebral palsy: a palsy arising prenatally, at birth, or early in life within the central nervous system, affecting large portions of the cerebral hemispheres, with extensive paralysis of many major muscles

hemiplegia: paralysis involving an arm and a leg on the same side of the body

palsy: a paralysis or partial paralysis involving loss of motor control, usually accompanied or followed by muscle weakness and muscle wasting over the affected area

parkinsonism: also called shaking palsy; a degenerative paralysis resulting from destruction of certain cells in the substantia nigra, a structure near the base of the cerebral hemispheres

quadriplegia: paralysis involving all four extremities more or less equally

spastic: characterized by uncontrollable spasms

substantia nigra: a clump of cells located near the base of the cerebral hemispheres that secrete the neurotransmitter dopamine

CAUSES AND SYMPTOMS

In general, the term "palsy" describes any type of dysfunction of the motor nerves that impairs or reduces the conscious control of muscles. The paralysis or loss of motor control is usually accompanied or followed by weakness and wasting of the muscles in the affected area.

The most common type of palsy is Bell's palsy, a paralysis of the seventh cranial nerve, or facial nerve, often accompanied by pain over part or all of the affected area. The number of muscles involved varies. The paralysis usually occurs on one side of the face at a time, with the result that the undamaged muscles of the opposite side pull the facial skin to that side. Typically, the eye on the affected side remains open all the time because the muscles that close it have been affected; attempts by the patient to close the eye merely result in the eyeball rotating upward. The rest of the face on the affected side generally droops but remains flat; the brow fails to wrinkle, and the cheeks never thicken. Smiles and other facial expressions are asymmetrically contorted.

Thorough neurological testing is needed to assess how much damage has been done and which branches of the facial nerve have been affected. If thedamage affects either hearing or taste, this finding indicates that the damage is closer to the root of the facial nerve, and the patient's chances for recovery are correspondingly much lower. If only a few muscles are involved, it indicates that the damage is further from the root of the nerve, which usually forecasts a better chance of recovery. In most cases, Bell's palsy is thought to arise from a reduced blood supply to the affected nerves. Viral infection by herpes simplex or herpes zoster (shingles) is also a frequent cause; the viral infections are believed to cause demyelination (deterioration of the myelin sheath that insulates nerves) of the affected parts of the facial nerve. Other causes include injuries to the area just below or in front of the external ear, resulting from blows to the head, surgery in this region, or other types of trauma.

Another common type of palsy is cerebral palsy, an impairment of movement and posture caused in most cases by injury, malformation, or other damage to the immature brain. Cerebral palsy is actually a group of paralytic disorders that begin during intrauterine development, at birth, or in early infancy. The extent of the paralysis may vary, often involving large groups of muscles while sparing others. Those muscles that are not totally paralyzed are often uncoordinated in their movements or poorly controlled; this is especially true of large muscle movements such as those of the limbs. In many cases, the patient exhibits a "scissors gait" in which the lower limbs are crossed and the one behind must be swung sideways before it is placed in front of the other limb. In addition to the lack of muscular control of the limbs, other symptoms variously include spasms, athetoid (slow, rhythmic, and wormlike) movements, or muscular rigidity. Speech is in many cases difficult or unclear if the muscles used in speaking are affected.

Mental deterioration may occur in some cases but not in others: Some patients with cerebral palsy are retarded, while others have managed to display brilliant artistic or literary talents with the use of whatever muscles still function in their bodies. Some cerebral palsy patients also suffer from seizure disorders such as epilepsy. Almost all cases of cerebral palsy are accompanied by some other type of neurological impairment, the nature of which varies greatly. In general, cerebral palsy is a nonprogressive type of disease; that is, it does not continually worsen. Afflicted individuals generally experience a normal life span, though with impaired motor functions.

The most common types of cerebral palsy are those that occur in infancy or earlier. Of this group, injuries received at birth (during forceps delivery, for example) form one of the largest and most well defined groups. Cerebral hemorrhage, a cause of many cerebral palsies, may occur either during intrauterine life or at birth. Cerebral palsy may also result from embryonic malformations, from injuries received during intrauterine life, or from injuries or other damage during the first two years of life. In addition to birth trauma, many other factors may contribute to a risk of cerebral palsy: premature delivery, breech delivery, toxemia of pregnancy, impairment of the baby's oxygen supply, maternal infection (especially rubella, also called German measles), premature detachment of the placenta during the birth process, and incompatibility between the Rh blood types of mother and child. Brain injuries caused by low oxygen levels (anoxia or hypoxia) can arise before, during, or after birth and can result from damage to the blood vessels, birth trauma, or infectious diseases such as meningitis or encephalitis.

Cerebral palsies are classified into two general types: pyramidal (or spastic) and extrapyramidal (or nonspastic). The pyramidal or spastic types show muscular spasms and other symptoms that persist with age and hardly vary with changes in emotion, tension, movement, or sleep. The pyramidal tracts of the brain stem are damaged in these forms of cerebral palsy. The extrapyramidal or nonspastic types are more variable and are subdivided into several subtypes according to the types of movement exhibited: none (rigid type), weak (dystonic type), rhythmic and wormlike (athetoid type), or uncoordinated shaking (ataxic type). The extrapyramidal tracts of the brain stem are damaged in all these forms of the disease. Most forms of cerebral palsy can also be described as hemiplegia (involving both extremities on one side of the body only), diplegia (involving both legs more than the arms), bilateral hemiplegia (involving the arms more than the legs), or quadriplegia (involving all four extremities more or less equally). Attempts to group the various forms of cerebral palsy by their causes have generally resulted in a lack of agreement among experts. One scheme divides the causes into subependymal hemorrhage among premature infants, damage from oxygen deprivation to the growing brain (the vast majority of cases), and developmental abnormalities of the nervous system.

The most common form of cerebral palsy is infantile spastic hemiplegia, which accounts for about one-third of all cerebral palsies. Most cases of spastic hemiplegia (about 65 percent) are thought to result from birth trauma, either from forceps delivery or from the difficult passage of a very large head through the mother's pelvic girdle. Another 30 percent arise after birth, during the first year of life, either from head injury or from infections such as meningitis and encephalitis. Only 5 percent of spastic hemiplegias arise before birth from embryonic malformations or from toxemia of pregnancy. The rate at which cerebral palsy occurs is higher for babies born prematurely than for those born at term. It is also higher for large babies that may suffer injury during a difficult passage through the birth canal. In the United States, there is a somewhat higher incidence rate among Caucasians than among African Americans.

Parkinsonism (also called Parkinson's disease, paralysis agitans, or shaking palsy) is a progressive or degenerative type of palsy. The disease usually produces a tremor which includes a distinctive "pill-rolling" movement of the thumb and forefinger; this tremor usually stops if a voluntary movement of some other kind is begun. Muscle weakness, stiffness, and muscular rigidity are common but intermittent symptoms that come and go; movements generally become slow and difficult. The muscles involved in chewing and swallowing are often affected in parkinsonism, so patients are often advised to eat high-calorie, semi-soft foods that require no chewing and are more easily swallowed than liquids. Involvement of the muscles of facial expression results in a masklike expression that does not alter with changes in emotion. Patients suffering from parkinsonism often have difficulty in initiating voluntary movements; this difficulty is often described by patients as a feeling of "being frozen in place."

The walking gait of Parkinson's disease patients is also very characteristic: The body above the waist leans forward, the head and shoulders droop, the feet shuffle slowly (and are barely lifted from the ground), and the arms are generally held slightly flexed and motionless rather than swinging. Many patients break into a trot or a run when they attempt to walk; as a result, parkinsonism patients often fall, most often forward. To prevent such falls, they frequently shuffle forward in very small steps. The shuffling gait is believed to result from a partial paralysis of the extrapyramidal motor system of neurons, which is generally responsible for controlling posture and co-ordinating motor activities.

Parkinsonism is known to result from a disorder in the production of dopamine, a neurotransmitter chemical normally secreted by certain parts of the brain. The affected parts of the brain are the basal ganglia deep within the cerebral hemispheres, and especially the substantia nigra, a deeper structure that sends dopamine-secreting nerve fibers to the basal ganglia. In patients with parkinsonism, cells of the substantia nigra are often degenerate and pale from the loss of normal pigments, but this may be a result, rather than a cause, of the primary defect: an impairment of the brain's ability to convert dopa (dihydroxyphenylalanine) into the neurotransmitter dopamine.

The chemical n-methyyl-4-phenyl-1,2,3,4-tetrahydropyridine has been found to produce in experimental animals a disease very similar to parkinsonism. For this reason, many researchers suspect that parkinsonism has an environmental cause that leads to the production of a related toxic chemical, one that presumably interferes with the production of dopamine.

Parkinsonism is uncommon before the age of forty, but it becomes so common in people over sixty that it is the leading neurological disorder in this age group. In the United States, the incidence rate is about 130 per 100,000 in the general population and is roughly the same in all races and ethnic groups. About 10 to 15 percent of those with parkinsonism show mental deterioration (dementia) as the disease progresses. Patients often experience depression, social withdrawal, and generalized apathy.

Other, less common palsies include brachial birth palsy, Erb's palsy, Klumpke's palsy, true or progressive bulbar palsy, pseudobulbar palsy, Féréol-Graux palsy, posticus palsy, lead palsy, scriveners' palsy, pressure palsy, compression palsy, and creeping or wasting palsy.

Brachial birth palsy is a paralysis of the infant's arm resulting from an injury received at birth, involving the whole arm, the upper arm only (Erb's palsy), or the lower arm only (Klumpke's palsy). Erb's palsy, a brachial birth palsy of the upper arm, is caused by an injury at birth to the brachial plexus or the posterior roots of the fifth and sixth cervical nerves; the muscles involved generally include the deltoideus, biceps brachii, and brachialis, impairing the raising of the upper arm, flexion of the elbow, or supination movements involving the forearm. In Klumpke's palsy, which results from an injury at birth, the muscles of the forearm and the small muscles of the hand undergo atrophy; this form is often accompanied by paralysis of the cervical sympathetic nerves.

True or progressive bulbar palsy, a palsy and progressive atrophy of the muscles of the tongue, lips, palate, pharynx, and larynx, often occurs late in life and is caused by degeneration of the motor neurons leading to these muscles. Twitching or atrophy of the tongue and other affected muscles causes drooling, difficulties in swallowing, and ultimately a respiratory paralysis which results in death. Many experts consider true bulbar palsy to be a manifestation of the same disease that causes amyotrophic lateral sclerosis (ALS), which is popularly known as Lou Gehrig's disease.

Pseudobulbar palsy ("laughing sickness") is a paralysis of the lips and tongue which mimics true or progressive bulbar palsy, but it arises in the brain itself and is accompanied by difficulties in swallowing and by spasmodic laughter at inappropriate times. Féréol-Graux palsy, a one-sided (unilateral) paralysis of the motor nucleus of the lateral rectus muscle of one eye and the medial rectus muscle of the other eye, results from damage to the medial longitudinal fasciculus and impairs the ability to direct either eye toward the affected side. Posticus palsy is a paralysis of the posterior cricoarytenoideus muscle (cricoary-tenoideus posticus), resulting in the vocal cords being held close to the midline.

Lead palsy is a paralysis of the extensor muscles of the wrist resulting from lead poisoning, while scriveners' palsy ("writers' cramp") is a repetitive motion disorder resulting in damage to the nerve controlling the small muscles of the hand. Pressure palsy is a paralysis caused by repeated or persistent compression of a nerve or nerve trunk. Compression palsy results from nerve compression, especially of the arm, caused by pressure from the use of a crutch (crutch palsy) or from compression of a nerve during sleep. Creeping palsy and wasting palsy are general terms for progressive muscle atrophy, such as that associated with ALS.

TREATMENT AND THERAPY

Bell's palsy is treated by various methods, including the application of warmth, the avoidance of cold drafts, or the administration of vasodilating drugs such as cortisone or antiviral drugs such as acyclovir. In unusual cases, surgery is performed to enlarge the passages through which the facial nerve passes, thus relieving compression on the nerve. In past generations, physicians often recommended treating eyes that could not be closed by taping them shut, especially in sleep. This treatment is no longer recommended. Instead, physicians usually advise patients who cannot close an affected eye to wear dark glasses during the day.

Many patients with Bell's palsy recover spontaneously on their own. The chances that a particular individual will spontaneously recover depend on the location of the damage and the extent of muscle involvement; the cases with the most favorable outcomes are those in which the damage is more peripheral and fewer muscles are involved. Frequent, repeated testing of each small group of facial muscles is needed to assess the extent of damage and the extent of any recovery.

Diagnosis of cerebral palsy is best made by a trained neurologist through observation of the patient's spontaneous motor movements and reflex actions. Infants who exhibit any reflex which persists beyond its appropriate age range, or any voluntary motor pattern that fails to develop at the appropriate age, should be examined more carefully for signs of nerve damage. For example, most babies can lift their heads by one month of age and their chests by two months. By three months of age, most babies can raise themselves up on their elbows, and by four months on their wrists. Newborn babies exhibit reflexes such as the Moro reflex, a flexion and "embracing" reflex in reaction to a sudden noise or other sudden stimulus or "startle"; however, the persistence of this reflex beyond six months of age (or its asymmetrical performance) may be indicative of some form of cerebral palsy. Another reflex often used in diagnosis is the "fencer" reflex, or asymmetric tonic neck reflex: Turning the baby's head toward one side usually causes extension movements in both the arm and leg on the side toward which the chin faces, while flexion movements usually take place on the opposite side of the body. This reflex is present at birth and disappears in a few months; its persistence after six months of age should be considered suspicious.

There is no cure for cerebral palsy. Treatment generally consists of physical rehabilitation and training the patient to use whatever muscles are still capable of being consciously controlled. This is a difficult form of therapy that must be tailored to the needs of each patient because individuals experience unique combinations of motor abilities and disabilities. Few patients with cerebral palsy are capable of walking on their own. Depending on the extent of impairment of muscle movements, some patients may require crutches or braces, while others use motorized wheelchairs. In cases in which there is speech impairment, speech therapy may also be needed to teach the patient to speak more clearly. Most types of cerebral palsy are already present during infancy; therapy for these types is always rather difficult because the patient is learning the necessary motor skills (such as walking or speaking) for the first time. On the other hand, palsies that arise during adolescence or adulthood respond differently to therapy because the patient is relearning skills that had already been mastered.

Treatment for parkinsonism includes the administration of a number of drugs that are chemically related to dopamine, the missing neurotransmitter. The drug most often used is levodopa, or L-dopa, a derivative of a naturally occurring amino acid in the brain. The drug carbidopa is also given to help deliver most of the levodopa into the brain. Dopamine agonists (enhancers) such as bromocriptine and pergolide are frequently given. The antiviral drug amantadine has also been shown to have effects that counter parkinsonism.

PERSPECTIVE AND PROSPECTS

The various palsies were identified in the nineteenth century. Bell's palsy was first described by Sir Charles Bell (1774-1842), a renowned Scottish anatomist. Parkinsonism was first described by James Parkinson (1755-1824), who called it "shaking palsy"; the understanding of the neurotransmitter dopamine and the use of L-dopa in the treatment of parkinsonism was a development of the late twentieth century. Cerebral palsy was first described in 1861 by a London physician, William J. Little; the famous psychoanalyst Sigmund Freud (1856-1939) published an account of this disease in 1883. The most thorough early work on this disease was published in 1889 by the distinguished Canadian physician Sir William Osler (1849-1919), who coined the term "cerebral palsies" to describe the several types of the disease.

Several types of cerebral palsy that were more common in the early twentieth century, such as those caused by the use of obstetrical forceps during delivery, have decreased in incidence as a result of improved medical procedures. For larger babies that formerly faced a greater risk of cerebral hemorrhage and other brain injury from passage through the mother's pelvic girdle at birth, the increased frequency of cesarean sections has greatly reduced the rates of cerebral palsy arising at birth.

—Eli C. Minkoff, Ph.D.

See also Bell's palsy; Cerebral palsy; Hemiplegia; Herpes; Motor neuron diseases; Nervous system; Neuralgia, neuritis, and neuropathy; Neurology; Neurology, pediatric; Paralysis; Paraplegia; Parkinson's disease; Physical rehabilitation; Quadriplegia; Shingles.

FOR FURTHER INFORMATION:

Adams, Raymond D., Maurice Victor, and Allan H. Ropper. *Adams and Victor's Principles of Neurology.* 7th ed. New York: McGraw-Hill, 2000. A good if somewhat technical text. Contains a nonstandard (and incomplete) classification of types of cerebral palsy according to their causes.

Behrman, Richard E., ed. *Nelson Textbook of Pediatrics.* 16th ed. Philadelphia: W. B. Saunders, 2000. The treatment of cerebral palsy is brief and to the point, including advice for diagnosis and treatment.

Chipps, E. M., N. J. Clanin, and V. G. Campbell. *Neurologic Disorders.* St. Louis: Mosby Year Book, 1992. Written for nurses, this reference work uses nontechnical language and an easy-to-read style.

Includes sections on Bell's palsy and parkinsonism, but does not cover cerebral palsy. Illustrations are provided.

Oski, Frank A., ed. *Oski's Pediatrics: Principles and Practice.* 3d ed. Philadelphia: J. B. Lippincott, 1999. Offers clear descriptions and illustrations, especially of the reflexes that are useful in the diagnosis of different types of cerebral palsy.

Rakel, Robert E., ed. *Conn's Current Therapy 2000: Latest Approved Methods of Treatment for the Practicing Physician.* Philadelphia: W. B. Saunders, 2000. Provides brief discussions of acute facial paralysis (including Bell's palsy) and parkinsonism.

Waxman, Stephen G. *Correlative Neuroanatomy.* 24th ed. Stamford, Conn.: Appleton and Lange, 2000. Balances basic information about functioning of nerves with clinical discussions. A readable treatment for college students.

PANCREAS

ANATOMY

ANATOMY OR SYSTEM AFFECTED: Abdomen, endocrine system, gastrointestinal system, glands, immune system

SPECIALTIES AND RELATED FIELDS: Endocrinology, gastroenterology, immunology, internal medicine

DEFINITION: A vital organ which produces enzymes used in the digestive process and hormones such as insulin, which regulates blood sugar levels.

KEY TERMS:

autoimmunity: a disorder in which the immune system starts to attack the body's cells as foreign matter

autosomal recessive gene: a gene (other than the X or Y chromosome) which must be on both chromosomes to be expressed

concordance: the inheritance of the same trait by both twins

duodenum: the initial part of the small intestine, where most of the digestion of food occurs

endocrine glands: ductless glands that secrete hormones directly into the bloodstream; these glands help to maintain homeostasis

exocrine glands: glands that excrete their products into tubes or ducts that empty onto the skin's surface

STRUCTURE AND FUNCTIONS

The pancreas is an organ about 15 to 18 centimeters long and weighing 100 grams that is located in the abdominal cavity. The head of the organ is situated in the loop of the small intestine that forms at the site where the small intestine joins the stomach. The pancreas is enclosed in a thin connective tissue capsule. As an accessory gland of the digestive system the pancreas is an exocrine gland. Scattered within the tissue of this exocrine gland, however, are small distinct regions known as the islets of Langerhans, which are a part of the endocrine system. The exocrine portion composes by far the greatest mass of tissue. For example, in the guinea pig about 82 percent of pancreatic cells are exocrine cells, while the endocrine portion is about 2 percent. The remaining cells are associated with the duct system and the blood vessels.

The exocrine pancreas is an arrangement of tubules that continue to branch until they form very fine ducts called the intercalated ducts. Along the edges of the intercalated ducts are the acinar cells. These cells produce the pancreatic juices that aid in the digestion of food in the small intestine and help neutralize the contents of the small intestine. The products drain from the ducts into the main collecting duct, which joins the common bile duct and empties into the duodenum.

The islets of Langerhans, as is the case with all endocrine glands, have a well-developed blood supply. The hormones produced by these endocrine cells are emptied into the surrounding capillaries. The hormones flow into the general circulation, where they are distributed to target cells throughout the body. Since the two portions of the pancreas are anatomically as well as functionally different, they will be considered independently.

The exocrine portion of the pancreas produces about 1 liter of aqueous fluid per day that is delivered directly to the duodenum. The two major components of the pancreatic juices are ions, which are used to neutralize the stomach contents as they enter the small intestine, and enzymes, which metabolize intestinal contents for absorption.

The various ions that are secreted include sodium, potassium, chloride, and bicarbonate ions. The sodium, potassium, and chloride are present in concentrations similar to their concentrations in the bloodstream. The bicarbonate ions act as the major buffer of the body. With only a few exceptions, the bloodstream and the contents of the body must be maintained at a pH of 7.4. Bicarbonate ions ensure that there is no change in pH.

The stomach is one of the areas of the body in which the pH varies. It may be as low as pH 1, which is highly acidic. The contents of the stomach empty directly into the duodenum, and while the cells of the stomach are capable of withstanding an acid environment, the cells of the small intestine are not. The acid must be rapidly neutralized in order to protect these cells. In addition, the enzymes that help to digest the food reaching the small intestine work optimally at about pH 7. If the pH varies significantly, the

The Pancreas

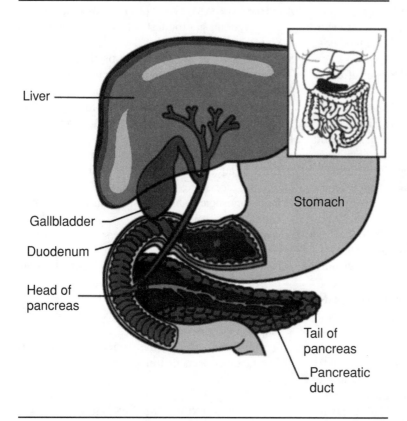

Liver

Gallbladder

Duodenum

Head of pancreas

Stomach

Tail of pancreas

Pancreatic duct

The pancreas is an unusual gland that contains both endocrine tissue and exocrine tissue; the inset shows the location of the pancreas within the gastrointestinal system.

food will not be properly digested and vital nutrients will not be absorbed by the intestinal cells.

The production of bicarbonate by the duct cells is controlled by a hormone called secretin. The contents of the small intestine become acidic as food moves into the area from the stomach. When the pH is lowered, the cells of the small intestine release secretin, which in turn stimulates the pancreas to produce more bicarbonate. As bicarbonate enters the small intestine, it neutralizes the acid, and the stimulus to produce secretin is removed.

The pancreas also produces a variety of enzymes that digest proteins, sugars, lipids, and nucleic acids. In order for protein to be absorbed by the cells of the small intestine, it must be broken down into its building blocks, amino acids. This breakdown is an enzymatic process that occurs only when the appropriate enzymes are present and at a pH near neutrality. The enzymes that digest proteins include trypsin, chymotrypsin, and carboxypeptidase. Like protein, sugars, nucleic acids, and lipids must be digested to their subunits if they are to be absorbed. Sugars are metabolized by amylase, nucleic acids by either ribonuclease or deoxyribonuclease, and fats by lipase, phospholipase, or cholesterol esterase.

The secretion of enzymes by the pancreas is controlled by the hormone cholecystokinin. As the content of protein and fat increases in the lumen of the duodenum, the duodenal cells release cholecystokinin, which acts on the acinar cells of the pancreas to release the enzymes. As the food is digested, the level of cholecystokinin decreases and the release of enzymes from the pancreas also decreases.

The islets of Langerhans have four different cell types and produce four different hormones. The alpha and beta cells produce glucagon and insulin, respectively. The delta cells produce somatostatin, which inhibits the secretion of hormones by the alpha and beta cells. The F cell produces pancreatic polypeptide, the function of which is not yet understood.

Insulin secretion is stimulated or inhibited by a large number of factors. Blood glucose levels are the most important factor in the release of insulin from the beta cells. If blood glucose increases, insulin is released until glucose levels return to normal. When insulin is released into the bloodstream, it stimulates the uptake of glucose by target cells. Although insulin is best known for its action on glucose, it also stimulates the uptake of amino acids and fatty acids from the bloodstream during periods of adequate nu-

trition. Glucagon is an antagonist of insulin. It is released in response to low levels of glucose and acts on cells to release glucose, amino acids, and fatty acids into the circulatory system.

DISORDERS AND DISEASES

Diseases of the pancreas can be divided into two basic categories: diseases of the exocrine cells of the organ and those diseases that effect the function of the endocrine portion, the islets of Langerhans. The exocrine cells of the pancreas can be affected by various conditions, including acute pancreatitis, chronic pancreatitis, cystic fibrosis, and carcinoma of the pancreas. Also, because the pancreas is a gland and glandular organs typically have a large blood supply, it is at risk of injury any time that circulation is impaired. The islets of Langerhans may be affected by diabetes mellitus.

Inflammation of the pancreas (pancreatitis) can be either acute or chronic. While some cases are mild, it is considered a serious disease and has a high mortality rate. Although the acute form is more serious, patients with chronic pancreatitis may suffer from acute episodes.

Acute pancreatitis may result from obstruction of the pancreatic duct (possibly by gallstones from the gallbladder or by mucous plugs, as in cystic fibrosis), bile reflux, acute intoxication by alcohol, shock, infection by the mumps virus, hypothermia, or trauma. The diagnosis, pathology, and prognosis are the same regardless of the cause.

The onset of the disease is usually quite sudden, with severe pain in the abdomen, nausea, and vomiting. Diagnosis is made by the presence of amylase in the blood serum. Amylase is an enzyme produced by the pancreas which is used to digest carbohydrates in the small intestine. The presence of elevated levels of the enzyme is an indication that it is not reaching the small intestine and is spilling over into the bloodstream.

The powerful enzymes produced by the pancreas are used to digest proteins, carbohydrates, and fats. If for any reason these substances are not released from the pancreas, they will digest the cells of the pancreas and destroy them. As pancreatitis progresses, it will cause tissue inflammation and will lead to swelling of the organ. In addition, the enzymes may start to digest the cells of the blood vessels in the immediate area, causing bleeding into the tissue. The inflammation, combined with the bleeding, may lead to greater swelling and further inflammation.

Acute pancreatitis can lead to complications in other tissue as well, such as fat necrosis leading to the release of fatty acids from adipose tissue. The fatty acids bind to circulating calcium and may cause tetanus of the skeletal muscle as a result of calcium deficiency. If the enzymes released from the exocrine cells destroy the endocrine cells, the resulting loss of hormone production will lead to hyperglycemia and the complications that stem from it. Cysts or abscesses may also result from acute pancreatitis. Although this disease is usually self-limiting, in many cases it will lead to death.

Chronic pancreatitis is a recurring disease that may also demonstrate acute episodes. It has generally been associated with chronic alcoholism, which seems to be the major cause. Chronic pancreatitis is primarily a disease of middle age and occurs more frequently in men than in women. The patient generally complains of abdominal or back pain, often after a large meal or excessive alcohol consumption. Because of the lack of enzymes for lipid digestion, patients often excrete large quantities of undigested lipids. Without fat absorption, many fat-soluble substances such as vitamins A, D, E, and K will not be absorbed.

Because the patient with chronic pancreatitis is often malnourished from inadequate digestion and absorption of food and from vitamin deficiencies, there is associated weight loss and muscular wasting. The exocrine portion of the pancreas is gradually replaced by fibrosis (scar) tissue, but the endocrine cells remain unaffected.

Disease of the pancreas can also be caused by cystic fibrosis. Cystic fibrosis, also known as mucoviscidosis, is an autosomal recessive disease of the exocrine glands. It occurs in about 1 in 2,500 live births of Caucasians but rarely occurs in blacks or Asians. Cystic fibrosis affects the mucus-secreting glands in the body and leads to the production of abnormally thick mucus. About 80 percent of these patients have involvement of the pancreas. The onset and severity of the disease vary widely, but most infants born with cystic fibrosis have a pancreas that appears to be normal. As the abnormal mucus is produced, however, it may block the ducts of the exocrine glands and lead to the destruction of the exocrine tissue. The glandular tissue is progressively replaced by fibrous or adipose tissue or by cysts. The loss of pancreatic activity may lead to malabsorption of nutrients and vitamins. Although the islets of Langerhans are not affected by the disease in its early stages, eventually they also may be destroyed.

Tumors of the pancreas are primary tumors; there is almost no incidence of tumors metastasizing to the pancreas from other locations in the body. The exocrine tumors are generally adenocarcinomas, a type of cancer which is increasing in frequency throughout the world. An association with cigarette smoking and diabetes mellitus has been established. The tumors most commonly occur in the area of the gland where the major ducts leave the pancreas. As the tumors enlarge, they may put excessive pressure on the common bile duct, which is located in the same region. This pressure leads to the backup of bile in the liver known as obstructive jaundice; this is one of the earliest signs of pathology. Tumors located at other sites will not be detected until much later because they do not produce symptoms. Metastases of these tumors may be to the liver or surrounding lymph nodes. Because diagnosis is usually after the disease has progressed, the prognosis is poor even in operable cases.

The most common disease of the endocrine portion of the pancreas is diabetes mellitus. Each year, about 35,000 patients die of diabetes in the United States. Diabetes is a chronic disorder affecting carbohydrate, fat, and protein metabolism. It may be further classified as insulin-dependent or juvenile diabetes (type I), non-insulin-dependent or adult-onset diabetes (type II), or secondary diabetes. All forms of diabetes have a common pattern in which insulin is present in insufficient quantities, is absent, or does not function normally—all of which lead to hyperglycemia. Both type I and type II diabetes are inherited. In identical twins, there is a 50 percent concordance rate for type I and a 90 percent concordance for type II. The latter figure indicates that heredity plays a more important role in type II diabetes.

Patients with type I diabetes are insulin-dependent. The disease starts at an early age and is sometimes referred to as juvenile diabetes. The decrease in insulin supply is caused by a decrease in functional beta cells in the islets of Langerhans. Evidence indicates that the beta cells are damaged or destroyed by an autoimmune reaction, which may follow a viral infection. Type I diabetics often have other endocrine disorders that are a result of autoimmunity. Type II diabetics produce at least some insulin, but not sufficient quantities. It appears that the tissues of these patients are resistant to insulin. The symptoms are less severe than those associated with type I. Secondary diabetes is a result of some other disease which causes injury or destruction of beta cells. Diseases such as chronic pancreatitis or carcinoma of the pancreas can interfere with insulin production. The severity of the three forms of the disease varies widely, as does the treatment. The type I diabetic requires insulin for survival, while in many type II diabetics the disease may be controlled by diet and exercise.

Although the presence of insulin has several effects on the body, the lack of insulin has the most pronounced effect on serum glucose levels. If insulin supply is diminished or if the cells do not respond to the insulin produced, there is a rise in blood glucose levels exceeding the amount that the kidney can retain. As a result, glucose is excreted in the urine along with large quantities of water. The loss of glucose and water may lead to hypoglycemia and dehydration. The problem is further complicated by the fact that if there is inadequate glucose available, the cells will metabolize fats. One of the by-products of fat metabolism is the production of chemicals known as ketones, which are acids. Thus the dehydration may be accompanied by a more acidic serum.

The symptoms described above are acute and demand immediate attention. In addition to these symptoms, many abnormalities may appear in patients who have diabetes for ten or more years. The cardiovascular system is highly vulnerable to the disease, and the cause of death in about 80 percent of diabetics is a cardiovascular abnormality.

PERSPECTIVE AND PROSPECTS

Since the pancreas is a vital organ, any disease or injury to it will have serious consequences. Problems with the pancreas may be magnified because the diseases associated with the exocrine portion of the gland are not easily detected. In acute cases of pancreatitis, the onset is sudden and requires immediate treatment to control the extent of the disease. Even when the disease is treated early, many patients die. Surgery is complicated by the inflammation and hemorrhaging that may have previously occurred.

Chronic pancreatitis and cancer of the pancreas are even more difficult to diagnose since many of the symptoms are common to other ailments and may not even be present until the disease has progressed to an acute stage. The chronic condition is complicated because the body cannot absorb nutrients and vitamins. By the time that the diagnosis has occurred, the patient is weakened by the loss of weight and muscular wasting from malnutrition.

Diabetes presents its own unique set of problems. In type I diabetes, the patient is often unable to follow the prescribed diet and must continually monitor his or her glucose levels to ensure that the insulin doses are appropriate. Assuming that the patient is able to follow the diet and takes the medication as prescribed, there will still be complications—particularly of the cardiovascular system, which may include renal damage.

Many advances have occurred which provide hope for the sufferers of diseases of the pancreas. Physicians are able to provide pancreatic transplants to patients who have no other recourse. The success rate is improving, and techniques are available that should continue to improve the prognosis for the patient. The limitation is the competition for the available organs and the expense of an organ transplant.

New techniques have been employed that are particularly promising for the type I diabetic. Instead of complete organ transplants, techniques are being perfected that will allow the transplantation of only the beta cells of the islets of Langerhans. As scientists become more adept at genetically altering cells, it may be possible to replace the defective genes with healthy ones.

There is also hope in the fact that scientists have become more successful in the treatment of autoimmune disease. With early diagnosis, it may be possible to treat children with type I diabetes with immunosuppressive drugs before the disease does any damage. It is likely that there will be significant progress with the treatment of diabetes as more becomes known about somatic gene therapy, cell transplants, immunosuppression, and the control of insulin receptors.

—*Annette O'Connor, Ph.D.*

See also Abdomen; Abscess drainage; Abscesses; Diabetes mellitus; Digestion; Endocrinology; Endocrinology, pediatric; Fetal tissue transplantation; Food biochemistry; Gastroenterology; Gastroenterology, pediatric; Gastrointestinal disorders; Gastrointestinal system; Glands; Hormones; Insulin resistance syndrome; Internal medicine; Metabolism; Pancreatitis; Stomach, intestinal, and pancreatic cancers; Systems and organs; Transplantation.

FOR FURTHER INFORMATION:

Goodman, H. Maurice. *Basic Medical Endocrinology.* 2d ed. New York: Raven Press, 1994. Contains good background information regarding endocrinology. There is a chapter on the endocrine activity of the pancreas and a thorough discussion of the physiological role of insulin and the other pancreatic hormones.

Marieb, Elaine N. *Essentials of Human Anatomy and Physiology.* 6th ed. Redwood City, Calif.: Benjamin/Cummings, 2000. This introductory anatomy and physiology textbook, easily accessible to those with little science background, is richly illustrated with diagrams and photographs that help to illuminate body systems and processes.

Pizer, H. F. *Organ Transplants: A Patient's Guide.* Cambridge, Mass.: Harvard University Press, 1991. An excellent treatment of organ transplants, with a chapter on pancreatic transplants. There is a wealth of general knowledge about such operations, including information on how candidates are chosen, the transplant team, antirejection drugs and side effects, and surgical procedures.

Underwood, J. C. E., ed. *General and Systematic Pathology.* Edinburgh, Scotland: Churchill Livingstone, 1992. A basic pathology book in an outline form. Although written for the scientist, it is not difficult to understand. The use of technical words is limited, and helpful illustrations accompany the text.

Valenzuela, Jorge E., Howard A. Reber, and Andre Ribet, eds. *Medical and Surgical Diseases of the Pancreas.* New York: Igaku-Shoin Medical, 1991. A well-written book that describes the diseases of the pancreas, with a clear description of the causes and treatment. Although written for the medical community, it is not too technical and should be clear to most readers.

Whitaker, Julian M. *Reversing Diabetes.* New York: Warner Books, 1987. A fine discussion of diabetes and an analysis of treatments for this disease. Written for the layperson, it contains much background information.

PANCREATIC CANCER. *See* STOMACH, INTESTINAL, AND PANCREATIC CANCERS.

PANCREATITIS
DISEASE/DISORDER

ANATOMY OR SYSTEM AFFECTED: Abdomen, endocrine system, gastrointestinal system, pancreas

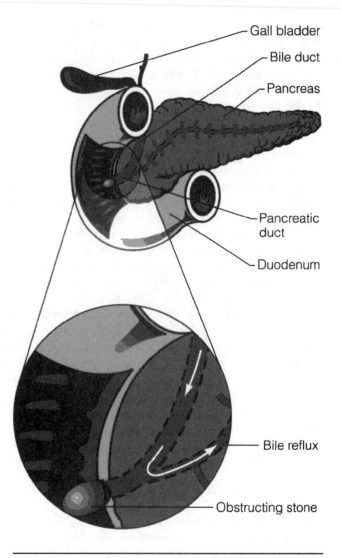

The pancreas, showing the pancreatic duct; when this duct is blocked, bile may reflux, leading to "autodigestion" of the pancreas.

SPECIALTIES AND RELATED FIELDS: Endocrinology, gastroenterology, internal medicine

DEFINITION: Inflammation of the pancreas, which may be acute or chronic.

CAUSES AND SYMPTOMS

Linked to the small intestines by the pancreatic duct, the pancreas contributes the enzymes necessary to digestion. When the pancreas is damaged or its duct is blocked, the enzymes may begin to digest the pancreatic tissue itself, a process called autodigestion.

Inflammation ensues, resulting in acute pancreatitis. Although there may be complications, most cases are self-correcting once the damaging agent is eliminated, and the pancreatitis does not recur. With continuing damage to the pancreas, however, the disease may become self-perpetuating and either break out periodically in attacks that mimic the acute form or cause few symptoms until much of the pancreas has been destroyed, a chronic form of pancreatitis that is difficult to treat. Either form can be fatal. Acute pancreatitis causes death in less than 5 percent of cases and generally does so because of complications, such as extensive tissue destruction and hemorrhage or infection. Complications from chronic pancreatitis can be fatal in as much as 50 percent of cases.

Medical science has not yet uncovered the exact biochemical processes responsible for pancreatitis. Although a variety of damaging agents are known to lead to the disease, in as many as 30 percent of cases no clear cause is detectable; doctors call these cases idiopathic pancreatitis. Of detectable causes, alcoholism and biliary tract disease account for about 80 percent of both acute and chronic cases in the United States and Europe (the percentages vary widely in other parts of the world). Alcohol is the most common toxic agent causing pancreatitis, although susceptibility varies and only a minority of heavy drinkers develop acute pancreatitis; however, a long history of steady drinking is by far the most common cause of chronic pancreatitis. Gallstones in the common bile duct, or any other stricture or obstruction that backs up bile into the pancreatic duct, can trigger pancreatitis. Because surgeons can correct this problem by removing the obstruction, it seldom leads to chronic pancreatitis. Other, rarer causes include traumatic injury (especially the damage done by the steering wheel or seat belt during an automobile accident), damage incurred during abdominal surgery or endoscopic procedures in the small intestine, reactions to some medicines, viral infections, very high levels of fats in the blood (hyperlipidemia), structural abnormalities in the pancreas, or hereditary disease.

Despite the variety in causes, patients present a fairly limited set of symptoms, at least during an acute episode. Usually (but not always), they initially complain of steady pain in the upper abdomen that in severe cases seems to bore into them and radiate to the back. They may also have an enlarged abdomen, run a fever, experience nausea, and vomit. The physician is likely to find the abdomen distended, while the patient feels tenderness when it is touched. In severe cases, the patient may develop signs of shock, unstoppable hiccuping, jaundice, discoloration around the navel, fluid buildup in the peritoneal cavity, and impaired bowel function. While abdominal pain is a prominent feature of chronic pancreatitis as well, the most common associated symptoms are diarrhea, fatty stool, weight loss from poor digestion, and the development of diabetes mellitus.

Because none of these symptoms belongs exclusively to pancreatitis, physicians must conduct tests to establish the diagnosis; however, no single test is conclusive. Only by carefully showing that other possible diseases, such as pancreatic cancer, are not responsible for the symptoms can doctors be sure that pancreatitis is the culprit. Blood tests that detect elevated levels of amylase and lipase (pancreatic digestive enzymes) support the diagnosis. X rays, ultrasonography, computed tomography (CT) scanning, and endoscopic inspection of the pancreas and common bile duct can identify both causes and complications of pancreatitis.

TREATMENT AND THERAPY

The treatment for pancreatitis depends on its cause. If the problem is abuse of alcohol or other drugs, physicians usually let an attack of acute pancreatitis run its course while the patient abstains from the offending substance. Nevertheless, even mild attacks frequently require hospitalization because painkillers and intravenous hydration therapy are needed. If gallstones are thought to be the problem, plans are made to remove them by surgery. Patients with severe acute pancreatitis are sent to the hospital's intensive care unit, since they urgently need supportive treatment to stay alive. There doctors insert a tube through the patient's nose and into the stomach to suck out excess gastric fluids and relieve pressure on the pancreas. They may give antibiotics if there is evidence of infection. Extra oxygen or mechanical assistance may be needed to support breathing. Surgery may rarely be called for even in pancreatitis not caused by gallstones in order to cut away dead, infected tissue or drain fluid accumulations known as pseudocysts. Following an attack and treatment, a patient may require intravenous nourishment for weeks before the pancreas is ready to resume its full function.

Continued alcohol abuse will generally spur recurrent bouts of pancreatitis. Sometimes, however, the alcohol (or, rarely, slowly developing biliary tract disease) causes more subtle, gradual impairment of pancreatic function with few symptoms; in fact, some patients do not go to the doctor until the damage has become extensive and permanently disabling. Others have intense, continual upper-abdominal pain that painkillers cannot reduce easily. (In fact, drug addiction from high dosages of painkillers often becomes a problem.) The doctor's first step is to stop the patient's alcohol intake. If gallstones or other obstructions are present, clearing the bile duct with surgery or endoscopic procedure will decrease pain. Sometimes, high doses of pancreatic enzymes may be helpful in relieving pain.

In cases of uncontrollable pain, however, surgery may be needed to block the sympathetic nerves or even to remove all or part of the pancreas. The chance of surviving some forms of pancreatic surgery is not high—as low as 50 percent—and the procedure often causes further complications. Because pancreatic function is destroyed, most chronic pancreatitis patients digest food poorly and require enzyme supplements to avoid continued weight loss. Since insulin is made in the pancreas, most such patients will also need treatment for diabetes, which may be difficult to manage.

—*Roger Smith, Ph.D.*

See also Alcoholism; Diabetes mellitus; Endocrine disorders; Endocrinology; Endocrinology, pediatric; Gallbladder diseases; Hypoglycemia; Obstruction; Pancreas; Stomach, intestinal, and pancreatic cancers; Stone removal; Stones.

FOR FURTHER INFORMATION:

Levine, Joel S., ed. *Decision Making in Gastroenterology*. 2d ed. Philadelphia: B. C. Decker, 1992. This text for physicians contains detailed information about the symptoms and development of cancers. Accompanying charts explain the sequence of examination, testing, and treatment, and dedicated laypersons can glean much of value from them.

Munoz, Abilio, and David A. Katerndahl. "Diagnosis and Management of Acute Pancreatitis." *American Family Physician* 62, no. 1 (July 1, 2000): 164-174. Acute pancreatitis usually occurs as a result of alcohol abuse or bile duct obstruction. A careful review of the patient's history and appropriate laboratory studies can help the physician identify the etiology of the condition and guide management.

Sachar, David B., Jerome D. Waye, and Blair Lewis, eds. *Pocket Guide to Gastroenterology*. Rev. ed. Baltimore: Williams & Wilkins, 1991. Discusses such topics as gastroenterology, the digestive organs, and digestive system diseases. Includes bibliographical references and an index.

PANIC ATTACKS
DISEASE/DISORDER

ANATOMY OR SYSTEM AFFECTED: Psychic-emotional system

SPECIALTIES AND RELATED FIELDS: Psychiatry, psychology

DEFINITION: Sudden attacks of intense apprehension, fear, doom, and/or terror.

CAUSES AND SYMPTOMS

The physical symptoms of panic attacks include shortness of breath, palpitations, chest pain, smothering sensations, tingling sensations, chills, nausea, sweating, and light-headedness. During attacks, individuals frequently report fears of "going crazy," losing control, or dying. A panic attack is a time-limited experience: Symptoms appear suddenly, build to a peak, and end in a period of ten minutes.

Panic attacks can be related to specific situations in which there is an almost invariable likelihood for a person to have an attack. They may also be partially related to situations, such that they occur in specific situations but not invariably or immediately. Finally, panic attacks may occur spontaneously, unrelated to specific cues or situations.

Agoraphobia, or anxiety about and active avoidance of specific panic-related situations, is often a complicating problem. The situations typically avoided are those from which escape or the attainment of assistance might be difficult. As a result, an individual's range of activities can become quite limited. The unpredictability of symptoms, and the patient's lack of ability to control them, can create a sense of helplessness. Additionally, agoraphobia often results in depression because of decreases in the number of pleasurable activities attempted.

The physical condition mitral valve prolapse (or mitral insufficiency) is also often associated with panic attacks. It is characterized by severe chest pain, palpitations, headache, giddiness, and a systolic murmur of the heartbeat. It is not a life-threatening condition; however, its presence in individuals who experience panic attacks is often associated with psychological distress. The symptoms of mitral valve prolapse are often misinterpreted as signs of cardiac arrest, leading to feelings of worry, distress, and sometimes panic. Because other conditions can also mimic panic attacks, the presence of such attacks requires medical evaluation. These conditions include hypoglycemia, temporal lobe epilepsy, pheochromocytoma, hyperthyroidism or hypothyroidism, and Cushing's syndrome.

Both biological and psychological theories attempt to explain the etiology of panic attacks. They are best understood, however, as being determined by a combination of these factors. Physically, panic attacks may result from normal "fight or flight" responses to dangerous situations or either constitutional or state-related hypersensitivity to physical and environmental stimuli. Hyperventilation has also been implicated as a cause of panic attacks. Similarly, drug withdrawal, drug effects, and drug intoxication can set the stage for attacks. Finally, physical conditions such as mitral valve prolapse that simulate the symptoms of panic can trigger panic attacks.

Panic attacks may result from behavioral and thought-related processes. Behaviorally, panic attacks may arise from conditioning, in which a person learns via association to experience panic in certain situations. In terms of thought processes, panic attacks may result from learned, maladaptive ways of interpreting and responding to physical and environmental cues. For example, a person might experience a tickling sensation in their chest, misinterpret it as a heart attack, and then begin to hyperventilate in response to this misinterpretation, setting the stage for a panic attack. In general, these types of cognitive distortions, combined with biological factors, seem to play a critical role in the development and maintenance of panic-related problems.

TREATMENT AND THERAPY

Four therapies are available to treat panic: bibliotherapies, pharmacotherapies, behavioral therapies, and cognitive therapies. Bibliotherapies involve dispensing information. Books are used at treatment initiation to provide corrective or background information. Bibliotherapy is also useful for individuals with mild panic disorders who are not in need of intensive therapy, as well as for the family members of individuals experiencing panic.

Pharmacotherapies are drug treatments. Historically, sedatives were used to treat panic-related problems. Once problems with dependence on such drugs were discovered, however, their use for this purpose was reduced. Instead, use of other antianxiety agents and certain antidepressant medications have become popular for treatment. Relatedly, the use of stimulating drugs (such as caffeine, diet pills, amphetamine, or cocaine) and hallucinogenic drugs (such as marijuana) is often discouraged in individuals complaining of panic attacks. The managed detoxification of drugs, where use or withdrawal is related to panic (such as alcohol or Valium use), is also a treatment strategy.

Other behavioral strategies include social and life skills training, relaxation, and desensitization. Desensitization helps individuals learn to relax in situations that would cause them to panic inappropriately. Behavioral therapies may also integrate family therapy to enlist support and/or to correct for the family-related aspects of a panic problem.

Finally, cognitive therapies focus on identifying irrational beliefs contributing to panic. Individuals work with therapists to identify maladaptive thinking styles. Such styles typically serve to heighten anxiety by magnifying patients' fears and/or minimizing their beliefs that they can cope with feared situations. Through therapy, individuals learn to identify and correct maladaptive thinking patterns, substituting more adaptive thinking where necessary.

PERSPECTIVE AND PROSPECTS

Panic attacks are experienced by both males and females in every culture, affecting 1 to 2 percent of the population each year. Women are disproportionately affected, with panic attacks being two to three times more prevalent. Understanding the origins and relevance of this apparent gender difference will be important to treatment advances. Similarly, understanding why panic disorders are more prevalent in some families than in others will be key in creating better behavioral and pharmacological therapies. Finally, though the incidence of panic attacks is higher in individuals between late adolescence and middle adulthood, both the very young and the very old endure problems related to panic attacks. Though the available therapies have promise for these groups, challenges are evident. Tailoring treatments to the dynamic physical, social, and cognitive developmental needs of children and the elderly will be critical.

—Nancy A. Piotrowski, Ph.D.

See also Anxiety; Factitious disorders; Hypochondriasis; Mitral valve prolapse; Neurosis; Palpitations; Phobias; Psychiatric disorders; Psychiatry; Psychiatry, child and adolescent; Psychiatry, geriatric; Psychoanalysis; Stress.

FOR FURTHER INFORMATION:

Markway, Barbara G., et al. *Dying of Embarrassment: Help for Social Anxiety and Phobia*. Oakland, Calif.: New Harbinger, 1992. This book provides clear and supportive instruction for assessing fears, practicing relaxation and deep breathing, and improving or developing new social skills.

Rachman, Stanley, and Padmal de Silva. *Panic Disorder*. Oxford, England: Oxford University Press, 1996. This concise volume covers many aspects of panic disorder. Includes bibliographical references and an index.

Root, Benjamin A. *Understanding Panic and Other Anxiety Disorders*. Jackson: University Press of Mississippi, 2000. Root explains physical and mental problems that can mimic panic disorders and that the differentiating diagnosis in an emergency room or clinic is often a major hurdle. Describes those likely to suffer from panic attacks and discusses drug and psychotherapy treatments.

Wolpe, Joseph, and David Wolpe. *Life Without Fear*. Oakland, Calif.: New Harbinger, 1988. Designed to dispel fear, this volume covers fears and phobias and offers guidelines for behavior therapy. Includes bibliographical references.

PARALYSIS

DISEASE/DISORDER

ANATOMY OR SYSTEM AFFECTED: Legs, muscles, musculoskeletal system, neck, nerves, nervous system, spine

SPECIALTIES AND RELATED FIELDS: Neurology, physical therapy

DEFINITION: Pronounced weakness or the inability to produce movement in a part of the body resulting from a variety of causes.

KEY TERMS:

brain cortex: the outer layer of the brain, or gray matter; divided into many areas, each with a different function such as motion (the motor cortex) or sensation (the sensory cortex)

central nervous system: a system consisting of the brain, the brain stem, the cerebellum, and the spinal cord

hemiplegia: paralysis of one side of the body

motor: referring to parts of the nervous system having to do with movement production

nerve cell: one of the cells that make up the brain, spinal cord, and all the nerves; some initiate nerve impulses, some transmit impulses from one nerve cell to another, some transmit impulses from nerve cells to muscle cells, and some function to regulate other impulses

nerve impulse: a weak, localized electrical current generated by the movement of charged particles across and along a nerve cell membrane

nerves: bands of nervous tissue that carry both motor and sensory nerve impulses between the central nervous system and the rest of the body

neurotransmitters: chemical substances, such as acetylcholine, that are released by nerve cells into synapses when the nerve is stimulated; they stimulate the next nerve cell to fire in turn, thus passing the impulse from cell to cell

paraplegia: paralysis of the legs and lower trunk

peripheral nervous system: a system consisting of the nerves not located in the central nervous system; these nerves carry impulses from the central nervous system to the target muscles and relay sensory impulses from the rest of the body to the central nervous system

quadriplegia: paralysis of all four limbs

spinal cord: a large collection of nerve cells that relay impulses between the brain and the rest of the body; sometimes the spinal cord initiates nerve impulses of its own, such as reflexes

NERVOUS SYSTEM FUNCTIONS

In order to understand the causes of paralysis, weakness, or the inability to move a part of the body, it is necessary to review briefly the motor nervous system and muscles. Following an action from initiation to completion through the motor nervous system may clarify this process. One may begin, for example, with a voluntary movement. An alarm clock rings early one morning. A sleeper hears the noise and decides to hit the "sleep" button. This decision is made in the cerebral cortex, which sends impulses to the nerves in the arm via the spinal cord.

The actual microscopic actions that result in a nerve impulse traveling from the motor cortex all the way to individual muscles will be briefly reviewed. An individual nerve cell, or neuron, comprises three parts: The dendrites, the cell body, and the axon. The cell body conducts the metabolism for the cell and otherwise keeps things in running order, but it has little direct involvement with the transmission of nerve impulses.

Dendrites are similar in appearance to the roots of plants. They are numerous and relatively short. Their function is to pick up impulses received either from sensory organs or from other cells. They do this when the receptors on their surface become activated by certain chemical signals released by neighboring nerve cells. Once these receptors are activated, they initiate a process known as depolarization.

In the most basic description, depolarization refers to the generation of a minute electrical charge on nerve cell membranes. It occurs through the motion of charged molecules, or ions, across the cell membrane. The specific ions involved include potassium, sodium, and calcium. Depolarization progresses down the length of the nerve cell. It passes through the dendrite to the cell body of the nerve cell and then to the axon. The axon is long and thin, some axons reaching lengths of three or more feet. Depending on its type and function, the axon may split into small filaments that go to several nerve or muscle cells, or it may remain single.

The sending axons do not touch the receiving cells when passing an impulse. Instead, they come close to the receiving cell's dendrites but leave a small gap (the synapse). Once a nerve impulse reaches the end of an axon, the axon releases chemical compounds called neurotransmitters.

Synthesized by the nerve cell, the neurotransmitter is collected and stored in small packets resting at the end of the axon. In response to depolarization, the small packets of neurotransmitter are released into the synapse, and the original electrical nerve impulse is converted into a chemical impulse. When the neurotransmitter is released, it diffuses across the gap and contacts specific receptors on the dendrite of the receiving nerve cell. The receiving nerve cell's receptors then depolarize the receiving nerve cell, converting the chemical impulse back into an electrical one.

The receiving nerve cell is forced to continue depolarizing until the neurotransmitter is no longer in contact with the receptor, or until the nerve cell itself becomes exhausted and cannot depolarize again. To allow the receiving nerve cell to stop firing and to prepare itself for another signal, the neurotransmitter must be removed rather quickly from the receptor. This can be done by the axon of the sending cell, which takes it back in, or by enzymes located within the synapse that actually destroy the neurotransmitter. The most common neurotransmitter is acetylcholine, and the most frequently encountered form of enzyme that destroys neurotransmitters is called acetylcholinesterase.

The transmission of the nerve impulses signaling the hand to press the alarm clock's sleep button involves passing the impulses through several nerves. They form synapses on nerve cells in the spinal cord before those cells pass the impulse down the spinal cord toward the arm to cause the desired action.

The spinal cord is protected inside the vertebral column, a hollow column of bone. This column is made up of a stack of vertebrae supported by solid bone in the front and a hollow ring of thinner bone in the back through which the spinal cord runs. The vertebrae are anchored to one another by bony connections; the facets and vertebral spines; fibrous ligaments to the front, back, and side; and the intervertebral disks. Disks are made up of soft, gelatinous material surrounded by fibrous tissue. The disks and joints in the vertebral column allow the spine to flex and turn, while the bony column surrounding the spinal cord provides protection.

When the nerve leaves the spinal cord, it travels in what is called the motor ramus, or "root." The ramus passes through an opening in the vertebral column called a foramen. While passing through the foramen, the ramus passes near the intervertebral disk. The motor nerve fibers (and consequently the nerve impulses sent out to turn off the alarm clock) in the motor ramus join with the sensory nerve fibers in the sensory ramus just outside the vertebral column, and together they form the spinal nerves. These spinal nerves regroup to form peripheral nerves.

A peripheral nerve is the part of the nervous system that finally contacts the muscles that turn off the alarm clock. Peripheral nerves carry both sensory and motor information in the same nerve. They are the only locations in which sensory and motor nerve fibers are so completely joined. Peripheral nerves must sometimes pass through relatively tight or exposed locations. An example of an exposed nerve is the "funny bone," the ulnar nerve, which causes an unpleasant sensation when struck. Nerves that pass through tight spaces may suffer entrapment syndromes. A common nerve entrapment syndrome is carpal tunnel syndrome, in which the median nerve is squeezed in the fibrous band around the wrist.

Finally, the arm muscles themselves become involved in the process of turning off the alarm. The muscles are made up of numerous muscle fibers, and each muscle fiber is made up of numerous muscle cells. Inside each muscle cell are two active protein filaments, actin and myosin, which pull together when activated, causing the muscle cell to shorten. When the majority of muscle cells "fire" at once, the whole muscle contracts. The signal from nerve to muscle cell is transmitted across a synapse. The sleep button is pushed, and the alarm ends. Finally, the signals to the arm end, and the filaments slide back to their initial positions, relaxing the muscle cells.

For actin and myosin to move well, there must be adequate blood flow and adequate concentrations of substances such as oxygen, glucose, potassium, sodium, and calcium. Many other substances are needed indirectly to keep muscle cells functioning optimally, including thyroid hormone and cortisone.

TYPES OF PARALYSIS

True paralysis is the inability to produce movement of a part of the body. Paralysis may result from problems at many locations in the body, such as the motor cortex of the brain, the spinal cord, the nerves in the arms or legs, the blood, or the muscle cells themselves. Doctors must determine the specific cause of paralysis or weakness since the treatment of each disease is different. The first task is to determine whether the weakness or paralysis is caused by a disease of the nervous system, the muscle cells, or one of the substances that interferes with nerve conduction or muscular contraction. Some characteristics of specific problems are helpful in this diagnosis.

Disease of the nervous system is most often associated with complete paralysis. Diseases affecting the muscle cells or the factors controlling them are usually associated with a partial rather than complete paralysis—there is weakness rather than a lack of movement. When weakness is severe, however, it may be mistaken for complete paralysis. The fact that diseases of the nervous system cause paralysis of one side or one part of the body is helpful in diagnosis. Paralyzing conditions that affect muscle cells tend to result in whole-body weakness, although some muscles may be more severely affected than others. Another aid in differentiation is that neurologic diseases are almost always associated with some degree of impairment in sensation, while muscular causes are never associated with sensory loss.

Damage to the central nervous system and to the peripheral nervous system can be differentiated by features of the dysfunction. Central nervous system problems affect either half of the body or one region of the body, while peripheral damage affects only the muscles controlled by the damaged nerve or nerves. Central nervous system damage leaves pronounced reflexes, while damage to peripheral nerves results in an affected area without any reflexes. There is some muscle wasting with either type of paralysis, but the wasting seen after a peripheral nerve disease appears more quickly and more severely. When central nervous system damage occurs, the muscles involved are generally tight (spastic paralysis). Conversely, in patients with peripheral nervous system damage, muscles are usually loose. Through attention to these differentiating features, the source of paralysis can usually be discovered.

In adults, the most common cause of paralysis is stroke. A stroke results from interruption of the blood supply to a part of the brain. After being cut off from blood flow, the affected area dies. Brain tumors may also cause paralysis. Unlike strokes, however, which cause most of their damage as soon as the blood supply is interrupted, the damage produced by tumors tends to increase slowly as the tumor grows. An interesting feature of brain tumors is that they are surrounded by an area of swelling called edema. The edema, not the tumor itself, causes most of the neurologic changes. This distinction is important because edema is usually responsive to medical treatment.

Subdural hematomas are collections of blood that are outside of the brain but inside the skull. They are seen most frequently in older people and alcoholics. To form a subdural hematoma, a small blood vessel becomes injured in such a way that blood slowly oozes from it, accumulates, and clots. Interestingly, the trauma may be so slight as to not be remembered by the patient. This clot may cause pressure on the motor cortex that results in paralysis. Generally, subdural hematomas are slow in onset.

Multiple sclerosis, a disease affecting the nervous system, causes scattered, multiple small areas of destruction virtually anywhere in the brain or spinal cord. The extent of paralysis depends on the sites and extent of the damaged areas. Patients often have impairments in vision, speaking, sensation, and coordination.

If the spinal cord is the cause, the extent and location of the paralysis and numbness depend on the size, location, and level of the lesion. Spinal cord paralysis may result from trauma, tumors, interruption of blood flow, blood clots, or infections such as abscesses. These disorders are similar, except for location, in most respects to the previously described conditions in the brain. One of the conditions, however, trauma of the spinal cord, is very different from trauma of the brain.

Significant trauma may result in fracture of the vertebral column. Spinal fractures may be classified as stable or unstable. Unstable fractures, unlike stable ones, are often associated with paralysis because unstable fractures allow subluxation to occur. Subluxation is a dislocation of the vertebral column that compresses the spinal cord. If it occurs in the neck, quadriplegia (paralysis of all four limbs) results. If it occurs lower down the spine, paraplegia (paralysis of both lower limbs) is seen. On occasion, through inadvertent or excessive movement, overenthusiastic rescuers cause permanent paralysis by converting a nonsubluxated fracture to a subluxated one during rescue attempts.

Another unique type of spinal cord trauma is the rupture of an intervertebral disk, which allows the gelatinous material to press on the spinal cord or on the rami leaving the spinal cord. In addition to causing severe pain, an intervertebral disk rupture may cause weakness or paralysis. It usually affects only one or two rami and spares the spinal cord itself. Trauma to the spinal cord is particularly dangerous to individuals with conditions that weaken the bony spine. These conditions include osteoporosis of all types and rheumatoid arthritis.

Peripheral nerve damage can occur through a number of conditions that may result in nerve degeneration, including diabetes mellitus, vitamin deficiencies, use or abuse of certain medications, and poisoning by toxins such as alcohol and lead. Sometimes, a temporary nerve degeneration called Guillain-Barré syndrome follows upper respiratory tract infections and may be quite serious if the respiratory muscles are affected. Peripheral nerves may also be damaged by direct trauma, or by pressure as it passes through a narrow compartment, as happens in carpal tunnel syndrome. Peripheral nerve conditions are accompanied by numbness, tingling, and weakness or paralysis of only the area served by the affected nerve.

Paralysis may complicate diseases affecting muscles, although in these cases the patients usually demonstrate weakness rather than paralysis. In muscular diseases, the paralysis (or weakness) tends to affect all the muscles of the body, although some may be more affected than others. The most frequent causes

of paralysis in children are inherited diseases such as muscular dystrophy. In adults, muscular diseases are mainly attributable to hormonal imbalances such as an underactive thyroid gland or an overactive adrenal gland.

Paralysis may result if the concentration of certain substances in the body is significantly altered, although weakness is a much more common occurrence. The concentration of potassium, sodium, calcium, glucose, and specific hormones may dramatically affect muscle strength. A specific, though uncommon, disease of this type is periodic hypokalemic paralysis, a condition that runs in families. In this disorder, the amount of potassium in the blood can be dramatically reduced for short periods of time, resulting in brief periods of severe weakness or paralysis. These episodes rarely have serious consequences.

Weakness or paralysis may result if the body is unable to produce adequate amounts of acetylcholine, or if this neurotransmitter is destroyed in the synapse before it can pass on its message. Myasthenia gravis is the most common example of this type of disorder. Affected patients initially have adequate strength, but they develop weakness and paralysis in muscles during periods of use because acetylcholine stores become depleted. The weakness in this condition tends to become more prominent as the day wears on. The most frequently used muscles are the most affected. This type of paralysis temporarily improves after rest or medication.

Another unique type of paralysis, called Todd's paralysis, may follow a generalized epileptic seizure. It happens only when the seizure has been so extensive and prolonged that the nerve cells in the brain are literally exhausted and no longer able to initiate the nerve impulses needed to generate movements. This paralysis is temporary.

Paralysis may be caused by a variety of psychiatric disorders, including hysteria, catatonic psychosis, conversion disorder, factitious disorder, and somatization disorder. In psychological paralysis, the patient's inability to move parts of the body is psychological. This paralysis is particularly common during periods of high stress such as combat. Psychological paralysis should be differentiated from malingering. In a psychological paralysis, the patients genuinely believe that they are paralyzed, whereas malingerers, though they deny it, know that they are not paralyzed. Malingering is usually seen when some benefit resulting from the paralysis is anticipated.

PERSPECTIVE AND PROSPECTS

Once a nerve cell has been destroyed, it cannot be repaired. This is the main reason that the outlook is quite poor when most types of paralysis occur. The only thing that doctors can do is to try to limit the extent of the paralysis. Improvements can be made only by training the neighboring cells to take over the functions of the lost cells.

After suffering a paralyzing event, a patient begins rehabilitation using a number of exercises. These activities are usually carried out with the help of physical therapists, occupational therapists, or kinesiotherapists. Unfortunately, progress is rather limited, and most patients are not able to resume their old lifestyle after suffering extensive paralysis.

It is very important to take seriously paralysis or weakness that is localized to a single muscle or single group of muscles. Doctors need to find out the cause of this weakness as soon as possible and take steps to minimize or reverse the damage prior to complete destruction of the nerve cells. Initial and subsequent stroke prevention, tumor treatments, hematoma evacuation, spinal alignment and stabilization, intervertebral disk surgery, toxin removal, hormonal manipulation, and ion correction are all currently available methods of dealing with paralysis.

Because of the poor prognosis for overcoming paralysis, research has focused on understanding how nerve cells grow. Some lower animals possess an ability to regenerate nerve cells when they are damaged. It is well known that a lobster which has lost one of its claws can regenerate that claw, as well as the nerves that control the claw's functioning. A lower animal nerve growth factor has been identified and is being examined by a number of researchers. It is likely that drugs which could aid regeneration of damaged nerve cells in higher animals will be discovered. Once available, these drugs will improve the outlook for recovery of patients with paralysis. These medications may also help with other conditions associated with nerve cell damage, such as Alzheimer's disease or Parkinson's disease.

Progress in medical treatment and an increased health awareness by the public will reduce the incidence of diseases such as diabetes mellitus and the intake of toxins, such as alcohol, that may cause paralysis. Seat belt laws and motorcycle helmet laws may reduce the incidence of paralysis by reducing the severity of injuries in motor vehicle accidents.

Progress in neurosurgery should also improve a patient's hope for recovery in trauma cases. Although dead nerve cells cannot regenerate, cut nerve filaments may be able to regenerate and reattach, which is why surgeons have been able to reattach severed limbs. With progressively finer techniques and equipment, the success rate should improve further. Future progress in neurosurgery may also benefit patients whose paralysis is attributable to causes other than trauma. Progress in genetic research may allow scientists to isolate the genes responsible for diseases causing paralysis. Diseases such as myasthenia gravis and muscular dystrophy could respond to treatment if genetic therapies are found.

—Ronald C. Hamdy, M.D.,
Mark R. Doman, M.D.,
and Katherine Hoffman Doman

See also Amyotrophic lateral sclerosis; Ataxia; Bell's palsy; Brain; Brain disorders; Cerebral palsy; Epilepsy; Fracture and dislocation; Guillain-Barré syndrome; Hemiplegia; Motor neuron diseases; Multiple sclerosis; Muscular dystrophy; Nervous system; Neuralgia, neuritis, and neuropathy; Neurology; Neurology, pediatric; Neurosurgery; Numbness and tingling; Palsy; Paraplegia; Parkinson's disease; Quadriplegia; Seizures; Spinal cord disorders; Spine, vertebrae, and disks; Strokes.

FOR FURTHER INFORMATION:

Andreoli, Thomas E., et al., eds. *Cecil Essentials of Medicine.* 5th ed. Philadelphia: W. B. Saunders, 2001. An excellent introductory text to medical problems. Contains basic reviews of anatomy and physiology, as well as an introduction to diagnosis and treatment. Easily read by those with some background in biology.

Goroll, Allan H., Lawrence A. May, and Albert G. Mulley, Jr. *Primary Care Medicine.* 4th ed. Philadelphia: J. B. Lippincott, 2000. One of the best resources for problem-oriented medical diagnosis and management. Can be used by physicians and laypersons alike.

Spence, Alexander P., and Elliott B. Mason. *Human Anatomy and Physiology.* 4th ed. St. Paul, Minn.: West, 1992. This reference work is a basic physiology and anatomy text used in some introductory college courses. Several other basic anatomy and physiology texts are available and may serve equally well.

MAGILL'S

MEDICAL GUIDE

ALPHABETICAL LIST OF CONTENTS

Entries by Anatomy or System Affected

Colitis
Colon and rectal polyp removal
Colon and rectal surgery
Colon cancer
Colon therapy
Colonoscopy
Computed tomography (CT)
    scanning
Constipation
Crohn's disease
Cystectomy
Diabetes mellitus
Dialysis
Diarrhea and dysentery
Digestion
Diverticulitis and diverticulosis
Endoscopy
Enemas
Enterocolitis
Fistula repair
Gallbladder diseases
Gastrectomy
Gastroenterology
Gastroenterology, pediatric
Gastrointestinal disorders
Gastrointestinal system
Gastrostomy
Giardiasis
Hernia
Hernia repair
Hirschsprung's disease
Ileostomy and colostomy
Incontinence
Indigestion
Internal medicine
Intestinal disorders
Intestines
Irritable bowel syndrome (IBS)
Kidney transplantation
Kidneys
Laparoscopy
Liposuction
Lithotripsy
Liver
Liver transplantation
Malabsorption
Nephrectomy
Nephritis
Nephrology
Nephrology, pediatric
Obstruction
Pancreas
Pancreatitis
Peristalsis

Peritonitis
Pregnancy and gestation
Prostate cancer
Pyloric stenosis
Reproductive system
Roundworm
Shunts
Splenectomy
Sterilization
Stomach, intestinal, and pancreatic
    cancers
Stone removal
Stones
Syphilis
Tubal ligation
Ultrasonography
Urethritis
Urinary disorders
Urinary system
Urology
Urology, pediatric
Worms

ANUS
Colon and rectal polyp removal
Colon and rectal surgery
Colon cancer
Colon therapy
Colonoscopy
Diaper rash
Endoscopy
Enemas
Episiotomy
Fistula repair
Hemorrhoid banding and removal
Hemorrhoids
Hirschsprung's disease
Intestinal disorders
Intestines
Irritable bowel syndrome (IBS)
Soiling
Sphincterectomy

ARMS
Amputation
Bones and the skeleton
Carpal tunnel syndrome
Fracture and dislocation
Fracture repair
Liposuction
Muscles
Pityriasis rosea
Skin lesion removal
Tendon disorders

Tendon repair
Thalidomide
Upper extremities

BACK
Arthritis, juvenile rheumatoid
Bone disorders
Bone marrow transplantation
Bones and the skeleton
Cerebral palsy
Chiropractic
Disk removal
Dwarfism
Gigantism
Kyphosis
Laminectomy and spinal fusion
Lumbar puncture
Muscle sprains, spasms, and
    disorders
Muscles
Osteoporosis
Pityriasis rosea
Sciatica
Scoliosis
Slipped disk
Spinal cord disorders
Spine, vertebrae, and disks
Spondylitis
Sympathectomy
Tendon disorders

BLADDER
Abdomen
Bed-wetting
Candidiasis
Catheterization
Cystectomy
Cystitis
Cystoscopy
Endoscopy
Fistula repair
Incontinence
Internal medicine
Lithotripsy
Schistosomiasis
Sphincterectomy
Stone removal
Stones
Toilet training
Ultrasonography
Urethritis
Urinalysis
Urinary disorders
Urinary system

Urology
Urology, pediatric

BLOOD
Anemia
Angiography
Arthropod-borne diseases
Bleeding
Blood and blood disorders
Blood testing
Bone marrow transplantation
Candidiasis
Circulation
Cytomegalovirus (CMV)
Dialysis
E. coli infection
Ebola virus
Fluids and electrolytes
Gulf War syndrome
Heart
Hematology
Hematology, pediatric
Hemolytic disease of the
   newborn
Hemophilia
Host-defense mechanisms
Hyperlipidemia
Hypoglycemia
Immunization and vaccination
Immunology
Ischemia
Jaundice
Jaundice, neonatal
Laboratory tests
Leukemia
Liver
Malaria
Nephrology
Nephrology, pediatric
Nosebleeds
Pharmacology
Pharmacy
Rh factor
Scurvy
Septicemia
Serology
Sickle-cell disease
Thalassemia
Thrombolytic therapy and TPA
Thrombosis and thrombus
Toxemia
Toxicology
Transfusion
Transplantation

Ultrasonography
Yellow fever

BLOOD VESSELS
Aneurysmectomy
Aneurysms
Angiography
Angioplasty
Arteriosclerosis
Bleeding
Blood and blood disorders
Blood testing
Bypass surgery
Catheterization
Cholesterol
Circulation
Claudication
Diabetes mellitus
Dizziness and fainting
Eclampsia
Edema
Electrocauterization
Embolism
Endarterectomy
Hammertoe correction
Heart
Heart disease
Heat exhaustion and heat stroke
Hemorrhoid banding and removal
Hemorrhoids
Hypercholesterolemia
Hypertension
Ischemia
Necrotizing fasciitis
Nosebleeds
Phlebitis
Shock
Strokes
Thalidomide
Thrombosis and thrombus
Umbilical cord
Varicose vein removal
Varicose veins
Vascular medicine
Vascular system
Venous insufficiency

BONES
Amputation
Arthritis
Bone cancer
Bone disorders
Bone grafting
Bone marrow transplantation

Bones and the skeleton
Bowlegs
Bunions
Cells
Cerebral palsy
Chiropractic
Cleft lip and palate
Cleft lip and palate repair
Craniosynostosis
Craniotomy
Disk removal
Dwarfism
Ear surgery
Ears
Estrogen replacement therapy
Ewing's sarcoma
Failure to thrive
Feet
Foot disorders
Fracture and dislocation
Fracture repair
Gigantism
Hammertoe correction
Hammertoes
Head and neck disorders
Heel spur removal
Hematology
Hematology, pediatric
Hip fracture repair
Hip replacement
Jaw wiring
Kneecap removal
Knock-knees
Kyphosis
Laminectomy and spinal fusion
Lower extremities
Marfan syndrome
Motor skill development
Neurofibromatosis
Nuclear medicine
Nuclear radiology
Orthopedic surgery
Orthopedics
Orthopedics, pediatric
Osgood-Schlatter disease
Osteochondritis juvenilis
Osteogenesis imperfecta
Osteomyelitis
Osteopathic medicine
Osteoporosis
Paget's disease
Periodontitis
Physical rehabilitation
Pigeon toes

Podiatry
Rheumatology
Rickets
Sarcoma
Sarcopenia
Scoliosis
Slipped disk
Spinal cord disorders
Spine, vertebrae, and disks
Sports medicine
Teeth
Temporomandibular joint (TMJ) syndrome
Tendon disorders
Tendon repair
Upper extremities

BRAIN

Abscess drainage
Abscesses
Addiction
Alcoholism
Altitude sickness
Alzheimer's disease
Amnesia
Anesthesia
Anesthesiology
Aneurysmectomy
Aneurysms
Angiography
Aphasia and dysphasia
Aromatherapy
Attention-deficit disorder (ADD)
Auras
Biofeedback
Brain
Brain disorders
Cluster headaches
Cognitive development
Coma
Computed tomography (CT) scanning
Concussion
Craniotomy
Creutzfeldt-Jakob disease and mad cow disease
Cytomegalovirus (CMV)
Dehydration
Dementias
Developmental stages
Dizziness and fainting
Down syndrome
Dyslexia
Electroencephalography (EEG)
Embolism

Emotions: Biomedical causes and effects
Encephalitis
Endocrinology
Endocrinology, pediatric
Epilepsy
Failure to thrive
Fetal alcohol syndrome
Fetal tissue transplantation
Fragile X syndrome
Galactosemia
Gigantism
Gulf War syndrome
Hallucinations
Head and neck disorders
Headaches
Hydrocephalus
Hypertension
Hypnosis
Jaundice
Kinesiology
Lead poisoning
Learning disabilities
Light therapy
Malaria
Melatonin
Memory loss
Meningitis
Mental retardation
Migraine headaches
Narcolepsy
Narcotics
Nausea and vomiting
Neurology
Neurology, pediatric
Neurosurgery
Nuclear radiology
Parkinson's disease
Pharmacology
Pharmacy
Phenylketonuria (PKU)
Poliomyelitis
Positron emission tomography (PET) scanning
Prion diseases
Psychiatric disorders
Psychiatry
Psychiatry, child and adolescent
Psychiatry, geriatric
Rabies
Reye's syndrome
Schizophrenia
Seizures
Shock therapy

Shunts
Sleep disorders
Sleeping sickness
Sleepwalking
Stammering
Strokes
Syphilis
Tetanus
Thrombolytic therapy and TPA
Thrombosis and thrombus
Tics
Tourette's syndrome
Toxicology
Toxoplasmosis
Trembling and shaking
Tumor removal
Tumors
Unconsciousness
Weight loss medications
Yellow fever

BREASTS

Abscess drainage
Abscesses
Breast biopsy
Breast cancer
Breast disorders
Breast-feeding
Breast surgery
Breasts, female
Cyst removal
Cysts
Estrogen replacement therapy
Glands
Gynecology
Gynecomastia
Klinefelter syndrome
Mammography
Mastectomy and lumpectomy
Mastitis
Sex change surgery
Tumor removal
Tumors

CELLS

Acid-base chemistry
Bacteriology
Biopsy
Cell therapy
Cells
Cholesterol
Conception
Cytology
Cytomegalovirus (CMV)

Cytopathology
Dehydration
DNA and RNA
E. coli infection
Enzymes
Fluids and electrolytes
Food biochemistry
Genetic counseling
Genetic engineering
Glycolysis
Gram staining
Gulf War syndrome
Host-defense mechanisms
Immunization and vaccination
Immunology
In vitro fertilization
Kinesiology
Laboratory tests
Lipids
Magnetic field therapy
Microbiology
Microscopy
Mutation
Pharmacology
Pharmacy
Toxicology

CHEST
Anatomy
Asthma
Bones and the skeleton
Breasts, female
Bronchiolitis
Bronchitis
Bypass surgery
Cardiac rehabilitation
Cardiology
Cardiology, pediatric
Chest
Choking
Common cold
Congenital heart disease
Coughing
Croup
Cystic fibrosis
Electrocardiography (ECG or EKG)
Embolism
Emphysema
Gulf War syndrome
Heart
Heart transplantation
Heart valve replacement
Heartburn
Hiccups

Interstitial pulmonary fibrosis (IPF)
Legionnaires' disease
Lung cancer
Lungs
Pacemaker implantation
Pityriasis rosea
Pleurisy
Pneumonia
Pulmonary diseases
Pulmonary medicine
Pulmonary medicine, pediatric
Respiration
Respiratory distress syndrome
Resuscitation
Sneezing
Thoracic surgery
Tuberculosis
Whooping cough

CIRCULATORY SYSTEM
Aneurysmectomy
Aneurysms
Angina
Angiography
Angioplasty
Apgar score
Arrhythmias
Arteriosclerosis
Arthritis, juvenile rheumatoid
Biofeedback
Bleeding
Blood and blood disorders
Blood testing
Blue baby syndrome
Bypass surgery
Cardiac rehabilitation
Cardiology
Cardiology, pediatric
Catheterization
Chest
Cholesterol
Circulation
Claudication
Congenital heart disease
Dehydration
Diabetes mellitus
Dialysis
Dizziness and fainting
Ebola virus
Eclampsia
Edema
Electrocardiography (ECG or EKG)
Electrocauterization
Embolism

Endarterectomy
Endocarditis
Exercise physiology
Heart
Heart attack
Heart disease
Heart failure
Heart transplantation
Heart valve replacement
Heat exhaustion and heat stroke
Hematology
Hematology, pediatric
Hemorrhoid banding and removal
Hemorrhoids
Hormones
Hypercholesterolemia
Hypertension
Ischemia
Kidneys
Kinesiology
Liver
Lymphatic system
Mitral valve prolapse
Motor skill development
Nosebleeds
Osteochondritis juvenilis
Pacemaker implantation
Palpitations
Phlebitis
Resuscitation
Reye's syndrome
Rheumatic fever
Septicemia
Shock
Shunts
Smoking
Sports medicine
Steroid abuse
Strokes
Systems and organs
Testicular torsion
Thrombolytic therapy and TPA
Thrombosis and thrombus
Transfusion
Transplantation
Varicose vein removal
Varicose veins
Vascular medicine
Vascular system
Venous insufficiency

EARS
Altitude sickness
Audiology

Auras
Biophysics
Cytomegalovirus (CMV)
Dyslexia
Ear infections and disorders
Ear surgery
Ears
Fragile X syndrome
Hearing aids
Hearing loss
Hearing tests
Ménière's disease
Motion sickness
Myringotomy
Nervous system
Neurology
Neurology, pediatric
Osteogenesis imperfecta
Otoplasty
Otorhinolaryngology
Plastic surgery
Quinsy
Sense organs
Speech disorders

ENDOCRINE SYSTEM
Addison's disease
Adrenalectomy
Biofeedback
Breasts, female
Contraception
Cretinism
Diabetes mellitus
Dwarfism
Eating disorders
Emotions: Biomedical causes and
    effects
Endocrine disorders
Endocrinology
Endocrinology, pediatric
Estrogen replacement therapy
Failure to thrive
Gigantism
Glands
Goiter
Hormone replacement therapy
Hormones
Hyperparathyroidism and
    hypoparathyroidism
Hypoglycemia
Klinefelter syndrome
Liver
Melatonin
Obesity

Pancreas
Pancreatitis
Parathyroidectomy
Postpartum depression
Prostate gland
Prostate gland removal
Sex change surgery
Sexual differentiation
Steroid abuse
Steroids
Systems and organs
Testicular surgery
Thyroid disorders
Thyroid gland
Thyroidectomy
Turner syndrome
Weight loss medications

EYES
Albinos
Arthritis, juvenile rheumatoid
Astigmatism
Auras
Blindness
Blurred vision
Cataract surgery
Cataracts
Chlamydia
Color blindness
Conjunctivitis
Corneal transplantation
Cytomegalovirus (CMV)
Diabetes mellitus
Dyslexia
Eye surgery
Eyes
Face lift and blepharoplasty
Galactosemia
Glaucoma
Gonorrhea
Gulf War syndrome
Jaundice
Laser use in surgery
Macular degeneration
Marfan syndrome
Microscopy, slitlamp
Motor skill development
Multiple chemical sensitivity
    syndrome
Myopia
Ophthalmology
Optometry
Optometry, pediatric
Pigmentation

Ptosis
Sense organs
Strabismus
Styes
Toxoplasmosis
Trachoma
Transplantation
Visual disorders

FEET
Athlete's foot
Bones and the skeleton
Bunions
Corns and calluses
Cysts
Feet
Flat feet
Foot disorders
Fragile X syndrome
Frostbite
Ganglion removal
Gout
Hammertoe correction
Hammertoes
Heel spur removal
Lower extremities
Nail removal
Nails
Orthopedic surgery
Orthopedics
Orthopedics, pediatric
Osteoarthritis
Pigeon toes
Podiatry
Sports medicine
Tendon repair
Thalidomide
Warts

GALLBLADDER
Abscess drainage
Abscesses
Cholecystectomy
Cholecystitis
Fistula repair
Gallbladder diseases
Gastroenterology
Gastroenterology, pediatric
Gastrointestinal disorders
Gastrointestinal system
Internal medicine
Laparoscopy
Liver transplantation
Malabsorption

Oncology
Pancreas
Pharmacology
Poisoning
Poisonous plants
Pulmonary diseases
Pulmonary medicine
Pulmonary medicine, pediatric
Rh factor
Rheumatology
Rubella
Sarcoma
Sarcopenia
Scarlet fever
Serology
Smallpox
Sneezing
Stress
Stress reduction
Systems and organs
Thalidomide
Toxicology
Transfusion
Transplantation

INTESTINES
Abdomen
Abdominal disorders
Appendectomy
Appendicitis
Bacterial infections
Bypass surgery
Celiac sprue
Colic
Colitis
Colon and rectal polyp removal
Colon and rectal surgery
Colon cancer
Colon therapy
Colonoscopy
Constipation
Crohn's disease
Diarrhea and dysentery
Digestion
Diverticulitis and diverticulosis
E. coli infection
Eating disorders
Endoscopy
Enemas
Enterocolitis
Fistula repair
Food poisoning
Gastroenterology
Gastroenterology, pediatric

Gastrointestinal disorders
Gastrointestinal system
Hemorrhoid banding and removal
Hemorrhoids
Hernia
Hernia repair
Hirschsprung's disease
Ileostomy and colostomy
Indigestion
Internal medicine
Intestinal disorders
Intestines
Irritable bowel syndrome (IBS)
Kaposi's sarcoma
Kwashiorkor
Lactose intolerance
Laparoscopy
Malabsorption
Malnutrition
Metabolism
Nutrition
Obesity
Obstruction
Peristalsis
Pinworm
Proctology
Roundworm
Salmonella infection
Soiling
Sphincterectomy
Stomach, intestinal, and pancreatic
    cancers
Tapeworm
Toilet training
Trichinosis
Tumor removal
Tumors
Ulcer surgery
Ulcers
Worms

JOINTS
Amputation
Arthritis
Arthritis, juvenile rheumatoid
Arthroplasty
Arthroscopy
Bursitis
Carpal tunnel syndrome
Cell therapy
Chlamydia
Cyst removal
Cysts
Endoscopy

Exercise physiology
Fracture and dislocation
Fragile X syndrome
Gout
Gulf War syndrome
Hammertoe correction
Hammertoes
Hip fracture repair
Kneecap removal
Lupus erythematosus
Lyme disease
Motor skill development
Orthopedic surgery
Orthopedics
Orthopedics, pediatric
Osteoarthritis
Osteochondritis juvenilis
Osteomyelitis
Physical rehabilitation
Rheumatoid arthritis
Rheumatology
Spondylitis
Sports medicine
Temporomandibular joint (TMJ)
    syndrome
Tendon disorders
Tendon repair

KIDNEYS
Abdomen
Abscess drainage
Abscesses
Adrenalectomy
Cysts
Dialysis
Galactosemia
Glomerulonephritis
Hanta virus
Hypertension
Internal medicine
Kidney disorders
Kidney transplantation
Kidneys
Laparoscopy
Lithotripsy
Metabolism
Nephrectomy
Nephritis
Nephrology
Nephrology, pediatric
Nuclear medicine
Nuclear radiology
Renal failure
Reye's syndrome

Fetal alcohol syndrome
Fistula repair
Genetic counseling
Genital disorders, female
Genital disorders, male
Glands
Gonorrhea
Gynecology
Hermaphroditism and
    pseudohermaphroditism
Hernia
Herpes
Hormone replacement therapy
Hormones
Human immunodeficiency virus
    (HIV)
Hydrocelectomy
Hypospadias repair and
    urethroplasty
Hysterectomy
In vitro fertilization
Infertility in females
Infertility in males
Internal medicine
Klinefelter syndrome
Laparoscopy
Menopause
Menorrhagia
Menstruation
Miscarriage
Multiple births
Mumps
Myomectomy
Obstetrics
Orchitis
Ovarian cysts
Pelvic inflammatory disease (PID)
Penile implant surgery
Precocious puberty
Pregnancy and gestation
Premature birth
Premenstrual syndrome (PMS)
Prostate cancer
Prostate gland
Puberty and adolescence
Reproductive system
Sex change surgery
Sexual differentiation
Sexual dysfunction
Sexuality
Sexually transmitted diseases
Sperm banks
Sterilization
Steroid abuse

Stillbirth
Syphilis
Systems and organs
Testicles, undescended
Testicular surgery
Testicular torsion
Tubal ligation
Turner syndrome
Ultrasonography
Urology
Urology, pediatric
Vasectomy
Warts

RESPIRATORY SYSTEM

Abscess drainage
Abscesses
Altitude sickness
Amyotrophic lateral sclerosis
Apgar score
Apnea
Asphyxiation
Asthma
Bacterial infections
Bronchiolitis
Bronchitis
Chest
Chickenpox
Childhood infectious diseases
Choking
Common cold
Coughing
Croup
Cystic fibrosis
Diphtheria
Edema
Embolism
Emphysema
Epiglottitis
Exercise physiology
Fluids and electrolytes
Fungal infections
Halitosis
Hanta virus
Head and neck disorders
Heart transplantation
Hiccups
Influenza
Internal medicine
Interstitial pulmonary fibrosis
    (IPF)
Kinesiology
Laryngectomy
Laryngitis

Legionnaires' disease
Lung cancer
Lung surgery
Lungs
Measles
Mononucleosis
Multiple chemical sensitivity
    syndrome
Nasopharyngeal disorders
Otorhinolaryngology
Oxygen therapy
Pharyngitis
Plague
Pleurisy
Pneumonia
Poisoning
Pulmonary diseases
Pulmonary medicine
Pulmonary medicine, pediatric
Respiration
Resuscitation
Rheumatic fever
Rhinitis
Roundworm
Sinusitis
Smallpox
Sneezing
Sore throat
Strep throat
Systems and organs
Thoracic surgery
Thrombolytic therapy and TPA
Thrombosis and thrombus
Tonsillectomy and adenoid removal
Tonsillitis
Toxoplasmosis
Tracheostomy
Transplantation
Tuberculosis
Tumor removal
Tumors
Voice and vocal cord disorders
Whooping cough
Worms

SKIN

Abscess drainage
Abscesses
Acne
Acupressure
Acupuncture
Age spots
Albinos
Allergies

Amputation
Anesthesia
Anesthesiology
Anthrax
Anxiety
Arthropod-borne diseases
Athlete's foot
Auras
Biopsy
Birthmarks
Bites and stings
Blisters and boils
Blood testing
Burns and scalds
Candidiasis
Cell therapy
Cells
Chickenpox
Cleft lip and palate repair
Corns and calluses
Cradle cap
Cryotherapy and cryosurgery
Cyst removal
Cysts
Dermatitis
Dermatology
Dermatology, pediatric
Dermatopathology
Diaper rash
Ebola virus
Eczema
Edema
Electrical shock
Electrocauterization
Face lift and blepharoplasty
Fifth disease
Frostbite
Fungal infections
Glands
Grafts and grafting
Gulf War syndrome
Hair loss and baldness
Hair transplantation
Hand-foot-and-mouth disease
Heat exhaustion and heat stroke
Hemolytic disease of the
    newborn
Hives
Host-defense mechanisms
Impetigo
Itching
Jaundice
Kaposi's sarcoma
Keratoses

Laceration repair
Laser use in surgery
Leishmaniasis
Leprosy
Lice, mites, and ticks
Light therapy
Lower extremities
Lupus erythematosus
Lyme disease
Malignant melanoma removal
Measles
Moles
Multiple chemical sensitivity
    syndrome
Nails
Necrotizing fasciitis
Neurofibromatosis
Numbness and tingling
Obesity
Otoplasty
Pigmentation
Pimples
Pinworm
Pityriasis alba
Pityriasis rosea
Plastic surgery
Poisonous plants
Porphyria
Psoriasis
Radiation sickness
Rashes
Ringworm
Rosacea
Roseola
Rubella
Scabies
Scarlet fever
Scurvy
Sense organs
Shingles
Skin
Skin cancer
Skin disorders
Skin lesion removal
Smallpox
Stretch marks
Sunburn
Tattoo removal
Tattoos and body piercing
Touch
Umbilical cord
Upper extremities
Warts
Wrinkles

SPINE
Anesthesia
Anesthesiology
Bone cancer
Bone disorders
Bones and the skeleton
Cerebral palsy
Chiropractic
Disk removal
Dystrophy
Fracture and dislocation
Head and neck disorders
Kinesiology
Laminectomy and spinal fusion
Lumbar puncture
Marfan syndrome
Meningitis
Motor neuron diseases
Multiple sclerosis
Muscle sprains, spasms, and
    disorders
Muscles
Muscular dystrophy
Nervous system
Neuralgia, neuritis, and neuropathy
Neurology
Neurology, pediatric
Neurosurgery
Numbness and tingling
Orthopedic surgery
Orthopedics
Orthopedics, pediatric
Osteoarthritis
Osteogenesis imperfecta
Osteoporosis
Paget's disease
Paralysis
Paraplegia
Physical rehabilitation
Poliomyelitis
Quadriplegia
Sciatica
Scoliosis
Slipped disk
Spina bifida
Spinal cord disorders
Spine, vertebrae, and disks
Spondylitis
Sports medicine
Sympathectomy

SPLEEN
Abdomen
Abdominal disorders

Abscess drainage
Abscesses
Anemia
Bleeding
Hematology
Hematology, pediatric
Immune system
Internal medicine
Jaundice, neonatal
Lymphatic system
Metabolism
Splenectomy
Transplantation

STOMACH
Abdomen
Abdominal disorders
Abscess drainage
Abscesses
Allergies
Botulism
Bulimia
Burping
Bypass surgery
Colitis
Crohn's disease
Digestion
Eating disorders
Endoscopy
Food biochemistry
Food poisoning
Gastrectomy
Gastroenterology
Gastroenterology, pediatric
Gastrointestinal disorders
Gastrointestinal system
Gastrostomy
Halitosis
Heartburn
Hernia
Hernia repair
Indigestion
Influenza
Internal medicine
Kwashiorkor
Lactose intolerance
Malabsorption
Malnutrition
Metabolism
Motion sickness
Nausea and vomiting
Nutrition
Obesity
Peristalsis

Poisoning
Poisonous plants
Pyloric stenosis
Radiation sickness
Roundworm
Salmonella infection
Stomach, intestinal, and pancreatic
    cancers
Ulcer surgery
Ulcers
Vagotomy
Vitamins and minerals
Weaning
Weight loss and gain

TEETH
Cavities
Crowns and bridges
Dental diseases
Dentistry
Dentistry, pediatric
Dentures
Endodontic disease
Fluoride treatments
Forensic pathology
Fracture repair
Gastrointestinal system
Gingivitis
Jaw wiring
Lisping
Nutrition
Orthodontics
Osteogenesis imperfecta
Periodontal surgery
Periodontitis
Root canal treatment
Teeth
Teething
Temporomandibular joint (TMJ)
    syndrome
Thumb sucking
Tooth extraction
Toothache
Veterinary medicine
Wisdom teeth

TENDONS
Carpal tunnel syndrome
Cysts
Exercise physiology
Ganglion removal
Hammertoe correction
Kneecap removal
Orthopedic surgery

Orthopedics
Orthopedics, pediatric
Osgood-Schlatter disease
Physical rehabilitation
Sports medicine
Tendon disorders
Tendon repair

THROAT
Auras
Bulimia
Catheterization
Choking
Croup
Epiglottitis
Fifth disease
Gastroenterology
Gastroenterology, pediatric
Gastrointestinal disorders
Gastrointestinal system
Goiter
Head and neck disorders
Hiccups
Laryngectomy
Laryngitis
Nasopharyngeal disorders
Nosebleeds
Otorhinolaryngology
Pharyngitis
Pulmonary medicine
Pulmonary medicine, pediatric
Quinsy
Respiration
Smoking
Sore throat
Strep throat
Tonsillectomy and adenoid removal
Tonsillitis
Tracheostomy
Voice and vocal cord disorders

URINARY SYSTEM
Abdomen
Abdominal disorders
Abscess drainage
Abscesses
Adrenalectomy
Bed-wetting
Candidiasis
Catheterization
Circumcision, male
Cystectomy
Cystitis
Cystoscopy

ENTRIES BY SPECIALTIES AND RELATED FIELDS

ALL
Accidents
Anatomy
Biostatistics
Clinical trials
Disease
Geriatrics and gerontology
Health maintenance organizations
  (HMOs)
Iatrogenic disorders
Imaging and radiology
Internet medicine
Invasive tests
Laboratory tests
Noninvasive tests
Pediatrics
Physical examination
Physiology
Preventive medicine
Screening
Self-medication
Systems and organs
Terminally ill: Extended care
Veterinary medicine

ALTERNATIVE MEDICINE
Acupressure
Acupuncture
Allied health
Alternative medicine
Antioxidants
Aromatherapy
Biofeedback
Cell therapy
Chronobiology
Club drugs
Colon therapy
Enzyme therapy
Healing
Herbal medicine
Holistic medicine
Hydrotherapy
Hypnosis
Magnetic field therapy
Massage
Meditation
Melatonin
Nutrition
Oxygen therapy
Pain management
Qi gong

Stress reduction
Supplements
Tai Chi Chuan
Yoga

ANESTHESIOLOGY
Acupuncture
Anesthesia
Anesthesiology
Catheterization
Cesarean section
Critical care
Critical care, pediatric
Dentistry
Hyperthermia and hypothermia
Hypnosis
Pain management
Pharmacology
Pharmacy
Surgery, general
Surgery, pediatric
Surgical procedures
Surgical technologists
Toxicology

AUDIOLOGY
Aging
Aging: Extended care
Audiology
Biophysics
Dyslexia
Ear infections and disorders
Ear surgery
Ears
Hearing aids
Hearing loss
Hearing tests
Ménière's disease
Motion sickness
Neurology
Neurology, pediatric
Otoplasty
Otorhinolaryngology
Sense organs
Speech disorders

BACTERIOLOGY
Anthrax
Antibiotics
Bacterial infections
Bacteriology

Blisters and boils
Botulism
Cells
Childhood infectious diseases
Cholecystitis
Cholera
Cystitis
Cytology
Cytopathology
Diphtheria
Drug resistance
E. coli infection
Endocarditis
Fluoride treatments
Gangrene
Glomerulonephritis
Gonorrhea
Gram staining
Impetigo
Infection
Laboratory tests
Legionnaires' disease
Leprosy
Lyme disease
Mastitis
Microbiology
Microscopy
Necrotizing fasciitis
Osteomyelitis
Pelvic inflammatory disease (PID)
Plague
Pneumonia
Salmonella infection
Scarlet fever
Serology
Shigellosis
Staphylococcal infections
Strep throat
Streptococcal infections
Syphilis
Tetanus
Tonsillitis
Toxemia
Tropical medicine
Tuberculosis
Typhoid fever and typhus
Whooping cough

BIOCHEMISTRY
Acid-base chemistry
Autopsy

Bacteriology
Cholesterol
Digestion
Endocrinology
Endocrinology, pediatric
Enzymes
Fluids and electrolytes
Fluoride treatments
Food biochemistry
Genetic engineering
Glands
Glycolysis
Gram staining
Histology
Hormones
Human Genome Project
Leptin
Lipids
Malabsorption
Metabolism
Nephrology
Nephrology, pediatric
Nutrition
Pathology
Pharmacology
Pharmacy
Respiration
Stem cell research
Steroids
Toxicology
Urinalysis

BIOTECHNOLOGY
Bionics and biotechnology
Biophysics
Cloning
Computed tomography (CT)
   scanning
Dialysis
Electrocardiography (ECG or
   EKG)
Electroencephalography
   (EEG)
Gene therapy
Genetic engineering
Human Genome Project
In vitro fertilization
Magnetic resonance imaging
   (MRI)
Pacemaker implantation
Positron emission tomography
   (PET) scanning
Sperm banks
Stem cell research

CARDIOLOGY
Aging
Aging: Extended care
Aneurysmectomy
Aneurysms
Angina
Angiography
Angioplasty
Anxiety
Arrhythmias
Arteriosclerosis
Biofeedback
Blue baby syndrome
Bypass surgery
Cardiac rehabilitation
Cardiology
Cardiology, pediatric
Catheterization
Chest
Cholesterol
Circulation
Congenital heart disease
Critical care
Critical care, pediatric
Dizziness and fainting
Electrocardiography (ECG or EKG)
Emergency medicine
Endocarditis
Exercise physiology
Geriatrics and gerontology
Heart
Heart attack
Heart disease
Heart failure
Heart transplantation
Heart valve replacement
Hematology
Hypercholesterolemia
Hypertension
Internal medicine
Ischemia
Kinesiology
Leptin
Marfan syndrome
Mitral valve prolapse
Muscles
Neonatology
Noninvasive tests
Nuclear medicine
Pacemaker implantation
Palpitations
Paramedics
Physical examination
Progeria

Rheumatic fever
Sports medicine
Thoracic surgery
Thrombolytic therapy and TPA
Thrombosis and thrombus
Transplantation
Ultrasonography
Vascular medicine
Vascular system
Venous insufficiency

CRITICAL CARE
Accidents
Aging: Extended care
Amputation
Anesthesia
Anesthesiology
Apgar score
Burns and scalds
Catheterization
Club drugs
Coma
Critical care
Critical care, pediatric
Electrical shock
Electrocardiography (ECG or EKG)
Electroencephalography (EEG)
Emergency medicine
Emergency medicine, pediatric
Geriatrics and gerontology
Grafts and grafting
Hanta virus
Heart attack
Heart transplantation
Heat exhaustion and heat stroke
Hospitals
Hyperthermia and hypothermia
Necrotizing fasciitis
Neonatology
Nursing
Oncology
Osteopathic medicine
Pain management
Paramedics
Psychiatry
Psychiatry, child and adolescent
Psychiatry, geriatric
Pulmonary medicine
Pulmonary medicine, pediatric
Radiation sickness
Resuscitation
Safety issues for children
Safety issues for the elderly
Shock

Circumcision, female, and genital
 mutilation
Circumcision, male
Cloning
Ethics
Euthanasia
Fetal tissue transplantation
Gene therapy
Genetic engineering
Gulf War syndrome
Hippocratic oath
Human Genome Project
Law and medicine
Malpractice
Münchausen syndrome by proxy
Sperm banks
Stem cell research

EXERCISE PHYSIOLOGY
Biofeedback
Bone disorders
Bones and the skeleton
Cardiac rehabilitation
Cardiology
Circulation
Dehydration
Electrocardiography (ECG or
 EKG)
Exercise physiology
Glycolysis
Heart
Heat exhaustion and heat stroke
Kinesiology
Lungs
Massage
Metabolism
Motor skill development
Muscle sprains, spasms, and
 disorders
Muscles
Nutrition
Orthopedic surgery
Orthopedics
Orthopedics, pediatric
Oxygen therapy
Physical rehabilitation
Physiology
Pulmonary diseases
Pulmonary medicine
Pulmonary medicine, pediatric
Respiration
Sports medicine
Steroid abuse
Vascular system

FAMILY PRACTICE
Abdominal disorders
Abscess drainage
Abscesses
Acne
Acquired immunodeficiency
 syndrome (AIDS)
Alcoholism
Allergies
Alzheimer's disease
Amyotrophic lateral sclerosis
Anemia
Angina
Anti-inflammatory drugs
Antioxidants
Arthritis
Arthritis, juvenile rheumatoid
Athlete's foot
Attention-deficit disorder (ADD)
Bacterial infections
Bed-wetting
Bell's palsy
Beriberi
Biofeedback
Birthmarks
Bleeding
Blisters and boils
Blurred vision
Bronchiolitis
Bronchitis
Bunions
Burping
Candidiasis
Chickenpox
Childhood infectious diseases
Chlamydia
Cholecystitis
Cholesterol
Chronic fatigue syndrome
Cirrhosis
Cluster headaches
Common cold
Constipation
Contraception
Coughing
Cradle cap
Cryotherapy and cryosurgery
Cytomegalovirus (CMV)
Death and dying
Dehydration
Depression
Diabetes mellitus
Diaper rash
Diarrhea and dysentery

Digestion
Dizziness and fainting
Domestic violence
Enterocolitis
Epiglottitis
Exercise physiology
Factitious disorders
Failure to thrive
Family practice
Fatigue
Fever
Fifth disease
Fungal infections
Ganglion removal
Genital disorders, female
Genital disorders, male
Geriatrics and gerontology
Giardiasis
Grief and guilt
Gynecology
Gynecomastia
Halitosis
Hand-foot-and-mouth disease
Headaches
Healing
Heart disease
Heartburn
Heat exhaustion and heat stroke
Hemorrhoid banding and removal
Hemorrhoids
Herpes
Hiccups
Hirschsprung's disease
Hives
Hyperadiposis
Hypercholesterolemia
Hyperlipidemia
Hypertension
Hypertrophy
Hypoglycemia
Incontinence
Indigestion
Infection
Inflammation
Influenza
Intestinal disorders
Laryngitis
Malabsorption
Measles
Mitral valve prolapse
Moles
Mononucleosis
Motion sickness
Mumps

Münchausen syndrome by proxy
Muscle sprains, spasms, and
    disorders
Myringotomy
Nasal polyp removal
Nasopharyngeal disorders
Nightmares
Nosebleeds
Nutrition
Obesity
Orchitis
Osgood-Schlatter disease
Osteopathic medicine
Otoplasty
Pain
Parasitic diseases
Pediatrics
Pharmacology
Pharmacy
Pharyngitis
Physical examination
Physician assistants
Pigeon toes
Pimples
Pinworm
Pityriasis alba
Pityriasis rosea
Pneumonia
Poisonous plants
Precocious puberty
Psychiatry
Psychiatry, child and adolescent
Psychiatry, geriatric
Ptosis
Puberty and adolescence
Quinsy
Rashes
Reflexes, primitive
Rheumatic fever
Ringworm
Rubella
Safety issues for children
Safety issues for the elderly
Scabies
Scarlet fever
Sciatica
Sexuality
Shingles
Shock
Sibling rivalry
Sinusitis
Skin disorders
Sneezing
Sore throat

Sports medicine
Sterilization
Strep throat
Stress
Styes
Sunburn
Supplements
Temporomandibular joint (TMJ)
    syndrome
Testicular torsion
Tetanus
Toilet training
Tonsillitis
Tourette's syndrome
Toxicology
Trachoma
Ulcers
Urology
Vascular medicine
Vasectomy
Viral infections
Vitamins and minerals
Weaning
Weight loss medications
Whooping cough
Wounds

FORENSIC MEDICINE
Autopsy
Blood and blood disorders
Blood testing
Bones and the skeleton
Cytopathology
Dermatopathology
DNA and RNA
Forensic pathology
Genetics and inheritance
Hematology
Histology
Human Genome Project
Immunopathology
Laboratory tests
Law and medicine
Pathology

GASTROENTEROLOGY
Abdomen
Abdominal disorders
Amyotrophic lateral sclerosis
Anthrax
Appendectomy
Appendicitis
Bulimia
Bypass surgery

Celiac sprue
Cholecystectomy
Cholecystitis
Cholera
Colic
Colitis
Colon and rectal polyp removal
Colon and rectal surgery
Colon cancer
Colonoscopy
Computed tomography (CT)
    scanning
Constipation
Critical care
Critical care, pediatric
Crohn's disease
Cytomegalovirus (CMV)
Diarrhea and dysentery
Digestion
Diverticulitis and diverticulosis
E. coli infection
Emergency medicine
Endoscopy
Enemas
Enterocolitis
Enzymes
Failure to thrive
Fistula repair
Food biochemistry
Food poisoning
Gallbladder diseases
Gastrectomy
Gastroenterology
Gastroenterology, pediatric
Gastrointestinal disorders
Gastrointestinal system
Gastrostomy
Giardiasis
Glands
Heartburn
Hemorrhoid banding and removal
Hemorrhoids
Hernia
Hernia repair
Hirschsprung's disease
Ileostomy and colostomy
Indigestion
Internal medicine
Intestinal disorders
Intestines
Irritable bowel syndrome (IBS)
Lactose intolerance
Laparoscopy
Liver

Down syndrome
Dwarfism
Embryology
Endocrinology
Endocrinology, pediatric
Enzymes
Failure to thrive
Fragile X syndrome
Galactosemia
Gene therapy
Genetic counseling
Genetic diseases
Genetic engineering
Genetics and inheritance
Grafts and grafting
Hematology
Hematology, pediatric
Hemophilia
Hermaphroditism and
    pseudohermaphroditism
Human Genome Project
Hyperadiposis
Immunodeficiency disorders
In vitro fertilization
Insulin resistance syndrome
Klinefelter syndrome
Laboratory tests
Leptin
Malabsorption
Marfan syndrome
Mental retardation
Motor skill development
Muscular dystrophy
Mutation
Neonatology
Nephrology
Nephrology, pediatric
Neurofibromatosis
Neurology
Neurology, pediatric
Obstetrics
Oncology
Osteogenesis imperfecta
Pediatrics
Phenylketonuria (PKU)
Porphyria
Precocious puberty
Reproductive system
Rh factor
Screening
Sexual differentiation
Sexuality
Sperm banks
Stem cell research

Tay-Sachs disease
Tourette's syndrome
Transplantation
Turner syndrome

**GERIATRICS AND
    GERONTOLOGY**
Age spots
Aging
Aging: Extended care
Alzheimer's disease
Arthritis
Bed-wetting
Blindness
Blurred vision
Bone disorders
Bones and the skeleton
Brain
Brain disorders
Cataract surgery
Cataracts
Corns and calluses
Critical care
Crowns and bridges
Death and dying
Dementias
Dentures
Depression
Domestic violence
Emergency medicine
Endocrinology
Estrogen replacement therapy
Euthanasia
Family practice
Fatigue
Fracture and dislocation
Fracture repair
Gray hair
Hearing aids
Hearing loss
Hip fracture repair
Hip replacement
Hormone replacement therapy
Hormones
Hospitals
Incontinence
Memory loss
Nursing
Nutrition
Ophthalmology
Orthopedics
Osteoporosis
Pain management
Paramedics

Parkinson's disease
Pharmacology
Psychiatry
Psychiatry, geriatric
Rheumatology
Safety issues for the elderly
Sarcopenia
Sleep disorders
Spinal cord disorders
Spine, vertebrae, and disks
Suicide
Visual disorders
Wrinkles

GYNECOLOGY
Abortion
Amenorrhea
Amniocentesis
Biopsy
Breast biopsy
Breast cancer
Breast disorders
Breast-feeding
Breasts, female
Cervical, ovarian, and uterine
    cancers
Cervical procedures
Cesarean section
Childbirth
Childbirth complications
Chlamydia
Circumcision, female, and genital
    mutilation
Conception
Contraception
Culdocentesis
Cyst removal
Cystectomy
Cystitis
Cysts
Dysmenorrhea
Electrocauterization
Endocrinology
Endometrial biopsy
Endometriosis
Endoscopy
Episiotomy
Estrogen replacement therapy
Genital disorders, female
Glands
Gonorrhea
Gynecology
Hermaphroditism and
    pseudohermaphroditism

Medicare
National Cancer Institute (NCI)
National Institutes of Health (NIH)
Sperm banks
Stem cell research
World Health Organization

ORTHODONTICS
Bones and the skeleton
Dental diseases
Dentistry
Dentistry, pediatric
Jaw wiring
Orthodontics
Periodontal surgery
Teeth
Teething
Tooth extraction
Wisdom teeth

ORTHOPEDICS
Amputation
Arthritis
Arthritis, juvenile rheumatoid
Arthroplasty
Arthroscopy
Bone cancer
Bone disorders
Bone grafting
Bones and the skeleton
Bowlegs
Bunions
Bursitis
Cancer
Chiropractic
Craniosynostosis
Disk removal
Dwarfism
Ewing's sarcoma
Feet
Flat feet
Foot disorders
Fracture and dislocation
Fracture repair
Geriatrics and gerontology
Growth
Hammertoe correction
Hammertoes
Heel spur removal
Hip fracture repair
Hip replacement
Jaw wiring
Kinesiology
Kneecap removal

Knock-knees
Kyphosis
Laminectomy and spinal fusion
Lower extremities
Marfan syndrome
Motor skill development
Muscle sprains, spasms, and
  disorders
Muscles
Neurofibromatosis
Orthopedic surgery
Orthopedics
Orthopedics, pediatric
Osgood-Schlatter disease
Osteoarthritis
Osteochondritis juvenilis
Osteogenesis imperfecta
Osteomyelitis
Osteopathic medicine
Osteoporosis
Paget's disease
Physical examination
Physical rehabilitation
Pigeon toes
Podiatry
Rheumatoid arthritis
Rheumatology
Scoliosis
Slipped disk
Spina bifida
Spinal cord disorders
Spine, vertebrae, and disks
Sports medicine
Tendon disorders
Tendon repair
Upper extremities

OSTEOPATHIC MEDICINE
Alternative medicine
Bones and the skeleton
Exercise physiology
Family practice
Holistic medicine
Muscle sprains, spasms, and
  disorders
Muscles
Nutrition
Osteopathic medicine
Physical rehabilitation

OTORHINOLARYNGOLOGY
Anti-inflammatory drugs
Aromatherapy
Audiology

Cleft lip and palate
Cleft lip and palate repair
Common cold
Croup
Ear infections and disorders
Ear surgery
Ears
Epiglottitis
Gastrointestinal system
Halitosis
Head and neck disorders
Hearing aids
Hearing loss
Hearing tests
Laryngectomy
Laryngitis
Ménière's disease
Motion sickness
Myringotomy
Nasal polyp removal
Nasopharyngeal disorders
Nausea and vomiting
Nosebleeds
Otorhinolaryngology
Pharyngitis
Pulmonary diseases
Pulmonary medicine
Pulmonary medicine, pediatric
Quinsy
Respiration
Rhinitis
Rhinoplasty and submucous
  resection
Sense organs
Sinusitis
Smell
Sore throat
Strep throat
Taste
Tonsillectomy and adenoid removal
Tonsillitis
Voice and vocal cord disorders

PATHOLOGY
Autopsy
Bacteriology
Biopsy
Blood testing
Cancer
Cytology
Cytopathology
Dermatopathology
Disease
Electroencephalography (EEG)

Jaw wiring
Laceration repair
Liposuction
Malignancy and metastasis
Malignant melanoma removal
Moles
Necrotizing fasciitis
Neurofibromatosis
Obesity
Otoplasty
Otorhinolaryngology
Plastic surgery
Ptosis
Rhinoplasty and submucous
    resection
Sex change surgery
Skin
Skin lesion removal
Surgical procedures
Tattoo removal
Tattoos and body piercing
Varicose vein removal
Varicose veins
Wrinkles

PODIATRY
Athlete's foot
Bone disorders
Bones and the skeleton
Bunions
Corns and calluses
Feet
Flat feet
Foot disorders
Fungal infections
Hammertoe correction
Hammertoes
Heel spur removal
Lower extremities
Nail removal
Orthopedic surgery
Orthopedics
Physical examination
Pigeon toes
Podiatry
Tendon disorders
Tendon repair
Warts

PREVENTIVE MEDICINE
Acupressure
Acupuncture
Aging: Extended care
Alternative medicine

Aromatherapy
Biofeedback
Cardiology
Chiropractic
Cholesterol
Chronobiology
Disease
Electrocardiography (ECG or
    EKG)
Environmental health
Exercise physiology
Family practice
Genetic counseling
Geriatrics and gerontology
Holistic medicine
Host-defense mechanisms
Hypercholesterolemia
Immune system
Immunization and vaccination
Immunology
Mammography
Massage
Meditation
Melatonin
Noninvasive tests
Nursing
Nutrition
Occupational health
Osteopathic medicine
Pharmacology
Pharmacy
Physical examination
Preventive medicine
Psychiatry
Psychiatry, child and adolescent
Psychiatry, geriatric
Qi gong
Screening
Serology
Spine, vertebrae, and disks
Sports medicine
Stress
Stress reduction
Tai Chi Chuan
Tropical medicine
Yoga

PROCTOLOGY
Colon and rectal polyp removal
Colon and rectal surgery
Colon cancer
Colonoscopy
Crohn's disease
Cystectomy

Diverticulitis and diverticulosis
Endoscopy
Fistula repair
Gastroenterology
Gastrointestinal disorders
Gastrointestinal system
Genital disorders, male
Geriatrics and gerontology
Hemorrhoid banding and removal
Hemorrhoids
Hirschsprung's disease
Internal medicine
Intestinal disorders
Intestines
Irritable bowel syndrome (IBS)
Physical examination
Proctology
Prostate cancer
Prostate gland
Prostate gland removal
Reproductive system
Urology

PSYCHIATRY
Addiction
Aging
Aging: Extended care
Alcoholism
Alzheimer's disease
Amnesia
Amyotrophic lateral sclerosis
Anorexia nervosa
Anxiety
Attention-deficit disorder (ADD)
Auras
Autism
Bipolar disorder
Bonding
Brain
Brain disorders
Breast surgery
Bulimia
Chronic fatigue syndrome
Circumcision, female, and genital
    mutilation
Club drugs
Delusions
Dementias
Depression
Developmental stages
Domestic violence
Eating disorders
Electroencephalography (EEG)
Emergency medicine

Emotions: Biomedical causes and effects
Factitious disorders
Failure to thrive
Family practice
Fatigue
Grief and guilt
Gynecology
Hallucinations
Hypnosis
Hypochondriasis
Incontinence
Intoxication
Light therapy
Masturbation
Memory loss
Mental retardation
Midlife crisis
Münchausen syndrome by proxy
Neurosis
Neurosurgery
Nightmares
Obesity
Obsessive-compulsive disorder
Pain
Pain management
Panic attacks
Paranoia
Penile implant surgery
Phobias
Postpartum depression
Post-traumatic stress disorder
Psychiatric disorders
Psychiatry
Psychiatry, child and adolescent
Psychiatry, geriatric
Psychoanalysis
Psychosis
Psychosomatic disorders
Schizophrenia
Separation anxiety
Sex change surgery
Sexual dysfunction
Sexuality
Shock therapy
Sleep disorders
Speech disorders
Steroid abuse
Stress
Stress reduction
Sudden infant death syndrome (SIDS)
Suicide
Toilet training
Tourette's syndrome

PSYCHOLOGY
Addiction
Aging
Aging: Extended care
Alcoholism
Amnesia
Amyotrophic lateral sclerosis
Anorexia nervosa
Anxiety
Aromatherapy
Arthritis, juvenile rheumatoid
Attention-deficit disorder (ADD)
Auras
Bed-wetting
Biofeedback
Bipolar disorder
Bonding
Brain
Bulimia
Cardiac rehabilitation
Cirrhosis
Club drugs
Cognitive development
Death and dying
Delusions
Depression
Developmental stages
Domestic violence
Dyslexia
Eating disorders
Electroencephalography (EEG)
Emotions: Biomedical causes and effects
Environmental health
Factitious disorders
Failure to thrive
Family practice
Forensic pathology
Genetic counseling
Grief and guilt
Gulf War syndrome
Gynecology
Hallucinations
Holistic medicine
Hormone replacement therapy
Hypnosis
Hypochondriasis
Kinesiology
Klinefelter syndrome
Learning disabilities
Light therapy
Meditation
Memory loss
Mental retardation

Midlife crisis
Motor skill development
Münchausen syndrome by proxy
Neurosis
Nightmares
Nutrition
Obesity
Obsessive-compulsive disorder
Occupational health
Pain management
Panic attacks
Paranoia
Phobias
Plastic surgery
Postpartum depression
Post-traumatic stress disorder
Psychosomatic disorders
Puberty and adolescence
Separation anxiety
Sex change surgery
Sexual dysfunction
Sexuality
Sibling rivalry
Sleep disorders
Sleepwalking
Speech disorders
Sports medicine
Steroid abuse
Stillbirth
Stress
Stress reduction
Stuttering
Sudden infant death syndrome (SIDS)
Suicide
Temporomandibular joint (TMJ) syndrome
Tics
Toilet training
Tourette's syndrome
Weight loss and gain
Yoga

PUBLIC HEALTH
Acquired immunodeficiency syndrome (AIDS)
Aging: Extended care
Allied health
Alternative medicine
Anthrax
Arthropod-borne diseases
Bacteriology
Beriberi
Biostatistics

Emergency medicine
Environmental diseases
Environmental health
Enzyme therapy
Food poisoning
Forensic pathology
Hepatitis
Herbal medicine
Homeopathy
Intoxication
Itching
Laboratory tests
Lead poisoning
Liver
Mold and mildew
Multiple chemical sensitivity
 syndrome
Occupational health
Pathology
Pharmacology
Pharmacy
Poisoning
Poisonous plants
Rashes
Snakebites
Toxemia
Toxicology
Toxoplasmosis
Urinalysis

UROLOGY
Abdomen
Abdominal disorders
Bed-wetting
Catheterization
Chlamydia
Circumcision, male
Cystectomy
Cystitis
Cystoscopy
Dialysis
E. coli infection
Endoscopy
Fluids and electrolytes
Genital disorders, female
Genital disorders, male
Geriatrics and gerontology
Gonorrhea
Hermaphroditism and
 pseudohermaphroditism
Hydrocelectomy
Hypospadias repair and
 urethroplasty
Incontinence

Infertility in males
Kidney disorders
Kidney transplantation
Kidneys
Lithotripsy
Nephrectomy
Nephritis
Nephrology
Nephrology, pediatric
Pediatrics
Pelvic inflammatory disease (PID)
Penile implant surgery
Prostate cancer
Prostate gland
Prostate gland removal
Reproductive system
Schistosomiasis
Sex change surgery
Sexual differentiation
Sexual dysfunction
Sexually transmitted diseases
Sterilization
Stone removal
Stones
Syphilis
Testicles, undescended
Testicular surgery
Testicular torsion
Toilet training
Transplantation
Ultrasonography
Urethritis
Urinalysis
Urinary disorders
Urinary system
Urology
Urology, pediatric
Vasectomy

VASCULAR MEDICINE
Amputation
Aneurysmectomy
Aneurysms
Angiography
Angioplasty
Anti-inflammatory drugs
Arteriosclerosis
Biofeedback
Bleeding
Blood and blood disorders
Bypass surgery
Catheterization
Cholesterol
Circulation

Claudication
Dehydration
Diabetes mellitus
Dialysis
Embolism
Endarterectomy
Exercise physiology
Glands
Healing
Hematology
Hematology, pediatric
Hemorrhoid banding and removal
Hemorrhoids
Histology
Hypercholesterolemia
Hyperlipidemia
Ischemia
Lipids
Lymphatic system
Mitral valve prolapse
Necrotizing fasciitis
Osteochondritis juvenilis
Phlebitis
Podiatry
Progeria
Shunts
Smoking
Strokes
Thrombolytic therapy and TPA
Thrombosis and thrombus
Transfusion
Varicose vein removal
Varicose veins
Vascular medicine
Vascular system
Venous insufficiency

VIROLOGY
Acquired immunodeficiency
 syndrome (AIDS)
Chickenpox
Childhood infectious diseases
Chlamydia
Chronic fatigue syndrome
Common cold
Creutzfeldt-Jakob disease and mad
 cow disease
Croup
Cytomegalovirus (CMV)
Drug resistance
Ebola virus
Encephalitis
Fever
Glomerulonephritis

Hanta virus
Hepatitis
Herpes
Human immunodeficiency virus
  (HIV)
Infection
Influenza
Laboratory tests
Measles
Microbiology
Microscopy

Mononucleosis
Mumps
Parasitic diseases
Pelvic inflammatory disease (PID)
Poliomyelitis
Pulmonary diseases
Rabies
Rheumatic fever
Rhinitis
Roseola
Rubella

Serology
Sexually transmitted diseases
Shingles
Smallpox
Tonsillitis
Tropical medicine
Viral infections
Warts
Yellow fever
Zoonoses